ESSENTIAL SURGERY

PROBLEMS, DIAGNOSIS AND MANAGEMENT

Publishers' note about the authors

George Burkitt obtained qualifications in dental surgery and community medicine before studying clinical medicine as a mature student in Cambridge. He is passionate about medical education and was a co-author of the first three editions of *Wheater's Functional Histology* and *Basic Histopathology*. He later returned to his native Australia where he has been involved in family practice, palliative care and men's health.

Clive Quick also trained as a dental surgeon before changing track to become a consultant general and vascular surgeon in Huntingdon. As an associate lecturer at Cambridge University, he teaches and examines clinical students in surgery and is involved in training junior surgeons. He has been a member of the Court of Examiners of the Royal College of Surgeons of England for the FRCS and the MRCS examinations, and is now part of the external quality control group for the MRCS.

Joanna Reed is a consultant general and upper gastrointestinal surgeon in Huntingdon where she is Clinical Director for surgery. She has a strong commitment to surgical training and teaches widely on practical laparoscopic courses at the Royal College of Surgeons of England, Addenbrooke's Hospital and elsewhere. She strongly believes a broad training in surgery is essential for any practising surgeon.

The artist, **Philip Deakin**, first trained in physiology and later in medicine and is now a family practitioner in Sheffield, England. He continues to prepare the drawings for each edition of *Wheater's Functional Histology* as well as for this book, employing his medical knowledge and artistic skill to achieve accuracy and immediacy whilst demonstrating an attractive economy and clarity of style.

Commissioning Editor: Laurence Hunter
Development Editor: Clive Hewat, Ruth Swan
Project Manager: Morven Dean
Senior Designer: Sarah Russell
Illustrator: Philip Deakin

FOURTH EDITION

ESSENTIAL SURGERY
PROBLEMS, DIAGNOSIS AND MANAGEMENT

H. George Burkitt
BDScHons (Queensland) FRACDS MMedSci (Nottingham) MB BChir (Cambridge) FRACGP FACPsychMed
General Medical Practitioner and Medical Author, Sydney, New South Wales, Australia

Clive R.G. Quick
MB BS (London) FDS FRCS (England) MS (London) MA (Cambridge)
Consultant General and Vascular Surgeon, Hinchingbrooke Hospital, Huntingdon; Associate Lecturer in Surgery, University of Cambridge; Former Examiner in Basic Sciences and Clinical Surgery for FRCS and MRCS (England), Royal College of Surgeons of England, London, UK

Joanna B. Reed
BMedSci (Hons), BM BS (Nottingham), FRCS (Eng)
Clinical Director for Surgery and Consultant Laparoscopic and Upper Gastrointestinal Surgeon, Hinchingbrooke Hospital, Huntingdon, UK

Illustrations by
Philip J. Deakin
BSc (Hons) MBChB (Sheffield)
General Medical Practitioner, Sheffield, UK

Foreword by
Andrew T. Raftery
BSc MD CIBiol MIBiol FRCS(Eng) FRCS(Ed)
Consultant Surgeon, Sheffield Kidney Institute, Sheffield Teaching Hospitals NHS Foundation Trust, Northern General Hospital, Sheffield; Member (formerly Chairman) Court of Examiners, Royal College of Surgeons of England; Member of Council, Royal College of Surgeons of Edinburgh; Honorary Senior Clinical Lecturer in Surgery, University of Sheffield, UK

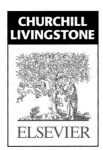

CHURCHILL LIVINGSTONE

ELSEVIER

EDINBURGH   LONDON   NEW YORK   OXFORD   PHILADELPHIA   ST LOUIS   SYDNEY   TORONTO   2007

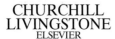

An imprint of Elsevier Limited

© 2007, Elsevier Limited. All rights reserved.

First published 1990
Second edition 1996
Third edition 2002
Fourth Edition 2007

Main Edition ISBN 9780443103452
International Student Edition ISBN 9780443103469

British Library Cataloguing in Publication Data
A catalogue record for this book is available from the British Library

Library of Congress Cataloging in Publication Data
A catalog record for this book is available from the Library of Congress

Note
Knowledge and best practice in this field are constantly changing. As new
research and experience broaden our knowledge, changes in practice,
treatment and drug therapy may become necessary or appropriate. Readers
are advised to check the most current information provided (i) on
procedures featured or (ii) by the manufacturer of each product to be
administered, to verify the recommended dose or formula, the method
and duration of administration, and contraindications. It is the
responsibility of the practitioner, relying on their own experience and
knowledge of the patient, to make diagnoses, to determine dosages and the
best treatment for each individual patient, and to take all appropriate
safety precautions. To the fullest extent of the law, neither the Publisher
nor the Authors assumes any liability for any injury and/or damage to
persons or property arising out or related to any use of the material
contained in this book.

The Publisher

ELSEVIER your source for books,
journals and multimedia
in the health sciences

www.elsevierhealth.com

Working together to grow
libraries in developing countries

www.elsevier.com | www.bookaid.org | www.sabre.org

ELSEVIER   BOOK AID International   Sabre Foundation

The
publisher's
policy is to use
**paper manufactured
from sustainable forests**

Printed in China

Foreword

When I wrote the foreword to the Third Edition, I commented that I had not thought that the First Edition could be improved upon. However, the Second Edition and the Third Edition were even more impressive and indeed I thought at the time it would be extremely difficult to improve on the Third Edition. I was wrong. The fact that there is a Fourth Edition attests to the popularity of this excellent textbook of surgery.

When the First Edition appeared in 1990 it was particularly impressive as only one of the authors (Clive Quick) was a Consultant Surgeon at the time of writing, whilst the other two (George Burkitt and Dennis Gatt—the latter having retired from the authorship after the Second Edition) were junior hospital doctors. George Burkitt, who was a mature medical student and already possessed a dental qualification, had written two successful medical textbooks as an undergraduate. I had the pleasure of teaching him as a clinical student in Cambridge and I like to think that I taught him some of the material presented in this book. In truth, I probably learned more from him than he did from me. Clive Quick is an outstanding surgical teacher and examiner and has been a colleague of mine for many years on the Court of Examiners of the Royal College of Surgeons of England. Phil Deakin, a family medical practitioner in Sheffield, has combined his medical knowledge with his considerable artistic skills to produce excellent diagrams which are easy to understand and interpret. The Fourth Edition has an additional author, Joanna Reed, who has provided a fresh perspective of a young Consultant Surgeon who has a particular interest in minimally invasive surgery. The Fourth Edition also benefits from the participation of Emma McGrath, a junior doctor who was involved in the preparation of this edition and provided a student's and junior doctor's perspective on the layout and presentation, as well as original contributions.

There has been a radical revision of the layout and text since the Third Edition. The text has been completely reordered and brought up-to-date, maintaining the approach of previous editions whilst adding new concepts where medical understanding has advanced. Many tables have been revised and new ones added. Illustrations have been used to emphasise important concepts. In particular, a new chapter on screening has been added and there is the added advantage of references to internet access to check facts and investigate trends. There is a welcome addition in Chapter 1, where Harold Ellis provides a historical perspective, reminding the reader of our surgical heritage. He comments on the introduction of basic sciences into surgery in centuries past, a ready reminder of their importance today, an importance which is accentuated in this book where the pathophysiological basis of surgical disease is presented in a way that bridges the gap between basic medical science and clinical surgery.

Essential Surgery is written in a different way from other standard surgical texts. The book describes sound principles of surgery on which to expand one's learning. The authors have employed a problem-solving approach to diagnosis and treatment where this has been practicable and have tried to view the practical management of patients through the eyes of a trainee or student.

This is an excellent book, providing a broad surgical education for both undergraduates and postgraduates. A wide variety of surgical topics is covered, together with some epidemiology and preventive medicine, which helps to integrate surgery into the healthcare and community setting. Although this book was primarily written for clinical medical students, there is sufficient in this book for the basic surgical trainee and some of the chapters will also provide excellent revision material for the higher surgical trainee, especially before sitting the UK Intercollegiate FRCS examination in general surgery.

It is a pleasure and privilege to have been asked to write the foreword for the Fourth Edition. This book goes from strength to strength and I believe that the reader will find it stimulating and will particularly enjoy the style of presentation. This book provides an excellent basis for surgical learning for both undergraduate and postgraduate alike. I wish it the success that it deserves.

Andrew T Raftery
Sheffield
2007   **v**

Preface

When we first set about writing this book, we felt we had something worthwhile to say about surgery and how it worked. We knew that if readers could acquire this knowledge and implement what they had learnt, the standard of surgical practice would rise and outcomes for patients would eventually improve.

We wrote the book in a completely different way from most other surgical books, determined to avoid propagating surgical myths and providing inadequate explanations. To achieve this, the authors sat down together to discuss each topic, employing first principles, basic science, current literature and surgical experience before writing an agreed version directly onto a computer screen. Many ideas were originated in the form of diagrams. Great credit goes to one of our former authors Dennis Gatt for much of this. We have continued this method for this new edition, with the added advantage of rapid internet access to check facts and investigate trends. We believe this approach has helped us understand the subjects better and put them across with exceptional clarity.

From the beginning, the authorship was unusual in that only Clive Quick was a consultant surgeon; George Burkitt was a junior doctor-cum-medical author and Dennis Gatt was a junior surgical trainee, later consultant surgeon. This mix enabled us to better address surgical problems from the viewpoint of the student and junior doctor. Emma McGrath, a junior trainee in paediatrics in Cambridge, has for this edition worked closely with the authors over long hours to help maintain the student perspective. She has provided constructive criticism as well as original contributions, including many ideas for graphical representation of complex problems.

Our overall concept has always been to produce an authored rather than an edited book, so as to retain uniformity of style and our own high standard of elucidation throughout. Nevertheless, an enormous amount of help has been generously given over the years by colleagues in specialist areas, both in original writing and illustration and in checking material already written. Their contributions have been integrated into the structure and edited to emphasise lucidity and ease of reading, with the intention that the reader could grasp the main ideas easily and effortlessly in one reading. Finally, the text is re-read by all the authors and given a concluding 'polish'. Writing in this style is time consuming but we feel it is worthwhile if the text proves enjoyable to read and draws the reader in, after the style of a good novel.

The continuing enthusiasm of students and teachers for the book has highlighted the need for this updated Fourth Edition. As in all previous editions, George Burkitt provided the perspective of an established medical author in agreeing content and structure and in ensuring clarity and harmony. Joanna Reed has joined us as an additional author for this edition, giving the fresh perspective of a young consultant surgeon who has a particular interest in minimally invasive surgery. We have undertaken a radical revision for this edition, endeavouring to build on the quality and content of the original without increasing its length; major changes represent the evolution and refinement of surgery over the five or so years since the previous edition. The content of each chapter has been carefully considered and some sections relocated to facilitate navigation. All of the text has been brought up to date, adding new concepts where medical understanding has advanced, for example *toll-like receptors* in innate immunity and *permissive hypotension* in managing acute blood loss. We have also added a new chapter on screening. The illustrations, one of the particular strengths of this book, have all been reviewed and updated or replaced. Since the last edition, consensus guidelines for managing common disorders have emerged, many from the UK National Institute for Clinical Excellence (NICE), and these have been incorporated where appropriate.

This book was written primarily for clinical medical students and aims to cover the whole field of general surgery with sufficient basic science for modern clinical courses. In addition general trauma surgery, cardiothoracic surgery and urology are covered in detail. We believe that *Essential Surgery* will continue to have the greatest appeal for readers who want to understand surgery rather than merely pass examinations. We have tried to present sometimes complex ideas in ways accessible to anyone with a moderate understanding of human biology, and yet still prove valuable to readers at a more advanced level. We believe this is why the book has a broad appeal beyond medical students, from nurses and trainees in professions allied to medicine, to dentists. It has proved indispensable as a textbook for many trainee surgeons taking examinations such as the MRCS, which require an understanding of applied basic sciences and the principles of surgery rather than extensive details of operative technique. In addition this book was designed to be a continuing reference text for doctors in other specialties, including family practice.

We have employed a problem-solving approach to diagnosis and treatment where practicable, believing that understanding how diagnoses are made and why particular treatments are used is more memorable than rote learning. With this in mind, we have tried to view the practical management of patients through the eyes of the trainee or student. In particular, the pathophysiological basis of surgical diseases and management is presented to bridge the gap between basic medical sciences and clinical problems.

Throughout the book we have used original illustrative material to emphasise important concepts, avoid unnecessary text and assist revision for exams. This includes photographs of clinical cases, operations and pathological specimens, radiographs, anatomical and operative diagrams, and tables and box summaries of the text. The clinical material is largely drawn from our day-to-day practice and we have generally chosen typical rather than gross examples so the reader can see how patients present most commonly.

We make no apology for including outlines of common surgical operations. This is to enable students and trainee surgeons to explain operations to patients, to participate intelligently in the operating department, to understand and thereby prevent complications as well as to help them perform certain minor operations themselves. Finally, there is a completely revised major section on accident surgery and head injuries as this is an important part of general surgical training and practice.

We do not pretend that surgery can be taught entirely in a problem-orientated way, so descriptions of individual diseases have also been covered in a more conventional manner. We hope our readers will continue to enjoy the book and will appreciate the continuing efforts we have made to keep pace with change. Above all, it remains our ambition to stimulate the reader to a greater enjoyment and understanding of the practice of surgery.

H. G. B.
C. R. G. Q.
Australia and UK 2007   J. B. R.

Acknowledgements

First, we gratefully acknowledge the huge contributions made to the First Edition of this book by Dennis Gatt, now a surgeon in Malta, and the late Leonard Beard, medical photographer. Other major contributors included Drs Graham Hurst and Catherine Hubbard, radiologists, Michael Williams, oncologist and the late Andrew Higgins, urologist. We also owe a tremendous debt to Jane Hailey, then a junior trainee and now a paediatrician in Canada, who helped turn our prose into an accessible and fluent text. Many others willingly assisted by providing material or images or checking our text for accuracy. To them and all subsequent contributors, we are extremely grateful; the book would not be what it is without their assistance.

There were numerous other contributors to the Second and Third editions, including Prof Ted Howard, paediatric surgeon, formerly of Great Ormond Street Hospital, Stephen Large, cardiothoracic surgeon at Papworth Hospital, Grant Williams urologist; and Mark Farrington, microbiologist and Richard Miller, colorectal surgeon, both at Addenbrooke's Hospital. Dr Paul Siklos, physician at West Suffolk Hospital and Course Director of the Cambridge Graduate Course in Medicine, thoroughly revised the chapter on medical management of surgical patients and has done so again for this new edition.

In preparing this Fourth Edition, we are once again grateful for the substantial and unstinting help we have received from colleagues and friends. They are based at Hinchingbrooke Hospital, Huntingdon unless otherwise stated. In particular, major contributions were made by radiologist Dr Tony Booth, updating Chapter 5 as well as reviewing all other radiographs and radiological procedures in the book. John Benson, breast surgeon, now of Addenbrooke's, radically revised the chapter on breast surgery to which Catherine Hubbard also contributed substantially. Stephen Tsui, consultant cardiothoracic surgeon at Papworth Hospital, revised the chapters on cardiac and thoracic surgery and Neville Jamieson, consultant general and transplant surgeon at Addenbrooke's hospital, revised his own original work on transplantation and hepatobiliary surgery. Andreas Karas, microbiologist, revised and updated the microbiological material, including disinfection and sterilisation, and Jeffrey Brain and Madan Samuel, paediatric surgeons at Addenbrooke's, radically revised chapters 50 and 51. Nimish Shah, urologist, updated the urology and the male genitalia chapters and Elizabeth Ambler, transfusion nurse and Katie Hoggarth, haematologist, transformed the chapter on blood transfusion. We are particularly grateful to Sue Clark, consultant colorectal surgeon at St Mark's Hospital, London for her help in revising all of the colorectal chapters. Paul Perkins, palliative care specialist, revised the chapter on cancer treatment and palliative care and Adrian Harris amended the chapters on oesophagogastric and pancreatic cancer. Dr Anita Gibbons, gastroenterologist, reviewed the chapter on inflammatory bowel disease. Olivia Will, specialist registrar and now PhD student at St Marks Hospital, provided invaluable help with the colorectal and trauma chapters and contributed an important table on non-trauma resuscitation. Antonia Wells, specialist registrar in surgery, provided valuable assistance for Chapter 15 on major trauma. Professor Harold Ellis provided an elegant and succinct Short History of Surgery in Chapter 1. Cedric Banfield, dermatologist, reviewed the skin chapter and Dr Suzanna Lishman, histopathologist, reviewed much of the pathology in the book and helped with renewing the histology slides.

Dr Helen Smith, anaesthetist at Addenbrooke's Hospital, reviewed the material on anaesthesia and perioperative pain relief and provided valuable advice on aspects of critical care. Once again David Adlam reviewed the oral and dental chapters. Nick Skelton, Surgical Nurse Practitioner, provided advice on preoperative assessment. Paul Hayes, vascular surgeon, reviewed all the vascular chapters and Roger Gray, ENT surgeon, provided an succinct summary of important ENT emergencies in diagrammatic form.

Other expert assistance has been provided by Dr Phil Roberts, gastroenterologist (nutrition), Colin Borland, physician (ECGs), Bassam Bekdash and Raqib Anwar (illustrations of stapled haemorrhoidectomy) and Dr Deepa Gopalan, radiologist at Papworth (thoracic radiographs). Finally, Mark Moughton, medical photographer, produced some excellent images.

A continuing debt of gratitude is owed to all those who have contributed to all of the editions of Essential Surgery, including of course all those whose names are not mentioned here. A substantial part of the book's success is due to them.

Contents

CONTENTS

Disease processes and diagnostic techniques

1

Surgery and the mechanisms of surgical disease

1

A SHORT HISTORY OF SURGERY

There can be no doubt that the first surgeons were the men and women who bound up the lacerations, contusions, fractures, impalements and eviscerations to which man has been subject since he appeared on Earth. Since man is the most vicious of all creatures, many of these injuries were inflicted by man upon man. Indeed, the battlefield has always been a training ground for surgery. Right up to the 15th century, surgeons dealing with trauma were surprisingly efficient. They knew their limitations—they could splint fractures, reduce dislocations and bind up lacerations, but were only too aware that open wounds of the skull, chest and abdomen were lethal and were best left alone, as were wounds involving major blood vessels or spinal injuries with paralysis. They observed that wounds would usually discharge yellow pus for a time; indeed this was regarded as a good prognostic sign and was labelled 'laudable pus'.

The 15th century heralded a new and dreaded pathology—the gunshot wound. These injuries would stink, swell and bubble with gas. There was profound systemic toxicity and a high mortality. Of course, we now know that this was the result of clostridial infection of wounds with the extensive anaerobic tissue damage caused by shot and shell. The surgeons of those times were shrewd clinical observers but they surmised that these malign effects were due to gunpowder acting as a poison, for it was not until centuries later that the bacterial basis of wound infection began to be understood. At that period the remedy was to destroy the poison with boiling oil or cautery. Boiling oil was the more popular since it was advocated by the Italian surgeon Giovanni da Vigo (1460–1525), the author of the standard text of the day, *Practica In Arte Chirurgica Compendiosa*. These treatments not only produced intense pain but also made matters worse by increasing the amount of tissue necrosis.

The first scientific departure from this barbaric treatment was taken by the great French military surgeon Ambroise Paré (1510–1590) who, while still a young man, revolutionised the treatment of wounds by using only simple dressings, abandoning cautery and introducing ligatures to control haemorrhage. He established that his results were much better than could be achieved by the old methods.

Ignorance of the basic sciences behind the practice of surgery was slowly overcome. The publications of *The Fabric of the Human Body* in 1543 by Andreas Vesalius (1514–1564) and of *The Motion of the Heart* by William Harvey (1578–1657) in 1628 were two notable landmarks.

Surgical progress however was still limited by two major obstacles. First, the agony of the knife: patients would only be prepared to undergo an operation to relieve intolerable suffering (for example from a gangrenous limb, a bladder stone or a strangulated rupture) and, of course, the surgeon needed to operate at lightning speed. Second, there was the inevitability of suppuration, with its prolonged disability and high mortality, which was often as high as 50% after amputation. Amazingly, both these barriers were overcome within a couple of decades of each other.

In 1846, William Morton (1819–1868), a dentist working in Boston, Massachusetts, introduced the use of ether as a general anaesthetic. This was followed a year later by chloroform, employed by James Young Simpson (1811–1870) in Edinburgh, mainly in midwifery. These agents were taken up with immense enthusiasm across the world in a matter of weeks.

The work of the French chemist Louis Pasteur (1822–1895) demonstrated the link between wound suppuration and microbes. This led Joseph Lister (1827–1912), who

3

was then a young professor of surgery in Edinburgh, to perform the first operation under sterile conditions in 1865. This was treatment of a compound fracture of the tibia in which crude carbolic acid was used as an antiseptic. The development of antiseptic surgery and, later, modern aseptic surgery progressed from there.

So at last, in the 1870s, the scene was set for the coming enormous advances in every branch of surgery whose breadth and successes form the basis of this book.

Prof. Harold Ellis CBE MCh FRCS

APPROACHES TO SURGICAL PROBLEMS

What do surgeons do?

Surgeons are doctors who do operations, i.e. cutting tissue to treat disease, the patient usually being under some form of anaesthesia. However, the range of work individual surgeons undertake varies widely, depending on the culture in which they work and the resources available, the nature and breadth of their specialisation, what other specialists are available, and the local needs. The principles of surgery—access, dissection, haemostasis, repair, reconstruction, preservation of vital structures and closure—are similar in all specialties.

A **general surgeon** usually means one who principally undertakes general surgical emergency work and elective abdominal gastrointestinal (GI) surgery. In geographically isolated areas and regions where resources are scarce, such a surgeon might also undertake some gynaecology, urology, paediatric surgery, orthopaedic and trauma surgery and perhaps basic ear, nose and throat (ENT) and ophthalmology, and even obstetrics. Conversely, in developed countries, there is an increasing trend towards greater specialisation. Gastrointestinal surgery, for example, is often divided into 'upper' and 'lower' GI surgery, and upper GI surgery itself may further divide into the subspecialties of hepatobiliary, laparoscopic, pancreatic and gastro-oesophageal cancer surgery.

Surgeons should not be thought of simply as 'cutting and sewing' doctors. The perceived drama of surgery may be superficially attractive but good surgery is rarely dramatic. Only when things go wrong does the drama increase, and this is often not comfortable. Surgery is an art or craft as well as a science, and judgement, coping under pressure, taking decisive action when necessary, teaching and training skills and people management skills are essential qualities. Operating skills can be learnt by most people, but the skills involved in deciding when it is in the patient's best interests to operate are absolutely essential and must also be actively learnt and practised.

Surgeons also play an important role in the diagnostic process, using both clinical skills and appropriate investigations as part of their armamentarium. In this context, many surgeons undertake various forms of diagnostic and therapeutic endoscopy. These include gastroscopy, colonoscopy, urological endoscopy, thoracoscopy and arthroscopy. In addition, the indications for laparoscopic surgery, supported by the outcomes of good quality clinical trials, continue to broaden as equipment and skills become increasingly sophisticated.

What sort of patients come to surgeons?

Different types of surgeon practise in very different ways, depending on their specialty and their level of responsibility for emergency work. In the UK, most patients are referred to surgeons by another doctor, e.g. family practitioner, accident and emergency (ER) officer or internal physician. The exceptions include patients suffering trauma who self-refer or are brought to a hospital by ambulance. In some other countries, patients are able to self-refer to the specialist they feel is most appropriate. Regardless of the route of referral, surgical patients fall into the following categories:

- **Emergency/acute**, i.e. symptoms lasting minutes to hours or up to a day or two—often obviously surgical conditions such as traumatic wounds, fractures, abscesses, acute severe abdominal pain or gastrointestinal bleeding
- **Intermediate urgency**—usually referrals from other doctors based on suspicious symptoms and signs and sometimes investigations, e.g. suspected colonic cancer, gallstones, renal or ureteric stones
- **Chronic conditions** likely to need surgery, e.g. varicose veins, hernias, arthritic joints, cardiac ischaemia or rectal prolapse

The diagnostic process

In order to manage surgical patients appropriately, a **working diagnosis** needs to be formulated to guide whether investigations are necessary and if so, their type and urgency, and to determine what intervention (i.e. treatment) is necessary. The process initially depends upon whether immediate life-saving intervention is required or, if not, the perceived urgency of the case. For example, a patient bleeding from a stab wound might need pressure applied to the wound immediately whilst resuscitation and detailed assessment are carried out. At the other end of the scale, if the symptoms suggest the patient has a rectal carcinoma, a systematic and timely approach is needed to obtain visual and histological confirmation of the diagnosis by **endoscopy** (colonoscopy plus biopsy) and radiological **imaging** (e.g. barium enema, CT scan). **Tumour staging** (see Ch. 13) endeavours to determine the extent of spread of a carcinoma in order to direct how radical treatment needs to be. Treatment may be **curative** (surgery, chemotherapy, radiotherapy) or **palliative** if clearly beyond cure (stenting to prevent obstruction, local tumour destruction using laser, palliative radiotherapy).

Formulating a diagnosis

The traditional approach to teaching surgical diagnosis is for the student to attempt to correlate a patient's symptoms and signs with recognised sets of symptoms and signs listed as characterising each disease. While most diagnoses match their 'classical' descriptions at certain stages in their evolution, this may not be so when the patient initially presents for treatment. Patients commonly present before a recognisable pattern has evolved or else at an advanced stage when the typical clinical picture has become obscured. The diagnostic process can also be confusing if all the symptoms and signs expected for a particular diagnosis are not present, or if some of the symptoms and signs seem inconsistent with the working diagnosis.

This book seeks to develop a more logical and reliable approach to diagnostic method than simple pattern recognition by attempting to explain how the evolving pathophysiology of the disease and its effect on the local anatomy bring about the various clinical features. The overall aim of this understanding is to target investigations and interventions that give the best chance of cure or symptom relief with the least harm to the patient.

PRINCIPAL MECHANISMS OF SURGICAL DISEASE

Surgical patients present with disorders resulting from inherited abnormalities, environmental factors or a combination of these in varying proportion. These are summarised in Box 1.1, providing a useful 'first principles' framework or *aide-mémoire* upon which to construct a differential diagnosis. This is particularly useful when the symptoms and signs do not immediately point to a diagnosis. This approach is often referred to as the 'surgical sieve'. However, it should not become a substitute for logical thought based on the clinical findings.

CONGENITAL CONDITIONS

The term **congenital** defines a condition that is present at birth, as a result of genetic changes and/or environmental influences in utero such as ischaemia or incomplete

---

Box 1.1 The surgical sieve

When considering the causes of a particular condition, it may be helpful to run through the range of causes listed here. However, this should be only a first step and not a substitute for thought. This approach gives no indication of the likely severity, frequency or importance of the cause.

Congenital
- Genetic
- Environmental influences in utero

Acquired
- Trauma—accidents in the home, at work or during leisure activities, personal violence, road traffic collisions
- Inflammation—physical or immunological mechanisms
- Infection—viral, bacterial, fungal, protozoal, parasitic
- Neoplasia—benign, premalignant or malignant
- Vascular—ischaemia, infarction, reperfusion syndrome, aneurysms, venous insufficiency
- Degenerative—osteoporosis, glaucoma, osteoarthritis, rectal prolapse
- Metabolic disorders—gallstones, urinary tract stones
- Endocrine disorders and therapy—thyroid function abnormalities, Cushing's syndrome, phaeochromocytoma

- Other abnormalities of tissue growth—hyperplasia, hypertrophy and cyst formation
- Iatrogenic disorders—damage or injury resulting from the action of a doctor or other health care worker; may be misadventure, negligence or, more commonly, system failure
- Drugs, toxins, diet, exercise and environment
  - Prescription drugs—toxic effects of powerful drugs, maladministration, idiosyncratic reactions, drug interactions.
  - Smoking—atherosclerosis, cancers, peptic ulcer
  - Alcohol abuse—personal violence, traffic collisions
  - Substance abuse—accidents, injection site problems
  - 'Western diet'—obesity, atherosclerosis, cancers
  - Lack of exercise—obesity, osteoporosis, aches and pains
  - Venomous snakes, spiders, scorpions and other creatures—local and systemic toxicity
  - Atmospheric pollution—pulmonary problems
- Psychogenic—Munchausen syndrome leading to repeated operations, problems of indigent living, ingestion of foreign bodies, self harm
- Disorders of function—diverticular disease, some swallowing disorders

developmental processes such as malrotation of the gut or maternal ingestion of drugs such as thalidomide. Congenital abnormalities of surgical interest range from minor cosmetic deformities such as skin tags right through to potentially fatal conditions such as some congenital heart defects, urethral valves and various gut atresias.

Congenital abnormalities may become manifest at any time between conception and old age, although the majority are evident at birth or appear in early childhood. Some disorders are diagnosed *antenatally*, for example, fetal gut atresias presenting during pregnancy with grossly excessive amniotic fluid (polyhydramnios). There are expanding specialist areas involving *intrauterine* surgical interventions or fetal surgery, for example for urinary tract obstruction or congenital diaphragmatic hernias. In the *neonatal* period, abnormalities such as urethral valves (which may present with obstructive renal failure) may become evident. During *infancy*, conditions such as congenital hypertrophic pyloric stenosis come to light. In *childhood*, incompletely descended testis may become evident, although this may be suspected much earlier. Finally, some congenital disorders may present at *any stage* from birth to early adulthood. For example, a patent processus vaginalis may be the precursor to an inguinal hernia even into late middle age.

Whilst many congenital abnormalities give rise to disease by direct **anatomical effects**, other abnormalities produce disease by more subtle **disruption of function**, with the underlying disorder only revealed on appropriate investigation. For example, ureteric abnormalities which allow urinary reflux from the bladder predispose to recurrent kidney infections.

ACQUIRED CONDITIONS

Acquired surgical disorders result from direct or indirect damage inflicted by trauma or disease or from the body's response to these, or else present as an effect or side effect of treatment. For example, obstruction of the bladder outlet may result from benign prostatic hypertrophy, from the fibrotic response to gonococcal urethritis or from damage inflicted during urethral instrumentation. The classification detailed here provides a framework to help consider the causes of surgical disease, but it should be remembered that particular conditions may fit under more than one heading, and that the mechanism behind some surgical disorders is still poorly understood.

Trauma

Tissue trauma, literally injury, includes in its wider sense damage inflicted by any physical means, i.e. mechanical, thermal, chemical or electrical mechanisms or ionising radiation. Common usage, however, tends to imply mechanical injury, either blunt or penetrating, as caused by accidents in industry or in the home, road traffic collisions, fights, firearm and other missile injuries or natural disasters such as floods and earthquakes. Damage varies according to the nature of the causative agent, and the visible surface injuries may give little indication of the extent of deep tissue damage as, for example, in head injuries or bullet wounds.

Inflammation

Many surgical disorders result from inflammatory processes, most often stemming from infection. However, inflammation may also result from physical irritation, particularly by noxious chemical agents, e.g. gastric acid/pepsin in peptic ulcer disease or pancreatic enzymes in acute pancreatitis.

Inflammation may also result from immunological processes which play a part in the inflammatory bowel disorders of ulcerative colitis and Crohn's disease. Whether they constitute cause or effect is not yet known. Autoimmunity, in which an immune response is directed at one or more of the body's own constituents, is recognised in a growing number of surgical diseases such as Hashimoto's thyroiditis and rheumatoid disease.

Infection

Primary infections commonly presenting to surgeons include soft tissue infections such as abscesses and cellulitis, primary joint infections and tonsillitis. Typhoid may cause caecal perforation, and abdominal tuberculosis may be discovered at laparotomy. Amoebiasis may cause ulcerative colitis-like effects. Preventing and treating infection is also an important factor in many surgical emergencies such as acute appendicitis or bowel perforation. Despite the rational use of prophylactic and therapeutic antibiotics, postoperative infection remains a common complication of surgery.

Neoplasia

Certain **benign tumours** such as lipomas are very common and are excised mainly for cosmetic reasons. Less commonly, benign tumours cause mechanical problems such as obstruction of a hollow viscus or surface blood loss, e.g. gastro-intestinal stromal tumours (GIST). Benign endocrine tumours may have to be removed because of excess hormone secretion (see *Endocrine disorders* later). Finally, benign tumours may be clinically indistinguishable from malignant tumours and are removed or biopsied to obtain a histological diagnosis.

Malignant tumours may present with signs and symptoms resulting from the primary tumour, the effects of metastases ('secondaries') and in some cases, systemic effects such as cachexia. Malignant tumours are responsible for a large part of the general surgical workload.

Vascular disorders

A tissue or organ becomes **ischaemic** when its arterial blood supply is impaired; **infarction** occurs when cell life can no longer be sustained. **Atherosclerosis** leads to progressive narrowing of arteries which often results in **chronic ischaemia**, causing symptoms such as angina pectoris or intermittent claudication. It also predisposes to **acute-on-chronic ischaemia** when diseased vessels finally occlude. Other common causes of acute arterial insufficiency are thrombosis, embolism and trauma involving blood vessels. Arterial embolism is a cause of acute ischaemia of limbs, intestine or brain; these emboli often originate in the heart. If the blood supply is restored after a period of ischaemia, for example by embolectomy, further damage can ensue as a result of **reperfusion syndrome**.

When a portion of bowel becomes strangulated, the initial mechanism of tissue damage is venous obstruction and this fairly rapidly progresses to arterial ischaemia and infarction.

An **aneurysm** is an abnormal dilatation of an artery resulting from degeneration of connective tissue. This may rupture, thrombose or generate emboli.

Chronic **venous insufficiency** in the lower limb causing local venous hypertension is responsible for the majority of chronic leg ulcers.

Degenerative disorders

This is an inhomogeneous group of conditions characterised by deterioration in one or more of the body tissues as life progresses. In the musculoskeletal system, **osteoporosis** decreases the density of bone and impairs its structural integrity, making fragility fractures more likely such as crush fractures of vertebrae or fractures of the femoral neck. Spinal disc and facet joint degeneration is common, causing back pain and disability, and osteoarthritis is widely prevalent, particularly in later life. The almost universal musculoskeletal aches and pains of later life are probably caused by degeneration of muscle, tendon, joint and bone.

Other degenerative disorders include age-related retinal macular degeneration, glaucoma, the inherited disorder retinitis pigmentosa, and certain neurological disorders (Alzheimer's, Huntington's and Parkinson's disease, bulbar palsy). Atherosclerosis and aneurysmal arterial diseases are often non-specifically labelled degenerative but their pathogenesis is gradually being elucidated.

Metabolic disorders

Metabolic disorders may be responsible for stones in the gall bladder (e.g. haemolytic diseases causing pigment stones) or in the urinary tract (e.g. hypercalciuria and hyperuricaemia causing calcium and uric acid stones respectively). Hypercholesterolaemia is a major factor in atherosclerosis and hypertriglyceridaemia is a rare but important cause of acute pancreatitis.

Endocrine disorders and hormonal therapy

Hypersecretion of certain hormones, as in thyrotoxicosis and hyperparathyroidism, may require surgical removal or reduction of glandular tissue. Endocrine tumours, both benign and malignant, may present with metabolic abnormalities such as hypercalcaemia caused by a parathyroid adenoma, Cushing's syndrome resulting from an adrenal adenoma or episodic hypertension caused by a phaeochromocytoma.

Diabetes mellitus, particularly when poorly controlled, may result in a range of complications of surgical importance, for example retinopathy and cataract formation, as well as predisposing to atherosclerosis.

Hormone replacement therapy in postmenopausal women brings mixed benefits: it slows osteoporosis and reduces the risk of colorectal cancer whilst slightly increasing the risks of breast and endometrial cancer. There is also some evidence of an increased rate of thromboembolism, as there is with higher oestrogen-containing oral contraceptive pills.

Other abnormalities of tissue growth

Growth disturbances such as **hyperplasia** (increase in the number of cells) and **hypertrophy** (increase in the size of cells) may give rise to surgical problems, in particular benign prostatic hyperplasia, fibroadenosis of the breast and thyroid enlargement (goitre).

In surgery, the term **cyst** is imprecisely used to describe a mass which appears to contain fluid because of its characteristic fluctuance and transilluminability. A cyst is defined as a closed sac with a distinct lining membrane that develops abnormally in the body. A variety of different pathological processes produce cysts. Most are benign but some may be associated with malignant change in the wall.

Iatrogenic disorders

Iatrogenic damage or injury is that resulting from the action of a doctor or other health care worker. It may be an unfortunate outcome of an adequately performed investigation or operation, e.g. perforated colon during colonoscopy or pneumothorax as a result of attempted aspiration of a breast cyst. This type of injury could be termed **surgical misadventure**. However, if the damage results from a patently wrong procedure, e.g. amputation of the wrong leg or removal of the wrong kidney, then **negligence** is likely to be proven. Such wrong site surgery is easily avoided by preoperative site marking. Other potentially negligent actions include retained surgical swabs after laparotomy or arterial trauma during central venous line insertion. Complications of bowel surgery such as anastomotic leakage may result from poorly performed surgery but can occur in expert hands; only carefully audited results can demonstrate whether the surgeon is proficient. Wrong drugs or doses are usually iatrogenic and are covered under the next heading.

It is unusual for iatrogenic problems to be simply due to one person's failure. More often it is a **system failure**, with inadequate checks and balances in the system.

Drugs, toxins and diet

Problems with prescribed drugs include unavoidable **toxic effects** of certain chemotherapeutic agents, e.g. neutropenia, and the **side effects** of drugs such as non-steroidal anti-inflammatory drugs (NSAIDs) causing duodenal perforation, or codeine phosphate causing constipation. Drug **allergy, idiosyncrasy** or **anaphylaxis** may result from individual responses to almost any drug, and **interactions** between drugs may cause adverse effects. In this respect warfarin is a prime culprit. Maladministration of drugs may also cause problems with, for example, the wrong drug being given for intrathecal chemotherapy causing paralysis.

In many countries, venomous creatures such as spiders, snakes or scorpions cause toxic and sometimes fatal harm.

Cigarette **smoking** is the biggest single preventable cause of death and disability in developed countries. Cigarette smoke is highly addictive and contains an array of carcinogens in the tar, vasoconstrictors in the form of nicotine, and carbon monoxide that preferentially binds to haemoglobin. Not surprisingly, it is a powerful factor in a huge range of diseases including cardiovascular disorders affecting the heart, limbs and brain, dysplasias and cancers of the lung, mouth and larynx, respiratory disorders such as pneumonias, chronic obstructive pulmonary disease (COPD) and emphysema via small airways inflammation, stillbirth and peptic ulcer disease. Smoking compounds the atherogenic effects of diabetes and is also strongly associated with premature skin ageing.

Environmental pollution almost certainly affects health: for example, micro-fine particles produced by diesel engines cause pulmonary inflammation.

Alcohol and substance abuse may have a surgical dimension: alcohol may lead to personal violence or road traffic collisions as a result of intoxication; cannabis smoke is carcinogenic and causes dysplasias and premalignant lesions of the oral mucosa as well as contributing to mental health problems of acute anxiety and psychotic-like paranoid thoughts. Misdirected injection of opioids and other drugs may cause abscesses, false aneurysms and even arterial occlusion.

The so-called 'Western diet' rich in fat and calories and low in vegetables, fruit and fibre is associated with a range of diseases including colorectal and breast cancers, obesity, dyslipidaemias, diabetes and hypertension. This is particularly so when combined with a sedentary life. Dietary fibre protects against colorectal adenomas and carcinomas as well as diverticular disease.

Psychogenic disorders

Psychogenic disorders are not often a source of surgical disease but Munchausen syndrome patients may present with abdominal pain and become subjects of repeated laparotomies, psychiatric patients living rough may suffer from exposure and frostbite, and others may repeatedly cause self harm or swallow foreign bodies, even such items as razor blades or safety pins.

Disorders of function

A range of common disorders are defined by the abnormalities of function they cause, although in most cases their pathogenesis remains ill understood. The gastrointestinal tract is particularly susceptible, with conditions such as idiopathic constipation, irritable bowel syndrome and diverticular disease.

Managing physiological change in the surgical patient

SYSTEMIC RESPONSES

FACTORS RESPONSIBLE FOR SYSTEMIC RESPONSES (Box 2.1)

Surgical patients are subject to a variety of major injuries and catastrophes that make massive demands on the body's ability to sustain life and maintain physiological equilibrium. Examples of such stressors include:

- **Major operations**—anaesthesia, tissue trauma, blood and fluid loss, healing and repair
- **Major trauma** including fractures and burns; head, abdominal and chest injuries
- **Major cardiovascular events**, e.g. myocardial infarction, pulmonary embolism, stroke
- **Haemorrhage and fluid infusion** including blood: fluid and electrolyte abnormalities
- **Infection, inflammation and sepsis**
- **Hypoxia**

The manner in which the body responds to major systemic insults depends on several factors—the **physiological reserve** of the patient's chief organ systems (i.e. basic fitness), the nature of the injurious process, the severity of physiological disruption and the virulence of any microorganisms involved. Several physiological systems are likely to be impacted upon simultaneously, evoking a range of complex homeostatic mechanisms. Each mechanism has evolved to allow the human organism to take care of one specific and usually isolated physiological disturbance of less than critical impact. In acute, life-threatening situations however, these mechanisms may interact or react excessively to complicate the situation rather than restore it to health. Careful evaluation and management (so-called 'critical care') is needed if the patient is to survive.

The aims of medical management are to recognise the problems early and to correct the abnormal physiology as rapidly and accurately as possible to prevent natural compensatory mechanisms becoming overwhelmed. If this happens in one organ system without being corrected, snowballing decompensation of other systems follows.

Management requires careful monitoring, often in a high-dependency or intensive care unit, and repeated checks on organ function and dysfunction. In most elective surgical operations, many of the responses discussed below can be mitigated by accurate fluid replacement, adequate analgesia, reducing psychological stress, preventing infection and using careful operative technique to minimise tissue trauma and blood loss. The result will then be minimal systemic upset with rapid recovery. Enhanced recovery programmes are gradually being introduced and these give special attention to all these factors (see below).

The individual factors responsible for systemic responses to severe injury or major surgery are summarised in Box 2.1.

Box 2.1 Factors responsible for systemic responses to severe injury or major surgery

- Direct and indirect tissue trauma
- Fall in intravascular volume, leading to a fall in cardiac output and reduced peripheral perfusion
- Local and spreading inflammation and infection
- Systemic inflammatory responses and sepsis
- Pain
- Psychological stress
- Excess heat loss
- Secondary effects on the blood
- Starvation

Box 2.2 Sources of excess fluid loss in surgical patients

Blood loss—traumatic or surgical

Plasma loss—burns

Gastrointestinal fluid loss—vomiting, nasogastric aspiration, sequestration in obstructed or adynamic bowel, loss through a fistula or an ileostomy, diarrhoea

Inflammatory exudate into the peritoneal cavity—generalised peritonitis or acute pancreatitis

Sepsis syndrome (septicaemia)—massive peripheral vasodilatation and third space losses due to increased capillary permeability causing relative hypovolaemia

Abnormal insensible loss—fever, excess sweating or hyperventilation

---

Direct and indirect tissue trauma

Tissue trauma leads to activation of local cytokine responses more or less in proportion to the degree of damage. This applies whether the damage is by cutting (surgical or traumatic), laceration or crushing, and is aggravated if the wounds are contaminated with debris and foreign bodies from without or by faeces from within. Tissue **ischaemia** caused by damage to the arterial supply causes indirect tissue trauma and also compounds the severity of the response to direct trauma.

Fall in intravascular volume (see Box 2.2)

This is one of the key factors that initiate systemic responses. Hypovolaemia results from:

- **Loss** of fluid as a result of haemorrhage or plasma exudation from the surface of burns
- **Interstitial sequestration** of fluid as oedema in damaged tissues themselves and more generally as a result of systemic hormonal responses. This process is amplified in systemic sepsis

- **Restricted oral intake** during any perioperative period or whilst in intensive care

A falling intravascular volume stimulates sympathetic activity by removing baroreceptor inhibition in an attempt to maintain blood pressure. This has the effect of boosting cardiac output and of increasing peripheral resistance. It also explains the mild tachycardia commonly seen in postoperative patients. This compensatory process is most effective in young fit individuals, but decompensation may occur more suddenly when losses reach a tipping point. **Catecholamines** also have profound metabolic effects in addition to their pressor effects, increasing the turnover of carbohydrates, proteins and lipids. Falling renal perfusion activates the **renin–angiotensin–aldosterone system**, increasing renal reabsorption of sodium and water. A centrally mediated increase in antidiuretic hormone (ADH) secretion promotes further conservation of water. Fluid replacement by infusion of only 750 ml of fluid also causes cytokine activation.

Reduced cardiac output and peripheral perfusion

Circulatory efficiency may be impaired by hypovolaemia, and myocardial contractility may be depressed by anaesthetic agents and other drugs. Less commonly, major events such as sepsis (septic shock), pulmonary embolism or myocardial infarction cause cardiovascular collapse.

Inflammation and infection

Products of tissue damage, inflammation and ischaemia cause systemic effects via release of cytokines and other humoral factors. The effects are similar to those involving infection (see Ch. 3).

Systemic inflammatory responses and sepsis

Surface proteins on invading microorganisms are recognised by specific Toll-like receptors on the outer surface of macrophages and this initiates the release of cytokines into the systemic circulation. The effect is to initiate systemic inflammation, which has beneficial effects when in proportion, but has a variety of adverse metabolic effects when in excess. This cytokine response can be initiated by a variety of adverse physiological insults and does not necessarily involve infection.

Pain

Pain causes increased catecholamine and adrenocorticotrophic hormone (ACTH) secretion. Blockade of pain (e.g. by regional anaesthetic procedures) at the time of surgery greatly reduces the adverse systemic effects of pain.

Stress

Psychological stress associated with injury, severe illness or elective surgery has an effect similar to pain on sympathetic function and hypothalamic activity.

Excess heat loss

This can occur during long operations and after extensive burns. Heat loss imposes enormous demands upon energy resources; if body core temperature falls, physiological processes such as blood clotting are impaired. Small babies are particularly vulnerable to heat loss. Heat loss in the operating theatre is counteracted as far as possible by raising the ambient temperature, wrapping exposed parts of the body with insulating material, using warm water underblankets or warm air 'bear-huggers' and by warming fluids during intravenous infusion.

Blood coagulation changes

General metabolic responses to injury activate thrombotic mechanisms and initially depress intrinsic intravascular thrombolysis. Thus the patient is in a **prothrombotic state** and may suffer intravenous thrombosis and consequent thromboembolism.

If substantial haemorrhage occurs, clotting factors eventually become exhausted, causing failure of clotting. The systemic inflammatory response syndrome (SIRS, see p. 16) may initiate widespread intravascular thrombosis, using up clotting factors and precipitating **disseminated intravascular coagulation (DIC)**, with failure of normal clotting or 'red ink syndrome'.

Starvation and stress-induced catabolism

Patients with major surgical conditions are often malnourished (see below, *Nutritional management in the surgical patient*). In particular, patients with upper gastrointestinal tumours, malabsorption syndromes or inflammatory bowel disease are likely to be in a state of chronic starvation before operation. Most surgical patients are starved for 6–12 hours before operation, even in uncomplicated elective surgery, and often do not start eating for 12–24 hours after operation. After major gastrointestinal surgery, food may be withheld for several days or much longer in the event of serious infective complications, anastomotic breakdown or fistula formation. Starvation increases susceptibility to infection and thus it is important to recognise it and, if possible, correct it in patients undergoing surgery.

METABOLIC RESPONSES TO PATHOPHYSIOLOGICAL STRESS

In severe trauma and extensive operative surgery, particularly if complicated by sepsis, the key factors in the systemic response are **increased sympathetic activity** together with increased **circulating catecholamines** and **insulin**. Cytokine responses signal other cells to prepare for action (e.g. polymorphs, T and B cells), to compensate for starvation, provide additional energy and building blocks for tissue repair, and conserve sodium ions and water.

There is also a massive attempt to increase glucose production by the process of **gluconeogenesis**. Adrenaline (epinephrine) and noradrenaline (norepinephrine) are released into the systemic circulation both from sympathetic nerve endings and from the adrenal medulla to play a central role in these particular systemic responses. In addition, there is enhanced secretion of ACTH, glucocorticoids (cortisol), glucagon and growth hormone, all of which contribute to the general **catabolic response**. At the same time increased aldosterone and ADH production mediate some of the fluid and electrolyte changes. **Insulin** acts as an antagonist of most of the above hormones and is secreted in increased amounts from the second or third day after injury.

The sum of these factors is to cause an intense but inevitable catabolism as well as potentially extreme changes in fluid balance and electrolyte concentrations. This results in the metabolic changes shown in Figure 2.1.

EFFECTS ON CARBOHYDRATE METABOLISM

The overall effect is a rise in blood glucose levels, often resulting in **hyperglycaemia** and a **pseudodiabetic state**. Blood glucose levels may reach 20 mmol/L and glucose may appear in the urine. This is in marked contrast to

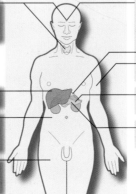

Increased secretion of growth hormone and thyroid hormones, both of which inhibit the effects of insulin and promote catabolism

Enhanced hepatic glycogenolysis and gluconeogenesis

Catecholamines and glucagon stimulate lipolysis in adipose tissue releasing fatty acids; these provide the major energy source for peripheral tissues

Breakdown of muscle protein releases amino acids, the main substrate for gluconeogenesis and the raw material for wound healing

Increased pituitary ACTH release induces a massive rise in circulating glucocorticoids; cortisol levels can increase tenfold immediately after surgery, remaining elevated for days or weeks.

Glucocorticoids also enhance gluconeogenesis and promote catabolism of muscle protein and liberation of amino acids

Increased insulin secretion but inhibition of its tissue effects which block cellular utilisation of glucose

Stimulation of glucagon secretion further enhances glycogenolysis and gluconeogenesis

Fig. 2.1 Metabolic responses to major systemic insults

simple fasting, in which glucose levels are normal or slightly depressed and glycosuria does not occur.

EFFECTS ON BODY PROTEINS AND NITROGEN METABOLISM

In the normal healthy adult, **nitrogen balance** is constantly maintained. Normal protein turnover results in the daily excretion of 12–20 g of urinary nitrogen and this is made good by dietary intake. In contrast, in a hypercatabolic state, nitrogen losses can increase three- or fourfold. Most importantly, the metabolic environment prevents proper utilisation of food or intravenous nutrition. There is therefore an enormous and inevitable daily destruction of skeletal muscle. This state of **negative nitrogen balance** contrasts markedly with simple starvation in which body protein is preserved.

EFFECTS ON LIPID STORES AND METABOLISM

The effects of major body insults upon lipid metabolism are little different from simple starvation; most of the energy requirements are met from fat stores.

Surgical catabolism only reverses as the patient recovers from the illness and therefore early parenteral nutrition has little effect, although carbohydrate administration may spare some protein loss.

Note that when patients have been severely ill, carbohydrate metabolism is minimal and energy comes from catabolism of protein and fat. Once feeding recommences, there is a danger of **refeeding syndrome** (see below), largely due to intracellular phosphate depletion; precautions need to be taken to anticipate and monitor the problem and to increase calorie intake slowly.

FLUID, ELECTROLYTE AND ACID–BASE MANAGEMENT

INTRODUCTION

Fluid, electrolyte and acid–base derangements can be minimised if high-risk patients are assessed before operation and their cardiovascular function and fluid balance closely monitored before and after operation. If abnormalities do develop, the diagnosis and management can be worked out with reasoning and common sense. Plasma urea and electrolytes should be checked at least once a day in patients undergoing major surgery or those receiving intravenous fluids.

Severely ill patients with abdominal infection, sepsis and fistulae are likely to suffer major problems of fluid balance (and nutrition, see below). These are best managed with the help of experienced anaesthetists in intensive care or high-dependency units, where monitoring and therapy can be rigorously managed. Patients with extensive **burns** are at particular risk of hypovolaemia and require early and vigorous fluid replacement before transfer to a specialist burns unit.

NORMAL FLUID AND ELECTROLYTE HOMEOSTASIS

The body of an average 70 kg adult contains 42 litres of fluid, distributed between the intracellular compartment, the extracellular space and the bloodstream (see Fig. 2.2). Fluid **enters** the body mainly by oral intake of fluids and food but about 200 ml of water is produced per day

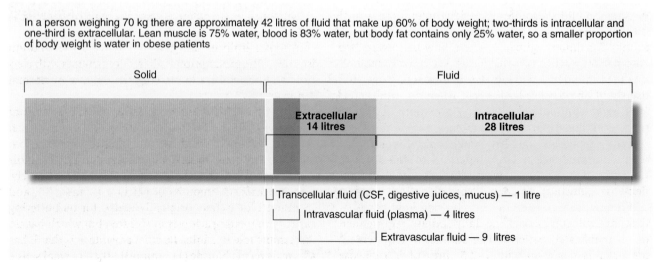

In a person weighing 70 kg there are approximately 42 litres of fluid that make up 60% of body weight; two-thirds is intracellular and one-third is extracellular. Lean muscle is 75% water, blood is 83% water, but body fat contains only 25% water, so a smaller proportion of body weight is water in obese patients

Table 2.1 Summary—normal daily fluid and electrolyte input and output

Normal daily intake	Normal daily output
Water	
Diet 2300 ml Metabolism 200 ml	Urine 1400 ml (minimum obligatory volume = 400 ml) Skin loss 500 ml (obligatory diffusion and vaporisation) *Note: sweating in pyrexia or a high ambient temperature can* *can cause several litres extra loss each day* Lung loss 500 ml (obligatory) Faecal loss 100 ml
Sodium	
Diet 150 mmol/day (range 50–300 mmol)	Stool 5 mmol/day Skin transpiration 5 mmol/day (in the absence of sweating) Urine 140 mmol/day (can fall down to 15 mmol/day if required)
Potassium	
Diet 100 mmol/day (range 50–200 mmol)	Stool 10 mmol/day (obligatory) Skin < 5 mmol/day Urine 85 mmol/day (rarely falls below 60 mmol/day)

as a by-product of metabolism. This same adult normally **loses** between 2.5 and 3 litres of fluid in 24 hours. About 1 litre of this is lost insensibly from skin and lungs, 1300–1800 ml are passed as urine (about 60 ml/hour or 1 ml/kg/hour) and 100 ml are lost in the faeces. About 100–150 mmol of sodium ions and 50–100 mmol of potassium ions are lost each day in the urine and this is balanced by the normal dietary intake (see Table 2.1).

When a patient is deprived of all oral intake, as occurs in the perioperative period or in coma, isotonic electrolyte solutions of appropriate types need to be given intravenously as replacement.

MAINTENANCE OF WATER AND SODIUM

In an uncomplicated patient, the daily water and sodium requirements can be administered as 2.5–3 litres of a standard **dextrose–saline** solution containing 4% dextrose and 0.18% sodium chloride (note: this has only one-fifth the salt content of 'normal', i.e. physiological, saline). This fluid regimen is often, however, prescribed automatically without considering the special requirements of individual patients. For this reason, its general use should be discouraged except when an intravenous infusion is required for only a day or two and there are no special fluid or electrolyte problems.

For most patients, the daily water and sodium requirements are best met by using appropriate quantities of **normal saline** solution (0.9% sodium chloride) and **5% dextrose** (glucose) solution. Normal saline contains 154 mmol each of sodium and chloride ions per litre. One litre will thus satisfy the daily sodium requirement of uncomplicated patients. The additional requirement for water is made up with 2–2.5 litres of 5% glucose (see Box 2.3). The small amount of glucose this contains

Box 2.3 Sample daily intravenous fluid regimens as a substitute for oral intake in uncomplicated cases

Prescription (1) for 24 hours (each bag to be given over 8 hours):

1000 ml 0.9% sodium chloride + 20 mmol KCl
1000 ml 5% dextrose + 20 mmol KCl
1000 ml 5% dextrose + 20 mmol KCl
Total: 154 mmol sodium and 60 mmol potassium

Prescription (2) for 24 hours (each bag to be given over 8 hours):

1000 ml dextrose–saline (i.e. 4% dextrose + 1.8% NaCl) + 20 mmol KCl
1000 ml dextrose–saline + 20 mmol KCl
1000 ml dextrose–saline + 20 mmol KCl
Total: 120 mmol sodium and 60 mmol potassium

contributes little to nutrition but renders the solution isotonic. This prescription is altered for patients with electrolyte abnormalities by varying the volume of normal saline given.

Note that **Hartmann's solution** (Ringer's lactate/compound sodium lactate) is often used without much thought as the sole fluid for intravenous infusion. However, it contains excessive levels of sodium (131 mmol/L) and too little potassium (5 mmol/L) if used exclusively, also insignificant amounts of calcium (2 mmol/L), and 29 mmol/L of lactate, originally added for its buffering capacity in treating acidosis in children but which has no discernible role in adults. Its chief advantage is that it has a lower level of chloride (111 mmol/L) than normal saline (154 mmol/L).

In children, water excretion is markedly reduced in the postoperative period as a result of increased ADH secretion. Maintenance fluids requirements are based on published guidelines and formulae but the volumes recommended have recently been reduced by 50%. It is still not clear whether paediatric dextrose–saline (5% dextrose plus 0.45% NaCl) plus KCl should be used or whether normal saline is better (see: http://www.nda.ox.ac.uk/wfsa/html/u19/u1914_01.htm).

MAINTENANCE OF POTASSIUM

Basic potassium requirements are met by infusing 60–80 mmol of potassium chloride in divided doses over each 24-hour period. Premixed intravenous fluids are generally available with 20 or 40 mmol of potassium chloride per 500 ml or 1000 ml infusion bags. If premixed solutions are not available, potassium chloride can be added to intravenous solutions but care must be taken to ensure thorough mixing. If concentrations of potassium chloride greater than 40 mmol in 500 ml are required, they should be given via an infusion in the intensive care unit, with cardiac monitoring. Bolus injections of KCl must *never* be given because rapid increases in plasma potassium can cause cardiac arrest.

Note that added potassium is not usually required in the first 24–48 hours after surgery because potassium is released from damaged cells and raises the plasma potassium concentration.

LIMITS OF COMPENSATORY MECHANISMS

The kidneys are normally able to maintain fluid and electrolyte homeostasis in spite of large variations of fluid intake from hour to hour and day to day. The same also applies to fluid and electrolytes given intravenously. Note that the kidneys' compensating capacity is reduced by renal parenchymal disease and by chronic renal insufficiency.

The total blood volume in an adult male is about 5 litres, of which about 55–60% is water (about 3.5 litres). Falls in blood volume which are not too rapid or extensive can be compensated by fluid movement from the extracellular compartment. This compartment has a volume of more than 10 litres. A deficit of more than 3 litres in whole body fluid volume cannot be sustained and intravascular volume inevitably becomes depleted. This is reflected in compensatory cardiovascular changes. Vasoconstriction causes cold peripheries: this is an important warning sign of hypovolaemia and more reliable than early tachycardia, particularly in children. Initially, there is a mild **tachycardia** but when the overall fluid deficit reaches about 3 litres, the pulse rate becomes very rapid and **hypotension** develops. Note that patients on beta-adrenergic blocking drugs or with cardiac conduction defects may not be able to increase the heart rate and will therefore decompensate earlier. With 4 or more litres of fluid deficit, the limit of cardiovascular compensation is reached and the patient develops **hypovolaemic shock**. Note that fit young people are able to sustain normal vital signs for longer than other patients but when they do decompensate, they do so abruptly.

In neonates, children, the elderly and the chronically ill, cardiovascular compensation capacity is greatly reduced. A relatively small fluid and electrolyte imbalance may cause life-threatening complications.

PHYSIOLOGICAL CHANGES IN RESPONSE TO SURGERY AND TRAUMA

The stresses of trauma or surgery cause a rise in the level of circulating **catecholamines**. Stress also stimulates the hypothalamo–pituitary–adrenal axis, which increases secretion of **cortisol** and **aldosterone**. These hormones promote renal conservation of sodium and water and cause a reduction in urine volume and urine sodium concentration.

Effects of a fall in renal perfusion

Any substantial reduction in the effective circulating volume may cause a fall in renal perfusion. Causes include haemorrhage, loss of oedema fluid into a site of trauma or operation, third-space or interstitial losses (see later), loss from vomiting or diarrhoea, excess insensible loss and sequestration within adynamic bowel. In addition, aortic surgery involving aortic clamping may alter the dynamics of renal artery flow, whilst raised intra-abdominal pressure (see abdominal compartment syndrome below) disrupts renal blood flow.

A fall in renal perfusion activates the renin–angiotensin–aldosterone mechanism to sustain the blood pressure. As glomerular filtration falls, **renin** release is stimulated from the juxtaglomerular apparatus of the kidney and this catalyses the conversion of **angiotensin I** to **angiotensin II** in the lungs. Angiotensin II has a powerful pressor effect on the peripheral vasculature, counteracting hypotension, as well as stimulating **aldosterone** release from the adrenal cortex. Aldosterone promotes active **reabsorption of sodium** ions from the distal convoluted tubules of the kidney; this is accompanied by passive reabsorption of water. Sodium reabsorption is linked to increased excretion of potassium and hydrogen ions.

The net effect is that in conditions causing renal perfusion to fall, the urine output falls by several hundred millilitres per day, and the urine that is produced is low in sodium (less than 40 mmol/L), high in potassium (greater than 100 mmol/L) and acidic. The loss of hydrogen ions causes a degree of **metabolic alkalosis.**

Other factors in water conservation

Water conservation is further enhanced by stress-mediated secretion of **antidiuretic hormone** (ADH), also known as vasopressin, from the posterior pituitary (neurohypophysis). Loss of water alone results in elevated plasma sodium concentration. This increases the plasma osmolality which is the most potent stimulator of ADH release, mediated by osmoreceptors in the hypothalamus. ADH binds to receptors in the distal renal tubules and promotes reabsorption of water. In the absence of ADH, the tubules are virtually impermeable to water and virtually none is reabsorbed. Release of ADH is also stimulated by falls in blood pressure and volume, sensed by stretch receptors in the heart and large arteries. Changes in blood pressure and volume are not nearly as sensitive a stimulator as increased osmolarity, but are potent in severe conditions. For example, loss of 15 or 20% of blood volume by haemorrhage results in massive secretion of ADH. Stress and pain probably also promote ADH release via other hypothalamic pathways.

Postoperative situation

At the site of trauma or major surgery, a volume of fluid is effectively removed from the circulation in the form of inflammatory oedema (isotonic local third-space losses). This displaced volume is compensated by fluid retained by the hormonal changes described above. More potassium is released from damaged cells than the excess lost by exchange in the kidney. Thus, the postoperative plasma **potassium level tends to rise** in the first day or two. This is particularly true if stored blood has been transfused as this releases potassium from elderly red cells. For these reasons, potassium supplements are not usually needed for the first few days after operation provided the preoperative plasma potassium level is normal and potassium-losing diuretics are not being prescribed.

It is important to recognise the **normal phase** of **relative oliguria** and **sodium retention** that inevitably occurs for up to 48 hours after major injury or surgery as this has an important bearing on fluid management. Like surgical catabolism, described earlier, these effects are resistant to external manipulation but resolve with recovery of the patient.

Abdominal compartment syndrome

(see http://ccforum.com/content/4/1/023)
Abdominal compartment syndrome, with the adverse effects it can cause on organ systems, is now recognised as an entity. Intra-abdominal pressure is normally less than 5 mmHg, but after surgery or trauma it may rise as high as 15 mmHg. Cardiac output begins to fall off at 10 mmHg, and hypotension and oliguria are likely between 15 and 20 mmHg. Anuria occurs with pressures over 40 mmHg.

The causes of abdominal compartment syndrome are often multifactorial and include **fluid accumulating** as a result of retroperitoneal haemorrhage, e.g. in ruptured abdominal aortic aneurysm, postoperative haemorrhage (particularly if clotting is disordered), organ trauma, pan-

creatitis, and interstitial oedema in sepsis or zealous fluid resuscitation. When the abdominal pressure exceeds the capillary pressure perfusing abdominal organs, dysfunction of these organs and eventually infarction is likely to occur.

Adverse effects include:

- Oliguria due to renal hypoperfusion and collapsed renal veins
- Respiratory embarrassment due to restriction and elevation of the diaphragm, as well as compression of the alveoli. This results in increased peak airways pressure, decreased tidal volume, hypoxaemia and hypercarbia
- Decreased venous return leading to falling cardiac output and hypotension
- Bowel ischaemia causing gastrointestinal bleeding

In patients with a distended and taut abdomen, measuring abdominal compartment pressure can help early recognition of organ dysfunction. Treatment involves reopening the abdomen and leaving it open until the risk of rising pressure subsides.

PROBLEMS OF FLUID AND ELECTROLYTE DEPLETION

LOSS OF WHOLE BLOOD OR PLASMA

Rapid and copious blood loss in traumatic injury or operative surgery initially depletes the intravascular compartment. Rapid loss of only 1 litre may cause hypotension or even hypovolaemic shock. When haemorrhage is less rapid, there is time for the extracellular compartment to replace the fluid loss, and greater volumes can be lost before the cardiovascular system becomes compromised. The lost blood is still a volume loss to the system even though it is compensated by extracellular fluid shift. The volume must be restored physiologically or by transfusion.

If blood loss has ceased, the need for transfusion is based on the estimated or measured volume lost and on the previous haemoglobin concentration. The possibility of further blood loss must of course be anticipated by ensuring good venous access and, if necessary, obtaining bank blood. Acute blood loss of 500–1000 ml is usually treated by transfusing crystalloids. Plasma substitutes such as **gelatin solutions** remain longer in the circulation but there is little evidence that they are better than crystalloids for treating acute blood loss. Larger volume losses are ideally replaced by transfusion of whole blood. However, this is becoming an increasingly rare commodity and packed red cells supplemented by normal saline to expand volume should be given. Slow chronic blood loss, e.g. from a peptic ulcer or hookworm infestation, does not lead to fluid balance problems but may cause symptoms and signs of anaemia. Transfusion is not usually required in such cases.

In **severe burns**, the amount of plasma likely to be lost should be calculated by using a standard formula based on the area burnt to guide fluid replacement (see Ch. 17). Infusion requirements can be seriously underestimated unless an accepted formula or a suitable alternative is used.

GASTROINTESTINAL FLUID LOSS

Between 5 and 9 litres of electrolyte-rich fluid is normally secreted into the upper gastrointestinal tract each day as saliva, gastric juice, bile, pancreatic fluid and succus entericus (small bowel secretions; see Table 2.2). Most of the fluid is reabsorbed in the large intestine.

Huge volumes of water and electrolytes may be lost from the body as a result of vomiting, nasogastric aspiration, diarrhoea, sequestration of fluid in obstructed or adynamic bowel or drainage to the exterior via a fistula or an ileostomy. If there is widespread **inflammation of the bowel** as in gastroenteritis or ulcerative colitis, inflammatory exudate may greatly increase the fluid lost as diarrhoea. Cholera can cause the loss of up to 10 litres of electrolyte-rich fluid in one day and this fluid loss is a frequent cause of death, particularly in children.

Abnormal fluid losses must be measured or estimated as accurately as possible and recorded on a fluid balance chart. In addition, observations should be regularly made for signs of fluid depletion including pulse rate, blood pressure, periodic urine output and, if necessary, central venous pressure (CVP). These measures enable intravenous replacement to be predicted and the adverse consequences of fluid and electrolyte depletion to be prevented.

From Table 2.2, it can be seen that **vomitus** and nasogastric aspirate usually contain about 120 mmol of sodium ions per litre and up to 10 mmol potassium ions per litre. Inflammatory **diarrhoea** contains a slightly lower concentration of sodium ions, but more than 40 mmol of potassium ions per litre. As a general rule, gastrointestinal fluid losses should be replaced by an equivalent volume of normal saline, with potassium chloride added as necessary. In intestinal obstruction or adynamic ileus, fluid sequestrated in the bowel is replaced in a similar manner, although volume requirements cannot be measured accurately and have to be estimated. Fistulae and overactive ileostomies cause chronic loss of fluid that is high in chloride and bicarbonate.

INTRA-ABDOMINAL ACCUMULATION OF INFLAMMATORY FLUID

Severe intra-abdominal inflammation may cause several litres of fluid rich in plasma proteins and electrolytes to be lost into the peritoneal cavity. This typically occurs in peritonitis or acute pancreatitis. Cytokine-induced **systemic inflammatory response syndrome** (SIRS) is likely to occur in these conditions. In SIRS, there is an important element of '**third-space loss**', i.e. fluid leached into the extracellular or interstitial space because of leaky capillaries. This is best replaced (as well as can be estimated) by physiological saline or other suitable crystalloids.

SYSTEMIC SEPSIS (SIRS AND MULTIPLE ORGAN DYSFUNCTION SYNDROME)

Systemic sepsis is associated with widespread endothelial damage and a large increase in capillary permeability mediated by a range of cytokines and other circulating substances. The result is extensive loss of protein and electrolyte-rich fluid from the circulation into the extracellular space, which, combined with a loss of peripheral resistance, results in cardiovascular collapse and shock. This fluid deficiency should be replaced as for fluid loss into the peritoneal cavity.

The required fluid volume is difficult to estimate and replacement is usually given so as to maintain cardiovascular stability (pulse rate and blood pressure) and urinary output (at least 0.5 ml/kg body weight/hour) whilst avoiding fluid overload and cardiac failure. In the severely ill patient, in whom the volume requirements are particularly difficult to judge, a central venous pressure line makes treatment safer and more precise. These patients

Table 2.2 Daily gastrointestinal secretions and electrolyte composition

Secretion	Volume (L)	Na⁺ (mmol/L)	K⁺ (mmol/L)	Cl⁻ (mmol/L)	HCO₃⁻ (mmol/L)
Saliva	1–1.5	20–80	10–20	20–40	20–160
Gastric juice	1–2.5	20–100	5–10	120–160	Nil
Bile	Up to 1	150–250	5–10	40–60	20–60
Pancreatic juice	1–2	120	5–10	10–60	80–120
Succus entericus (small bowel secretions)	2–3	140	5 (increases up to 40 in inflammatory diarrhoea)	Variable	Variable

are best managed in high-dependency or intensive care units. Transoesophageal ultrasound may prove to be a more accurate method of assessing precise fluid replacement needs (see *Enhanced Recovery Programmes*, below).

ABNORMAL INSENSIBLE FLUID LOSS

Abnormal insensible fluid loss can greatly increase overall fluid loss, particularly in the seriously ill patient. Insensible losses must be included in the fluid balance equation, especially if losses are sustained for more than a short period. **Pyrexia** increases insensible loss by approximately 20% for each degree Celsius rise in body temperature, mainly in the form of exhaled water vapour. A pyrexia of 38.5°C for 3 days would therefore cause an extra litre of fluid loss. **Sweating** causes loss of sodium-rich fluid which can be easily overlooked in patients with fever and when the ambient temperature rises in summer. The elderly are particularly vulnerable when denied oral fluids before operation.

PREVENTING ACUTE RENAL FAILURE

Maintaining fluid balance in surgical patients depends on anticipating problems before they cause adverse effects and put the patient at risk of acute renal failure. Acute renal failure is a serious complication with a high mortality in surgical patients. Prevention involves the same strategy in all patients at risk, namely:

- Observing changes in vital signs—pulse rate, blood pressure and CVP if appropriate
- Checking hourly urine output is adequate
- Measuring fluid losses to guide replacement
- Seeking clinical signs of fluid imbalance (both dehydration and overload)
- Regularly estimating plasma urea and electrolytes

In patients with cardiac failure or shock, monitoring and treatment is best carried out in an intensive care or high-dependency unit, using invasive monitoring to help determine the required volume of fluid replacement.

COMMON FLUID AND ELECTROLYTE PROBLEMS

INTERMEDIATE ELECTIVE OPERATIONS AND UNCOMPLICATED EMERGENCY OPERATIONS

Most operations fall into this category. Patients are generally in fluid and electrolyte equilibrium before operation, although some have problems caused by diuretic therapy (for cardiac failure, hypertension or chronic renal failure). For these, plasma urea and electrolytes should be checked before operation. Note that loop and thiazide diuretics may cause **hypokalaemia** whilst potassium-sparing

diuretics such as spironolactone may cause **hyperkalaemia**. If serious abnormalities are found, operation must be postponed until the problem is corrected. Hypokalaemia can usually be treated by oral potassium supplements or by adding a potassium-sparing diuretic. Hyperkalaemia is usually corrected by substituting a loop or thiazide diuretic.

Mild renal dysfunction (plasma urea up to about 15 mmol/L and creatinine up to about 170 mmol/L) is not usually a contraindication to surgery. These patients tend to be mildly dehydrated, however, and oral fluid intake should be strongly encouraged.

Management

For elective surgery, the patient is often kept 'nil by mouth' for 6–12 hours before operation, although there is a trend towards encouraging clear fluids by mouth up to 3 hours before operation. The patient is likely to take very little oral fluid for up to 6 hours after operation and a fluid deficit of 1000–1500 ml is therefore common. Mild fluid deficits can usually be accommodated and are quickly made up once the patient is drinking normally. Intravenous fluid replacement is therefore not required for most uncomplicated intermediate operations in adults. For patients with **mild renal failure**, an infusion should be set up at the outset of the 'nil by mouth' period to prevent the dire consequences of acute-on-chronic renal failure. Occasionally, and despite the use of anti-emetics, patients vomit after operation and intravenous fluids should be employed if vomiting is prolonged.

Children and especially infants and neonates are much more vulnerable to fluid deprivation because of their small total body fluid volume and disproportionate insensible losses. Even relatively minor operations can cause dehydration and intravenous fluids may be necessary, with the rate and volume calculated according to body weight and measured blood loss.

As a rule, the sooner the body can assume control over its own fluid and electrolyte homeostasis the better. Intravenous fluids should be discontinued as soon as normal oral intake has been resumed and urine output is satisfactory.

MAJOR OPERATIONS

Major elective or emergency operations, especially those involving bowel, pose particular problems with fluid management. The principal reasons are:

- Patients are often elderly and are likely to have a diminished cardiovascular reserve. They may have pre-existing fluid and electrolyte abnormalities
- Preoperative vomiting and restricted fluid intake may have caused dehydration and electrolyte abnormalities
- Blood loss during and after operation may be substantial

- Operations may take several hours with consequent insensible losses from the open wound
- Third-space losses of 500–1000 ml can occur after major surgery or trauma as a result of systemic responses to trauma
- The recovery period when oral intake is nil or restricted may become extended—several days following complicated bowel surgery or peritonitis (e.g. perforated diverticulitis or an anastomotic leak)

Careful preoperative and postoperative assessment of patients undergoing major surgery is crucial so that problems can be recognised early. This should include clinical examination for evidence of **dehydration** (dry mouth and loss of normal skin turgor) or **overhydration** (elevated jugular venous pressure or cardiac failure). Plasma urea and electrolytes, creatinine and full blood count should be measured daily. An elevated urea concentration with little elevation of creatinine is characteristic of dehydration. An abnormally high haemoglobin concentration (providing polycythaemia is not present) also indicates dehydration, especially if it was normal beforehand.

ENHANCED RECOVERY PROGRAMMES

In recent years, clinicians in surgery have been attempting to shorten hospital stays and reduce complication rates by developing structured systems that reduce the stress response to enhance recovery. These involve attention to all facets of surgical care, so-called 'multimodal optimisation' or 'fast track recovery'. This includes particularly careful attention to perioperative fluid management, the use of minimal access surgical techniques and mechanisms to preserve postoperative organ function, including:

- Preoperative assessment and improved education and preparation of patients so that they understand what will happen and cope with planned early discharge
- Home care arrangements to cope with early discharge
- Improved methods of fluid replacement that ensure the patient remains normovolaemic within narrow limits, preventing hypovolaemia and fluid overload. Current methods are somewhat arbitrary, relying on insensitive measures such as blood pressure and pulse rate and sometimes CVP. Transoesophageal ultrasound monitoring of aortic blood flow may prove to be a useful assessment technique: in preliminary trials its use appears to shorten hospital stays and reduce complication rates
- Planned and assisted early postoperative mobilisation
- Early enteral nutrient challenge and the use of gut-specific nutrients such as glutamine, antioxidants and synbiotics (nutritional supplements that improve the balance of intestinal microflora). Methods that enable earlier return of gut function may be

fundamental to rapid recovery. Gastrointestinal gut-associated lymphoid tissue (GALT) forms more than half the body's immunological cell mass and is believed to play a key role in the stress response to surgery. Sustaining the nutrition of the small bowel wall from within the lumen may prevent the breakdown of intestinal barrier function. Healthy bowel function enables earlier tolerance of food, less postoperative ileus and less postoperative nausea and vomiting

- Avoiding opiates by using epidural analgesia
- Delivering high concentrations of inspired oxygen

ABNORMALITIES OF INDIVIDUAL ELECTROLYTES (see Table 2.3 for a summary of causes and effects)

ABNORMALITIES OF PLASMA SODIUM CONCENTRATION

Plasma sodium abnormalities are usually discovered incidentally on regular measurement of electrolytes.

Hyponatraemia

A low plasma sodium level may be real or spurious. Spurious results commonly arise when blood is taken from an arm receiving an intravenous infusion; less commonly, false laboratory results can occur if there is **lipaemia** resulting from parenteral nutrition. If in doubt, the test should be repeated with appropriate precautions.

In hyponatraemia (except in severe hyperglycaemia or infusion of mannitol), the plasma becomes **hypotonic**. This causes cellular overhydration which in severe cases results in cerebral oedema. Mild hyponatraemia is symptomless but when the plasma sodium falls below about 120 mmol/L, patients often become confused. Convulsions and coma occur when sodium concentrations fall below about 110 mmol/L. If hyponatraemia is confirmed biochemically, the next step is to clinically assess the **state of hydration** (i.e. the extracellular fluid volume) and this will guide therapy.

There are three possibilities:

- **Water deficit with a larger sodium deficit** (clinical signs—dry mouth, poor skin turgor, poor urine output, high urine osmolality): sodium insufficiency is usually due to diuretic therapy, vomiting, diarrhoea or other excessive losses of body fluids with inadequate replacement. Treatment involves rehydration with appropriate sodium-containing intravenous fluids
- **Sodium normal with a larger water excess** (clinical signs—weight gain, ankle swelling, raised jugular venous pressure): this usually results from organ dysfunction. Cardiac failure is the most common

Table 2.3 Causes and effects of sodium and potassium deficiency and excess

Electrolyte abnormality	Causes	Adverse effects
Hyponatraemia	Diuretics (especially thiazides) Water excess (ingested or intravenous) Diarrhoea Vomiting Losses from intestinal fistula Renal failure Syndrome of inappropriate antidiuretic hormone secretion (SIADH) Addison's disease Nephrotic syndrome Liver failure	Confusion Seizures Hypertension Cardiac failure Muscle weakness Nausea Anorexia
Hypernatraemia	Fluid loss without water replacement, e.g. diarrhoea, vomiting, burns Saline excess (usually iatrogenic) Diabetes insipidus Diabetic ketoacidosis Primary aldosteronism (Conn's syndrome)	Thirst Dehydration Confusion Coma Seizures
Hyperkalaemia	Sampling artefact (haemolysis of sample or delayed processing) Drugs, e.g. ACE inhibitors, spironolactone, suxamethonium Digoxin poisoning Excess potassium chloride (iatrogenic) Massive blood transfusion Burns Rhabdomyolysis Tumour lysis syndrome Renal failure Aldosterone deficiency Addison's disease Metabolic acidosis	Cardiac arrhythmias Sudden death
Hypokalaemia	Vomiting Diarrhoea Losses from intestinal fistula Diuretics Purgative abuse Renal tubular failure Cushing's disease, exogenous steroids or ACTH Metabolic alkalosis Primary hyperaldosteronism (Conn's syndrome) Secondary hyperaldosteronism	Cardiac arrhythmias Muscle weakness Hypotonia Muscle cramps Tetany

cause, followed by renal, liver and respiratory failure. Overhydration is compounded by excessive intravenous fluid administration. Management is based primarily on treating the organ failure, e.g. diuretics for cardiac failure

- **Water excess**: this is uncommon and is usually due to **inappropriate antidiuretic hormone (ADH) secretion**. This is rare on a surgical ward except for TUR syndrome in which excess fluid is absorbed during transurethral resection of the prostate. It can also occur following head injury or neurosurgery, or may occur in pneumonia, empyema, lung abscess or oat-cell carcinoma of the lung. Excess ADH increases water reabsorption by the renal tubules independently of sodium. The result is water

overload and dilutional hyponatraemia. Inappropriate ADH secretion is the most likely diagnosis if the urine osmolality is found to be high and the plasma osmolality low. Hyponatraemia caused by inappropriate ADH secretion is managed by restricting fluid intake to 1 litre per day

Hypernatraemia

This is an uncommon problem and is often iatrogenic in the surgical patient. The usual cause is either excess administration of sodium via intravenous fluids or inadequate water replacement. Hypernatraemia is more likely to occur after operation because increased aldosterone secretion causes sodium to be conserved by the kidney.

19

Very rarely, hypernatraemia is caused by **Conn's syndrome** (primary hyperaldosteronism).

Treatment involves encouraging the patient to drink more water, or infusing fluids with a low sodium content.

ABNORMALITIES OF PLASMA POTASSIUM CONCENTRATION

Acid–base abnormalities (see below) can have a profound effect on plasma potassium concentration but are likely to correct spontaneously as the acid–base problem is treated.

Hypokalaemia

In the preoperative patient, hypokalaemia usually results from poor dietary intake, diuretic therapy, chronic diarrhoea, losses from a malfunctioning ileostomy or, rarely, excess mucus secretion from a rectal villous adenoma. Rarely, hypokalaemia may be caused by **primary hyperaldosteronism** (Conn's syndrome).

Postoperatively, hypokalaemia is usually caused by inadequate potassium supplementation in intravenous infusions. The lack of intake is compounded by increased urinary losses from stress-induced **secondary hyperaldosteronism**.

Hypokalaemia causes skeletal muscle weakness and reduces gastrointestinal motility, with paralytic ileus in extreme cases. When severe, there is also a risk of sudden cardiac arrhythmias or even cardiac arrest. Hypokalaemia can usually be corrected with oral potassium supplements (effervescent or slow-release tablets). For patients on intravenous fluids, potassium supplements are added as appropriate. The infusion rate should not generally exceed 15–20 mmol per hour, but larger quantities may be required following operations involving cardiopulmonary bypass.

Hyperkalaemia

This is less common in surgical patients than hypokalaemia but may require urgent correction. In the preoperative patient, it is most commonly caused by chronic renal failure, high doses of ACE inhibiting drugs or potassium-sparing diuretics. Occasionally, non-steroidal anti-inflammatory drugs cause hyperkalaemia. Postoperative hyperkalaemia is usually iatrogenic, caused by excessive intravenous potassium administration, although it may be associated with acute renal failure or large transfusions of old stored blood.

Patients with a potassium of > 6.5 are at risk of ventricular fibrillation and sudden death. Typical ECG changes occurring in hyperkalaemic patients are:

Early ECG changes:

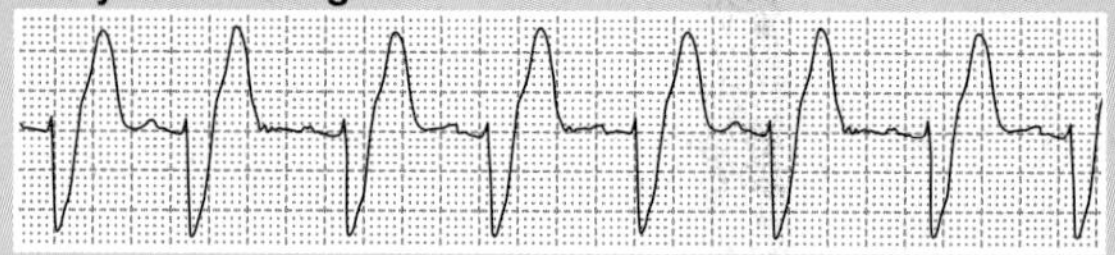

tall 'tented' T waves
flat P waves
increased P–R interval

Late ECG changes:

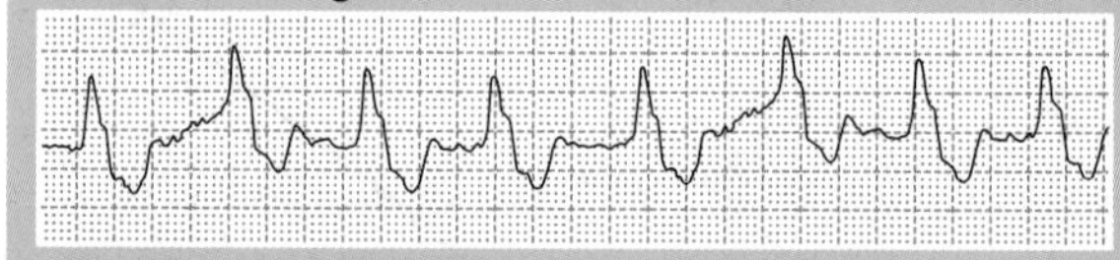

widening of the QRS complex
sinusoidal pattern
ventricular tachycardia/ventricular fibrillation

Emergency management of hyperkalaemia

1. Cardioprotection
Calcium gluconate (10 ml of 10%) is given intravenously over 2 minutes. The dose can be repeated if necessary

2. Drive potassium into the cells
Give insulin and glucose (e.g. 20 units of insulin and 50 ml of 50% dextrose) ± nebulised salbutamol (usually 2.5 mg)

3. Deplete total body potassium
Polystyrene sulfonate resin is given orally or rectally to bind potassium. Haemodialysis or peritoneal dialysis may also be required

Fig. 2.3 Emergency management of hyperkalaemia

Hyperkalaemia is asymptomatic in the early stages but there is a high risk of sudden death from asystole when the plasma potassium concentration reaches about 7.0 mmol/L. The emergency management of hyperkalaemia is shown in Figure 2.3. Potassium concentration at this level is a medical emergency, especially if there are typical ECG changes (i.e. peaked T-waves), and it should be treated initially by intravenous infusion of insulin and glucose (after a cardioprotective dose of calcium gluconate). This causes a shift of potassium from the extracellular to the intracellular fluid compartment. Severe renal failure may require haemofiltration.

ACID–BASE DISTURBANCES (see Fig. 2.4 and Table 2.4)

Major acid–base abnormalities are rare in uncomplicated surgery and usually arise in seriously ill patients. In a nutshell, when breathing is inadequate, carbon dioxide builds up and combines with water to produce carbonic acid ('respiratory acid') which contributes to an acidic pH. Treatment is to lower the PCO_2 by assisted breathing. In addition, when normal metabolism is impaired, oxidative metabolism declines and lactic acid accumulates.

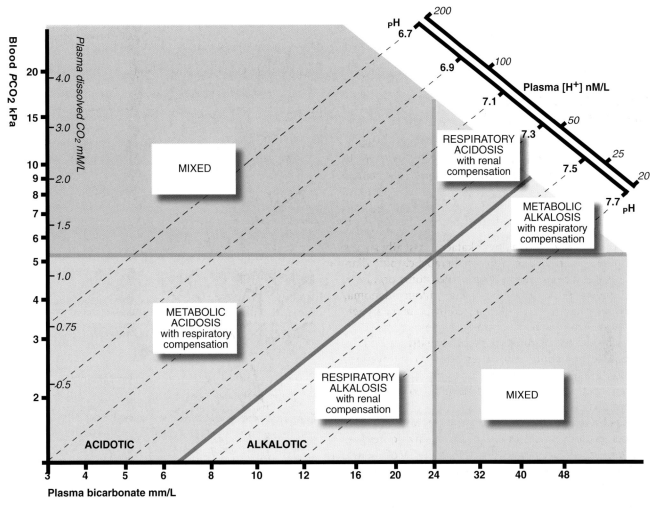

Fig. 2.4 Interpretation of blood gas analyses in the patient with acid–base disturbances

Table 2.4 Acid–base disorders

Acid–base status	Blood gas analyses		
	pH	PCO_2	HCO_3^-
Respiratory acidosis	↓ or normal (if compensated)	↑↑	↑ (if compensated)
Respiratory alkalosis	↑ or normal (if compensated)	↓↓	↓ (if compensated)
Metabolic acidosis	↓ or normal (if compensated)	↓ (if compensated)	↓↓
Metabolic alkalosis	↑ or normal (if compensated)	↑ (if compensated)	↑↑

Treatment is directed at the cause of metabolic impairment, e.g. sepsis, together with organ support therapy, e.g. oxygen, intravenous fluids and antibiotics.

METABOLIC ACIDOSIS

Metabolic acidosis usually follows an episode of severe tissue hypoxia resulting from hypovolaemic shock, myocardial infarction or systemic sepsis. The most common cause is inadequate tissue oxygenation leading to accumulation of lactic acid. In surgical patients, the onset of metabolic acidosis is often an indicator of serious intraabdominal problems such as an anastomotic leak. Metabolic acidosis is also seen in acute renal failure and uncontrolled diabetic ketoacidosis. Clinically, patients have rapid, deep, sighing 'Kussmaul' respirations as they hyperventilate to blow off carbon dioxide (a respiratory compensatory mechanism). Arterial blood gas estimations show the characteristic picture of raised hydrogen ion concentration and low standard bicarbonate with a low arterial PCO_2. Plasma potassium concentration is elevated because of a shift from the intracellular compartment to the extracellular compartment.

Treatment is directed at the underlying cause. Bicarbonate infusion was formerly considered appropriate in severe cases but this does not address the underlying cause and is rarely used.

RESPIRATORY ACIDOSIS

This results from carbon dioxide retention in respiratory failure. The usual causes in surgical patients are underlying chronic respiratory disease made worse by postoperative chest complications or prolonged respiratory depression due to sedative, hypnotic or narcotic drugs. Plasma hydrogen ion concentrations and PCO_2 are elevated but standard bicarbonate is initially normal. A degree of metabolic compensation may occur as the kidneys excrete excess hydrogen ions and retain bicarbonate. Treatment is directed at the underlying cause and to providing assisted ventilation.

METABOLIC ALKALOSIS

Metabolic alkalosis is usually caused by severe and repeated vomiting or prolonged nasogastric aspiration for intestinal obstruction. The latter classically occurs in pyloric stenosis with gross loss of gastric acid. The patient becomes severely dehydrated and depleted of sodium and chloride ions; the condition is thus known as **hypochloraemic alkalosis** or **chloride-sensitive alkalosis**. The kidney attempts to compensate by conserving hydrogen ions but this occurs at the expense of potassium ions lost into the urine. Patients become hypokalaemic not only from excess urinary loss but also because potassium shifts into the cells in response to the alkalosis. Treatment of hypochloraemic hypokalaemic alkalosis involves rehydration with normal saline infusion with potassium supplements; large volumes (up to 10 litres) are often required. Renal excretion of bicarbonate ions eventually corrects the alkalosis.

RESPIRATORY ALKALOSIS

This occurs when carbon dioxide is lost via excessive pulmonary ventilation. The usual cause in surgical practice is prolonged mechanical ventilation during general anaesthesia or in the intensive care unit without adequate monitoring.

NUTRITIONAL MANAGEMENT IN THE SURGICAL PATIENT

ESSENTIAL PRINCIPLES

Malnutrition can be defined as a wasting condition resulting from energy (i.e. calorie) and protein deficiency, sometimes with vitamin and trace element deficiency as well. Recognising and treating pre-existing malnutrition and preventing postoperative starvation are important aspects of surgical management that are often neglected. In fact, there is remarkably little research published on this topic. Basic evaluation for malnutrition should be a standard part of assessing surgical patients (see Box 2.4) because untreated malnutrition predisposes to a range of problems that substantially increase morbidity and mortality rates and delay recovery (see Box 2.5).

Causes of malnutrition include **reduced food intake** (anorexia, fasting, pain on swallowing, physical or mental impairment), **malabsorption** (impaired digestion or absorption, or excess loss from gut) and **altered metabolism** (trauma, burns, sepsis, surgery, cancer cachexia). Patients with any of these predisposing factors need to be scrutinised more thoroughly for malnutrition.

In practice, most surgical patients have no special nutritional requirements and easily withstand the short period of starvation associated with their illness and operation. All hospitalised patients should be screened using a recognised screening tool (a variety of local versions have been produced) and if they are found to be malnourished, steps should be taken to improve nutrition before operation.

However, many major surgical operations are required urgently and there may be conflict between the need to get on with the operation and the need to optimise the patient's nutritional state. In any case, optimal nutritional support should be provided after operation.

Nutritional support in general can range upwards in complexity from encouraging the patient to eat regularly, offering easily prepared but tasty oral diets (e.g. liquidised normal food), through concentrated **sip feeds** (e.g. Fortisip) and various types of supplementary **enteral nutrition** given via tube, to **total parenteral nutrition (TPN)** for patients unable to absorb nutrients from the gastrointestinal tract. In many hospitals, a **nutrition support team** is available for advice and help and should be consulted early if likely to be needed.

RECOGNISING THE PATIENT AT RISK

Malnutrition is common in surgical patients and it often goes unrecognised. Studies have shown that as many as 50% of surgical inpatients suffer from mild malnutrition and 30% from severe malnutrition. Simple clinical assessment helps determine the state of nutrition; other indices can also be used (see Box 2.4) but none has been shown to be better than clinical assessment.

For patients found to be malnourished, studies have shown that simple pretreatment with regular proprietary sip feeds can stave off postoperative muscle weakness,

> **Box** 2.4   **Assessing patients for malnutrition**

Clinical assessment

- Lack of nutritional intake for 5 days or more
- Clinical appearance ('end-of-bedogram')—does the patient look malnourished?
- Unintentional weight loss of more than 10% from usual body weight within previous 6 months indicates malnutrition. More than 20% is likely to represent severe malnutrition
- Body mass index (BMI)—less than 18.5 suggests malnutrition

Anthropometric assessment

- Triceps skin fold thickness—technically difficult to perform but provides a good proxy for body density and hence overall fat content
- Mid arm circumference—unreliable because of technical measurement artefact and lack of dependable data upon which to base measurements
- Hand grip strength—easy to perform but lack of reproducible baseline data limits application to research projects

Blood indices

- Reduced plasma albumin, prealbumin or transferrin. In critically ill patients, plasma albumin of less than 35 g/L is associated with a 5-fold increase in complications and a 10-fold increase in death rate. Note that low plasma albumin alone is not an accurate marker of malnutrition but may be caused by other metabolic abnormalities
- Reduced lymphocyte count. If plasma albumin and lymphocyte count are both low, there is a 20-fold increase in death rate

> **Box** 2.5   **Adverse effects of protein/calorie depletion in surgical patients**

- Protein deficiency leads to impaired wound healing and higher rates of wound breakdown
- Protein depletion seriously impairs immune function and the ability to combat infection
- Skeletal muscle mass is lost, reducing muscular strength and general physical activity as well as causing fatigue. This increases the risk of thromboembolism and pressure sores
- Thoracic muscle mass depletion depresses respiratory efficiency and increases risk of pneumonia
- Albumin becomes depleted leading to generalised oedema
- Small bowel mucosal atrophy reduces its ability to absorb nutrients and may lead to bacterial translocation into the bloodstream because of loss of mucosal integrity
- Impaired mental function leads to apathy, depression and low morale
- Postoperative complication rates are higher—twice the rate of minor complications, three times the rate of major complications and three times the mortality compared with well-nourished patients
- Combinations of these factors lead to prolonged recovery times and longer hospital stays

reduce fatigue and markedly lessen complication rates. However, for more complex and prolonged endeavours to improve nutrition by the parenteral route (for example in oesophageal cancer), the evidence of clinical benefit is weak. Even if it is impracticable to improve the pre-operative nutritional state, malnutrition still needs to be recognised and attention given to the problem in the postoperative period. The duration of starvation should be kept as short as possible and appropriate nutrition provided. This contributes to healing, improves resistance to infection and reduces complications caused by muscle weakness (see Box 2.5).

EFFECTS OF STARVATION

SIMPLE STARVATION

During simple starvation (i.e. in the absence of illness or trauma), blood glucose concentration is maintained by a lowering of insulin secretion and an increase in glucagon production. Liver glycogen becomes exhausted within 24 hours but **gluconeogenesis** in the liver and kidneys is enhanced, utilising amino acids from protein breakdown and glycerol from lipolysis as substrates. Much of the glucose thus produced is used by the brain, as most other tissues are able to metabolise fatty acids and ketones derived from adipose tissue. Overall energy demands fall in simple starvation and energy is obtained largely from body fat. Protein is conserved until a late stage.

TRAUMA, SURGERY OR SEPSIS

In severe trauma or major surgery and particularly in sepsis, energy requirements increase by 20–100% of normal resting levels. As in simple starvation, lipid is more and more used as a fuel source; this decreases glucose utilisation, but note that fatty acids other than glycerol cannot be used for glucose synthesis. Hepatic glucose production increases, and at the same time peripheral glucose utilisation is impaired, often leading to hyperglycaemia. This feeds tissues that have obligate glucose requirements such as inflammatory cells in wounds and areas of infection.

Skeletal **muscle proteolysis** and urinary nitrogen excretion increase enormously compared with the fasted state. Protein from skeletal muscle is catabolised to release amino acids (particularly alanine), lactate and pyruvate. The stimulus for proteolysis is likely to be macrophage cytokines, particularly interleukins IL1 and IL6 and tumour necrosis factor (TNF). IL1 reduces hepatic albumin synthesis in favour of more urgently needed **acute-phase proteins** and gluconeogenesis. Amino acids are also used directly in wound healing and in haemopoiesis.

In **sepsis**, there is a progressive inability at mitochondrial level to fully oxidise substrates for energy generation, leading to a fall in oxygen consumption as sepsis worsens. Fatty acids are mobilised to an increasing extent from adipose tissue, manifesting as hypertriglyceridaemia; mobilisation is governed by raised levels of glucagon, catecholamines, cortisol and TNF. Fatty acids are oxidised for adenosine triphosphate (ATP) production in order to fuel synthesis of new glucose and proteins. If liver failure develops, amino acid clearance deteriorates and plasma concentrations rise. Some amino acids are then metabolised into false neurotransmitters which promote the vasodilatation and hypotension seen in sepsis and cause septic encephalopathy.

SUPPLEMENTARY NUTRITION

Supplementary nutrition other than liquidised diets and sip feeds is a complicated and sometimes expensive process with distinct risks of complications. It should not be undertaken without proper assessment. Deciding whether a patient is likely to benefit from supplementary nutrition depends on determining:

- That the patient is malnourished or will be deprived of nutrition for at least 5 days
- That the patient is likely to benefit—certain conditions make supplemental nutrition ineffective (e.g. enteral feeding in entero-cutaneous fistula; parenteral feeding in sepsis) but may be worth trying in carefully considered cases
- Whether there is an appropriate route for administration, e.g. suitable gut function or problems with venous access

Nutritional support is generally recommended in well-nourished patients who are unable to tolerate oral feeding for 7–10 days, or 5–7 days if already malnourished.

METHODS OF GIVING SUPPLEMENTARY NUTRITION

Box 2.6 summarises the range of nutritional regimens and their main surgical indications. The gastrointestinal tract should be used whenever possible for supplementary nutrition because any form of enteral feeding is intrinsically safer than parenteral nutrition and is much cheaper. In addition, the small intestinal mucosa tends to atrophy when not used. Enteral feeding supports the **gut-associated immunological shield** and prevents microorganisms translocating into the circulation, reducing the chances of blood-borne infection. Contraindications

---

Box	2.6	**Special methods of nutrition and their indications**

1. **Selective diets for specific indications**, e.g. diabetic, low-protein (renal and liver failure), low-fat (gallstones), high-fibre (constipation, diverticular disease) or weight reducing (obesity)
2. **Liquidised normal diet**—for patients with partial oesophageal obstruction (e.g. stricture, tumour or oesophageal intubation for cancer)
3. **High-protein, high-calorie dietary supplements 'sip diet'**—for chronically malnourished patients capable of a normal diet or debilitated convalescent patients
4. **Polymeric liquid diet** via tube—short chain peptides, medium chain triglycerides and polysaccharides plus vitamins and trace elements These contain the full range of nutritional requirements often including fibre. Used for nutritional support of patients unable to eat or drink such as the unconscious, ventilated and seriously ill patient in intensive care or patients unwilling to take adequate nutrition following major surgery or trauma
5. **Elemental diet** via tube, containing L-amino acids and simple sugars requiring no digestion and minimal absorptive capacity—for patients with minimal remaining bowel after massive resection. These are expensive and unpalatable and the high osmolarity can cause diarrhoea
6. **Peripheral parenteral nutritional support** for patients unable to have tube feeding but needing specific energy or protein supplementation
7. **Total parenteral nutrition (TPN)**, i.e. comprehensive intravenous nutrition—for patients with prolonged ileus or a very proximal fistula

---

to enteral feeding include intestinal obstruction, high-output intestinal fistula, intractable vomiting or diarrhoea, and severe malabsorption.

Sip feeds

If the patient is able to eat, fluid diets can be given orally, either as the sole means of nutrition or as dietary supplements, usually with advice from a dietician. Proprietary sip feeds containing easily absorbed calories, protein, minerals and vitamins are available in a variety of formulations and flavours and are well tolerated, particularly if cooled. These can be freely offered to patients able to swallow and absorb food.

Tube feeds

Certain patients are unsuitable for sip feeding but can be fed by one of a range of tube feeding routes. Indications include patients with swallowing difficulties (including overspill and lack of cooperation), anorexia, lack of palatability of liquid feeds, the need for a higher volume of feed than the patient can comfortably manage and anticipated substantial delay in resuming oral feeding after operation.

Even if the patient is unable to swallow (for example, because of bulbar palsy, unconsciousness or facial fractures), complete enteral nutrition can be delivered by means of a **fine-bore nasogastric tube**. These tubes can be negotiated into the jejunum endoscopically or radiologically (**naso-jejunal tube**) for patients who require post-pyloric enteral feeding, e.g. in acute pancreatitis. They cause minimal annoyance to the patient and can be left in place for long periods. A fluid diet is planned and formulated for the individual and is delivered at a controlled rate using a pump, often overnight.

Feeding tubes can also be placed percutaneously into the stomach or jejunum, either at operation (where feeding problems are anticipated) or with endoscopic or laparoscopic help. Gastrostomies are often employed in patients after stroke or in those with upper gastrointestinal anastomoses or obstructing lesions. The usual technique nowadays is by **percutaneous endoscopic gastrostomy (PEG)** in which a combination of gastroscopy and percutaneous placement is used. PEG tubes are contraindicated in peritonitis, ascites and prolonged ileus.

For **jejunostomy** placement, the tube is tunnelled submucosally for a distance before entering the bowel lumen using a wide-bore needle; this minimises the risk of leakage. Jejunostomy tubes must be placed under direct vision at operation after, for example, total gastrectomy, or laparoscopically. Nutrition is delivered as for fine-bore nasogastric tubes.

Certain patients not requiring full enteral or parenteral feeding may benefit from vitamin supplements, for example, folic acid and thiamine supplements for alcoholics, or vitamin K injections for patients on prolonged antibiotic therapy where disturbance of gut flora may impair intestinal absorption of vitamin K.

TOTAL PARENTERAL NUTRITION (TPN)

Parenteral nutrition should be reserved for appropriate cases of intestinal failure, i.e. where the amount of functioning gut is below the minimum necessary for adequate digestion and absorption of nutrients, and should not be embarked upon lightly.

TPN formulations principally contain a mixture of glucose, amino acids, lipids, minerals and vitamins. Standard supplements of vitamins and minerals are usually incorporated into the mix. Amino acids are complemented by non-nitrogenous sources of energy in the form of glucose and lipids which have a **protein-sparing** effect and minimise the consumption of protein as energy.

The osmolality of the mixture is usually high so that administration needs to be via a dedicated central venous line to minimise the risk of venous thrombosis; formulations for peripheral infusion are available but the technique is losing favour. The usual aim of TPN is to provide sufficient nitrogen and energy to offset the catabolic demands of surgery and/or trauma and their complications and, if possible, compensate for any pre-existing malnutrition.

In calculating requirements, protein intake should be matched to the estimated nitrogen losses; this can be calculated by measuring urinary nitrogen losses as urea or else a standard formula (which also estimates other requirements) can be employed. For example, basic adult daily requirements are 100 g protein (in the form of amino acids), 350 g glucose and 50 g lipid to provide energy. These quantities need to be adjusted according to individual requirements.

Excessive nutrition can be a problem. Hyperglycaemia can be corrected with modest doses of insulin but in the longer term disturbances of liver function may reflect intrahepatic cholestasis caused by fatty infiltration. In intrahepatic cholestasis blood tests show elevated plasma alkaline phosphatase and gamma glutaryl transferase.

Indications for total parenteral nutrition

Parenteral nutrition should be reserved for patients who are already malnourished (or who are likely to become malnourished), in whom the gastrointestinal tract is not functional or is inaccessible and is likely to remain so for a substantial number of days or weeks. Note that in major sepsis, the metabolic changes described earlier mean that TPN brings little benefit.

Indications may include:

- Entero-cutaneous fistula
- Intra-abdominal infection
- Short bowel syndrome where there is insufficient residual absorptive capacity after massive small bowel resection
- Multiple injuries involving viscera

Methods of giving TPN

Parenteral nutrition is largely delivered into the superior vena cava via the internal jugular or subclavian vein. This is so that the high venous flow rapidly dilutes the hyperosmolar TPN solution, minimising the risk of thrombosis. If long periods of nutritional support are anticipated, a **tunnelled line** with the skin access point remote from the venous entry point is usually employed to minimise the risk of line infection. A frequently used type is the Groshong line. Feeding lines must only be used for that purpose and not for blood transfusion, drug administration or other fluid infusions.

The choice and quantity of nutrients starts from a standard baseline related to body weight and is then varied (with specialist advice) according to individual needs as regards amino acids, glucose and additives, as mentioned earlier. Nowadays, a whole day's requirement is prepared in the hospital pharmacy in a single 3 litre bag.

Box 2.7 Monitoring of parenteral nutrition

8-hourly

- Blood glucose (finger-prick stix)

2–4 times daily

- Temperature and pulse rate

Daily

- Fluid balance charts and body weight
- Inspection of line entry site (blood cultures on any sign of local or systemic infection)
- Plasma urea, electrolytes until stable

Twice-weekly

- Creatinine and liver function tests

Weekly

- Plasma calcium, phosphate, magnesium (if risk of refeeding syndrome, should be measured daily until stable)
- Zinc and selenium can be measured initially and then every 2–4 weeks

---

Box 2.8 Complications of parenteral nutrition

Catheter problems (10% of central lines develop substantial complications)

- Central venous line placement problems, e.g. failure to cannulate, trauma to great arteries or veins, pneumothorax, haemothorax, brachial plexus injury, loss of Seldinger wire into vein
- Line infection—a common cause of fever and tachycardia likely to progress to systemic sepsis. If suspected, blood cultures should be taken from the line. If positive, line must be removed and tip cultured
- Blockage, breakage or leakage of catheter
- Air embolism
- Central venous thrombosis

Metabolic problems (5% develop metabolic derangements)

- Hypophosphataemia ($PO_4 < 0.5$ mmol/L)
- Hypernatraemia (Na > 150 mmol/L)
- Hyponatraemia (Na < 130 mmol/L)
- Hyperglycaemia
- Overnutrition
- Long-term—fatty degeneration of the liver
- Trace element and folate deficiency
- Deranged liver function tests
- Linoleic acid deficiency

Parenteral nutrition is costly in materials and in staff time and is prone to complications; it should not be used unless required for 7 days or more and should be discontinued as soon as nutrition can be supplied by an enteral route. Patients on TPN need close and regular monitoring for a range of problems including line problems, local and systemic infection, fluid balance and deficiencies of electrolytes (see Box 2.7). Complications of TPN are detailed in Box 2.8.

REFEEDING SYNDROME

Refeeding syndrome was first described in prisoners in the Far East after the Second World War who developed cardiac failure when starting to eat after prolonged starvation. When there is reduced carbohydrate intake, insulin secretion falls and fat and protein are catabolised in place of carbohydrate. This results in loss of intracellular electrolytes, particularly phosphate, which becomes depleted. Phosphate is essential for generating adenosine triphosphate and for other vital phosphorylation reactions.

When enteral or parenteral feeding is restarted after starvation of any kind, there is a sudden reversion from fat to carbohydrate metabolism. As a result, insulin secretion rises and cellular uptake of glucose, phosphate, potassium and water increases. This can lead to profound hypophosphataemia, often in association with hypokalaemia and hypomagnesaemia, with potentially serious consequences. Note that all extracellular fluid is affected by declining levels of these electrolytes. In the starved state, there is total body depletion of electrolytes but plasma concentrations can be misleadingly normal because of renal compensation.

Refeeding syndrome occurs when the plasma phosphate falls to less than 0.50 mmol/L. Clinical features include **cardiac and respiratory failure, arrhythmias, rhabdomyolysis, white cell dysfunction, seizures, coma and sudden death.** The early signs may go unrecognised in patients at risk; the plasma phosphate may not be measured or the significance of grossly abnormal results may not be recognised.

Malnourished patients at risk of refeeding syndrome need to be identified so that artificial feeding can be started with a quarter to half of the expected calorie requirements. Plasma phosphate, magnesium, calcium, potassium, urea and creatinine concentrations should be measured before feeding and daily for 4 days afterwards because of the expected rapid falls which require electrolyte replacement. Thiamine must also be replaced in these patients.

Established cases require treatment with intravenous phosphate. Patients can be managed on general wards by giving 50 mmol of intravenous phosphate over 24 hours. This is successful in most cases but continued close monitoring is needed as low phosphate levels can recur.

Immunity, inflammation and infection

3

IMMUNE RESPONSES

INTRODUCTION

The **innate immune response** constitutes the first line of defence against invading microorganisms. Surprisingly, many elements of this important mechanism were not understood until the 1990s. The key mechanism is that Toll-like receptors (TLRs) on the surface of dendritic cells recognise various classes of molecules produced by groups of pathogens and trigger inflammatory responses to limit the invasion. The better known **adaptive immune system,** which involves T and B cells, is much more organism specific. During the course of an infection, it evolves to deal optimally with the microorganism involved. Once produced, some of the specially trained T and B cells remain, priming the body for any later attack by the same organism. Vaccines operate by promoting this adaptive system.

INNATE IMMUNITY

The innate system produces a semi-specific response to organisms the body has not previously encountered. It is also essential to the process of triggering the adaptive response by means of signalling cytokines. Without innate immunity, adaptive immune responses simply do not occur. **Macrophages** and **dendritic cells** patrol the body's tissues searching for foreign proteins likely to indicate infection. Invaders bearing foreign proteins are engulfed and destroyed. Antimicrobial molecules are produced and the **complement system** activated. Once engaged, the Toll-like receptors also prompt the cells to unleash particular suites of cytokines which recruit additional macrophages, dendritic cells and other immune cells to wall off and non-specifically attack the microbe. **Dendritic** cells containing engulfed protein then head to the lymph nodes where they present fragments of the pathogen's protein to an array of T cells and also release more cytokines. **Lipopolysaccharide** (LPS) produced by Gram-negative bacteria is a particularly powerful immune stimulator. It prompts inflammatory cells to release **tumour necrosis factor alpha (TNF-alpha)** and **interleukin-1 (IL1)**. These two cytokines are probably the most significant in controlling the inflammatory response, and also, if left unchecked, in causing autoimmune disorders, e.g. rheumatoid arthritis.

Ten human varieties of Toll-like receptors have been discovered since 1997. They act in specific pairs of receptors which project from the dendritic cell surface. Each pair

27

binds to a different class of protein that is characteristic for a type or group of organisms, e.g. lipopolysaccharide from Gram-negative bacteria, single-stranded DNA viruses or flagellin. TLR3 and TLR7 sense the presence of viruses and induce the production and release of **interferon**. Meanwhile, the released cytokines generate the typical symptoms of infection—fever and flu-like symptoms.

Overactivity of this innate system, particularly of TLR4, can lead to potentially fatal **sepsis**. TLRs may also be implicated in **autoimmunity** by responding inappropriately, for example to products from damaged cells. A range of **drugs** that activate particular TLRs are in advanced stages of testing, e.g. as vaccine adjuvants or antiviral agents. Inhibitors are being developed for treating sepsis, inflammatory bowel disease and autoimmune diseases, so far with limited success.

ADAPTIVE IMMUNITY

Macrophages and other cells, having chopped up a pathogen, display pieces of it on their surface. This ultimately activates those B and T cells that recognise that fragment to proliferate and then launch a powerful and highly focused attack on the particular invader. Activated B cells secrete antibody molecules that bind to antigen components unique to a given invader and then destroy the invader or mark it for destruction. T cells recognise antigens displayed on cells. Some activate more B and T cells whilst others directly attack infected cells. Following the initial infection, enough **memory T and B cells** remain to deal effectively with the organism should it return. This can occur so quickly that inflammation may not occur at all.

INFLAMMATION

ACUTE INFLAMMATION

INTRODUCTION

Acute inflammation is the principal mechanism by which living tissues respond to injury. The purpose of the inflammatory response is to neutralise the injurious agent, to remove damaged or necrotic tissue and to restore the tissue to useful function. The central feature of acute inflammation is the formation of an inflammatory exudate. This has three principal components: **serum**, **leucocytes** (predominantly neutrophils) and **fibrinogen**.

Formation of the inflammatory exudate involves local vascular changes which are collectively responsible for the four **'cardinal signs of Celsus'**—rubor (redness), tumor (swelling), calor (heat) and dolor (pain)—as well as loss of function. These vascular phenomena are described in Figure 3.1.

OUTCOMES OF ACUTE INFLAMMATION

The outcomes of acute inflammation are summarised in Figure 3.2.

Resolution

If tissue damage is minimal and there is no actual tissue necrosis, then the acute inflammatory response eventually settles and the tissue returns virtually to normal with no evidence of scarring. A good example is the resolution of mild sunburn or transient peptic gastritis.

Abscess formation (Fig. 3.3)

An abscess is a collection of pus (dead and dying neutrophils plus proteinaceous exudate) walled off by a zone of acute inflammation. Acute abscess formation particularly occurs in response to certain **pyogenic** microorganisms that attract neutrophils and yet are resistant to phagocytosis and lysosomal destruction. Abscesses also form in response to highly localised tissue necrosis and to some organic foreign bodies (e.g. wood splinters, linen suture material), although infection may also be involved in these cases. The main pyogenic organisms of surgical importance are *Staphylococcus aureus*, some streptococci (particularly *Strep. pyogenes*), *Escherichia coli* and related Gram-negative bacilli ('coliforms'), and *Bacteroides* species (spp).

Without treatment, abscesses eventually tend to 'point' spontaneously to a nearby epithelial surface (e.g. skin, gut, bronchus), and then discharge their contents. If the injurious agent is thereby eliminated, spontaneous drainage leads to healing. If an abscess is remote from a surface (e.g. deep in the breast), it progressively enlarges causing much tissue destruction. Sometimes local defence mechanisms are overwhelmed, leading to runaway local infection (**cellulitis**) and sometimes systemic sepsis.

Even with small and well-localised abscesses, showers of bacteria enter the general circulation (**bacteraemia**) but are mopped up by the phagocytic cells of the liver and spleen before they can proliferate. This process is responsible for the **swinging pyrexia** that is characteristic of an abscess. A typical temperature chart is shown in Figure 3.4. The abscess site may not be clinically evident if it is very deep-seated (e.g. subphrenic or pelvic abscess) and the patient may be otherwise well. In the presence of an abscess, the number of neutrophils in the bloodstream rises dramatically as they are released in large numbers from the bone marrow; thus, a marked **neutrophil leucocytosis** (i.e. white cell count greater than 15×10^9/L with more than 80% neutrophils) usually indicates a pyogenic infection. Severe infection with an excessive cytokine response spilling over into the systemic circulation

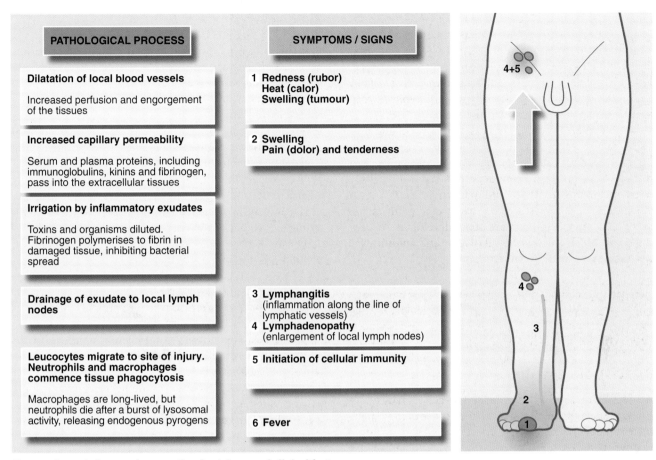

Fig. 3.1 Acute inflammation—pathophysiology and clinical features

causes **systemic sepsis** and rapid clinical deterioration (see p. 54).

The chronic state (see Chronic inflammation, p. 30)
If spontaneous drainage of an abscess does not eliminate the injurious agent, the neutrophil response persists and pus continues to be formed, resulting in a **chronic abscess**. This may be manifest as a continuously discharging sinus or a surface abscess which intermittently forms, discharges and then heals. Alternatively a chronic abscess may be suspected only because of its systemic effects (e.g. a swinging pyrexia). From the foregoing, it follows that the essential principle of managing any abscess is to establish complete **drainage**, usually by incision or aspiration. Any residual necrotic or foreign material should be eliminated by curettage or excision. Indeed, before the antibiotic era, abscesses were a major cause of hospital admission and the principle of drainage was well known, with most hospitals having a separate 'septic' ward.

Antibiotics and abscesses
Antibiotics are often misused to treat abscesses. Once an abscess has fully formed, antibiotics seldom effect a cure because the pus and foreign or necrotic material remain and the drug cannot gain ready access to the bacteria within the pus. Nevertheless, antibiotics may halt expansion or even sterilise the pus; the residual sterile abscess is sometimes known as an **antibioma**. If appropriate antibiotics are given early enough in an infection, organisms can be eliminated before the stage of abscess formation. For example, staphylococcal breast infections are common during lactation and if untreated often lead to breast abscesses. This formerly common surgical problem is now rare because of timely antibiotic treatment by family practitioners. Likewise, in surgical operations where there is known to be a particular risk of infection, **prophylactic antibiotics** can dramatically reduce the incidence of postoperative abscess formation and other infective complications.

Organisation and repair

The most common sequel to acute inflammation is **organisation**, in which dead tissue is removed by phagocytosis and the defect filled by vascular connective tissue known as **granulation tissue**. This granulation tissue is gradually 'repaired' to bring about a **fibrous scar**. In some cases the original tissue may regenerate, i.e. rebuild its specialised cells and structure.

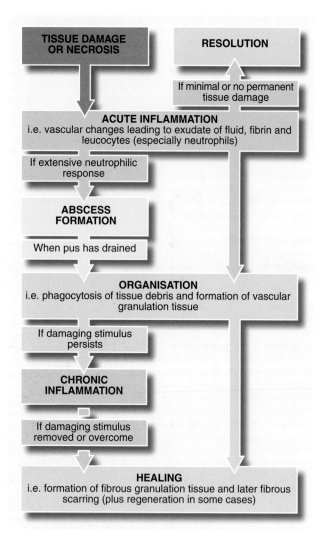

Fig. 3.2 Acute inflammation and its sequelae

WOUND HEALING

Healing by primary intention

The simplest example of organisation and repair is healing of an uncomplicated skin incision (see Fig. 3.5). In this case, there is no necrotic tissue and the margins of the wound are brought into apposition with sutures. An acute inflammatory response develops in the immediate vicinity of the incision, and by the third day granulation tissue bridges the dermal defect. In the meantime, proliferating surface epithelium rapidly restores the epidermis from the wound edges. Fibroblasts invade the granulation tissue, laying down collagen so the repair will be strong enough to permit suture removal after 5–10 days. At this stage the scar is still red but the blood vessels gradually regress and it becomes a pale linear scar within a few months. This process is known as **healing by primary intention.**

Healing by secondary intention

If tissue loss prevents the wound edges from coming together, the healing process has to make good the deficiency. The defect is initially filled with blood clot. This later becomes invaded by a mass of vascular granulation tissue from the healthy wound base. Inflammatory exudate solidifies at the surface forming a protective scab. Fibroblasts invade the granulation tissue and collagen is laid down in the extracellular spaces; after about a week, some fibroblasts differentiate into **myofibroblasts** and contraction of their myofibrils eventually shrinks the wound defect by 40–80%, beginning about 2 weeks after the insult. Over the succeeding weeks and months, the blood vessels regress and more collagen is formed, leaving a relatively avascular scar; gradual contraction of the mature collagen (cicatrisation), combined with wound contraction, ensures that the final scar is much smaller than the original defect. The overlying epidermal defect is gradually bridged by epithelial proliferation from the wound margins. Epithelial cells slide over each other beneath the edges of the scab upon the surface of the granulation tissue and the scab is eventually shed. This whole process is known as **healing by secondary intention** (see Fig. 3.5).

Factors impairing wound healing

The rate and success of wound healing may be impaired by a variety of local, regional and systemic factors (see Fig. 3.6).

CHRONIC INFLAMMATION

In certain circumstances, an injurious agent persists over a long period causing continuing tissue destruction. The body attempts to deal with both the original and the continuing tissue damage by the processes of acute inflammation, organisation and repair, all at the same time. In these cases, the damaged area may display several pathological processes at once, i.e. tissue necrosis, an inflammatory response, granulation tissue formation and fibrous scarring. This whole process is known as chronic inflammation and is characterised histologically by a predominance of **macrophages** (sometimes forming giant cells) which are responsible for the phagocytosis of necrotic debris. Lymphocytes and plasma cells are also present, indicating the involvement of immunological mechanisms in chronic inflammation.

Chronic inflammation represents a tenuous balance between a persistent injurious agent and the body's reparative responses. Healing only takes place if the injurious agent is removed. Healing can then proceed in the usual manner but often results in much more scarring.

A wide range of agents can lead to chronic inflammation. The clinical patterns of disease can be grouped into three broad categories:

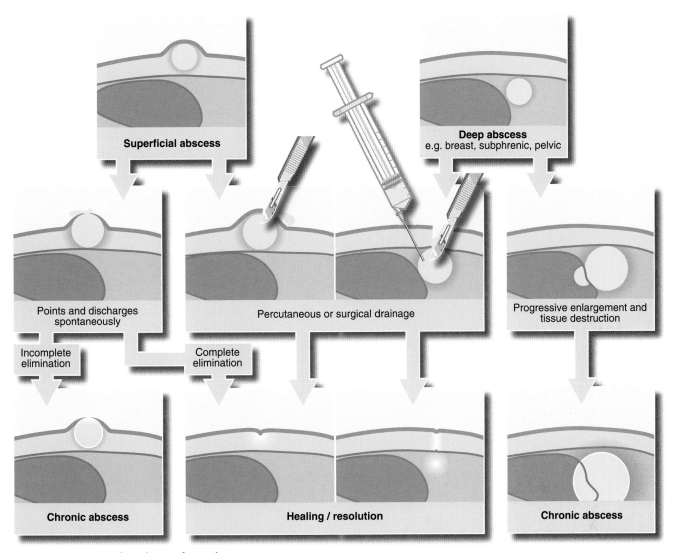

Fig. 3.3 Outcomes after abscess formation

- Chronic abscesses
- Chronic ulcers
- Specific granulomatous infections and inflammations

CHRONIC ABSCESSES

As described earlier, a chronic abscess arises if the agent causing an acute abscess is not fully eliminated. Pus continues to be formed and the abscess either persists or discharges continuously via a **sinus** or else 'points' and discharges periodically with the sinus healing over between times. The wall of a chronic abscess consists of fibrous scar tissue lined with granulation tissue resulting from attempts at healing.

Causes of chronic abscesses include the following:

- **Infected foreign bodies.** These are probably the most common cause of chronic abscesses in modern surgical practice. Foreign bodies may have been implanted deliberately and then become infected (e.g. synthetic mesh for inguinal hernia repair, prosthetic hip joint) or have become embedded during an accident (e.g. glass fragments)
- **Dead (necrotic) tissue** of any sort can act as a foreign body, forming a nidus for infection. For example, diabetes may be complicated by deep infections in the foot with necrosis of tendon and bone leading to chronic abscesses and ulcers. Hairs deeply implanted in the skin of the natal cleft may be responsible for a pilonidal sinus or abscess. An infected dead tooth or root fragment may intermittently discharge via an associated 'gum boil' (see Fig. 3.7). Chronic osteomyelitis is associated with remnants of dead bone known as **sequestra**
- **Deep abscesses.** A chronic abscess can arise without a foreign body if the abscess is so deep and well circumscribed as to prevent spontaneous drainage. The best example is a subphrenic abscess

31

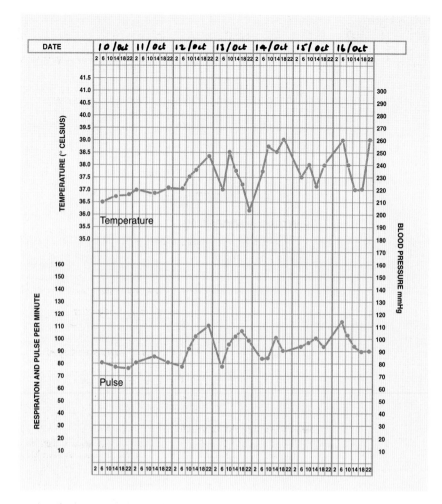

Fig. 3.4 Temperature chart showing swinging pyrexia

CHRONIC ULCERS

An ulcer is defined as a persistent defect in an epithelial or mucosal surface. Except for malignant ulcers, ulceration usually results from a combination of low-grade mechanical or chemical injury to epithelium and supporting tissue, together with an impaired reparative response. For example, elderly and debilitated patients are susceptible to **pressure sores** ('bed sores') which develop over bony prominences such as the sacrum and heels. In these cases, the patient does not regularly and automatically shift position to relieve the pressure of body weight. This is because of immobility and perhaps diminished protective pain responses. Tissue necrosis results and healing is impaired by the presence of necrotic tissue and continuing pressure ischaemia. Other factors may include poor tissue perfusion (from cardiac or peripheral vascular disease) and malnutrition.

Another common ulcer is the longstanding leg ulcer in chronic venous insufficiency; this fails to heal because of local nutritional impairment induced by the high venous pressure and oedema. The problem is often exacerbated by secondary infection. Ischaemic leg ulcers fail to heal because of insufficient arterial blood flow.

A chronic peptic ulcer results from *Helicobacter pylori* infection of gastric or duodenal mucosa combined with persistent acid–pepsin attack (Fig. 21.1). The lesion persists because the infection remains and the body's response is insufficient to tip the balance towards repair. In infected mucosa, an ulcer is often initiated and then exacerbated by aspirin or other non-steroidal anti-inflammatory drugs (NSAIDs) or excess alcohol. On the other hand, healing can be initiated by antibiotic therapy for *H. pylori*, at the same time blocking acid production with H_2 antagonists or proton pump inhibitors.

In summary, any chronic ulcer represents an unresolved balance between persistent damaging factors and inadequate reparative responses. The principle of managing any ulcer is therefore to diminish or remove the damaging factors and to promote the healing mechanisms.

THE SPECIFIC GRANULOMATOUS INFECTIONS AND INFLAMMATIONS

Certain microorganisms such as *Mycobacterium tuberculosis*, *Mycobacterium leprae* and *Treponema pallidum* (causing tuberculosis, leprosy and syphilis respectively) excite a minimal acute inflammatory response whilst stimulating

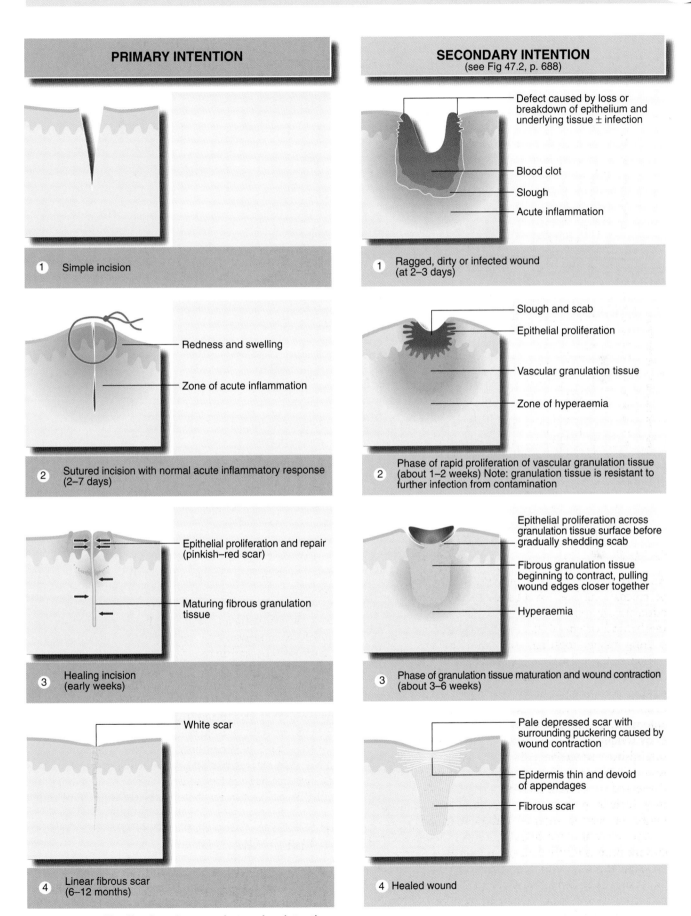

Fig. 3.5 Wound healing by primary and secondary intention

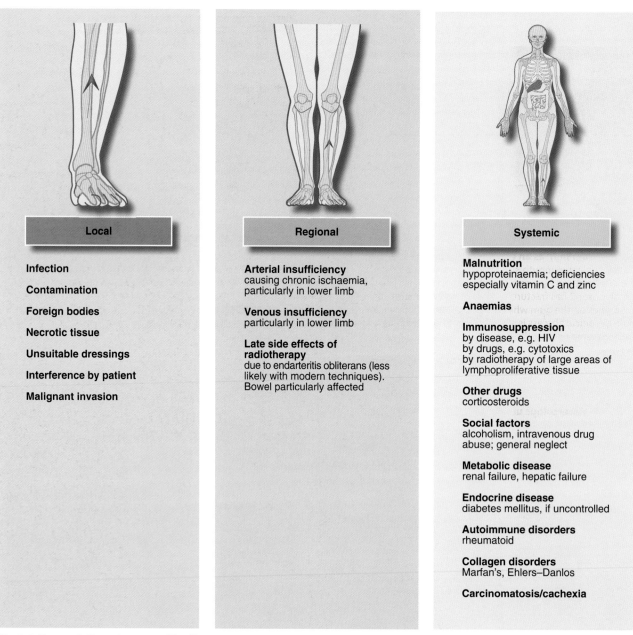

Local	Regional	Systemic
Infection	**Arterial insufficiency** causing chronic ischaemia, particularly in lower limb	**Malnutrition** hypoproteinaemia; deficiencies especially vitamin C and zinc
Contamination		**Anaemias**
Foreign bodies	**Venous insufficiency** particularly in lower limb	**Immunosuppression** by disease, e.g. HIV
Necrotic tissue	**Late side effects of radiotherapy** due to endarteritis obliterans (less likely with modern techniques). Bowel particularly affected	by drugs, e.g. cytotoxics by radiotherapy of large areas of lymphoproliferative tissue
Unsuitable dressings		**Other drugs** corticosteroids
Interference by patient		**Social factors** alcoholism, intravenous drug abuse; general neglect
Malignant invasion		**Metabolic disease** renal failure, hepatic failure
		Endocrine disease diabetes mellitus, if uncontrolled
		Autoimmune disorders rheumatoid
		Collagen disorders Marfan's, Ehlers–Danlos
		Carcinomatosis/cachexia

Fig. 3.6 Factors influencing wound healing

a chronic inflammatory response almost from the outset. The lesions are characterised by accumulation of macrophages which form into **granulomas**, and from these, the diseases are known as the **specific granulomatous infections**.

A tuberculous **cold abscess** is a pus-like accumulation of liquefied caseous material containing the occasional mycobacterium. In contrast to a pyogenic abscess, the lesion is cold to the touch since there is no associated acute inflammatory vascular response. Tuberculous abscesses were once common in developed countries but are now rare. Cervical lymph node tuberculosis ('scrofula') often produced a 'collar-stud' abscess, i.e. a superficial fluctuant abscess communicating with a deep (and often larger) lymph node abscess via a small fascial defect. Tuberculosis

of the thoraco-lumbar spine causes local destruction and deformity and may track down beneath the inguinal ligament within the psoas sheath, presenting as a '**psoas abscess**' in the groin. A tuberculous ulcer overlying tuberculous inguinal nodes is shown in Figure 3.8.

Certain extremely fine particulate materials such as talc and beryllium produce similar granulomatous reactions known as **foreign body granulomas**. Talc was traditionally used as a lubricant powder in surgical gloves. Occasionally, after laparotomy, it aroused an intense, diffuse granulomatous peritoneal reaction causing widespread bowel adhesions. Talc was abandoned and replaced by starch, which itself has been incriminated in causing starch granulomas. For this reason, when body cavities are opened, best practice is to use gloves without powder.

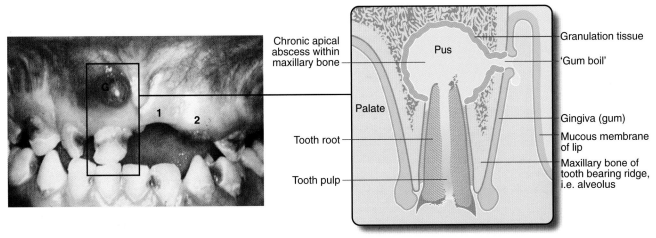

Fig. 3.7 'Gum boil' as an example of a chronic abscess

Grossly neglected mouth showing widespread dental caries. There is an inflammatory swelling on the buccal (cheek) aspect of the alveolus **G** caused by a chronic apical dental abscess on the upper right incisor. Note the left central incisor 1 is missing and the left lateral incisor 2 has fractured at gum level because of caries. Sagittal section through 'gum boil' of upper incisor tooth. The gum boil is in fact a sinus on the gum which discharges either chronically or intermittently. Exposed to infection, the tooth pulp has become necrotic while the apical abscess is slowly expanding due to the continued presence of infected necrotic tissue (i.e. the tooth pulp). The tooth root is all that remains after the crown has fractured due to dental caries.

Fig. 3.8 Tuberculous ulcer

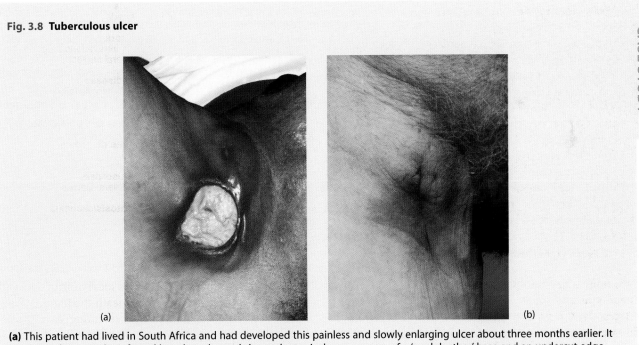

(a)   (b)

(a) This patient had lived in South Africa and had developed this painless and slowly enlarging ulcer about three months earlier. It originates from nearby infected lymph nodes and shows the typical appearances of a 'wash leather' base and an undercut edge. Diagnosis was based on a biopsy and treatment involved draining the involved lymph nodes visible above the ulcer and a course of antituberculous chemotherapy. **(b)** The healed lesion 2 months later.

INFECTION

GENERAL PRINCIPLES

It is important to distinguish between colonisation, infection and sepsis:

- **Colonisation** is when bacteria are present in or on a host but do not cause an immune response or signs of disease
- **Infection** occurs when this relationship changes and there is a sustained local attack by microorganisms, provoking an immune response and signs of disease, for example when normal commensal bacteria in the colon such as *E. coli* contaminate the peritoneal cavity
- **Sepsis** (systemic sepsis) is essentially the result of an excessive and inappropriate production of cytokines in response to particular types of severe infection (or other provoking agent such as a gangrenous limb) that causes organ dysfunction and progressive organ failure

Clinically significant infection arises when the size of an inoculum or the virulence of a microorganism is sufficient to overcome the general resistance offered by protective surface mechanisms and non-specific tissue defences, as well as any specific immune responses. The **virulence** of an organism depends on its qualities of adherence and invasiveness and its ability to produce toxins. **Tissue invasion** of microorganisms may be enhanced by their secretion of enzymes (e.g. hyaluronidase and streptokinase), by mechanisms to avoid phagocytosis (e.g. encapsulation or spore formation), by inherent resistance to lysosomal destruction or by their ability to kill phagocytes. Toxins may be secreted by the organism (**exotoxins**) or released upon the death of the organism (**endotoxins**). In either case the toxin may produce local tissue damage (e.g. gas gangrene) or cause distant toxic effects (e.g. tetanus) or it may activate cytokine systems to cause systemic sepsis, sometimes including disseminated intravascular coagulopathy.

Infections may be **community-acquired** (e.g. pneumococcal lobar pneumonia in a fit young adult) or **hospital-acquired**. The latter are also known as **nosocomial** infections and are defined as infections that were not present or incubating at the time of admission. Nosocomial infection may be acquired by cross-infection from infected patients, from contaminated equipment or furnishings, or from '**carriers**' among staff by means of inhalation, ingestion or contamination of intravenous cannulas or urinary catheters, for example. These infections are often caused by antibiotic-resistant bacteria such as meticillin-resistant *Staphylococcus aureus* (**MRSA**). Risk of such infections can be drastically reduced by the simple measure of everyone in contact with patients cleansing their hands with alcohol-based gel between **every patient contact**. Testing bacterial swabs for MRSA from staff and

from patients before admitting them to hospital further reduces the risk. Of course, all hospital areas must be clean and high-risk areas monitored for MRSA. Known MRSA-infected patients or carriers should be isolated when in hospital. Patients having operations where infection carries very high risk should ideally be treated in areas separated from sick patients, especially emergency admissions from long-term care institutions. Particular risk is associated with eye surgery, joint replacements and prosthetic vascular grafts.

Postoperative patients are at particular risk of nosocomial infections (e.g. pneumonias, urinary tract infections) because host defences are impaired by the surgical assault. Particular physiological **protective mechanisms** may be disrupted allowing infection to gain ascendancy. For example, neutropenia predisposes to infection, and smokers are more liable to develop bronchopneumonia following immobility or general anaesthesia. The surgical patient's **general resistance** may be further impaired by malnutrition, malignancy, rheumatoid disease, corticosteroid therapy or other immunosuppressive drugs.

In **post-surgical** ('surgical site') infections, organisms gain entry to the tissues via an abnormal breach of epithelium. This may be surface damage (such as a surgical or traumatic wound or an injection) or result from a perforated viscus. In many cases, the infecting organisms are part of the patient's normal skin, bowel or respiratory tract flora or are normally present in the external environment. They cause disease by virtue of their unwelcome presence in sites where they are not meant to be. For example, *Staph. epidermidis* is commonly present on skin but causes serious chronic infection of implanted arterial grafts.

METHODS OF CONTROL OF NOSOCOMIAL INFECTION

Environment

Patient areas in hospitals must be clean and free from contaminating bacteria, especially areas where invasive procedures occur such as operating theatres and high-dependency units. Special precautions are taken in theatres (see Ch. 11)

Contaminated dressings, bed linen and equipment must be disposed of or sent for processing without risking transfer of infection to other patients.

Staff

Staff must be vaccinated against hepatitis B and should not be carriers of MRSA. HIV-positive individuals should not undertake any invasive procedures. Open wounds must be securely covered and those staff with infective skin lesions should avoid patient contact. Universal blood and body fluid precautions should be taken to prevent viral transmission (see below) and guidelines followed for dealing with needle-stick injuries.

Medical and nursing staff must cleanse their hands (e.g. with alcohol gel) before touching any patient or their surroundings in order to minimise cross-infection.

Patients

Surgery should be deferred if possible on patients with acute respiratory or urinary tract infections. Patients known to have transmissible infections or to be carriers, e.g. of MRSA, should be nursed in isolation. Patients should receive bacterial swabbing to assess MRSA status before major surgery, e.g. hip replacements, arterial grafts.

Procedures

Equipment—including syringes, needles, theatre gowns and drapes—must be sterile, ideally in secure packaging or as single-use disposable items. Other important principles include:

- Minimising surgical site infection and avoiding systemic sepsis by thorough debridement of contaminated wounds plus appropriate antibiotic treatment
- Early recognition and treatment of bowel-related infection, e.g. acute appendicitis, peridiverticular abscess
- Drainage of abscesses
- Appropriate use of prophylactic antibiotics (see various sections below and Ch. 11)
- Early recognition and treatment of infective complications—wound infections, pneumonias and urinary tract infections

UNIVERSAL BLOOD AND BODY FLUID PRECAUTIONS

Increasing awareness of blood-borne viral infections such as hepatitis B and C and the prevalence of HIV has led to the concept of **universal blood and body fluid precautions** in combatting cross-infection between patients and staff. Staff often try to be vigilant with known carriers of HIV or hepatitis and other high-risk patients but relax at other times. However, research has shown that this extra care soon lapses; this may explain publicised cases of unexpected transmission from patient to doctor, doctor to patient and patient to patient. For this reason, every patient should be assumed to be a potential carrier of blood-borne infection, and precautions should be employed whenever skin is likely to be breached and whenever instruments contaminated with blood or other body fluids are handled. Transmission of infection can occur in obvious situations such as a needle-stick injury (see below) as well as with less obvious events such as splashes of infected material into the eye.

Disposable gloves should be worn for all medical procedures and physical examinations except for palpating skin where there is no obvious open lesion in either patient or examiner. Staff with broken skin should apply occlusive dressings. The integrity of skin affected by minor scratches or grazes can be checked with an alcoholic skin wash, wipe or swab which causes stinging if the skin is broken. Protective **eyewear** should be worn during invasive procedures to prevent conjunctival splashes with potentially contaminated material.

Hepatitis B vaccination

Staff directly involved in patient care should be vaccinated against hepatitis B. This involves three intramuscular injections: the initial injection, then an injection 1 month and 5 months later, with booster doses at 5-yearly intervals thereafter. Hepatitis B serology should be checked 2 months after completion of vaccination. Around 5% of healthy young people fail to seroconvert and should be revaccinated. Half of these will seroconvert and the remainder are genetic non-responders.

Needle-stick and other penetrating injuries

Sharps injury, especially from a contaminated hollow needle, may lead to transmission of an infection if the patient carries a blood-borne virus. A needle-stick injury occurs when a needle already used for a patient inadvertently penetrates the skin of a health care worker. Such injuries are capable of transmitting hepatitis B and C but the risk for HIV is much lower because the viral concentration in HIV-positive fluids is much lower and the volume of blood transmitted by needle-stick injuries is small.

This common injury is largely avoidable: resheathing of used needles causes about 40% of needle-stick injuries and this practice should be avoided. Venepuncture is a high-risk procedure and should be performed with caution. An ignored needle removed from a cannula left beside a patient might prove lethal to an unsuspecting staff member. Needles, scalpel blades and other disposable instruments contaminated with blood should be handled with great care and disposed of immediately after use into special plastic 'sharps' containers. These should be available wherever sharps are used so that instruments need not be passed from person to person nor carried from one place to another. **Note that it is the sole responsibility of the user to dispose of sharps properly**.

Viral infection following sharps (needle-stick) injury

If a definite sharps injury has occurred that involves blood being transmitted from an infected person, the risk of hepatitis B infection to the recipient is about 25%. For hepatitis C the risk is 2% and for HIV 0.5%. There is also a very high risk after sharps injury in a recreational environment (e.g. needles left on the beach by intravenous drug users) since hepatitis B and HIV survive well in warm, moist conditions, especially in serum and tissue debris. Thus all sharps injuries should be treated with the utmost concern. A recommended protocol is shown in Box 3.1.

Box 3.1   **Protocol for managing 'sharps' injuries**

1. Wash injured area immediately and encourage blood to flow from wound
2. Record names of people involved and all details of incident
3. Test injured person (*the recipient*) serologically for HIV, hepatitis B and hepatitis C
4. Test person whose blood/body fluids contaminated the sharp (*the donor*) for HIV, hepatitis B and hepatitis C
5. If hepatitis B status of recipient or donor is uncertain and cannot be determined reliably within 48 hours of injury (e.g. over a weekend), administer the following to the recipient as soon as possible:
   - hepatitis B immunoglobulin (0.06 ml/kg body weight)
   - hepatitis B vaccine—first dose
6. The immune status of donor and recipient dictates further management as follows:
   - recipient hepatitis B immune—no further action (or may give hepatitis B booster)
   - recipient hepatitis B non-immune (or non-responder) and donor positive or unknown—give hepatitis B immunoglobulin and start course of hepatitis B vaccination
   - recipient hepatitis B non-immune and donor negative—start course of hepatitis B vaccination
   - donor HIV antibody positive or in high-risk group (e.g. homosexual, intravenous drug user, prostitute, heterosexual patients from high HIV incidence countries)—consult infectious diseases physician for post-exposure prophylaxis
   - counsel recipients on safe sex procedures to prevent possible infection of their sexual partners
7. Follow up recipients with serological testing after 3 months (hepatitis B, hepatitis C, HIV), 6 months (hepatitis B and C) and 12 months (hepatitis C); ensure completion of hepatitis B vaccination courses instituted earlier

---

After a significant exposure to HIV, antiretroviral drugs should be given promptly for post-exposure prophylaxis, ideally within 24 hours. A combination of antiretroviral drugs is given for 4 weeks. Side effects are often very unpleasant and include bone marrow suppression, nausea and other gastrointestinal symptoms, and headache. For health care workers exposed to hepatitis C, no vaccination or preventative treatment can yet be recommended. Guidelines for post-exposure management are to enable early identification of infection and specialist referral.

USE OF MICROBIOLOGICAL TESTS IN MANAGING SURGICAL INFECTIONS

Surgical infection should be diagnosed on clinical grounds and the laboratory used to define the nature of the infection and to guide antibiotic therapy. Keen but inexperienced junior medical or nursing staff often take microbiological swabs from wounds or ulcers, which grow organisms in the laboratory, without realising that this may represent **colonisation** rather than clinically important infection. The clinical picture should always be the factor which determines a decision to begin treatment, although certain organisms such as *Strep. pyogenes* may require treatment to prevent cross-infection even if the lesion is clinically mild.

The results of specimens taken from dirty contaminated sites must be interpreted with caution. Superficial slough or discharge often contains colonising organisms of little significance. For example, in osteomyelitis caused by *Staph. aureus*, the sinus opening may be colonised by *Proteus* or *Pseudomonas* spp. The infecting organism may not be grown unless the wound is first carefully cleaned with saline and then the lesion swabbed deeply. If larger quantities of infected material are available, a syringe of pus or an excised segment of infected tissue should be sent to the laboratory for culture. Where possible, samples should be taken before antibiotics are given.

For best results, microbiological specimens should be transported quickly to the laboratory and certainly within 2 hours. If this is not possible, the specimen should be kept at 4°C. Blood culture specimens should be placed in an incubator at 35°C.

PRINCIPLES OF TREATMENT OF SURGICAL INFECTION

REMOVAL OF INFECTED FOCI

An infected area that is poorly vascularised is effectively isolated from the body's humoral and cellular defence mechanisms as well as from circulating antibiotics. Retained infected material may overactivate cytokine mechanisms and thus precipitate systemic sepsis and its sequelae. A vital first step therefore is to remove any infected necrotic tissue and drain collections of pus. This principle should not be ignored on the grounds that the patient is too ill for operation because the very ill patient may recover dramatically after this type of surgery. Common examples include draining abscesses, amputating infected necrotic limbs, removing infected foreign bodies (e.g. cannulae, prostheses, trauma debris) and draining the infected contents of hollow viscera such as bile ducts, kidneys and ureters.

ANTIBIOTIC THERAPY (see Table 3.1)

Empirical antibiotic therapy

If treatment is urgent, antibiotics should be chosen according to the common pathogens most likely in a given situation, together with knowledge of the local antibiotic

Table 3.1 **The main surgical infections, their common microbial causes and suggested empirical therapy**

Clinical condition	Common pathogen	Commonly used antibiotics
Gastrointestinal tract		
Gastroenteritis	**Bacterial:** *Campylobacter* *Salmonella* *Shigella* and others **Viral:** SRSV Adenovirus Rotavirus **Travel associated:** *Entamoeba histolytica*	Antibiotics not normally required If severe or lasting > 48 h, give ciprofloxacin Metronidazole
Pseudomembranous colitis (hospital-acquired)	*Clostridium difficile*	Metronidazole orally Vancomycin orally second line
Peritonitis Biliary tract	Coliforms Anaerobes *Enterococcus* spp. *E. coli* *Klebsiella* *Bacteroides* *Enterococcus* *Pseudomonas* Clostridia	Cefuroxime (ciprofloxacin for peripancreatic infections) + metronidazole or ampicillin + gentamicin + metronidazole
Oesophageal perforation	*Candida*	Fluconazole or itraconazole + cefuroxime and metronidazale
Superficial and wound infections		
Breast abscess or mastitis	*Staphylococcus aureus*	Flucloxacillin or cefradine or erythromycin
Carbuncle, furunculosis	*Staphylococcus aureus*	Avoid antibiotics unless signs of systemic infection Flucloxacillin or cefradine or erythromycin If recurrent, mupirocin/Naseptin nasal cream
Cellulitis	*Staphylococcus aureus* *Streptococcus pyogenes* (group A Strep.)	Cefradine or erythromycin If diabetes mellitus, add ciprofloxacin or gentamicin
Gas gangrene	*Clostridium perfringens* & other spp. *Bacteroides* spp. and other anaerobes Coliforms	Surgery essential Penicillin + clindamycin
Infected surgical wound 6–72 hours 3–7 days > 7 days	*Streptococcus pyogenes* (group A) *Clostridium* *Staphylococcus aureus* *Streptococcus pyogenes* (group A) *Pseudomonas aeruginosa* Coliforms	Surgery essential Co-amoxiclav Co-amoxiclav Drainage/debridement if necessary. Antibiotics if spreading infection
Infected traumatic wound	*Staphylococcus aureus* *Streptococcus pyogenes* (group A)	Cefradine or erythromycin
Necrotising fasciitis	*Streptococcus pyogenes* (group A) Mixed infection with anaerobes and coliforms	Surgery essential Penicillin + clindamycin Co-amoxiclav
Bites (cat, dog, human)	Anaerobes *Pasteurella* spp. *S. moniliformis*	Co-amoxiclav or doxycycline
Lungs		
PNEUMONIAS Community-acquired	*Staphylococcus* *Pneumococcus* *Chlamydia psittaci* *Mycoplasma* *Legionella*	Amoxicillin or cefuroxime Add erythromycin if 'atypical' pneumonia suspected Rifampicin

Table 3.1 The main surgical infections, their common microbial causes and suggested empirical therapy—cont'd

Clinical condition	Common pathogen	Commonly used antibiotics
Hospital-acquired pneumonia (severe)	Streptococcus pneumoniae Coliforms (resistant) Pseudomonas aeruginosa	Penicillin G + ciprofloxacin Add metronidazole if risk of aspiration Use vancomycin if MRSA risk
Hospital acquired pneumonia (non-severe)	Other resistant Gram-negative bacilli Staphylococcus aureus (MRSA) Legionella pneumophila	Piperacillin/tazobactam Ciprofloxacin + metronidazole Meropenem Add vancomycin if MRSA risk
Aspiration pneumonia	Coliforms Oral flora (Streptococcus spp., anaerobes) Streptococcus pneumoniae Staphylococcus aureus	Cefuroxime + metronidazole
ENT		
Acute tonsillitis Otitis media	Strep. pyogenes Strep. pneumoniae Haemophilus influenzae	Penicillin or erythromycin Amoxicillin or erythromycin
Genito-urinary system		
Urinary catheter infection	Coliforms (resistant) Pseudomonas aeruginosa Other resistant Gram-negative bacilli Candida spp.	No treatment unless signs of systemic infection Consult microbiology for treatment advice as pathogen often antibiotic resistant
Asymptomatic bacteriuria	Coliforms Staphylococcus saprophyticus Enterococcus spp. Pseudomonas aeruginosa	Norfloxacin or cefalexin
Pyelonephritis	Coliforms including Pseudomonas aeruginosa	Cefuroxime or ciprofloxacin
Prostatitis—acute and chronic	Coliforms and Pseudomonas aeruginosa Staphylococcus aureus & spp. Enterococcus spp. Mycoplasma spp. and Ureaplasma spp. (if chronic, consider Corynebacterium spp., Mycobacterium tuberculosis)	Ciprofloxacin
Prostatitis—age under 35 yrs	Chlamydia trachomatis Neisseria gonorrhoeae Mycoplasma spp. and Ureaplasma spp. Herpes simplex	Ciprofloxacin + azithromycin Aciclovir
Cardiovascular system		
Acute native valve endocarditis	Staphylococcus	Flucloxacillin + rifampicin Vancomycin if MRSA
Sub-acute native valve endocarditis	Streptococcus	Benzyl penicillin + gentamicin (vertically centred) Enterococcus
Prosthetic valve endocarditis	Staphylococcus	Vancomycin + rifampicin + gentamicin
Central nervous system		
Meningitis	Meningococcus Pneumococcus Haemophilus influenzae Listeria	Cefotaxime ciftriaxone Amoxicillin + gentamicin
Musculoskeletal system		
Osteomyelitis or septic arthritis	Staph. aureus Coliforms, Pseudomonas	Flucloxacillin Vancomycin if MRSA risk + ciprofloxacin if diabetic/immunocompromised
Eye		
Purulent conjunctivitis	Staph. aureus Haemophilus influenzae Strep. pneumoniae and Pseudomonas aeruginosa	Chloramphenicol eye drops Gentamicin eye drops

sensitivity profiles. A Gram stain performed on material from a usually sterile site can guide initial therapy until culture and sensitivity results are available. In an abdominal wound infection where hollow viscera have not been opened, *Staph. aureus* is the likely infecting organism and an anti-staphylococcal penicillin such as flucloxacillin can be commenced. If, however, the patient is known to carry meticillin-resistant *Staph. aureus* (MRSA), vancomycin may be indicated. If bowel has been opened, Gram-negative organisms including anaerobes are likely and an antibiotic regimen is chosen to include these bacteria.

Specific antibiotic therapy

Once microbiological test results are available, therapy is modified to deal with the particular organisms grown and their antibiotic sensitivities. Specific 'narrow-spectrum' therapy is more effective and has fewer side effects than broad-spectrum 'shotgun' therapy. It also minimises the possibility of superinfection with organisms such as *Clostridium difficile* and yeasts.

NUTRITIONAL SUPPORT

Major infection and sepsis result in severe catabolism (see Ch. 2) and may be associated with hypoalbuminaemia and wasting. Relatively simple measures such as naso-gastric tube feeding should be considered if the patient is unable to swallow. The more complex procedure of total parenteral nutrition may be appropriate in other situations (see Ch. 2).

BACTERIA OF PARTICULAR SURGICAL IMPORTANCE

STAPHYLOCOCCI

PATHOPHYSIOLOGY

Staphylococci are **Gram-positive cocci**, of which the main pathogenic species is *Staph. aureus*. The organism can be part of the normal human bacterial flora, with about 30% of the general population being nasal carriers and 10% carrying it on the perineal skin. *Staph. aureus* typically produces pustules, boils, breast abscesses, wound infections and osteomyelitis. Part of its virulence is due to its production of a variety of enzymes and toxins. A few patients harbour particularly virulent strains that produce the toxic shock syndrome toxin (TSST-1). Infection with these produces **toxic shock syndrome** with serious systemic effects such as fever, hypotension, shock and multi-organ failure. *Staph. epidermidis*, (formerly *Staph. albus*), a **coagulase-negative** staphylococcus, is a universal skin commensal which rarely produces significant clinical infection or merits antibiotic therapy, except when it causes infections associated with exogenous materials such as prosthetic implants and intravenous cannulae.

Some strains such as meticillin-resistant *Staph. aureus* (MRSA), see below, can be passed from patient to patient on staff hands if care is not taken with hand washing after every patient contact.

ANTIBIOTIC SENSITIVITIES

Most strains of staphylococci were sensitive to penicillin in the early antibiotic era but more than 85% are now resistant in both family practice and hospital. This is largely due to their ability to produce **penicillinase**. Most *Staph. aureus* strains remain sensitive to a reasonable range of commonly used antibiotics, e.g. **flucloxacillin** (a **penicillinase-resistant** penicillin), **erythromycin** and some of the **cephalosporins. Gentamicin** is also active against *Staph. aureus*.

The last decade has seen the emergence of strains of *Staph. aureus* resistant to flucloxacillin and all cephalosporins. Some are also resistant to gentamicin, erythromycin and chloramphenicol and in general are sensitive only to the glycopeptide antibiotics, **vancomycin and teicoplanin**, and these have to be given parenterally. These strains are known by the term **meticillin-resistant *Staph. aureus* (MRSA)**. Meticillin is the drug employed in the laboratory to predict flucloxacillin and cephalosporin resistance. MRSA now accounts for up to half of all *S. aureus* isolates in hospitals and is also emerging as a problem in the community, with the emergence of community-acquired MRSA (CA-MRSA). Ward areas at greatest risk of MRSA infection are burns units, intensive care units, cardiothoracic surgical wards, neonatal units, orthopaedic wards and geriatric wards. It is often erroneously believed that MRSA is inherently more pathogenic than other *Staph. aureus* strains. In fact, the organisms excite similar inflammatory responses aimed at their elimination; the difference is that MRSA infections are more difficult to treat. MRSA may be sensitive in vitro to aminoglycoside antibiotics such as gentamicin but this is rarely of much value in clinical practice. In some cases, oral treatment with **tetracycline, co-trimoxazole** or a **combination of rifampicin and fusidic acid** is appropriate; the combination prevents rapid development of antibiotic resistance to each agent alone.

A particularly worrying development is the emergence of vancomycin-insensitive *Staph. aureus*, **VISA**, which is of intermediate sensitivity (i.e. relatively resistant) to vancomycin. Inappropriate use of vancomycin must be avoided to prevent selection of such mutants. A number of new antibiotics that are active against MRSA and VISA have been developed recently. These include linezolid, which can also be given orally, and daptomycin.

STREPTOCOCCI

PATHOPHYSIOLOGY

Streptococci are **Gram-positive** coccoid organisms which were first described in infected surgical wounds by Billroth in 1874.

Streptococci may be classified by their oxygen requirements into **aerobic, anaerobic** and **microaerophilic** (i.e. grow best in reduced oxygen concentrations) and further subdivided by their ability to produce different patterns of **haemolysis** on agar culture plates containing red blood cells.

Alpha-haemolytic streptococci cause partial haemolysis with a green discolouration; important pathogens in this group include the *viridans* group of streptococci and *Strep. pneumoniae.*

Beta-haemolytic streptococci produce complete haemolysis and may be grouped serologically into **Lancefield groups** A to O. The important human pathogens are group A streptococci (*Strep. pyogenes*—of major surgical importance) and group B streptococci (*Strep. agalactiae*—a common cause of serious neonatal sepsis). Streptococci in groups C and G are occasional causes of cellulitis and bacteraemia. Some streptococci and most enterococci carry a group D antigen. Microaerophilic streptococci such as *Strep. milleri* carry a group F antigen.

Some streptococci are non-haemolytic and these were formerly known as gamma-haemolytic streptococci.

STREPTOCOCCI OF PARTICULAR SURGICAL SIGNIFICANCE

Strep. pyogenes (groups and haemolytic streptococcus)

This is the main human pathogenic streptococcus and is carried in the upper respiratory tract by about 10% of children but less often by adults. It can cause cellulitis and, less commonly nowadays, erysipelas. *Strep. pyogenes* is also a common cause of sore throat as well as post-streptococcal syndromes such as rheumatic fever which itself predisposes to cardiac valvular damage and subsequent risk of infective endocarditis.

In acute **cellulitis**, a locally spreading infection involves the dermis and hypodermis, facilitated by production of hyaluronidase and streptokinase. In limb infections, organisms draining towards regional lymph nodes via lymphatics may produce perilymphatic inflammation and painful red streaks along the limb, i.e. **lymphangitis.** The regional nodes react vigorously, becoming enlarged,

painful and tender, a condition known as **lymphadenitis**. This may also occur in staphylococcal infections. Severe tissue damage may be caused by certain highly invasive strains of *Strep. pyogenes* leading to one variety of **necrotising fasciitis,** a deep-seated infection of the subcutaneous tissue that progressively destroys fascia and fat. If the infecting strain produces certain exotoxins a life-threatening **streptococcal toxic shock syndrome** may develop. This syndrome is associated with fulminant soft tissue infection, shock, adult respiratory distress syndrome and renal failure; 30–70% of patients die in spite of aggressive modern treatments.

Viridans streptococci

The *viridans* group of streptococci are oral commensals of low virulence but are the most common organisms causing infective endocarditis. This may occur as a complication of certain surgical procedures in the presence of pre-existing cardiac abnormalities; the subject is described in detail in Chapter 8.

Strep. pneumoniae (pneumococcus)

This organism is the most common cause of lobar pneumonia and can also cause bronchopneumonia in susceptible post-surgical patients. *Strep. pneumoniae* is a common cause of middle ear infections (otitis media); it is also involved in acute exacerbations of chronic bronchitis. Pneumococcal meningitis may occur in the young and elderly and may complicate head injury. Severe pneumococcal sepsis is particularly likely after splenectomy but may be prevented by vaccination and penicillin prophylaxis.

Strep. milleri (anginosus group)

Many of the *Strep. milleri* group have microaerophilic culture requirements. They are often found in abscesses in the appendix area, the liver, lung and brain.

Anaerobic streptococci

Members of this group are bowel commensals and may form part of the mixed flora in many intraperitoneal abscesses and infection associated with necrotic tissue, e.g. diabetic foot ulcers.

ANTIBIOTIC SENSITIVITIES

Penicillin is the drug of choice for most streptococcal infections. In seriously ill patients, **benzylpenicillin** is given parenterally. For less serious infections in patients able to tolerate oral therapy, **penicillin V (phenoxymethylpenicillin)** or **ampicillin/amoxicillin** are the drugs of choice. Many streptococci are also sensitive to **macrolides** (e.g. **erythromycin, clarithromycin**). Some pneumococci are now partially resistant to penicillin. Most infections, however, are still cleared with high-dose penicillin although meningitis needs alternative antibiotics such as ceftriaxone or vancomycin.

ENTEROCOCCI

PATHOPHYSIOLOGY

The enterococci are **Gram-positive cocci** closely related to streptococci. *E. faecalis* (formerly *Strep. faecalis*) is the most common species. Enterococci form part of the normal bowel flora and may cause infection where bowel has been opened or infect the urinary or genital tracts.

ANTIBIOTIC SENSITIVITIES

Penicillin, **ampicillin**, **amoxicillin** or **vancomycin** are used for enterococcal infections. In serious infections such as endocarditis, a combination of high-dose penicillin and gentamicin is used to ensure bactericidal activity.

The cephalosporins are all ineffective. In hospitals where broad-spectrum (third-generation) cephalosporins are used as empirical therapy for bowel-related infections or septicaemia, enterococci are a frequent cause of nosocomial (hospital-acquired) infection. Vancomycin-resistant enterococci (VRE) are now being found. They are usually low-grade pathogens but can infect intravascular lines, nearly always in transplant and haematology patients and on intensive care units. Endocarditis caused by VRE is difficult to treat, but the newer Gram-positive antibiotics linezolid, daptomycin and quinupristin/dalfopristin are active against most strains of VRE.

ENTEROBACTERIACEAE

PATHOPHYSIOLOGY

The Enterobacteriaceae are a large family of **Gram-negative bacilli** (i.e. rods) which usually make up about 1% of the normal intestinal flora (see Table 3.2); these organisms are commonly referred to as **coliforms**. The organisms can be cultured under aerobic and anaerobic conditions and, like other members of the bowel flora, grow in media containing bile salts such as MacConkey or CLED agar; this helps in their identification.

Infections of surgical importance with Enterobacteriaceae are usually opportunistic in nature with the bacteria almost always arising from the patient's own bowel. Infection results from direct contamination from perforated or surgically opened bowel, perineal spread (to nearby wounds or urinary tract) or haematogenous spread. These and other Gram-negative organisms contain the sugar **lipopolysaccharide** (LPS), a powerful stimulator of inflammation and production by macrophages of the cytokines TNF-alpha and interleukin-1.

Escherichia coli is the most common pathogen of the Enterobacteriaceae and is responsible for many surgical

Table 3.2 Bacteria of the family enterobacteriaceae

Organism	Clinical infection
Primary gut pathogens	
Salmonella, e.g. *S. typhi*, *S. enteritidis* *Shigella*, e.g. *S. dysenteriae*, *S. sonnei* Some *Escherichia coli* strains, e.g. O157 : H7	Typhoid fever Gastroenteritis Dysentery Traveller's diarrhoea Haemolytic uraemic syndrome
Gut colonisers that can cause infections	
Escherichia coli *Klebsiella* *Proteus* *Enterobacter* *Morganella* *Citrobacter*	Peritonitis and intraperitoneal abscesses (usually mixed infection with anaerobes) Septicaemia Urinary tract infections Ascending cholangitis (May also cause hospital-acquired infections, e.g. after instrumentation, central venous catheters, pneumonia in intensive care)
Gut colonisers that rarely cause infection	
Enterobacter *Serratia* *Morganella* *Citrobacter*	Usually hospital-acquired infections, e.g. after instrumentation, central venous catheters, in intensive care

infections, often in synergy with other bacteria. *E. coli* is the most common cause of urinary tract infections (about 80% of all UTIs) and **Gram-negative sepsis**. Coliform bronchopneumonia occasionally occurs in debilitated, immunosuppressed or seriously ill patients. *Klebsiella*, *Enterobacter* and *Serratia* are being isolated more often in surgical bowel-related infections. *Proteus* is a common cause of urinary tract infections but occasionally causes other surgical infections, usually originating from the urinary tract.

ANTIBIOTIC SENSITIVITIES

Many coliforms are now resistant to ampicillin (and amoxicillin) and first-generation cephalosporins, e.g. cefalothin, but most are sensitive to **second- and third-generation cephalosporins**, e.g. **cefuroxime, cefotaxime**. Gentamicin is still a very effective and cheap agent against coliforms. Many coliforms are sensitive to the fluoroquinolones (ciprofloxacin, levofloxacin, moxifloxacin) but resistance is emerging. For prophylaxis in bowel and biliary tract surgery and for treating related local and systemic infections, gentamicin or a second-generation cephalosporin (e.g. cefuroxime) is recommended, together with metronidazole for its activity against anaerobes. Antibiotic and beta-lactamase inhibitor combination antibiotics such as co-amoxicillin–clavulanate and piperacillin–tazobactam are also very active against bowel flora and can be used without metronidazole as they have good activity against anaerobes. Anaerobes are the main colonisers of the bowel and often accompany Enterobacteriaceae in infections but are not part of this group.

Resistant strains of Enterobacteriaceae are much more frequent in hospitals than in the community. They are often found on intensive care units or causing urinary tract infection in catheterised patients who have had repeated courses of antibiotics. Strains of *E. coli* and *Klebsiella* spp. that are multi-drug resistant have emerged in hospitals all over the world since the 1980s. They produce enzymes that can destroy second- and third-generation cephalosporins (extended spectrum beta-lactamase enzymes or ESBL), and are also often resistant to quinolones and most aminoglycosides. The only antibiotics active against these ESBL strains are the **carbapenems** (meropenem, imipenem, ertapenem) and amikacin. The carbapenems are very broad spectrum, but are expensive antibiotics that can only be given parenterally. Their use in most hospitals is restricted to prevent resistance developing.

'NON-SURGICAL' ENTEROBACTERIACEAE

Other members of the Enterobacteriaceae family produce primary bowel infections, although these only occasionally enter the province of the surgeon. For example, *Salmonella typhi* causes **typhoid** which may cause bowel perforations and *Shigella* causes **bacillary dysentery**. Rarely, *Salmonella* is incriminated in acute appendicitis and primary 'mycotic' aneurysms. An increasingly important cause of **acute haemorrhagic colitis** is *E. coli* O157 : H7 and other verotoxin-producing *E. coli*. This is clinically indistinguishable from acute ulcerative colitis and should be sought bacteriologically in all cases of haemorrhagic colitis. These *E. coli* strains have caused large outbreaks of food-borne disease and produce a verotoxin (Shiga-like toxin or SLT) that is responsible for the haemolytic uraemic syndrome (HUS) resulting in acute renal failure. *Yersinia* sometimes produces an acute inflammation of the ileum which may mimic the clinical picture of acute appendicitis. At laparotomy it appears similar to Crohn's disease of the terminal ileum. *Campylobacter jejuni*, the most common cause of food-borne infection, can also cause a pseudoappendicitis by initiating a terminal ileitis and inflammation of mesenteric lymph nodes.

PSEUDOMONAS

PATHOPHYSIOLOGY

The main pathogen in this group of **aerobic Gram-negative rods** is *Pseudomonas aeruginosa*, an uncommon cause of surgical infection. It tends to cause infections in debilitated, hospitalised patients. The organism is found in a wide variety of habitats including soil, water, plants and animals, which reflect its predilection for moist environments. It is commonly found on hospital and cleaning equipment and even in chemical disinfectants and antiseptics. In about 10% of the population, *Ps. aeruginosa* is a normal commensal of the human intestine and is primarily an in-hospital (nosocomial) pathogen. The organism is resistant to many antibiotics and therefore tends to proliferate when other flora have been suppressed by broad-spectrum antibiotic therapy.

Pseudomonas is a common colonising organism in long-standing wounds such as compound fractures, chronic leg ulcers and indwelling urinary catheters but its presence is not always clinically significant. In wounds and ulcers, *Pseudomonas* can be recognised by the characteristic blue-green discharge. The organism often colonises burns and may become pathogenic when burns are extensive, giving rise to fatal sepsis. *Pseudomonas* infection can be a serious complication of ophthalmic surgery and may lead to loss of the infected eye. It is also often responsible for chronic and recurrent external ear infections (otitis externa). Finally, *Ps. aeruginosa* may be responsible for hospital-acquired pneumonias in ventilated patients or for fatal systemic sepsis in terminally ill patients.

ANTIBIOTIC SENSITIVITIES

When considering antibiotic therapy, true infection must, as ever, be distinguished from colonisation. Treatment of colonisation is not indicated and encourages the development of resistance. *Pseudomonas aeruginosa* is intrinsically resistant to most antibiotics but antibiotics that have activity include the **aminoglycosides** (**gentamicin** and **tobramycin**), some extended-spectrum beta-lactam antibiotics (**ceftazidime** or **cefepime**), the combination of **piperacillin** and **tazobactam** and the carbapenems (**imipenem** or **meropenem**). The quinolones, **ciprofloxacin** and **ofloxacin**, are the only effective oral antipseudomonal agents.

ANAEROBES

Anaerobic bacteria make up a major part of the indigenous flora in the gastrointestinal tract, outnumbering *E. coli* and related coliforms by about 1000 to 1. Many parts of the body are colonised by anaerobes, even those exposed to air, including skin, mouth, upper respiratory tract, external genitalia and vagina. These colonising organisms are very important in the aetiology of surgical infections because creating breaks in anatomical barriers during surgery allows contamination and predisposes to infection. Other important factors in setting conditions that allow anaerobes to grow include intestinal obstruction, tissue destruction and hypoxia as in burns and vascular insufficiency, and the presence of foreign bodies. Anaerobes often cause life-threatening disease, and surgical management of anaerobic infections is often required treatment. Some anaerobes such as the clostridia cause toxin-related diseases including tetanus. The most commonly encountered anaerobes are:

- **Gram-negative bacilli**—*Bacteroides fragilis* and other *Bacteroides* species (spp.), *Porphyromonas* spp., *Prevotella* spp., *Fusobacterium* spp. and *Bilophila wadsworthia*
- **Gram-positive cocci**—*Peptostreptococcus* and microaerophilic streptococci
- **Gram-positive bacilli**—*Clostridium* spp. (spore forming), *Actinomyces* spp., *Propionibacterium* spp. and *Bifidobacterium* spp.

ANTIBIOTIC SENSITIVITIES

Most anaerobes are highly sensitive to **metronidazole**. Metronidazole can be given orally, intravenously or rectally, with the last giving blood levels equivalent to intravenous administration. Metronidazole is routinely given preoperatively as standard prophylaxis before appendicectomy and large bowel surgery, and its use has dramatically reduced the incidence of postoperative peritoneal and wound infections. Other antibiotics with a good broad anaerobic activity are **amoxicillin/clavulanic acid** (Augmentin), piperacillin/tazobactam (Tazocin), the carbapenems (imipenem and meropenem) and chloramphenicol.

BACTEROIDES

Pathophysiology

Bacteroides is important surgically for causing pyogenic infections after faecal contamination of the peritoneal cavity, usually in combination with other gut commensals. It also occasionally causes sepsis in debilitated patients. These organisms were not identified as pathogens until the early 1970s because their strictly anaerobic culture requirements had not been recognised. Indeed *Bacteroides* spp. were probably responsible for many so-called 'sterile' intra-abdominal abscesses in the past. The importance of *B. fragilis* as a cause of surgical infection is probably still underestimated.

CLOSTRIDIA

Clostridia are Gram-positive rods which are widely distributed in the soil and as intestinal commensals. The organisms form **spores** which are resistant to drying, heat and antiseptics and can survive for long periods. Clostridia are mostly **obligate anaerobes** which can only proliferate in the absence of oxygen; they are responsible for much of the putrefaction and decay of animal material in

nature. The main pathological effects of clostridial infections are caused by powerful **exotoxins**. The infections of surgical importance are **gas gangrene**, **tetanus** and **pseudomembranous colitis**.

Gas gangrene

Gas gangrene results when *Clostridium perfringens* (formerly called *C. welchii*) and other anaerobes (e.g. *Bacteroides* spp. and anaerobic streptococci) proliferate in necrotic tissue, secreting powerful toxins. These spread rapidly and destroy nearby tissues, generating gas at the same time which gives rise to the characteristic clinical sign of crepitus ('crackling') on palpation and the typical X-ray appearance shown in Figure 3.9. Deep traumatic wounds involving muscle, and wounds contaminated with soil, clothes or faeces are most susceptible. The condition is particularly common in battle wounds—gas gangrene was responsible for vast numbers of deaths during the First World War.

In surgical practice, the highest risk of gas gangrene is in **lower limb amputations** performed for ischaemia (infection from the patient's own bowel) and in high-

Fig. 3.9 Gas gangrene

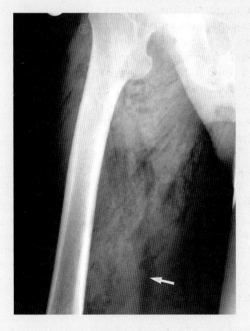

This 46-year-old man sustained extensive contaminated lacerations of the medial right thigh (arrowed) in a road traffic collision. Gas gangrene developed, rapidly involving all the muscles of the thigh because the condition was not recognised early and necrotic muscle was not excised immediately and completely. Note the widespread streaks of radiolucent gas bubbles tracking along the muscle planes. This patient died of toxaemia despite antibiotics, surgery and hyperbaric oxygen therapy.

velocity **gunshot wounds** (infection from the patient's own perforated bowel or by external contamination). Gas gangrene occasionally occurs in other surgical wounds where ischaemic tissue has become contaminated with bowel flora. The area of muscle necrosis may be small at first. Gas gangrene is recognised when the overlying skin turns black and the process spreads at an alarming rate. Within hours the underlying necrosis rages along the muscle planes. Later the skin breaks down and a thin, foul-smelling purulent exudate leaks from the wound. Toxins are absorbed into the general circulation and cause rapid clinical deterioration and death within 24–48 hours unless the process can be halted by timely and vigorous intervention.

C. perfringens is very sensitive to **benzylpenicillin** which should be given prophylactically by injection immediately after a traumatic injury involving muscle, or less than an hour before amputation of an ischaemic limb (metronidazole can be used for patients allergic to penicillin). Preventing clostridial infection in the surgery of contaminated wounds requires meticulous excision of all necrotic tissue followed by packing of the wound rather than suturing. Further excisions are likely to be needed and delayed primary closure can be performed when risk of infection is over, a few days later.

Treatment of gas gangrene

Treatment of established gas gangrene is urgent and must proceed vigorously if there is to be any hope of survival. Treatment is with penicillin and radical excision of necrotic tissue. High doses of penicillin are given intravenously to kill organisms in viable and vascularised tissue. Emergency surgery is performed to remove all necrotic tissue. This involves carving back the necrotic muscle to healthy bleeding tissue; the affected muscle is recognised by its brick-red colour and failure to contract on cutting.

Hyperbaric oxygen therapy may be used to raise the oxygen tension in the necrotic tissues, inhibiting growth of the organisms. The patient is placed in a high-pressure chamber with pure oxygen at about 3 atmospheres pressure for several hours daily. However, gas gangrene may continue to spread despite these measures, necessitating further heroic surgical interventions. Even with all this intensive treatment, the prognosis for established gas gangrene remains bleak.

Tetanus

Tetanus is caused by *Clostridium tetani* which infects dirty wounds in a similar manner to gas gangrene. The size of the entry wound may be minute, perhaps caused by a rose thorn or splinter. The organism produces an **exotoxin** which has little local effect but, even in minute quantities, has powerful remote neuromuscular effects causing widespread muscular spasm. The first signs are often **acute muscle spasms** and **neck stiffness** or **trismus** (**'lockjaw'**). If untreated, these progress to **opisthotonus** (arching of the back due to extensor spasm), generalised convulsions and eventually death from exhaustion and respiratory failure several days later.

Tetanus is now rare in developed countries because of widespread immunisation with **tetanus toxoid** during childhood, followed by boosters at 10-year intervals. In the UK the recommendation is now that boosters are no longer needed if a person has completed his or her initial five-dose vaccination schedule as a child. In Australia and New Zealand a single booster at age 45–50 is recommended. The annual incidence of tetanus in developed countries is about one per million population and is most common following trivial gardening injuries in the elderly, who are least likely to have been properly immunised. If there is doubt about satisfactory immunisation status following a major contaminated injury, **benzylpenicillin** should be given prophylactically as well as passive immunisation with **tetanus immune globulin** collected from people with known high titres. Treatment of established tetanus usually requires artificial ventilation with drug paralysis, in addition to the usual antibiotics and passive immunisation. Mortality remains high, especially in the elderly.

Globally, tetanus remains a massive problem after trauma. A particular local problem in some developing countries is neonatal tetanus resulting from the practice of applying cow dung as a dressing to the umbilical stump.

Pseudomembranous colitis

Pseudomembranous colitis can be the most serious form of **antibiotic-associated diarrhoea** (see Ch. 28) and is caused by overgrowth of a toxigenic *Clostridium difficile*. The organism gets its name from the difficulty of growing it in culture. Infection results in the formation of a thick fibrinous 'membrane' on the large intestinal mucosa, within which the organism proliferates. Its toxins cause a profound watery and sometimes bloody diarrhoea, leading to dehydration and loss of electrolytes.

Although pseudomembranous colitis is uncommon, it may develop after only a single dose of almost any antibiotic. Clindamycin and lincomycin were the most commonly implicated drugs but these are rarely used now; cephalosporins and ciprofloxacin are now the most common cause. Diagnosis can be made by sigmoidoscopy and biopsy in the 50% of patients with left-sided colonic involvement. The best method of diagnosis is to **detect the specific toxin in the stool**; this can be performed by looking for a cytopathic effect on cells cultured in vitro. *C. difficile* can also be cultured from the stool. Although the organism is sensitive to penicillin, this fails to penetrate the pseudomembrane. **Oral metronidazole** is effective in most patients but takes at least 2 days before clinical response is observed. Relapses are common in the elderly and oral **vancomycin**, which is not absorbed from the gastrointestinal tract, can be used for relapses and when metronidazole treatment fails. Oral vancomycin must be used only as a second line agent because of concerns about promoting the growth of vancomycin-resistant organisms.

VIRUSES OF PARTICULAR SURGICAL IMPORTANCE

Chronic blood-borne viral infections such as **hepatitis B and C** and **human immunodeficiency virus (HIV)** are important in surgical practice because of the risk of virus transmission from the patient to the surgeon during operation and vice versa, as well as cross-infection between patients. Preventative measures to be adopted by medical and nursing staff and the management of needle-stick injuries are discussed earlier in this chapter. Patients may also need surgical intervention for complications of hepatitis or HIV infection.

HUMAN IMMUNODEFICIENCY VIRUS (HIV)

CLASSIFICATION OF HIV INFECTIONS

The human immunodeficiency virus causes a chronic infection that usually progresses to the **acquired immune deficiency syndrome (AIDS)** over a period of 7 or more years. The illness evolves through several stages or groups, classified by the Centers for Disease Control Classification, 1986:

- (Group I) the **acute seroconversion illness**. Seroconversion occurs as long as 3 months after infection has been acquired, and as many as 70% of infected patients are asymptomatic at the time of seroconversion. Patients usually test negative for antibodies against HIV both before and during the initial seroconversion illness
- (Group II) the **asymptomatic period** during which the patient usually feels completely well
- (Group III) as the disease progresses, the patient may develop generalised lymphadenopathy and wasting (**AIDS-related complex**)
- (Group IV) **AIDS** is manifest by development of unusual opportunistic infections (e.g. *Pneumocystis* pneumonia, cytomegalovirus (CMV) infections, cerebral toxoplasmosis, atypical mycobacterial infections), certain malignant diseases (Kaposi's sarcoma, generalised or cerebral lymphoma, aggressive invasive uterine cervical cancer) and neurological disease (**AIDS dementia complex**)

The use of combinations of antiretroviral drugs ('high activity antiretroviral therapy') has had a dramatic effect on the natural history of the disease, with a large sustained drop in mortality from opportunistic infections.

SURGICAL INVOLVEMENT IN HIV CASES

Surgeons may be involved in diagnosing bowel-related problems (e.g. oesophageal candidiasis) by oesophago-gastro-duodenoscopy (OGD). In late-stage disease, cytomegalovirus (CMV) infection may involve any part of the gastrointestinal tract, ranging from mouth ulcers, to ulcers in the jejunum that may perforate, to colitis. For AIDS colitis, colonoscopy and biopsy are often required for diagnosis. Treatment involves intravenous antiviral drugs.

AIDS patients may develop severe perianal herpes with secondary anal fistula or abscess formation. In a patient with known AIDS, perianal lesions should be assumed to be herpes until proven otherwise as the presentation is often atypical. Kaposi's sarcomas (see Ch. 46) may require local excision.

Surgeons may also become involved with HIV-infected patients who in late-stage disease require a long-term central venous catheter with a subcutaneous infusion port (e.g. Hickman line). Surgeons may also be asked to place a percutaneous endoscopic gastrostomy (PEG) for feeding purposes. Orthopaedic surgeons may be exposed to the virus when performing joint replacements in HIV-infected haemophiliacs.

VIRAL HEPATITIS

Viral hepatitis manifests clinically with anorexia, nausea and sometimes abdominal discomfort in the right upper quadrant followed by jaundice. There are many viruses that cause hepatitis, often with different modes of transmission, incubation times, prognosis and complications. These include CMV, Epstein–Barr and the hepatitis viruses. Hepatitis A and E are spread by the faecal–oral route whereas hepatitis B and C can be acquired by blood and some body fluids and therefore represent a potential risk to the surgeon.

HEPATITIS A

Hepatitis A is transmitted by the faecal–oral route. It has an incubation period of 2–6 weeks but rarely causes fulminating disease and never leads to chronic hepatitis or cirrhosis. Its only surgical importance is when considering the differential diagnosis of jaundice. A vaccine for preventing hepatitis A is now available.

HEPATITIS B

Hepatitis B is transmitted by blood or body fluids, including sexual intercourse, or from mother to fetus or baby (termed **vertical transmission**). Incubation is from 6 weeks to 6 months. Hepatitis B infection leads to chronic hepatitis and cirrhosis in 5–10% of cases; this variety of cirrhosis commonly progresses to **hepatocellular carcinoma** (the most common cause of hepatocellular carcinoma world-wide). Hepatitis B is preventable by vaccination and this is indicated for neonates of mothers who carry the virus, all health care workers and people living in high-risk areas.

Exposure to hepatitis B virus has several possible outcomes:

- **Acute fulminant hepatitis**—this is rare but fatal
- **Acute hepatitis**—clearing of the virus leads to lifelong immunity
- **Chronic infection**—this may lead to chronic hepatitis/ cirrhosis (and possibly hepatocellular carcinoma)
- **Chronic carrier state**—this is mainly due to infection at birth but can occur later with development of immune tolerance and no obvious active disease

Diagnosis of hepatitis B

The hepatitis B surface *antigen* (**HBsAg**) can be detected in blood in the early stages of the disease. Patients later develop *antibodies* to the viral core (**anti-HBc**) which does not confer immunity but is a marker of exposure to the virus. Later still, with clearance of the virus, patients develop surface *antibodies* (**anti-HBs**) which confer lifetime immunity. Patients who do not clear the virus remain surface *antigen* (HbsAg) positive and may become **chronic carriers**, i.e. remain infectious to other people and prone to risk of complications themselves.

Patients who are HBsAg-positive may transmit the virus if there is recipient exposure to sufficient material, e.g. by blood transfusion. The special case of **e antigen positivity** (HBeAg) indicates patients with high infectivity.

Hepatitis B vaccines contain recombinant inactivated surface *antigen* and induce immunity by stimulating production of surface *antibody*; this is the only serological marker that is positive in people who have been vaccinated.

Treatment of hepatitis B

Hepatitis B DNA can now be detected in blood, giving a definitive diagnosis and an estimate of the quantity of virus in the bloodstream (viral load) to guide treatment. Therapy with interferon and lamivudine has been partially successful in treating chronic hepatitis B infections, reducing its infectivity and also the risk of developing hepatocellular carcinoma. Chronic carriers failing therapy should be monitored for hepatocellular carcinoma by annual estimation of **serum alpha-fetoprotein** and undergo liver ultrasound scanning every 2 years, as partial hepatectomy can sometimes cure early cases.

HEPATITIS C

Hepatitis C is transmitted via the same routes as hepatitis B but sexual transmission is believed to be less common. The incubation period is approximately 2 months. Chronic liver disease develops in a higher proportion of cases (30–50%) but is often of low-grade activity. Hepatitis C is also an important cause of hepatocellular carcinoma world-wide.

Serological diagnosis is troublesome because HCV antibody tests often give false positives. Seroconversion occurs late, often weeks to months after the acute illness. Definitive diagnosis is made by detecting hepatitis C RNA in serum. As in hepatitis B, viral load assays are used to monitor response to therapy and infectivity, and treatment with interferon and ribavirin has also been partially successful. In most cases a positive hepatitis C antibody test is likely to mean continuing infection.

HEPATITIS D

This is a defective virus that requires hepatitis B surface antigen for full expression and occurs only as a co-infection with hepatitis B. It can be prevented by vaccination for hepatitis B.

SEPSIS

MULTIPLE ORGAN DYSFUNCTION AND THE SYSTEMIC INFLAMMATORY RESPONSE SYNDROME

Multiple organ dysfunction syndrome or MODS (also known as multi-organ failure or MOF) came to be recognised as a distinct clinical entity in the mid-1970s when it became widely recognised that any major physiological insult could lead to failure of one or more organs remote from the initiating disease process. Later it was conceived that the underlying condition was an unrestrained systemic inflammatory response (**systemic inflammatory response syndrome, SIRS**), initiated by a range of adverse events such as trauma, infection, inflammation, ischaemia or ischaemia–reperfusion injury. MODS is the most common reason for surgical patients to stay longer than 5 days in intensive care (see Box 3.2).

Sepsis (also known by or incorporated within the terms **septic shock, systemic sepsis, septicaemia and sepsis syndrome**) describes the clinical features which

Systemic inflammatory response syndrome (SIRS)

Present if two or more of the following are found:

- Temperature > 38°C or < 36°C
- Heart rate > 90 beats/min
- Respiratory rate > 20 breaths/min or $PaCO_2$ < 4.3 kPa
- White cell count > 12 000 cells/mm³ or < 4000 cells/mm³ or more than 10% immature forms

Multiple organ dysfunction syndrome (MODS)

Present if SIRS is associated with organ dysfunction, e.g. oliguria, hypoxia

Sepsis (or systemic sepsis)

Defined as SIRS in association with bacterial infection proven by culture

Severe sepsis

Defined as sepsis associated with signs of organ dysfunction, e.g. renal failure

Septic shock

Defined as SIRS associated with hypotension refractory to volume replacement and requiring vasopressors

---

occur when infection is the initiating factor of MODS. At an early stage, the condition may be reversible. Note that the term sepsis is *not* synonymous with infection and should be reserved for the systemic process described here. In MODS, the sequence of failure of individual organs often follows a predictable pattern with **pulmonary failure** occurring first, followed by hepatic, intestinal, renal and finally cardiac failure. Pulmonary failure is associated with acute (formerly 'adult') respiratory distress syndrome (**ARDS**). In hepatic failure, patients have a rising bilirubin, serum glutamic oxaloacetic transaminase (SGOT) and lactate dehydrogenase (LDH). Intestinal failure is recognised by **stress bleeding** requiring blood transfusion, renal failure by rising plasma creatinine and low urine output, and cardiac failure by low cardiac output and hypotension. Altered mental states such as confusion also occur (cerebral failure) as may disseminated intravascular coagulopathy (DIC).

The mortality of MODS is directly related to the number of organs that fail. With one organ the mortality rate is 40%; with two, 60%; and with three organs, more than 90%.

PATHOPHYSIOLOGY OF SIRS AND MODS

SIRS involves widespread changes including inflammatory cell activation leading to cytokine release, endothe-

lial injury, disordered haemodynamics and impaired tissue oxygen extraction. It thus represents a grossly exaggerated activation of innate immune responses intended as host defences. An excessive unregulated release of inflammatory mediators, however, does much more harm than good by causing the widespread microvascular, haemodynamic and mitochondrial changes that eventually lead to organ failure.

Following initial tissue injury, a local inflammatory response occurs with cytokine induction (see *Immunity* at the start of this chapter). The primary response to this is to mobilise other inflammatory cells including macrophages and neutrophils which diapedese into the tissues. In addition, cytokines signal systemic elements of inflammation to occur, including activation of endothelium, the complement system and blood coagulation, thus amplifying the primary inflammatory response. All of this is normal and appropriate. However, if the injury is severe or persistent, the localised reaction may spill over excessively into the systemic circulation producing a systemic inflammatory response, or if initiated by infection, producing the sepsis syndrome.

Mediators of SIRS and MODS

SIRS and MODS involve complex interactions of endogenous and sometimes exogenous mediators. A range of cytokines is released from activated macrophages as well as from endothelial and other reticulo-endothelial cells. The suite of cytokines released depends on the nature of the provoking agent and is governed by the type of Toll-like receptors that recognise the aggressor. Cytokines released include **tumour necrosis factor-alpha** (TNF-alpha), the **interleukins** (particularly IL1 but also IL2, IL6) and platelet activating factor. Individually, these mediators cause responses similar to those found in SIRS when injected into volunteers. Attempts have been made to suppress this excess cytokine response with drugs but to date these have been ineffective or have produced serious side effects.

Sepsis

The classic septic response, with a hyperdynamic circulation, systemic signs of inflammation and disrupted intermediary metabolism, can be induced in healthy volunteers by injecting **lipopolysaccharide** (derived from the cell walls of Gram-negative bacteria) or the cytokines TNF-alpha or IL1. In Gram-negative sepsis, the lipopolysaccharide component of the organisms powerfully activates Toll-like receptors on dendritic cells and hence the whole inflammatory cascade. This results in endothelial activation which increases vascular permeability and neutrophil–endothelial interaction. The final common pathway may involve migration of activated neutrophils into the interstitial space of the affected organ and the development of tissue hypoxia. In sepsis, these and other circulating factors working in synergy bring about the devastating effects of MODS.

CLINICAL CONDITIONS LEADING TO SIRS AND MODS

These include infection and endotoxaemia (Gram-negative sepsis) in 50–70% of cases, retained necrotic tissue and shock. Any of these can initiate distant organ failure by the following mechanisms:

- Inducing excessive release of endogenous cytokines
- Disrupting oxygen delivery to the tissues
- Impairing intestinal barrier function allowing **translocation** of intestinal bacteria and endotoxin to the portal and systemic circulations
- Damaging the reticulo-endothelial system

Organ failure induced by acute pancreatitis is caused by a combination of these factors.

Infection

The source of infection that leads to MODS may be **acquired** (e.g. intra-abdominal abscess) or **endogenous**, i.e. from the patient's own bowel. Local infection, especially with Gram-negative bacteria, stimulates the release of powerful inflammatory cytokines. A similar response is provoked by a substantial volume of necrotic tissue, e.g. gangrenous leg, and is made much worse if the tissue is infected. These **paracrine responses** are beneficial in a local sense, combating infection by increasing blood flow and vascular permeability to allow influx of dendritic cells and macrophages, as well as activating neutrophils to degranulate and release cytotoxic oxygen radicals. If the stimulating factor is so great that inflammatory mediators spill over into the systemic circulation in large quantities, a cascade is initiated which leads to sepsis and MODS. Superoxide radicals and other circulating factors then damage cells elsewhere in the body, causing widespread vasodilatation and increased vascular permeability leading to hypotension and circulatory collapse. The myocardium is depressed and cellular metabolic functions are disrupted.

Endogenous sources of infection

Bowel is a reservoir for bacteria and endotoxin which are normally safely contained. If the **intestinal barrier** is breached by splanchnic ischaemia, impoverished luminal nutrition of enterocytes or altered intestinal flora, then **translocation** of bacteria into the portal circulation can occur in as little as 30 minutes. If the liver Kupffer cells are also impaired, intestinal bacteria and endotoxin are not prevented in the normal way from reaching the systemic circulation. This may explain the potential for renal failure in jaundiced patients undergoing operation (hepato-renal syndrome). This endogenous source of sepsis probably explains the 30% or so of patients who

suffer organ dysfunction without an obvious source of infection. Typically, such patients are affected after prolonged hypotension (hypovolaemic or cardiogenic shock) or hypoxaemia (e.g. multiple trauma victims), or as a result of direct visceral ischaemia (e.g. prolonged aortic clamping and hypotension in a patient with a ruptured aortic aneurysm).

PREVENTION OF SEPSIS AND MODS

Prevention and early treatment of MODS is summarised in Box 3.3.

Surgical aspects

When multiple organ dysfunction occurs in surgical patients, it often results from a complication such as a bowel anastomotic leak ('septic') or from severe acute pancreatitis (which may be sterile but becomes devastating if associated with pancreatic infection). Extensive tissue necrosis following trauma or death of an ischaemic limb may also precipitate the syndrome in one form or another.

Organ dysfunction often has an insidious onset. At an early stage, subclinical organ dysfunction is often suspected and may be confirmed by investigation; at this stage active resuscitation and dealing with causative factors such as a necrotic limb are likely to have beneficial effects. By 7–10 days without effective treatment, pulmonary failure (ARDS) and hepatic and renal failure appear; MODS is now present and the prognosis becomes substantially worse.

Prevention of sepsis and early management of major gut-related infection before it provokes the SIRS–MODS

Box 3.3 Prevention and early treatment of multiple organ dysfunction syndrome

General prevention

- Rapid resuscitation and early definitive treatment of major injuries
- Good surgical technique
- Appropriate use of prophylactic and therapeutic antibiotics
- Early diagnosis and treatment of infective surgical complications, e.g. leaking anastomoses
- Early and thorough excision of necrotic and infected tissue

Prevention for at-risk patients and treatment of early signs

- Rapid cardiovascular resuscitation and prevention of shock (minimise splanchnic ischaemia)
- Optimisation of oxygen delivery (measure arterial PO_2 and pH and correct metabolic acidosis)
- Nutritional support via an enteral route (to nourish enterocytes)

---

cascade is vital. Appropriate use of **prophylactic antibiotics** in bowel surgery or trauma is important, but intraoperative and postoperative **errors in technique** or clinical judgement are major contributing factors in more than 50% of patients with multiple organ dysfunction. Good clinical judgement, effective resuscitation, good operative technique, effective excision of necrotic tissue, minimising bacterial contamination and preventing accumulation of postoperative fluid collections (serum or blood) are all necessary factors in prevention. The purpose is to eliminate the local environment in which bacteria multiply and improve the delivery of host antibacterial defences.

Surgical complications with septic potential should be treated early, usually by definitive surgery, e.g. removal of necrotic tissue (including amputation of necrotic lower limbs), drainage of abscesses and control of peritoneal contamination by exteriorising leaking anastomoses. This helps reduce the circulating level of inflammatory mediators and limits the period of stress. In many cases it is better to perform a laparotomy on suspicion and find it normal than to 'wait and see' and risk rapid deterioration and death.

Other preventive factors in at-risk patients

Adequate and early **fluid resuscitation** is essential in patients with hypovolaemia, whether in trauma victims, acute pancreatitis or bowel obstruction, because the loss of intravascular volume leads to deficient tissue perfusion (i.e. shock) and splanchnic ischaemia. Maintaining tissue oxygenation is also vital; at-risk patients must have arterial blood gases and pH estimated and be given supplemental oxygen or assisted ventilation as required. To help prevent intestinal bacterial translocation, enterocytes and colonocytes are best supported by **enteral feeding**, if necessary by a feeding jejunostomy or a fine-bore nasogastric tube. Glutamine, arginine and omega-3 fatty acids are believed to be particularly important components.

TREATMENT OF SEPSIS AND MODS

Septic patients need managing and careful monitoring in an intensive care unit. The longer the process continues, the more widespread and irreversible the damage; the sooner treatment is initiated, the better the chances of success. The general principles of treatment include search for and elimination of infective foci, appropriate antibiotic treatment, fluid and blood maintenance, oxygenation and enteral feeding. Treatment with new drugs designed to manipulate the endotoxin–cytokine axis has so far been unsuccessful, possibly because the agents need to be given at the onset of the cascade of sepsis. Specific organ support is given as required: for example, for ARDS and renal failure. Despite all of this, the prospects for established MODS remain grim.

4 Shock and resuscitation

THE PATHOPHYSIOLOGY OF SHOCK

The term 'shock' can be defined as **acute circulatory failure of sufficient magnitude to compromise tissue perfusion**, which, if untreated, proceeds rapidly to irreversible organ damage and death of the patient. Deficient delivery of oxygen and nutrients to vital organs leads to cellular hypoxia and disruption of metabolic functions.

Any form of additional hypoxia in the shocked patient compounds the problem of oxygen delivery. Such hypoxia may be caused by mechanical airways obstruction, impaired gas exchange in pneumonia or pulmonary embolism, hypoventilation as a side effect of drugs such as morphine, or delayed recovery from anaesthetic drugs.

There are several different mechanisms of shock:

- **Hypovolaemic shock** (preload insufficiency) occurs when the effective blood volume is insufficient
- **Cardiogenic shock** occurs when the pump function of the heart is impaired
- **Septic shock** arises as a result of microvascular changes and cardiac depression caused by systemic inflammation
- **Anaphylactic shock** is an acute hypersensitivity reaction to an allergen

The classical symptoms and signs of shock are found in **hypovolaemic** and **cardiogenic** shock and to a degree in anaphylactic shock. These include hypotension, hyperventilation, a rapid weak pulse, cold clammy cyanotic skin and oliguria. Mental changes also occur, with a sense of great anxiety and foreboding, confusion and sometimes combativeness. In addition, there is a metabolic acidosis, low oxygen saturation and low central venous pressure. In contrast, in **septic shock** there is marked peripheral vasodilatation rather than vasoconstriction, but the classical metabolic abnormalities are present.

Shock has been described as progressing through three stages. Initially, in stage I, there are attempts at **compensation** with skin and splanchnic vasoconstriction. Symptoms and signs are minimal but recognisable. In stage II, **decompensation** occurs, with body mechanisms unable to ensure that vital organs receive sufficient oxygen despite working at full capacity. Urgent intervention is needed at this stage. By stage III the changes are essentially **irreversible**, with prolonged shock having caused severe damage to major organs. Successful treatment depends crucially on **early recognition** of shock and its precursors, together with quick and accurate diagnosis and treatment of the underlying cause to halt progression; at the same time measures must be taken to support vital organ function.

EARLY RECOGNITION OF SHOCK

Shock may be encountered in surgical patients at any stage: before their arrival at hospital, in the emergency department, whilst being prepared for urgent surgery, during operation or at any time through to final recovery.

When surgical patients in hospital deteriorate catastrophically, it is often found retrospectively from charts that vital signs had been deteriorating for some time but that clinical staff had failed to respond with appropriate levels of intervention. Early recognition and intervention in such cases is crucial because failure of one organ leads to synergistic failure of other organs; the longer the

Table 4.1 Modified Early Warning Score (MEWS)*

Score	3	2	1	0	1	2	3
Respiratory rate (bpm)		< 9		9–14	15–20	21–29	≥ 30
Heart rate (bpm)		< 40	41–50	51–100	101–110	111–129	≥ 130
Systolic blood pressure (mmHg)	< 70	71–80	81–100	101–199		≥ 200	
Temperature (°C)		< 35		35–38.4		≥ 38.5	
AVPU score				**A**lert	Reacting to **V**oice	Reacting to **P**ain	**U**nresponsive

*MEWS is one form of bedside scoring that can help early identification of patients likely to need urgent assessment (score 3 or more). A score of 5 or more indicates that the patient is likely to require critical care, usually in a high dependency or intensive care unit

process is allowed to continue, the more advanced and irreversible the damage becomes.

To rationalise and formalise the process of recognising these patients early, various structured scoring systems have been developed for bedside use, seeking to follow the simplicity, reliability and clinical usefulness of the Glasgow Coma Score (Ch. 16, p. 246). These systems generally employ routinely recorded physiological data and most are modifications of the **Early Warning Score** (Table 4.1). These have proved useful in both 'medical' and surgical patients for spotting those at risk of deterioration likely to need urgent medical attention. For example, a Modified Early Warning Score (MEWS) of 3 can be an indication for urgent medical review. A score of 5 or more has been shown to be associated with 5–10 times the risk of potentially preventable death and is often regarded as a critical indicator that the patient needs admission to the intensive care or high-dependency unit (ICU/HDU). MEWS scoring is often employed as part of the standard care of surgical inpatients, with nursing staff collecting the data twice daily on a dedicated data chart until the patient recovers. High scores trigger graded clinical responses. The **respiratory rate** in particular has been found to be a valuable predictor of deterioration but it is important that the rate is counted over a full minute.

TYPES OF SHOCK

HYPOVOLAEMIC SHOCK (PRELOAD INSUFFICIENCY)

Preload is defined as the rate of venous return of blood to the heart. Preload insufficiency reduces the diastolic filling pressure and volume and leads to low cardiac output. The underlying problem may be an inadequate total volume of blood that results in underfilling of the venous compartment, i.e. **absolute hypovolaemia** (hypovolaemic shock). Alternatively, the problem may be **relative hypovolaemia** (distributive shock) caused by an increase in capacity of the venous compartment or widespread opening up of capillary beds relative to blood volume. Preload insufficiency is responsible for about 75% of cases of shock encountered in hospital and most of these are due to hypovolaemia. Note that loss of up to 10% of effective circulating volume may not cause changes in heart rate or mean arterial pressure. Figure 15.1 (p. 222) shows the changes in vital signs associated with increasing amounts of blood loss.

Hypovolaemic shock

The main causes of fluid loss leading to hypovolaemic shock are:

- 'Revealed' haemorrhage, e.g. deep lacerations, large haematemeses (vomiting of blood) from a peptic ulcer, continued blood loss from a surgical wound drain indicating internal bleeding
- 'Concealed' haemorrhage, e.g. intra-abdominal bleeding from ruptured spleen or aortic aneurysm, haemorrhage from a duodenal ulcer into the small intestine, intramuscular blood loss from fractures
- Extensive burns, resulting in massive loss of serum into blisters or weeping from the skin surface
- Severe vomiting or diarrhoea, or prolonged fluid loss from a small bowel fistula or ileostomy
- Excessive urinary fluid loss, e.g. diabetic ketoacidosis, diuretic phase of acute tubular necrosis, powerful diuretics
- Sequestration of fluid in bowel caused by bowel obstruction
- Massive loss of fluid into interstitial tissues ('third space losses') as occurs in sepsis
- Major accumulation of fluid in the peritoneal cavity in acute pancreatitis, ascites or generalised peritonitis

Distributive shock

Relative hypovolaemia occurs if there is inappropriate expansion of the circulatory capacity in relation to blood volume; it may result from failure of normal peripheral resistance mechanisms and/or venodilatation of the large veins. Peripheral resistance normally maintains cardiac afterload and is controlled predominantly by the tone of smooth muscle arteriolar and capillary sphincters. About 80% of capillaries are normally closed, and any mechanism that causes inappropriate opening produces excess circulatory capacity. In septic shock, both arteriolar dilatation and an increase in venous volume play a part. Simple fainting (syncope) is caused by a transient form of rapid vasodilatation in which spontaneous recovery occurs rapidly if the patient lies down or falls down. Fainting in fright may be due to arteriolar relaxation.

SEPTIC SHOCK

Septic shock results from overactivation of the innate immune system. The term **sepsis syndrome** describes the same process but septic shock implies a more advanced state; however, the distinction is imprecise. The terminology is also confusing because the triggering injury is not necessarily infective; it may be traumatic or surgical, or it may involve local inflammation, infection, severe burns or the presence of necrotic tissue, e.g. a gangrenous leg. If immune responses escape local control, this spillover provokes a complex cellular response and mediator cascade that leads to progressive clinical manifestations including the **systemic inflammatory response syndrome** and, later, **multiple organ dysfunction**. Mediator responses involve the complement system, acute phase proteins and cytokines (particularly tumour necrosis factor (TNF)-alpha and the interleukins IL1-beta and IL6); once triggered, the inflammatory response cascade is difficult to control or suppress.

Septic shock is a combination of distributive shock and organ dysfunction induced by cytokines and other mediators and sometimes bacterial toxins. Systemic inflammatory responses to severe **infections** typically cause septic shock, especially those involving certain staphylococci or Gram-negative bacilli, e.g. from a colonic anastomotic leak. Bacterial toxins and cell wall components activate cytokine systems and other defensive mechanisms to produce a variety of tissue effects. A similar process occurs with the other causes of septic shock. The net result of this **immune burst** is that oxygen usage declines, metabolic acidosis develops and multiple organ dysfunction ensues. Failure of oxygen usage is the result of the triad of cardiorespiratory impairment, microcirculatory imbalance and, at the cellular level, mitochondrial dysfunction.

Septic shock itself can be thought of in three phases. Initially there is extensive peripheral vasodilatation including venodilatation in which nitric oxide is implicated, causing relative hypovolaemia. In phase 2 there is widespread endothelial damage causing greatly increased capillary permeability and massive fluid leakage into the interstitial space, and in phase 3 there is depression of myocardial contractility. The overall effect of septic shock is inadequate blood pressure and multiple organ dysfunction in the presence of a normal or even increased cardiac output.

The inflammatory burst also upsets normal blood coagulation by downregulating normal anticoagulants such as alpha-1-antitrypsin, and stimulating procoagulants such as **tissue factor** as well as inhibiting fibrinolysis. The result may be **disseminated intravascular coagulation** with microvascular occlusion, large vessel thrombosis and ischaemia, all contributing to organ dysfunction.

Toxic shock syndrome is a particular form of septic shock associated with staphylococcal or streptococcal infection occurring with the use of super-absorbent tampons.

PUMP FAILURE (CARDIOGENIC SHOCK)

Cardiogenic shock describes a drastic reduction in cardiac output resulting from any form of 'pump failure' caused by direct myocardial damage, mechanical abnormality or malfunction of the heart. This most commonly arises from an **acute myocardial infarction** or an **acute ventricular arrhythmia**. Myocardial infarction may cause papillary muscle ischaemia or infarction which produces acute mitral regurgitation. A large **pulmonary embolus** may also obstruct blood flow through the lungs and cause secondary cardiac failure. Other causes include cardiac (pericardial) tamponade and tension pneumothorax.

ANAPHYLACTIC SHOCK

Anaphylactic shock is a generalised form of a type I hypersensitivity reaction, occurring in response to an antigen to which the patient has previously become sensitised. The antigen binds with antibodies attached to the surface of mast cells, triggering degranulation and release of histamine and other vasoactive amines. The predominant effect is extensive **dilatation of the venous compartment** causing marked hypovolaemia; the heart is working normally and there is a normal amount of blood. Fluid rapidly moves into the tissues and remains there as oedema. The systemic effects are compounded by intense bronchoconstriction and often laryngeal oedema which, together, effectively halt ventilation.

In surgical practice, anaphylactic shock usually results from drug administration, particularly via the intravenous route. **Antibiotics**, particularly penicillins, are the most common culprits. Anyone administering a drug must ensure the patient is not known to be sensitive. Anaphylactic reactions may also occur after intravenous injections of **radiological contrast media**. Insect bites (wasps, bees and hornets) and ingested nuts are also important causes and may be encountered in the emergency department.

CLINICAL FEATURES OF SHOCK

The essential feature of any type of shock is a **precipitate fall in arterial blood pressure** with systolic pressure dropping by at least 40 mmHg from usual levels to less than 90 mmHg. The immediate homeostatic response is **intense sympathetic activity** and catecholamine release. The heart rate increases dramatically in an attempt to increase cardiac output. Except in septic shock, there is intense cutaneous and visceral vasoconstriction in an attempt to restore intravascular volume by increasing peripheral resistance. Sudomotor activity causes profuse sweating. Hypoxic tissues revert to anaerobic respiration, producing lactic acid sufficient to cause a metabolic acidosis, and the respiratory rate rises in an attempt at compensation. The clinical picture is a cold, pale, clammy, hypotensive patient with a rapid thready pulse and increased respiratory rate.

Septic shock presents a contrasting clinical picture in which cytokine-mediated peripheral vasodilatation is unresponsive to circulating catecholamines. The patient's skin is flushed and hot and cardiac output is increased to fill the dilated periphery. The pulse is typically 'bounding' in quality. Temperature may be above normal or even below normal.

In all forms of shock, the circulatory system cannot support the main organ systems without treatment, and the organs fail (i.e. decompensate) one by one in a synergistic rather than simply an additive manner. Pulmonary failure leads to **adult respiratory distress syndrome** (ARDS), and cerebral hypoxia soon causes confusion and eventually coma. Inadequate renal perfusion causes a dramatic fall in urinary output (oliguria) which, if not rapidly corrected, leads to acute tubular necrosis and renal failure. If shock persists, reduced coronary flow and heart failure cause death. In septic shock, organ damage is exacerbated by an intense inflammatory burst and deterioration is inevitable unless the source of infection can be rapidly eliminated and effective support instituted.

SPECIFIC TREATMENTS FOR SHOCK

HYPOVOLAEMIC SHOCK

Identifying the cause of the fluid loss is the top priority. Immediate measures should be taken to control blood loss, e.g. pressure on a swab over a bleeding wound, endoscopic injection of bleeding peptic ulcer, or laparotomy for ruptured spleen. Fluid replacement should be equivalent to estimated fluid loss but adjusted according to the response of pulse rate, blood pressure, central venous pressure and urine output. If available, transoesophageal ultrasound helps assess cardiac output. Where possible, fluids of similar composition to those lost should be used: whole blood for haemorrhage, colloids after major burns. In general, however, it is not what is given but how quickly that matters. Fluids should be given in rapid boluses, e.g. 250 ml at a time, and the response observed. If inadequate, the bolus is repeated until shock is controlled or other measures to control fluid loss are employed.

CARDIOGENIC SHOCK

The management of cardiogenic shock is best reviewed in a medical textbook; the management of pulmonary embolism (which may present as cardiogenic shock) is discussed in Chapter 12. Fluid overload is a significant hazard in cardiogenic shock and must be avoided.

SEPTIC SHOCK (see SIRS and MODS, p. 48)

Systemic sepsis leading to septic shock usually originates from a specific focus of infection or from the patient's own intestinal organisms. The source may be obvious but, if not, a careful search must be made, bearing in mind the common sites. In surgical practice, septic shock is most commonly a result of **faecal peritonitis** following large bowel perforation or **anastomotic breakdown**. In a patient who has had bowel surgery, intraperitoneal infection is the prime suspect but bladder or chest infection or an otherwise 'silent' infection of a central venous cannula is often the cause. Debilitated patients, uncontrolled diabetics and infants are particularly vulnerable to acute sepsis; in such cases the source of infection may not be found. Gangrene of a leg is also a potent cause. The damaging effects of the underlying poor organ perfusion are increased by direct and indirect bacterial exotoxic and endotoxic tissue damage.

Treatment of septic shock is urgent and involves fluid resuscitation, oxygenation, administration of appropriate antibiotics and the tracing and eliminating of the source of infection.

Blood cultures must be taken and intravenous antibiotics administered on a 'best-guess' basis. Experience has shown that a broad-spectrum combination of gentamicin, benzylpenicillin and metronidazole is an effective starter regimen which can be modified later if resistant organisms are isolated.

In the meantime, intravenous plasma expanders are given and the rate and volume adjusted according to pulse rate, blood pressure, central venous pressure and urine output. Because of interstitial losses, volumes given may have to be large. Volume expansion helps to sustain cardiac output and tissue perfusion. Corticosteroids are known to stabilise cell membranes but evidence of their effectiveness in septic shock is lacking.

If the diagnosis of septic shock is correct, resuscitative measures should produce dramatic improvement in the patient's condition within 1–2 hours. By that time, the patient should be ready for immediate operation if an abscess, bowel perforation or other surgically remediable cause appears to be the culprit. It is important to emphasise that the source of infection must be urgently eliminated if the septic cascade is to be reversed.

DISSEMINATED INTRAVASCULAR COAGULATION

Another major problem in sepsis is generalised activation of the clotting cascade causing disseminated intravascular coagulation (DIC), see earlier. This exhausts the supply of platelets and clotting factors V, VIII and fibrinogen (**consumption coagulopathy**) and activates the intrinsic fibrinolytic mechanisms. DIC manifests as spontaneous bleeding or bruising and uncontrollable haemorrhage from any operation site. Diagnosis is made by finding low **fibrinogen** levels and high levels of D-**dimers** which are cleaved from fibrin by plasmin and provide evidence of fibrin lysis. Treatment includes managing the initiating cause, giving intravenous heparin to arrest the coagulation process and transfusing appropriate clotting factors, e.g. fresh-frozen plasma, cryoprecipitate.

ANAPHYLACTIC SHOCK

Anaphylaxis or anaphylactic shock is caused by massive histamine release and requires urgent treatment. Initiating allergens include food, medications (typically blood products, antibiotics, aspirin/other NSAIDs, heparin and neuromuscular blocking drugs), insect venoms and latex. Immediate treatment includes securing the airway and giving oxygen, laying the patient flat and raising the feet and administering 500 mg of intramuscular adrenaline (epinephrine), i.e. 0.3 ml of 1 : 1000 solution. This dose may be repeated at 5 minute intervals if necessary. An antihistamine (e.g. chlorphenamine (chlorpheniramine) 10–20 mg) should be given by slow intravenous injection and continued for up to 48 hours to stabilise mast cells. Hydrocortisone 100–300 mg should also be given intravenously but it takes several hours to block the histamine receptors that mediate much of the peripheral vascular response and so should not be regarded as contributing to the emergency treatment. Intravenous fluids may also be needed to treat the hypovolaemia.

Because of the risk of anaphylactic shock, a doctor should always check that the patient is not sensitive and administer the first dose of any intravenous agent, including radiological contrast agents and radioisotopes. A doctor should also be available whenever parenteral drugs (including vaccinations) are being administered. Note that the doctor giving the treatment is legally responsible for ensuring that resuscitation drugs and equipment are immediately available and must check this beforehand, particularly if working in an unfamiliar ward or department.

RESUSCITATION OF THE 'COLLAPSED' NON-TRAUMA PATIENT

PRINCIPLES OF MANAGING SHOCK BY RESUSCITATION

In the collapsed trauma patient, initial resuscitation essentially focuses on the airway and replacement of blood loss. In contrast, shocked non-trauma patients often have multiple comorbidities, both medical and surgical, which combine to produce the similar clinical picture of shock. Whatever the cause, the aim is to restore tissue perfusion and oxygenation by resuscitative measures while the diagnosis is being made and before specific treatment begins.

Early management, ideally within 24 hours of acute deterioration, can be summarised as follows:

- **Treat the cause of shock**—this can have the effect of shutting down the inflammatory response. Treatment may mean an operation to exteriorise a leaking anastomosis (i.e. bring the bowel ends to the skin surface) or to excise infected and necrotic tissue or drain pus
- **Treat infection**—if infection is apparent or suspected, institute antibiotic therapy using potent agents chosen on clinical suspicion until definitive microbiological results become available
- **Support vital organs** during the time it takes surgery or antibiotics to work. Airway and breathing support (e.g. oxygen administration, intubation, ventilation) benefits most patients, but the most critical concern is to optimise the cardiovascular and haemodynamic system, aiming for a central venous pressure between 8 and 12 mmHg, a mean arterial pressure over 65 mmHg and a urine output of at least 0.5 ml/kg/hour.
- **Monitor and assess the response**

A SCHEME FOR MANAGING THE ACUTELY ILL OR SHOCKED PATIENT

This scheme is given in note form as an aide mémoire for clinicians.

RECOGNITION OF THE ACUTELY UNWELL PATIENT (see Table 4.1)

The cardinal signs in a patient likely to need critical care in a high-dependency or intensive care unit include:

- Substantially increased or decreased respiratory rate
- Bradycardia or tachycardia
- Low blood pressure
- Hypo- or hyperthermia
- Decreased level of consciousness

SEQUENCE FOR ACTION IN THE PATIENT AT RISK

In summary this includes the following steps, which are detailed below:

A. Initial assessment
B. Broad diagnosis
C. Immediate care
D. Monitoring and reassessment
E. Investigation to narrow the diagnosis
F. Definitive treatment

A. Initial assessment

The aim is to rapidly establish the urgency and severity of the situation. If vital signs are poor and the patient unresponsive, a cardiac arrest or crash call may be needed to bring more hands to assist. If an early warning score is above a predetermined threshold, consultation is needed to arrange transfer to a critical care unit.

History

As much history should be gleaned as time permits, e.g. the context of the acute deterioration, medical state before deterioration, past medical history including allergies, and recent treatments including operations. Check drug charts.

Vital signs

Nurses can help gather information while assessment continues; vital signs should be monitored at frequent intervals. Observations include respiratory rate, temperature, pulse rate, systolic blood pressure and level of consciousness (the AVPU scale is simple and reproducible—A means the patient is fully Alert, V means responds to Voice, P means responds to pain and U is unresponsive).

Initial tests include oxygen saturation, blood glucose estimation, blood gas analysis and ECG for evidence of myocardial infarction. Note that new onset atrial fibrillation or flutter on ECG is often an indicator of sepsis. A bounding pulse and flushed extremities may suggest septic shock.

Examination—the initial survey
General impression including skin
- Intravenous lines and fluids, drug treatments being given via syringe driver, catheters, etc.
- Peripheral perfusion, hydration, oedema, anaemia, jaundice, bruising, rashes, nutritional state

Head and neck
- Stridor—obstruction of upper airway, e.g. bleed into thyroid lesion/mediastinal mass (?metastases); inhaled foreign body; inhaled vomitus
- Mouth and throat—evidence of abscess, e.g. peritonsillar abscess (quinsy), Ludwig's angina

Chest
- Localised poor air entry—infection, atelectasis, pneumothorax
- Generalised poor air entry—asthma, large pleural effusions
- Expiratory wheeze—anaphylaxis or cardiac failure
- If acutely breathless, consider thromboembolism

Heart
- New onset chest pain—myocardial infarction (MI)
- Cardiac murmurs—infective endocarditis, MI, acute valve prolapse
- Elevated jugular venous pressure—acute cardiac failure due to MI
- If cardiac problem suspected, check ECG for changes of ischaemia, arrhythmias

Abdomen including rectal and/or vaginal examination if necessary
- Localised tenderness—localised intra-abdominal infection, renal colic (loin)
- Generalised tenderness—peritonitis
- Distension—bowel obstruction, intraperitoneal or retroperitoneal bleed, ascites
- Melaena or fresh blood per rectum—gastrointestinal bleed
- Lump—strangulated hernia, intra-abdominal mass

Limbs
- Unilaterally (or bilaterally) pale and cold with or without necrosis—acute ischaemia
- Globally pale, cold—peripheral shutdown due to shock
- Swollen and blue—deep venous thrombosis (in patient with suspected pulmonary embolism)
- Red—cellulitis, diabetic foot infection with systemic sepsis

Neurology
- Conscious level
- Signs of unilateral palsy—stroke

B. Broad diagnosis

Priorities for immediate treatment and further investigation need to be decided following initial assessment, if necessary from a single major finding. Priorities change as evidence is collected snd depending on the response to treatment.

Examples are:

- *Respiratory*—upper airways obstruction, e.g. thyroid enlargement/haemorrhage into nodule
- *Vascular events*—abdominal aortic aneurysm rupture, aortic dissection, pulmonary embolism, acute coronary syndromes including MI, stroke and lower limb gangrene (usually causes insidious rather than acute development of shock)
- *Abdominal problems*
  - **Blood loss**—upper or lower gastrointestinal bleeding, intra- or retro-peritoneal bleed
  - **Gastrointestinal obstruction including strangulation**—gastric, small bowel or large bowel, hernia, volvulus
  - **Generalised peritonitis**—perforation of an abdominal viscus (appendix, peptic ulcer, diverticular disease); acute pancreatitis
  - **Abdominal colic**—ureteric, biliary, intestinal
  - **Intra-abdominal infection**—gastroenteritis, acute appendicitis, diverticulitis, cholecystitis; urinary tract infection
  - **Obstetric and gynaecological**—ruptured ectopic pregnancy/ovarian cyst/pregnancy/salpingo-oophoritis
- *Other infections*—infected central venous line, abscesses, cellulitis, diabetic foot, limb gangrene, gastroenteritis including antibiotic-associated colitis
- *Metabolic*—surgical disease can precipitate or be complicated by hypoglycaemia in diabetics; consider Addison's disease (adrenal insufficiency) if the patient is hypotensive

C. Immediate care

Inform a senior doctor about the urgency of the case if appropriate.

Oxygen

Immediately secure a mask delivering 100% oxygen. The comatose patient may need to be intubated and positive-pressure ventilation commenced.

Fluid management

Haemodynamic optimisation is very important and is based on clinical signs and monitoring of central venous pressure and urine output.

- Take **venous blood** for haemoglobin, haematocrit, urea and electrolytes, glucose, amylase and blood grouping/ordering of blood for transfusion if necessary. Take an arterial sample for blood gas estimation and acid–base status; get blood cultures if septic shock is suspected

- Set up an **intravenous infusion** and administer i.v. fluids/drugs, guided by vital signs and findings. For example, if the patient is hypotensive, give crystalloid or colloid solutions (at least 1 litre rapidly); if cardiogenic shock is likely, the circulating volume must not be expanded rapidly
- **Blood transfusion** if necessary
- **Urinary catheter** to monitor hourly output; urine dipstix

Drugs

- Analgesia if in pain—i.v. morphine
- Infection—antibiotics
- Low blood glucose—dextrose

D. Monitoring and reassessment

Monitoring

The most useful guides to the success of resuscitation are respiratory rate (unless ventilated), central venous pressure (CVP), hourly urinary output and plasma lactate.

- Central venous line—often required to monitor central pressure and response to fluids
- Arterial line if necessary
- Nasogastric tube if vomiting; include fluid aspirated on the fluid balance chart
- Request a cardiac ECG monitor if a cardiac problem is suspected

Reassessment

Check the response to therapy: respiratory rate, pulse rate, blood pressure, CVP and plasma lactate. Consider moving the patient to a critical care bed and surgical intervention if the response to therapy is inadequate.

E. Investigation to narrow the diagnosis

Consider the most likely diagnosis and quickest route to confirming the initial 'best guess':

- Check blood results
- If there is infection: blood culture, sputum culture
- Chest problems: chest X-ray, CT pulmonary angiogram if pulmonary embolism is suspected
- Cardiac problems: troponin blood levels, echocardiogram
- Abdomen: plain X-ray/ultrasound or CT scan/ endoscopy if the clinical diagnosis is equivocal

F. Definitive treatment

Give definitive treatment as required according to the diagnosis.

Imaging and interventional techniques in surgery

5

INTRODUCTION

This chapter gives an overview of imaging and endoscopic procedures commonly used for investigating patients (including percutaneous methods of obtaining tissue for histological examination), together with related minimal access therapeutic procedures. The basis for each method is described, together with its main indications and shortcomings. The growing field of **interventional radiology** comprises active procedures carried out using image guidance. They are performed by radiologists, other clinicians or both together, and are intended to make a diagnosis or treat a diagnosed condition. Examples include ultrasound- or CT-guided biopsy and endoscopic placement of biliary stents. The principles of these techniques are described here and a summary of these and other therapeutic applications is given in Table 11.4, page 166.

PLAIN RADIOLOGY

The various tissues and constituents of the body absorb X-rays by amounts related to the cube of the atomic number of their constituent elements. This results in differential penetration by X-rays through the body and proportionate exposure of the silver salts in traditional **X-ray films** or activation of sensors in a filmless rig. A radiograph is in effect a 'shadow' picture.

On a plain radiograph, gas and fat absorb little X-irradiation and appear as **radiolucent** (dark) areas on the image. Bone and other calcified tissues absorb most of the X-rays directed at them and are thus poorly penetrated; they appear as **radiopaque** (white) film images. For this reason, calcified lesions such as most urinary tract stones, some gallstones, old tuberculous lymph nodes and heavily calcified atheromatous deposits are also radiopaque.

Some **foreign bodies** in wounds are radiopaque; these include metal and most glass fragments but wood and plastic fragments are radiolucent and invisible on X-rays. Gauze swabs used in operating theatres are radiolucent but have a radiopaque strand woven into them so they can be located radiographically if inadvertently left inside a wound (see Fig. 5.1).

Certain X-ray investigations, known as **contrast studies**, obtain their diagnostic information by imaging structures outlined with highly absorptive fluid **contrast media**.

Fig. 5.1 Plain abdominal X-ray showing retained surgical swab

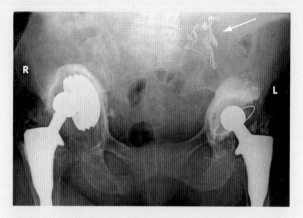

This 83-year-old woman had persistent pain in the left iliac fossa after a left hip replacement. This pelvic X-ray was taken to investigate the new joint. However, a radiopaque marker was spotted (arrowed) indicating a surgical swab that had been left in the abdomen after a laparotomy for perforated duodenal ulcer 8 years previously. The swab was removed uneventfully at a second laparotomy.

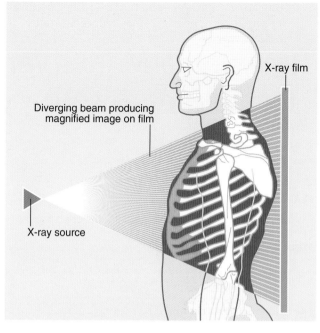

Fig. 5.2 Radiological projection

PERSONAL RADIATION PROTECTION

Ionising radiation is potentially both mutagenic and carcinogenic. Irradiation of patients and observers must therefore be kept to the minimum. This is achieved by the following:

- Giving training in radiation protection to all staff using and working near X-ray equipment
- Ensuring that every investigation helps with the management of the patient and that none is performed merely as 'routine'
- Improving design of X-ray equipment to minimise radiation dose whilst preserving diagnostic detail. In addition, X-ray **scatter** is minimised and unwanted types of radiation removed by filters
- Physical barriers to X-rays are built into radiology suites or provided to protect staff. These include barium plaster in walls, lead-glass windows and lead-rubber aprons
- Workers involved in taking X-rays should keep away from the direct line of the beam and maintain a good distance from the X-ray source during exposure. Note that the inverse square law determines the fall-off of radiation with distance
- All involved in radiography should wear X-ray-sensitive **film badges** which need to be regularly monitored for excess radiation

GENERAL PRINCIPLES OF RADIOLOGY

There are several important factors involved in producing a useful radiographic image:

- **X-ray power and exposure time** are chosen to give a diagnostically useful exposure without excess dosage. Good quality images have a range of densities appropriate to the anatomical area. For example, thoracic spine views require a larger dose than lung fields
- **Different projections (views)** produce different images of the same subject. Since the X-ray tube is effectively a point source and produces a diverging beam (see Fig. 5.2), the subject is inevitably magnified. This size distortion least affects the side of the patient closest to the film, which is thus shown most clearly. Since the projection has important consequences for interpretation, it should be recorded on the film, e.g. a frontal chest film might be labelled PA (postero-anterior) or AP (antero-posterior), indicating the direction of the beam. With lateral exposures, the side nearest the film is indicated, e.g. a 'Rt' lateral chest X-ray (CXR) has the right side of the chest nearest the film
- **Patient position** during exposure (i.e. supine, prone, oblique or erect) affects the image because of the effect of gravity upon organs and other body contents such as gas or fluid. Most films are taken with the patient lying supine with the X-ray beam aimed vertically downwards. A horizontal X-ray beam is sometimes needed to demonstrate fluid

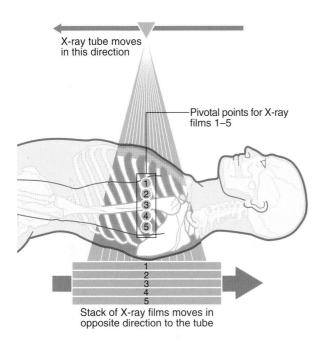

X-ray tube moves
in this direction

Pivotal points for X-ray
films 1–5

1
2
3
4
5

1
2
3
4
5

Stack of X-ray films moves in
opposite direction to the tube

Fig. 5.3 The principle of tomography

levels in a cavity or in bowel (lateral decubitus), or free gas under the diaphragm

TOMOGRAPHY

Some body structures that would be obscured by overlying or underlying tissues on conventional X-rays can be seen more clearly by tomography. In tomography, the X-ray tube and film are moved in opposite directions during exposure, with the pivot point between the two centred on the structure under investigation (see Fig. 5.3). A transverse slice at the chosen depth is thus defined clearly on the film, and tissues superficial or deep to this layer are blurred into obscurity (e.g. soft tissue, bowel gas, faeces or bones). The technique has largely been superseded by other imaging modalities but is still occasionally used in intravenous urography when gas or faeces obscure the field of interest. If a stack of films is used, one exposure can give a set of 'cuts' at predetermined distances from the surface. Computerised tomography (CT) is an important development of this principle.

ELECTRONIC RECORDING TECHNIQUES

X-ray, magnetic resonance (MRI), ultrasound and isotope scan images are increasingly being recorded electronically in **digital** form, as opposed to the **analogue** form of conventional radiographic film. Digital images can be processed to optimise the available information; this includes enhancing the contrast between tissues, magnifying areas of special interest and abstracting the most relevant parts

from a series of images. Electronic **storage** has a number of advantages over conventional film:

- Substantial cost saving on film and processing chemicals
- Reduced physical space needed for storage
- Reduced staff costs—no need to file or retrieve films
- Better availability of images—no need to obtain physical films; several viewers can see the same images simultaneously
- Substantially reduced numbers of missing examinations
- Easy transmission of images from one institution to another—by portable storage media (CD-ROM) or electronic links

'Filmless' X-ray departments are already becoming the norm, with images displayed on terminals dispersed around the hospital. In some cases, images can be accessed remotely by family practitioners and other clinicians.

EXAMPLES OF PLAIN RADIOLOGY

CHEST X-RAY

Interpreting plain chest X-rays requires a methodical approach. Several long and learned documents have been written on the subject, e.g. http://www.studentbmj.com/issues/00/09/education/316.php, and no attempt will be made to produce a short but incomplete version here.

PLAIN ABDOMINAL RADIOLOGY

Most abdominal films are taken with the patient lying supine with the X-ray beam passing vertically downwards. Bowel is visible when it contains gas (see Figs 5.4–5.6); normal **small bowel** is less than 3 cm wide and tends to occupy the centre of the abdomen in the supine position. When dilated, it can be recognised by the prominent transverse folds (**plicae circulares**) which completely cross the lumen (Fig. 5.4). The colon usually lies peripherally in the abdomen and is recognised by its **haustrations**; these are folds that only partly traverse the lumen (Fig. 5.5). Normal colon is less than 6 cm wide and is often seen to contain lumps of faeces with a mottled radiolucent and radiopaque appearance. Further reading about this topic is available from http://www.studentbmj.com/topics/clinical/imaging_techniques.php.

Free intraperitoneal gas

Free gas is diagnostic of **bowel perforation** unless the patient has undergone a recent laparotomy. The most useful method of demonstrating it is on a chest or upper abdominal X-ray taken with a horizontal beam and the patient **erect**. This usually (but not always) reveals a radiolucent gas layer beneath the diaphragm (see Fig. 19.9, p. 308). This layer can be very small (and easily

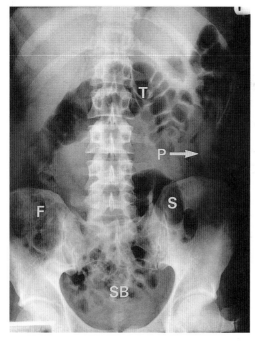

Fig. 5.4 Normal supine abdominal X-ray
There is gas in most parts of the colon (transverse colon **T** and sigmoid colon **S**) and a few small bowel loops **SB** in the pelvis. Radiopaque lumps of faecal matter **F** are seen in the caecum and ascending colon. A normal pro-peritoneal fat line **P** is present on the patient's left; this would disappear if there was retroperitoneal inflammation.

Fig. 5.5 Abdominal X-ray

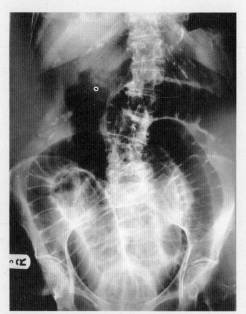

Supine plain abdominal film showing gross small bowel dilatation. At laparotomy, the cause proved to be an obstructing carcinoma of the caecum.

Fig. 5.6 Abdominal X-ray

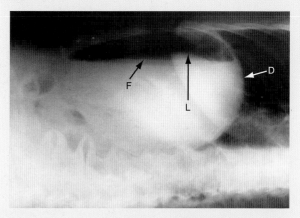

This 78-year-old woman presented with a sudden onset of severe abdominal pain. Erect chest X-ray failed to show free abdominal gas but a perforation was clinically suspected so this **lateral decubitus X-ray** was performed. The right side is raised and the head is to the right of the picture; the X-ray beam was horizontal. Free intraperitoneal gas is seen above a fluid level **F** beneath the diaphragm **D** and 'floating' over the liver **L**. At laparotomy, the cause proved to be a perforated duodenal ulcer.

missed) but more often it is obvious. Where the result is doubtful or if the patient is too ill to sit or stand, the patient should be placed in the **right-side raised lateral decubitus position** (i.e. lying on the left side) for 10 minutes. A horizontal beam abdominal X-ray is then taken across the table. As little as 2 ml of gas may then be demonstrable above the lateral border of the liver (see Fig. 5.6).

Plain abdominal films

In the standard supine film free gas indicating bowel perforation usually collects in the right upper quadrant but can also be confidently diagnosed in the rare instances when both the inside and outside of the bowel wall are outlined by radiolucent shadows (Rigler's sign, Fig. 32.8). The kidneys may be outlined by a radiolucent border of perinephric fat. However, overlapping bowel gas and faeces often obscure the renal outlines. Also, in a post-nephrectomy patient, the former 'renal outline' may still be visible and the kidney appears to be present. Small urinary tract stones are easily obscured by overlying bowel gas or faeces. The liver may be visible but its size cannot be accurately estimated.

When examining an abdominal X-ray, the important features to look for are:

- Calcification in areas prone to stone formation, e.g. kidney, ureters, bladder or biliary tree (see Fig. 5.7a)

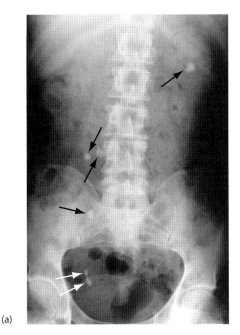
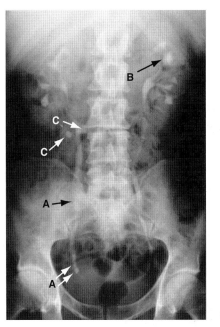

(a)   (b)

Fig. 5.7 Plain abdominal X-ray and IVU compared
(a) A plain abdominal film and **(b)** an intravenous urogram (IVU) of the same patient showing urinary tract stones. In the plain film, several calcified opacities (arrowed) are seen. From the IVU, in which the pelvicalyceal systems and ureters contain contrast material, it can be seen that three stones **A** lie within the lower right ureter and stone **B** lies within the upper calyces of the left kidney. On the right side, two other opacities **C** are seen to lie outside the urinary tract, probably representing calcified lymph nodes in the small bowel mesentery.

- Dilated bowel (stomach, small bowel or large bowel)
- Free intraperitoneal gas indicating bowel perforation. Note the importance of the patient's position when the film was taken
- Gas in abnormal places (e.g. biliary tree or urinary tract) suggesting a fistula connecting with bowel
- Non-biological objects, e.g. foreign bodies, surgical tubes or pieces of metal
- Pathological calcification, e.g. aortic aneurysm, pancreas, adrenals or uterine fibroids

The limitations of plain abdominal radiography are summarised in Box 5.1.

Box	5.1	**The limitations of plain abdominal radiography**

- Intraperitoneal structures are not visualised unless they contain gas themselves, displace gas-filled bowel or indent structural fat
- Stones that are not calcified (90% of gallstones, 10% of urinary tract stones) are not visible
- Bowel gas and faeces easily obscure stones
- Phleboliths, calcified abdominal lymph nodes and costal cartilages readily mimic stones
- Liver and spleen size cannot be estimated accurately
- Free intraperitoneal gas is not usually visible on a supine film (a horizontal beam film is needed)

CONTRAST RADIOLOGY

When plain radiography is unsuitable for studying the area of interest, a highly X-ray-absorbing **contrast medium** can often be employed to opacify it. Contrast media work in two ways: they outline anatomical structures **directly** or else are concentrated physiologically in the organ they are designed to show. The latter is known as **indirect imaging.**

Direct contrast studies can be made in a variety of ways: contrast material can be swallowed, instilled into body orifices, sinuses (sinogram) or fistulae (fistulogram), or injected into blood vessels or hollow viscera. Commonly used direct contrast studies are barium enemas for examining the large bowel and arteriograms for investigating the arterial system.

Indirect contrast studies depend on contrast being concentrated in the organ under investigation. For example, in intravenous urography, contrast injected intravenously is excreted in the urine to display the renal tract.

CONTRAST MATERIALS

Barium sulphate is the most satisfactory agent for directly outlining the gastrointestinal tract. It is insoluble in water and is not absorbed. An aqueous suspension is non-irritant and very radiodense. **Gastrografin** is a water-soluble contrast medium employed if contrast material is likely to leak from the bowel into the peritoneal cavity, for example when checking a recent rectal anastomosis after resection. If Gastrografin is inadvertently inhaled, however, it causes pulmonary oedema and should not therefore be used by mouth in patients with intestinal obstruction. Barium investigations of the upper and lower gastrointestinal tracts have been superseded to a large degree by endoscopic investigations but are still occasionally employed when other investigations are inappropriate.

Water-soluble **iodinated benzoic acid derivatives** can be injected into blood vessels to opacify the circulating blood. When injected, there is also almost immediate excretion of the contrast through the kidneys into the urine. Thus, two different functions can be achieved: direct opacification of arteries or veins (arteriography or venography), and indirect demonstration of kidneys, collecting systems and bladder (intravenous urography). Note that direct venography is rarely used nowadays having been replaced by colour duplex ultrasound.

Injectable contrast media have been improved over the years to make them safer but they remain potentially nephrotoxic in patients with renal failure. In diabetic patients taking metformin who also have renal failure, lactic acidosis can develop. In these at-risk patients, alternative methods of imaging should be sought or else great care taken to use minimal doses of contrast and ensure that the patient is well hydrated and renal function is carefully monitored.

Finally, care should be taken to ensure in advance that the patient is not sensitive to the contrast medium as sensitivity may provoke an anaphylactic reaction. Resuscitation equipment and drugs should always be on hand when contrast media are injected.

EXAMPLES OF CONTRAST RADIOLOGY

BOWEL CONTRAST RADIOLOGY

Any part of the gastrointestinal tract can be demonstrated using contrast techniques but the diagnostic yield varies from high (barium enema) to low (small bowel follow-through). In the early days of barium examinations, a single contrast technique was used. Barium was given alone and radiographs taken. However, the dense column of barium obscured much of the finer detail. Most barium studies nowadays use a **double contrast** method. Following the barium, air or carbon dioxide is used to distend the bowel, or effervescent tablets are given to distend the stomach. Air or other gas separates the barium-coated bowel walls and acts as a second radiolucent contrast agent (see Fig. 5.8b). An anticholinergic agent such as hyoscine butylbromide (Buscopan) is sometimes given at the same time to relax the bowel wall muscle and abolish spasm, thereby further improving the image.

Barium should be avoided if substantial peritoneal spillage is likely, as when there may be a perforation or anastomotic leak. In these cases, **water-soluble contrast medium** is best given initially, and if no leak is seen, barium is substituted. This is because water-soluble materials are less radiopaque and less effective at coating the bowel wall and show less surface detail than barium. For the same reasons, barium may reveal a tiny leak from the bowel which is invisible with water-soluble contrast.

Preparation for bowel contrast studies

For upper gastrointestinal studies, patients should be fasted overnight except for water. For small bowel studies, laxatives are sometimes given the day before to empty the colon. This may hasten transit of contrast through the small bowel. For a barium enema, bowel preparation is performed with laxatives (e.g. sodium picosulfate) and sometimes bowel washouts, so that artefacts are removed (faecal lumps look very similar to polyps) and small mucosal defects are not obscured. Thorough preparation of the colon is vital if important pathology is not to be missed. If a barium enema reveals inadequate preparation, further efforts should be made to clear the colon and the examination repeated. If a right-sided colonic lesion is suspected and other methods have failed, CT scanning may show the region satisfactorily.

Upper gastrointestinal tract

For examining the upper gastrointestinal tract, barium suspension is given orally (**barium swallow** for oesophagus and **barium meal** for stomach and duodenum), although for most purposes, upper gastrointestinal endoscopy is preferred nowadays. Progress of the contrast is observed by **screening**, with a moving image displayed on a screen. The radiologist can select representative **spot films** to summarise the examination. Screening for 1 minute gives the patient an X-ray dose equivalent to one standard X-ray film. Screening is useful to study rapid gastrointestinal motility as in swallowing; the images can be studied later in slow motion.

Large bowel

The **large bowel** is examined by means of contrast material given rectally (**barium enema**). The lower rectum is not always well shown on this examination so a prior rectal examination and sigmoidoscopy is recommended to ensure low lesions are not missed. Figure 5.8 illustrates the differences between a single contrast and a double contrast barium enema (air and barium) in the same patient.

Fig. 5.8 Single and double contrast barium enemas

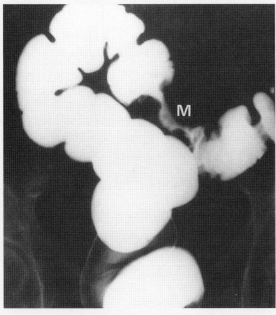 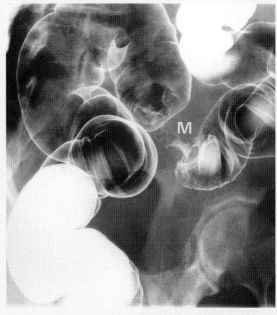

(a) (b)

Typical annular carcinoma of the proximal sigmoid colon in a woman of 72. **(a)** Single contrast barium enema showing the malignant stricture **M**. Note all mucosal detail in the colon is obscured by barium. **(b)** Double contrast barium enema of the same patient also showing the stricture, but mucosal detail is outlined with a thin coating of barium. The bowel has been inflated with air.

With improved technology, **CT** is being increasingly used for large bowel examination. The examination can be performed without laxative preparation where it would be acceptable to miss small polyps, for example in suspected obstructing carcinoma. For a more complete examination, **CT colonography** involves full bowel cleansing and insufflation with air or carbon dioxide (double contrast); the technique is sensitive enough to detect polyps and other lesions larger than 1 cm. The procedure is quicker and less unpleasant than a conventional barium enema and may eventually supplant barium enema examination altogether. Three-dimensional images of the bowel can be constructed from the CT data to produce a virtual 'walk-through' of the colon. This technique is still evolving and holds promise for the future.

Small bowel

For **small bowel** examination, a barium meal may be 'followed through' the small bowel, or contrast can be instilled directly into the proximal jejunum via a nasal or oral tube. In either case, the diagnostic yield is poor and these techniques are likely to be replaced by the more reliable capsule endoscopy (see below).

COMPLICATIONS OF BARIUM CONTRAST STUDIES

The limitations of barium contrast studies are summarised in Box 5.2. In particular, caution is needed in patients

Box 5.2 The limitations of barium contrast studies

- It is often impossible to distinguish between different types of pathological lesion, e.g. between malignant and inflammatory colonic stenosis, or between malignant and peptic ulcer of the stomach
- Fine mucosal detail is not shown, e.g. gastric lesions such as inflammation, shallow ulceration or early cancer, or angiodysplasias of the colon. In acute gastrointestinal bleeding, barium meal may miss the bleeding lesion
- Small bowel is difficult to examine in detail because of contrast dilution by bowel contents and loops of bowel overlying each other
- The luminal outline of obstructed bowel cannot be satisfactorily demonstrated with contrast; barium in a follow-through does not reach the site of complete obstruction. 'Instant' or unprepared barium enema examination is useful in distinguishing mechanical large bowel obstruction from pseudo-obstruction but does not demonstrate the bowel proximal to an obstruction
- Barium taken orally may turn an incomplete colonic obstruction into complete obstruction, as may barium given rectally
- Major abnormalities may be concealed because of tissue overlap. Multiple projections, double contrast techniques and tube angulation reduce this deficiency

Fig. 5.9 Inhalational pneumonitis after barium meal

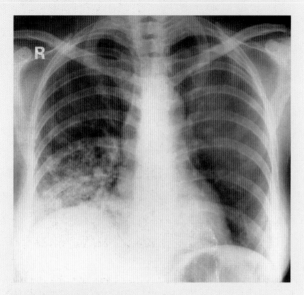

This man of 68 had undergone a laparotomy several days previously and a small bowel mass was resected. Recovery of bowel function was delayed and this barium follow-through examination was attempted to demonstrate a cause. However, the patient vomited during the investigation and aspirated barium into the lung. The film shows right lower lobe consolidation resulting from aspiration of stomach contents including barium.

with bowel obstruction because barium dehydrates and solidifies within the bowel and this can turn incomplete obstruction into complete obstruction. A barium follow-through is sometimes performed in suspected small bowel obstruction, but there is a risk that contrast material may be vomited and aspirated into the bronchial tree, causing aspiration pneumonitis (see Fig. 5.9). CT scanning is often a safer investigation and is likely to provide more useful information.

Some radiologists prefer not to perform barium enema examination for several days after high rectal biopsies because of a potential risk of perforation.

BILIARY RADIOLOGY

Some biliary investigations described in previous editions of this book (e.g. oral cholecystography and intravenous cholangiography) have largely been superseded because of improved equipment and experience in ultrasound and increased availability of **endoscopic retrograde cholangio-pancreatography** (ERCP, see p. 68 below) and **magnetic resonance cholangio-pancreatography** (MRCP). Magnetic resonance cholangiography now produces images that rival the quality of ERCP.

Oral cholecystography

Until the mid-1980s oral cholecystography was the standard investigation for gall bladder disease but has now been replaced by high-resolution ultrasound which is rapid, reliable, requires no contrast material and is unaffected by jaundice. Cholecystography required the patient to absorb oral contrast, excrete it via the liver and concentrate it in the gall bladder. Images were taken 12 hours after ingestion. The investigation was no value in obstructive jaundice or a severely diseased gall bladder because insufficient contrast was excreted or concentrated to register an image.

Intravenous cholangiography

Intravenous cholangiography (IVC) used to be the standard investigation for suspected biliary stones but has largely been replaced by ERCP and direct contrast injection into the biliary tree. Image resolution with IVC is poor and the contrast often causes nausea and vomiting. Nevertheless, IVC has found renewed favour with some surgeons for seeking bile duct stones before laparoscopic cholecystectomy.

Magnetic resonance cholangiopancreatography (MRCP) (Fig. 5.10 e and f)

MRI differentiates tissues and organs by their varying content of water. Bile and pancreatic juice are mostly water, hence MRCP gives clear images of bile in the gall bladder and ducts and outlines the pancreatic duct, even in the jaundiced patient. It also reveals filling defects caused by stone. MRCP can identify bile leaks, gallstones in the bile ducts, and duct obstruction from any cause. There are no known hazards. MRCP is beginning to replace HIDA scanning (cholescintigraphy) and ERCP for pancreatico-biliary investigation.

Indications for MRCP include:

- Suspected retained bile duct stones, particularly if within the liver
- Bile duct strictures, particularly if within the liver—post-surgical, cholangiocarcinoma
- Suspected sclerosing cholangitis
- Acute pancreatitis of unknown aetiology—MRCP reveals anatomical duct abnormalities
- Biliary-type pain with abnormal liver function tests in younger women in the absence of stones on ultrasound
- Choledochal cysts
- Patients unsuitable for ERCP because they are intolerant of the procedure or have had previous gastrectomy

Percutaneous transhepatic cholangiography (PTC)

Percutaneous cholangiography is rarely used for diagnosis but has occasional therapeutic indications. A long fine

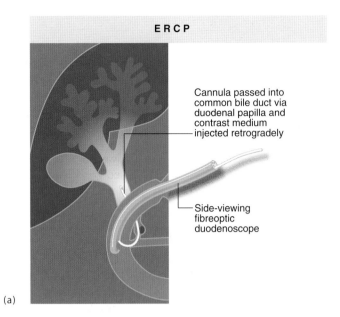

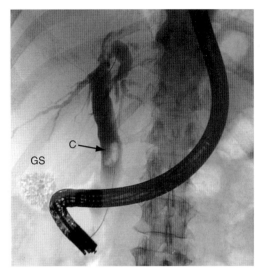

(a) (b)

(a) and (b) Endoscopic retrograde cholangiography
The patient is sedated and a side-viewing gastroscope passed down so the tip reaches the second part of the duodenum. The ampulla of Vater is cannulated under direct vision and contrast medium injected to outline the bile ducts. **(b)** A large gallstone **C** is seen within the dilated common bile duct and a collection of radiopaque gallstones **GS** is seen in the gall bladder.

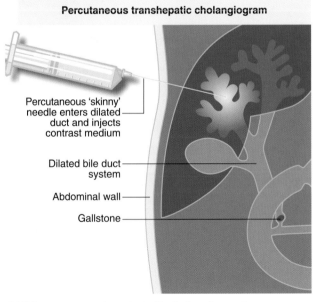

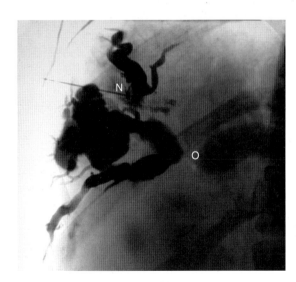

(c) (d)

(c) and (d) Percutaneous transhepatic cholangiography
A needle **N** is passed into the liver until it encounters a dilated duct. Contrast medium is then injected to outline the ducts. **(d)** Case study—this deeply jaundiced 57-year-old woman has grossly dilated intrahepatic ducts and complete obstruction of the proximal common bile duct in the porta hepatis at **O**. This was due to lymph node metastases from carcinoma of stomach. This method is employed less often nowadays because of the superior safety of other methods described here.

Fig. 5.10 Some techniques for demonstrating the biliary system

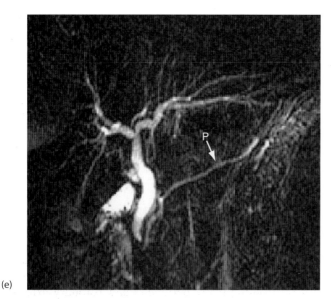

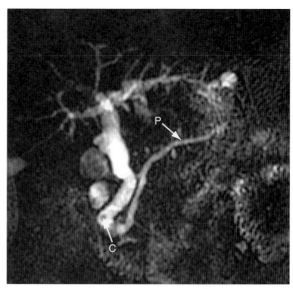

(e)

(f)

(e) and (f) Magnetic resonance cholangio-pancreatography (MRCP)
The technique produces images of static fluid, thus the images are of native biliary and pancreatic secretions. Each image was obtained in one second using a thick slab 'projection' method that generates images very similar to ERCP. The pancreatic duct in each image is labelled **P**. **(e)** An example of normal biliary and pancreatic duct systems. **(f)** A small calculus, **C**, in the distal common bile duct. There is also mild dilatation of the pancreatic duct with some side branches visible.

Fig. 5.10, cont'd

(22 G) 'Chiba' needle is passed percutaneously, directly into dilated intrahepatic ducts, and contrast is injected to display the duct system (see Fig. 5.10c). The test can be useful to show the position and configuration of extra-hepatic duct obstruction from the proximal direction. Occasionally, PTC is employed to drain obstructed bile ducts after failure of endoscopic placement of a drain or stent (sometimes because of duodenal obstruction or previous surgery). Disordered blood clotting is likely in jaundiced patients so vitamin K injections should be given and a **clotting screen** and platelet count performed before PTC.

Endoscopic retrograde cholangio-pancreatography (ERCP)

This investigation is described below (see *Diagnostic and therapeutic duodenoscopy*); its use in obstructive jaundice is described in detail in Chapter 19. The basic technique is illustrated in Figure 5.10 a and b.

Operative cholangiography and choledochoscopy

It is standard practice to perform operative cholangiography during open cholecystectomy. For laparoscopic cholecystectomy, some surgeons routinely perform operative cholangiography, whilst others prefer preoperative assessment using intravenous cholangiography, ERCP or MRCP for those cases deemed likely to have duct stones.

Operative cholangiography serves several purposes. It allows the (highly variable) biliary anatomy to be demon-

strated, it demonstrates stones in the major ducts and it shows whether contrast flows freely into the duodenum. To perform the procedure, a fine plastic cannula is introduced into a small hole cut in the side of the cystic duct and then passed into the common bile duct. Water-soluble contrast material is injected in two or three stages to outline the duct system and fluoroscopic images or X-ray films are taken. If stones are demonstrated in the bile ducts, they are usually retrieved surgically. At open cholecystectomy, this is via a longitudinal incision in the common bile duct (**exploration of the common bile duct**). At laparoscopic surgery, these may be removed by laparoscopic methods. A further cholangiogram is often done afterwards to ensure the duct has been cleared. Stone removal may however be deferred and performed later at ERCP. However, ERCP carries significant risk of complications including biliary leakage and acute pancreatitis.

Many surgeons also inspect the inside of the bile ducts after operative stone removal using a **choledochoscope**. At open surgery, this can be a rigid L-shaped instrument with attachments for grasping stones, or a flexible instrument around 5 mm in diameter that can also be used at laparoscopic surgery. Choledochoscopy can markedly reduce the incidence of residual stones after exploring the bile ducts.

T-tube cholangiography

Following exploration of bile ducts for stones, a T-tube is often left in situ to drain the duct. The transverse limb of the T lies in the duct and the long limb drains out through an opening in the duct to the exterior. About 1 week after operation, contrast can be injected along the T-tube to outline the biliary tree and show abnormalities such as residual stones, bile leakage and duct stenoses as well as confirming free drainage into the duodenum.

VASCULAR RADIOLOGY (ANGIOGRAPHY)

General principles and hazards of arteriography and venography

The general principles of vascular radiology are described here; further detail about applications is given in Chapter 41.

The veins or arteries of a particular anatomical region can be opacified by intravenous or intra-arterial injection of contrast media. This is known as **angiography** and includes both arteriography and venography. In **arteriography**, a specialised catheter is passed over a previously placed guide-wire to enter a vessel some distance away from the target site; the guide-wire is removed and the catheter advanced and the tip manipulated into the correct position. Favoured entry points are the femoral artery in the groin, the brachial artery above the elbow and, more recently, the radial artery at the wrist using smaller diameter catheters.

If there is any suspicion of a bleeding disorder, **clotting studies** should be performed before vascular radiology to predict potential haemorrhagic complications from the vessel puncture site.

The contrast material is the same as is used for intra-venous urography and therefore carries similar hazards (see *Urography* below). In addition, there is the risk of complications from the arterial or venous cannulation, particularly trauma to the vessel or loss of part of the catheter into the vessel lumen. Vessel trauma may cause bleeding or thrombosis and, for arteries, wall dissection, arteriovenous fistula or false aneurysm formation.

Arteriography

Digital subtraction is an electronic process that is now standard for contrast vascular studies. The unchanging opacities of a plain radiographic image (particularly bone and gas) are **subtracted** in real time from the radiological image produced after intra-arterial injection of contrast material. The advantages are that lower doses of contrast media produce better quality images. In some cases, intra-venous contrast alone can produce useful images. In addition, the image can be processed electronically to enhance definition, change contrast or concentrate on particular areas.

In **lower limb arteriography** the usual access point is via the femoral artery but this route is not accessible if the aorto-iliac system is occluded and femoral pulses are undetectable. A catheter can then be placed via the radial or brachial artery but magnetic resonance angiography (MRA) is often preferred if available. In conventional arteriography, water-soluble contrast is injected directly into the artery and images recorded on rapid-sequence films or electronically. Thus stenoses or occlusions due to thrombosis, atheroma or embolism can be demonstrated. Occasionally, the aorta has to be punctured directly using a long needle from the left lumbar region with the patient lying prone. This is known as **translumbar aortography**; it gives poorer views of the distal lower limb vessels and carries a greater risk of complications than femoral or brachial arteriography.

Endovascular techniques

Percutaneous transluminal angioplasty (PTA) or balloon angioplasty

Balloon angioplasty under local anaesthesia has rapidly become established as a less invasive alternative to surgery for overcoming many peripheral and coronary arterial stenoses. In general, short stenoses in large vessels are most suitable for this approach. The method is particularly useful for lower limb atherosclerosis (especially of the iliac and superficial femoral arteries) and for coronary artery disease and, to a lesser extent, renal artery stenoses. Carotid artery disease is also suitable for angioplasty in some cases; filters are usually placed above the stenotic segment before dilatation to reduce the risk of embolism to the brain.

Major complications of angioplasty are rare in experienced hands but there is a small risk of precipitating acute ischaemia. Thus, surgical salvage should be readily available should complications develop. Unfortunately, 25–40% of angioplastied lesions undergo restenosis or occlusion within 1 year, but the process can usually be repeated. Where stenoses fail to remain open at the time of angioplasty, expandable stents can be placed within the treated lesion. Peripheral arterial stents are most often used to treat iliac occlusive disease and have been shown to improve the long-term patency. Overall, angioplasty causes minimal interventional and anaesthetic stress to the patient and is often performed on a day-case basis. Angioplasty can often be offered when open bypass surgery is not indicated.

Techniques of percutaneous angioplasty. Angioplasty is usually performed under local anaesthesia (Fig. 5.11). A needle is first inserted percutaneously into an accessible artery (usually femoral, brachial or radial) and a short flexible guide-wire passed into the artery. A working sheath with a valved side-arm is passed over the **guide-wire** and advanced about 15 cm into the artery. A long guide-wire is then substituted for the first and manipulated up to and through the stenosis using contrast injections and X-ray fluoroscopic control. An **angioplasty catheter** with a plastic inflatable balloon at its end is then passed over the guide-wire and manipulated into position across the stenosis. Current synthetic angioplasty

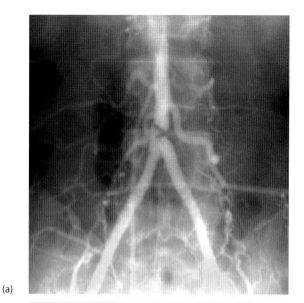

(a)

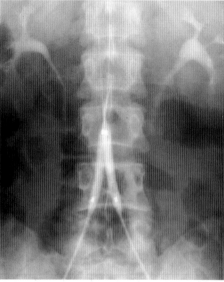

(b)

Fig. 5.11 Percutaneous transluminal angioplasty
This man of 55 presented with bilateral calf and thigh
claudication. **(a)** A localised severe stenosis of the distal
abdominal aorta. **(b)** The 'kissing balloon' technique used to dilate
the stenosis. Two balloons, shown inflated, are used to prevent
asymmetrical dilatation which might compromise the opposite
common iliac artery.

balloons are now no wider than the catheter before inflation and inflate to a fixed diameter even at high pressure.
Before dilatation, the arterial pressure above and below
the stenosis can be measured via the catheter to determine any significant pressure gradient. The balloon is
then inflated to a pressure of between 3 and 12 atmospheres to dilate the stenosis and further contrast is
injected to check the result. The pressure gradient can be
remeasured and the differential across the stenosis should
have been eliminated. Angioplasty equipment has progressively improved and, as experience with the technique has increased, many patients can now return to
near-normal life after minimal intervention.

Longer stenoses and occlusions are being tackled by
subintimal angioplasty. The balloon catheter is deliberately passed beneath the intima/inner media, outside the
obstructing material and along its entire length, before
re-entering the lumen distally. The obstruction is then
angioplastied in the standard way.

Many more patients with claudication or coronary
heart disease than would formerly have been offered
reconstructive arterial surgery are now considered for
angioplasty because of its minimally invasive nature and
low complication rates.

Local arterial thrombolytic therapy

An artery freshly occluded by thrombosis and causing
ischaemia can be recanalised by local intra-arterial infusion of thrombolytic agents. High local concentrations
with limited systemic spill-over were intended to avoid
the serious bleeding and allergic complications of systemic thrombolysis. However, experience has shown that
the risk of major haemorrhage still exists, some episodes
of which have been fatal. Examples include intracerebral
haemorrhagic strokes and bleeding from recent surgical
wounds. For this reason, the treatment is now rarely used.
Thrombolytic agents include **streptokinase**, **urokinase**
and **recombinant tissue plasminogen activator** (R-tPa).
R-tPa acts more quickly and does not have the frequent
allergic effects of streptokinase, though it is more
expensive.

The main indication for thrombolysis used to be the
acutely ischaemic limb where arteriography demonstrated
acute thrombosis superimposed upon pre-existing atherosclerotic narrowing. Most of these cases are treated
nowadays by angioplasty or bypass grafting. For recent
acute embolic ischaemia, surgical embolectomy remains
the best treatment.

Thrombolytic therapy can be employed for treating
pulmonary embolism but the indications and efficacy are
not yet well established.

Therapeutic embolisation

Highly vascular lesions such as certain haemangiomas
that would be difficult or impossible to treat by surgery
alone can have their arterial supply reduced or obliterated
by embolisation. The main supplying artery is identified
by selective arteriography and a catheter manoeuvred
into it, close to the lesion. A small quantity of occlusive
material is injected via the catheter so as to impact in the
artery at a point where it narrows. The usual materials for
embolisation are **gelatin foam, lyophilised human dura
mater, minute steel coils** or **cyanoacrylate glue**. The
process is repeated for all the feeding vessels.

Embolisation is sometimes used to reduce the vascularity of other lesions prior to difficult surgery (e.g. carotid
body tumour) or to palliate lesions not amenable to

surgery (e.g. hepatic metastases or extensive arteriovenous malformations).

Minimal access graft placement

Increasing experience in endovascular techniques such as angioplasty and stent placement has stimulated progress towards more ambitious minimally invasive treatments, particularly **endovascular stent-grafts** for abdominal aortic aneurysm. A Dacron graft with integral metal stent is passed proximally via a femoral arteriotomy until it lies within the neck of the aneurysm. A balloon is inflated to expand the stent into position to retain the graft. A similar mechanism is used to secure the distal limbs. Devices continue to improve and clinical trials are giving promising results; however, some doubt remains about long-term outcomes. Particular problems include **endoleakage**, i.e. continued slow bleeding into the aneurysm sac caused by failure of the graft to exclude blood from the aneurysm, and **graft migration**. The late complication rate is about 10% per year, considerably greater than that for open aneurysm grafting, but this rate is falling with improving techniques.

Venography

Colour duplex Doppler ultrasound scanning has largely replaced contrast venography for diagnosing **deep vein thrombosis** (DVT), as well as for demonstrating reflux from deep to superficial vessels in varicose veins. A skilled operator can demonstrate the patency or otherwise of all the lower limb veins and the presence of fresh or old thrombus. The competence of valves in deep and superficial veins and perforating veins can be shown. In addition, vein wall irregularity associated with previous DVT can be displayed. Contrast venography can sometimes be helpful in defining the anatomy of complex superficial varicose veins and very occasionally to diagnose or exclude calf vein DVT where duplex is inconclusive.

Placement of vena caval filters

After venous thromboembolism, a few patients experience **recurrent pulmonary embolism** despite adequate anticoagulation. In others, anticoagulation therapy is contraindicated and other methods of preventing pulmonary embolism must be found, e.g. in pregnancy, after a haemorrhagic stroke, in patients with a high risk of falling or those with certain bleeding disorders. In both of these groups, the risk of pulmonary embolism can be markedly reduced by placing a filter in the inferior vena cava, above or below the renal veins. This still allows venous blood to return to the heart but traps any substantial embolic material in the flowing blood. In the past, various methods of interrupting venous return have been tried, including ligation of femoral veins or the inferior vena cava but both cause lower limb oedema. Partial interruption of the inferior vena cava using suture plication or caval clips

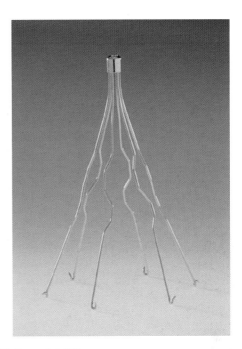

Fig. 5.12 Greenfield filter
This is one type of filter employed in patients suffering recurrent pulmonary embolism despite adequate anticoagulation. It is placed percutaneously via a femoral or jugular vein to lodge in the inferior vena cava. Here it traps emboli travelling from the limb and pelvic veins, allowing them to dissolve without complication. Photograph by permission of Boston Scientific.

reduced the oedema rate but caused caval occlusion in more than 30%. Since the mid-1960s a range of filtration devices have been developed that can be inserted relatively simply using a catheter via the femoral or jugular vein. A typical example is the Greenfield filter (see Fig 5.12). Studies have shown a zero rate of caval occlusion and a 4% rate of pulmonary embolism, none of which has been fatal.

Minimally invasive treatment of varicose veins

Several new methods of ablating the long or short saphenous vein have appeared recently including foam sclerotherapy and laser or radiofrequency ablation. These are described in Chapter 43.

UROGRAPHY

General principles

Urography is a radiological technique for examining the kidneys and urinary collecting systems. It uses intravenous contrast that is concentrated and excreted by the kidneys. A plain abdominal **control film** is taken before contrast injection so that any calcified opacities can be compared with films taken after contrast. This helps to identify whether an opacity lies within the renal tract and hence whether it is likely to be a stone (see Fig. 5.7a, p. 63).

In an intravenous urogram (IVU), films are taken at intervals after injection and the urinary tract is examined sequentially from kidneys to bladder. The renal parenchyma normally opacifies almost immediately. Contrast then flows successively into the renal pelvis, ureters and bladder. The kidneys can be shown in greater detail by **tomography**. This is sometimes used in conjunction with ultrasound when investigating adults with haematuria.

Special precautions with intravenous urography

Intravenous contrast is potentially nephrotoxic in patients with impaired renal function; patients with diabetic nephropathy are at particular risk. When requesting urography, conditions which might be associated with renal parenchymal disease should be specified on the request form to help the radiologist plan the safest investigation. Alternative imaging tests such as ultrasound, unenhanced CT or occasionally MR should be considered. The important disorders are:

- Diabetes mellitus
- Renal failure (include results of renal function tests on the request form)
- Multiple myeloma
- Heart failure

CT urography

Unenhanced CT scanning of the renal tract is increasingly being used instead of intravenous urography to diagnose renal or ureteric colic. It is more sensitive for detecting stones and is a quicker test to perform than IVU; however, it usually gives a higher dose of radiation. CT combined with intravenous contrast is occasionally used to investigate persistent haematuria when other tests are normal.

Percutaneous techniques

The renal pelvis can be punctured percutaneously with a needle guided by ultrasound or CT scanning. The tract is then dilated to allow tubes of various sizes and types to be inserted. Gaining access to the kidney in this way is known as **percutaneous nephrostomy**. It can be employed to remove stones from the renal pelvis, to urgently but temporarily relieve acute distal urinary obstruction and drain the kidney over a few days ahead of a definitive procedure (nephrostomy drainage), or to conduct sophisticated pressure and flow measurements in suspected pelviureteric junction obstruction.

MEDICAL ULTRASOUND

Medical ultrasound developed from sonar used for the detection of submarines in the Second World War. However, the technology remained an official secret until the 1960s. Since then, the principle has found many applications, from identifying shoals of fish to non-invasive imaging of body organs.

Medical ultrasound was pioneered in obstetrics where it has long been an important part of prenatal assessment. As technology and electronics have improved the resolution and discrimination, surgical applications have become ever wider. An important advance was **grey scale ultrasound**, which enables a whole range of tissue echogenicities to be displayed on the screen rather than just black and white.

Interpreting ultrasound depends very much on the dynamic picture the operator sees during the examination rather than what is recorded on the static films. The film record may mean little to anyone but the operator who performed the study!

GENERAL PRINCIPLES OF MEDICAL ULTRASOUND

Ultrasound is non-invasive, painless and almost certainly safe. An ultrasound probe containing the transducer is applied to the skin over the area of interest and the image of deeper structures is displayed on a screen. The probe must be 'coupled' to the skin with jelly to exclude an air interface and is then moved in different directions and at different angles to best display the organs of interest and any abnormalities. 'Spot' films are taken to record the examination.

The transducer consisting of piezo-electric crystals both transmits and receives the ultrasound. A one-microsecond pulse of ultrasound is emitted every millisecond, and the transducer then 'listens' for reflected ultrasound echoes over the next 999 microseconds. An image representing a slice through the body is generated electronically, with reflections showing as bright spots on a dark screen. This is known as **B-mode** (brightness mode) and the intensity of each spot is proportional to the sound reflectivity of the tissue interfaces. The moving image is displayed on a video screen as the examination proceeds and is thus described as **real time ultrasound**.

The length and breadth of organs or lesions displayed on the screen can be accurately determined by electronically measuring the image. Furthermore, the **volume** of some structures such as the urinary bladder or the left ventricle can be estimated. This can give useful functional information, for example, the volume of residual urine in the bladder in chronic retention, or the completeness of left ventricular emptying in cardiac failure.

Bone, stones and other calcified tissues cause an abrupt and marked change in acoustic impedance, resulting in virtually complete reflection of ultrasound. Thus the surface of hard tissue such as a gallstone is revealed by its echogenicity and also by the **acoustic shadow** it casts (see Fig. 20.4, p. 320). A similar, though lesser change in acoustic impedance occurs at gas/soft tissue interfaces such as that of bowel wall and its gas-filled lumen.

Minimal patient preparation is needed for ultrasound examination. For biliary examinations, the patient should be fasted to minimise bowel gas shadows and to reduce gall bladder contraction. For examination of the pelvis, the bladder should be full of urine. This provides a fluid-filled, non-reflective 'window' for the ultrasound to reach the pelvic organs.

Duplex scanning is a technological advance for studying blood flow). In this, both B-mode and Doppler shifted ultrasound are employed. A further improvement is **colour duplex** in which the image has false colour added to show the direction and approximate volume of flow, with red indicating one direction and blue the opposite direction of flow.

Special ultrasound transducers

Special ultrasound probes have been developed for inserting into various body orifices and body cavities via endoscopic instruments, percutaneous cannulae and laparoscopes. These devices are placed closer to the organ being examined than conventional surface probes and this allows higher-frequency sound to be used. This type of sound has lower penetration but greater spectral resolution giving a more detailed display. These transducers are often combined with biopsy devices to enable tissue sampling of the organs studied.

Rectal probes are used for examining the rectal wall and prostate gland in detail and **vaginal probes** for investigating the pelvic organs. **Endoscopic probes** (e.g. trans-oesophageal) can examine and monitor the heart, upper gastrointestinal organs and adjacent tissues. **Laparoscopic probes** can be applied directly to viscera to seek the extent of tumour spread and the presence of metastases, e.g. pancreas, liver. They give a high-resolution image and provide a more reliable diagnosis of liver metastases than percutaneous ultrasound or cross-sectional imaging.

APPLICATIONS OF ULTRASOUND IN GENERAL SURGERY

DIAGNOSTIC B-MODE (BRIGHTNESS MODE) ULTRASOUND

Ultrasound has replaced cholecystography for diagnosing gall bladder disease and largely replaces intravenous urography for examining the urinary tract. In children and women of child-bearing age, ultrasound should be considered in preference to other tests where appropriate because it avoids the use of potentially damaging ionising radiation.

Ultrasound is useful for:

- Reliably distinguishing **solid** from **cystic** lesions, e.g. a thyroid cyst from solid nodule, renal or pancreatic cyst from solid tumour
- Assessing palpable **abdominal masses** in the upper abdomen or pelvis
- Detecting **abnormal tissues** in a homogeneous organ, e.g. liver metastases or renal adenocarcinoma
- Detecting **damage to solid organs after trauma**, e.g. splenic or liver rupture
- Detecting **abnormal fluid collections**, e.g. pseudocyst of pancreas, ascites, pleural effusions, abscesses
- Obtaining information about the nature of lesions from the way the **echo texture** contrasts with the normal, e.g. distinguishing liver secondaries from benign lesions or normal liver
- Detecting **movement**, such as pulsation of an aneurysm, contraction of the heart (echo shows valve morphology and movement, ventricular wall movement) and fetal anatomy and movement
- Detecting upper urinary tract **dilatation** (hydronephrosis)
- **Measuring physical dimensions**, e.g. the diameter of an abdominal aortic aneurysm or a dilated bile duct, or the volume of residual urine in the bladder after micturition
- Investigating the **biliary system** for gallstones, thickened gall bladder wall, dilated ducts, masses in the head of the pancreas or porta hepatis
- **Guiding percutaneous interventional procedures** for tissue sampling, e.g. aspiration or biopsy of liver metastases, pancreatic tumours or retroperitoneal masses, or drainage of fluid collections
- Investigating **breast lumps**, e.g. distinguishing cystic from solid lesions, suspected malignant lesions, guided cyst drainage, guiding fine-needle aspiration (FNA) for cytology, or core biopsy

The limitations of diagnostic ultrasound are summarised in Box 5.3.

DOPPLER-SHIFTED ULTRASOUND

Ultrasound can be used for detecting and studying blood flow by applying the Doppler principle. Simple hand-held equipment is cheap and portable, and is invaluable in the vascular clinic (see Fig. 5.13). Using a special probe coupled to the skin with conduction gel, a beam of ultrasound is directed at an artery or vein. Ultrasound is reflected from the moving red cells and this causes a shift in sound frequency related to the blood velocity. The reflected ultrasound is used to generate an audible signal (for detecting blood flow) or else is electronically processed to reveal information about the nature of flow. The pitch of the audio signal is related to blood **velocity** and

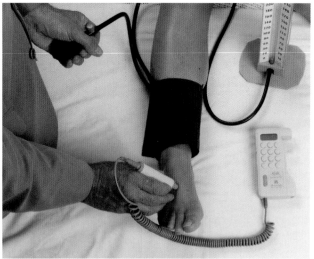

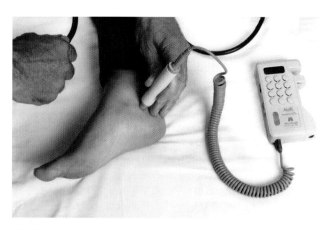

(a) (b)

Fig. 5.13 Measuring ankle systolic pressure using a hand-held Doppler flowmeter
(a) A standard sphygmomanometer cuff is placed around the ankle just above the malleoli. Ultrasound conducting gel is applied to the tip of the probe and the probe placed lightly over the likely position of the dorsalis pedis (DP) pulse, between the first two metatarsals. The probe is moved a tiny amount at a time so as to obtain the strongest signal, then the cuff is inflated until the pulse disappears. The cuff is then released gradually and the systolic pressure recorded at the point of return of signal. **(b)** The same process is repeated at the posterior tibial pulse (PT), using the midpoint of a line between the heel and the medial malleolus to find the pulse. Note that accurate measurements require considerable experience, especially when the pressure is low. **Headphones** are recommended to reduce interference.

Box	5.3	The limitations of diagnostic ultrasound

- Bone almost completely reflects ultrasound and, as a result, obscures any tissues beyond it. Ultrasound is therefore of little use for examining the brain and spinal cord, although it is valuable in examining the heart (echocardiography) and for fluid collections in the chest; special **transcranial** Doppler probes are used for monitoring during neurosurgery and carotid artery surgery
- Bowel gas partly reflects ultrasound, which may prejudice the examination. Starving the patient and giving laxatives may help
- A thick layer of fat degrades the ultrasound image. Thus ultrasound is less accurate (but still the first choice) for investigating suspected gall bladder disease in obese patients
- Ultrasound is unreliable for showing stones at the lower end of the common bile duct

---

provides some qualitative assessment of whether flow is normal or abnormal. Colour flow Doppler requires much more complicated and expensive equipment (see below).

Main applications of hand-held Doppler ultrasound

- Measuring systolic blood pressure when it is low. This includes brachial pressure in shocked patients or in infants, and reduced ankle systolic pressures in lower limb ischaemia. For this purpose, a sphygmomanometer cuff is placed around the arm or ankle and a portable Doppler flow detector is used as an electronic stethoscope by applying it to an artery beyond the cuff (Fig. 5.13)
- Detecting the fetal heart rate
- Simple detection of reflux of venous blood at the sapheno-femoral or sapheno-popliteal junction in varicose veins, particularly in recurrent varicosities after surgery

DUPLEX DOPPLER ULTRASOUND SCANNING

Duplex Doppler scanning combines frequency spectral analysis of blood flow using Doppler ultrasound with real time B-mode imaging of the vessel. **Colour flow Doppler** is a more advanced variant which adds false colour to show the direction of blood flow (red one way, blue the other) and gives qualitative information about blood volume.

Duplex equipment is complex and expensive, and the diagnostic process is time-consuming and requires special training. However, it adds a new dimension to the investigation of blood vessels and blood flow and has largely superseded established methods in some areas, for example replacing venography for deep venous insufficiency and arteriography for carotid artery disease. Blood vessels can be imaged in longitudinal or transverse section to reveal the direction of blood flow, the velocity of flow (this rises as blood passes through a stenosis) and the presence of abnormal vessel walls or mature thrombus in the lumen.

Cardiac echo investigation (transthoracic echocardiography) employs similar instruments and provides comprehensive information about cardiac structure and function. As with ultrasound generally, images are best viewed as moving pictures. Echocardiography allows the study of pathological anatomy, patterns of blood flow, cardiac wall movement, cardiac output and valve movements. The most common reason for requesting an echo is to study **left ventricular function**, particularly when symptoms suggest heart failure. Echo can determine the severity as well as the underlying cause of heart failure, e.g. ischaemic left ventricular dysfunction, dilated cardiomyopathy, valve dysfunction or right ventricular dysfunction. In addition, ischaemic regional wall movement abnormalities can be identified. These include **hypokinesis** (diminished movement), **akinesis** (absent movement) and **dyskinesis** (passive outward bulging in systole suggesting ventricular aneurysm). The **ejection fraction** (ratio between stroke volume and end-diastolic volume) can easily be assessed.

Echo is the investigation of choice for **valve abnormalities**. It can define the cause of a heart murmur, assess the severity of valvular stenosis or reflux and determine the need for antibiotic prophylaxis in patients with a murmur. In patients with **atrial fibrillation**, echo can detect underlying structural defects and guide the need for anticoagulation or cardioversion. In patients with **systemic embolism**, echo rarely shows intracardiac thrombus but is likely to show any underlying cardiac defect that is the source of embolism, such as mitral valve disease or vegetations, left ventricular aneurysm or a patent foramen ovale.

Applications of duplex Doppler

- **Deep vein thrombosis**—when available, this is the method of choice for detecting postoperative DVT. Thrombus more than 24 hours old can be seen and venous flow changes detected. However, the profunda vein and small calf veins are often poorly seen

- **Chronic lower limb deep venous insufficiency**— patency and valvular competence in deep veins (e.g. femoral and popliteal) can be determined dynamically; perforator incompetence can also be detected
- **Varicose veins**—duplex ultrasound is useful for detecting and guiding marking of the short saphenous/popliteal junction before operation and for detecting communications between superficial veins and the sapheno-femoral junction in 'recurrent' long saphenous varicose veins. Recent work shows there are advantages to performing ultrasound in all varicose vein patients before treatment to clarify the diagnosis
- **Carotid artery disease**—duplex has now become the standard test for investigating extracranial vascular disease in preference to carotid angiography (which carries distinct risks). Duplex shows the morphology of diseased arteries and the velocity of flow, allowing the percentage of stenosis to be calculated. The severity of stenosis determines whether operation is required. Duplex is useful for evaluating asymptomatic bruits and following up patients after carotid endarterectomy, including the early postoperative period
- **Femoro-popliteal bypass grafts**—duplex is used for marking out the saphenous vein graft before surgery and for graft surveillance after surgery to detect remediable vein graft stenoses
- **Aorto-iliac and femoro-popliteal occlusive disease**—duplex is proving valuable for estimating the sites and severity of stenoses and occlusions and replaces arteriography in some circumstances
- **Deeper blood vessels**—these can be imaged for blood flow and obstruction, e.g. superior mesenteric and renal arteries, and renal veins for spread from renal cell carcinoma
- **Cardiac disease**—echocardiography is used for detecting abnormal anatomy and function including heart failure, ventricular dysfunction, valvular abnormalities including stenoses, congenital cardiac defects including septal defects, and intracardiac abnormalities predisposing to embolism

CROSS-SECTIONAL IMAGING

COMPUTERISED TOMOGRAPHY (CT SCANNING)

GENERAL PRINCIPLES OF CT SCANNING

Computerised tomography involves X-raying a series of thin transverse 'slices' of the patient's head, body or limbs. A precise fan-shaped beam of X-rays is repeatedly pulsed from successive angles around the circumference of each

slice and the transmitted radiation is electronically recorded on the opposite side (see Fig. 5.14).

Since CT was first introduced, the pace of development has been rapid. Modern machines capture images in a continuous spiral around the patient (**spiral CT**). This has been further developed into **multislice CT** which enables several slices to be captured simultaneously with each revolution of the X-ray tube. The most modern machines now generate 64 slices for each turn. The result is more

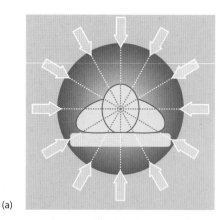

(a)

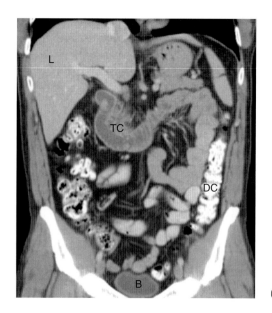

(c)

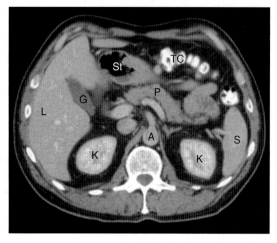

(b)

Fig. 5.14 Computerised tomography
(a) Principle of CT scanning. All images are fed into a computer and a single image of each slice produced. **(b)** Normal transverse CT scan. Liver **L**, gall bladder **G**, stomach **St**, kidneys **K**, aorta **A**, pancreas **P**, spleen **S**. **(c)** Normal CT scan reconstructed in the coronal plane. Liver **L**, bladder **B**, transverse colon **TC**, descending colon **DC**.

rapid image capture of thinner slices at higher resolution. Spiral multislice CT scanning can now produce images of the chest and abdomen in less than 1 minute. The data quality also allows images to be accurately reconstructed in three dimensions or in any chosen plane, e.g. sagittal, coronal or oblique, to improve the detection of abnormalities.

The X-ray beam is attenuated in proportion to the density of the tissue it traverses. The numerous radiation counts for each point in the slice are built up and analysed by a computer using complex mathematical processes to construct a picture of tissue densities in the slice. Each picture element is called a **pixel** and each volume element is known as a **voxel**. The images are displayed on a screen where they can be electronically edited and then recorded on film or electronically. Note that the best CT images are obtained in well-nourished patients because some fat lies between the organs, enabling them to be differentiated more precisely than in very thin patients.

Further information can often be gained by performing CT after or during contrast enhancement. For example, oral or rectal contrast clearly outlines bowel, whilst intravenous contrast can show blood vessels, kidneys, damage to the blood–brain barrier or areas of absent blood flow in pancreatic necrosis.

At present CT and MRI are rivalling each other for first place in the cross-sectional imaging stakes. However it is likely that each modality will prove to have intrinsic advantages in different areas of the body.

APPLICATIONS OF CT SCANNING

Pathological anatomy can be studied in great detail by computerised tomography and a huge array of information can be obtained non-invasively to assist with surgical diagnosis. In many cases the information is more accurate than could be obtained by exploratory operation. This is outstandingly so in brain injury after trauma where the management of serious head injuries has been transformed by head scanning. The technique enables timely and appropriate surgical intervention and avoids unnecessary exploratory operations.

As CT becomes more available, cheaper and technically better, it is often being used earlier in the diagnostic process, particularly in emergency cases, and for an increasing range of clinical conditions.

Some indications for CT scanning are:

- Investigating areas difficult to examine by standard radiology or ultrasound. Examples include the retroperitoneal area and pancreas (deep inside the body), the lungs and mediastinum, and the brain and spinal cord (encased in bone)

- Investigating acute abdominal pain—early CT misses fewer serious diagnoses and may reduce mortality and shorten hospital stay (see below)
- Investigating abdominal pathology when ultrasound has proved unsatisfactory or as an alternative to more intrusive investigations such as barium enema examination for suspected large bowel cancer
- Pre-treatment planning and follow-up of malignant tumours being treated with radiotherapy and/or chemotherapy, e.g. for staging lymphomas (replaces laparotomy)
- Planning surgery, e.g. establishing the extent of local invasion of oesophageal carcinoma, identifying the upper level of an aortic aneurysm, investigating the extent of lateral spread in rectal or prostatic cancer, preoperative assessment of intrathoracic tumours including retrosternal thyroid enlargement
- Assessing solid organ damage in abdominal or thoracic trauma
- Guiding needles during biopsy of masses, drainage of fluid collections or obtaining aspiration cytology specimens
- More recently, diagnosis of pulmonary embolism, renal tract calculi and arterial disease. In the future, multi-slice CT may replace conventional diagnostic coronary arteriography

MAGNETIC RESONANCE IMAGING (MRI)

GENERAL PRINCIPLES OF MAGNETIC RESONANCE IMAGING

Magnetic resonance imaging (MRI), formerly known as nuclear magnetic resonance, was introduced into clinical practice in the early 1980s. MRI involves applying a powerful magnetic field to the body which causes the protons of all hydrogen nuclei to become aligned. The protons are then excited by pulses of radio waves transmitted at a frequency which causes them to resonate and emit radio signals; these are recorded electronically. Sophisticated computation then produces images which can be viewed in any plane, transversely, longitudinally or at any obliquity (see Fig. 5.15).

Lipids have a particularly high hydrogen content and are clearly seen on MRI. For this reason, the initial applications of MRI were in examining the brain and spinal cord. The technique is increasingly employed for investigating joints such as the knee, shoulder, hip and ankle, and in some cases replaces the need for arthroscopy. Modern equipment has meant that examination times have fallen and good-quality images of chest, abdomen and pelvis can now be obtained. However, MRI is unsuitable for imaging gas-filled organs and dense bone.

Disadvantages of MRI

Some patients are unable to tolerate MRI because of claustrophobia but the main technical drawback is the effect of magnetism on metal. Thus metallic foreign bodies, especially in the eyes, may move in the magnetic field and cause damage. MRI cannot be used with cardiac pacemakers and some metallic implants, and patients being artificially ventilated require machines made of non-ferrous materials. Scanning times are still longer than for CT and so MRI is less suitable for young children, the elderly or confused, patients in pain, ventilated patients and emergency patients with active bleeding. All of these disadvantages are being addressed and are likely to disappear as newer machines become available. The diagnostic applications of MRI continue to expand in parallel with the technical improvements.

APPLICATIONS OF MAGNETIC RESONANCE IMAGING

General surgical diagnosis

MRI is especially useful for assessing soft tissue tumours, biliary anatomy and pelvic disease. MRI is valuable in planning surgery for soft tissue tumours of the extremities. It can demonstrate the true extent of the tumour and its relationship to vital structures, so that excision margins can be decided before operation.

MRI is becoming more useful for imaging the biliary tree as speed and resolution improve. This is known as **magnetic resonance cholangio-pancreatography (MRCP)**. Compared with ERCP, the technique has the advantages that there is no risk of causing pancreatitis and sedation is not required. However, therapeutic manoeuvres cannot be carried out as they can with ERCP.

Pelvic MRI is invaluable for assessing the sites and anatomical complexity of **anorectal fistulae** as well as the extent of some **pelvic malignancies**. There is also an evolving role for MRI in **breast cancer**. Contrast enhanced MRI may be shown to have advantages over mammography in distinguishing benign from malignant disease and in assessing multifocal disease. In young women with a strong family history or genetic predisposition to breast cancer, screening may have to begin at an age before mammography would be likely to have sufficient discrimination. MRI may accomplish this screening role without using irradiation.

Blood flow

An exciting development is the ability to demonstrate **blood flow** in the heart and blood vessels, i.e. **magnetic resonance angiography (MRA)**. Blood vessels can be visualised without the need for contrast injection and abnormalities detected as in conventional angiography. In addition, volume flow in particular vessels can be

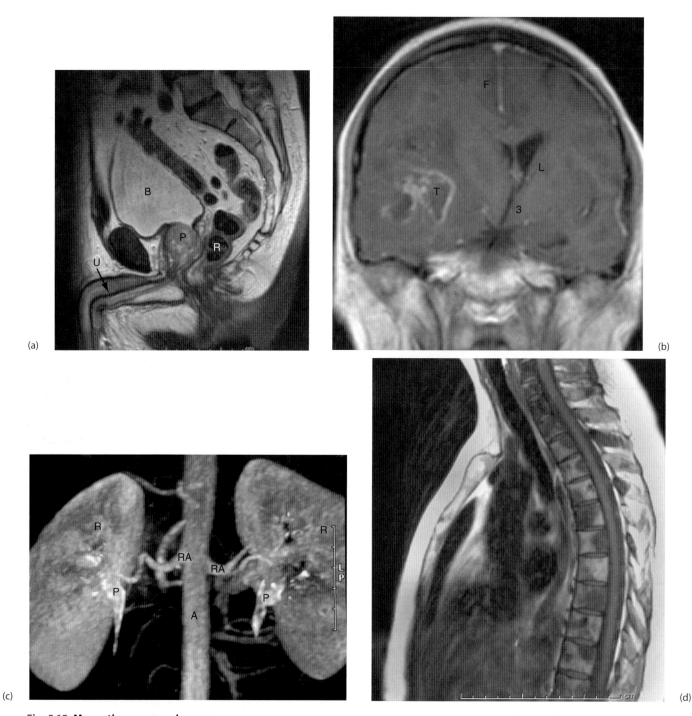

Fig. 5.15 Magnetic resonance images

(a) Sagittal view of male pelvis showing bladder **B**, prostate **P**, urethra **U** and rectum **R**. **(b)** Gadolinium enhanced T1-weighted coronal MRI of the brain. Note enhancement of a tumour **T**, mid-line shift with compression of the right lateral ventricle **L**. The falx **F** and third ventricle **3** are also labelled. **(c)** Magnetic resonance angiogram of normal kidneys showing aorta **A**, renal arteries **RA**, renal substance **R** and renal pelvis **P**. **(d)** T1-weighted sequence sagittal MRI of the thoracic spine in a patient with known prostate cancer, back pain and an elevated prostate specific antigen. The image demonstrates bony metastases as dark areas in the vertebral bodies and spines; the white areas are normal fat in the marrow.

calculated. Spatial resolution can be improved by injecting paramagnetic materials such as compounds containing **gadolinium**. MRI is playing an escalating role in diagnosing cardiac and arterial disease and may in time replace diagnostic coronary angiography.

POSITRON EMISSION TOMOGRAPHY (PET)

PET measures physiological function by looking variously at blood flow, metabolic rates of tissues and the distribution of neurotransmitters and radio-labelled drugs. The method depends on detecting radioactivity emitted from the target organ after a small amount of radioactive tracer is injected into a peripheral vein (usually oxygen-15, fluorine-18, carbon-11 or nitrogen-13). PET is usually combined with CT (**PET-CT**) to enable accurate anatomical location of any abnormality discovered.

PET is commonly used to measure the rate of **glucose consumption** in different parts of the body. The isotope ^{18}F replaces some of the oxygen in glucose to produce fluorodeoxyglucose (FDG). As this sugar is metabolised, more radioactivity is emitted from the more active cells. Cancer cells are often metabolically very active, and this principle enables **FDG-PET** to detect malignancy and differentiate between malignant and benign tissue in many cases; PET can be more sensitive than CT or MRI for detecting cancer. Whole body PET scanning is beginning to be employed to stage some cancers before attempting curative surgery, e.g. oesophagus and lung, or to distinguish recurrent tumours from radiation necrosis or scar tissue.

Blood flow and oxygen consumption in the **brain** can be examined using PET to help understand strokes and dementias and to track chemical neurotransmitters such as dopamine in Parkinson's disease.

INTERVENTIONAL RADIOLOGY

Many of the conventional X-ray, ultrasound and CT techniques already described have been adapted to guide needles to obtain biopsy material, to place drains, to dilate diseased arteries and many other techniques, thus enabling less invasive therapeutic manoeuvres than were formerly required. Some of these techniques have revolutionised treatment and established the interventional radiologist as a front-line clinician, and the field is still growing. Some of the main surgical applications are described in the text of this chapter or in the relevant sections of the book. The remainder are described below.

TISSUE SAMPLING

Fine needle aspiration cytology (FNA) and core biopsy

A fine needle (22 gauge) can be safely passed through most organs or small bowel to aspirate small fragments of tissue from a suspicious lesion. Larger-diameter needles can be used for direct core biopsy of masses. The depth and direction of the needle can be accurately guided by ultrasound or CT to ensure a representative sample is taken. For example, pancreatic masses can be reached by transfixing bowel lying in front of the pancreas; this causes remarkably few side effects. Where practicable, many surgeons and pathologists prefer the larger specimens obtainable with **core biopsy** techniques using specially designed needles such as the **Trucut**, which is available in various configurations and dimensions.

Minimally invasive applications in breast disease include ultrasound- or mammographically-guided fine needle aspiration (FNA) or core biopsy of asymptomatic abnormalities detected on mammography, including those found on screening. **Stereotactic** apparatus can be

employed to make this process more accurate. Mammographic guidance is also sometimes used to place a hooked wire close to an impalpable abnormality to locate it before surgical excision (**mammographic localisation**).

Guided core biopsy or FNA techniques are also important in the diagnosis of thyroid lumps, for sampling liver nodules and for taking renal biopsies in diffuse renal disease.

DRAINAGE OF ABSCESSES AND FLUID COLLECTIONS

Ultrasound and CT are often used to guide percutaneous drainage of well-defined fluid collections in the abdomen or chest, e.g. pancreatic pseudocysts, or abscesses, e.g. paracolic or subphrenic. Ultrasound or CT can demonstrate the site and the dimensions of the fluid collection and can guide the least harmful route for drainage. Fluid can be drained via a needle on a once-only basis or else a self-retaining 'pigtail' drain can be put in place and drainage allowed to continue. In the first category, a subphrenic or other localised abscess can be drained; in the second category, a drain can be placed into a pseudocyst of the pancreas or locally to drain a biliary leak after surgery or to drain a gaseous diverticular perforation. In this way, many major surgical interventions can be avoided.

DILATATION OF GASTROINTESTINAL STRICTURES

Large balloon catheters similar to angioplasty catheters can be used to dilate benign oesophageal strictures secondary to oesophagitis. For **achalasia**, balloon dilatation is now a standard technique. Balloon dilatation is sometimes used for benign rectal strictures such as may occur at an anastomosis site, provided they are not caused by recurrent tumour.

Cloth-lined expanding metal stents are now successfully employed for oesophageal, gastric outlet and colonic strictures caused by malignancy. They are usually placed endoscopically, often after contrast radiology. However, stenting is not indicated as a permanent solution for benign conditions.

RADIONUCLIDE SCANNING

GENERAL PRINCIPLES OF RADIONUCLIDE SCANNING

Radionuclide or isotope scanning is the application of nuclear medicine techniques for diagnosis by identifying sites of abnormal physiology, e.g. the presence of pus, abnormal phagocytic activity or areas of excessive bone turnover. Isotope scanning, however, gives poor anatomical detail. Suitable tracer agents combine a substance taken up physiologically by the target tissue and a **radioactive label**, usually technetium-99m (^{99m}Tc).

The tracer is concentrated in a specific type of tissue (such as iodine in the thyroid gland) or else in tissues with similar physiological or pathological activity such as reticulo-endothelial cells or areas of inflammation.

In the early days of nuclear medicine, tracer was detected in the body using a rectilinear scanner which tracked back and forth over the patient for an hour or more to build up the image. Nowadays, a **gamma camera** consisting of multiple detector units simultaneously collects and counts the level of radioactivity across the area of interest. This produces a complete image in one exposure (see Fig. 5.16). Several views are taken from different directions (usually anterior, posterior and oblique), providing more diagnostic information than a single view.

Some pathophysiological functions can be investigated by **dynamic imaging**. For this, detection of isotope continues for a period and the changing level of radioactivity is recorded for later computer analysis. Examples of this include estimating renal blood flow and studying renal clearance.

APPLICATIONS OF RADIONUCLIDE SCANNING

LUNG SCANNING

The most important application of lung scanning is the diagnosis of pulmonary embolism. Now that multi-slice CT is becoming available, lung scanning is used less often for this purpose. CT is also a better option if the patient has a history of lung disease such as emphysema or if the chest radiograph is abnormal, as lung scintigraphy is almost always equivocal in these cases.

The principle of lung scanning for pulmonary embolism is that pulmonary emboli tend to obliterate patchy areas of the pulmonary arterial circulation but do not interfere with lung ventilation. This is the opposite of what happens with pulmonary infection. Ideally, a **ventilation scan** and a **perfusion scan** should be performed, the two together being known as a **ventilation/perfusion scan** or **V̇/Q̇ scan**. The ventilation scan is performed first. The patient inhales a gaseous radioactive tracer such as an aerosol of technetium-labelled DTPA or xenon-133 and the lungs are imaged from front and back. Then technetium-labelled albumin microspheres are injected intravenously for the perfusion scan. These lodge in the pulmonary capillaries after traversing the chambers of the right side of the heart.

The two scans are compared for **ventilation/perfusion mismatch**, i.e. areas that are ventilated but not perfused (embolism) and areas that are perfused but not ventilated (consolidation or collapse). An example is shown in Chapter 12 (Fig. 12.9). V̇/Q̇ scanning may give either a strongly positive or strongly negative indication of pulmonary embolism, but all too often the results are equivocal.

BONE SCANNING

Phosphate-based agents (phosphates or biphosphonates) labelled with technetium are usually used for bone scan-

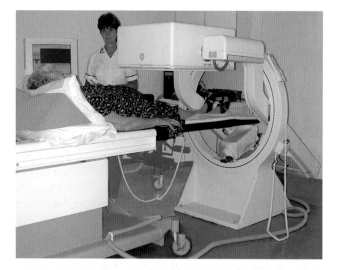

Fig. 5.16 Isotope scanning using a gamma camera
The patient has received an intravenous injection of radiolabelled tracer. The pattern of uptake is imaged by the detector array and transmitted electronically to be displayed on a monitor.

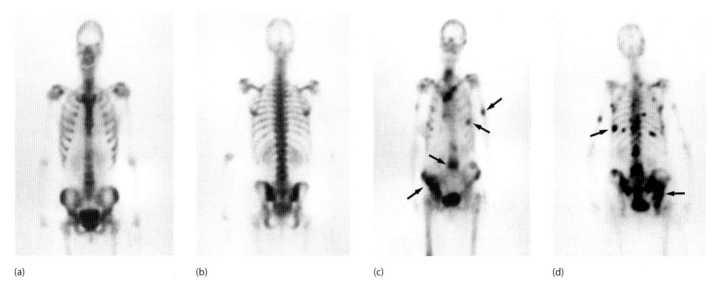

(a)   (b)   (c)   (d)

Fig. 5.17 Isotope bone scans
(a) Anterior view of normal bone scan. **(b)** Posterior view of normal bone scan. **(c)** Anterior view of bone scan in a patient with multiple bony metastases (arrowed) from breast cancer. **(d)** Posterior view of bone scan in the same patient as **(c)**.

ning. The tracer is taken up in areas of increased bone deposition and resorption, indicating sites of bone growth and repair (see Fig. 5.17). These include **growth plates, some primary tumours, secondary tumours, foci of bone infection, healing fracture sites, active arthritis** and **Paget's disease**. Bone scanning is highly sensitive but interpretation of the scans requires caution because it lacks specificity.

The tracer agent is injected intravenously and becomes distributed throughout all body fluids. The highest concentration collects at sites of osteogenesis about 6 hours later and the patient is then scanned. The tracer is also taken up in areas of **dystrophic calcification** and may sometimes reveal an unsuspected carcinoma of breast, an old myocardial infarction scar or a uterine fibroid.

The main indications for bone scanning are:

- Suspected bone metastases (e.g. staging breast carcinoma) or investigation of bone pain
- Biochemical abnormalities suggesting bone disease (e.g. hypercalcaemia or raised plasma alkaline phosphatase)
- Suspected occult (stress) fractures of bone
- Suspected osteomyelitis
- Localising abnormalites in unexplained skeletal pain

RENAL SCANS

Renal scanning is an important method of investigating the urinary tract. It can obtain information that is not available from any other source, is quick and simple to perform and allows the function of each kidney to be assessed individually.

There are three main varieties of renal scan, using different isotopes. DTPA (diethylene tetramine penta-acetic acid) is excreted in the urine like urographic contrast, while DMSA (dimercapto-succinic acid) and MAG3 remain in cortical tissue. (Aide-mémoire: DT 'Pee' A, excreted in urine; D 'Meat' SA, retained in cortical tissue). Examples are shown in Figure 5.18.

DTPA scanning is used to follow up children with reflux nephropathy. The isotope is instilled into the bladder; the child then voids urine while being scanned and any vesico-ureteric reflux is demonstrated. DTPA is also used to diagnose ureteric obstruction and to distinguish obstructed from merely capacious non-obstructed renal tracts.

When unilateral renal parenchymal disease is being investigated, both DMSA and DTPA can give an estimate of excretory activity. The two agents can be used to estimate differential renal function when investigating renal artery stenosis or the function of a transplanted kidney. DMSA is used specifically to image the renal parenchyma to demonstrate renal scars or tumours.

SCANNING FOR GASTROINTESTINAL BLEEDING

Scanning using the patient's own isotopically **labelled red cells** may be employed to locate a source of continuing or intermittent gastrointestinal bleeding. This is useful where the rate of bleeding is relatively slow or in a patient with recurrent haemorrhage, particularly where the source cannot be identified by endoscopy or arteriography.

The patient's blood is labelled with radioactive technetium; this may be performed ex vivo or else in vivo by injecting first pyrophosphate, which binds to red cells, then technetium, which binds to pyrophosphate. The abdomen is scanned at intervals over the next 24 hours or so for 'hot spots' indicating accumulating recent

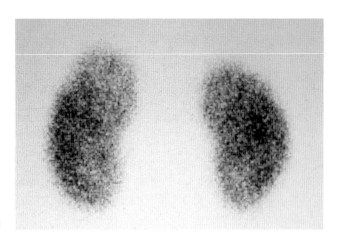

(a)

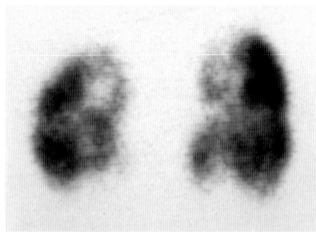

(b)

Fig. 5.18 Renal DMSA isotope scans
(a) Normal and **(b)** abnormal showing patchy scarring due to episodes of pyelonephritis. In this case, there had been bilateral reflux of urine in childhood.

gastrointestinal haemorrhage. If the rate of bleeding is more than about 0.1 ml per minute, the scan usually reveals activity concentrated in one part of the bowel. This indicates the general area of haemorrhage rather than the precise location but does enable the surgical search to be focused, for example on the distal stomach and duodenum or the right side of the colon. Radionuclide scanning has the advantage of detecting an accumulation of blood over a period, whereas the alternative investigation of **selective angiography** is less sensitive and requires a higher rate of active bleeding at the moment of injection; however, it can reveal the site of bleeding more precisely.

In children, rectal bleeding may be due to bleeding from a Meckel's diverticulum. This is usually caused by ulceration of ectopic gastric mucosa. A radionuclide compound of technetium that is concentrated in gastric mucosa may be employed in cases of suspected bleeding Meckel's diverticulum.

LEUCOCYTE SCANNING FOR INFLAMMATION AND INFECTION

When an abscess or other infected focus is suspected but cannot be localised, the patient's own white blood cells can be labelled with indium-111 or gallium-67 citrate, then reinjected; the patient is then scanned. Typical indications for this are patients with a high swinging pyrexia after operation, or patients with sepsis of unknown origin. The process is relatively expensive because it requires a cell separator but it has a high degree of specificity and sensitivity. There is a small proportion of false negative tests, however, where an occult abscess is not revealed by the scan.

Leucocyte scanning is also useful to determine the extent of bowel involvement in inflammatory bowel disease, both ulcerative colitis and Crohn's disease. Tc-

hexamethylpropyleneamine oxime (HMPAO)-labelled leucocytes migrate towards areas of inflamed bowel which are then revealed on imaging.

THYROID SCANS

Thyroid scanning is described in Chapter 49. Its use is declining in favour of fine needle aspiration and cytology except in specific disorders of thyroid function.

CARDIOVASCULAR IMAGING

A multiple gated acquisition (MUGA) scan can provide information about the function of the ventricles of the heart. This can be useful following myocardial infarction or for patients receiving doxorubicin (Adriamycin) chemotherapy which can damage heart muscle. Radionuclide lymphangiography can also demonstrate the patency and capacity of lower limb lymphatics in chronic lymphoedema.

LIVER AND SPLEEN SCANS

Hepatobiliary imaging (HIDA scanning)

Technetium-labelled imido-diacetic acid (IDA) derivatives are concentrated by hepatocytes and are excreted into bile even in the presence of jaundice. This provides a means of testing the patency of the biliary tree and cystic duct.

Hepatobiliary imaging can be used for:

- Demonstrating cystic duct obstruction in suspected acute cholecystitis
- Demonstrating whether bile ducts are obstructed in jaundiced patients. This is often employed in neonates with jaundice. If there is unequivocal evidence of intestinal excretion of the radiolabel, the patency of the extrahepatic biliary system is confirmed

FLEXIBLE ENDOSCOPY

PRINCIPLES OF FLEXIBLE ENDOSCOPY

Strictly speaking, endoscopy applies to any method of looking into the body through an instrument, either via an orifice such as the nose or mouth, or via an artificially created opening (e.g. laparoscopy, thoracoscopy or arthroscopy). Endoscopy using simple tubular instruments has been used for many years and a few of these methods are still in regular use, e.g. rigid sigmoidoscopy. Developments in fibreoptics first led to a major improvement in illumination for conventional rigid endoscopes and later to the construction of flexible instruments. These greatly extended the range and sophistication of diagnostic and therapeutic endoscopic techniques. The unqualified term **endoscopy** is now often employed to mean gastrointestinal endoscopy using flexible instruments with fibreoptic illumination and video image transmission.

Fibreoptic illumination

Rigid endoscopes and the early flexible instruments were illuminated by tiny incandescent bulbs which were prone to failure. The amount of light they could emit was limited by the production of waste heat. These were superseded by **fibreoptic light guides** in both rigid and flexible endoscopes. Fibreoptic light guides are used to channel light from a powerful, fan-cooled light source remote from the patient to the distal end of an endoscope. The light guides are made up of thousands of parallel glass fibres, each with total internal reflection, so that very little light is lost in transmission and no heat is transmitted. A powerful, cool light beam thus emerges from the distal end of even the longest endoscope.

Image transmission

The second development that was crucial in the design of early flexible endoscopes was the manufacture of **coherent viewing bundles**. In these, the orientation of fibres at the distal end exactly matched that at the proximal viewing end. Each fibre thus transmitted a tiny part of the distal scene to the viewing end where it could be inspected or photographed with a still or video camera. The distal end of most endoscopes allowed a viewing angle of over 100°, and the lenses gave a remarkable depth of focus. The image was so clear that accurate diagnosis could often be made on inspection alone.

A later development was the charge-coupled device (CCD) **video camera**, a light- and colour-sensitive microchip positioned at the distal end of a flexible endoscope. The image is transmitted via an electrical cable and is viewed on a colour monitor and not through an eyepiece. This system has now largely replaced the older direct viewing system.

Structure of flexible endoscopes

Most flexible endoscopes include a mechanism to steer the distal end in four directions (except for specialised ultra-slender scopes), a distal imaging chip for video endoscopy, one or two fibreoptic light guides, a suction channel and a channel for inflating the hollow viscus under inspection with air, doubling as a lens washing channel (see Fig. 5.19). The suction channel is also used to pass slender flexible operating tools such as tiny forceps for taking biopsies, grasping forceps for retrieving foreign bodies, laser guides for therapy (haemostasis or tumour destruction), snares for excision of polyps, diathermy wires, scissors for cutting sutures and needles for injecting haemostatic agents.

APPLICATIONS OF FLEXIBLE ENDOSCOPY

Flexible endoscopes were first used to inspect the stomach in the late 1960s and the range of instruments has progressively expanded since then. There are now instruments available to inspect and cannulate the duodenal papilla, to examine all or part of the large bowel, to inspect the interior of the bile ducts at operation and to examine the bladder interior using only local anaesthesia.

Choledochoscopes are rigid or flexible instruments used to inspect the interior of the bile ducts at open or laparoscopic operation to ensure that any stones are cleared. Their use has improved the rate of stone clearance during exploration of the common bile duct.

Narrow fibreoptic **bronchoscopes** can be passed under topical anaesthesia. They are used to inspect bronchi for disease and can be used to aspirate mucus plugs responsible for postoperative lobar collapse.

Further applications of flexible endoscopy will undoubtedly appear as endoscopes become smaller and more sophisticated.

DIAGNOSTIC UPPER GASTROINTESTINAL ENDOSCOPY

Oesophago-gastro-duodenoscopy, also known as **OGD** or **gastroscopy**, involves inspection of the upper gastrointestinal mucosa using a steerable, flexible fibreoptic endoscope. It is usually carried out under intravenous sedation and local anaesthetic spray on a day-case basis. Among other applications, gastroscopy enables the whole area prone to peptic ulcer disease and cancer to be directly and comprehensively examined.

Flexible endoscopy has the following advantages over gastrointestinal contrast radiology:

- Structural abnormalities such as chronic ulcers can be inspected directly whereas radiology provides only

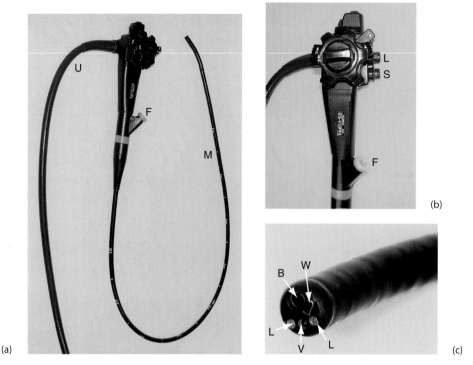

Fig. 5.19 Flexible fibreoptic gastroscope
(a) This end-viewing gastroscope is composed of a flexible main shaft **M** which is 1 m long and marked at 10 cm intervals; the distal 10 cm can be flexed in four directions to steer the instrument in order to advance it and to obtain the best view. There is also an 'umbilical cord' **U** which is plugged into the control box. This carries air to inflate the viscus, water to wash the viewing lens and suction to aspirate fluid from the lumen. There is a flush tube **F**, through which fluid can be injected to wash the stomach wall. The steering controls are better seen in **(b)**. **(b)** The steering controls consist of two concentric wheels labelled respectively **D** and **U** (down and up) and **L** and **R** (left and right). The channel **F** is also used to pass instruments; buttons control suction **S** and air inflation and lens washing **L**. **(c)** shows the tip of the instrument in detail. The two light guides are marked **L**, **V** is the lens for the imaging chip, **W** is the exit for the inflation air and lens washing water and **B** is the channel for passing instruments and for suction. Note that the video image is transmitted up the 'scope and along the umbilical cord to the processor unit, from where it is displayed on a video monitor.

a two-dimensional image with little information about surface characteristics

- Benign ulcers and early malignancies are often indistinguishable on radiology whereas at endoscopy, suspicious lesions such as ulcers can be inspected and biopsied
- Shallow mucosal abnormalities invisible on radiology such as superficial ulceration or vascular malformations can be inspected at endoscopy
- Bile reflux through the pylorus may be visible at endoscopy
- Fibrosis and anatomical distortions from previous disease or surgery interfere much less with recognition of what is abnormal on endoscopy than on radiology
- Endoscopy can often identify the exact site of the lesion causing acute upper gastrointestinal haemorrhage and give an indication of the rate of haemorrhage and the likelihood of rebleeding. Tracing the source is often impossible radiologically
- During endoscopy, therapy may be applied during the same procedure, e.g. injection of the source of acute bleeding, retrieving swallowed foreign body, placement of feeding gastrostomy tube

THERAPEUTIC UPPER GASTROINTESTINAL ENDOSCOPY

Treatment of upper gastrointestinal haemorrhage

First-line therapy for upper gastrointestinal haemorrhage caused by bleeding ulcers typically involves injection of the ulcer base with adrenaline solution alone or in combination with sclerosants. Other treatments such as laser or direct heat coagulation have proved less effective, but are sometimes used. With such techniques, the need for urgent surgery for bleeding has been substantially reduced. Patients who have their acute haemorrhage from benign lesions arrested by these methods can often be managed in the long term without resort to surgery. The subject is discussed in more detail in Chapter 19. Haemorrhage due to oesophageal varices is now best treated in most cases by endoscopic rubber-band ligation or injection sclerotherapy rather than surgery.

Treatment of oesophageal strictures

Endoscopic methods are often used for dilating benign oesophageal strictures. The endoscope is passed until the stricture is visible and then a flexible wire is passed through it into the stomach. The endoscope is removed, leaving the wire in situ. Plastic or metal dilators of increasing size are then passed over the wire which guides them safely through the stricture until sufficient dilatation has been achieved. The technique is relatively safe, can easily be repeated and avoids the need for a general anaesthetic. There is a small risk of oesophageal perforation but this is uncommon (see Fig. 5.20).

Dysphagia caused by an inoperable malignant stricture can be improved by creating a pathway through the tumour with endoscopically guided **laser fulguration**. Unfortunately the tumour inevitably recurs and multiple treatments are likely to be necessary. However, swallowing can be maintained and the patient's quality of life thereby improved without major surgery. In other cases, a **stent** can be placed endoscopically to keep the oesophagus open. This involves first dilating the stricture as for a benign stricture and then pushing a collapsed metal expanding stent covered with cloth down the oesophagus until it lies across the stricture. The cover is removed from the stent as it is deployed and it expands outwards. It also avoids a risky operation and may provide worthwhile palliation for an obstructing tumour.

DIAGNOSTIC AND THERAPEUTIC DUODENOSCOPY

A side-viewing duodenoscope can be used to inspect the duodenal papilla and guide insertion of a cannula or a variety of therapeutic tools. Cannulation allows injection of contrast material into the common bile duct and separately into the pancreatic duct. The technique is known as ERCP (**endoscopic retrograde cholangio-pancreatography**) (see Fig. 5.21 and Ch. 11) and is now an important

Fig. 5.20 Pneumomediastinum following perforation of an oesophageal tumour during endoscopy

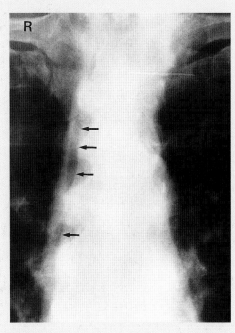

This 56-year-old man who was being investigated for difficulty in swallowing complained of chest pain after the examination. Crepitus was found in the neck due to surgical emphysema resulting from oesophageal air leaking out of the perforation and tracking up the mediastinum into the neck.

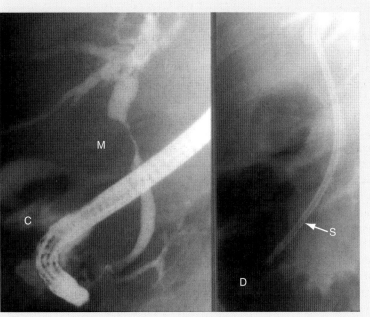
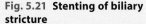

Fig. 5.21 Stenting of biliary stricture
(a) This 54-year-old man developed painless, unremitting obstructive jaundice. This ERCP shows a malignant stricture of the common bile duct **M** due to cholangiocarcinoma. Contrast has been injected to outline the bile ducts and has leaked back into the duodenum **C. (b)** A stent **S** was placed endoscopically across the stricture for palliation. The second part of the duodenum is outlined by gas **D.**

(a)

(b)

part of gastroenterological investigation. It is used to image the biliary duct system in preference to percutaneous transhepatic cholangiography.

ERCP can be both diagnostic and therapeutic. Indications for diagnostic ERCP may be decreasing as newer and safer techniques such as MRCP (**magnetic resonance cholangio-pancreatography**) become available. Therapeutic ERCP allows many disorders of the bile ducts that would previously have required difficult, time-consuming and dangerous operations to be managed by minimal access techniques, with short hospital stays. For example, bile duct stones can often be removed endoscopically by slitting the sphincter at the lower end (**sphincterotomy**) and retrieving them with a balloon catheter or a Dormia basket. Other therapeutic measures include insertion of bile duct stents for palliation of malignant biliary obstruction (cancer of pancreatic head, bile duct or duodenum) and for managing postoperative bile leaks.

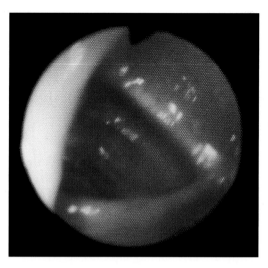

Fig. 5.22 Colonoscopic view of normal transverse colon
When seen colonoscopically, the transverse colon is typically triangular in cross-section; the taenia coli form the apices.

ENTEROSCOPY

Barium follow-through, CT and MRI have low rates of positive diagnosis in small bowel disorders. Direct small bowel visualisation used to be achieved by 'push' enteroscopy (with a 2 m endoscope that could examine up to a metre beyond the duodeno-jejunal flexure) or by operative enteroscopy via a laparotomy. Later, a technique of double-balloon enteroscopy appeared, with an endoscope passed via the mouth and then coaxed along the small bowel using attached balloons as counter-traction. None of these methods was convenient or reliable.

The latest development for small bowel investigation is **capsule endoscopy**, first introduced in 1999. This enables visualisation of the entire 3–5 metres of small bowel with relative ease. The process involves the patient swallowing a capsule which is propelled through the gastrointestinal tract by peristalsis. An imaging device continually transmits images to sensors on the abdominal wall and the capsule-camera then passes out in the stool.

One device, the PillCam SB capsule endoscope, is only 26 × 11 mm, weighs under 4 g and costs about £300. It contains a battery, light-emitting diodes, an imaging chip camera that captures images at 2 frames a second and a radio transmitter that passes images to a sensor array for up to 8 hours. The camera has an image field of 140°. If obstruction is suspected, a different model with a body made of lactose can be used. This disintegrates in less than 48 hours if arrested.

Capsule endoscopy has a positive diagnosis rate of around 65% compared with around 20% for other methods. In obscure gastrointestinal bleeding, there is a positive diagnostic yield of 45–75% in patients who have already had a normal upper and lower gastrointestinal endoscopy. Typical findings include angiodysplasia, tumours, varices and ulcers. Other indications include suspected small bowel Crohn's disease, particularly in children, assessment of coeliac disease, screening in familial polyposis syndromes and diagnosis of Barrett's oesophagus (by attaching a string). Biopsies cannot yet be taken.

LARGE BOWEL ENDOSCOPY (COLONOSCOPY)

Flexible endoscopes of different lengths are available for large bowel examination (see Fig. 5.22). The shortest, the **fibreoptic sigmoidoscope**, is about 60 cm long. It is simple to use and allows examination of the rectum, sigmoid colon and descending colon with minimal bowel preparation. Longer colonoscopes enable inspection of the entire large bowel, and vary in stiffness to assist intubation to the caecum. Other techniques also help reach the caecum, including insufflation with carbon dioxide rather than air, and releasing seed oil from the tip to lubricate the instrument.

Colonoscopy allows inspection of pathological lesions, biopsy of suspicious lesions and resection of lesions such as polyps. Colonoscopy is also employed in surveillance and follow-up of patients treated for colorectal cancer or polyps. New tumours or polyps (metachronous lesions) are looked for and the original site of surgery can be examined. Similar examinations are also used for surveillance of patients with longstanding ulcerative colitis; multiple biopsies are taken to examine for dysplasia and the entire large bowel is inspected for adenomas or carcinomas. Acutely bleeding angiodysplastic lesions in the large bowel can be treated with diathermy.

Colonoscopy is the most reliable method of screening asymptomatic people for colorectal carcinoma. However its value is limited by the lack of trained endoscopists, by cost and by lack of patient compliance.

UROLOGICAL ENDOSCOPY

Endoscopic urology is becoming a progressively larger part of urological surgery. Most is still performed with rigid instruments but flexible instruments are now being used for diagnostic cystoscopy and ureteroscopy.

Cystourethroscopy (cystoscopy) using a rigid instrument is the main diagnostic and therapeutic tool for disease of the urethra, prostate and bladder. Transurethral resection of the prostate has virtually eliminated the need for open retropubic prostatectomy and most early bladder tumours can be treated endoscopically. Laser enucleation of prostatic adenomas is an exciting development. An instrument similar to the cystoscope (but longer), the **ureteroscope**, can now be used to retrieve stones from the lower half of the ureter.

Endoscopic methods of percutaneous stone removal from the renal pelvis have become widely available (**percutaneous nephrolithotomy**). These involve creating a channel from the skin into the renal pelvis and dilating it until an endoscope can be passed. When the stone is seen, various instruments can be used to fragment it and achieve its removal.

Diagnostic and therapeutic laparoscopy is covered in Chapter 11.

6 Screening for adult disease

GENERAL PRINCIPLES OF SCREENING

INTRODUCTION

Medical screening is a public health activity that involves examining or testing asymptomatic, apparently healthy people for the purpose of detecting disease at an earlier stage than would otherwise be the case. Measures can then be taken to prevent the disease altogether (if there is a precursor stage), treat the disease at an early stage (with an improved chance of cure), or at least offer treatment to delay the development of advanced disease. For example, colonic screening can detect adenomas and carcinomas; removing adenomas prevents the well-recognised adenoma–carcinoma sequence, and actual cancers detected tend to be at an earlier and more curable stage. Unfortunately, for the types of cancer that do not have an easily detected precursor stage such as breast or prostate cancer, these beneficial outcomes are elusive.

Screening can also be used to detect disorders that predispose to other diseases, for example, high blood pressure or elevated cholesterol levels, to discover people at increased risk of atherosclerotic heart disease and stroke. Screening is also useful for infection control, e.g. preoperative screening of patients living in residential homes for meticillin-resistant *Staphylococcus aureus* (MRSA) carrier status to make elimination therapy possible before operation.

Screening can be directed at an entire population (**mass screening**) but is more usually **targeted** at particular risk groups within a population. Selection might be on the basis of age, gender or risk factors for cardiovascular disease, for example (Box 6.1). **Opportunistic screening** involves a more random approach, such as screening patients who happen to attend a particular clinic.

ASSESSING THE POTENTIAL BENEFITS OF SCREENING

Several groups subscribe to the simplistic view that screening must by definition be 'a good thing'. These groups include most of the lay public, people associated with particular distressing diseases, populist politicians and people with vested financial interests. Poorly conceived screening however may consume inordinate amounts of medical and financial resources to identify just a small number of new cases and bring about little clinical benefit, e.g. CT scanning for lung cancer. Worse still, early diagnosis of a condition for which early intervention brings no substantial advantage may cause suffering. People can be prematurely placed in an anxiety-provoking sick role where unrealistic treatment expectations are raised. These same people may also be subjected to unnecessary treatments that have potentially severe side effects, e.g. treatment of some breast or prostate cancers that might never have progressed to invasive disease.

As with any other public health measure, any medical and social benefits accruing from a particular screening programme need to be rigorously evaluated and the process separated entirely from the incentive to screen for profit. Whole-body scanning by CT or MRI is currently being strongly marketed on the basis that a scan will show unsuspected abnormalities and allow early treatment. Abnormalities are bound to be discovered by such exten-

proved successful despite the difficulty of engaging many women at high risk. Sadly, the natural history of untreated dysplastic cervical cellular abnormalities was not properly established before the impact of widespread screening made this ethically impossible. This severely hampered the scientific study of the disease, its early diagnosis and best treatment.

Criteria for assessing a screening programme

Many years ago the World Health Organization (WHO) realised that even beneficial screening could be expensive, unpleasant, inaccurate and unproductive, and could have adverse effects on psychological or physical well-being. In 1968, they published a list of criteria for effective screening programmes (Box 6.2); these include attributes of the disease, the test and the treatment. The WHO principles are still highly relevant today and have been added to by the UK National Screening Committee and other groups. Box 6.3 shows a summary of these modified criteria.

Evolution of screening programmes

Once instituted, any screening programme must remain under constant evaluation and then modified or discontinued when appropriate criteria are no longer being met. For example, in the 1950s and 1960s, screening for pulmonary tuberculosis (TB) by mass miniature chest X-ray was highly successful but it was appropriately disbanded in the 1970s when the number of new cases fell below a level at which the unit cost per new case could be justified; interestingly, by this time, the yield of new cases of lung cancer from screening began to exceed that of TB, but at the time there was virtually no effective treatment for it.

sive screening, but more often than not it is difficult to reliably determine which ones signify serious disease and which (if any) should be treated. Doctors should not perform unproven screening tests any more than they should use unproven drugs, and they should resist patient pressure for inappropriate screening.

Premature introduction of screening

Politicians can play a part in initiating inappropriate screening programmes. When UK prime minister, Margaret Thatcher sanctioned large-scale nationwide breast screening in 1988 two weeks before a general election; some believe this was to garner the women's vote. The decision was premature and based on insufficiently validated evidence from the Swedish two counties study and the Forrest report. In the 1970s, screening for cancer of the uterine cervix was widely introduced, also before its efficacy had been fully evaluated. Fortunately, it has

Box 6.3 Summary of attributes of a good screening programme

The disease

- Important health problem
- Detectable truly early stage
- Predictable biological behaviour
- Long period between first detectable stages and overt disease

The diagnostic test

- Valid (sensitive and specific)
- Simple and cheap
- Safe and acceptable
- Reliable and reproducible

Diagnosis and treatment

- Effective, acceptable and safe treatment available
- Evidence of better outcomes if treated early
- Benefits of screening must outweigh risks
- Treatment facilities must be adequate
- Screening overall must be cost effective
- Screening must be sustainable

CRITERIA FOR AN EFFECTIVE SCREENING PROGRAMME

In order to implement any national screening programme, certain criteria must be fulfilled. Initially there must be a perceived need in the medical community or in the wider public. Pilot studies are then carried out. If outcomes are promising, **prospective randomised controlled trials (RCTs)** need to be performed on a large scale so that there is robust evidence upon which to base implementation. This is critically important because once a screening programme has been introduced, it is often extremely difficult politically to stop it later, even when the evidence shows little or no benefit, e.g. breast screening (Nordic Cochrane Collaboration 2001 and 2006).

The disease

- The condition being screened for should be an important health problem. This may be because it is a common disease such as lung or prostate cancer or one that has potentially serious but preventable consequences such as carotid artery disease or abdominal aortic aneurysm (AAA). The **prevalence** (the proportion of cases already in a population) and the **incidence** (the proportion of new cases) of the disease in the population at risk are likely to be known from pilot studies
- There should be a truly early stage at which treatment outcomes are better than at a late stage.

Colorectal adenomas and early colorectal cancers are particularly good examples

- The biological behaviour or natural history of the disease should be well understood, including how latent disease progresses to clinical disease, and the course of the disease should be reasonably predictable. For example, AAAs are known to expand smoothly for the most part and rarely rupture until they are large. The risks associated with untreated disease also need to be understood
- There should be a long period between the first detectable stages and overt disease

The diagnostic test

- The test must be valid, i.e. reliable in detecting the disease. This is defined by two factors, **sensitivity** and **specificity**. Sensitivity is the capability of the test to identify affected individuals in the screened population, i.e. the proportion of people who have the disease and are detected by the test. A test with a high rate of false negative results is insensitive and thus unreliable. Specificity is the degree to which a positive test can be relied upon to prove the disease is present; in other words, the higher the false positive rate, the lower the specificity of the test
- The test must be simple and cheap and it must identify the disease at an early stage by a method that is reliable, validated and reproducible. The distribution of test values should be understood well enough to define normality or relative risk associated with particular stages, e.g. for an AAA, the diameter at which there is a high risk of rupture. Intervals for repeating the test should be worked out for normal subjects and for those with positive results close to the threshold
- The complete screening programme must be clinically safe and acceptable socially and ethically to health professionals and the public. This includes not only the test itself but also any diagnostic procedures and treatments or interventions the screening initiates. For example, if a test is perceived as unpleasant, e.g. colonoscopy, uptake is low and the benefits are proportionally smaller
- The overall benefits should be greater than the risks; this includes any physical and psychological harm caused by the test, the diagnostic procedures and the treatment

Diagnosis and treatment

- Cases identified by the test must be amenable to effective, acceptable and safe, detailed diagnostic procedures
- The potential benefits of medical or surgical intervention prompted by earlier diagnosis need to be understood

- There should be clear evidence from high-quality randomised controlled trials (RCTs) that early treatment produces better outcomes than treatment initiated at later stages, i.e. 'cure' should be more likely, survival longer, or earlier treatment easier. Treatment should have minimal side effects. There also needs to be agreement about who should be offered treatment and what treatments should be offered; this evidence may emerge from RCTs
- The overall benefits of screening must outweigh the risks. This includes any physical and psychological harm caused by the test, the diagnostic procedures and the treatment
- Treatment facilities must be adequate and health services must have the capacity to deal with the extra clinical workload resulting from screening
- Screening overall must be cost effective compared to other health care interventions and demands. Costs include the testing, further diagnosis and treatment, administration, staff training and quality assurance. For example, because of its high unit cost, CT screening for any condition is unlikely to ever be effective unless proved extremely effective in early diagnosis of a common, highly remediable life-threatening condition. In a world of competing public health measures, debate continues about what is an acceptable cost per life year saved: £100—£5000—£35 000?
- The screening programme must be sustainable in terms of management, monitoring and agreed quality standards
- High-quality, realistic unbiased information needs to be offered to potential participants about the possible consequences of testing, investigation and treatment to help them decide whether or not to go ahead
- Ideally, any appropriate primary prevention interventions for the disease should have been implemented before or at least in parallel with the screening programme

LIMITATIONS OF SCREENING

Screening is conceptually and ethically different from usual clinical practice in that the process is aimed at the population as a whole, although achieved by dealing with apparently healthy individuals within that population. Participants expect that the diagnosis of the presence or absence of disease will be accurate, and that if disease is found, the outcome will be favourable. However, there can be no guarantee of protection because there will always be a small number of false positive and false negative results, however good the screening test. In addition, the disease may progress unexpectedly rapidly in the interval between screenings. This emphasises the importance of good education programmes for the population

and informed consent for individuals engaging in the programme.

Bias

A number of phenomena can foster mistaken claims for efficacy of a screening programme:

- **Lead time bias**—screening relies on the principle that potentially serious or fatal disease can be diagnosed at a specific and early stage in its natural history, and that this will definitively improve the morbidity and mortality compared with later diagnosis. However, if early diagnosis and treatment as a result of screening does not actually alter the course of the disease, that 'earlier' diagnosis gives the statistical illusion of prolonged survival. It also makes affected patients aware of the presence of their disease for a longer period
- **Selection bias** occurs where more health conscious people (often at lower risk of the disease in question) choose to undergo screening in contrast to those in the target population who do not attend for screening
- **Length bias** occurs when the screening test detects less aggressive disease (with a more benign natural history) than the type of disease that the screening programme was set up to discover. Length bias is frequently cited in the context of breast cancer screening

Participation rates

Universal participation in a screening programme is not usually necessary to achieve measurable community benefit and cost effectiveness. This is because community benefit is no more than the sum of the individual benefits (except when screening for infectious diseases such as tuberculosis). If a validated screening programme has low set-up costs, the benefits are usually proportional to the costs. For colorectal cancer screening, for example, cost effectiveness has been shown to fall off only at extremely low levels of participation.

OTHER ASPECTS OF SCREENING

Cost effectiveness

Within any debate about the desirability of screening for a particular condition, imponderables such as the economic value of saving a human life or of enhancing a period of survival need to be considered. All screening studies have a financial cost in detecting cases and treating them. The cost effectiveness of a screening programme is usually reported in terms of **cost per life year saved** or the cost of an increase in 'quality adjusted life years' (**QALYs**). However, the acceptable financial cost to a population of life year saved is a matter for debate;

somewhere between £12 000 and £30 000 is often quoted as acceptable in developed countries.

Research benefits

Screening a population at risk can teach the clinical community and the public much about the natural history and the progression of a disease, its aetiology and its various associations, for example the link between abdominal aortic aneurysm and smoking. Different investigations and treatments can be trialled in large groups of affected individuals, to the ultimate good of the population at large.

Consent

Organisers of screening programmes are obliged to provide participants with reliable and unbiased information about the benefits and risks of any particular screening process and its consequences. There must not, of course, be any form of coercion to participate. Much current information tends to overemphasise the benefits of screening and minimises the risks, often not clearly indicating that participation is voluntary. Breast cancer screening in the UK has been criticised in this respect.

SCREENING FOR CANCER

EARLY DETECTION OF CANCER

As a general principle, the earlier in its natural history that malignancy is diagnosed and treated, the better the prognosis. The ideal would be to detect cancer before invasion or metastasis had occurred, i.e. during the pre-invasive stage. However, many cancers invade and spread before they reach a detectable size or produce any tumour markers. Where true early detection is possible, health education can play an important part in alerting the public to early symptoms and warning signs. In the case of skin and testicular tumours, this should include regular self-examination. Self-examination is still promoted for breast cancer but there is little evidence that it is useful.

The common cancer killers are shown in Table 6.1, with carcinoma of the bronchus still leading the field. Unfortunately, this disease does not fit the criteria for screening, having no detectable early stage; attempts at screening have been uniformly ineffective.

In women, breast cancer is a huge public health problem, followed by carcinoma of the cervix and ovary. In men, prostate cancer is a large and growing problem.

Colorectal cancer is common and evenly matched in frequency in both sexes in the UK; 30 000 new cases are detected each year and 16 000 die of it. Gastric and pancreatic cancers are also big killers but screening is of little value except in areas of exceptionally high incidence. In China, high-risk areas for oesophageal cancer have been identified and brush cytology without gastroscopy has proved beneficial.

Several genetic predispositions to cancer have been identified, e.g. polyposis coli for colorectal cancer and BRCA1 and BRCA2 for breast and other cancers. Genetic screening is not covered in this chapter but individual disorders are described in other chapters.

CERVICAL CANCER

Pilot screening trials using cervical smears and Papanicolaou staining began in the UK in the mid-1960s and national screening started in 1988. Nearly all reports indicate that early detection and treatment prevents 80–90% of invasive cervical cancers and has greatly reduced the cervical cancer mortality. The International Agency for Research on Cancer (IARC) indicated that yearly screening between the ages of 25 and 64 reduces the incidence of invasive cancer by 94%, 3-yearly screening reduces it by 91%, 5-yearly by 84%, and 10-yearly by 64%. These figures provided the basis for the present UK policy—that yearly screening is unnecessarily frequent and 3- or 5-yearly screening is best.

In the UK, 4 million women are screened annually and 82% of the 14 million eligible women have been screened in the previous 5 years. The programme costs £150 million a year, which amounts to £37.50 per screen.

British data show that about a quarter of all cervical cancers occur in each of the four age groups 25–39, 40–54, 55–69 and 70+ years but there are problems with recruiting young women and women from lower socioeconomic strata. Both of these groups have been shown to be at higher risk. In a study from Hawaii in 2003, only 1 in 12 eligible women had not been screened in the pre-

Table 6.1 Most frequent deaths from cancer, England and Wales 2002

	Female	Male
Bronchus	11 500	17 500
Breast	11 500	80
Genital	7000	9000
Colorectal	5000	5000
Stomach and pancreas	5000	6500
Total	40 000	38 080

ceding 5 years, but this small group accounted for two-thirds of the invasive cancers in the community. Thus there are very real concerns that those at greatest risk are not being tested. In addition, those with positive results may not be being treated effectively. Recent recommendations in the UK are that women should first be invited for screening at age 25. They should then be screened 3-yearly until 49 and 5-yearly from 50 to 64. Women of 65+ only need screening if they have not been screened since age 50 or a recent abnormality has been found.

A recent cost effectiveness study from Peru, India, Kenya, Thailand and South Africa indicates that a single screen (and treatment if necessary), employing testing for human papillomavirus in cervical cells or visual inspection of the cervix after swabbing with acetic acid rather than a cervical smear is a cheap and effective way to reduce a woman's lifetime risk by 25–36%. Two rounds of screening, at 35 and 40 years, could reduce lifetime risk by a further 40%. If screening were introduced across the developing world then the global incidence of cervical cancer could fall by up to 50%.

BREAST CANCER

Screening for breast cancer by mammography was introduced nationally in the UK in the late 1980s following the Forrest report of 1986. Most developed countries employed a similar strategy following results from the HIP study of New York, the Swedish two-county study and the Canadian National Breast Screening Study. These studies appeared to demonstrate a 30% reduction in mortality from breast cancer in screened women. In the Swedish study, there was also a significant 13% reduction in all-cause mortality.

Mammographic screening detects breast cancers of smaller size than those presenting clinically, with around 30% being either carcinoma in situ or invasive cancers less than 0.5 cm in diameter. A high proportion are node negative—only about 20% have axillary spread compared with 40% for symptomatic cancer. As a result of detecting small lesions, screening substantially increases the reported incidence of invasive breast cancer. This might be expected to cause a fall in the incidence of new cases in later years, as prevalent cases would have been removed from the population at risk. In Norway and Sweden this has proved not to be the case, suggesting that screening is not picking up most of the clinically important cases that will progress to become invasive or metastasise.

In any population of women with breast cancer, there will be lesions at different stages of development and pathological potential. These may be grouped into three categories as follows:

- **Biologically early cancers**—these include lesions too small to be detectable but nevertheless with the potential to metastasise

- **Small cancers and carcinoma in situ**—these are predominantly non-aggressive lesions which may never metastasise
- **Large or advanced tumours**—these will usually be symptomatic and quickly fatal

Large trials have concluded that as many as one-third of cancers detected by screening would never have presented clinically in a patient's lifetime.

The sensitivity of breast screening for clinically significant cancers is poor; in particular, lobular or mucinous cancers and some rapidly proliferating, high-grade tumours may not be detectable. This is illustrated by the high proportion of **interval cancers** that present clinically between screening visits. In one representative series, 38% of all breast cancers presented as interval cancers. These tended to occur in younger patients with dense breasts and with a higher usage of hormone replacement therapy (HRT) or the oral contraceptive pill.

On the basis of tumour doubling times, it has been estimated that breast cancers detected clinically have been present for an average of 8 years, whereas mammographically detected lesions have been present for approximately 6 years—a long period in which to metastasise. This perhaps explains the failure of screening to increase the cure rate for the clinically significant cancers, and does call into question the political pressure for patients with suspected breast cancers to be evaluated within a very short time.

EFFECTIVENESS OF MAMMOGRAPHIC SCREENING

Mammographic screening every 2 years has been estimated to avert only 2 deaths in 1000 women aged between 50 and 59 over a period of 10 years. To achieve this requires 5000 screens and 242 recalls, and for 64 women to have at least one biopsy. Five women will have a ductal carcinoma in situ detected, some of which may never have progressed to invasive cancer. Less than 1% of women invited for screening will benefit from it; a much larger percentage have to endure the problems of false alarms, unnecessary surgery and inappropriately being labelled as having cancer.

In the USA, the independent Health Services/Technology Assessment Text (HSTAT) reviewed the published clinical trials and concluded that 'in absolute terms, the mortality benefit shown with mammography screening was small enough that biases in the trials could erase or create the observed mortality reduction'.

The Cochrane view of breast screening

The Cochrane Collaboration is an international non-profit organisation that rigorously and dispassionately reviews published research evidence and provides up-to-date information about the effects of health care. Over

11 000 articles have been published in the last 20 years on the subject of breast screening. The Nordic Cochrane Centre reviewed all RCTs in this area in 2001 and found that astonishingly few were of sufficient rigour to reliably determine whether screening reduced morbidity and mortality. Seven RCTs were identified, of which only two were regarded as being of sufficiently high quality. Evidence from the adequately randomised Canadian and Malmö trials showed that screening had no significant effect. The other five trials, in which randomisation was regarded as inadequate, found that screening decreased the risk of death by about 25%. However, these trials showed a slight **increase** in risk for screened women for death from any cause. A further Cochrane review was published in 2006, which reanalysed data from previously published trials.

Both Cochrane reviews found little detectable benefit from breast screening and stated in 2006 that the absolute risk reduction for breast cancer as a result of screening was only 0.05%. They also found that screening led to substantial over-diagnosis and over-treatment. They concluded: 'the currently available reliable evidence does not show a survival benefit of mass screening for breast cancer, and the evidence is inconclusive for breast cancer mortality'. These controversial conclusions imply that breast screening does no good, causes actual harm and probably should be abandoned. This, however, is unlikely to happen.

Why breast screening is claimed to improve survival

Several factors can explain how breast screening could appear to reduce mortality, as follows:

- Lead time bias, with over-detection of clinically insignificant lesions, increases the apparent number of breast cancer cases. These cases do well
- Breast cancer mortality can occur over a very long period; at 35 years after treatment, the commonest cause of death in a Cambridge UK series was still breast cancer. Thus screening studies need to be prolonged
- Parallel improvements in breast cancer treatment take place over the period of the main trials. Tamoxifen and perhaps better chemotherapy undoubtedly extended survival between the early and late 1980s in absolute terms. Over a similar period, reductions were also seen in other cancers for largely unknown reasons. Thyroid cancer incidence fell by 12%, testis by 17% and melanoma by 23%
- Subjectivity, unrealistic optimism and perhaps vested interests may lead to misleading presentation of statistics and unsustainable claims for the industry of breast screening

OTHER BENEFITS FROM BREAST SCREENING

The experience gained from breast screening and managing patients detected in this way has brought about rapid improvements in mammographic equipment, technique and interpretation as well as perhaps a more sensitive approach to breast disease. In addition, it has generated much scientific study of the management of early breast cancer. All of this will eventually bring about benefits for all women with breast cancer and for people with other types of cancer.

For the future, there is interest in using magnetic resonance imaging (MRI) as a screening test, particularly among high-risk women, as MRI detects significantly more cancers than mammography and is better able to discriminate between cancer and a scar. However, any role MRI might have in breast cancer screening has yet to be established.

COLORECTAL CANCER

Colorectal cancer is a major health hazard which kills 16 000 people a year in the UK; only about 10% are diagnosed early. Early cancers have survival rates of more than 90% but the all-stage overall 5-year survival rate of 35% has hardly improved despite advances in treatment, as most cases present late. Nine out of 10 cases occur in people over 50.

Screening for colonic cancer has a good chance of being effective. It fulfils many of the criteria required for a screening programme. In particular there is a clearly recognised sequence of adenoma progressing to adenocarcinoma. In addition, early cancers are detectable and are known to progress steadily to advanced cancers. About 75% of colorectal cancers arise sporadically, most likely in pre-existing adenomas. Thus a window of opportunity exists for detecting adenomatous polyps at a premalignant stage or cancers at an early invasive stage (i.e. pathologically less advanced than those with symptoms), at which stage they are potentially curable. The transition phase from benign to malignant is long, as shown by the cumulative risk of cancer in polyps 10 mm or greater being only 8% at 10 years.

However, detection methods are the stumbling block. The **sensitivity** of faecal occult blood (FOB) testing is no better than 50% and the **specificity** is also low. With 2-yearly FOB testing alone, there are also a high number of **interval cancers**: as many as 30–40% of cancers and as many as 80% of polyps are missed. However, both sensitivity and interval cancer rates can be improved by adding flexible sigmoidoscopy. Unfortunately, both faecal occult blood (FOB) testing and flexible endoscopy are distasteful and patient participation in these methods of screening is low. Better forms of screening would undoubtedly improve participation rates.

Despite the drawbacks of FOB testing, meta-analysis of four RCTs has shown that FOB screening can reduce mortality from colorectal cancer by 16% for those allocated to screening and by 23% of those actually screened. On this basis, a 2-yearly FOB screen offered to 10 000 people aged over 40 with two-thirds attending for at least one test would prevent 8.5 deaths (CI: 3.6–13.5) from colorectal cancer over 10 years, a mortality reduction of 23% (RR 0.77, CI: 0.57–0.89); 2800 participants would have a colonoscopy and there would be 3.4 major complications from this, i.e. perforation or haemorrhage (Cochrane). The cost of screening was £5290 per cancer detected and an estimated £1584 per life year gained.

Reports of pilot screening studies suggest screening could improve mortality by 33%, and national screening with FOB testing every 2 years has been approved for implementation in the UK. This started in April 2006 for men and women aged 60–69 (50–74 in Scotland) and is to be rolled out over 3 years. In addition, large-scale pilots of endoscopic colorectal screening are being trialled in patients in their late 50s.

PROSTATE CANCER

Prostate cancer is rapidly becoming the most common cause of cancer deaths in men. Unfortunately, as yet the prospects for prevention are poor. The problem is not so much in detecting the disease but in detecting it early enough (and accurately staging it) and predicting which early cancers are likely to progress. Many cancers remain forever dormant, as demonstrated by post mortem studies in men who have died of something else. Foci of prostate cancer occur in 70% of 70-year-olds, 60% of 60-year-olds and 50% of 50-year-olds. These patients die with the disease rather than from it and offering radical treatment for this type of disease is clearly inappropriate.

In the USA, uncontrolled screening using prostate specific antigen (PSA) has spawned an apparent epidemic of prostate cancer. The chairman of the UK National Screening Committee has stated that 'the scientific evidence is that screening for prostate cancer does not reduce mortality, and causes actual harm by exposing people to a procedure which has side effects of incontinence and impotence and where there is no evidence that they will benefit'.

The UK government sponsored a Health Technology Assessment on prostate screening in 1997, which stated that the criteria for a population screening programme had not been met. Their findings were that:

- The epidemiology and natural history of the disease were ill understood
- Screening tests were inaccurate and staging was unreliable
- There was poor evidence of the effectiveness of treatment
- Little research had been conducted into the complications and quality of life after radical treatment
- On present evidence, there was no justification for PSA testing in primary care and there was insufficient evidence to support national screening
- PSA testing should be limited to symptomatic men, to monitoring prostate cancer treatment and to randomised trials investigating screening

LUNG CANCER

A Cochrane review of all randomised controlled trials showed that no screening test had an impact on the treatment or deaths from lung cancer. Tests examined include chest X-ray, sputum tests and CT scanning.

SCREENING FOR CARDIOVASCULAR DISEASE

HYPERTENSION

Hypertension is an important cause of myocardial infarction and stroke. Lowering elevated blood pressure substantially lowers the risk. However, blood pressure on its own has proved to be a poor screening tool; in one large study, the 10% with the highest blood pressures suffered only 21% of the ischaemic cardiac events and only 28% of the ischaemic strokes. Even after adding other risk factors to the equation, including low-density lipoprotein (LDL) cholesterol, diabetes and smoking history, the top 5% had only 28% of the deaths from myocardial infarction. Advancing age or a previous cardiovascular event are probably the best predictors of future cardiovascular events, thus all patients with risk factors should receive best advice and appropriate treatment.

ABDOMINAL AORTIC ANEURYSM

INTRODUCTION

Ruptured abdominal aortic aneurysm (AAA) causes at least 6000 deaths each year in the UK and 1.4% of all deaths in men over 65. The peak mortality is between 65 and 85 years and the risk of rupture is roughly proportional to the diameter; when this reaches 6 cm, the risk rises sharply. A ruptured aortic aneurysm is nearly always an acute emergency and carries a very high mortality. About half the cases never reach hospital and die at home or in transit to hospital. Half of the remainder (25%) die without an operation and half of those undergoing operation die. Thus the true mortality rate is 85–90%. An emergency operation requires a trained vascular surgeon, ties up an emergency team for 3 or more hours, requires an intensive care bed for 3 or more days, uses large quantities of bank blood, and costs 25% more than an elective procedure, whether or not the patient survives. Detecting aortic aneurysms before they rupture means that less risky elective interventional procedures, which have a mortality of 5% or less, can be employed.

APPROPRIATENESS OF SCREENING FOR AAA

By WHO criteria, AAA is a near ideal candidate for screening. It is an important health problem, the natural history regarding expansion and rupture is fairly well understood, there is an easily detectable early stage, and treatment at an (appropriately) early stage is of greater benefit than at a later stage (i.e. ruptured). Ultrasound is a suitable and highly reliable test for the early stage and the test is acceptable, with an average of 80% of those invited attending. Appropriate intervals for repeating the test have been determined by randomised trials. There is adequate health service provision for the extra clinical workload resulting from the screen: a screening programme has been estimated to generate approximately 6 extra aneurysm repairs per year per surgeon.

Several trials have shown that the risks are less than the benefits, with up to 75% reduction in rupture rate, a low elective operative mortality, no excess psychological morbidity in those screened, and survival of those operated upon electively being little different from an unaffected population. Costs appear to be balanced against the benefits, with trials estimating the cost per life year saved at between zero (Huntingdon and Danish studies) and £12 500 (2006 figures from the UK Multicentre Aneurysm Screening Study).

TRIALS OF AAA SCREENING

Several large studies have published data, with a remarkable concordance between the results. The prevalence of AAA, the age distribution, the attendance rates among those invited, the reduction in AAA mortality and the cost effectiveness calculations from studies in Chichester, Gloucester, Huntingdon, Denmark, Western Australia and the large UK Multicentre Aneurysm Screening Study all concur.

Only one study, from Chichester, has randomised women into screening. The prevalence of AAA was six times lower in women (1.3%) than in men (7.6%). Over 5- and 10-year follow-up intervals, the incidence of rupture was the same in the screened and the control groups. Screening women for AAA was considered to be neither clinically indicated nor economically viable.

The Danish study

A Danish study randomised 12 500 men of 65 and over to AAA screen or nothing. Seventy five per cent attended and 4% had aneurysms. Screening reduced the rate of emergency surgery by 75% (CI: 51–91%), 59 were operated on electively with a 5.1% mortality. As regards cost effectiveness, 352 needed to be screened to save one life 4 years after screening. The screened population was rescreened after 5 years: 30% of those with aortas 25–29 mm developed an aneurysm but none of those originally less than 25 mm did so. People with aortas of 25 mm or more in diameter need periodic rescreening.

The Huntingdon study

In the Huntingdon study, 15 000 men of 50 and over were screened over the course of 7 years: 540 were found to

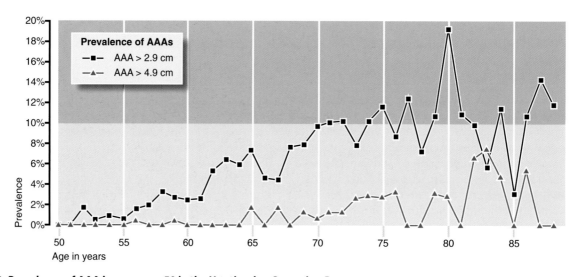

Fig. 6.1 Prevalence of AAA in men over 50 in the Huntingdon Screening Programme
The graphs show the percentage of those screened found to have small aneurysms (black line) and large aneurysms (green line). Note that the lines are approximately parallel, suggesting that small AAAs become large AAAs some years later.

have an AAA larger than 2.9 cm, and 69 an AAA larger than 4.9 cm (Fig. 6.1). Very few small and no large aneurysms were found under the age of 60, an important factor when planning a screening programme. Over the age of 70, there was virtually a 10% incidence of small AAAs. In this study, AAA mortality also fell by 75% and the number needed to be invited to save one life was 600.

The UK MASS study

Screening was undertaken in four centres and 68 000 people were randomised to screening or no screening, beginning in 1997. Ninety eight per cent of people in both groups were matched with national mortality statistics. After 7 years, 21% of men had died. There was a 76% attendance rate among those invited (27 147 were screened) and 4.9% were found to have an aortic diameter of 3 cm or greater. There was a reduction in all-cause mortality of 4% in those invited for screening and a 47% risk reduction for AAA deaths in this group. The cost of screening and treating detected aneurysms was £12 500 per life year saved and no adverse effects were found on quality of life. The 30-day mortality for elective cases was 6%; for emergency cases operated upon, mortality was 37%. It was calculated that if screening were offered to a population, only 6% of the AAA workload would eventually be ruptures compared with around 30% at present.

THE CONSEQUENCES OF SCREENING FOR AAA IN AN AREA

There is a rise in elective AAA surgery during the first 5–7 years as the existing but as yet undiagnosed cases are progressively detected. This is gradually offset by a fall in rupture rates and a reduction in surgical referrals of symptomatic and incidentally discovered aneurysms. This first becomes apparent 4 years after screening commences and continues rising until the entire population has been screened. The cost per life year saved compares favourably with colonic and cervical cancer.

PERIOPERATIVE CARE

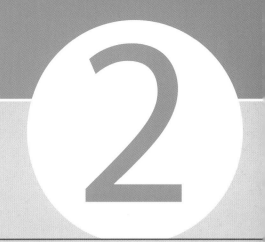

Preoperative assessment

7

INTRODUCTION

When a patient requires hospital admission for surgical investigation or treatment, a detailed history and examination (**clerking**) is usually undertaken and the findings recorded in the hospital notes. This forms an essential document for passing important information to others involved in the patient's care and is also a permanent record for medico-legal purposes should things go wrong. It is important that the notes are accurate and legible, that entries are dated and signed, and that the doctor's name is identifiable.

Where treatment is elective and can be planned, clerking is often performed at a separate **pre-assessment visit**. This process is concerned mainly with anticipating potential complications, both medical and social, and taking necessary preventive action rather than with diagnosing the primary disorder, although certain aspects of that should be checked at the same time (Box 7.1). Assessment may be performed by a junior doctor or a specially trained surgical or anaesthetic assistant. An anaesthetist (anaesthesiologist) will additionally make his or her own assessment, particularly where there is significant comorbidity.

For emergency admissions, clerking is often a layered process, with the most junior doctor performing the initial assessment and reporting to more senior doctors. For major trauma, however, senior staff are usually mobilised in advance of the arrival of the ambulance and are poised to apply the principles of the Advanced Trauma Life Support system in the resuscitation room. When clerking emergencies, diagnosis of the primary disorder is the prime purpose, but comorbidity and other complicating factors are sought at the same time.

PRINCIPLES OF ASSESSMENT

The essence of preoperative assessment is to pinpoint potential problems associated with the anaesthetic and operation, as well as social aspects of the admission, by careful questioning and examination. The next step is to optimise the patient's condition, taking the urgency of the surgical intervention into account. In preparing a patient for operation, the doctor needs to answer a series of questions which are summarised in Box 7.1. Findings from the history and examination may disclose the need for tests or some other action. Most surgical cases are straightforward but preventable disasters will occur unless a thorough and systematic approach is used. The history and examination will identify patients with medical comorbidity at particular risk of specific problems in the perioperative period. Part of the process is to review current treatment of comorbidity, e.g. diabetes, hypertension. Investigations may be needed to identify and characterise particular problems and to provide baseline information against which later changes can be measured, e.g. echocardiography in heart failure. The common problems of high-risk groups of patients are summarised in Table 7.1.

> **Box 7.1   Preoperative assessment and planning**
>
> **1. Diagnosis**
>
> - What is the (provisional) diagnosis and how confident is the diagnosis?
> - What are the important facets of the history?
> - What are the findings on examination?
> - What are the results of investigations already performed?
> - If appropriate, have tissue diagnoses been obtained before admission to hospital?
> - Are any further investigations needed to confirm the primary diagnosis?
>
> **2. Operation**
>
> - What operation or procedure is planned?
> - Have any circumstances changed relating to the planned operation?
> - Has the patient got better or worse?
> - Has any new diagnostic information appeared? (e.g. pulmonary metastases on a chest X-ray)
> - Is the planned operation still appropriate?
> - Are there any special risks attending this particular operation, intraoperative or postoperative? (e.g. risk of DVT after pelvic surgery)
> - Are there any standard procedures that need to be performed in relation to the operation? (e.g. ordering blood if heavy blood loss is anticipated)
> - Are there operation-specific actions that need to be performed? (e.g. examining vocal cord movement before thyroid surgery, arranging peroperative radiology for cholangiogram during cholecystectomy)
>
> **3. Anaesthesia**
>
> - What type of anaesthesia is to be employed?
> - Can any anaesthetic complications be anticipated? (e.g. risk of postoperative chest infection after thoracotomy or upper
>
> abdominal surgery, risk of a patient with bowel obstruction inhaling vomitus during anaesthetic induction)
>
> **4. Fitness for operation**
>
> - Are there any intercurrent diseases and are they currently being appropriately treated, e.g. insulin-dependent diabetes, or any that might pose special problems? e.g. rheumatoid arthritis with cervical spine involvement
> - Are any preoperative investigations or treatments needed for intercurrent disease? (e.g. lung function tests and physiotherapy for chronic bronchitis, cervical spine radiology for rheumatoid arthritis)
> - Does the surgical condition itself pose special problems? (e.g. fluid or electrolyte disturbances as a result of recent vomiting)
> - Is the patient taking any drugs which might cause problems with anaesthesia or operation? (e.g. monoamine oxidase inhibitors or corticosteroids)
> - Is the patient fit for the planned anaesthetic and operation?
>
> **5. High risk**
>
> - Is this patient particularly predisposed to anaesthetic or surgical complications (Table 7.1)?
>
> **6. After the operation**
>
> - Can any special problems be anticipated for this patient during the postoperative period and after discharge from hospital? (e.g. elderly patients living alone)
> - Are there any problems specific to this anaesthetic or operation with respect to recovery and rehabilitation, and is any special planning required? (e.g. prostheses after mastectomy, stoma care, limb fitting and rehabilitation following amputation)

ESSENTIALS OF PREOPERATIVE ASSESSMENT

Although procedures vary in different hospitals, certain basic steps must be taken to ensure the greatest safety of a patient before operation (see Box 7.2). These steps depend on the nature and urgency of the operation and the condition of the patient.

EXPLANATIONS TO THE PATIENT AND INFORMED CONSENT

The surgeon or a trained assistant must carefully explain the diagnosis and the proposed operation and any appropriate alternatives to the patient beforehand. Patients often absorb very little of what has been said initially, however, and are unable to comprehend the full implications. This is because most have little understanding of

how their body works and they are often anxious about their condition and the treatment and are overwhelmed by the clinic visit.

For **elective operations**, consent should be a two stage process, the initial explanation and options being discussed well in advance, without the pressure of an imminent operation, and then the patient's understanding of what's to be done and his or her consent confirmed before operation. The patient should be given information leaflets at an early stage, and perhaps given guidance about reliable and accurate internet sites. The doctor must adopt a sympathetic and unhurried approach and must often explain things more than once. By this means, the surgeon can ensure the patient is giving informed consent as far as this is possible. This also requires an account of poten-

Table 7.1 High risk groups for perioperative complications

Group	Particular risks	Management
Premature or tiny babies, neonates and infants	Fluid and electrolyte loss Heat loss in operating theatre	Careful measurement and replacement Warming blanket, temperature monitoring
Patients over 60	Cardiovascular disease	Chest X-ray and ECG preoperatively if indicated by guidelines, and monitoring during operation
Very elderly patients	Confusion Hyponatraemia Immobility	Multifactorial—see Chapter 8 Preoperative electrolyte estimations and correction Good nursing and rehabilitation
Smokers	Postoperative chest infection and atelectasis Increased risk of myocardial infarction	Stop smoking before operation—ideally at least four weeks beforehand Preoperative chest X-ray Preoperative and postoperative physiotherapy Preoperative ECG; avoid hypoxia during and after operation; postoperative oxygen therapy
Obese patients	Increased risk of DVT Increased risk of other complications, e.g. wound infection Reduced mobility	DVT prophylaxis (see Ch. 12) Preoperative counselling during consent process Early mobilisation with assistance Encoorage patients to lose weight prior to surgery
Patients with intercurrent medical disease	Depends on medical condition	Early referral to anaesthetist and/or medical specialist

Box 7.2 Essential steps in preoperative assessment and preparation

- History taking
- Physical examination
- Collating pre-admission information about diagnosis
- Arranging any further diagnostic investigations
- Making special preparations for the particular operation
- Investigating any intercurrent or occult illness suggested by medical clerking or enlisting appropriate specialist help
- Discussing the operation and the recovery period with the patient and obtaining signed consent
- Marking the operation site
- Making arrangements for the operation with the operating theatre staff
- Arranging and informing the anaesthetist
- Prescribing medication, prophylactic antibiotics and treatment to prevent thromboembolism, as appropriate
- Planning rehabilitation and convalescence

tial complications with more than a 1–5% risk as a result of the procedure, or of any less common but serious procedure-specific risks such as recurrent laryngeal nerve injury in thyroid surgery.

For **emergency surgery**, there may not be time to go through this entire process, nor may it be clear what might be found at operation, but clear explanations by the surgeon or a surgeon capable of performing the operation should be given as far as possible, and if necessary include close relatives. It should be remembered that patients trust doctors for the most part and seek their guidance on what should be done. For many conditions, the doctor will be unambiguous about what treatment he or she recommends, but must be prepared to discuss alternatives and offer equivalent options, even if it means referral to another specialist. Patients tend to be attracted to treatments perceived as modern, often involving 'keyhole surgery' and lasers, but a balanced view must be presented, with the doctor understanding the risks and benefits of each procedure.

PLANNING THE RECOVERY PERIOD

If the immediate postoperative period is likely to be unpleasant or unfamiliar, such as admission to an intensive care unit, it is prudent to forewarn the patient and arrange a visit to the unit beforehand. Patients with learning difficulties and the elderly have particular difficulty in adapting to changing circumstances and care should be taken to familiarise them with facilities and staff.

Plans for rehabilitation and convalescence should be discussed with the patient and relatives in advance. The patient should be advised about the likely rate of recovery and the level of activity possible on discharge. In this way, social, business and domestic arrangements can be made in good time. If necessary, domestic or home nursing help can be arranged. Uncertainty about these matters often causes anxiety and hampers recovery.

MARKING THE OPERATION SITE

At the time of obtaining final consent, the surgeon should **mark the operation site** on the patient's skin with an indelible pen. This is particularly important if the operation could be performed on either side of the body, for example an inguinal hernia or limb amputation. It is even more important if the patient is likely to be turned prone (face down) in theatre as this often results in confusion as to the side of operation, and failure to mark the site represents a disaster in waiting. This marking procedure also gives the patient an opportunity to agree which operation is to be done and on which side. Careful checking processes for identity, type of operation, side and marking should be in place at several stages during the patient's journey to the operating theatre. Of course, the surgeon needs to be entirely clear what is to be done on the anaesthetised patient presented to him or her!

IMMEDIATE PREOPERATIVE STARVATION AND FLUID RESTRICTION

Any patient about to undergo general anaesthesia must have an empty stomach to minimise the risk of aspiration of gastric contents into the lung on induction of anaesthesia or during early recovery. Local practice varies to a degree but, in general, no solid food or drinks containing milk should be taken for 6 hours before surgery. Clear fluids may be taken for up to 3 hours before surgery in adults or 2 hours in children. In patients at particular risk of inhalation, e.g. with gastro-oesophageal reflux disease, gastric outlet obstruction or hiatus hernia, the anaesthetist may prescribe acid suppressing and prokinetic drugs.

LIAISON WITH ANAESTHETIST

For elective cases, the anaesthetist should be informed in advance of the proposed operation or list of operations. Pre-assessment will often have been done already and potential problems anticipated. For emergency cases, the anaesthetist needs to know which operation is intended for which patient, how urgent the procedure is, and the condition of the patient and the state of resuscitation. The anaesthetist visits the patient to anticipate problems, discuss the planned anaesthetic procedures and prescribe premedication if appropriate. The anaesthetist is ultimately responsible for ensuring that the patient is fit for the operation and usually assists in the process of resuscitation.

OPERATING THEATRE ARRANGEMENTS

For elective and emergency cases, the house surgeon (intern) is usually responsible for informing the operating department about the operation(s) and the need for any special arrangements. A formal **operating list** should be prepared, giving full details of the name, age, sex, ward, and proposed operation for each patient. The side of the body to be operated on should be clearly (and correctly!) indicated. In addition, any special requirements for instruments, intraoperative radiography or patient positioning must be noted on the list. The presence of meticillin-resistant *Staphylococcus aureus* (MRSA) infection or a carrier state should be recorded, as well as any significant allergies, e.g. to latex or iodine. In some hospitals, the amount of bank blood ordered for a patient is also noted on the list. If changes are made to the list, a complete new list should replace the old to avoid confusion.

PLANNING THE ORDER OF AN OPERATING LIST

For an elective operating list, several elements govern the order in which patients are best operated upon:

1. **Latex allergy**—the theatre needs to have all latex containing products removed and be 'purged', i.e. pressure ventilated, for several hours beforehand
2. **Paediatric cases**—to minimise the period of starvation and to reduce anxiety
3. **Diabetic patients**—to make perioperative diabetes management as smooth as possible, minimise the period of starvation and return rapidly to normal diet and treatment
4. **Adult day cases**—to maximise the amount of available recovery time before discharge
5. **In-patients** with no special theatre requirements
6. **Contaminated, infected cases, colorectal cases, gangrenous limbs**—so as not to infect later cases on the list
7. **Patients with transmissible infections**, e.g. MRSA, blood-borne viral infections requiring barrier nursing—non-essential equipment and personnel are removed from theatre; disposable items replace recyclable items of linen, and theatre can be cleaned before next list

PREPARATION FOR MAJOR OPERATION—CASE HISTORY

This case history illustrates the way a patient might be prepared for a major operation and the considerations that guide the preoperative management. This account is a full record that would be recorded in the hospital notes.

HISTORY

James Brown, a 70-year-old retired farmer, with a proven carcinoma at the rectosigmoid junction admitted electively for an anterior resection of the rectum.

Present complaint

Seen urgently in outpatient clinic 3 weeks ago with a 5-week history of loose stools three to five times a day, without blood or mucus. GP reported three stool specimens were positive for occult blood. Lost about 4 kg in weight over the last 3 months, but has been trying to lose weight anyway.

Results of outpatient investigations

- Flexible sigmoidoscopic examination—obvious fungating tumour of upper rectum. Scope could not be passed beyond it. Biopsies confirmed adenocarcinoma
- Contrast enhanced CT scan of abdomen and pelvis—no other synchronous colonic cancers seen; liver free of metastases
- Chest X-ray—normal, no metastases
- Transrectal ultrasound for local staging—no spread outside the bowel wall
- Blood tests: full blood count—haemoglobin 11.6 g/L, otherwise normal. Urea and electrolytes, liver function tests—normal

Systems enquiry

Generally well, but recent onset of shortness of breath after walking 200 metres on flat ground and occasional fast palpitations. No other cardiorespiratory symptoms. Poor stream on micturition. Nil else on systemic enquiry.

Past medical history

Appendicectomy aged 14; no anaesthetic complications. Serious farming injury to left elbow aged 20. Jaundiced during the Second World War in Asia, nil since. Hypertensive for 10 years and on drug treatment for 5 years. Diabetes discovered 3 years ago on routine urine testing, controlled by diet alone.

Family history

Mother was obese; died age 55 from complications of diabetes (gangrene). Older brother had major stroke at 64 but partially recovered. No family history of bowel cancer.

Social history

Widowed for 2 years, wife died of breast cancer. Has one son and one daughter, both married with young children but living far away. Lives in own house with an upstairs lavatory, on a smallholding with a few stock animals. Lives independently, and uses car for shopping. Smoked 20 cigarettes a day since age 15; alcohol intake averages 4 units a day.

Drug history

Takes atenolol 50 mg (a beta-blocker) and bendroflumethiazide 2.5 mg (a diuretic) once a day in the morning for hypertension. Takes aspirin 75 mg daily 'for his heart'. Told in the past not to have penicillin, but cannot recall why; does not remember when he last had penicillin. Not allergic to iodine.

EXAMINATION

General. Fit-looking man of 70, not obviously anxious. Tanned; not evidently anaemic; no cyanosis, jaundice, lymphadenopathy or clubbing; no thyroid enlargement. Fingers tobacco stained. Not febrile. (Continued on p. 107.)

Table 7.2 Example of preoperative assessment of a patient admitted for a major operation (case history given above)

Problem	Surgical significance	Plan of action for each problem
1. 'Mild' diabetes mellitus	No such thing as mild diabetes! Is it under good control?	All urine samples to be tested for glucose Fasting blood glucose estimation and HbA1c May need sliding scale insulin perioperatively
2. Obesity	Multiple potential problems Lifting and handling on the ward and in the operating theatre May make access difficult at operation Predisposes to wound infection Increased risk of deep vein thrombosis or pulmonary embolism	Early referral to anaesthetist Is special bed or operating table required? Availability of hoist postoperatively Ensure adequate theatre time available plus at least two assistants Consider delayed primary closure of wound if contaminated Prophylaxis, e.g. low dose heparin plus graduated compression stockings
3. Hypertension	How well is hypertension controlled on present medication? Is elevated BP on admission just due to anxiety? Are there other complications of hypertension such as ventricular hypertrophy or dilatation?	Monitor blood pressure 4-hourly on admission and then decide about drug therapy Check pulse rate and BP at intervals over several hours Perform (and check) ECG and chest X-ray. Echocardiography if indicated

Table 7.2 Example of preoperative assessment of a patient admitted for a major operation (case history given above)—cont'd

Problem	Surgical significance	Plan of action for each problem
4. Recent shortness of breath on exertion and palpitations	Are these merely symptoms of anxiety about the diagnosis or do they represent significant cardiac or respiratory disease?	Consult cardiologist re palpitations ECG and chest X-ray Possibly needs lung function tests Recheck Hb—has anaemia worsened since outpatient visit?
5. Poor urinary stream and enlarged prostate	Possible carcinoma of prostate Possible difficulty with catheterisation that will be required at operation Risk of postoperative urinary retention when catheter removed	Transrectal ultrasound; biopsy if necessary Measure plasma PSA Anticipate—may need suprapubic catheterisation kit in theatre Anticipate
6. Jaundice in the past	History suggestive of hepatitis	Serological tests needed if hepatitis B or C is likely
7. Smoker	Possible occult lung cancer Possible impaired lung function Increased risk of postoperative chest infections Increased risk of myocardial infarction	Chest X-ray Respiratory function tests Preoperative physiotherapy and breathing exercises Postoperative oxygen therapy
8. Left elbow injury	May cause inconvenience during operation	Inform theatre staff about need for careful positioning on the operating table
9. Diuretic therapy	Are electrolytes and renal function normal?	Plasma urea, electrolytes and creatinine estimations
10. Aspirin therapy	Could gastric irritation partly account for the mild anaemia? May cause excess bleeding at operation	Use non gastric irritant analgesics Anticipate—stop 10–14 days before surgery if practicable
11. Possible penicillin allergy	A penicillin is often used for prophylaxis or treatment of postoperative infections	Record possible penicillin allergy; alternative drugs may have to be used
12. Cardiac murmur	Is this clinically significant? Is cardiac antibiotic prophylaxis necessary?	Consult anaesthetist or cardiologist; consider echocardiogram Consult guidelines, e.g. BNF
13. Lives alone, looks after animals	Who will look after his animals while he is in hospital? Who will look after him when he returns home?	Discuss domestic arrangements and convalescence plans with medical social worker
14. Low haemoglobin	Not low enough to need preoperative transfusion but there is less reserve for the operation Potentially extensive operation—may have large blood loss	Cross-match at least two units of blood to cover operation Cross-match extra blood, i.e. at least 4 units in all
15. May need temporary or even permanent colostomy	What does he understand about stomas? Will he be able to cope?	Refer to stoma nurse for counselling and possible preoperative 'trial' of colostomy appliance (see Ch. 27)
16. Bowel will be opened during operation	Potential for faecal contamination of abdominal cavity and wound	Likely to need preoperative bowel preparation and will need perioperative prophylactic antibiotics
17. Lesion at pelvic brim	Does it involve the ureter?	Consider ultrasonography of kidneys to exclude hydronephrosis
18. Varicose veins	Increases risk of DVT (already high because of major pelvic operation and age 70)	Give prophylaxis—low dose heparin, antiembolism stockings Early mobilisation

Cardiovascular and respiratory system. Pulse 68 beats per minute and regular. BP 150/110 mmHg. Soft systolic murmur at the left sternal edge. No ankle swelling and JVP not elevated. Extensive bilateral varicose veins. Chest examination unremarkable apart from a few crepitations which do not clear with coughing.

Abdomen. Moderately obese. Appendicectomy scar. Soft to palpation. No organomegaly. Possible mass in left iliac fossa—not indentable (i.e. not faeces). No groin hernias. External genitalia normal. Rectal examination— moderately enlarged smooth prostate and normal-coloured stool.

Central nervous system and locomotor system. Fixed flexion deformity of left elbow at 90°, otherwise normal.

SUMMARY

A 70-year old man with proven rectosigmoid carcinoma without obvious dissemination, admitted for anterior resection of the recto-sigmoid.

A problem list was constructed from this information, which led to further investigations and a management plan. The reasoning is shown in Table 7.2.

8 Medical problems

INTRODUCTION

'Medical' disorders appear in surgical practice in four main ways:

- A pre-existing medical condition may precipitate a surgical admission because of exacerbation, progression or complications of the condition: for example, foot problems in patients with diabetes
- A pre-existing medical condition may be made worse by operation. In chronic obstructive pulmonary disease for example, general anaesthesia and postoperative sputum retention may precipitate a life-threatening pneumonia
- A surgical condition may be complicated by an unrelated medical disorder. For example, a patient with rheumatoid arthritis on steroid therapy is vulnerable to impaired healing and recurrent infection
- An occult condition can become manifest under the stress of anaesthesia and operation. For example, perioperative or postoperative myocardial infarction can be caused by occult ischaemic heart disease

CARDIAC AND CEREBROVASCULAR DISEASE

Many surgical patients are elderly and thus have an increased risk of cardiovascular disease. Cardiovascular disease and respiratory disorders account for most postoperative medical (as opposed to surgical) complications.

Emergency surgery in patients with cardiac disease is about four times more likely to result in death than the same operation done electively. Thus, preoperative assessment is particularly important in emergency patients so any cardiac condition can be stabilised, electrolyte imbalanced corrected and appropriate anaesthesia, surgical technique, monitoring and aftercare employed to minimise risk.

1. ISCHAEMIC HEART DISEASE

The most common clinical manifestations of ischaemic heart disease are:

- Angina and previous myocardial infarction
- Cardiac failure
- Arrhythmias, e.g. atrial fibrillation

Asymptomatic myocardial ischaemia may progress to infarction under the various stresses of anaesthesia and operation. These stresses include laryngoscopy and endotracheal intubation, pain, hypoxia, rapid blood loss, anaemia, hypotension, hypocarbia and fluid overload. For major operations, general anaesthesia and spinal anaesthesia carry similar risks. Local anaesthesia is far safer wherever it is practicable.

Clinical problems

a. Unstable coronary syndromes

Stable angina poses little increased risk during operation but unstable or severe angina or myocardial infarction within the previous 3 months is a major risk factor and indicates the need for intensive management and, if practicable, delaying the operation. Nitrates, which dilate the coronary arteries and reduce preload and left ventricular work, may reduce cardiac ischaemia during general anaesthesia and should not be stopped in the perioperative period. A transdermal nitrate patch is a useful alternative to tablets or sprays. Beta-adrenergic blockers, which reduce cardiac work and oxygen demand, should be continued unless non-ischaemic cardiac failure develops.

b. Myocardial infarction

Myocardial infarction associated with surgery usually occurs during the first few days after operation, particularly on the second to fourth postoperative nights, rather than during the operation. Typical chest pain is not always a feature; postoperative infarction may present 'silently' (i.e. painlessly) with hypotension, cardiac failure, arrhythmias or cardiac arrest, particularly in patients with diabetes. Diagnosis can usually be made by typical electrocardiograph (ECG) changes, especially if a preoperative ECG is available for comparison. A troponin I level taken between 14 and 18 hours after the insult is a very sensitive and specific indicator of myocardial infarction.

Preoperative assessment of ischaemic heart disease

The cardiac history should include questions about previous myocardial infarction, angina and particularly exercise tolerance, e.g. on stairs. Exercise functioning is by far the most important indicator of the patient's ability to tolerate anaesthesia and surgery.

An ECG should be performed before operation on all patients over 60 years of age and on any patient with cardiac symptoms or signs. Preoperative ECGs may show arrhythmias, ischaemic changes or evidence of previous infarction. They are also worth their weight in gold during the 3 a.m. assessment of a postoperative patient with chest pain or other features suggesting acute myocardial damage!

In patients undergoing major surgery, a preoperative exercise ECG test may give useful information. However, it should be remembered that symptoms of angina and ECG changes come relatively late in the evolution of myocardial ischaemia, so if there is concern from the history or the resting or exercise ECG that there may be a major risk of cardiovascular disease, then coronary angiography with appropriate revascularisation (if possible) is the best course of action. Patients with ischaemic heart disease will usually be taking low dose aspirin (and sometimes clopidogrel) and the risks of increased bleeding have to be balanced against the risks of stopping anti-platelet therapy.

2. CARDIAC FAILURE

The condition of patients with cardiac failure should be optimised before operation, but even so it is important to be aware that there is still a substantially increased mortality rate after major surgery of up to 5%. The causes, symptoms and signs of cardiac failure are shown in Figure 8.1.

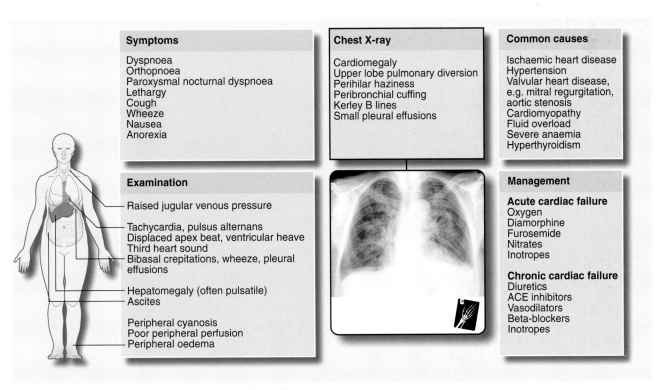

Symptoms

Dyspnoea
Orthopnoea
Paroxysmal nocturnal dyspnoea
Lethargy
Cough
Wheeze
Nausea
Anorexia

Examination

Raised jugular venous pressure

Tachycardia, pulsus alternans
Displaced apex beat, ventricular heave
Third heart sound
Bibasal crepitations, wheeze, pleural effusions

Hepatomegaly (often pulsatile)
Ascites

Peripheral cyanosis
Poor peripheral perfusion
Peripheral oedema

Chest X-ray

Cardiomegaly
Upper lobe pulmonary diversion
Perihilar haziness
Peribronchial cuffing
Kerley B lines
Small pleural effusions

Common causes

Ischaemic heart disease
Hypertension
Valvular heart disease,
e.g. mitral regurgitation,
aortic stenosis
Cardiomyopathy
Fluid overload
Severe anaemia
Hyperthyroidism

Management

Acute cardiac failure
Oxygen
Diamorphine
Furosemide
Nitrates
Inotropes

Chronic cardiac failure
Diuretics
ACE inhibitors
Vasodilators
Beta-blockers
Inotropes

Fig. 8.1 The causes, symptoms and signs of cardiac failure
The chest X-ray is of a 60-year-old woman with a history of ischaemic heart disease. The signs are indicative of congestive heart failure.
Note: some of these changes are very subtle and do not reproduce well in illustrations.

Clinical problems

a. Cardiac failure before operation

Surgery should be postponed until cardiac failure has been treated and stabilised. Hasty preoperative diuretic therapy is dangerous because it may provoke dehydration and electrolyte abnormalities. Plasma urea, electrolytes and creatinine should be measured before operation because patients taking diuretics and angiotensin-converting enzyme (ACE) inhibitors may have abnormalities of fluid and electrolytes, such as chronic dehydration or hypokalaemia.

Over-treatment with diuretics may cause:

- Low serum potassium (usually due to potassium-losing diuretics prescribed without potassium supplements)
- Low serum sodium concentration
- Raised serum urea and creatinine with raised serum potassium (particularly if taking an ACE inhibitor and spironolactone)
- Thirst
- Anorexia
- Postural hypotension

b. Cardiac failure developing during or after operation

This problem most often results from poor tolerance of intravenous fluids or unaccustomed supine posture. Cardiac failure can also result from myocardial infarction or ischaemia in the perioperative period, or arrhythmias induced by the stresses of surgery and anaesthesia, for example at laryngoscopy or with poor pain control. Prompt and vigorous diuretic therapy with intravenous furosemide is required to prevent worsening cardiac failure, hypoxia, renal failure or other potentially lethal complications. In addition, treatment of any precipitating factors should be instituted such as reducing cardiac stress by giving good pain relief. Postoperative cardiac failure is best managed in an intensive care unit, using a central venous pressure (CVP) line to guide fluid replacement.

Preoperative assessment of cardiac failure

Chest X-ray will demonstrate cardiomegaly and may show signs of pulmonary oedema including upper lobe diversion, hilar congestion, septal Kerley B lines and pleural effusions (see Fig. 8.1). ECG may show an arrhythmia, myocardial ischaemia, ventricular hypertrophy, left bundle branch block or loss of R waves. Left ventricular function can be assessed by echocardiography and documented more precisely by radionuclide studies using multiple gated acquisition (MUGA). If there is any doubt about the fitness of a patient for operation, a cardiological opinion should be sought.

3. CARDIAC ARRHYTHMIAS

Clinical problems

a. Atrial fibrillation (Fig. 8.2)

This is usually secondary to ischaemic heart disease but may be caused by mitral valve disease or thyrotoxicosis. Atrial fibrillation with a controlled ventricular rate (i.e. a pulse rate of less than 90 beats per minute at rest) causes minimal extra risk. An uncontrolled ventricular rate may cause perioperative cardiac failure. Atrial fibrillation (even with a controlled ventricular response) increases the risk of **arterial embolism** from any thrombus present in the left atrium. Adequate control of ventricular rate should be achieved before operation with digoxin, occasionally supplemented with verapamil, amiodarone or beta-adrenergic blockade. Digoxin can be given intravenously if rapid control is necessary but potassium levels need to be monitored closely as digoxin given in the presence of hypokalaemia leads to a variety of further arrhythmias. If the patient is anticoagulated with warfarin, there is a small risk of excessive bleeding at operation; stabilising the international normalised ratio (INR) between 1.5 and 2.5 may be the safest option. Another alternative is to stop warfarin and change to intravenous heparin. Although theoretically more precise, it is difficult to manage safely in practice.

Common causes in surgical patients	Diagnosis	Management

Acute causes
  Anastomotic leakage after bowel resection
  Myocardial infarction
  Pneumonia
  Pulmonary embolism
 	
Chronic causes
  Ischaemic heart disease
  Heart failure
  Hypertension
  Mitral valve disease
  Hyperthyroidism
  Alcohol abuse
	Examination
	Pulse irregularly irregular
	Apex rate is greater than radial pulse rate
	
	ECG
	Absent P waves
	Irregular QRS complexes
	Atrial fibrillation
		1 Treat any reversible precipitating factors
		2 Control ventricular rate.
		  Drugs commonly used include:
		    Digoxin
		    Beta-blockers
		    Verapamil
		    Amiodarone
		3 Consider cardioversion to sinus rhythm (if acute onset)
		4 Anticoagulation to prevent emboli

Fig. 8.2 Atrial fibrillation—causes, diagnosis and management

b. Bradycardia

Bradycardia is common in young fit athletic patients and is not a problem. In patients taking beta-blockers or digoxin, if the apex rate is below 60 beats per minute, that day's dose should be omitted and the regular dose reviewed.

Bradycardia may be caused by **complete heart block**, easily diagnosed on electrocardiography. This requires urgent **transvenous pacing** unless the block results from acute (usually inferior) myocardial infarction without haemodynamic compromise. In this case, the situation may be observed as the heart block may rapidly resolve spontaneously. If the onset of atrial arrhythmia (particularly atrial fibrillation) is associated with right bundle branch block on the ECG, this suggests a diagnosis of pulmonary embolism.

If a patient has a **cardiac pacemaker**, it is important to know the reason for its insertion: is the patient pacemaker dependent, has the pacemaker been checked recently, what type of pacemaker has been inserted? Surgical diathermy, particularly monopolar diathermy, can interfere with the pacemaker if the current flows close to the heart. Ideally, bipolar diathermy should be used if diathermy is required. In addition a strong magnet should be available; if placed over the pacemaker this will revert the rate to 100 beats/min.

c. Other arrhythmias

Bifascicular block, in which conduction is impaired down two of the three main fascicles (right bundle plus anterior or posterior divisions of the left bundle), may progress to complete heart block (and low cardiac output) under anaesthesia. For these patients, a prophylactic temporary transvenous pacemaker should be seriously considered before operation.

4. HYPERTENSION

About one in four patients coming to surgery is either hypertensive or is receiving antihypertensive therapy. Most have **'essential' hypertension**, but other causes include oral contraceptives, renal parenchymal disease, renal artery stenosis and phaeochromocytoma (Fig. 8.3).

Clinical problems

a. Mild-to-moderate essential hypertension

Patients with a systolic pressure of less than 180 mmHg and a diastolic less than 110 mmHg are at minimal risk of cardiac complications unless there is some other cardiovascular disease. Sometimes, anxiety about the operation contributes to the hypertension. A labile blood pressure or systolic hypertension at any time may, however, indicate widespread atherosclerosis.

b. Treated hypertension

Diuretic therapy may cause fluid and electrolyte abnormalities. These should be corrected before operation.

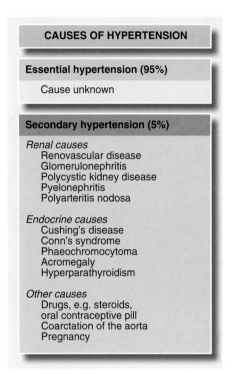

Fig. 8.3 Causes of hypertension

Most common antihypertensive drugs are cardioprotective and should not be stopped prior to general anaesthesia. Despite the patient being 'nil by mouth' in the immediate preoperative period, the normal dose of oral antihypertensive drugs should usually be given with a small amount of water. Sudden withdrawal of antihypertensive drugs may cause rebound hypertension. Withdrawal of beta-blockers may trigger autonomic hyperactivity and lability of blood pressure. Postural hypotension may occur after operation, especially if there is dehydration.

c. Severe or poorly controlled hypertension

If the diastolic BP is ≥ 110 mmHg, then treatment needs to be instituted and any non-urgent operative procedure delayed. During anaesthesia the untreated hypertensive patient has a very labile BP and is at high risk of perioperative myocardial infarction, cardiac failure or stroke.

Preoperative assessment of hypertensive patients

Chest X-ray may identify cardiomegaly or cardiac failure, both of which increase the perioperative morbidity and mortality. An ECG may reveal signs of ventricular hypertrophy and ischaemia. Serum urea and electrolytes should be measured in all patients taking diuretics or ACE inhibitors and in any patient with suspected chronic renal failure.

5. CEREBROVASCULAR DISEASE

A patient has cerebrovascular disease if there is a **history of stroke or transient ischaemic attacks (TIAs)**.

Cerebral atherosclerosis may render the blood flow to the brain precarious, with an increased risk of perioperative stroke from hypoxia, hypotension or increased blood viscosity resulting from dehydration.

Patients with **ischaemic heart disease** or **peripheral vascular disease** should also be assumed to have cerebrovascular disease and, as a minimum, the carotid arteries should be auscultated for bruits. In high-risk patients, a duplex Doppler examination of the carotids should ideally be performed, and patients with a stenosis greater than 70% considered for carotid endarterectomy before the planned operation if conditions permit. The anaesthetist should be warned of any signs or symptoms suggestive of carotid artery disease so that special care can be taken to avoid hypotension during surgery.

After a **stroke**, operation should be avoided for at least 2 months, if practicable. This is because autoregulation of cerebral blood pressure becomes disrupted after a stroke, so that cerebral arterial pressure becomes directly related to systemic arterial pressure. Brain perfusion thus loses the buffering effect of autoregulation on peaks and troughs of blood pressure that tend to occur during anaesthesia and surgery. If operation cannot be delayed, it is important to prevent hypertension and hypotension in the perioperative period.

There are few other measures likely to reduce cerebrovascular complications in patients with cerebrovascular disease, although there is an argument for prescribing low-dose **aspirin** (75 mg daily) to inhibit platelet aggregation. The surgeon needs to be involved in any decision to stop or start aspirin; in any case, this needs to be stopped at least a week before major surgery to reduce the risk of excessive bleeding.

6. VALVULAR HEART DISEASE (Fig. 8.4)

The common valvular abnormalities are listed here in decreasing order of frequency: mitral regurgitation, aortic stenosis, aortic regurgitation and mitral stenosis. Any of these may dangerously alter cardiovascular dynamics, but stenotic lesions are more serious than regurgitant ones, as the cardiac output tends to be fixed.

Under perioperative stress, valvular disease may precipitate acute myocardial ischaemia, hypotension, cardiac failure, arrhythmias or thromboembolism. Valvular heart disease also predisposes to infective endocarditis. Thus certain operations need to be covered by antibiotic prophylaxis.

Aortic stenosis

Aortic stenosis is potentially the most serious valvular disorder in a surgical patient because it limits the cardiac output and reduces blood flow to the coronary arteries. Indeed, the patient may already be functioning close to the limit with almost no reserve. Perioperative hypotension and tachycardia can be life threatening in such cases.

Aortic sclerosis produces a similar ejection systolic murmur and is caused by a fixed, rigid arterial tree. The perioperative risk is substantially lower in aortic sclerosis.

In a patient with an ejection systolic murmur, any associated **cardiac symptoms** may help identify the murmur as pathological, e.g. a history of syncope, angina or shortness of breath on exertion. Note, however, that any systolic murmur is difficult to categorise clinically, particularly in the elderly. Ideally, an **echocardiogram** should be performed to identify the valvular cause and offer an assessment of severity.

Clinical signs of aortic stenosis are:

- Slow rising upstroke of the carotid pulse
- A harsh ejection systolic murmur radiating into the neck
- Hyperdynamic apex beat indicating left ventricular hypertrophy. (*Note:* the apex beat is only displaced laterally if aortic stenosis coexists with aortic regurgitation or is complicated by cardiac failure)
- Left ventricular hypertrophy on ECG

If aortic stenosis is suspected, an echocardiogram with Doppler assessment of the gradient across the valve is an important part of preoperative assessment. The degree of stenosis and the left ventricular function can be quantified.

Preoperative assessment of valvular heart disease

The patient with valvular heart disease may or may not have a cardiac murmur. When a murmur is present, it may be the innocent flow murmur of a hyperdynamic circulation associated with anxiety or pregnancy. Previously identified murmurs have often been assessed and any functional deficit documented. If not, specialist preoperative cardiological assessment is essential. In most patients, there is no special risk for general anaesthesia or surgery but antibiotic prophylaxis must be considered.

Symptomatic valvular disease is potentially dangerous and requires full preoperative assessment and treatment. Major valvular heart disease may be discovered in recent immigrants from developing countries where **rheumatic heart disease** is prevalent. Patients with valvular heart disease undergoing general anaesthesia require monitoring of cardiac function during operation and probably intensive care afterwards.

Prosthetic replacement valves carry the greatest risk of **infective endocarditis**. For these patients, antibiotic prophylaxis is required for most invasive procedures. Patients with mechanical valves are usually maintained on permanent warfarin anticoagulation and it is important to maintain this to prevent valve thrombosis, a potentially fatal condition. Patients with bioprosthetic valves (pig valves) do not usually require anticoagulation.

Anticoagulation should be continued wherever possible to prevent thrombotic complications. It should be

Valvular defect	Common causes	Clinical features	Comments
Mitral stenosis 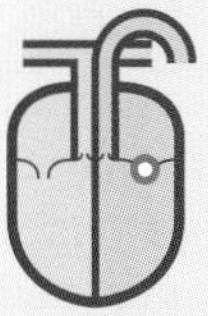	Rheumatic fever Congenital Prosthetic valve	Malar flush Low volume pulse Tapping undisplaced apex beat Mid-diastolic murmur	A common cause of atrial fibrillation
Mitral regurgitation 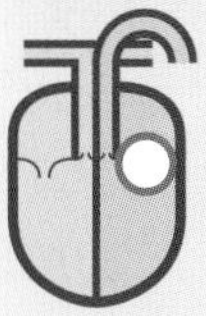	Left ventricular dilatation Annular calcification Rheumatic fever Infective endocarditis Ruptured chordae tendineae Connective tissue disorders, e.g. Marfan's Cardiomyopathy	Displaced hyperdynamic apex beat Right ventricular heave Apical pansystolic murmur radiating to axilla	
Aortic stenosis 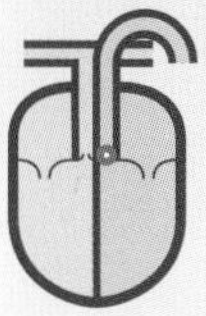	Age-related calcification Congenital bicuspid valve	Slow rising pulse Narrow pulse pressure Heaving undisplaced apex beat Left ventricular heave Ejection systolic murmur radiating to the carotids	Risk of sudden death if hypotensive under anaesthesia
Aortic regurgitation 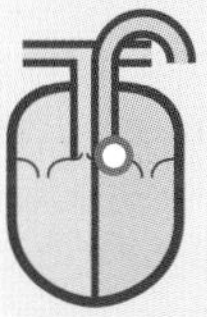	Congenital Rheumatic fever Infective endocarditis Rheumatoid arthritis Hypertension Aortic dissection Trauma Marfan's syndrome	Collapsing pulse Wide pulse pressure Displaced dynamic apex beat Early diastolic murmur	
Tricuspid stenosis 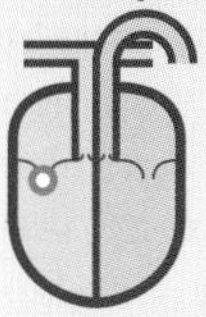	Rheumatic fever	Opening snap Early diastolic murmur	Usually occurs with mitral or aortic valve disease
Tricuspid regurgitation 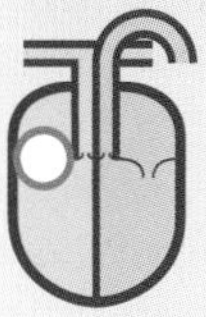	Pulmonary hypertension Rheumatic fever Infective endocarditis Congenital	Right ventricular heave Pansystolic murmur Pulsatile hepatomegaly	
Pulmonary stenosis 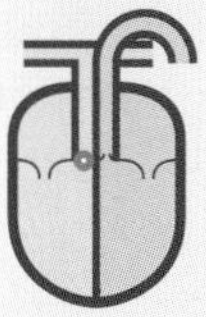	Congenital Rheumatic fever	Right ventricular heave Ejection systolic murmur	
Pulmonary regurgitation 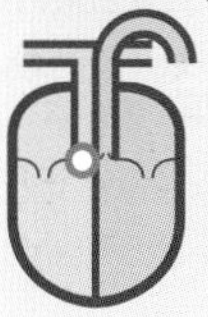	Pulmonary hypertension	Early diastolic decrescendo murmur	

Fig. 8.4 Valvular heart disease

remembered that warfarin is intended to minimise intra-vascular thrombosis and does not affect the extrinsic thrombotic mechanisms. For many operations it is safe to continue warfarin therapy as long as the INR is maintained in the lower therapeutic range (INR 1.5–2.5). Agreement with a haematologist or the patient's anticoagulant clinic is advisable. For major surgery where much bleeding is anticipated, some surgeons prefer to stop warfarin 2 days before operation and substitute subcutaneous heparin or an intravenous infusion. For patients with mitral valve prostheses where the risk of thrombosis is high, full heparinisation must be carefully maintained throughout the perioperative period. However, heparin anticoagulation is more brittle than warfarin and carries a greater risk of over-anticoagulation and potential haemorrhage. For other patients, heparin can be stopped 12 hours before operation and restarted once the danger of bleeding is over. The advantage of heparin over warfarin is that its effects can be quickly reversed by stopping the infusion or with **protamine** if bleeding is excessive. However, rapid reversal may precipitate thrombosis.

Infective endocarditis and indications for antibiotic prophylaxis

When blood is forced under pressure through a narrow orifice, laminar flow is disrupted and eddy currents predispose to local thrombus formation and deposition of circulating bacteria. The vegetations of infective endocarditis are thus formed on the low-pressure side of the jet of blood passing through a damaged valve or a ventricular septal defect. The left side of the heart is more susceptible than the right because of the higher pressures and greater potential for turbulence.

Streptococcus viridans is the most common causative organism of infective endocarditis. Other bacteria such as coliforms or fungi such as *Candida* may also be responsible. Many types of operation and some invasive investigations cause a transient bacteraemia. Although the incidence of infective endocarditis following such procedures is small, the consequences may be catastrophic. The efficacy of prophylactic antibiotics is not absolutely proven, but they are all that is available. The relative risks associated with various cardiac and valvular lesions are summarised in Figure 8.5. The procedures most likely to cause bacteraemia are also shown in Figure 8.5.

The choice of prophylactic antibiotics and the dose regimen depend on the anticipated organisms and the operative procedure. Local protocols may be available. Alternatively, a hospital microbiologist may be consulted or a regimen from a formulary such as the *British National Formulary* employed.

RESPIRATORY DISEASES

Respiratory complications (mainly atelectasis and pneumonia) occur in as many as 15% of surgical patients and are the leading cause of postoperative mortality in the elderly. The risk of a respiratory complication increases with the increasing duration of anaesthetic and is amplified by pre-existing respiratory disease such as chronic obstructive pulmonary disease, asthma or bronchiectasis. Other important factors include smoking, cardiac failure, obesity, old age and general debility. Good postoperative pain relief allows the patient to breath deeply and cough, which, along with effective physiotherapy, helps reduce the risk of respiratory complications.

CLINICAL PROBLEMS

a. Chronic obstructive pulmonary disease (COPD; also known as chronic obstructive airway disease and chronic bronchitis)

COPD is common and strongly predisposes to post-operative chest complications, particularly bronchopneumonia, lobar collapse and pneumothorax. There is often a degree of reversible **bronchoconstriction**, and this can be assessed before operation by measuring peak expiratory flow before and after treatment with a bronchodilator.

Other chronic lung diseases include bronchiectasis, pneumoconiosis, pulmonary fibrosis, sarcoidosis and pulmonary tuberculosis.

The complication rate in chronic lung diseases can be greatly improved by careful preoperative assessment, including lung function tests, and treatment designed to bring the patient into optimum physical condition.

b. Cigarette smoking

Smokers of cigarettes have a five times greater risk of postoperative respiratory problems than non-smokers. This is partly due to pre-existing smoking-related respiratory disease but also to the fact that smokers have a highly reactive airway. This increases the intraoperative risk of laryngeal spasm and bronchospasm.

Smoking should be stopped at least 4 weeks before operation and ideally 8 weeks before if any benefit is to be achieved. This gives time for recovery of physiological respiratory functions such as bronchial ciliary activity. Stopping smoking just before surgery may actually be detrimental because it causes an increase in bronchial mucus production.

c. Current respiratory infections

Acute upper respiratory tract infections (usually viral) are common and such patients have a reduced resistance to surgical trauma and infection. This alone may be grounds for postponing an elective operation.

Conditions associated with chronic infection such as bronchiectasis and cystic fibrosis are more difficult problems. Elective operations should be carried out during periods of remission where possible, with intensive physiotherapy and prophylactic antibiotics perioperatively.

Cardiovascular lesions at risk of infective endocarditis and indications for perioperative antibiotic prophylaxis

High-risk conditions

Prosthetic valve or other intracardiac surgery
Rheumatic valve disease
Congenital heart disease
    (structural valve defects, atrial and ventricular septal
    defects) and aortic coarctation, whether or not corrected
Degenerative valve disease
Previous infective endocarditis

Low-risk conditions

Mitral valve prolapse
Haemodialysis shunts
Transvenous pacemakers
Ventriculo-atrial and ventriculo-peritoneal
shunts for hydrocephalus

Minimal-risk conditions

Coronary bypass grafts
Closed patent ductus arteriosus
Closed atrial septal defect
Established prosthetic arterial grafts

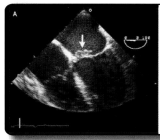

Echo image of mitral and tricuspid valves, showing vegetations on the anterior leaflet of the mitral valve (arrowed)

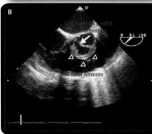

Echo image of aortic valve, showing perforation of valve leaflet (arrow) and an abscess around the valve root (triangles)

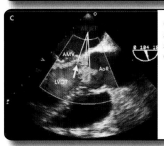

Colour duplex image of aortic valve area showing turbulent flow due to valve vegetations

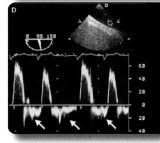

Doppler flow pattern showing reflux through damaged valve (arrowed)

Procedures frequently associated with bacteraemia and requiring antibiotic cover in patients at risk of bacterial endocarditis

Surgical operations

Dental extractions and other procedures involving the gums
Tonsillectomy
Oesophageal dilatation
All gastrointestinal and biliary tract surgery
Most urological procedures including endoscopy, catheter
insertion and removal, transrectal prostatic biopsy
Hysterectomy, dilatation and curettage, termination of
pregnancy
Surgery of infected wounds and tissues
Cardiac surgery

Other procedures

Sigmoidoscopy, colonoscopy, barium enema and liver biopsy
—prophylaxis is only required for patients at high risk, e.g.
prosthetic valves

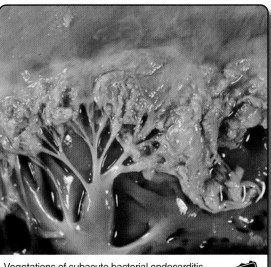

Vegetations of subacute bacterial endocarditis on mitral valve at post mortem

Fig. 8.5 Infective endocarditis

d. Asthma

Asthma is common in children and adolescents but may occur later in life, particularly as a component of COPD. The main elements of asthma are airway hyper-reactivity (with constriction), bronchial wall oedema, excessive mucus production and airway plugging. All these factors predispose to atelectasis, infection and hypoxia.

Asthmatic problems can be exacerbated by the following factors associated with general anaesthesia and surgery:

- Endotracheal intubation—causes increased airways sensitivity
- Increased airways secretions—caused by instrumentation or the autonomic side effects of anaesthetic drugs such as muscle relaxants
- Dehydration—increases mucus viscosity
- Limitation of movement and posture because of pain—inhibits clearance of secretions
- The direct effects of other drugs, e.g. bronchoconstriction caused by beta-blockers or respiratory depression associated with morphine

In asthmatic patients, the usual medication should be continued in the perioperative period if practicable. Alternatively, inhaled preparations may be given via a nebuliser for the first 24 hours. The operation should be postponed during acute exacerbations.

e. Previous pulmonary embolus or deep venous thrombosis

These patients have a greatly increased risk of recurrent thromboembolism. Prophylactic measures are mandatory for all but the most minor procedures.

PREOPERATIVE INVESTIGATION OF RESPIRATORY DISEASE

A chest X-ray should be performed on any patient with symptoms or signs of chest disease. There is no need to take 'routine' chest X-rays on all preoperative patients as studies have shown that undirected screening of asymptomatic patients has an extremely low yield of abnormalities likely to influence surgical outcome. Guidelines for when to take a chest X-ray are available locally and from radiological societies.

Appropriate **lung function tests** should be performed in patients with chronic lung disease. Peak flow measurements are useful to determine the extent of airflow limitation. The reversible element of bronchospasm can be assessed using peak flow measurements before and after bronchodilators. Blood gas measurements are indicated if hypoxaemia or carbon dioxide retention is likely.

PERIOPERATIVE MANAGEMENT OF RESPIRATORY DISEASE AND HIGH-RISK PATIENTS

The following measures will maximise respiratory function and reduce the risk of postoperative complications:

- **Preoperative physiotherapy**—helps to prevent postoperative chest complications. Physiotherapy should include teaching the patient breathing exercises and correct posture
- **Drug therapy**—may need to be adjusted to achieve the optimum respiratory function. Theophyllines may be added to the therapy of patients with asthma, and nebulised bronchodilator drugs (such as salbutamol) may improve the reversible component of COPD and may help to prevent an exacerbation of asthma perioperatively. Adequate hydration reduces the risk of retained secretions which might cause airways obstruction. Prophylactic antibiotics are not recommended for COPD
- **Encouragement of smokers to quit**—should be started at time of booking for elective surgery. Smoking should be stopped at least 4 weeks before operation to achieve the optimum beneficial effect
- **Alternative methods of anaesthesia—local, regional or spinal**—should be considered for patients with chronic respiratory disorders but they are not necessarily the best solution. With the use of newer anaesthetic drugs and techniques, these patients may be better off with endotracheal intubation and ventilation using short-acting muscle relaxants. These techniques allow good bronchial toilet at the end of operation. Certain abdominal operations are technically more difficult under spinal anaesthesia, for example if a patient with chest trouble coughs persistently during the procedure; general anaesthesia avoids this
- **Early postoperative physiotherapy**—aims to enhance deep breathing, coughing and general mobility, reducing the incidence of respiratory complications

GASTROINTESTINAL DISORDERS

The main gastrointestinal conditions giving rise to complications in surgical patients are malnutrition, dental problems, peptic ulcer disease, gastro-oesophageal reflux and inflammatory bowel disease. Previous abdominal surgery may also complicate inpatient treatment.

MALNUTRITION

Many surgical patients are malnourished because of reduced food intake, malabsorption and changes in metabolism (in trauma, burns and sepsis). Studies have shown that 50% of patients undergoing gastrointestinal surgery are mildly malnourished and 30% are moderately or severely malnourished. The severity of malnourishment increases postoperative morbidity and mortality proportionately. For example, severely malnourished patients experience 8 times the rate of complications and 3 times the expected mortality following gastrointestinal surgery. Wound healing is delayed, immune resistance is impaired and muscles are weakened.

Nutritional assessment

There is no universal tool for assessing malnutrition but the combination of a BMI of less than 18.5 kg/m^2 with weight loss exceeding 5% of usual body weight over the preceding 1–2 months) and a serum albumin level below 35 g/l (in the absence of renal or hepatic disease) indicates significant malnutrition. Other tools include measuring mid upper arm circumference, skin fold thickness and grip strength.

Indications for nutritional support

If enteral support (i.e. supplemental nutrition into the gastrointestinal tract) is practicable before operation, certain patients have been shown to benefit from it in terms of reduced mortality and morbidity. Indications published by the British Society of Gastroenterology include patients with severe anorexia, with moderate or severe malnutrition unable to eat or swallow sufficient by mouth, with recent weight loss of 10% or more, with intestinal failure and also patients not anticipated to resume oral intake for 10 or more days after operation. Nutritional support is best given as supplements by mouth if possible or else via a fine-bore nasogastric tube.

DENTAL PROBLEMS

Teeth and artificial fixed crowns and bridges are vulnerable to damage during intubation. This causes not only cosmetic and medico-legal problems, but also exposes the patient to the risk of aspirating foreign bodies into the bronchial tree. Similarly, infected material from carious (decayed) teeth or inflamed gums may be aspirated. This causes a particularly grave aspiration pneumonia. Dentures must be removed before operation for the same reason and they must be labelled so the patient can retrieve them afterwards! In unconscious trauma victims, the possibility of aspiration, swallowing or pharyngeal obstruction by a dental prosthesis should always be considered.

PEPTIC ULCER DISEASE

Peptic ulcer disease may be a surgical problem in its own right, but patients admitted for other surgical reasons may have an active peptic ulcer that can be exacerbated by the stresses of hospital admission. These include

serious illness and trauma, operations, and drugs such as aspirin, NSAIDs and corticosteroids. The result may be a sudden catastrophic **haemorrhage** (presenting as haematemesis or melaena), or occasionally **perforation**. Bleeding may also result from acute stress ulceration in the seriously ill patient. Note that stress ulceration is distinct from chronic peptic ulcer disease.

Patients with known peptic ulcer disease or strongly suggestive symptoms should receive perioperative prophylaxis with H$_2$-receptor antagonists or proton pump inhibitors. NSAIDs and irritant oral drugs should be avoided.

Previous gastrectomy can be associated with a number of long-term side effects. These include anaemia (due to deficiency of iron, vitamin B$_{12}$ and occasionally folate) and, rarely, osteomalacia. A full blood count should be included in the preoperative assessment of these patients.

GASTRO-OESOPHAGEAL REFLUX DISEASE (GORD)

Patients with GORD are at risk of aspirating acidic gastric contents during induction of anaesthesia and should receive preoperative treatment with proton pump inhibitors. Aspiration may cause interstitial lung damage which, in its severe form, is known as **Mendelson's syndrome**.

INFLAMMATORY BOWEL DISEASE

Patients with chronic inflammatory bowel disease may be anaemic or malnourished if the disease is active. Patients may also be **steroid dependent** because of adrenal suppression from long-term steroid therapy, requiring perioperative administration of hydrocortisone. Occasionally immunosuppressive drugs such as azathioprine are being taken and may increase the predisposition to infection.

HEPATIC DISORDERS

Pre-existing liver disease may have important consequences in the surgical patient and generally increases the risk of postoperative morbidity and mortality. A history of jaundice must be evaluated as it may be a clue to serious risks for both patient and medical staff.

CLINICAL PROBLEMS

a. History of jaundice

A past history of jaundice raises the possibility that the patient may be a carrier of hepatitis B or C and this can readily be transmitted to health care staff. The main danger is from needle-stick injuries. Vaccination against hepatitis B is now mandatory for health workers at occupational risk of infection.

Most previously jaundiced patients will have suffered acute infective hepatitis (hepatitis A) and this poses no risk to staff because the infective agent does not cause a chronic carrier state. In contrast, lifetime **chronic hepatitis** develops in 5–10% of those infected with hepatitis B virus (HBV) and in 80% of those infected with HCV. These diseases should be suspected if the illness associated with the previous jaundice was prolonged or serious. Jaundice contracted in developing countries should be regarded with particular suspicion because hepatitis B and C are often endemic. Hepatitis C is becoming more common and, because of its chronicity, causes a high rate of cirrhosis in the long term, although it often develops slowly over many years; some patients with cirrhosis due to hepatitis B and C progress to hepatocellular cancer. Antiviral chemotherapy is showing promise in preventing these late complications. Hepatitis B and C are also common among male homosexuals and intravenous drug abusers who share syringes. The history taking should include questions to determine whether the patient falls into a high-risk group. Clinical examination should include a search for intravenous injection sites characteristic of drug abuse. In high-risk patients, screening for hepatitis B surface antigen (HBsAg) and hepatitis C antibody should ideally be performed before any other blood test (see Ch. 3).

b. Presence of obstructive jaundice

Surgery in this situation is usually performed to relieve an obstruction in patients where endoscopic stenting of the bile ducts is inappropriate, has failed or is unavailable. This surgery carries a number of special risks and management problems which are described in Chapter 18. These include ascending cholangitis, clotting disorders, deep vein thrombosis and acute renal failure.

c. The patient with known hepatitis

Patients with any form of hepatitis, whether viral or alcoholic, tolerate general anaesthesia and surgery badly and there is a distinct mortality risk. Surgery should be avoided unless absolutely essential. If alcoholism is suspected, a CAGE questionnaire (Box 8.1) should be completed. Positive answers to two or more of the four questions suggest a drinking problem.

Box 8.1 CAGE questionnaire for assessing possible alcoholism

- Have you ever felt you ought to **Cut down** on your drinking?
- Have people **Annoyed** you by criticising your drinking?
- Have you ever felt bad or **Guilty** about your drinking?
- Have you ever had a drink first thing in the morning to steady your nerves or get rid of a hangover (**Eye-opener**)?

An elevated serum gamma glutaryl transferase level is a fairly good indicator of excessive alcohol intake. Mean corpuscular red cell volume (MCV) may also be raised, and should alert the doctor to the possibility of concealed alcoholism.

d. The patient with known cirrhosis

Patients with cirrhosis have a high risk of perioperative morbidity and mortality. The main factors are:

- Anaemia
- Portal hypertension
- Defective synthesis of clotting factors and thrombocytopenia
- Malnutrition
- Electrolyte disturbances (particularly hyponatraemia)
- Defective energy metabolism (gluconeogenesis and glycogenolysis)
- Abnormal drug metabolism and distribution (due to hypoalbuminaemia)
- Ascites

The main postoperative complications of cirrhosis are excessive bleeding, defective wound healing, hepatocellular decompensation leading to encephalopathy, and susceptibility to infection.

Excessive bleeding results from several factors:

- Defective synthesis of clotting factors (all but factor VIII are synthesised in the liver)
- Thrombocytopenia (due to hypersplenism and depressed platelet production)
- Abnormal polymerisation of fibrin
- Portal hypertension (greatly expanded intra-abdominal venous network under high pressure). This, together with numerous vascular adhesions, makes dissection in the abdominal cavity tedious, difficult and bloody

Portal hypertension may initially be discovered because of ascites or splenomegaly or an acute upper gastrointestinal haemorrhage. (Note that only about half of such episodes of haematemesis/melaena in patients with portal hypertension are due to oesophageal varices. The rest are largely caused by gastroduodenal ulcers, Mallory–Weiss tears or gastric erosions.) If a patient with known oesophageal varices requires an operation, preoperative endoscopic assessment and sclerotherapy or banding may be appropriate.

Preoperative assessment and management

Preoperative blood tests for patients with liver disease are listed in Box 8.2. If the prothrombin ratio is prolonged, intravenous vitamin K injections are given for several days before operation. If this fails to correct the abnormal clotting (as in severe hepatocellular impairment), **fresh-**

Box 8.2 Preoperative blood tests for patients with liver disease

Initial tests

- Serological testing for hepatitis B and C
- Consider HIV testing

Further tests

- Full blood count
- Clotting screen
- Consider blood group and cross-match if excess bleeding anticipated
- Plasma urea and electrolytes
- Bilirubin
- Transaminases
- Gamma glutaryl transferase
- Albumin
- Calcium
- Phosphate

Fig. 8.6 Cimino–Brescia arteriovenous fistula

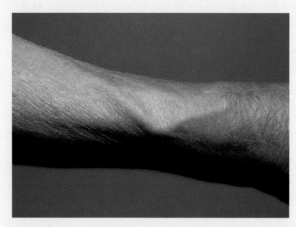

This recently constructed fistula was performed for chronic renal failure in a diabetic woman of 56. It involved dividing the cephalic vein and suturing the proximal end to the side of the radial artery. It was performed under local anaesthesia via the incision visible on the wrist. The wrist veins are already dilating and will soon be usable for renal dialysis.

frozen plasma is given during the operation. If the patient is thrombocytopenic, platelet transfusion may also be required.

RENAL DISORDERS

Renal impairment is commonly encountered in general surgical patients. It is characterised by impaired homeostasis of fluid and electrolytes and reduced excretion of nitrogenous compounds. The risk of perioperative complications increases with the degree of renal failure. Patients can be divided into two groups: mild chronic renal failure (CRF) and severe chronic renal failure. Acute renal failure is usually a postoperative complication, often with several contributory causes including hypovolaemia, and is described in Chapter 12. Patients with pre-existing renal disease are particularly vulnerable to acute renal failure ('acute-on-chronic renal failure').

CLINICAL PROBLEMS

a. Mild chronic renal failure

This is common in the elderly and may be caused by hypertension. The main management problems in surgical patients are:

- **Impaired excretion of drugs**—drugs handled in this way must therefore be given in smaller doses or less frequently, as documented in drug formularies such as the *British National Formulary*. In practice, digoxin and gentamicin pose the main problems
- **Fluid and electrolyte homeostasis**—only becomes a problem in mild chronic renal failure if fluid balance is not monitored carefully enough in the

perioperative period. Monitoring should include regular checks of serum urea, electrolytes and creatinine, especially if the patient is receiving diuretic therapy

- **Reduction in renal reserve**—even mild renal failure implies a drastic reduction in renal reserve. For example, major reconstructive surgery to the abdominal aorta in a patient with mild renal failure may interfere with renal function because of aortic cross-clamping near the renal arteries. This is exacerbated by transient hypotension caused by blood loss. The lack of renal reserve in these patients may then progress to acute renal failure.

b. Severe chronic renal failure (CRF)

These patients are usually under the care of specialist physicians who should be involved in perioperative management. Patients may be receiving regular haemodialysis or ambulatory peritoneal dialysis; in such patients, surgery is usually for renal transplantation.

The main perioperative problems of severe CRF are:

- **Fluid overload**—this is caused by impaired glomerular filtration and may require correction with large doses of diuretics and fluid restriction and haemofiltration if necessary
- **Regulation of serum osmolality**—this is disordered in patients with severe CRF who are particularly vulnerable to hypo- and hyper-natraemia. Care must be taken that the sodium content of intravenous fluids is appropriate

- **Hyperkalaemia**—this is a particular risk in advanced CRF. Patients with lesser degrees of CRF are vulnerable to an increase in potassium load (due to transfusion, tissue damage or hypoxia) or changes in glomerular filtration rate (caused by cardiac failure or hypotension). Hyperkalaemia may cause cardiac arrest and susceptibility to this is best assessed by monitoring the ECG. To minimise this risk, the preoperative plasma potassium level should be stabilised below 5.0 mmol/L

- **Metabolic acidosis**—this tends to develop in chronic renal failure but it is usually compensated by respiratory alkalosis. This compensation is disrupted by general anaesthesia and also by additional metabolic acidosis resulting from tissue ischaemia or hypoxia

- **Chronic normochromic normocytic anaemia**—this results from decreased erythropoietin production by the kidney. Cardiovascular function is usually well adapted to this anaemia and preoperative transfusion is unnecessary. If the haemoglobin concentration is substantially below 10 g/dl, the patient is usually treated with **erythropoietin**

PREOPERATIVE ASSESSMENT

Patients with severe renal failure should be asked about their daily urine volume, as those who are oliguric are at risk of over hydration. The state of hydration should be assessed clinically by looking for evidence of dehydration or fluid overload (particularly jugular venous pressure). Plasma urea, electrolytes, creatinine and bicarbonate should also be checked for abnormalities. Full blood count is checked for anaemia.

DIABETES MELLITUS

Both severe hypoglycaemia and hyperglycaemia are life-threatening conditions. The blood glucose levels of a diabetic surgical patient need to be closely monitored and treated as appropriate.

Patients with diabetes are at special risk from general anaesthesia and surgery for the following reasons:

- Certain complications of diabetes are associated with a higher perioperative risk. These are summarised in Box 8.3
- Stress (including surgery, trauma and infections) causes increased production of catabolic hormones which oppose the action of insulin (see Ch. 2). This makes diabetic control more difficult
- General anaesthesia, surgery, deprivation of oral intake and postoperative vomiting disrupt the delicate balance between dietary intake, exercise (energy utilisation) and diabetic therapy
- Diabetic ketoacidosis may cause an elevated leucocyte count and raised amylase level, which may confuse the

---

Box 8.3 Specific perioperative problems in patients with diabetes

Predisposition to ischaemic heart disease
- Greater risk of perioperative myocardial infarction, which has a substantially higher mortality in diabetics, particularly females
- Infarction may be painless or 'silent' (possibly due to autonomic neuropathy)

Increased danger of cardiac arrest
- Due to autonomic neuropathy

Renal problems
- Predisposition to diabetic nephropathy
- Tendency to chronic renal failure

Predisposition to peripheral vascular disease
- Greater risk of perioperative strokes and lower limb ischaemia

Predisposition to heel pressure sores
- Especially if there is peripheral neuropathy

Increased incidence of postoperative infection
- In the wound, chest or urinary tract

Obesity
- Particularly common in type 2 diabetes
- Associated with increased operative morbidity

---

diagnosis of an acute abdomen. Indeed, ketoacidosis may sometimes present with abdominal pain
- Diabetic patients are at greater risk of hospital-acquired infection, which may be elusive as a cause of deterioration

CLINICAL PROBLEMS

Preoperative assessment in patients undergoing major surgery should include evaluation of current diabetic control by serial blood glucose and **glycosylated haemoglobin** measurements. Potential cardiovascular and renal complications should be assessed by performing an ECG (with Valsalva manoeuvre to look for autonomic neuropathy) and measuring plasma urea and electrolytes.

Perioperative management aims to maintain blood glucose level between 4 and 10 mmol/L, but it is particularly important to avoid hypoglycaemia. Surgery may have to be deferred if the blood glucose cannot be stabilised below 13 mmol/L. Above this level, the risk of ketoacidosis or a hyperosmolar non-ketotic state is unacceptable unless surgery is critically urgent. If the patient is unwell and ketones are present in the urine in large quantities, consider postponing surgery. Surgery in the presence of

---

Box 8.4 Perioperative management of insulin-dependent diabetes

Before operation

1. Arrange preoperative outpatient stabilisation of diabetes with diabetes physician and specialist nurse in advance, if available
2. Admit patient to hospital at least one day before operation if outpatient preparation is unavailable or unsatisfactory
3. Establish optimal preoperative control—may need advice from patient's diabetic management team
4. Monitor blood glucose throughout the day, e.g. before and after meals and at bedtime
5. Check blood glucose and electrolytes before operating list commences—postpone if glucose level greater than 13 mmol/L or electrolyte abnormalities are found
6. Arrange for the operation to take place as early as possible in the day

Operation day

1. Starve from midnight and omit first dose of insulin
2. Commence intravenous dextrose and insulin infusions
3. Check blood glucose and electrolytes at conclusion of operation (or at 1–2-hour intervals in a long operation)
4. Adjust concentration of infusions and rate of administration as required

After operation

1. Check glucose hourly initially and electrolytes 6–12 hourly and adjust infusion as indicated
2. Continue infusion until full oral diet is established, then reintroduce subcutaneous insulin, using the preoperative regimen

---

Box 8.5 Perioperative management of diabetics using insulin infusion

1. Intravenous 5% or 10% dextrose infusion at 125 ml per hour
2. Constant pump-controlled intravenous soluble insulin infusion. This is adjusted according to 2–4-hourly blood glucose estimations
3. If there is a need to limit fluids—use 20% dextrose solution and infuse at 50 ml per hour

---

- Add potassium to the dextrose infusion
- Monitor blood glucose and electrolytes frequently throughout the operative and early postoperative period

A typical management protocol is given in Box 8.4 and a recommended insulin infusion regimen in Box 8.5. The key to successful management of diabetes is adjusting the dose of insulin against frequent measurements of blood glucose. Finger-prick tests on the ward are adequate, provided they are performed correctly by properly trained staff. The insulin dose is adjusted hourly according to the blood glucose results.

b. Diabetics controlled on oral hypoglycaemic drugs

Many of these patients are receiving short-acting sulphonylureas such as glipizide. Patients on long-acting drugs such as metformin should be changed several days before operation to a short-acting sulphonylurea. If this fails to provide adequate control, an insulin regimen can be used as above.

On the morning of the operation, the patient is starved in the usual manner and the short-acting sulphonylurea omitted. This drug is reintroduced when oral intake is resumed. Blood glucose should be monitored regularly as for insulin-dependent patients because it may still reach unacceptable levels despite the lack of carbohydrate intake. If glucose rises above 13 mmol/L, it can be controlled by small subcutaneous doses of short-acting insulin, e.g. 6 units of soluble insulin. If a major operation is planned or if postoperative 'nil by mouth' is likely to be prolonged, it is best to use insulin and glucose infusions as for insulin-dependent diabetics.

c. Diabetics controlled by diet alone

If preoperative control is adequate, these patients require no special perioperative measures; they do not become hypoglycaemic and blood glucose rarely drifts above acceptable levels. Finger-prick blood glucose measurement may be used if there is any doubt.

d. Diabetics poorly controlled on emergency admission

Any diabetic patient may present with uncontrolled diabetes, particularly if admitted as an emergency. This may

---

ketoacidosis has a high mortality and should be avoided if possible until the acidosis is under control, i.e. until bicarbonate is greater than 20 or pH > 7.3.

For the purposes of perioperative management, patients with diabetes fall into three groups: those who are **insulin dependent**, those taking **oral hypoglycaemic** medication and those who are **diet controlled**.

a. Insulin-dependent diabetics

Insulin-dependent diabetics depend for their metabolism on administered insulin. If the blood glucose level is low, insulin is not withheld but glucose infusion is increased. The general principles of perioperative management are:

- Establish good diabetic control before operation
- Give insulin as a continuous intravenous infusion during the operative period
- Give an infusion of dextrose (glucose) throughout the operative period to balance the insulin given and to make up for lack of dietary intake

Fig. 8.7 Thyrotoxic eye signs

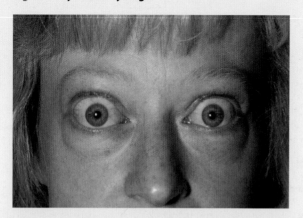

This woman of 36 presented with a typical history of primary thyrotoxicosis (Graves' disease), with weight loss, irritability and menstrual irregularity. In addition her eyesight had become blurred. She had fairly florid exophthalmos with protruding eyeballs (proptosis) and lid lag. She was barely able to close her eyelids and would soon be at risk of corneal drying.

be due to infection or vomiting. The diabetes must first be brought under control with rehydration and then infusions of insulin (using a 'sliding scale' with the dosage proportionate to the blood glucose, see p. 121), glucose and potassium.

THYROID DISEASE

THYROTOXICOSIS

Thyroid or non-thyroid surgery for a patient with uncontrolled thyrotoxicosis carries a risk of thyrotoxic crisis and this carries a high mortality. Thus any patient with features of thyrotoxicosis should have thyroid function tests (usually TSH) included in the preoperative assessment.

In surgery for hyperthyroidism, the patient should be rendered euthyroid before operation using antithyroid drugs (propylthiouracil is useful in this respect as it also blocks peripheral conversion of T4 to the active T3) and beta-blocking drugs. Non-selective beta-blocking drugs rapidly control the cardiovascular effects of thyrotoxicosis and can be used for urgent preoperative preparation.

HYPOTHYROIDISM

Untreated hypothyroid patients are at moderate risk when undergoing surgery. They are more sensitive to CNS depressants, have a decreased cardiovascular reserve, and are also susceptible to electrolyte disorders (particularly water retention). Severe infection, especially accompa-

nied by trauma, a cold environment or depressant drugs, may precipitate myxoedema coma which, though very rare, is often fatal.

If there is clinical suspicion of hypothyroidism, operation should be postponed and thyroid function checked by measuring free thyroxine (T4) and thyroid stimulating hormone (TSH) levels. If hypothyroidism is diagnosed, oral replacement therapy is commenced. If surgery must be performed urgently, it is usually best to proceed with the operation and begin oral treatment later.

DISORDERS OF ADRENAL FUNCTION

ADRENAL INSUFFICIENCY

The most common cause of adrenal insufficiency is hypothalamo–pituitary–adrenal suppression by long-term corticosteroid therapy. It is occasionally caused by primary adrenal failure (**Addison's disease**) or pituitary ablation (due to tumour or surgery). Very rarely, it results from previous adrenalectomy which was sometimes employed for palliation of breast cancer, treatment for a hypersecretion syndrome or surgery for bilateral primary adrenal tumours.

In primary or secondary adrenal failure, the patient is usually already taking oral steroid replacement therapy, but the lack of additional adrenal response to the stresses of trauma, surgery or infection may cause acute postoperative cardiovascular collapse with hypotension and shock (**Addisonian crisis**).

Perioperative 'steroid cover'

Patients with potential adrenal insufficiency must be given steroid cover during the perioperative period. This is usually in the form of intravenous hydrocortisone, e.g. 25–50 mg prior to the operation and 50 mg daily until recovery. It is better to give prophylactic hydrocortisone in doubtful cases than risk acute hypo-adrenalism. For any steroid-dependent patient, a doctor should write clearly in the notes 'Treat any unexplained collapse with hydrocortisone.'

CUSHING'S SYNDROME

Cushing's syndrome results from excess secretion of cortisol. This may be in response to excess adrenocorticotropic hormone (ACTH) secretion by a pituitary tumour, ectopic ACTH secretion (usually by a malignant tumour) or rarely due to a primary tumour of an adrenal gland. The most common cause of Cushingoid features is long-term steroid therapy for conditions such as rheumatoid arthritis or asthma. Clinically the patient may be plethoric, moon-faced, hypertensive, hirsute and obese with abdominal striae and have a characteristic 'buffalo hump'. The main surgical problems in Cushingoid patients are hypertension,

Fig. 8.8 Subluxation of the atlanto-axial joint in rheumatoid arthritis

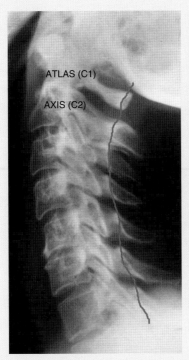
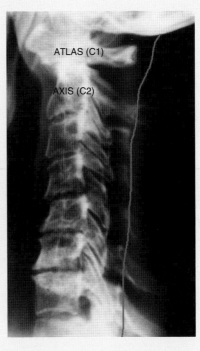

(a)

(b)

This 62-year-old woman with longstanding severe rheumatoid arthritis required a major abdominal operation. Cervical radiographs were taken before operation to anticipate problems during anaesthesia. **(a)** Cervical spine in extension. **(b)** The same patient in flexion. On each X-ray, a red line is drawn along the posterior limit of the spinal canal. Anterior subluxation (i.e. partial dislocation) is most obvious if the most posterior part of the spine of the atlas is compared with the line and with that of the axis in the two pictures. This mobility is caused by destruction of the transverse axial ligament of the odontoid by pannus (excessive granulation tissue) from the synovial joint. Under general anaesthesia, muscle relaxation may allow exaggeration of the subluxation, causing damage to the cervical cord.

hyperglycaemia, poor wound healing, infection and peptic ulceration. If the condition is due to steroid therapy, there is an additional risk of secondary adrenal insufficiency.

MUSCULOSKELETAL AND NEUROLOGICAL DISORDERS

Musculoskeletal and neurological disorders influence the outcome of surgery in two main ways. First, any condition which hinders mobility predisposes to chest infection, deep venous thrombosis and pulmonary embolism, aspiration pneumonitis and pressure sores. The last is even more likely if there is also sensory impairment due to stroke or diabetic peripheral neuropathy. Second, specific aspects of these disorders must be considered in relation to general anaesthesia, positioning of the patient on the operating table and the use of drugs.

RHEUMATOID ARTHRITIS

Rheumatoid arthritis poses special problems related to chronic anaemia, drug therapy and spinal complications.

(Note that some of these problems are shared by other collagen disorders):

- **Normochromic normocytic anaemia**—common in chronic inflammatory disorders, including rheumatoid arthritis. The anaemia is refractory to iron therapy and there is no benefit from preoperative transfusion unless haemoglobin concentration is extremely low
- **Gastrointestinal disorders**—most rheumatoid patients are taking aspirin or other NSAIDs, all of which predispose to peptic ulceration, ulceration and perforation of small and large bowel and small bowel strictures. Long-term steroid therapy may contribute to peptic ulceration. Chronic low-grade bleeding from the upper gastrointestinal tract may exacerbate the existing anaemia in these patients. Operative stress may also precipitate acute gastrointestinal haemorrhage
- **Long-term steroid therapy**—may result in adrenal insufficiency under stress. Gold and penicillamine cause renal parenchymal damage and bone marrow depression; NSAIDs may exacerbate chronic renal failure

- **Other medications**—a range of powerful drugs is now used to treat rheumatoid arthritis including chloroquine, methotrexate, sulfasalazine and cytokine inhibitors. Refer to standard formularies for potential problems
- **Odontoid subluxation** (Fig. 8.8)—if rheumatoid arthritis involves the atlanto-axial joint, the transverse ligament may be destroyed, allowing the odontoid process to sublux. During general anaesthesia, the protective reflexes are lost. If the neck is hyperextended during intubation, there is a serious risk of injury to the spinal cord by the unrestrained odontoid

Preoperative assessment of the rheumatoid patient

Full blood count is essential to check for non-specific anaemia or iron deficiency anaemia. Serum urea, electrolytes and creatinine are measured if there is any suspicion of chronic or drug-induced disturbance of renal function. Preoperative assessment must include clinical examination of neck movements and cervical spine X-rays.

EPILEPSY

Epilepsy is common and many elective surgical patients will therefore be taking anticonvulsive drugs. Fortunately, there is no particular risk from general anaesthesia or surgery. Indeed, the central depressive effect of general anaesthetic drugs is a powerful anticonvulsant!

HAEMATOLOGICAL DISORDERS

ANAEMIAS

Severe anaemias are associated with increased perioperative morbidity and mortality. General anaesthesia poses the greatest single problem. For elective surgery, the haemoglobin concentration should ideally be above 10 g/dl before operation but long-standing chronic anaemias probably pose little increased risk.

Management of anaemic patients depends on the cause of the anaemia. Whether or not to transfuse before operation depends on the level of anaemia (trigger levels have come down in recent years as a response to the shortage of blood for transfusion, see local guidelines), whether the anaemia is acute and on the expected blood loss during the operation. Transmission of human immunodeficiency virus (HIV) and other infective agents by transfusion is a very small risk in developed countries where sophisticated screening of donors is usual, but remains a serious risk in countries without such precautions. Even so, it is good policy to transfuse donor blood only when strictly necessary. Transfusion for anaemia can usually be avoided in young, fit patients but elderly or very ill patients with less cardiorespiratory reserve are more likely to need transfusion. Transfusions should be given at least 24 hours before operation to allow fluid balance to stabilise and to ensure optimal red cell function. For diagnosed deficiency anaemias, treatment as appropriate with iron, vitamin B_{12} or folate may be all that is necessary before operation. Treatment with erythropoietin (EPO) is expensive but effective and is likely to become more available.

HAEMOGLOBINOPATHIES

Patients with sickle-cell disease and beta thalassaemia have a high operative mortality and morbidity, particularly if the condition is unrecognised, e.g. in emergency situations. They require intensive perioperative management with particular attention to avoiding hypoxia, infection, acidosis, dehydration and hypothermia. Patients with sickle-cell trait are at much lower risk and develop complications only if they become severely hypoxic. Sickle-cell trait and disease occur amongst black and mixed race people, who should always be asked specifically about a history of sickle-cell disease. A sickle-cell test must be performed before operation on any black patient so that the anaesthetist can be prepared.

POLYCYTHAEMIA

Polycythaemia may be caused by a primary myeloproliferative disorder such as **polycythaemia vera** or be secondary to chronic cardiac or pulmonary disease or heavy cigarette smoking. There is an increased red cell mass in both primary and secondary polycythaemia which causes a high haematocrit and increased blood viscosity. In primary polycythaemia, the platelet count may be increased which, paradoxically, is associated with defective haemostasis as well as the risk of thrombosis.

The main complications of polycythaemia vera are **haemorrhage** and **arterial or venous thrombosis**. The risk increases once the haematocrit rises above 50%. In general, operation should be postponed to allow treatment by venesection or myelosuppression. If possible, the cardiovascular system should be allowed to stabilise for about 1 month after treatment. In an emergency, the haematocrit may be reduced by preoperative venesection, restoring the volume by colloid infusion.

LEUKAEMIA, LEUCOPENIA AND THROMBOCYTOPENIA

Patients with these haematological disorders may need surgery for unrelated conditions. Prophylactic antibiotics may be required in neutropenia, and haematologists give specific advice in patients at risk because of chemotherapy. In thrombocytopenia, haemorrhage can be minimised by transfusing platelet concentrates.

BLEEDING DISORDERS

Bleeding diatheses such as thrombocytopenia, von Willebrand's disease (abnormal platelet function and factor VIII deficiency) and haemophilia are occasionally encountered in general surgical practice. Most surgical bleeding problems, however, are caused by poorly controlled anticoagulant therapy, liver disease, aspirin therapy and sometimes vitamin K malabsorption. The last occurs in obstructive jaundice and malabsorption syndromes.

A history of abnormal bleeding or factors which may predispose to abnormal bleeding should be sought from every surgical patient as follows:

- Excessive bleeding from simple cuts, previous surgery, dental extractions or childbirth
- Current use of anticoagulant drugs or aspirin
- A family history of bleeding disorders
- Intercurrent haematological or liver disease, cystic fibrosis or other malabsorption syndromes
- Recent jaundice
- Previous intestinal resection or bypass surgery

Any clotting abnormality may lead to excessive bleeding at operation or early in the postoperative period. Preoperative recognition and treatment of a clotting problem is vital because runaway haemorrhage can easily occur, leading to clotting factors becoming depleted. At this point, bleeding may be very difficult to control even with transfusion of clotting factors.

If a bleeding disorder is suspected, a **platelet count** and **clotting screen** must be performed. A clotting screen includes prothrombin time or ratio and activated partial thromboplastin time. If an abnormality is revealed, further investigations such as assays of individual clotting factors may be necessary. Operation should be deferred if possible until the problem is overcome.

Clinical problems of bleeding disorders

a. Inherited clotting disorders
Haemophilia occurs in males. The disorder is an X-linked deficiency of factor VIII or, less commonly, factor IX. The appropriate specific antihaemophilic factor is administered before operation and for up to 2 weeks after operation until the danger of secondary haemorrhage is over. **Von Willebrand's disease** is an autosomal dominant condition with abnormalities of both factor VIII and platelet function. It is managed perioperatively with replacement of the specific factors.

b. Anticoagulant therapy
Long-term anticoagulant therapy with warfarin is commonly used in venous thromboembolism, for patients with mechanical heart valve prostheses and in older patients with atrial fibrillation. Patients on anticoagulants have a small extra risk of perioperative haemorrhage, particularly if control is poor. For most patients, some form

of anticoagulation needs to be continued, particularly if a mechanical heart valve is in situ. Many doctors prefer to continue oral warfarin, reducing the prothrombin ratio somewhat during the perioperative period. An alternative approach is to discontinue warfarin about 2 days before operation and convert to intravenous heparin infusion. This can be closely adjusted or even reversed but is more volatile and difficult to manage.

If anticoagulation is for venous thromboembolism, some doctors prefer to discontinue warfarin before operation and cover the perioperative period with prophylactic subcutaneous low-dose heparin (see Ch. 12).

c. Liver disease
Bleeding disorders in cirrhosis are described earlier in this chapter, and disorders in the jaundiced patient are described in detail in Chapter 18.

d. Aspirin therapy
Aspirin has an irreversible inhibitory effect on platelet aggregation which persists clinically for at least 10 days. The effect is reversed only when the affected platelets have been replaced by the bone marrow. Most NSAIDs act on platelets in the same way. A similar but short-lived effect is also produced by high doses of intravenous penicillin. Aspirin ingestion, even in low doses, tends to result in oozing during and after operation, although this is rarely serious. For major elective arterial surgery, aspirin should ideally be stopped about 2 weeks before operation.

e. Malabsorption of fat-soluble vitamins
Vitamin K absorption may be impaired in pancreatic dysfunction, after resection of the proximal ileum or in malabsorption syndromes. The problem is readily overcome by preoperative injections of vitamin K.

PSYCHIATRIC DISORDERS

MENTAL ILLNESS AND LEARNING DISABILITY

Behavioural problems associated with mental illness and learning disability can be minimised by a sympathetic and consistent approach from medical and nursing staff. Any procedure or investigation must be explained to the patient as far as possible in terms that can be understood, ideally in the presence of a carer or relative. Patients should not be moved from bed to bed around the ward as this produces disorientation.

Monoamine oxidase inhibitors (used as antidepressants) interact with sympathomimetic amines and opiate analgesics to cause severe hypertension. Although rarely used nowadays, they should be discontinued at least 2 weeks before operation. Tricyclic antidepressants and phenothiazines also have a wide range of interactions. Serum urea, electrolytes and thyroid function should be checked in patients taking **lithium** (usually for bipolar disorder), which may cause renal parenchymal damage and disturbed thyroid function.

ALCOHOLISM AND DRUG ADDICTION

Alcoholics are prone to cirrhosis, malnutrition and peripheral neuropathies. Drug addicts are at risk of hepatitis, HIV/acquired immunodeficiency syndrome (AIDS) and other infections. Alcohol potentiates general anaesthetic agents, and an inebriated patient needs smaller doses. In contrast, chronic alcohol abuse induces liver enzymes which break down anaesthetic agents. This also increases tolerance to central nervous system depressants and higher doses of anaesthetic agents are needed. Similarly, larger doses of intravenous sedatives are required for procedures such as gastrointestinal endoscopy. Opiate addiction leads to similar dosage problems. Alcohol is the cause of, and complicates, many traumatic injuries. For example, a patient smelling of drink may have altered consciousness because of cerebral injury, not just inebriation.

Problems of drug withdrawal

Withdrawal symptoms may develop unexpectedly during the postoperative period if drug or alcohol addiction has been concealed. Alcohol withdrawal is characterised initially by irritability and tremors. Convulsions may develop after 24–48 hours. Full-scale **delirium tremens** may appear as long as 10 days after alcohol withdrawal. It is characterised by confusion and visual hallucinations accompanied by fever, tachycardia, pallor, vomiting and sweats. Similar symptoms and signs also occur in a range of other postoperative complications and alcohol withdrawal can be easily overlooked.

Alcoholic cirrhosis may cause episodic hypoglycaemia, the symptoms of which may be confused with those of delirium tremens. Hypoglycaemia should be excluded by measuring blood glucose.

Mild alcohol withdrawal states may be managed with regular oral doses of clomethiazole or benzodiazepines. Parenteral B vitamins are usually given daily. Opiate withdrawal symptoms are broadly similar to those of alcohol. Treatment is usually with a substitute drug such as methadone.

DEMENTIA

Patients with even mild dementia become even more confused when subjected to the strange and ever-changing environment of the surgical ward. They tolerate the stress of general anaesthesia and operation poorly and so the potential benefit of any elective procedure should be carefully weighed against the possible adverse effects.

Sudden deterioration in mental state or increasing confusion may be provoked by infection, dehydration, electrolyte disturbances, hypoxia or overdose of drugs such as digoxin, hypnotics and sedatives. All these potential causes should be considered in any patient who undergoes deterioration in mental state in the perioperative

Table 8.1 Surgical complications of obesity

Complication	Factors
Cardiopulmonary complications such as cardiac failure and chest infections	Predisposing factors are atherosclerosis, increased demands on the cardiovascular system, decreased chest wall compliance, inefficient respiratory muscles and shallow breathing
Wound complications such as infection, infection, dehiscence	Poor-quality abdominal wall musculature with fat infiltration. Large 'dead space' in which fat predisposes to haematoma formation
Venous thromboembolism—increased risk of deep venous thrombosis and pulmonary embolism	Poor peripheral venous return; delayed return to normal mobility
General anaesthesia complications	Anatomical problems, e.g. intravenous cannulae are difficult to insert and intubation is more difficult. Clinical signs of dehydration and hypovolaemia are more difficult to elicit Physiological problems: metabolic problems, e.g. altered distribution of drugs
Predisposition to various **medical disorders**	Hypertension, ischaemic heart disease, type 2 diabetes, gallstones, gout
Operative difficulties	Operations take longer to perform because of difficult access and vital structures obscured by fat. This leads to a higher incidence of anaesthetic and surgical complications, particularly involving the wound
Problems of manual handling of patients who are markedly overweight	Weight and size limitations of standard equipment including CT scanners, operating tables, beds Need for hoists, powered beds Risks to staff involved in lifting and handling

---

Box 8.6   Potentially dangerous drugs in the surgical patient*

- Glucocorticoids
  - Predispose to peptic ulceration, delayed wound healing and infection
  - Adrenal atrophy caused by long-term steroid therapy may lead to acute adrenal insufficiency causing cardiovascular collapse
- Antihypertensive and anti-anginal drugs
  - Should not be stopped. Hazardous if abruptly stopped, which may cause rebound hypertension or angina
- Antidepressants
  - MAOIs are rarely used but should be stopped 2 weeks before surgery. Tricyclic antidepressants need not be stopped but carry risks of arrhythmias, hypotension and interaction with vasopressor drugs. Selective serotonin reuptake inhibitors should be continued. Lithium should be stopped 24 hours before major surgery but not minor surgery
- Oral contraceptives and hormone replacement therapy (HRT)
  - Mildly increased risk of deep venous thrombosis and pulmonary embolism. HRT should be stopped two weeks before major surgery. Stopping OCP risks pregnancy
- Anticoagulants and anti-platelet drugs
  - Predispose to haemorrhage and need careful management
- Diuretics
  - May cause electrolyte abnormalities and dehydration. Potassium sparing diuretics should be stopped on the morning of surgery

*Note that formularies such as the *BNF* carry details of drug interactions with anaesthetic agents.

---

period. Such deterioration is best estimated by using a score derived from a mini-mental test questionnaire.

OBESITY

Gross obesity carries 2–3 times the normal risk of perioperative death or morbidity, as outlined in Table 8.1. Whenever possible, weight should be reduced before operation, particularly if the operation is not urgent. Referral to a dietician may be helpful although self-help groups often provide stronger motivation. Preoperative investigations for obese patients include blood glucose measurement and ECG, even if the patient is asymptomatic.

CHRONIC DRUG THERAPY

Many drugs prescribed for long-term treatment of 'medical' conditions may complicate management of the surgical patient. Note that the risk of stopping long-term medication before surgery is often greater than the risk of continuing it throughout surgery and the early postoperative period. Drugs that should not normally be stopped include antiepileptics, antiparkinsonian drugs, antipsychotics, anxiolytics, bronchodilators, cardiovascular drugs, glaucoma drugs, immunosuppressants, drugs of dependence and thyroid or antithyroid drugs. The most important of these commonly encountered in practice are summarised in Box 8.6.

Blood transfusion

PRINCIPLES OF BLOOD TRANSFUSION

The ability to safely transfuse blood and blood products revolutionised the outcomes of major trauma. It also facilitated extraordinary advances in areas of surgery that involve heavy blood loss such as arterial reconstruction, open-heart surgery and organ transplantation.

Nevertheless, blood transfusion carries a range of potential **hazards**, for example from transfusion reactions, transmission of infection, clerical errors leading to the transfusion of incompatible products, and potential immunosuppression in cancer patients. The problem of infection has been tragically highlighted by the development of HIV/AIDS in haemophiliacs and of a few cases of vCJD after unwitting transfusion of infected blood.

For replacing blood loss, stored blood has the advantage over gelatin and electrolyte solutions that it remains within the vascular compartment. However, most 'blood' for transfusion consists only of concentrated red cells with all other useful components such as platelets and clotting factors removed. This paucity of useful factors coupled with the many potentially lethal side effects mean that a decision to transfuse blood or blood products is a serious one that must be based on very clear indications and after considering alternatives (see *Reducing the need for bank blood transfusion*, p. 130). Alternatives include:

Preoperative
- Tolerating lower haemoglobin concentration
- Iron therapy for iron deficiency anaemia
- Treatment with erythropoietin before or after operation, using recombinant human erythropoietin (rHuEPO)

Intraoperative
- Using alternative infusions for hypovolaemia such as gelatin solutions

- Techniques of autologous blood transfusion (i.e. recycling the patient's own blood during operation)

The types of transfusion components currently available and the general indications for their use are summarised in Box 9.1.

LABORATORY ASPECTS OF BLOOD TRANSFUSION

BLOOD GROUPING AND COMPATIBILITY TESTING

Transfusion of ABO incompatible blood may be fatal. Transfusion practice has been developed to minimise this risk and involves two main steps: first, the patient's ABO and Rhesus groups are determined; second, the patient's blood (and each unit of donor blood) is screened for antibodies. Traditionally, each unit of group-compatible donor blood intended for transfusion has been directly **cross-matched** against the patient's serum to ensure complete compatibility. Fortunately, in donor blood shown to be antibody-free, 99% is completely compatible with a group-matched recipient and can safely be transfused without cross-matching. Thus grouped and antibody screened blood can quickly be supplied from a prepared pool of units, rather than individually preparing blood units for each patient. This practice saves time and money and an increasing number of hospitals are adopting it.

After transfusion of approximately 10 units of blood (e.g. for massive haemorrhage from liver trauma), the patient's own antibodies are so depleted that further group-compatible blood is usually given without cross-matching. In an emergency (e.g. obstetric haemorrhage) where group-compatible blood is not available, then group O, Rh-negative blood can be given with comparative safety, but there is a long-term risk of antibodies emerging which would make future cross-matching difficult.

| Box | 9.1 | **Types of transfusion and indications for their use** |

Whole blood

Very rarely used because of the demand for separate blood components. Whole blood also carries greater risks of adverse reactions owing to the presence of leucocytes

Packed or concentrated red cells (the most common transfusion product)

For use in substantial haemorrhage and anaemia. Whole blood is collected then centrifuged to separate the red cells (and platelets and plasma). Packed/concentrated red cells are then suspended in a preservative solution ready for reinfusion. A bag of red cells is approximately 300 ml and raises the haemoglobin concentration by approximately 1 g/dl

Human albumin solution, available as 4.5% and 20% solutions

Albumin is expensive and is derived from human donor blood. In terms of efficacy, mortality and cardiorespiratory function, there is little evidence that albumin solutions are better than plasma substitutes or normal saline for resuscitating patients with **traumatic** or **septic shock** or requiring large peroperative volume replacement

Transfusion of albumin solutions should probably be restricted to patients with hypoproteinaemic oedema with nephrotic syndrome or with ascites in chronic liver disease. Other uses are difficult to justify in the absence of scientifically proven benefit

Fresh-frozen plasma (FFP)

Plasma is separated from fresh whole blood and then frozen. FFP contains near normal amounts of all clotting factors and other plasma proteins. It should be blood group compatible when possible and should not be used simply for volume replacement. FFP is often used to replace clotting factors exhausted during major haemorrhage (due to a combination of consumption of clotting factors by attempted haemostasis and the lack of clotting factors in transfused blood). This is likely when blood loss exceeds 1.5 times the blood volume, and the loss has been replaced rapidly with red cells and crystalloids or colloids. Clotting studies usually demonstrate a coagulopathy

FFP is also used to replace coagulation factor deficiencies when there is continued bleeding and the necessary specific factor concentrates are unavailable. This may occur in liver disease, thrombotic thrombocytopenic purpura (TTP) and acute disseminated intravascular coagulation (DIC)

Platelet concentrates

Used for platelet exhaustion during major haemorrhage (e.g. ruptured abdominal aortic aneurysm) and in thrombocytopenia. Indicated if the platelet count is $< 50 \times 10^9$/L, or massive blood loss is occurring. Platelets should be avoided in autoimmune platelet disorders except in the presence of life-threatening haemorrhage

Cryoprecipitate, fibrinogen and other specific clotting factor concentrates

Used for various specific coagulation deficiencies, e.g. severe hypofibrinogenaemia, haemophilia. These should only be used in consultation with a haematologist

Plasma substitutes

These are solutions of macromolecules with colloid osmotic pressure and viscosity characteristics similar to plasma. Gelatin solutions (e.g. Haemaccel, Gelofusine) and etherified starch solutions (e.g. hetastarch) are used for initial restoration of circulating volume in haemorrhage or burns and to maintain volume, blood pressure and renal perfusion intraoperatively where blood transfusion is not indicated.

STORAGE AND USEFUL LIFE OF BLOOD

Blood and blood products have exacting requirements if their quality is to be preserved. Their usefulness is easily impaired if they are handled inappropriately.

Packed red cells are stored between 2° and 6°C, and have a shelf life of 35 days. Improvements in preservative solutions mean red cell quality deteriorates little during storage but pH changes can occur and potassium leaches out of the cells. Luckily, this is only clinically significant in neonates undergoing exchange transfusion or in patients with renal failure.

Blood must not normally be frozen, although expensive techniques for freezing patients' own blood in glycerol for later autotransfusion have been developed for patients with rare blood groups or unusual antibodies.

To ensure vitality, blood should not be removed from the designated blood refrigerator until immediately before use. If blood has been out of the refrigerator for more than 30 minutes and has not been transfused, it should be returned to the laboratory for disposal because of the increased risk of bacterial proliferation. The laboratory should be informed as soon as it becomes apparent that blood products are not required so they can be made available for other patients. Empty used blood packs should be retained for 48 hours so that they can be examined and tested in the event of a transfusion reaction.

BLOOD TRANSFUSION IN CLINICAL PRACTICE

BLOOD TRANSFUSION AND ELECTIVE SURGERY

Attitudes to transfusion in elective surgery are becoming more conservative. Blood is an expensive commodity and its use is not risk-free. In elective surgery, patients usually fall into one of three categories: transfusion not anticipated (e.g. hernia repair), transfusion possible but unlikely (e.g. cholecystectomy), and transfusion probable (e.g. major arterial reconstruction). For patients in the second category, a blood sample should be sent in advance for ABO and Rhesus grouping and antibody screening, and the serum retained in the laboratory for further compatibility testing if required later ('group and save'). For patients in the third category, an appropriate number of units of blood are requested to be available for transfusion at the time of operation; many hospitals operate a maximum surgical blood ordering schedule (MSBOS), which should be followed to ensure appropriate ordering of blood for surgical patients. In patients for whom blood is ordered, the blood group and antibody screen is performed on receipt of the request and the blood is prepared a day or so before operation. If a further transfusion is required more than 72 hours later, a further blood sample must be tested for new antibodies that may have developed.

To guard against the disaster of blood being given to the wrong patient, scrupulous attention must be paid to correct and complete labelling of transfusion blood samples **whilst in the presence of the patient**. Hospitals still relying on a 'paper system' generally specify that all transfusion samples must be hand labelled. Immediately before transfusion, the label of each unit of the supplied blood must be carefully checked against the identity and blood group of the patient (along with the compatibility slip if used), in the presence of the patient.

VOLUME AND RATE OF TRANSFUSION

The volume of blood required and the rate of transfusion depend on the age of the patient, the indications for transfusion and the patient's general and cardiovascular condition.

Volume and rate in haemorrhage (see Table 9.1)

Haemorrhage can be classified clinically according to the response to initial colloid or crystalloid resuscitation. If there is no response, such as in torrential obstetric haemorrhage from placenta previa, a red cell transfusion is required. If there is no cross-matched blood available, group O Rh-negative blood can be transfused in an emergency so as to maintain adequate blood pressure and a positive central venous pressure. It is important to order blood for transfusion at the same time, as most hospitals have only a limited supply of emergency O negative blood. As soon as the group is known, it is best to administer group-specific rather than O negative blood, followed by cross-matched or antibody screened blood when available. If the response to resuscitation with colloid or crystalloid is satisfactory, immediate transfusion is not indicated.

If rapid transfusion is required, an inflatable pressure infuser can be wrapped around the blood pack to increase the pressure. Blood warming devices are potentially hazardous but are indicated for **adults** likely to receive blood at a rate of more than 50 ml/kg/h (approximately 10 units an hour in a 75 kg adult), **infants** undergoing exchange transfusions and patients with clinically significant **cold agglutinins**.

Volume and rate in anaemia

Surgery can usually be performed safely on patients whose haemoglobin is greater than 10 g/dl. In addition, compensated anaemia down to 8 g/dl in a young person may be tolerated with no increase in morbidity or mortality. Older patients are less tolerant of this level of anaemia unless it is chronic and little surgical blood loss is expected. In elective surgical patients found to be anaemic, the cause of anaemia should be investigated beforehand where possible and treatment with haematinics begun where appropriate. If preoperative transfusion proves necessary, it should be given at least 2 days before surgery if possible so as to maximise the beneficial effects of the blood and allow fluid balance to stabilise.

REDUCING THE NEED FOR BANK BLOOD TRANSFUSION

Deaths and serious reactions still occur from incompatible blood transfusions (particularly when blood products

Table 9.1 Recommendations for fluid replacement in haemorrhage by the British Committee for Standards in Haematology (BCSH) guidelines 2001

Amount of blood loss	Fluid replacement required
15–30% of blood volume (800–1500 ml in an adult)	Transfuse crystalloids or synthetic colloids; red cell transfusion **unlikely** to be needed unless the patient has pre-existing anaemia, reduced cardio-respiratory reserve or if blood loss continues
30–40% of blood volume (1500–2000 ml in an adult)	Volume replacement with crystalloids or synthetic colloids; red cell transfusion **likely** to be required
> 40% of blood volume (> 2000 ml in an adult)	**Rapid volume replacement** including red cell transfusion required

are administered under general anaesthesia). In addition, serious infections such as hepatitis, malaria and HIV can be transmitted from apparently fit but infected donors with chronic latent carrier states, despite careful screening of donors and donations. Variant Creutzfeldt–Jakob disease (vCJD) is an increasing concern with several cases of transfusion-transmitted vCJD identified. The risk of side effects and complications increases in parallel with the number of units transfused. Risks can be reduced by strict scrutiny of the indications for transfusion.

Non-transfusion methods of reducing bank blood transfusion have been discussed earlier. Transfusion methods involve 'recycling' the patient's own blood (**autologous transfusion**) by one of the following methods:

Preoperative autologous donation (PAD)

In a pre-deposit programme, up to 4 units of blood can be collected at weekly intervals from a patient planned for major elective surgery. Pre-donation can be safely achieved even in the elderly and those with cardiac disease. There are several drawbacks: the collection, storage and checking system is costly and complicated to administer and patients must be prepared well in advance of operation. Note that pre-donation does not prevent incompatible blood being transfused as a result of clerical errors. Erythropoietin may be given to increase the bone marrow response and shorten the donation programme, but at present it is too expensive for routine use.

Pre-donation is particularly useful for patients with rare antibodies who are difficult to cross-match and those patients who consistently refuse to receive homologous blood. In the UK, hospitals wishing to carry out PAD require approval from the National Blood Service (NBS).

Acute normovolaemic haemodilution (ANH)

This involves collecting whole blood from the patient immediately before surgery and replacing it afterwards if necessary. At the time of collection, normovolaemia is restored with colloid or crystalloid. The technique has the advantages of autologous transfusion but without the disadvantages of pre-donation or the need for intraoperative cell washing and collecting equipment. Up to 2 litres of blood can safely be removed from adults without cardiac disease around the time of induction of anaesthesia.

The procedure reduces the venous haematocrit and increases cardiac output. When about 300 ml of low-haematocrit blood has been lost at operation, re-infusion of the autologous blood is begun. If total blood loss is less than 2 litres, additional blood is rarely needed. The procedure is inexpensive, convenient for the patient and flexible as regards operation scheduling. The blood is fresh and contains functioning platelets and clotting factors. The collected blood is not removed from the operating theatre, minimising the risk of ABO incompatible transfusion due to clerical error. The technique has been used extensively in cardiac and vascular surgery but could be extended to other types of surgery where there is a potential blood loss of more than 20% of the blood volume. It can also be used in conjunction with other methods of blood conservation (see below).

Intraoperative cell salvage (IOCS)

UK government directives and national guidelines have endorsed intraoperative cell salvage as an effective technique, particularly appropriate in cardiac, vascular and orthopaedic surgery.

Intraoperative cell salvage involves collecting blood spilled at operation by suction, processing it and reinfusing it. There are two main techniques:

- In manual (unwashed) salvage, blood is collected into a reservoir containing anticoagulant before being reinfused via a fine filter
- In the more sophisticated washed systems, an automated cell saver collects, washes, concentrates and re-suspends salvaged red cells in physiological solution

This blood, with a packed cell volume of 50%, is then available for reinfusion. Some Jehovah's Witnesses will allow intraoperative cell salvage, as the blood is regarded as never having left the body.

In malignant disease the technique remains controversial even though clinical studies have so far failed to demonstrate dissemination of metastases.

Postoperative cell salvage (POCS)

This technique salvages blood lost in the postoperative period. It is collected via a specially filtered wound drain and is then transfused via another filter back into the patient. This is suitable for use in procedures with an expected and 'clean' postoperative blood loss such as total knee replacements.

HAZARDS AND COMPLICATIONS OF BLOOD TRANSFUSION

FEBRILE NON-HAEMOLYTIC TRANSFUSION REACTIONS (FNHTR)

These reactions are usually caused by leucocyte rather than red cell incompatibility and have become rare since universal leucodepletion of blood products has become regularly employed. Febrile reactions are more common in multi-transfused or parous women. An increase in temperature of one degree above baseline and shivering during or after the transfusion indicates a FNHTR. Symptoms can usually be managed by stopping the transfusion for 15–30 minutes and administering an antipyretic and

> **Box** **9.2** **Clinical features of a haemolytic transfusion reaction**
>
> - Rapidly developing pyrexia at onset of transfusion
> - Dyspnoea, constrictive feeling in chest, intense headache
> - Severe loin pain
> - Hypotension
> - Acute oliguric renal failure with haemoglobinuria (due to obstruction of tubules with haemoglobin, hypotension causing acute tubular necrosis)
> - Jaundice (developing hours or days later)
> - Disseminated intravascular coagulation with spontaneous bruising and haemorrhage

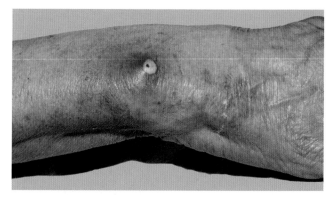

Fig. 9.1 Infected cannula site at the wrist

an antihistamine. This type of reaction of itself is rarely life threatening, but fever with or without rigors may be the prelude to a more serious reaction.

HAEMOLYTIC REACTIONS

If there is major ABO incompatibility, massive haemolysis will occur and this can be fatal. Incompatibility in minor determinants causes a lesser degree of haemolysis. Almost all haemolytic reactions are caused by human error resulting in transfusion of incompatible blood. The clinical features of a haemolytic reaction are summarised in Box 9.2. The diagnosis is confirmed by finding hyperbilirubinaemia and a positive Coombs' test in the patient's blood, and by demonstrating a new antibody on repeat screening. With massive intravascular haemolysis, haemoglobinaemia and haemoglobinuria may occur. The transfusion must be halted immediately and the patient resuscitated. Oliguria is treated by osmotic diuresis (e.g. mannitol), aided by a loop diuretic if appropriate.

ALLERGIC REACTIONS

Allergic reactions to transfusion occasionally occur and manifest as fever, pruritus (itching), skin rashes, wheals or angio-oedema (periorbital, facial and laryngeal swelling) and, rarely, anaphylaxis. Mild allergic reactions can usually be managed by slowing or stopping the transfusion for 30 minutes and administering an antihistamine. Recurrent severe allergic reactions require antihistamine premedication and, occasionally, the use of saline washed cells. Investigation of the cause of such allergic reactions is required. Note that latex allergy is an increasingly common problem and the effect may be wrongly interpreted as a transfusion reaction.

INFECTION

Infection may arise from three sources: present in the donor, contamination during the process of blood prepa-

ration and storage, or from the giving set or cannula site (Fig. 9.1).

Infections transmitted by donor blood or blood product transfusion

Donated blood can now be screened for most significant transmissible infectious agents. Many of the tests, however, rely on detecting antibodies to viruses and cannot detect disease acquired too recently for the antibody response to develop.

Donor infections are most likely to be transmitted when a **chronic latent carrier state** exists in the donor. Diseases that can cause this state include:

- **Viral infections**—hepatitis B, C and D; HIV I and II; HTLV I and II; cytomegalovirus; Epstein–Barr virus
- **Bacterial infections**—syphilis; brucellosis
- **Protozoal infections**—malaria; Chagas' disease and babesiosis
- **Prions**—variant Creutzfeldt–Jakob disease (vCJD)

The more frequent of these infections are discussed below.

Hepatitis viruses

Donors have been screened for hepatitis B virus (HBV) by all transfusion services in the developed world since the late 1960s and this has dramatically reduced the incidence of transfusion-related hepatitis B. Despite screening, infections occasionally occur because the surface antigen HBsAg, which is the first marker to appear, may be absent in the early days after infection. For this reason, patients needing multiple transfusions or blood products should be vaccinated against hepatitis B. In carriers or infected individuals, hepatitis B virus is present in the plasma and is therefore transmitted by all blood products except those subject to viricidal treatment.

Hepatitis C used to be transmitted twice as often via blood transfusion as hepatitis B. The illness associated with hepatitis C is often mild but up to half of all cases progress to chronic hepatitis (10% for hepatitis B) and 10% develop cirrhosis or hepatoma or both. Since 1991 all donations in the UK have been screened for hepatitis C and the incidence of post-transfusion hepatitis C has fallen from 1.3 per 1000 units transfused to 0.1. However, it is recognised that the 'window' after infection for the appearance of HCV antigen can be up to 3 months. Antiviral chemotherapy is now available to eliminate or suppress hepatitis C in patients known to have the infection.

Human immunodeficiency virus (HIV)

In 1981, the HIV epidemic and its link with blood transfusion began to be recognised with reports of opportunistic pneumonias in transfused haemophiliacs. By the mid 1980s, the risk of HIV transmission via transfused blood in the USA was as high as 1 in 2500. Luckily, transmission via blood transfusion associated with surgery has been rare in the UK. Haemophiliacs were much less fortunate, being infected via clotting factor VIII preparations, often collected abroad.

In the UK, all blood donors and donations have been screened for HIV antibody since 1985. About 5 per million donors in the UK have been found to be HIV positive. Current HIV antibody detection methods are very reliable but there is a 'window' period lasting 1–3 months after infection when antibody may be undetectable. The most effective method of reducing the risk in countries where donors are unpaid is donor self-exclusion. Potential donors have the risks of infection transfer explained and are asked not to donate blood if they know they have transmissible infections or fall into high-risk categories. When combined with a low prevalence of HIV in the donor pool (as in the UK), the risk of transmitting HIV via a screened blood or blood component donation is small but not negligible.

Cytomegalovirus

Infection with cytomegalovirus is widespread, with the virus remaining latent in leucocytes. The risk of infection is significant only in immature neonates and immunosuppressed patients who are CMV seronegative. To minimise the risk, donated blood for these groups should be screened for CMV-specific antibody.

Protozoal infection—malaria

Transfusion-transmitted malaria remains rare in developed countries. In endemic areas, however, it is common and the majority of healthy blood donors will be potentially infectious. The disease should be considered if a patient becomes ill after transfusion.

Variant Creutzfeldt–Jakob disease (vCJD)

vCJD was first described in 1996 in the UK. Note that it differs from the familial forms of CJD. Scientific evidence shows that vCJD in humans is closely linked to bovine spongiform encephalopathy in cattle (BSE) and is thought to be acquired through the ingestion of infected meat.

There are currently 12–15 new cases of vCJD per annum in the UK, but the number of individuals incubating the disease is unknown.

It is now known that vCJD is transmissible through blood products. In the UK, several precautions have been taken to minimise the risk such as universal leucodepletion of blood products and the sourcing of plasma for fractionation from non-UK sources.

There is currently no screening method, diagnostic tool or treatment for this disease. Avoiding unnecessary blood transfusion is the only way to minimise the potential risk.

Contamination of blood or giving sets with microorganisms

Low-grade contamination of blood packs from the environment rarely has serious consequences because of the low temperature of blood storage and the self-sterilising properties of blood. However, microorganisms may proliferate if storage conditions are inadequate or blood is left unchilled before transfusion.

Transfusion of bacterially infected blood products is rare but it can be catastrophic, leading to death within a very short time. Platelet transfusions have been most commonly incriminated. Gram-negative aerobic bacilli, particularly *Pseudomonas* and *Salmonella* species, have been identified. Accumulation of exotoxins or endotoxins may also lead to life-threatening complications.

Giving sets may become contaminated unless strict aseptic technique is maintained during the setting-up or changing of any component of transfusion equipment. Finally, peripheral intravenous cannulae, and particularly central venous lines, may become infected by opportunistic skin commensals (e.g. coagulase-negative staphylococci) or contaminating pathogens (e.g. *Staph. aureus*, *E. coli*) causing local infection (see Fig. 9.1), bacteraemia or even systemic sepsis. Cannula sites should be inspected daily and changed at least every 72 hours. The same vein can then later be reused for a new infusion. In a patient with a central venous line and pyrexia of unknown origin, the line should be removed and tested bacteriologically.

The clinical result of transfusing a bacterially contaminated donation resembles that of a haemolytic reaction, with fever, chills, hypotension, nausea and vomiting, oliguria and disseminated intravascular coagulation. If a patient develops these adverse symptoms, investigations should include culture of the patient's blood and the blood product as well as rechecking compatibility.

IMMUNOSUPPRESSIVE EFFECTS OF BLOOD TRANSFUSION

Blood transfusion has been demonstrated to have a potential for immunosuppression, which may influence recurrence of certain cancers. For this reason, transfusion may have an adverse influence on postoperative infection rates. Nevertheless, data are contradictory in both of these areas and as yet there is no definite evidence of an important clinical effect. In some patients, the potential immunosuppressive effects of blood transfusion may bring benefit, for example those undergoing renal transplantation.

FLUID OVERLOAD

Fluid overload is rarely a problem of blood transfusion in healthy adults but may readily develop if the cardiovascular system is already compromised or if particularly large volumes are given. Overload is a particular risk when transfusing babies and small children.

TRANSFUSION-RELATED ACUTE LUNG INJURY (TRALI)

Transfusion, particularly of a plasma-containing product, may be followed by acute and rapid onset of shortness of breath and cough. Typically there is a 'white-out' on chest X-ray. TRALI is treated in the same way as acute respiratory distress syndrome (ARDS) from any other cause; it usually requires intensive care admission and mechanical ventilation. The injury is caused by the donor's antibodies reacting with the patient's leucocytes. Implicated donors are usually multiparous women and it is vital that the central or National Blood Service is informed to exclude the particular donor from the panel.

DELAYED TRANSFUSION REACTIONS

Post-transfusion purpura (PTP)

This is fortunately rare as it is a potentially fatal side effect. It is more common in female patients and is caused by platelet-specific allo-antibodies. Symptoms usually occur about a week after transfusion, with the patient developing thrombocytopenia with bleeding. PTP is treated with high doses of intravenous immunoglobulins, which gives a favourable response in around 85% of cases.

Transfusion-associated graft versus host disease (Ta-GvHD)

In certain cases, transfused donor lymphocytes, even though compatible with the recipient, can recognise the recipient's cells as foreign and initiate **graft versus host disease**. Patients most at risk are those with defective cell-mediated immunity. This may be inherited or acquired, e.g. in Hodgkin's disease. Irradiation of blood products is needed to inactivate T-cells likely to cause GvHD in susceptible patients. The mortality rate of Ta-GvHD is 75–90% as there is no effective treatment.

Diagnosis and management of common postoperative problems

10

INTRODUCTION

Despite the best endeavours at each stage (preoperative assessment, surgical technique and perioperative management) unexpected symptoms and signs arise in the postoperative period which may herald a postoperative complication. Many complications can be detected early by regular and close postoperative patient observation and treated before they become established. For example, daily auscultation of the chest after major surgery may reveal pneumonia before the symptoms appear.

Managing the common problems such as pain, fever or collapse requires accurate diagnosis and early treatment. Diagnosing the cause can be difficult for the doctor on the spot who is called to see a postoperative patient with problems and who may not know the patient or his or her history. The difficulty is compounded if the patient is anxious, in pain or not fully recovered from an anaesthetic. It is essential to conduct a thorough and systematic clinical assessment and if necessary, arrange investigations, whatever the hour, for potentially serious but often remediable complications.

The following problems are often seen in the early postoperative period, frequently 'after hours', and are usually the immediate responsibility of junior surgical doctors.

POSTOPERATIVE PAIN

Pain can be expected from most surgical wounds but in most cases this can be controlled by planned analgesia. It gradually subsides over the first few days after operation. Some types of wound are more painful than others, for example vertical abdominal incisions and skin graft donor sites. Postoperative analgesia is far better managed nowadays, with the recognition that it is better to prevent pain than to react to established pain.

METHODS OF PERIOPERATIVE PAIN RELIEF

Postoperative pain can be reduced by preoperative counselling, peroperative measures and postoperative analgesia. Counselling involves letting the patient know in advance what to expect after the operation in terms of wounds, intravenous lines, catheters and so on. The patient should also be told the likely extent of pain, the plans for pain relief and the degree of mobility he or she might expect after operation. During operation, a great deal can be achieved by using **pre-emptive analgesia**. This involves a variety of methods to ensure that pain does not become established.

Pre-emptive analgesia may involve:

- Long-acting analgesic drugs given intravenously
- Local anaesthetic infiltration into the wound edges at the end of the operation with long-acting **bupivacaine**
- Regional nerve blocks (e.g. intercostal nerves for upper abdominal surgery)
- Epidural analgesia using morphine and local anaesthetic agents during and after abdominal and pelvic surgery
- Non-steroidal analgesic agents given before the patient awakes by means of suppository or intravenous injection. With non-steroidal agents, care must be taken not to give them to patients with known **allergy** to aspirin or other NSAIDs, a history of severe asthma or angio-oedema, bleeding disorders, renal impairment, hypovolaemia or pregnancy. Mild asthma is not a contraindication. It is also unwise to use these drugs in operations that carry a high risk of haemorrhage, e.g. major arterial surgery

Commonly used oral and parenteral analgesic drugs are listed in Box 10.1. Postoperative analgesia is discussed in the next two sections.

Box 10.1 Postoperative analgesics and their indications (approximate ascending order of analgesic strength)

Mild-to-moderate pain:

- Paracetamol
- Compounds of paracetamol and low-dose codeine, e.g. co-codamol
- Milder non-steroidal anti-inflammatory drugs (NSAIDs), e.g. ibuprofen

Moderate pain:

- Paracetamol
- Codeine or dihydrocodeine 30–60 mg
- Stronger NSAIDs as tablets or suppositories, e.g. diclofenac

Moderate-to-severe pain:

- Other opiate analgesics stronger than codeine, e.g. oxycodone, tramadol
- Non-steroidal anti-inflammatory drugs by intravenous injection, e.g. diclofenac
- Morphine slow-release tablets
- Morphine or diamorphine—patient-controlled intravenous injection

ANALGESIA FOR MINOR AND INTERMEDIATE SURGERY

Patients vary greatly in their tolerance of pain and their need for analgesics. For minor and intermediate surgery, pre-emptive techniques described above usually mean that simple analgesic tablets are sufficient. However, the amount of analgesia must be tailored to individual need. Anxiety, exhaustion and sleep deprivation may greatly reduce pain tolerance; these should be considered in any patient who fails to respond to a reasonable amount of analgesia.

ANALGESIA FOR MAJOR SURGERY AND TRAUMA

Many hospitals now provide an **acute pain service**, usually run by a specialist nurse and one or more anaesthetists. This team can plan an analgesic strategy for individual patients and ensure it is carried out with at least twice-daily ward visits. The team also serves an important educational function, making sure clinicians and nurses are pain-relief aware as well as helping to deal with individual problems as they arise. True objective rating is difficult to achieve but some form of visual analogue scale upon which the patient places his or her immediate experience of pain can be helpful (Fig. 10.1).

Following major abdominal and many perineal operations **epidural analgesia** using drugs such as bupivacaine

and morphine can be invaluable. A single dose can be given to provide anaesthesia for the operation, e.g. transurethral prostatectomy, and can provide several hours of complete postoperative analgesia. For more extensive surgery, e.g. abdominal aortic aneurysm grafting, an epidural cannula can be left in situ to allow 'topping-up' for prolonged postoperative analgesia. These patients need to be carefully observed for signs of toxicity or severe hypotension and respiratory depression. Traditionally, this took place in a high-dependency unit, but specific nurse training has allowed it to be extended on to normal wards. Note that moderate hypotension is merely an indication of a satisfactory sympathetic blockade.

For major surgery and trauma where epidural analgesia is inappropriate, the dose of analgesic needs to be sufficient to eliminate the pain without dangerous side effects, and the drug needs to be given frequently enough to maintain continuous pain relief. The old practice of writing up intermittent intramuscular opiates 'at 4-hourly intervals, as required' has been recognised as inadequate and ineffective for relieving pain associated with major surgery. Given the enormous variation in analgesic requirements, standard regimens of this type are too inflexible and usually inadequate. Much more effective pain control can be achieved by allowing patients to give themselves small intravenous increments of opiates as soon as they are needed using a **patient-controlled analgesia** (PCA) device (Fig. 10.2). This allows presetting of the incremental dose (often 1 mg of morphine), with a 5 minute lockout to prevent it being given too frequently, as well as control of the total dose given. Continuous effective pain relief is thus easily achieved and, paradoxically, the total dose of drug used is often less than with intermittent injections. Furthermore, this technique causes minimal sedation and respiratory depression while maintaining excellent continuous analgesia, although it can cause opiate-induced nausea.

EXCESSIVE POSTOPERATIVE PAIN

If the pain is not controlled by what appears to be an adequate dose and frequency of analgesia, complications should be suspected. The dose should be reviewed in relation to the expected severity of pain and the weight of the patient

- **Local postoperative complications** should be considered. Wound pain may be caused by pressure from a **haematoma**. In limb trauma, bleeding into a fascial compartment must be diagnosed before ischaemia ensues ('**compartment syndrome**'). Wound pain increasing after the first 48 hours may be caused by **infection**. The wound will be unusually tender even before redness and induration develop. There is usually a pyrexia. Other complications to consider with lower limb pain include deep vein

Fig. 10.1 **Pain measurement scales**

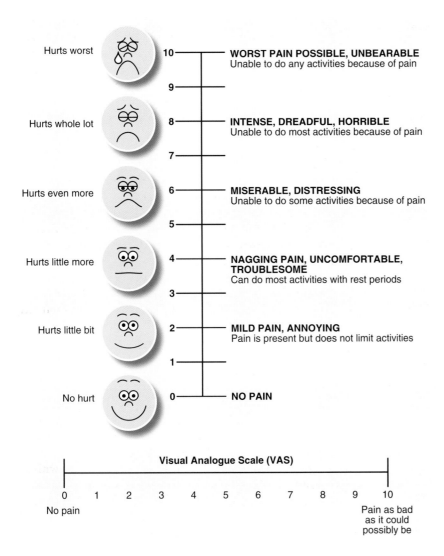

Hurts worst	10	**WORST PAIN POSSIBLE, UNBEARABLE** Unable to do any activities because of pain
	9	
Hurts whole lot	8	**INTENSE, DREADFUL, HORRIBLE** Unable to do most activities because of pain
	7	
Hurts even more	6	**MISERABLE, DISTRESSING** Unable to do some activities because of pain
	5	
Hurts little more	4	**NAGGING PAIN, UNCOMFORTABLE, TROUBLESOME** Can do most activities with rest periods
	3	
Hurts little bit	2	**MILD PAIN, ANNOYING** Pain is present but does not limit activities
	1	
No hurt	0	**NO PAIN**

Visual Analogue Scale (VAS)

0   1   2   3   4   5   6   7   8   9   10
No pain   Pain as bad
                                          as it could
                                          possibly be

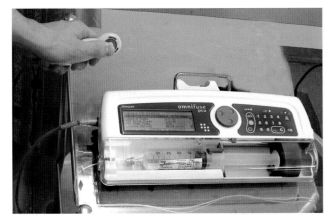

Fig. 10.2 Patient-controlled analgesia
This microprocessor-controlled device prevents overdosage by locking out if used too frequently. The patient's control handset is seen on the left.

thrombosis and acute ischaemia. Lastly, major comorbid conditions may be the cause of pain, for example myocardial ischaemia, or a fractured neck of femur may follow a fall from a bed

- **Major complications** in the area of the operation may need to be considered. After an abdominal operation, excessive pain may be caused by intra-abdominal complications. These include haemorrhage, anastomotic leakage, biliary leakage, abscess formation, gaseous distension due to ileus or air swallowing, intestinal obstruction, urinary retention and bowel ischaemia. Constipation may also cause late postoperative pain. These complications are all described in Chapter 12.

As a general rule, serious complications cause deterioration in the patient's general condition, whereas the patient remains well in the presence of less serious complications such as urinary retention or constipation.

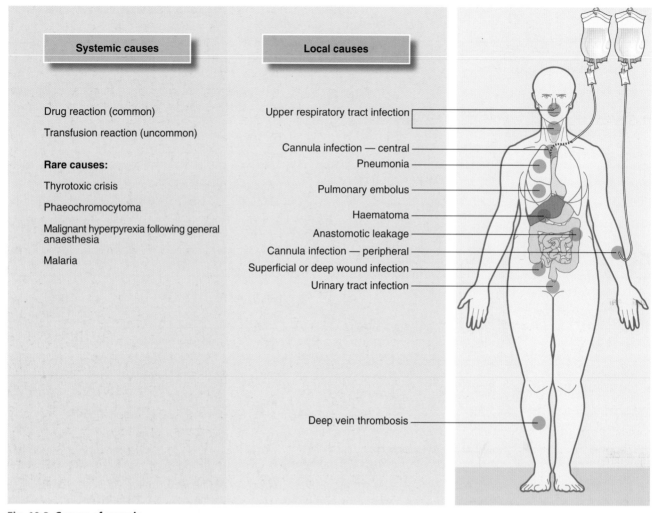

| Systemic causes | Local causes |

Drug reaction (common)

Transfusion reaction (uncommon)

Rare causes:

Thyrotoxic crisis

Phaeochromocytoma

Malignant hyperpyrexia following general anaesthesia

Malaria

Upper respiratory tract infection

Cannula infection — central
Pneumonia

Pulmonary embolus

Haematoma
Anastomotic leakage
Cannula infection — peripheral
Superficial or deep wound infection
Urinary tract infection

Deep vein thrombosis

Fig. 10.3 Causes of pyrexia

PYREXIA (see Fig. 10.3)

Fever is a common postoperative observation which is not always caused by infection. Pyrexia within the first 48 hours after operation is usually caused by basal atelectasis of the lungs and should be treated with physiotherapy and mobilisation. After this period, a search should be made for a focus of infection. The common ones are **superficial** or **deep wound infection, chest infection** (pneumonia), **urinary tract infection** and infection of an **intravenous cannula site**. If there is a central venous line, infection of this should always be suspected in a patient with unexplained pyrexia. Unfortunately, this can only be properly diagnosed by removing the line and culturing the tip for organisms. Blood cultures are often positive in such cases but do not reveal the source of infection. Patients usually recover spontaneously once the cannula is removed.

Unrelated infections such as viral **upper respiratory tract infections** are easily overlooked. **Malaria** should be considered in a recent immigrant or traveller from an endemic area.

Common non-infective causes of pyrexia include **transfusion reactions, wound haematomas, deep venous thrombosis** and **pulmonary embolism**. Pyrexia is sometimes the only sign of an idiosyncratic or allergic **drug reaction**. Other rare causes of pyrexia include thyrotoxic crisis, phaeochromocytoma and malignant hyperpyrexia following general anaesthesia.

TACHYCARDIA

Tachycardia (rapid heart rate) may simply indicate **pain** or **anxiety** but it is also a feature of **infection, circulatory disturbances** and **thyrotoxicosis**. Mild tachycardia may be a sign of incipient **hypovolaemic shock** as a result of haemorrhage or dehydration. It may also herald **cardiac failure** which, if missed, may progress to a life-threatening state. Tachycardia may be a sign of recent onset **atrial fibrillation or flutter**; this is confirmed by electrocardiography, and may indicate the patient has suffered a myocardial infarction (Fig. 10.4). In postoperative bowel surgery patients, this change is often a sign of **anastomotic leakage**, presumably mediated by cytokines released as a result of the leakage.

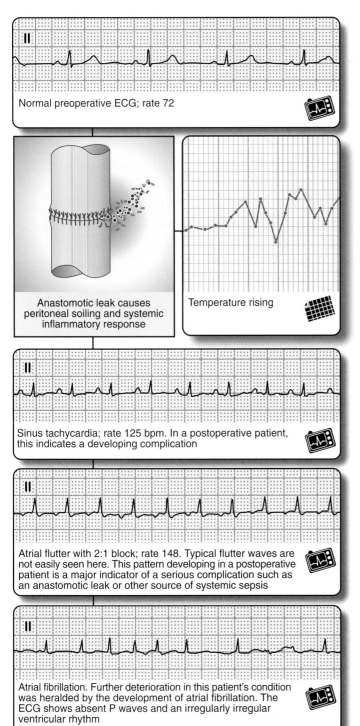

Normal preoperative ECG; rate 72

Anastomotic leak causes peritoneal soiling and systemic inflammatory response

Temperature rising

Sinus tachycardia; rate 125 bpm. In a postoperative patient, this indicates a developing complication

Atrial flutter with 2:1 block; rate 148. Typical flutter waves are not easily seen here. This pattern developing in a postoperative patient is a major indicator of a serious complication such as an anastomotic leak or other source of systemic sepsis

Atrial fibrillation. Further deterioration in this patient's condition was heralded by the development of atrial fibrillation. The ECG shows absent P waves and an irregularly irregular ventricular rhythm

Fig. 10.4 Early consequences of a bowel anastomotic leak

COUGH, SHORTNESS OF BREATH AND TACHYPNOEA

These symptoms are often associated with an overt respiratory problem such as **acute bronchopneumonia, aspiration of gastric contents, lobar collapse, pneumothorax** or an exacerbation of a **pre-existing chronic lung disorder**. Clinical examination and chest X-ray will rapidly diagnose most of these.

Shortness of breath and rapid shallow breathing are a feature of alveolar collapse (**atelectasis**) which may not be detected by clinical examination or chest X-ray. Atelectasis usually responds to chest physiotherapy. **Abdominal distension** may also cause rapid shallow breathing by inhibiting diaphragmatic movement. Shortness of breath and tachypnoea may be early features of **cardiac failure** or **fluid overload** but there are usually other clues such as tachycardia and basal crepitations.

A sudden onset of shortness of breath and tachypnoea, often associated with collapse, may indicate **pulmonary embolism**. This must be recognised, investigated and treated vigorously. **Acute respiratory distress syndrome** may occur in chest trauma, acute pancreatitis or systemic sepsis and should be anticipated in these patients. Finally, respiratory symptoms may be due to **hyperventilation** induced by pain, anxiety or hysterical reaction to stress.

COLLAPSE OR RAPID GENERAL DETERIORATION

The doctor on call is commonly asked to deal with a patient who has 'collapsed' or 'gone off' in a non-specific way. To make matters more difficult, the patient is often under the care of another surgical team. The more serious general possibilities are summarised in Box 10.2.

In practice, the problem is tackled in the following order, which usually leads to a logical diagnosis:

- Brief history of the collapse and postoperative course to date
- Rapid clinical appraisal—check Airway, Breathing and Circulation first, then changes in temperature, pulse, blood pressure and respiratory rate. Review urinary output and fluid balance
- Review of:
  —Reason for admission and preoperative state
  —Other pre-existing comorbid conditions
  —The nature and extent of surgical operation, including any particular operative problems
  —Extent of perioperative blood and other fluid losses (including sequestration in bowel)
  —Adequacy of fluid replacement
  —Drug therapy—what drugs have been prescribed? Have important drugs been given or omitted?
- Detailed physical examination
- Check blood glucose using reagent strips
- Special tests as suggested by clinical findings, e.g. ECG, chest X-ray, serum electrolyte estimation, arterial blood gas analysis, full blood count, urinalysis

Cardiovascular

- Myocardial infarction
- Other cause of rapid deterioration of cardiac function, e.g. sudden arrhythmia or fluid overload
- Pulmonary embolism
- Stroke (may be without obvious limb paralysis)

Respiratory

- Failure to reverse anaesthesia adequately (early)
- Drug-induced respiratory depression
- Hypoxia due to a respiratory disorder or respiratory depressant drugs

'Surgical' and infective

- Hypovolaemic shock from acute blood loss, or sudden decompensation in unrecognised hypovolaemia
- Bowel strangulation or obstruction
- Systemic sepsis (often caused by anastomotic leakage)
- Severe localised infection, e.g. chest or operation site

Metabolic

- Electrolyte disturbances, e.g. hyponatraemia
- Hypoglycaemia or hyperglycaemia associated with diabetes
- Adrenal insufficiency, e.g. adrenal suppression by steroids; causes hypotension

Drug effects

- Drug reactions, e.g. anaphylaxis

NAUSEA AND VOMITING

DRUGS AS A CAUSE

Nausea and vomiting are common postoperative problems. The usual causes are side effects from drugs used for premedication, general anaesthesia and postoperative analgesia. The major culprits are **opiates**. Anti-emetics such as prochlorperazine or metoclopramide are usually given with opiates and are prescribed 'as required' for the early postoperative period. Nausea and sometimes vomiting later in the postoperative period may also be caused by drugs. The worst offenders are the antibacterial agents erythromycin and metronidazole when given orally, and **digoxin** overdosage (which should be anticipated in the elderly and in chronic renal failure).

CAUSES IN THE IMMEDIATE POSTOPERATIVE PERIOD

- Vigorous handling of the patient in moving around the operating department and in the recovery room may stimulate vestibular input causing motion sickness
- Oropharyngeal stimulation—caused by a nasogastric (NG) tube or postoperative aspiration of secretions
- Hypoxia
- Hypotension
- Pain
- Anxiety

BOWEL OBSTRUCTION CAUSING NAUSEA AND VOMITING (see Ch. 12)

Serious or sustained vomiting 48 hours or more after operation is usually caused by failure of normal peristalsis of stomach, small bowel or large bowel. This may be caused either by **mechanical obstruction** or by **adynamic bowel**. **Acute gastric dilatation**, an adynamic problem, may follow any abdominal operation and any patient who vomits should be examined for a 'succussion splash'. If present, immediate nasogastric intubation is necessary; 2 or more litres of fluid may need to be aspirated which might otherwise be vomited and inhaled. Aspiration of gastric contents can cause mild or severe aspiration pneumonia (Mendelson's syndrome). If massive aspiration occurs, it can effectively drown the patient causing sudden death. Other adynamic bowel problems may be a response to local factors (e.g. bowel handling, a bowel-wall haematoma or a collection of pus in contact with bowel) or to systemic abnormalities, particularly **hypokalaemia**. Adynamic large bowel (**pseudo-obstruction**) sometimes occurs in a debilitated patient with a severe non-abdominal illness such as fractured neck of femur. Finally, **faecal impaction** is a common problem in the elderly or immobile patient. It may cause vomiting from what amounts to physical obstruction plus adynamic bowel.

Mechanical obstruction, usually of small bowel, may follow any abdominal operation. Early obstruction due to fibrinous adhesions occurs within 4 days of operation and may respond to conservative treatment but often requires a further operation.

SYSTEMIC DISORDERS CAUSING NAUSEA AND VOMITING

Electrolyte disturbances, uraemia, hypercalcaemia and other systemic disorders may cause vomiting via their central effects. Centrally mediated vomiting also occurs with raised intracranial pressure. This must be considered following head injuries, neurosurgical operations or in patients with cerebral metastases.

HAEMATEMESIS

Elderly postoperative patients sometimes produce a small quantity of **'coffee ground' vomitus** which is positive for blood on 'stick' testing. This rightly causes concern to nurses but rarely indicates a major haematemesis. It probably results from trivial bleeding from mild, stress-related gastritis or reflux oesophagitis. No special treatment is usually required but the patient should be closely observed for signs of internal bleeding, and antacid preparations such as an H_2 antagonist or a proton pump inhibitor given.

Occasionally, a major upper gastrointestinal haemorrhage occurs in the postoperative patient. If there has been forceful vomiting, a Mallory–Weiss oesophageal tear at the oesophago-gastric junction may be the cause. Major bleeding may also arise from exacerbation of a peptic ulcer or even oesophageal varices. Seriously ill patients and the victims of burns and head injuries are susceptible to **acute stress ulceration**, which may cause catastrophic gastrointestinal haemorrhage (see Ch. 21).

DISORDERS OF BOWEL FUNCTION

The main bowel function disorders that develop in the postoperative period are adynamic bowel problems and intestinal obstruction (covered earlier in this chapter), diarrhoea and finally constipation.

DIARRHOEA

Transient diarrhoea frequently follows abdominal operations, and should be regarded as normal early in the recovery phase following bowel resections or operations to relieve intestinal obstruction.

Diarrhoea may also complicate **antibiotic therapy**. Several days after the onset of treatment, loose, frequent stools are passed for a short period, probably as a result of bacterial or fungal overgrowth. Less commonly, **antibiotic-associated diarrhoea** may develop and even become life threatening. This is characterised by severe and persistent diarrhoea, sometimes containing blood (see Ch. 12).

After surgery of the abdominal aorta, blood-stained diarrhoea may sometimes occur a few days postoperatively. This may indicate **large-bowel ischaemia** due to surgical interference with the blood supply of the sigmoid colon by ligating the inferior mesenteric artery. This is a dangerous complication and requires urgent investigation and surgical exploration.

CONSTIPATION

Constipation is common and becomes apparent several days after operation. It usually represents a failure to re-establish normal bowel function. The causes include restriction of oral fluids and fibre, difficulty or reluctance in using a bed pan, slow recovery of normal peristalsis and general lack of mobility. **Anal pain** is a powerful disincentive to defaecation following surgery for anal conditions. Constipation causes great distress, especially in the elderly. It should be anticipated and prevented if practicable by prescribing **bulk-forming agents** (e.g. methylcellulose or ispaghula husk preparations), **osmotic laxatives** (e.g. lactulose) or **lubricant laxatives** (e.g.

liquid paraffin). Irritant laxatives and bowel stimulants can be used if there is still no progress.

For colonic surgery, large-bowel cleansing procedures (enemas, osmotic laxatives and restriction of solid foods) are usually carried out beforehand to prevent solid faecal matter disrupting the anastomosis. Bowel cleansing also reduces the risk of faecal contamination during operation and may help recovery of normal bowel habit afterwards.

Impacted faeces in any patient may result in **overflow incontinence** which must not be confused with diarrhoea from other causes. Thus any patient with abnormal bowel function must undergo digital rectal examination to exclude faecal impaction.

POOR URINE OUTPUT

RETENTION OF URINE

Abnormally low urinary output or complete failure to pass urine is a frequent postoperative problem. The most common cause is urinary retention, which usually occurs in males. It is readily diagnosed if there is a palpable suprapubic mass which is dull to percussion. Retention can readily be confirmed by ultrasound examination or more invasively by passing a urinary catheter.

BLOCKED CATHETER

If the patient is already catheterised, the catheter may have become blocked. The catheter can be checked for patency using a bladder syringe and flushed or replaced as necessary.

DIMINISHED URINE PRODUCTION

Poor urine output commonly results from poor renal perfusion due to **hypotension** during the operation or **hypovolaemia** caused by inadequate fluid replacement. If untreated, this may progress to acute renal failure. Renal failure from other causes, e.g. systemic sepsis, should also be considered.

If **hypovolaemia** is suspected, then an intravenous **fluid challenge** of 250 ml of dextrose-saline or Hartmann's solution should be given over 15 minutes or so, while monitoring urine output (Fig. 10.5). This can usually be repeated once after 30 minutes. If the patient is **hypotensive**, the cause (cardiac failure or hypovolaemia, for example) must be identified and treated as soon as possible. If oliguria persists or worsens, then a urinary catheter should be inserted to ensure that the bladder is emptying and to enable hourly measurement of urine output. If urine output is still poor, a central venous line should be placed for monitoring of CVP. If CVP is satisfactory, many patients will respond to a small intravenous dose of a loop diuretic, e.g. 40 mg of furosemide. If these simple measures fail to improve urine output, then acute renal failure must be suspected and investigated.

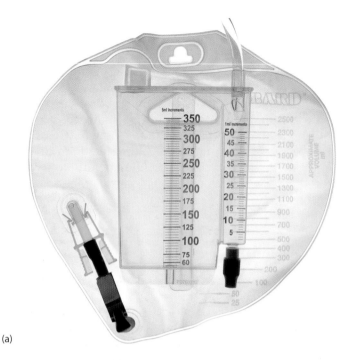

(a)

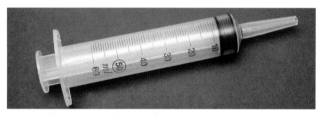

(b)

Fig. 10.5 Urine burette and bladder syringe
(a) Urine burette for precise measurement of urine output. Urine first enters the narrow compartment on the right to enable small quantities to be measured. It is then tipped into the main container to measure running totals.
(b) Bladder syringe used to flush urinary catheters suspected of blockage with debris. The nozzle is specially shaped to fit the end of a Foley urinary catheter. Note that full sterile precautions must be employed to reduce the risk of urinary infection.

Lastly, bilateral ureteric obstruction should be considered (or unilateral if only one kidney is present). This is extremely rare as a cause of postoperative low urine output. It can be diagnosed by renal ultrasound which will usually reveal bilateral hydronephrosis.

CHANGES IN MENTAL STATE

Marked mental changes may occur in the early postoperative period and are most common in older patients. These changes are often loosely called 'confusion'. Common phenomena include clouding of consciousness, perceptual disturbances, incoherent speech and agitation or destructive behaviour, such as pulling out cannulas or catheters. Other features are loss of orientation, apathy and stupor, and stereotyped movements such as plucking at the bedclothes.

ELDERLY PATIENTS

The elderly are vulnerable to dementia and cerebrovascular insufficiency. There may thus be little tolerance of systemic insults that can tip the balance against cerebral equilibrium.

Factors which predispose to postoperative mental changes in the elderly include:

- Disorientation brought about by rapid changes of environment (from ward to operating theatre and on to ITU, for example)
- Dehydration
- Hyponatraemia
- Hypoxia (from pneumonia or cardiac failure, for example)
- Infection (especially of the urinary tract)
- Drugs (particularly opiates and hypnotics)
- Uraemia
- Hypoglycaemia

In addition, pain, anxiety and sleep deprivation may precipitate confusion.

OTHER CAUSES OF MENTAL CHANGE

Marked alterations in behaviour, particularly in younger patients, may indicate alcohol withdrawal or craving for drugs such as cocaine or heroin. The history has usually been concealed at the time of admission. Patients with a recent history of head injury may behave abnormally if hypoxic or if intracerebral bleeding develops.

JAUNDICE

GENERAL CAUSES

Jaundice may develop several days after operation in a patient with no history of biliary disease. In these patients, the cause is usually a prehepatic or hepatic disorder. Causes of **prehepatic jaundice** include large blood transfusions, absorption of large haematomas or exacerbation of a haemolytic disorder such as thalassaemia or sickle-cell trait (exacerbated by postoperative hypoxia, dehydration or hypothermia).

Hepatic causes are less common. They include cholestasis (caused by infection near the liver or drug idiosyncrasy), hepatitis and liver cell toxicity from drug idiosyncrasy and visceral ischaemia caused by shock.

CAUSES RELATED TO BILIARY OR LIVER SURGERY

Patients subjected to biliary tract or liver surgery may become jaundiced after operation. The most likely cause is **obstruction** of the extrahepatic bile ducts due to retained stone, unrecognised surgical trauma or inadvertent duct ligation. Other causes include **infection** such as ascending cholangitis, and systemic absorption of an intra-abdominal collection of bile (biliary peritonitis).

Principles of operative surgery

11

INTRODUCTION

This chapter describes the operating environment and outlines the essential principles of operative surgery including those employed in 'minor' surgical techniques. These principles should be understood by all doctors, not just by surgeons, so as to give them an appreciation of the scope of surgery, to enable them to provide adequate explanation to patients before and after surgery and to help them participate intelligently at the operating table. Furthermore, most doctors are required to perform minor operations, emergency department procedures or invasive investigations at one time or another and these require a knowledge of appropriate techniques.

Various suffixes derived from Greek and Latin are used in describing certain surgical techniques; these are summarised in Box 11.1.

PRINCIPLES OF ASEPSIS

INTRODUCTION

The main bacteria and viruses involved in surgical infections have already been described in Chapter 3. The chief sources of infection are the patients themselves (particularly bowel flora), less commonly the hospital environment, food or cross-infection from other patients, and only occasionally bacteria and viruses carried by theatre personnel. Rare sources of infection are contaminated surgical instruments or equipment, dressings or parenteral drugs and fluids. The viruses causing hepatitis B and C and particularly human immunodeficiency virus (HIV) pose sinister risks of transmitting infection from patient to operating staff and vice versa; there is also the risk of patient-to-patient transmission. These risks of transmitting potentially serious viral diseases make it mandatory to observe **universal blood and body fluid precautions** described in Chapter 3.

The risk of postoperative bacterial infection depends upon the extent of contamination of the wound or body cavity that occurs at operation or, in the case of intestinal perforation, before operation. Bacteria enter a wound by five possible routes:

- Air-borne bacteria-laden particles
- Direct inoculation from instruments and operating personnel
- From the patient's skin
- From the flora of the patient's internal viscera, especially the large bowel
- Via the bloodstream

Modern operating theatre design and correctly observed aseptic procedures minimise wound contamination but infections do still occur. Their results can be devastating, especially in relation to artificial prostheses, skin grafts,

Box 11.1   Surgical terminology

— *oscopy* = examination of a hollow viscus, body cavity or deep structure employing an instrument specifically designed for the purpose, e.g. gastroscopy, colonoscopy, laparoscopy, arthroscopy, bronchoscopy. The general term is endoscopy

— *ectomy* = removal of an organ, e.g. gastrectomy, orchidectomy (i.e. removal of testis), colectomy

— *orrhaphy* = repair of tissues, e.g. herniorrhaphy

— *ostomy* = fashioning an artificial communication between a hollow viscus and the skin, e.g. tracheostomy, colostomy, ileostomy. The term may also apply to artificial openings between different viscera, e.g. gastro-jejunostomy, choledocho-duodenostomy (i.e. anastomosis of duodenum to common bile duct)

— *otomy* = cutting open, e.g. laparotomy, arteriotomy, fasciotomy, thoracotomy

— *plasty* = reconstruction, e.g. pyloroplasty, mammoplasty, arthroplasty

— *pexy* = relocation and securing in position, e.g. orchidopexy (for undescended testis), rectopexy (for rectal prolapse)

bone and the eye. Furthermore, some patients are particularly vulnerable to infection, notably neonates, the immunosuppressed, the debilitated and the malnourished. Note that treatment of established infection is no substitute for prevention.

The use of preoperative prophylactic antibiotics began in the 1970s and has revolutionised the scope and outcome of certain types of operative surgery in a manner comparable to the changes heralded by Lister's introduction of antisepsis in the late nineteenth century.

THE OPERATING ENVIRONMENT

Modern **operating theatre design** plays a major role in the control of air-borne wound contamination. This is important mainly for staphylococci carried on air-borne skin scales.

The main factors influencing air-borne operating theatre infection rates are:

- The concentration of organisms in the air
- The size of bacteria-laden particles
- The duration of exposure of the open wound

The first two are influenced mainly by theatre design and air supply, and the last one can be minimised by avoiding unnecessarily long procedures. Operating theatre complexes are laid out so as to minimise introduction of infection from elsewhere in the hospital via air, personnel or patients. Air is drawn from the relatively clean external

environment, filtered and then supplied to the operating theatres at a slightly higher pressure than outside to ensure a constant outward flow. **Air turnover** is the most important factor; the aim is to ensure 3–15 air changes per hour which 'scrubs out' the theatre air by dilution. Standard air delivery systems aim to achieve a constant flow of clean air towards the operating table, which is then exhausted from the theatre. Despite this, convection currents allow some recirculation of air, which may have been contaminated, into the operation site.

The crucial importance of preventing infection in joint replacement surgery led to the development of sophisticated **ultra-clean air delivery systems**. These reduce postoperative infection two- to fourfold but the cost is very high. Their cost effectiveness is very much lower than can be achieved with prophylactic antibiotics, which lower infection rates by at least five times more than ultra-clean air systems. Enclosure of the patient in a sterile tent in which the surgeons wear space-type suits can reduce infection rates by a further 5–7.5% but these measures are probably not warranted except perhaps in highly specialised joint replacement units.

MINIMISING INFECTION FROM OPERATING THEATRE PERSONNEL

Studies of bacterial types in wound infections have shown that only a modest proportion of wound infections are derived from theatre personnel. Bacteria reach the wound via the air or by direct inoculation. About 30% of healthy people carry *Staphylococcus aureus* in the nose but pathogenic organisms may also be present in the axillae and perineal area, the latter probably being the most important source. In addition, minor skin abrasions are usually infected, as are skin pustules and boils; thus personnel with these lesions must ensure that they are effectively covered with occlusive dressings or else should not enter the operating area.

Air-borne, personnel-derived infection is reduced by changing from potentially contaminated day clothes to clean theatre clothes and shoes which should not then be worn outside the theatre complex. Trouser cuffs should be elasticated or tucked into boots. Some studies suggest that females should wear trousers instead of dresses, in order to reduce 'perineal fallout'. **Face masks** are worn to deflect bacteria-containing droplets in expired air, but most types become ineffective after a relatively short period, especially if they become wet. With the exception of nasal *Staph. aureus* (particularly important in infection of prostheses), bacteria derived from the head do not generally cause wound infection. The effectiveness of wearing masks and hair coverings to reduce infection is unknown.

Sterile gloves and gowns are worn by surgeons and staff directly involved in the operation to prevent direct inoculation of bacteria. Gloves are impermeable to bacteria but hands and forearms are washed before gloving and gowning with antiseptics which persist on the skin. This minimises bacterial contamination if a glove is punctured or the sleeve of the gown becomes wet. **Thorough washing** with soap and water removes extraneous contaminants but not resident flora, the numbers of which can be considerably reduced by using detergent solutions containing antiseptics such as **chlorhexidine** and **povidone–iodine**; disinfection is further improved by a final **alcohol rinse**. These are most effective if they are not rinsed off but merely dried with a sterile towel. The traditional ritual of scrubbing with a brush for 3 minutes is actually less effective than washing the hands thoroughly because it causes microtrauma to the hands and brings more bacteria to the surface.

Despite the protection given by wearing gloves and gown, the less the wound is handled the better. This principle applies particularly when aseptic conditions are less than ideal. On the ward, minor procedures such as bladder catheterisation or insertion of a chest drain should be performed using standard sterile precautions and a **no-touch technique**. Catheters, for example, should not be handled directly but only within their wrapper or by using instruments.

MINIMISING INFECTION FROM THE PATIENT'S SKIN

The patient's skin, especially the perineal area, is the source of up to half of all wound infections. These can be minimised by the following measures:

- **Removing body hair**—body hair was thought to be an important source of wound contamination but this is no longer believed. Hair is removed only to allow the incision site to be seen and the wound to be closed without including hair. Shaving produces numerous small abrasions which rapidly become infected with skin commensals. If shaving is required, it should be done as close to the time of surgery as possible. Most surgeons now restrict hair removal to clipping away just enough to provide adequate skin access. An effective alternative is to use depilatory creams which avoid trauma. For small operations on the head, hair is not usually removed
- **Painting the skin with antiseptic solutions**— povidone–iodine or chlorhexidine in alcoholic or aqueous solution is applied to a wide area around the proposed operation site ('skin prep'); this is now done only when the patient is on the operating table, but in the past patients were subjected to ineffective applications of antiseptics such as gentian violet for several days beforehand!
- **Draping the patient**—the standard procedure used to be to isolate the operating area by placing sterile drapes made of cotton or synthetic cloth over all but

the immediate field of operation. However, these drapes are permeable to bacteria, especially when soaked with blood or other body fluids. Nowadays, disposable impermeable self-adhesive paper drapes are preferred by many users, particularly for high-risk surgery such as joint replacements or arterial grafting. However, they may cost more than conventional drapes
- **Investing the skin** at the operation site with a thin film of adherent clear plastic—the skin incision is then made through the plastic film so that little bare skin is exposed. This method has proved counterproductive because bacteria multiply beneath the film. Films impregnated with povidone–iodine may be more effective

REDUCING INFECTION FROM INTERNAL VISCERA

The large bowel teems with potentially pathogenic bacteria and the peritoneal cavity inevitably becomes contaminated in any operation at which the large bowel is opened. Pathogenic bacteria are also found in obstructed small bowel. The same applies to the stomach and small bowel of patients on H_2-receptor blocking drugs or proton pump inhibitors where the normal bactericidal effect of gastric acid is lost. Great care should be taken at operation to minimise this contamination. Bowel preparation of the colon before operation may help this process. All of these patients should be given appropriate prophylactic antibiotics before operation.

STERILISATION OF INSTRUMENTS AND OTHER SUPPLIES (see Table 11.1)

In modern surgical practice, infection from instruments, swabs, equipment and intravenous fluids has been virtually eliminated by the supply of sterile packs from central sterile supply departments (CSSD). Reusable instruments and drapes are sterilised by high-pressure steam autoclaving according to strict regulations. Most disposable items are purchased in pre-sterilised, sealed packs. Sterilisation in small autoclaves near the operating theatre should only be performed if instruments in short supply are required for successive operations. Sterilisation by any method is likely to be ineffective unless all organic material is removed from instruments first by thorough cleaning.

Problems are posed by sterilising instruments which would be damaged by heat. These include plastics, cystoscopic lenses, flexible endoscopes and electrical equipment. These can be sterilised using a variety of chemical methods such as ethylene oxide gas. Glutaraldehyde in a 2% concentration is commonly used for endoscopic instruments that need to be reused several times during an endoscopy session. They must be immersed in sterile water before use. Special precautions are required to prevent chemical injury to staff.

Table 11.1 Time and temperature requirements for sterilisation by different methods

Method	Equipment to be sterilised	Temperature	Time
Steam autoclave	Unwrapped instruments and bowls Instrument sets, dressings and rubber	123°C 126°C	10 min 3 min
Ethylene oxide gas	Heat-sensitive materials; plastics, endoscopes, electrical equipment	55°C	2–24 hr
Liquid glutaraldehyde	Cystoscopes and other urological equipment, plastics and heat-sensitive equipment required urgently	Room temperature	10 min

World-wide, many surgical instruments are prepared by boiling water 'sterilisers'. Boiling water is markedly inferior to other methods of sterilisation but is included here as it may be the only practical method in developing countries because of cost and technical difficulties. Boiling water kills most vegetative organisms within 15 minutes but spores are not killed by this method. All organic debris should, as always, be scrupulously removed first, then the instruments immersed in visibly boiling water, returned to the boil and boiled continuously for at least 30 minutes to ensure hepatitis and human immunodeficiency viruses are destroyed.

SURGICAL TECHNIQUE

Surgical technique plays an important part in minimising the risk of operative infection. Non-vital tissue and collections of fluid and blood are particularly vulnerable to colonisation by infecting organisms, which may enter via the bloodstream even if direct contamination has been avoided by aseptic technique. Tissue damage should be kept to the minimum in the course of surgery by careful handling and retraction and by avoiding unnecessary diathermy coagulation. Haematoma formation is minimised by careful attention to haemostasis and placing drains into potential sites of fluid collection; **closed-drainage** or **suction-drainage** systems reduce the risk of organisms tracking back into the wound from the ward environment.

During extensive resections of bowel, early ligation of its blood supply allows bacteria to permeate the wall (**translocation**) and this may contaminate the peritoneal cavity.

Gross faecal contamination is associated with a high risk of infection and great care is taken in operations where the bowel is opened. In emergency operations for large bowel perforation, free faecal matter is meticulously removed. A planned **'second look' laparotomy** after 48 hours is often advisable to deal with remaining contamination and new abscesses even if the patient appears well.

After performing an anastomosis involving large bowel, a drain is often placed in the vicinity, intended to remove collections of blood and other fluids and perhaps to minimise the danger of general peritoneal contamination should the anastomosis leak. Evidence now shows this is ineffective and possibly harmful.

PREVENTION OF CROSS-INFECTION (NOSOCOMIAL INFECTION)

Cross-infection is the term used to describe infection transmitted from other patients in the nearby hospital environment and it is rare. It should be distinguished from **colonisation** with other patients' bacteria, which is common. Cross-infection is mainly spread via food, staff, medical equipment or ward furnishings. Whenever there is patient contact which might result in transfer of infection, the principles of asepsis used in the operating department must be applied, although the achievable level of aseptic technique is lower. Doctors are probably the worst offenders as regards transfer of infection—by removing dressings to inspect wounds in the open ward, by failing to cleanse hands between patients and by careless aseptic technique when performing ward procedures such as bladder catheterisation. Minimising patient movements between wards and hospital units also decreases cross-infection rates.

A patient with an infection that is potentially dangerous to other patients should be isolated and barrier-nursed in a single room. These infections include *Streptococcus pyogenes*, open tuberculosis and infective diarrhoeas. Infection with meticillin-resistant *Staph. aureus* (MRSA) requires a patient to be transferred to an isolation area in the ward or, if the patient is in intensive care, transferred to an isolation room within the unit to avoid having to close to new admissions (see Ch. 1).

PROPHYLACTIC ANTIBIOTICS

Despite the best aseptic techniques, some operations carry a high risk of wound infection as well as other infective complications; these can be reduced dramatically by using prophylactic antibiotics. The chosen antibiotics should be matched to the organisms likely to occur in the

Risk 2–5%

Clean operations with no preoperative infection and no opening of gastrointestinal, respiratory or urinary tracts (e.g. inguinal herniorrhaphy, breast lump excision, ligation of varicose veins)

Risk less than 10%

Clean operations with gastrointestinal, respiratory or urinary tracts opened but with minimal contamination (e.g. elective cholecystectomy, transurethral resection of prostate, excision of minimally inflamed appendix)

Risk about 20%

Operations where tissues inevitably become contaminated but without pre-existing infection (e.g. elective large bowel operations, appendicectomy where the appendix is perforated or gangrenous, fresh traumatic skin wounds (except on the face))

Risk greater than 30%

Operations in the presence of infection (e.g. abscesses within body cavities, small bowel perforation, delayed operations on traumatic wounds)

Risk greater than 50%

Emergency colonic surgery (bowel unprepared) for perforation or obstruction

- A single dose of antibiotic is adequate for most purposes.
- Never continue prophylaxis for more than 48 hours
- Dose should be administered immediately before the procedure
- If the patient is already suspected of having an infection, go straight to treatment

area of the operation and should be bactericidal rather than bacteriostatic (see Table 11.2). The relative risk of postoperative infection in different types of operation is summarised in Box 11.2.

As a general principle, prophylactic antibiotics are indicated if the anticipated risk of infection exceeds 10%, i.e. all emergency abdominal surgery, all elective colonic operations, and upper gastrointestinal operations for malignancy. Prophylactic antibiotics are also used by many surgeons for operations in the 5–10% risk category, e.g. cholecystectomy. In addition, prophylactic antibiotics are indicated in inherently low-risk cases where the consequences of infection would be catastrophic, e.g. operations employing prosthetic implants, or in patients with mitral stenosis or other cardiac defects at risk of infective endocarditis. Prophylactic antibiotics can reduce postoperative infection rates in high-risk cases by 75%, and may almost entirely eliminate infection in lower-risk cases.

In the great majority of wound-related infections, the organisms are introduced during the operation and become established during the next 24 hours. Thus, if prophylactic antibiotics are to be effective, high blood levels must be achieved during the operation, at the time contamination occurs. To achieve this, the first dose of antibiotic should be given either 1 hour before operation or preferably intravenously at induction of anaesthesia; prophylactic antibiotics should not be given any earlier as this may encourage resistant organisms to proliferate. A single preoperative dose of antibiotic is probably sufficient provided it is rapidly bactericidal and the inoculum of bacteria is small; long operations with heavy blood loss, e.g. ruptured abdominal aortic aneurysm, merit a second perioperative dose of antibiotics. Many surgeons prefer to give two additional doses postoperatively but there is little evidence of additional benefit. Longer courses of prophylactic antibiotics are certainly of no advantage.

In general, intravenous antibiotics provide the most predictable blood levels; peak tissue levels are achieved within 1 hour of injection. However, for prophylaxis against anaerobes, metronidazole administered rectally gives equivalent blood and tissue levels to intravenous administration although these are not reached until 2–4 hours after administration. Oral metronidazole is usually inappropriate because of unreliable absorption and enforced perioperative starvation.

Operations involving bowel and biliary system

Patients having these operations are at risk mainly from a mixture of Gram-negative bacilli (Enterobacteriaceae family), faecal anaerobes (*Bacteroides fragilis*) and *Staph. aureus*. Less commonly, enterococci cause surgical infection, notably *E. faecalis* (formerly *Strep. faecalis*).

The most commonly used prophylactic antibiotic regimens are shown below. A more comprehensive list is given in Table 11.2:

- For biliary surgery—a cephalosporin alone (e.g. cefuroxime)
- For colonic and other bowel surgery—either a combination of a cephalosporin (as for biliary surgery) and metronidazole or else a combination of gentamicin, benzylpenicillin (or ampicillin) and metronidazole. The latter combination is often preferred for bowel-related prophylaxis as it covers enterococci as well as the other organisms expected
- For appendicectomy—rectal metronidazole alone, given 2 hours before operation; this has proved as

Table 11.2 Recommended antimicrobial prophylaxis for surgical procedures and clinical conditions

	Likely organisms	Antibiotic
Abdominal surgery		
Severe acute pancreatitis	Coliforms Anaerobes	Ciprofloxacin 400 mg i.v. + metronidazole 500 mg i.v. or meropenem 1 g i.v.
Colonic and other bowel surgery	Coliforms Anaerobes *Staphylococcus aureus* *Streptococcus pyogenes* *(Group A Strep.)*	Cefuroxime 1.2 g i.v. + metronidazole 500 mg i.v.
Appendicectomy	Anaerobes	Rectal metronidazole suppository 1 g or proportionately less in children
Endoscopic gastrostomy Gastroduodenal surgery Oesophageal surgery	Anaerobes *Staphylococcus aureus* *Streptococcus pyogenes* *(Group A Strep.)* Coliforms *Candida* spp	Cefuroxime 1.2 g i.v. + metronidazole 500 mg i.v. + fluconazole 50 mg i.v.
Inguinal or other hernia repair with mesh	*Staphylococcus aureus* *Staphylococcus epidermidis* (coagulase-negative) *Streptococcus pyogenes* *(Group A Strep.)* Coliforms	Cefuroxime 1.2 g i.v.
Other hernia repair without mesh		Not recommended
Laparoscopic cholecystectomy		Cefuroxime 1.2 g i.v. (but no clinical evidence of efficacy)
Orthopaedic surgery		
Total hip replacement or prosthetic knee joint	*Staphylococcus aureus* *Staphylococcus epidermidis* (coagulase-negative) *Streptococcus pyogenes* *(Group A Strep.)* Coliforms	Cefuroxime 750 g i.v. 8-hourly for 3 doses If MRSA risk factors or known MRSA: add vancomycin 1 g i.v. 12-hourly for 2 doses
Trauma with contaminated wounds	*Staphylococcus aureus* *Streptococcus pyogenes* *(Group A Strep.)*	Cefuroxime 750 mg i.v. 3 doses *or* doxycycline 100 mg orally If heavily contaminated or dead tissue, add metronidazole 500 mg i.v. for 2 doses
Elective orthopaedic surgery without prosthetic device		Not recommended
Vascular surgery		
Lower limb amputation or vascular surgery, abdominal and lower limb	*Staphylococcus aureus* *Staphylococcus epidermidis* (coagulase-negative) *Streptococcus pyogenes* *(Group A Strep.)* Coliforms	Cefuroxime 1.2 g i.v. + metronidazole 500 mg i.v. If MRSA, **add** vancomycin 1 g i.v.
ENT surgery		
Head and neck surgery	*Staphylococcus aureus* *Streptococcus pyogenes* *(Group A Strep.)* Coliforms Anaerobes	Cefuroxime 1.2 g i.v. + metronidazole 500 mg i.v. If MRSA, **add** vancomycin 1 g i.v.
Ear, nose, sinus Tonsillectomy		Not recommended
Urology		
Transrectal prostate biopsy Shock wave lithotripsy Transurethral resection of prostate (TURP)	Coliforms *Enterococcus*	Amoxicillin 1 g i.v. + gentamicin 120 mg i.v. *or* ciprofloxacin 200 mg i.v.

effective as any other regimen. The evidence for the beneficial effect of metronidazole in preventing infection after appendicectomy is now so strong that it may be negligent not to use it

The choice of antibiotics for prophylaxis must be kept under review because organisms change their sensitivities. An important consideration in this regard is that aminoglycosides such as gentamicin do not alter the bowel flora because their concentration in the lumen is low; this is in contrast to the cephalosporins and ampicillin. In consequence, there is a rising tide of beta-lactam-resistant bowel organisms insensitive to cephalosporins and ampicillin but sensitive to aminoglycosides. If resistant staphylococci are a problem, vancomycin or other newer antibiotics may become necessary for prophylaxis.

Operations involving implantation of prostheses

Vascular grafts and joint replacements are at particular risk from *Staph. aureus* infection. Coagulase-negative staphylococci (e.g. *Staph. epidermidis*) are also a common source of chronic infection. Coliforms are a very rare cause. Flucloxacillin is the agent of first choice for prophylaxis but gentamicin is usually added for extra protection. Rifampicin is used to soak vascular grafts as it is effective against *Staph. epidermidis*. Cephalosporins are often used but they are less efficacious against staphylococci than flucloxacillin or gentamicin. Meticillin-resistant *Staph. aureus* (MRSA) is becoming a more common cause of prosthetic infection. In areas where the risk is substantial, prophylaxis with vancomycin is appropriate.

Operations where ischaemic or necrotic muscle may remain

Lower limb amputations for arterial insufficiency and major traumatic injuries involving muscle are susceptible to gas gangrene and tetanus. **Clostridia** are highly sensitive to benzylpenicillin and metronidazole, one of which should be given in high dose as early as possible after major trauma and before major amputations for ischaemia.

BASIC SURGICAL TECHNIQUES

ANAESTHESIA

GENERAL PRINCIPLES

Some form of anaesthesia is required for almost every surgical procedure, with the aim of preventing pain in all cases, minimising stress for the patient in most, and providing special conditions for some operations, e.g. muscular relaxation in abdominal surgery. The choice of anaesthetic techniques includes **topical (surface) anaesthesia, local anaesthetic infiltration or peripheral nerve block, spinal or epidural anaesthesia** and **general anaesthesia**. Methods other than general anaesthesia may be supplemented with intravenous sedation if the patient is anxious or agitated (e.g. with benzodiazepines). Intravenous sedation with these drugs produces relaxation, anxiolysis and amnesia whilst retaining protective reflexes. However, unconsciousness can also be produced by these drugs and they must be carefully titrated to produce the desired effects. Intravenous sedation of this type does not provide pain relief; if needed, this must be achieved by local anaesthesia or intravenous analgesics.

CHOICE OF ANAESTHETIC TECHNIQUE

Combining local or regional anaesthesia (for pain relief) with a light general anaesthetic can minimise postoperative respiratory and cardiovascular depression compared with general anaesthesia alone, thus reducing postoperative morbidity. An example is the use of caudal anaesthesia in perineal operations. Local or regional anaesthesia using bupivacaine or levobupivacaine can also be used during an operation to provide postoperative pain relief; for example, intercostal nerve blocks after an abdominal operation allow more comfortable breathing and coughing, reducing the likelihood of respiratory complications. Another common example is wound infiltration with the same long-acting local anaesthetic agents. The main factors influencing choice of anaesthesia are summarised in Box 11.4.

Careful selection of appropriate drug combinations for each case and close liaison between surgical and anaesthetic staff before, during and after operation greatly enhance postoperative recovery. The use of a **'high-dependency' recovery area**, where at-risk patients can be intensively nursed and monitored immediately postoperatively, also plays an important part in early recovery from major surgery.

INCISION TECHNIQUE

CHOICE OF INCISION

The purpose of most skin incisions is to gain access to underlying tissues or body cavities. The first consideration when planning a surgical incision must be to achieve good access. Furthermore, the incision should be placed in a position which will allow it to be extended if necessary. The incision should also be made in a position and in such a way as to enable it to be effectively closed to give the best chance of primary healing and the lowest chance of an incisional hernia forming later. Despite

Box 11.4   Choice of anaesthetic technique

1. Local anaesthesia

In general, used for calm and rational patients when no autonomic discomfort is anticipated:

- Minor operations, e.g. excision of small skin lesions or dental operations
- Minor but painful procedures, e.g. insertion of chest drain, siting of peripheral venous cannulae
- Unavailability of general anaesthetic expertise, e.g. in developing countries
- Patients unfit for general anaesthesia, e.g. cardiac and respiratory cripples
- Ambulatory ('day case') surgery especially if comorbidity
- Patients unwilling to undergo general anaesthesia
- Use of combined local anaesthetic and vasoconstrictor to provide a relatively bloodless operative field (note: this must never be used in the extreme peripheries, i.e. digits, penis, nose)

2. Regional nerve block

- Minor surgery requiring wide field of anaesthesia, e.g. femoral nerve block for varicose vein surgery, pudendal block for forceps delivery
- When it is undesirable to inject local anaesthetic into the operation site, e.g. drainage of an abscess (local anaesthesia works less well in inflamed tissue)
- To avoid tissue distortion from local infiltration in delicate surgery
- Short-lived, wide-field ambulatory anaesthesia for reduction of forearm fractures or hand surgery (Bier's intravenous regional anaesthesia)

3. Epidural and spinal anaesthesia

- Lower limb surgery, e.g. amputations
- Lower abdominal, groin, pelvic and perineal surgery, e.g. Caesarean sections, inguinal hernia repair, prostatectomy, bladder and urethral surgery

4. Intravenous sedation or intravenous analgesia alone

- Short-lived uncomfortable procedures where local anaesthesia is impractical, e.g. gastrointestinal endoscopy, musculoskeletal manipulation

5. Intravenous sedation combined with local anaesthesia

- Potentially unpleasant procedures despite adequate local anaesthesia, e.g. wisdom tooth extraction, toenail operations, siting of central venous lines

6. Regional analgesia with light general anaesthesia

- Caudal epidural plus general anaesthesia for operations in the perineal area, e.g. transurethral prostatectomy or resection of bladder tumours, haemorrhoidectomy, circumcision. This provides perioperative and postoperative analgesia

7. General anaesthesia

- Where all of the above are unsuitable or difficult to achieve
- Severe patient apprehension or patient preference for general anaesthesia
- Major or prolonged operations
- Abdominal or thoracic operations requiring muscle relaxation
- Where it is necessary to secure the airway by intubation
- Special indications, e.g. neurosurgery

---

patients' impressions, the length of an incision (and the number of sutures required for closure) has little bearing on the rate of healing, and the success of an operation should not be put at risk by inadequate access.

Secondary considerations in the choice of incision are as follows:

- **Orientation of skin tension lines (based on Langer's lines) and skin creases**—wherever possible, incisions should be made parallel to the lines of skin tension determined by the orientation of dermal collagen (e.g. a 'collar' incision for thyroid operations) as the wound is less likely to break down, there is minimal distortion, and healing occurs with little scar tissue to give a better cosmetic result
- **Strength and healing potential of the tissues**—the nature and distribution of muscle and fascia, particularly in different parts of the abdominal wall, influences the strength of the repair. For example, a vertical lower midline incision situated in the linea alba where the abdominal wall consists of a strong layer of fascia is less prone to incisional herniation than a paramedian incision lateral to the midline
- **The anatomy of underlying structures, particularly nerves**—the incision line should run parallel to, but some distance away from, the expected course of underlying structures, reducing the risk of damage. For example, to gain access to the submandibular gland, the incision is made parallel to and 2 cm below the lower border of the mandible to avoid the mandibular branch of the facial nerve
- **Cosmetic considerations**—wherever possible, incisions should be placed in the least conspicuous position such as in a skin crease or a site that will later be concealed by clothing, e.g. a transverse suprapubic (**Pfannenstiel** or bucket-handle) incision below the 'bikini' line for operations on the bladder, uterus or ovary, a peri-areolar incision for breast biopsy

DISSECTION AND HANDLING OF DEEPER TISSUES

The skin consists of thin **epidermis** and dense, somewhat thicker **dermis**, as well as the underlying fatty **hypodermis** which may be as much as 10 cm thick in an obese individual.

Once the skin incision has been made, the scalpel is mainly reserved for incising fascia and other fibrous structures like breast tissue. The purpose of dissection is to protect structures which might be damaged by bold incisions and to preserve blood supply and venous drainage. Anatomical detail is exposed and displayed by a combination of blunt and sharp dissection. **Blunt dissection** involves teasing or stripping tissues apart using fingers, swabs or blunt instruments, following natural tissue planes. **Sharp dissection** with scissors and forceps or scalpel is used where tissues have to be cut and also to display small structures. Some surgeons prefer sharp to blunt dissection in general, believing it causes less tissue trauma. Most dissection, however, involves a combination of both.

PRINCIPLES OF HAEMOSTASIS

Bleeding is an unavoidable part of surgery. Blood loss should be minimised because bleeding obscures the operative field and hampers operative technique (the finer the surgery, the more continued bleeding interferes with visibility and quality of outcome), and because the loss has to be made up later. Excessive bleeding can be averted by judicious dissection with control of bleeding as the operation proceeds, and by minimising the area of raw tissue exposed at the operation site by accurately siting the incision and by avoiding opening unnecessary tissue planes.

CLIPPING, LIGATION AND UNDER-RUNNING

Ligation is obligatory when large vessels are divided and is desirable for vessels larger than about 1 mm calibre (see Fig. 11.1). If the end of a bleeding vessel cannot be grasped by haemostat forceps, a suture can be used to encircle the vessel and its surrounding tissues, a technique often described as **under-running**. It is particularly useful for a bleeding artery in the fibrous base of a peptic ulcer.

DIATHERMY

Diathermy achieves haemostasis by local intravascular coagulation and contraction of the vessel wall caused by heating (-*thermy*) generated by particular electrical waveforms. However, enough heat is also produced to burn the tissues and these may be needlessly damaged by

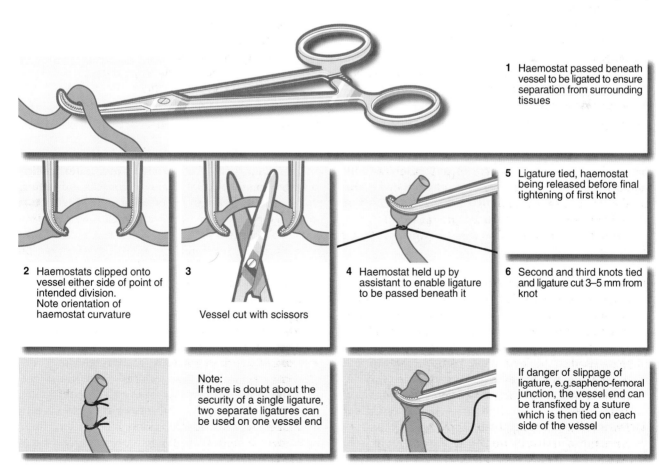

1 Haemostat passed beneath vessel to be ligated to ensure separation from surrounding tissues

2 Haemostats clipped onto vessel either side of point of intended division. Note orientation of haemostat curvature

3 Vessel cut with scissors

4 Haemostat held up by assistant to enable ligature to be passed beneath it

5 Ligature tied, haemostat being released before final tightening of first knot

6 Second and third knots tied and ligature cut 3–5 mm from knot

Note:
If there is doubt about the security of a single ligature, two separate ligatures can be used on one vessel end

If danger of slippage of ligature, e.g. sapheno-femoral junction, the vessel end can be transfixed by a suture which is then tied on each side of the vessel

Fig. 11.1 Techniques of haemostasis

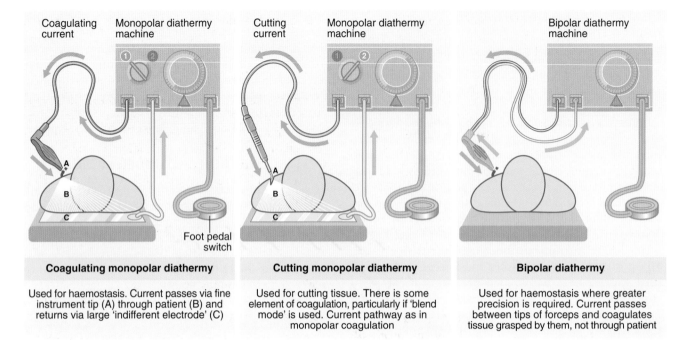

Fig. 11.2 Three modes of diathermy

Coagulating monopolar diathermy	Cutting monopolar diathermy	Bipolar diathermy
Used for haemostasis. Current passes via fine instrument tip (A) through patient (B) and returns via large 'indifferent electrode' (C)	Used for cutting tissue. There is some element of coagulation, particularly if 'blend mode' is used. Current pathway as in monopolar coagulation	Used for haemostasis where greater precision is required. Current passes between tips of forceps and coagulates tissue grasped by them, not through patient

careless use, particularly near the skin or nerves. Diathermy is ineffective for large vessels, which should be ligated. There are three main variants of diathermy, illustrated in Figure 11.2, and all three modes are available on modern diathermy machines.

Monopolar diathermy is the most widely used for operative haemostasis but there is wide dispersion of the coagulating and heating effects, making it unsuitable for use near nerves and other delicate structures. Since the current passes through the patient's body, there is a risk of coagulating vessels en passant (e.g. monopolar diathermy used in circumcision may cause penile thrombosis), as well as provoking arrhythmias in patients with cardiac pacemakers. Monopolar diathermy may also result in skin burns at the **indifferent electrode plate** if skin contact is poor or if the plate becomes wet during operation. Current recommendations to improve contact include shaving hair from the skin where the plate is placed and using disposable self-adhesive diathermy plates.

Bipolar diathermy is used mainly for finer surgery. The current passes only between the blades of the forceps and it requires fairly accurate grasping of the bleeding vessel. It uses low levels of electrical power, there is almost no electrical dispersion from the tip of the forceps and much less heat is generated. The main advantages are minimal tissue damage around the point of coagulation and safety in relation to nearby nerves, blood vessels and cardiac pacemakers.

Cutting diathermy is mainly used for dividing large masses of muscle (e.g. during thoracotomy or access to the hip joint) and cutting vascular tissues (e.g. breast).

The intention is a form of sharp dissection, at the same time coagulating the numerous small blood vessels as the tissue is cut; unfortunately this is not always wholly effective. A blend of cutting and coagulation is sometimes used.

TOURNIQUET AND EXSANGUINATION

This technique is used in surgery of the limbs and hands where a bloodless field is particularly desirable. For the whole limb, a pneumatic tourniquet is placed proximally around the limb. The limb is exsanguinated by elevation and spiral application of a rubber bandage (Esmarck) or ring exsanguinator from the periphery; the tourniquet is then inflated. Upper limb tourniquets must not be left inflated for more than 30 minutes and lower limb tourniquets for more than about 1 hour to avoid the risk of necrosis.

PRESSURE

Pressure is a useful means of controlling bleeding until platelet aggregation, reactive vasoconstriction and blood coagulation take over. It can be used for emergency control of severe arterial or venous bleeding but is equally useful for controlling diffuse small-vessel bleeding from a large raw area, e.g. liver bed after cholecystectomy. Pressure is usually applied with gauze swabs which must be kept in position for at least 10 minutes. Even if bleeding is not arrested completely, this process usually allows a clearer view and allows haemostasis by standard means.

For intractable bleeding which is not amenable to ligature, diathermy or suture, various resorbable packing materials, e.g. oxidised cellulose, can be left in position until haemostasis occurs, allowing the wound to be closed. If bleeding simply cannot be controlled—for example, after liver injury—the bleeding cavity can be packed with gauze swabs which are left in situ and removed 48–72 hours later at a further operation. Bleeding, once controlled by this method, rarely recurs.

When a raw cavity has been created beneath the skin, external pressure dressings are sometimes a useful method of controlling potential postoperative oozing and minimising haematoma formation, e.g. after breast lump excision.

HYPOTENSIVE ANAESTHESIA

This method of anaesthesia is sometimes employed when marked diffuse bleeding is anticipated, e.g. prostatectomy, or where a bloodless field is desirable for fine dissection but where a tourniquet is impossible, e.g. parotid surgery. The anaesthetist achieves controlled hypotension by the judicious infusion of drugs such as nitroprusside.

SUTURING AND SURGICAL REPAIR

TYPES OF SUTURE MATERIAL AND NEEDLES

Numerous types of suture are available (see Box 11.5), the most important distinction being between **absorbable** and **non-absorbable** materials. This clear-cut difference has been blurred by the advent of **slowly absorbed sutures**, e.g. polydioxanone (PDS). The groups can be subdivided into **natural** and **synthetic** materials (although natural materials are being gradually phased out) and further subdivided into **monofilament** and **polyfilament** (braided) materials. The choice of suture material depends upon the task at hand, the handling qualities and personal preference.

Absorbable versus non-absorbable materials

The strength of absorbable sutures declines at a predictable rate for each type of material, although the suture material remains in the wound long after it has any useful ability to hold tissues together.

In increasing duration of useful strength, the main absorbable materials are:

- Plain catgut and chromic catgut—useful strength 3 and 5 days respectively (no longer available in many countries)
- Modified polyglactin (Vicryl Rapide)—useful strength about 6 days
- Polyglycolic acid (Dexon) and polyglactin (Vicryl)—useful strength about 10 days
- Poliglecaprone 25 (Monocryl)—useful strength about 20 days
- Polydioxanone (PDS)—retains its strength for at least 28 days

The strength of catgut declines even more quickly in the presence of infection or gastric acid, but this is not true of the synthetic absorbable sutures.

The eventual elimination of absorbable materials from the body overcomes the problem of a permanent foreign body which can harbour infection. Absorbable sutures are often used in the skin to avoid the need for removal; typical applications are minor skin operations, median sternotomies, surgery in children, circumcisions and vasectomies. Catgut sutures give a poorer cosmetic result because of the inflammatory response they provoke, but polyglycolic acid/polyglactin (undyed) gives good results as the sutures are removed by hydrolysis without inflammation. The newer, modified, short-lived polyglactin seems to have ideal properties for skin closure where short suture life is required, e.g. inguinal hernia repair, and the monofilament poliglecaprone 25 (Monocryl) is ideal for situations when longer wound support is required.

Non-absorbable sutures retain most of their strength indefinitely. They are used where the repair will take a long time to reach full strength (e.g. abdominal wall closure) or will be inherently weak (e.g. inguinal and incisional hernia repairs, arterial anastomoses). Non-absorbable sutures are also widely used for skin closure;

> ### Box 11.5 Suture materials and their characteristics
>
> Typical brand names are given in brackets
>
> **Absorbable**
> - Plain catgut—natural monofilament
> - Chromic catgut—natural monofilament
> - Polyglycolic acid-synthetic braided (Dexon)
> - Polyglactin—synthetic braided (Vicryl)
> - Polydioxanone—synthetic monofilament (PDS, Maxon)
>
> **Non-absorbable**
> - Silk—natural braided
> - Linen—natural braided
> - Stainless steel wire—monofilament or braided
> - Nylon—synthetic, usually monofilament (Ethilon)
> - Polyester—synthetic braided (Ticron, and others)
> - Polypropylene—synthetic monofilament (Prolene)
> - Polytetrafluoroethylene (PTFE)—synthetic 'expanded' monofilament (Goretex)

synthetic monofilament sutures give good cosmetic results and are easily and painlessly removed. Subcuticular sutures, which do not penetrate the epidermis, give excellent cosmetic results.

Natural versus synthetic materials

Catgut has been used as a suture and ligature material since before Roman times, derived from the material used for musical instrument strings. It consists mainly of collagen and is actually made from the dried small bowel submucosa of sheep or cattle. Catgut was widely used but is gradually being replaced with synthetic materials. Silk and linen also have a long and distinguished history but their use is minimal. Many surgeons believe that silk has the best handling and knotting properties of any material, but it provokes a strong inflammatory response exceeded only by linen. Silk is sometimes used for skin sutures, where its softness means there are no sharp ends to prick nearby skin. In general, natural materials are about half the price of the synthetics, a factor of importance in developing countries.

The main advantages of synthetic absorbable suture materials are that they are stronger than catgut and provoke little or no inflammatory reaction. There is no risk of biological contamination with prions or viruses and they can be designed to meet specific requirements of absorbability, period of retention of strength, and handling properties.

Non-absorbable synthetic materials, similarly, do not provoke inflammatory reactions. Polyesters, nylon and polypropylene all retain virtually all of their strength over long periods in the tissues; this is particularly important when they are used to suture arterial prostheses where healing alone would not retain the prosthesis. All natural materials deteriorate over time and silk used for arterial prostheses had a high long-term failure rate leading to false aneurysm formation.

Monofilament versus polyfilament sutures

Monofilament materials have a smooth surface and can be pulled through the tissues with minimal friction; this makes them easier to insert and remove than polyfilament braided materials. On the other hand, monofilament materials are stiff, springy and more difficult to knot. Braided materials have the best handling qualities, but their interstices provide a haven for bacteria. When used at a surface (e.g. skin or bowel wall) they tend to act as a 'wick', drawing infected material in. This problem is partly overcome by the manufacturers' application of surface coatings.

Wire sutures

Metal wire sutures have largely been displaced by non-absorbable synthetics. Stainless steel wire is, however, extensively used in orthopaedic surgery for bone fixation and sometimes for closure of sternotomy wounds in cardiac surgery. It is virtually inert but its main disadvantages are high rates of glove penetration and late breakage due to metal fatigue.

GAUGE OF SUTURE MATERIAL

The gauge of suture chosen for a particular task depends largely on practical experience. This takes into account the following factors:

- Strength of repair required
- Number of sutures to be placed—the greater the number, the finer can be the gauge
- Type of suture material being used—for a given gauge, the various materials have different strengths; catgut is the weakest
- Cosmetic requirements—multiple fine sutures give a better cosmetic result than fewer heavier sutures

The traditional method of describing suture gauge (US Pharmacopoeia) is confusing for the newcomer and derives from the time when sutures were much thicker than those used today. The finest suture then was designated gauge 1, with gauge 2 and upwards applying to heavier sutures. As finer and finer sutures came into use, the scale had to be taken progressively backwards from 1, i.e. gauges 0, 00 (i.e. 2/0), 000 (3/0) and so on. Nowadays, the finest suture is 10/0, which is used for extremely delicate surgery such as in the eye. A more rational metric gauge, based on suture diameter, is in use but the traditional gauge is still widely used. A simple guide to the use of different gauges is outlined in Box 11.6.

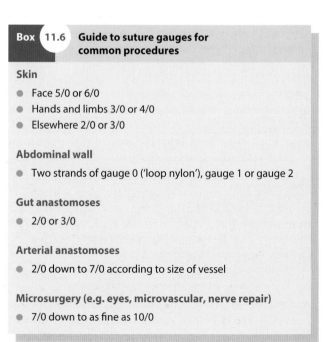

Box 11.6 Guide to suture gauges for common procedures

Skin
- Face 5/0 or 6/0
- Hands and limbs 3/0 or 4/0
- Elsewhere 2/0 or 3/0

Abdominal wall
- Two strands of gauge 0 ('loop nylon'), gauge 1 or gauge 2

Gut anastomoses
- 2/0 or 3/0

Arterial anastomoses
- 2/0 down to 7/0 according to size of vessel

Microsurgery (e.g. eyes, microvascular, nerve repair)
- 7/0 down to as fine as 10/0

1. **Method of use**
- Hand-held needles—routine for skin suturing; sometimes used for abdominal wall closure
- Instrument-held needles—necessary for deeper access and fine control

2. **Shape of needle**
- Straight—skin suturing
- Curved—half-circle used for most purposes, quarter-circle for microvascular anastomoses, three-quarter-circle for hand closure of abdominal wall

3. **Length of needle**
- Range from 2 to 60 mm—according to depth of penetration and delicacy of surgery

4. **Tissue penetration characteristics**
- Round-bodied with smooth pointed tip—most soft tissues, e.g. gut, fat, muscle
- Trocar point (semi-cutting)—moderately tough tissues, e.g. atherosclerotic arteries, fascia
- Cutting point—tough tissues, e.g. skin, breast tissue

5. **Means of attachment of suture to needle**
- Needles with an eye requiring suture material to be threaded by hand—mainly used in developing countries so that needles can be reused
- 'Atraumatic' needles with suture material already attached (swaged into the end)—there is no double thickness of suture material to cause extra drag and trauma as it is pulled through the tissues, and the suture material does not detach from the needle during use

TYPES OF SUTURE NEEDLE

Vast ranges of needles have been designed to accommodate both the breadth of different demands of general and specialist surgery and the stringent requirements of microsurgery. Characteristics of needles and broad indications for their use are summarised in Box 11.7 and illustrated in Figure 11.3.

METHODS OF SKIN SUTURING

The objective of skin suturing is to approximate the cut edges so they will heal rapidly, leaving a minimal scar. Edges to be apposed should have been cut in a clean line and perpendicular to the skin surface; ragged or angled edges should be trimmed. The cut edges should be capable of being brought together neatly and without tension; otherwise the wound may break down or the scar slowly stretch, giving an ugly result. To achieve this, it may be necessary to insert a layer of subcutaneous sutures or even mobilise the skin by undercutting in the fatty layer (see Fig. 11.4). Undue laxity should also be avoided by trimming excess skin.

There are many techniques of skin closure, the choice being governed by the nature and site of the operation and by the surgeon's personal preference. In general, facial wounds are closed with multiple fine sutures which are removed after 4 or 5 days. Abdominal and chest wound sutures are generally removed after 7 days, while sutures for wounds on the back are best left in situ for 14 days to minimise wound stretching.

Subcuticular sutures, either non-absorbable or absorbable, are often used for longer wounds in cosmetically sensitive areas, provided the risk of infection is low. Elsewhere, the choice is between interrupted and continuous suture techniques. Interrupted sutures are indicated if there is a risk of infection; if infection develops, some sutures can be removed early to facilitate drainage. If the risk of infection is high, e.g. large bowel perforation, skin wounds are better left open and closed 48–72 hours later by **delayed primary closure**. The commonly used methods of skin suturing are illustrated in Figure 11.5.

Clips and staples

Stainless steel clips (e.g. Michel clips) have been used for several decades for closing skin wounds and are popular for neck incisions after thyroidectomy as they are haemostatic. As the clips do not penetrate skin yet give good edge apposition, the cosmetic result is excellent. Staples are a relatively recent development in surgery and various instruments are used for both skin closure and bowel surgery. The skin closure devices are similar in concept to ordinary paper staplers, with staples stored in a magazine and applied singly instead of sutures (Fig. 11.6). More complex devices, which apply multiple staples simultaneously, either in a linear or circular fashion, are available for bowel anastomoses and closure of tubular viscera. Some of these devices have revolutionised surgical practice, e.g. re-anastomosis of colon to rectum after Hartmann's resection or bronchial stump closure. When used for internal viscera, the staples remain in place indefinitely.

POSTOPERATIVE WOUND MANAGEMENT

Once a wound has been closed, the doctor has three main responsibilities: choosing the dressing, monitoring the progress of healing and deciding when to remove the sutures.

The purposes of dressings for surgical wounds are as follows:

- To maintain the wound in a warm and moist state most conducive to healing

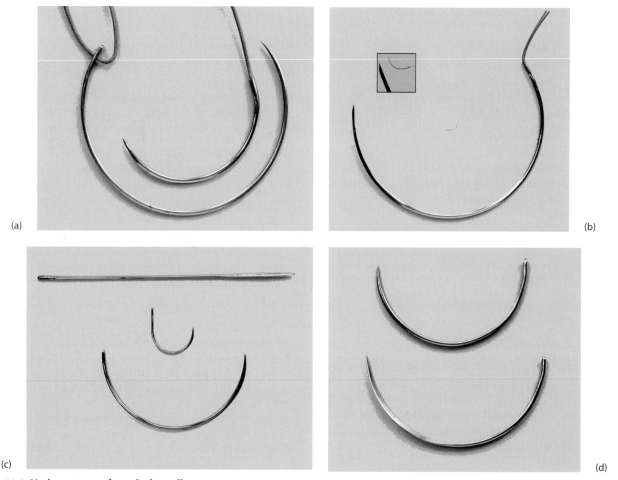

Fig. 11.3 Various types of surgical needles
(a) Two half-circle round-bodied needles, the larger with a threaded 'eye', and the smaller with the suture material swaged into it (*'atraumatic' needle*). Note the braided nature of the suture material. **(b)** The largest and smallest needles in common use. The larger needle is a 5/8-circle needle with a semi-cutting point, used in the hand for abdominal wall closure. Note the two strands of nylon swaged into the end. The smaller needle is used in ophthalmic surgery and has 10/0 suture material (enlarged in the inset). **(c)** Three shapes of needle. The straight needle has a cutting point and is used for skin suturing. The J-shaped needle is used mainly for femoral hernia repairs, and the large half-circle needle is for abdominal wall closure. **(d)** Two large needles showing the difference between 'round-bodied' (above) and 'cutting' ends (below).

- To absorb or contain any superficial bleeding or inflammatory exudate
- To protect the delicate healing tissue from trauma, bacterial contamination and interference
- To prevent sutures catching on clothing or other objects
- To conceal the wound from view
- To apply pressure to the wound if haematoma formation is likely

TYPES OF WOUND DRESSING

For small surgical wounds, particularly on the face, a dressing is often unnecessary as the linear crust of inflammatory exudate performs this task admirably. For other simple wounds, plastic spray dressing is suitable, e.g. Opsite. In most other cases, **prepacked adhesive dressings** are used, incorporating an absorbent pad with non-stick film in contact with the wound surface. While convenient, these dressings may conceal accumulations of blood, inflam-matory exudate or infected discharge. Wound inspection then requires painful removal of the dressing which can be an opportunity for infection to enter. Transparent **semipermeable plastic film dressings** neatly overcome this problem but are unsuitable for discharging wounds.

Paraffin gauze (**tulle gras**) is used mainly for covering raw areas (e.g. skin-graft donor sites). However, its non-stick paraffin content rapidly declines and blood clot and tissue proliferation soon incorporate the dressing via its open weave. As removal tends to damage the delicate new epithelium, a better alternative dressing is a flexible poly-amide net coated with soft silicone (e.g. Mepitel). This has very low wound adherence and is usually easy to remove when necessary. Other dressings include saline-soaked gauze, **calcium alginate** (seaweed origin), **hydrocolloids** and **hydrogels**. Newer dressings offer a better wound environment with increased hydration, fewer dressing changes and greater comfort. Cost effectiveness is an issue yet to be resolved.

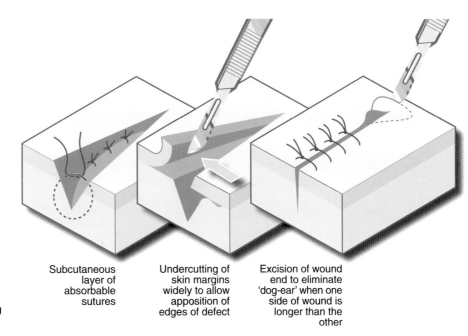

Subcutaneous layer of absorbable sutures

Undercutting of skin margins widely to allow apposition of edges of defect

Excision of wound end to eliminate 'dog-ear' when one side of wound is longer than the other

Fig. 11.4 Methods of approximating skin edges

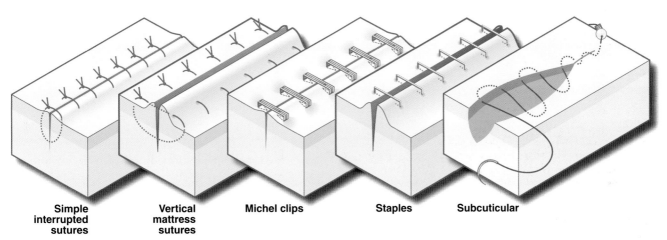

Simple interrupted sutures

Vertical mattress sutures

Michel clips

Staples

Subcuticular

Fig. 11.5 Commonly used skin closure techniques

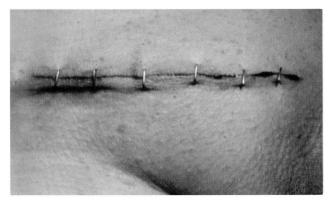

Fig. 11.6 Inguinal hernia wound closed with staples

Gamgee is a thick cotton wool dressing material enveloped in a thin layer of gauze; this is variously used for padding sites vulnerable to trauma (e.g. amputation stumps), as pads beneath pressure bandages or as absorbent dressings for leaking wounds. **Dry dressings** are wads of dressing material (e.g. cotton gauze), usually taped or bandaged in place. Dry dressings need regular replacement and may be prevented from sticking by first placing a piece of non-adherent dressing material (e.g. Melolin, N/A dressing) against the wound. If dry dressings are used for infected wounds, exudate must not be allowed to permeate to the surface as bacteria rapidly spread from here into the environment ('**strike-through**').

REMOVAL OF DRESSINGS AND SUTURES

Provided the dressing remains clean and dry and the patient afebrile and generally well, there is no need to inspect clean surgical wounds until the time of suture removal. If wound complications are suspected, the dressing should be removed and the wound checked and redressed as appropriate. If infection is apparent, a wound swab should be taken for culture and sensitivity. Localised abscess formation requires suture removal and probing to effect drainage, whilst spreading cellulitis requires antibiotic therapy in addition.

Skin sutures should be removed as soon as the wound is strong enough to remain intact without support. On the back and around joints, this can take 14 days; on the abdomen, it takes about 7 days (longer in the case of steroid therapy or infection). On the face and neck healing is rapid and less influenced by functional stresses. Here, sutures can be safely removed after 3–5 days, giving a better cosmetic result.

MANAGEMENT OF DRAINS IN THE POSTOPERATIVE PERIOD

Abdominal drains provide a potential route for infection to enter the abdomen even though the intra-abdominal pressure nearly always exceeds the external pressure. The risk can be minimised by ensuring the drain opens into a sterile environment such as a drainage bag (**closed drainage**) and by removing the drain as soon as its task is completed. Decisions about removal of drains should rest with the operating surgeon who will undoubtedly have personal preferences.

The general principles of drain management are as follows:

- Suction drains help to collapse down spaces left in the tissues at operation as well as to drain blood and inflammatory exudate. These drains are mainly used after extensive excisional surgery where a large enclosed raw surface remains, e.g. after mastectomy, thyroidectomy or excision of the rectum. High-vacuum suction drains, however, should not be used near bowel for fear of suction perforation. A suction drain is usually retained only for 24 hours after operation unless substantial drainage (e.g. > 30 ml/24 hours) persists
- Non-suction drains (e.g. large-bore silicone or rubber tubes, or corrugated drains) are mainly used for bowel and biliary anastomoses and in abscess drainage. In this case, the drain is left in place for about 5 days. Some surgeons prefer to withdraw the drain in stages so that the deep part of the drainage tract can collapse progressively, reducing the risk of leaving a deep pool of fluid

SOFT TISSUE SURGERY

METHODS OF OBTAINING TISSUE FOR DIAGNOSIS

BIOPSY

If major surgery or other therapy is being contemplated for a suspected malignant lesion, an accurate **tissue diagnosis** should be made wherever possible.

Skin lesions can be **biopsied** by incision under local anaesthesia. Rectal lesions can be biopsied without anaesthesia using forceps through a rigid sigmoidoscope, while gastric and colonic lesions can be biopsied via a flexible endoscope. Breast lumps or suspicious mammographic lesions can be sampled using percutaneous core needle biopsy or by fine needle aspiration cytology (see below).

Enlarged lymph nodes can often be diagnosed by **incision biopsy** or by removing one or more completely for histological examination (**excision biopsy**), although many units can now obtain satisfactory results by needle biopsy. Lymphadenectomy often requires general anaesthesia, particularly for lumps in the neck.

Biopsy guided by ultrasound or CT scanning

Abdominal masses such as liver metastases or pancreatic lesions can be biopsied percutaneously with the aid of ultrasound or CT scanning. The suspicious lesion is first located as an image and then a biopsy needle is guided into it with the help of further imaging. Guided biopsy techniques have greatly assisted surgical diagnosis and have saved many patients from unnecessary exploratory laparotomy in the case of benign lesions and inoperable tumours. The technique can be used to sample abdominal masses or suspicious para-aortic lymph nodes in staging lymphomas or following treatment for testicular germ cell tumours.

CYTOLOGY

Special staining techniques for malignant cells can be applied to material obtained by fine needle aspiration. Cytological diagnosis requires special laboratory skills but often permits accurate diagnosis (e.g. of malignancy), which renders more invasive investigations unnecessary. A negative cytological result, however, must be interpreted with great caution because it may be due to sampling error.

Cytological diagnosis can be useful for the following:

- Examining cells aspirated from solid masses. This is particularly useful for thyroid nodules (see Ch. 49), breast lumps and mammographically detected lesions and pancreatic masses
- Examining ascitic fluid obtained from the abdomen by **paracentesis**, or pleural effusions aspirated from the chest. Fluid may also be sent for microbiological analysis

- Examining cellular material scraped from surfaces, e.g. uterine cervical smears, or fluid obtained from within hollow viscera, e.g. urine, pancreatic secretions, sputum

'MINOR' OPERATIVE PROCEDURES

Many skin lesions are amenable to simple excision or biopsy, often under local anaesthesia. These may be performed in family medical practice or in dermatological or surgical outpatient departments. A strict aseptic technique must be employed.

LOCAL ANAESTHESIA FOR SKIN LESIONS

The usual method of administration is by infiltration (injection) of local anaesthetic agents (e.g. lidocaine (lignocaine) 0.5% or 1%) into the skin surrounding the lesion. Between 1 and 10 ml of solution is usually required, but care must be taken to remain within recommended maximum safe dosages (see Table 11.3). A vasoconstrictor (e.g. adrenaline 1 in 200 000) may be incorporated to reduce vascularity in the operative field, but this must never be used on the extreme peripheries, i.e. fingers, toes, penis or nose, because of the high risk of ischaemic necrosis. The injecting needle should be as fine as possible and inserted into the skin as few times as possible to avoid causing unnecessary pain. Before each injection, aspiration is attempted to ensure that the solution is not injected directly into a blood vessel as intravascular injection may cause systemic toxicity. Methods of infiltration of local anaesthetic are illustrated in Figure 11.7.

BIOPSY TECHNIQUES

Excision biopsy

The technique of excision biopsy illustrated in Figure 11.8 is appropriate for most small lesions not considered to be malignant. The lesion is removed with a fusiform piece of normal skin, with the long axis orientated along skin creases and tension lines. The specimen should include a millimetre or two of normal skin on either side of the lesion and should include the full depth of the dermis down to the subcutaneous fat.

Incision biopsy

Incision biopsy is a technique of obtaining a tissue sample from a lesion that is too large or anatomically unsuitable for excision biopsy, e.g. a skin rash or a suspected malignant tumour. Major surgical procedures or radiotherapy should not be performed without histological confirmation of the diagnosis. The objective is to obtain a representative sample of the full depth of the lesion, including an area of the margin and adjoining normal tissue (see Fig. 11.9).

Destruction of lesions by diathermy, electrocautery, cryocautery or curettage

These techniques are used for small lesions where there is no clinical suspicion of malignancy or for small basal cell carcinomas where a histological diagnosis is not required; the lesion is destroyed in the process of removal. Local infiltration of anaesthetic is necessary except for cryocautery, which is relatively painless.

Removal of cysts

A cyst is a fluid-filled lesion, lined by epithelium and usually encapsulated by a condensation of surrounding fibrous tissue. The aim of treatment is to remove the whole epithelial lining because any remnant will lead to recurrence. The technique of removal is outlined in Figure 11.10. Ideally, the cyst is dissected out intact without puncturing the cavity. If this occurs, the cyst collapses, making it difficult to identify and remove the epithelial

Table 11.3 Maximum safe doses of local anaesthetic agents for infiltration in fit patients

Lidocaine (lignocaine)	Bupivacaine (Marcain) or levobupivacaine (Chirocaine)
2% lidocaine is probably no more effective for achieving anaesthesia than 1% or even 0.5% so use lowest concentration needed; 10 ml of 1% lidocaine contains 100 mg	0.5% bupivacaine is probably no more effective than 0.25% 10 ml of 0.5% bupivacaine contains 50 mg
The maximum safe dose of **plain lidocaine** is 4 mg/kg body weight	The maximum safe dose of **plain bupivacaine** is 2 mg/kg body weight
For a fit 60 kg adult, the maximum safe dose of 1% *plain* lidocaine is 16–24 ml	For a fit 60 kg adult, the maximum safe dose of 0.5% bupivacaine is 24 ml
With adrenaline, this dose can be increased to 7 mg/kg body weight	Addition of adrenaline does **not** increase the safe dose of bupivacaine and there is little point in using it for infiltration except to provide vasoconstriction
For a fit 60 kg adult, the maximum safe dose of 1% lidocaine *with adrenaline* is 30–40 ml	No increase

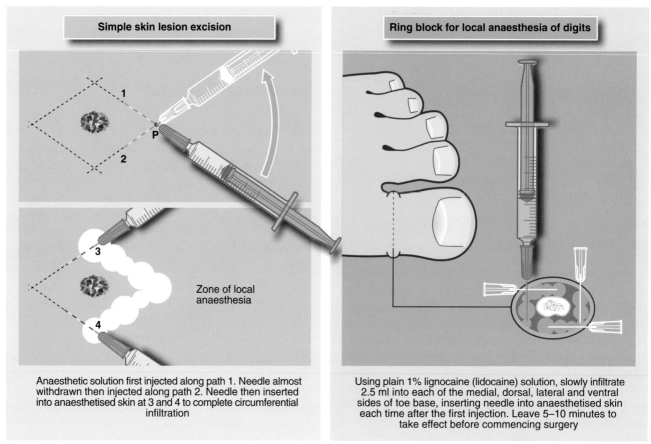

Simple skin lesion excision	Ring block for local anaesthesia of digits
Anaesthetic solution first injected along path 1. Needle almost withdrawn then injected along path 2. Needle then inserted into anaesthetised skin at 3 and 4 to complete circumferential infiltration	Using plain 1% lignocaine (lidocaine) solution, slowly infiltrate 2.5 ml into each of the medial, dorsal, lateral and ventral sides of toe base, inserting needle into anaesthetised skin each time after the first injection. Leave 5–10 minutes to take effect before commencing surgery

Fig. 11.7 Local anaesthetic infiltration techniques

lining. Inflamed cysts are best simply drained and excised later when the inflammation has settled.

Marsupialisation

This technique is usually employed for the treatment of cysts or other fluid-filled lesions which are too large, inaccessible or technically difficult to remove. It is rarely appropriate for skin lesions but is often used for large salivary retention cysts in the floor of the mouth, cysts in the jaw and pancreatic pseudocysts. The technique is illustrated in Figure 11.11. The surgeon removes a disc from the wall of the cavity and sutures the lining to the overlying epithelium around the cut edge. This leaves a pouch, which slowly fills from below once the pressure of the cyst contents has been removed.

SURGERY INVOLVING INFECTED TISSUES

MANAGEMENT OF ABSCESSES

The first principle of managing an abscess is to establish drainage of the pus. When an abscess is 'pointing' to the surface, surgical drainage involves a skin incision at the site of maximum fluctuance followed by blunt probing with sinus forceps or a finger (usually under general anaesthesia) to ensure that all loculi are drained; necrotic material is removed at the same time by curettage.

After drainage, small abscesses need only a dry dressing, the cavity filling in rapidly from beneath. Larger and deeper abscesses need a method of keeping the skin opening patent until the cavity has filled with granulation tissue. A corrugated drain, which is gradually withdrawn ('shortened') over a few days, will achieve this or else the cavity may be packed with ribbon gauze soaked in saline or antiseptic solution; these packs are usually changed daily or every other day. Good analgesia is required in the early stages. When the cavity is granulating, a silicone foam dressing may be used. This is poured into the wound as a liquid where it rapidly foams and sets. The dressing is absorbent and can easily be removed, washed and replaced. New dressings are made as the wound shrinks.

MANAGEMENT OF INFECTED SURGICAL WOUNDS

Grossly infected surgical wounds must be opened up to ensure free drainage, and cleaned. All necrotic tissue is excised leaving only healthy tissue, and the wound packed daily afterwards with saline-soaked gauze. The wound is usually allowed to heal by secondary intention,

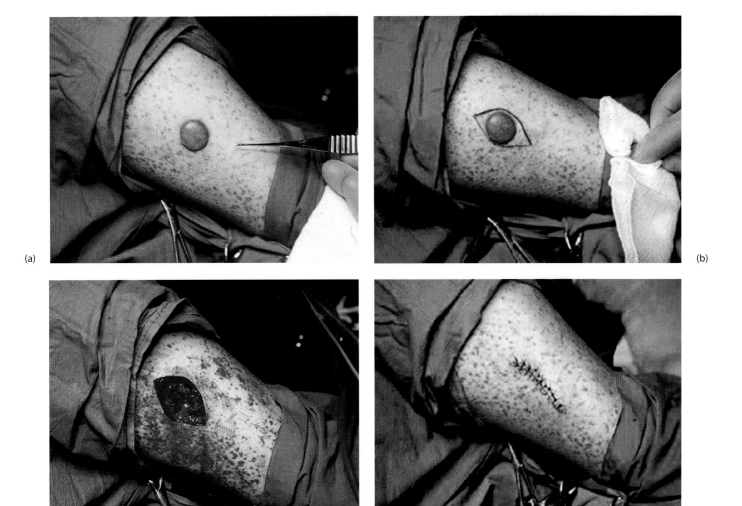

(a)

(b)

(c)

(d)

Fig. 11.8 Excision biopsy technique

although a large wound can be sutured later when infection is no longer a problem (**delayed primary closure**). In the case of deep, slowly healing wounds, a silicone foam dressing can be employed.

MANAGEMENT OF DIRTY OR CONTAMINATED WOUNDS

Major soft tissue injuries result in crushing and tearing of tissues, leaving devascularised areas and deep impregnation with soil, road grit or fragments of clothing. If such a wound is merely sutured, pyogenic infection is certain, and there is a serious risk of gas gangrene or tetanus.

The principles of managing these wounds were first established during the First World War, as follows:

- Thorough removal of all foreign material from the wound (sometimes called '**debridement**')
- Excision of all non-viable tissue ('**necrosectomy**')
- Loose open packing of the wound with dry cotton gauze without suturing

- Inspection of the wound under anaesthesia 2–4 days later, plus drainage of any new abscesses and removal of any newly apparent non-viable tissue
- Suturing of the wound when it looks clean and granulating, but avoiding tension; this is known as **delayed primary closure**. Alternatively, split skin grafting may be employed without wound closure

PRINCIPLES OF PLASTIC SURGERY

The discipline of plastic surgery was born during the First World War in response to the appalling disfigurement caused by blast injuries and burns. Since then, specialised techniques of skin reconstruction have progressed much further, especially in the fields of axial flap design and microvascular reconstructive surgery. The scope of modern plastic surgery is outlined in Box 11.8. There is a considerable degree of overlap and collaboration between the field of plastic surgery and other surgical specialties, especially ear, nose and throat, maxillofacial and orthopaedic surgery.

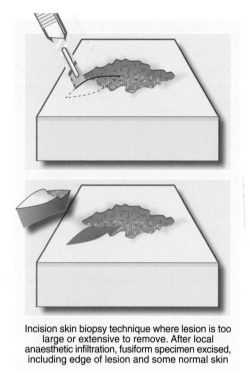

Incision skin biopsy technique where lesion is too large or extensive to remove. After local anaesthetic infiltration, fusiform specimen excised, including edge of lesion and some normal skin

Fig. 11.9 Incision skin biopsy technique

TISSUE TRANSFER TECHNIQUES

Obtaining satisfactory skin cover is one of the major problems in plastic surgery, and other tissues such as fat and muscle could not be satisfactorily transferred without revascularisation. Free transplantation of full-thickness skin (other than tiny grafts) or any other tissue other than bone without revascularisation is usually unsuccessful.

Tissue transfer can be achieved in three main ways:

- Skin grafts
- Vascularised flaps
- Free flaps

Skin grafts

Split skin (Thiersch) grafting involves transplanting a very thin layer of skin consisting of little more than epidermis, which has no blood supply of its own. It depends for nutrition on the recipient bed for its survival. Split skin grafts are commonly employed for burns and after wide excision of skin lesions, provided there is a recipient base of healthy tissue. The donor site heals rapidly since small islands of epithelium are left behind (see Fig. 11.12). The donor site is potentially more painful than the recipient but pain is well controlled if the donor site is dressed immediately with hydrogel or similar dressings. These may be left in position for several days until the wound has epithelialised. Creating a 'mesh' of the graft with a device to make multiple regular perforations helps the graft attach in certain circumstances as it allows free

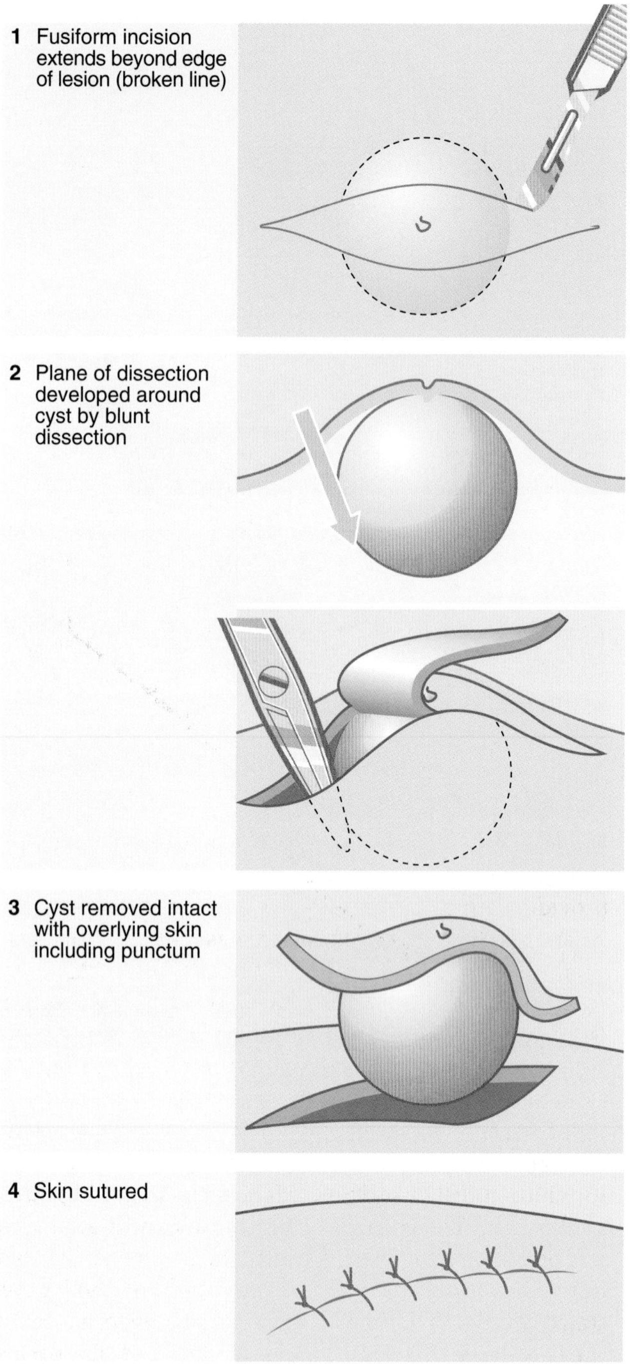

1 Fusiform incision extends beyond edge of lesion (broken line)

2 Plane of dissection developed around cyst by blunt dissection

3 Cyst removed intact with overlying skin including punctum

4 Skin sutured

Fig. 11.10 Technique of excision of an epidermal (sebaceous) cyst

drainage through the perforations. Meshing also allows a graft to be expanded to a greater area. Small full thickness (Wolfe) grafts may survive in certain circumstances. Examples include skin from behind the ear transferred to a severed finger tip and pinch grafts for leg ulcers.

Vascularised flaps

A flap has a blood supply of its own; a flap is not a graft. The blood supply reaches the flap via its base, known as

1 Cyst 'de-roofed'

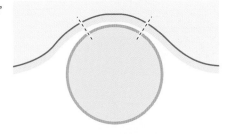

2 Cyst edge
sutured to
overlying
epithelium

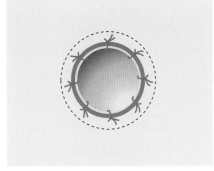

Fig. 11.11 Marsupialisation of a cyst

Congenital problems

- Correction of congenital defects, e.g. cleft lip and palate, syndactyly and polydactyly, prominent ears, hypospadias, vascular malformations, craniofacial deformities, congenital skin conditions, e.g. 'port-wine stains'

Trauma

- Reconstruction after mutilating surgery or trauma, e.g. skin cover for compound lower limb fractures, vascularised bone transfer
- Management of facial soft tissue trauma
- Management of burns—grafting, management of scars and deformities
- Hand trauma—tendon repairs, microsurgical nerve and artery repairs, replantation surgery, e.g. digits and limbs

Elective hand surgery

- Dupuytren's contracture, nerve decompressions, joint replacements in rheumatoid disease

Cancer

- Cutaneous malignancies—excision and reconstruction with grafts or local flaps
- Major cancer surgery of the head and neck—excision and reconstruction with free tissue transfer
- Breast reconstruction after mastectomy

Aesthetic (cosmetic) surgery

- Scar removal, breast reduction and augmentation, 'face-lifts', eyelid skin reduction, nasal adjustment including after trauma
- Surgery for obesity, e.g. abdominal skin reduction, liposuction, apronectomy (for pendulous abdomen)

Miscellaneous, including reconstruction of large defects

- Reconstruction for facial palsy, decubitus (pressure) sores, soft tissue sarcoma excision, leg ulcers, reconstruction of skin after radiotherapy, destructive infections, e.g. necrotising fasciitis, compartment syndromes

the vascular pedicle. Flaps can be advanced, rotated or transposed into the defect to be filled and this may provide sufficient mobility to close a moderate-sized defect. If a new defect is produced as a result of flap rotation, this clean area can usually be covered with a small split skin graft. Most flaps now employed are **axial flaps** which use established anatomical sites to ensure a blood supply running the length of the long axis of the flap. The early **random flaps**, devised by Gillies, were limited in scope because there was no dominant blood supply and this prevented construction of a flap that was longer than its width. Another early technique was the use of **pedicle flaps** in which a flap of skin was raised and formed into a tube while remaining attached to its site of origin at both ends. Later, one end of the tube was divided and transposed to the recipient site; later still the other end of the tube was divided and the flap opened out, shaped and sutured at the recipient site to reconstruct the defect. This, however, was a prolonged procedure necessitating long periods in hospital and uncomfortable immobilisation of the parts involved.

Axial flaps are selected according to the site of the defect and the tissues needed. A series of flaps are now described, based on detailed anatomical studies of blood supply. Flaps may be **cutaneous** (e.g. forehead flap), **fascio-cutaneous** (e.g. the 'Chinese' radial forearm flap), **myocutaneous** (e.g. latissimus dorsi, pectoralis major), **TRAM** (transverse rectus abdominis myocutaneous—often used for breast reconstruction), and **osseous** (e.g. fibula, radius, iliac crest and rib).

Free flaps

In free tissue transfer, a carefully planned piece of tissue is first dissected out, complete with at least one main artery and vein; axial flap sites are often suitable. The whole flap is then relocated to the recipient site where the vessels are connected to a suitable local artery and vein by microvascular anastomoses. The donor site can often be closed primarily or else covered with a split skin graft. Examples are the **radial forearm flap** which supplies bone, muscle and skin, and the big toe which can be used to replace a lost thumb.

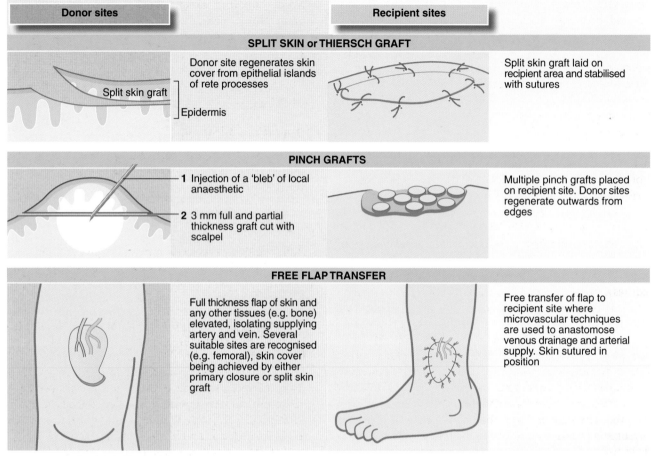

Donor sites		Recipient sites

SPLIT SKIN or THIERSCH GRAFT

Split skin graft

Donor site regenerates skin cover from epithelial islands of rete processes

Epidermis

Split skin graft laid on recipient area and stabilised with sutures

PINCH GRAFTS

1 Injection of a 'bleb' of local anaesthetic

2 3 mm full and partial thickness graft cut with scalpel

Multiple pinch grafts placed on recipient site. Donor sites regenerate outwards from edges

FREE FLAP TRANSFER

Full thickness flap of skin and any other tissues (e.g. bone) elevated, isolating supplying artery and vein. Several suitable sites are recognised (e.g. femoral), skin cover being achieved by either primary closure or split skin graft

Free transfer of flap to recipient site where microvascular techniques are used to anastomose venous drainage and arterial supply. Skin sutured in position

Fig. 11.12 **Methods of skin grafting**

LAPAROSCOPIC SURGERY

MINIMAL ACCESS SURGERY

The last two decades have seen an explosion in interest and rapid development of techniques to achieve accurate diagnosis and provide treatment with the least possible tissue injury and trauma to patients (Table 11.4). Laparoscopic surgery was the first to catch the surgical profession's imagination but other techniques such as lithotripsy, percutaneous stone removal and angioplasty advanced more or less in parallel. Initially called **minimally invasive surgery**, the principle of minimal access surgery is that if less tissue is damaged by avoiding or minimising surgical incisions, then less pain is likely to be experienced afterwards and the physiological responses to injury which slow recovery will be reduced. The result is intended to cause less patient suffering and allow a more rapid return to normal life. It is important to realise that the greatest benefits of laparoscopic surgery are evident in operations when the amount of tissue injured in obtaining access to the abdomen at open surgery is much more than the surgical trauma involved in the actual operation. In addition, patients

need to be informed that even with short-stay laparoscopic surgery, there will still be a period of physiological recovery.

Gynaecologists led the way with laparoscopic diagnosis and procedures, particularly tubal ligation, but little development in instrumentation occurred until laparoscopic cholecystectomy emerged as a viable and popular option. The pioneers stimulated the interest of general surgeons, and enthusiasm for these novel techniques was shared by popular media and the public. As interest and demand grew, commercial companies invested heavily to develop and improve laparoscopic equipment. 'Chip' CCD cameras appeared which allowed superior full-colour images, and practical courses proliferated rapidly to teach the techniques to surgeons.

An example of rapid progress in minimal access surgery is provided by cholecystectomy. Early laparoscopic cholecystectomy was hampered by poor equipment, poor imaging and lack of experience. Now that equipment is first class, training and experience have disseminated and audit is in place, the indications, contraindications and risks have largely become clear; as a result, laparoscopic cholecystectomy has become the gold standard for removal of the gall bladder.

Interest in minimal access techniques is increasingly spreading through the surgical specialties, prompting surgeons to seek new ways of performing operations that cause less trauma to their patients. Thus orthopaedic surgeons perform many operations **arthroscopically** and even joint replacements are being performed through smaller incisions allowing rapid mobilisation. **Thoracoscopy** is a variation on laparoscopy and uses similar instruments for diagnostic and therapeutic applications in the thorax (see details in Ch. 31). Endocrine surgeons now perform parathyroidectomy through very small incisions using special microscopes and retractors, although the benefits are less evident than for other procedures. Breast surgeons now perform **sentinel lymph node biopsy** using dye or radioactive marker techniques. Many urological procedures such as nephrectomy and ureteric procedures are now undertaken laparoscopically, and vascular surgeons have even performed part of aortic aneurysm operations laparoscopically. In fact there is probably no abdominal operation that has not been attempted laparoscopically, although the difficulties of many larger procedures make them impractical for routine use. Laparoscopic techniques have proved most useful in areas of the body with limited access, such as the gastro-oesophageal junction, the adrenal gland and the pelvis, allowing delicate instruments to be used in confined spaces with excellent views unhampered by the surgeon's hands.

LAPAROSCOPY

Laparoscopy or peritoneoscopy has been in wide use clinically by gynaecologists since the early 1970s for diagnosing pelvic disorders and for sterilisation by tubal ligation. In the early days, laparoscopy had limited application in general surgery and was largely confined to visually guided liver biopsies. The first therapeutic gastrointestinal procedure was probably an appendicectomy performed by Semm in 1983. In 1987, Mouret first removed a diseased gall bladder laparoscopically in France. Since then, the techniques have been adopted on a broad scale by general and thoracic surgeons as a method of performing abdominal and thoracic operations via a series of small punctures rather than through large incisions.

ADVANTAGES OF LAPAROSCOPIC SURGERY

The advantages of laparoscopic surgery go well beyond simply avoiding large painful wounds to give better cosmesis and less postoperative pain:

Surgical advantages

- Improved access and vision in difficult areas, e.g. pelvis and gastro-oesophageal junction

- Avoids handling, exposure, desiccation and cooling of abdominal tissues, which may result in reduced adhesion formation
- Reduced contact with patient's blood and body fluids for health care professionals
- Fewer wound infections, dehiscences and incisional hernias

Postoperative advantages

- Fewer postoperative chest complications
- Less postoperative analgesia and shorter hospital stays

RISKS AND COMPLICATIONS

Certain complications are common to open and laparoscopic surgery, but laparoscopic operations carry their own particular risks. Problems specific to laparoscopic techniques include:

- The induction of the pneumoperitoneum (inflating the abdomen with gas) may cause subcutaneous emphysema or injury to bowel or major blood vessels and must be performed with care, preferably using an open technique rather than a Veress needle
- The ensuing trocar insertion may cause injury to the abdominal wall (including the diaphragm), intra-abdominal organs and blood vessels. It must be performed under direct vision, being alert to structures that may potentially be damaged
- The raised intra-abdominal pressure and head-down position mean that patients have to be ventilated at higher inflation pressures. This reduces venous return and cardiac output and may cause circulatory compromise in patients with cardiac ischaemia. To mitigate this, intra-abdominal pressures should be kept to the minimum necessary for the procedure to be performed safely, i.e. 8–12 mmHg; patients should not be placed in extreme head-up or head-down positions for prolonged periods
- The diaphragm is 'splinted' by the pneumoperitoneum and this can precipitate cardiorespiratory complications in patients with respiratory problems. Again, minimising inflation pressures reduces this effect
- The pneumoperitoneum compresses intra-abdominal veins and reduces venous return. This predisposes to thrombo-embolic complications such as deep venous thrombosis. Patients should receive appropriate prophylaxis at all times
- Inadvertent injury can occur to a range of structures during dissection, diathermy or laser instrumentation, often through excess heating. The damage may go unrecognised if the damage occurs out of the sight of the laparoscope, leading to late complications

Table 11.4 Summary of minimally invasive/minimal access approaches to diagnosis and treatment

Specialty area (in alphabetical order)	Diagnostic applications	Therapeutic applications
Abdomen CT or ultrasonography (note laparoscopy is covered in the adjoining text and Boxes 11.9 and 11.10)	• Diagnosis of fluid collections, e.g. ascites, pancreatic pseudocyst, abscess • Percutaneous guided biopsy of enlarged lymph nodes, liver or pancreatic masses, other masses • Diagnosis of acute or chronic abdominal symptoms including detection of colorectal cancer	• Guiding drainage of fluid collections by aspiration or drain insertion • Guiding sampling of suspected pancreatic necrosis for infection in acute pancreatitis • Stent placement for obstructing colonic lesions
Anal canal	• Proctoscopy to inspect the anal canal and, if necessary, biopsy lesions	• Injection or banding of haemorrhoids • Perineal operations for rectal prolapse • Transanal resection of tumours—'TART'
Arterial	• Conventional arteriography or magnetic resonance angiography—demonstrating the sites, severity and morphology of arterial obstruction or aneurysms—selective or highly selective angiography for detecting the source of acute intestinal bleeding or bleeding after pelvic fracture, or determining the blood supply of an organ • Ultrasound or CT diagnosis of aortic and other aneurysms • Duplex Doppler ultrasound scanning—for carotid artery disease, peripheral arterial disease, femoro-popliteal and other graft surveillance	• Angioplasty of arterial stenoses (percutaneous transluminal angioplasty—PCTA) • Stenting of obliterative arterial disease • Intraluminal stent grafting for aneurysms • Percutaneous thrombolysis • Embolisation for bleeding/tumours/arteriovenous malformations/preoperative treatment of vascular lesions to reduce vascularity
Biliary (see also Pancreas)	• Distal duodenoscopy for ampullary tumours • Diagnostic ERCP for suspected bile duct stones or strictures, or for suspected duct damage after surgery	• Endoscopic sphincterotomy to retrieve bile duct stones, e.g. in obstructive jaundice • Stent placement across bile duct strictures, traumatic leaks or tumours
Breast	• Detection and fine needle aspiration cytology or needle biopsy of solid lumps • Stereotactic fine needle aspiration or biopsy of mammographically detected lesions suspected of malignancy	• Ultrasound guided aspiration of cysts
Cardiac	• Endomyocardial biopsy for detecting rejection in heart transplants	• Angioplasty and stenting of obstructed coronary arteries • Off-pump coronary artery bypass—OPCAB (under evaluation) • Small incision or thoracoscopic approaches to standard cardiac operations using cardio-pulmonary bypass or without, e.g. via partial sternotomy (under evaluation)
Chest	• Ultrasound diagnosis of fluid collections • Thoracoscopic pleural or lung biopsy • Mediastinoscopic node biopsy	• Thoracoscopic cervico-dorsal sympathectomy for hyperhidrosis of the hands • Pleurectomy or lobectomy for benign disease
Gynaecology	• Laparoscopic diagnosis for infertility • Diagnosis of cause of acute abdomen in suspected pelvic inflammatory disease, tubal pregnancy, ovarian problems	• Laparoscopic sterilisation (tubal clipping) • Laparoscopic assisted hysterectomy (but carries 2.5 times the risk of urinary tract injuries compared with abdominal or vaginal) • Laparoscopic oophorectomy for palliation of breast carcinoma • Laparoscopic obtaining of eggs for in vitro and other forms of assisted fertilisation • Laparoscopic pelvic lymphadenectomy for radical cancer surgery • Laparoscopic operations for urinary stress incontinence

Table 11.4 Summary of minimally invasive/minimal access approaches to diagnosis and treatment—cont'd

Specialty area (in alphabetical order)	Diagnostic applications	Therapeutic applications
Oesophagus	● Diagnostic oesophagoscopy and biopsy—flexible instruments usually used	● Dilatation of benign oesophageal strictures ● Pulsion (pushing) placement of luminal tubes and cloth-covered stents for obstructing carcinoma ● Palliative laser ablation of obstructing tumours—'reboring' ● Injection of bleeding ulcers ● Balloon compression and endoscopic sclerotherapy injection of varices ● Balloon dilatation of narrow cardia in achalasia ● Thoracoscopic myotomy for achalasia (Heller's operation) ● Laparoscopic anti-reflux surgery
Orthopaedics	● Diagnostic arthroscopy—hip, knee, ankle, shoulder, elbow and wrist	Therapeutic arthroscopy: ● Knee—removal of loose bodies; articular cartilage and meniscal surgery; cruciate reconstruction; irrigation for infection ● Shoulder—impingement decompression; shoulder stabilisation; rotator cuff repair ● Hip, elbow and ankle—removal of loose bodies; articular cartilage surgery ● Wrist—percutaneous screw for scaphoid fracture
Pancreas	● Endoscopic pancreatography for suspected duct abnormalities ● Endoscopic collection of exocrine secretions for cytology ?malignancy	● Early sphincterotomy and trawling of biliary and pancreatic ducts to relieve stone-induced pancreatitis
Rectum and colon	● Diagnostic flexible sigmoidoscopy or colonoscopy (including biopsy) for bleeding, suspected tumour, inflammatory bowel disease and surveillance after polyp or cancer removal ● Endoluminal ultrasound imaging for staging rectal cancer and determining sphincter damage ● Magnetic resonance imaging for detailing the anatomy of complex fistulae	● Snare excision of polyps and adenomas ● Diathermy to bleeding angiodysplasias ● Diathermy loop resection of inoperable rectal tumours for palliation, or benign rectal strictures
Stomach and duodenum	● Diagnostic inspection for ulcers and cancer ● Biopsy of ulcers and tumours ● Biopsy to diagnose *Helicobacter* infection as a cause of ulceration	● Injection treatment of acutely bleeding ulcers ● Endoscopic retrieval of foreign bodies ● Combined percutaneous and endoscopic placement of feeding gastrostomy tubes ('PEG')
Urology *Endoscopic—* usually rigid but latterly flexible	● Haematuria (staging, treatment and follow-up of bladder tumours) ● Poor urinary stream (assessment of bladder neck and prostatic obstruction) ● Ureteric obstruction (ureteroscopy or retrograde ureterography)	● Fulguration or resection of bladder tumours ● Resection of bladder neck or prostate (TURP) ● Laser enucleation of prostate ● Stenting of ureter to relieve stone obstruction, strictures or external compression ● Balloon dilatation of stenosed pelvi-ureteric junction via transurethral route
Percutaneous		● Direct endoscopic stone destruction and removal; indirect stone destruction using lithotripsy ● Placement of suprapubic catheters
Venous system	● Duplex Doppler ultrasound scanning—for diagnosing deep and superficial venous insufficiency	● Percutaneous ablation of long or short saphenous vein in varicose veins using foam sclerotherapy, radiofrequency or laser ablation ● Subfascial endoscopic perforator surgery (SEPS) for treating venous ulceration

● Postoperatively, bowel may strangulate through peritoneal defects, and incisional hernias can occur through port sites. The latter should be carefully closed under direct vision to minimise this risk

TECHNIQUE OF LAPAROSCOPY

Laparoscopy is usually performed under general anaesthesia, most often with full muscle relaxation to allow full and safe insufflation of the abdominal cavity. A **pneumoperitoneum** is first created by introducing carbon dioxide under controlled pressure to lift the abdominal wall away from the viscera, allowing inspection of the peritoneal cavity.

Gas is most safely introduced via a blunt cannula placed by an open technique which enables direct visualisation of the peritoneal contents. The technique is steadily replacing 'blind' insufflation via a Veress needle which has a small but significant risk of major vascular injury. The gas pressure should be kept as low as possible while maintaining a satisfactory view, in order to minimise the cardiac and respiratory risks. A 5 or 10 mm diameter working laparoscope with video camera is then introduced into the abdominal cavity, displaying the image on monitors.

Most laparoscopic procedures need additional cannulae (trocars) through which to pass instruments such as diathermy hooks, graspers, needle holders, clip appliers and linear staplers. These secondary trocars are inserted through new access points under direct vision from within the abdomen to prevent injury to bowel and other viscera. Different operations each require various port placements. Preferences vary from surgeon to surgeon and port siting also depends on the particular conditions of the operation; for example cholecystectomy in an obese patient necessitates different port sites from those used in a slim patient.

The laparoscopic operation is performed by an operator and one or more assistants, all observing progress on video monitors. Sharp or blunt dissection may be employed as in open surgery. Sharp dissection uses laparoscopic scissors whilst blunt dissection is carried out using fine dissecting forceps ('Petolins' or 'Marylands'), laparoscopic gauze pledgets or the tip of a suction probe. Blunt dissection tears rather than cuts small vessels, deliberately causing minor tissue damage that rapidly activates the coagulation cascade and causes spontaneous cessation of bleeding. This is a safer technique than sharp dissection which may require (potentially excessive) use of diathermy. Haemostasis still requires diathermy and this must be cautiously used to prevent arcing of the current to adjacent organs. Increasingly, safer alternatives are being used such as **bipolar** diathermy forceps or the **harmonic scalpel**, which uses ultrasound to coagulate and cut vessels and tissue.

Grasping forceps, probes, hooks, flexible retractors or folding 'fans' are used for retraction. Larger blood vessels that would be ligated at open surgery can be clipped with metal or plastic locking devices using clip applicators. Larger vessels can be stapled with vascular staplers. Repairs and other operative procedures are completed using laparoscopic sutures or staples, and bowel resections performed using linear or circular staplers. In laparoscopic-assisted surgery, for example colectomy, a large part of the dissection is performed laparoscopically, then a small abdominal incision is made to deliver the resected specimen.

After operation, patients experience abdominal discomfort at trocar insertion sites and shoulder discomfort from retained gas in the peritoneal cavity. Few restrictions are placed on the patient after discharge; he or she can return to work as soon as comfortable, often after a few days. Overall pain experienced is less than open surgery but cost:benefit ratios for many operations remain to be evaluated.

ROBOTIC-ASSISTED SURGERY

The first generation of surgical 'robots' is on trial in a few operating theatres around the world. These robots are not autonomous but aid the surgeon who sits at a remote console (which may be close to the patient or far away). The surgeon controls very precisely the robotic manipulation of laparoscopic instruments, previously inserted into the anaesthetised patient by an assistant, via the surgical arm unit. The imaging system provides 3-D vision, and robotic mechanisms transmit the surgeon's precise hand movements to the laparoscopic instruments. The da Vinci system allows manipulation of all instruments necessary whilst other simpler systems just control the camera.

Potential benefits include increased precision of movement with 'smoothing' of any tremor, prevention of fatigue in long operations and perhaps eventually the need for fewer assistants in the theatre. In the longer term, a surgeon could operate on a patient many kilometres away by **tele-surgery**. Disadvantages of robotic surgery include the high capital cost (currently around $1 000 000), complete lack of any tactile feedback for the surgeon and long set-up times for individual patients.

APPLICATIONS OF LAPAROSCOPY

Laparoscopy in general surgery has both **diagnostic** and **therapeutic applications**. The diagnostic applications are well recognised and are increasingly employed as first-line investigative procedures. The advantages and potential complications of laparoscopic biliary tract surgery are now well understood despite its having been introduced without the usual rigorous clinical trials. However, some of the results of this uncontrolled experiment have been catastrophic in inexperienced hands. Following laparoscopic cholecystectomy, other applications such as appendicectomy, inguinal hernia repair, laparoscopic-assisted colectomy and many others have been introduced more slowly and with better evaluation of the risks and benefits compared with traditional open techniques.

Thorough training and supervised experience are essential for would-be laparoscopic surgeons. The lack of 'feel' inherent in laparoscopic surgery and the two-dimensional view remove much of the feedback of open surgery and novel techniques have to be learned. Patients undergoing laparoscopic surgery sometimes have to be 'converted' to open surgery if visibility is impaired or if complicating factors such as bleeding or adhesions make it too difficult to evaluate the anatomy. This means that any surgeon undertaking laparoscopic procedures must have the necessary experience to perform the procedure 'open'. As more surgery is performed laparoscopically, available experience becomes scarce and this represents a potential problem for the future.

DIAGNOSTIC LAPAROSCOPY

Diagnostic laparoscopy has long been used by individual surgeons for assessing chronic liver disease and ascites of unknown origin. Recent advances in instrumentation and imaging now allow surgeons to perform abdominal exploration almost as thoroughly as is possible via a long laparotomy incision. A key application is for staging gastric or pancreatic cancer to assess operability. This is achieved by inspection, obtaining peritoneal washings for cytology and performing biopsies. By this method, patients with incurable disease are spared the trauma of exploratory open surgery (Box 11.9). Diagnostic laparoscopy is a valuable investigation that is increasingly being used for assessing right iliac fossa pain, particularly in women of menstruating age. The procedure allows more accurate assessment of the gynaecological organs, improves diagnostic accuracy and minimises negative appendicectomy rates.

THERAPEUTIC LAPAROSCOPY

Laparoscopic cholecystectomy is already the gold standard operation for removal of the gall bladder, both in the elective and the emergency situation (described in Chapter 20). Other procedures described below and listed in Box 11.10 are rapidly becoming standard operations in the armoury of specialist laparoscopic surgeons.

Laparoscopic appendicectomy

Open appendicectomy for acute appendicitis is one of the most frequently performed operations by general surgeons, and laparoscopic appendicectomy is swiftly becoming a regular operation for surgical trainees. Laparoscopic appendicectomy offers improved diagnostic accuracy with the ability to examine the entire abdomen if the appendix is normal, a lower rate of wound complications, reduced postoperative pain and hospital stay, and perhaps more rapid return to normal activities. Laparoscopic appendicectomy may offer a lower rate of pelvic adhe-

---

Box 11.9   Potential indications for diagnostic laparoscopy

- Evaluation of acute or chronic abdominal pain, e.g. suspected appendicitis, gynaecological pain
- Diagnosis and staging of intra-abdominal malignancies (including evaluating the results of chemotherapy or radiotherapy on intra-abdominal malignancies)
- Assessing blunt or penetrating abdominal trauma in stable patients with proven free intra-abdominal fluid
- Evaluation of acute or chronic liver disease
- Diagnosis of ascites of unknown cause
- As a 'second-look' procedure in patients operated on for mesenteric ischaemia
- Exclusion of acute acalculous cholecystitis after major trauma or surgery in intensive care patients

---

Box 11.10   Current therapeutic applications of laparoscopy

- Cholecystectomy (described in Ch. 20) and common bile duct exploration
- Appendicectomy
- Colonic resections and colostomy formation—benign and malignant disease
- Abdominal operations for rectal prolapse
- Division of symptomatic adhesions
- Inguinal, femoral, Spigelian and incisional hernia repairs
- Small bowel surgery—including resection and enteral access procedures
- Peptic ulcer disease (plugging of duodenal perforations)
- Symptomatic hiatus hernias and oesophageal reflux (Nissen fundoplication and other anti-reflux operations)
- Nephrectomy, pyeloplasty and other ureteric procedures
- Splenectomy and adrenalectomy
- Laparoscopic liver biopsy and deroofing of liver cysts
- Distal pancreatectomy
- Laparoscopically assisted oesophagectomy and gastrectomy
- Laparoscopic drainage of pancreatic pseudocysts and pancreatic necrosectomy
- Laparoscopic surgery for obesity
- Laparoscopically assisted total hysterectomy and all tube and ovarian procedures including marsupialisation of ectopic pregnancy

sions because of reduced trauma; this is an advantage in young women.

Laparoscopic inguinal hernia repair

The standard open techniques for inguinal hernia repair are based on Bassini's extraperitoneal groin approach described in 1884. Open transabdominal repairs were performed in the 1930s but carried the increased morbidity associated with abdominal operations. Renewed interest has arisen in both transperitoneal and extraperitoneal approaches via a laparoscopic route. Both techniques involve less dissection than the open groin approach and both are believed to reduce the likelihood of damage to testicular vessels and the ilio-inguinal nerve (particularly for recurrent hernias), resulting in a lower incidence of long-term chronic groin pain.

Laparoscopic inguinal hernia repair requires a great deal of supervised experience for a surgeon to achieve consistent results. The procedure is now widely performed, and controlled trials show that it can have better results in some respects than open hernia repair techniques. Evidence about long-term recurrence rates is equivocal but early data suggest that outcomes in experienced hands are comparable to open surgery. Laparoscopic repair is of particular value for recurrent hernias, allowing surgery to be performed in tissue planes free from scarring. It is also recommended for treatment of bilateral hernias, when both sides can be repaired through three small incisions.

Laparoscopic fundoplication

Laparoscopic fundoplication can be employed for patients suffering from large hiatus hernias or gastro-oesophageal reflux disease resistant to medical management. The technique involves dissection of the gastro-oesophageal junction at the hiatus, repair of the crura and wrapping of the gastric fundus around the lower oesophagus (Nissen-type wrap). Clinical trials show that it offers more rapid return to normal activity and results are as durable as open fundoplication.

Laparoscopic management of duodenal ulcer perforation

Duodenal ulcers usually perforate anteriorly and the perforation can readily be seen with the laparoscope. Under laparoscopic visualisation, the ulcer is closed in the same way as at open operation, with part of the greater omentum secured to the duodenum to seal the perforation with laparoscopically placed sutures. The peritoneal cavity is irrigated with a pressure irrigator and the fluid aspirated.

Laparoscopic placement of enterocutaneous jejunostomy tube

In patients requiring long-term enteral feeding in whom a gastrostomy is unsuitable, a fine-bore feeding tube can be placed into the jejunum using laparoscopic techniques, thus avoiding the need for laparotomy.

Laparoscopic splenectomy

As with cholecystectomy, laparoscopic splenectomy has become the gold standard for elective splenectomy, particularly in haematological conditions. Substantially enlarged spleens can be removed laparoscopically but the risk of conversion to open operation rises steeply once the spleen weighs over 1 kg (such spleens usually reach the costal margin). At operation, the patient lies on the right side for best access and vision, and the hilar vessels are divided between clips or with vascular staplers. The spleen is placed in a laparoscopic retrieval bag and broken up or liquidised to enable removal via one of the small port incisions.

Laparoscopic adrenalectomy

Laparoscopic adrenalectomy has proved a useful procedure, allowing adrenal tumours of all sizes to be removed safely and with much less trauma than the muscle-cutting flank incisions previously employed. It is particularly useful in **phaeochromocytoma** where very delicate handling of the tumour is needed. This includes precise delineation and clipping of the vessels in the appropriate order to avoid catecholamine surges.

Laparoscopically assisted colectomy

Laparoscopic techniques were first used to perform simple colorectal procedures such as rectopexy and formation of colostomies. Early experience with colorectal cancer showed port site metastases appearing more commonly than wound metastases at open surgery. This led to concern that the cancer was being disseminated by the pneumoperitoneum. However, further research and refinement of 'no touch' techniques have laid these fears to rest. Laparoscopically assisted resection of benign and malignant colonic lesions is becoming more commonplace, although the learning curve is steep and prolonged training is necessary. Furthermore, substantial benefits have not yet been demonstrated.

Laparoscopic surgery for obesity

In recent years there has been a major expansion in laparoscopic surgery for obesity (**bariatric surgery**). The most common technique involves placing an adjustable restrictive silicone band around the upper part of the stomach to create a small proximal pouch that causes early satiety. Results are excellent in carefully selected, well-motivated patients who have good support and follow-up. Recently, more radical bariatric operations such as gastric bypass and bilio-pancreatic diversion (BPD) operations are also being performed laparoscopically. These operations achieve greater weight loss but may carry higher rates of morbidity and mortality.

Complications of surgery

12

INTRODUCTION

Any operation, major trauma or other surgical admission may be attended by one or more complications, many of which are preventable. Complications cause added pain and suffering and may even put the patient's life at risk. Furthermore, patients with complications often need high-dependency care and need longer hospital admissions, thus imposing extra costs on already overstretched budgets. For example, an anastomotic leak or a wound dehiscence can double the cost of an elective colonic resection.

While some complications are to some extent inherent in the condition being treated (e.g. deep venous thrombosis following multiple lower limb fractures) or arise from some comorbid (pre-existing) condition such as myocardial ischaemia, others arise from failure to visit or examine a patient when called, errors of judgement (e.g. misdiagnosis), poor nursing practice (e.g. allowing pressure sores to develop) or even frank negligence (e.g. operation on the wrong side). Many complications can be traced to **system failure** rather than individual poor practice, and rigorous examination of serious complications by surgeons and others, in an environment where no blame is attached, can help correct failures in the system.

For example, a complication might be attributed to lack of appropriate training or the absence of a clear local guideline (or a failure to follow it). **Poor communication** between hospital staff members is a frequent cause of avoidable complications, e.g. failing to record important events occurring in the patient's treatment (and the date or name of the doctor), or failure to record a drug allergy in the case record, or neglecting to inform the operating department about a late change to an operating list.

Even in an ideal system, a large proportion of complications can be prevented or minimised by appropriate anticipation, by taking particular prophylactic measures, by careful attention to detail and by early recognition and treatment of problems as they develop. With potentially serious complications (e.g. bowel anastomotic leak), early diagnosis and reoperation is crucial, as delay often leads to catastrophic 'snowballing' sepsis and multi-organ failure. Once two or more body systems become impaired, survival falls to only about 50%. If, for example, acute respiratory distress syndrome (ARDS) and renal failure complicate an operation for obstructive jaundice in a patient with liver impairment, the odds are heavily stacked against the patient's survival.

In respect of operative surgery, complications can be divided into the **general** complications of any operation

Box **12.1** **Principal categories of surgical complications**

1. Complications predisposed to by intercurrent 'medical' disorders, whether symptomatic or occult, e.g. ischaemic heart disease, chronic respiratory disease or diabetes mellitus (discussed in Ch. 8)
2. Complications of anaesthesia
3. General complications of operations, e.g. haemorrhage or wound infection
4. Complications of any surgical condition, e.g. pulmonary embolism, pneumonia or urinary tract infection
5. Complications of specific disorders and operations (complications of operations involving bowel are discussed here; the rest are discussed in Chs 18–51, as relevant)

and the **specific** complications of individual operations. Both groups of complications can be subdivided into **immediate** (during operation or within the next 24 hours), **early postoperative** (during the first postoperative week or so), **late postoperative** (up to 30 days after operation) and **long-term**.

The complications of surgery can be divided into five broad categories as shown in Box 12.1. This chapter covers categories 2, 3, 4 as well as the complications of abdominal surgery from category 5; 'medical' complications are discussed in Chapter 8. The complications associated with specific operations are discussed in Chapters 18–51, as appropriate.

COMPLICATIONS OF ANAESTHESIA

Complications as a result of anaesthesia are usually the responsibility of the anaesthetist, although the surgical team is involved in predicting problems. The exception is local anaesthesia, which is usually administered by the surgeon. Before general anaesthesia, a junior member of the surgical team or a specialist nurse usually makes the first preoperative assessment of the patient and by predicting potential complications, can help prevent them. The main complications of anaesthesia are summarised in Box 12.2.

GENERAL COMPLICATIONS OF OPERATIONS

The main complications that can affect the outcome of any operation are: inadvertent trauma to the patient in the operating department, haemorrhage, surgical damage to related structures, infection and problems with wound healing.

- Excess pressure on the calf causing deep venous thrombosis
- Excess heel pressure causing pressure sores
- Cardiac pacemaker disruption by diathermy equipment

INADVERTENT TRAUMA IN THE OPERATING DEPARTMENT

Patients are at risk of injury when being transported and transferred in the operating department, especially when under anaesthesia. In addition, staff involved in patient handling are at risk of injury, e.g. to the back. Special 'lifting and handling' training should be given all who handle patients in operating departments to minimise these risks.

The most common complications caused by trauma in the operating theatre are:

- Injuries resulting from falls from trolleys or from the operating table during positioning
- Injury to diseased bones and joints from manipulation or positioning. These include dislocation of a rheumatoid atlanto-axial joint and dislocation of a prosthetic hip joint
- Ulnar, lateral popliteal and other nerve palsies resulting from pressure
- Electrical burns from wet or poorly contacting diathermy pads or misuse of the diathermy probe

HAEMORRHAGE

PERIOPERATIVE HAEMORRHAGE

Haemorrhage occurring during an operation (**primary haemorrhage**) should be controlled by the surgeon before the operation is completed; the methods are described in Chapter 11.

EARLY POSTOPERATIVE HAEMORRHAGE

Haemorrhage during the immediate postoperative period usually indicates inadequate operative haemostasis or a technical mishap such as a slipped ligature or unrecognised trauma to a blood vessel. Occasionally it is due to a bleeding disorder.

If an operation involves major blood loss that requires large volume transfusion of stored blood, postoperative haemorrhage may be perpetuated by **consumption coagulopathy**, in which platelets and coagulation factors have been 'consumed' in a vain attempt at haemostasis. **Disseminated intravascular coagulopathy** (DIC) can be

Box 12.2 **Complications of anaesthesia**

Local anaesthesia

- Injection site—pain; haematoma; delayed recovery of sensation (direct nerve trauma); infection
- Vasoconstrictors—ischaemic necrosis (if used in digits or penis)
- Systemic effects of local anaesthetic agent
  —Toxicity due to excess dosage (see Ch. 11) or inadvertent intravenous injection. Same effect produced by premature release of a Bier's block cuff
  —Toxic effects include: dizziness, tinnitus, nausea and vomiting, fits, central nervous system (CNS) depression, bradycardia and asystole
  —Idiosyncratic or allergic reactions (very rare)

Spinal, epidural and caudal anaesthesia

- Failure of anaesthetic—anatomical difficulties or technical failure
- Headache after operation—loss of cerebrospinal fluid because of dural puncture
- Epidural or intrathecal bleeding—increased risk if patient on anticoagulants
- Unintentionally wide field of anaesthesia
  —In **epidural** anaesthesia, injection into wrong tissue plane may give a spinal anaesthetic
  —In **spinal** anaesthesia, respiratory paralysis occurs if the anaesthetic agent flows too far proximally
- Permanent nerve or spinal cord damage—injection of incorrect or contaminated drug
- Paraspinal infection—introduced by the injection
- Systemic complications—autonomic block may cause severe hypotension or postural hypotension

General anaesthesia

Postoperative nausea and vomiting

- Usually a response to anaesthetic or analgesic drugs. Individual sensitivity varies. Antiemetics usually administered before end of anaesthesia

Pain

- Analgesics usually administered during operation (e.g. intravenous opiates or paracetamol, diclofenac suppositories) plus local/regional anaesthetic techniques

Problems with drugs and fluids

- Fluid and electrolyte imbalance—too little, too much or inappropriate intravenous infusion
- Inappropriate choice of drugs or dosage in relation to age or the requirements of day surgery

- Idiosyncratic or allergic reactions to anaesthetic agents
  —Minor effects, e.g. nausea and vomiting
  —Major effects, e.g. cardiovascular collapse, respiratory depression, halothane jaundice
- Unexpected drug interactions—a wide range of adverse effects may occur
- Inherited disorders
  —Malignant hyperpyrexia (MH): any inhalational anaesthetic or suxamethonium may trigger MH
  —Pseudocholinesterase deficiency produces prolonged apnoea after succinylcholine
- Slow recovery from anaesthetic—many reasons including inadequate reversal
- 'Awareness' during anaesthetic—effective paralysis but ineffective anaesthesia (medico-legally very expensive!)

Cardiovascular complications

- Myocardial ischaemia/infarction/failure, arrhythmias, hypo/hypertension, tachy/bradycardias

Respiratory complications

- Laryngospasm/bronchospasm, atelectasis, upper or lower respiratory tract infections

Renal complications

- Particularly in patients with comorbid renal impairment—pre-renal, renal or post-renal

Hypothermia (Note: neonates and small infants are especially vulnerable to hypothermia)

- Long operations with extensive fluid loss
- Large-volume transfusion of cold blood

Inadvertent trauma

- Dental problems and prostheses
  —Teeth (particularly decayed or loose), crowns and bridges are vulnerable during intubation. Damage risks aspirating a foreign body into a bronchus and causes cosmetic and medico-legal problems
  —Infected material from carious (decayed) teeth or inflamed gums may be aspirated and cause a particularly grave aspiration pneumonia
  —Dentures must be removed before operation and labelled. Unconscious accident victims may aspirate or swallow a dental prosthesis or obstruct the pharynx with it
- Corneal abrasions
- Pressure injury to nerves (especially ulnar, radial and lateral popliteal)
- Diathermy pad burns
- Initiation of pressure sores

one facet of the systemic inflammatory response syndrome with widespread intravascular thrombosis and exhaustion of clotting factors. Occasionally bleeding results from the preoperative use of aspirin or aspirin-like drugs (responses vary greatly between patients), uncontrolled anticoagulant drugs or, less commonly, a pre-existing but unrecognised bleeding disorder. Any patient giving a history of excess bleeding should have a platelet count and a coagulation screen checked before operation.

Operations at particular risk of early postoperative haemorrhage include the following:

- Major operations involving highly vascular tissues such as the liver or spleen
- Major arterial surgery, especially ruptured aortic aneurysm (large volume blood loss may occur, and the patient may be heparinised during operation)
- Operations which leave a large raw surface such as abdomino-perineal resection of the rectum

This type of postoperative haemorrhage has been traditionally described as **reactionary haemorrhage** in the belief that it was a 'reaction' to the recovery of normal blood pressure and cardiac output. This concept is probably misleading and should now be discarded, especially since it may hinder the decision to reoperate as a matter of urgency.

Management of early postoperative haemorrhage

It should be remembered that early postoperative haemorrhage is really a form of primary haemorrhage and, if it is substantial, the patient must be surgically re-explored and the source of haemorrhage treated as at the original operation. It is wise to perform a clotting screen (including platelet count) and order an appropriate amount of bank blood as a preliminary measure. Good intravenous access should be ensured and a central venous pressure catheter inserted for monitoring. If heparin has been used at the original operation, **protamine** can be given to reverse any residual activity. If the clotting screen is abnormal, infusions containing clotting factors such as fresh-frozen plasma or platelet concentrates should be given. Many of these patients will stop bleeding with supportive measures and blood transfusion but re-exploration must be seriously considered at every stage.

LATER POSTOPERATIVE HAEMORRHAGE

Haemorrhage occurring several days after operation is usually related to infection which has eroded blood vessels close to the operation site; this is known as **secondary haemorrhage**. Treatment involves managing the infection, but exploratory operation is often required to ligate or suture the bleeding vessels.

SURGICAL INJURY

UNAVOIDABLE TISSUE DAMAGE

Anatomical structures, particularly nerves, blood vessels and lymphatics, may be **unavoidably damaged** during operation. This is particularly true in cancer surgery, illustrated by facial nerve excision during total parotidectomy. If anticipated, the probability must be discussed with the patient beforehand (ideally by the surgeon performing the operation) and may have to be accepted as part of the operative risk. Sometimes the integrity or location of vulnerable structures can be established before operation, thus allowing better planning of the operation. For example, intravenous urography (IVU) may be carried out to identify the course of the ureters in patients with colonic cancer, or indirect laryngoscopy may be done to assess vocal cord integrity prior to thyroid surgery.

INADVERTENT TISSUE DAMAGE

Structures may be **inadvertently damaged** during operation. Examples include recurrent laryngeal nerve damage during thyroidectomy, and trauma to the bile ducts during laparoscopic cholecystectomy. The main factors are inexperience, anatomical anomalies, attempts at arresting precipitate haemorrhage and the obscuring of tissue planes by inflammation or malignancy. Signs of damage to structures at risk during specific operations should be sought in the postoperative period; for example, hoarseness after thyroidectomy or jaundice after cholecystectomy.

INFECTION RELATED TO THE OPERATION SITE

MINOR WOUND INFECTIONS

The most common operative infection is a superficial wound infection occurring within the first postoperative week. This relatively trivial infection presents as localised pain, redness and a slight discharge. The organisms are usually staphylococci derived from the skin. The infection usually settles without treatment. The exception is the patient in whom a prosthesis such as an arterial graft or artificial joint has been inserted. For these patients, antibiotics must be given to prevent the devastating consequences of infection around the prosthesis.

WOUND CELLULITIS AND ABSCESS

More severe wound infections occur most commonly after bowel-related surgery, when staphylococci (both meticillin sensitive and resistant varieties) or faecal organisms are usually incriminated. The majority present in the first postoperative week but they may occur as late

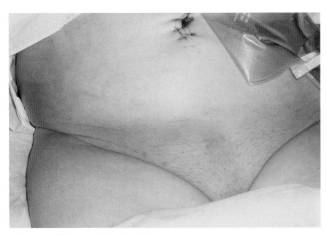

Fig. 12.1 Abdominal cellulitis
This woman of 73 presented with faecal peritonitis caused by a diverticular perforation of the sigmoid colon. She was resuscitated and underwent a laparotomy and sigmoid loop colostomy (note bag), without resection of the perforation. She remained toxic with a high fever and tachycardia, and developed spreading cellulitis in the left groin and flank. This proved to be due to continuing leakage from the perforation. Nowadays, a Hartmann's operation or resection and primary anastomosis is often performed so there is no longer a perforation leaking faecal matter into the peritoneal cavity.

as the third postoperative week, sometimes after the patient has left hospital. These infections commonly present first with a pyrexia; examination of the wound reveals either a spreading **cellulitis** or localised **abscess formation** (Fig. 12.1)

Cellulitis is treated with appropriate antibiotics after taking a wound swab for culture and sensitivity, whereas a wound abscess is treated by surgical drainage. This may simply involve suture removal and probing of the wound, but deeper abscesses are likely to require re-exploration under general anaesthesia. In either case, the wound is left open afterwards to heal by secondary intention (see Fig. 12.2).

Intra-abdominal infection is discussed under complications of abdominal and bowel surgery later in this chapter.

GAS GANGRENE

Gas gangrene is an uncommon, acute, life-threatening wound infection, in which the anaerobic organisms multiply in necrotic tissue, particularly muscle (see Ch. 3).

Fig. 12.2 Deep wound infection drained and allowed to heal by secondary intention

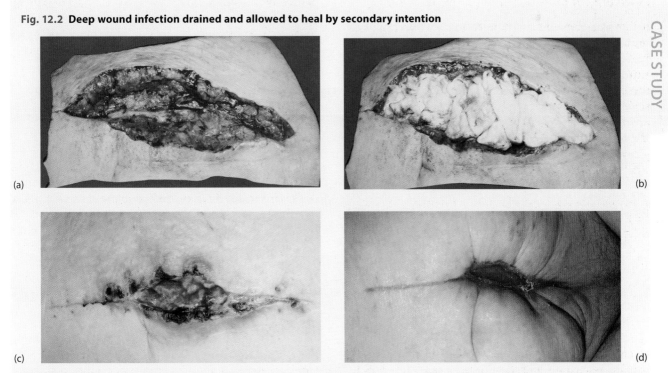

(a)

(b)

(c)

(d)

CASE STUDY

This 80-year-old diabetic woman underwent laparotomy and the wound became infected with *Staphylococcus aureus*. This resulted in a wound abscess and necrosis of the wound edge. **(a)** The wound after all necrotic tissue has been excised. **(b)** The wound packed with gauze and allowed to heal by secondary intention. **(c)** and **(d)** The wound at 3 weeks and 8 weeks. It was completely healed after 2 further weeks. Note the degree of wound contraction, which plays a major part in overcoming the tissue defect.

LATE INFECTIVE COMPLICATIONS

A late infective complication of surgery is a chronically discharging **wound sinus** which emanates from a deep chronic abscess. It usually relates to foreign material such as a non-absorbable suture or mesh or sometimes necrotic fascia or tendon. These sinuses commonly follow wound infections where healing is delayed and incomplete. Wound sinuses occasionally appear after apparent normal healing, particularly after insertion of a prosthesis.

Sinuses rarely heal spontaneously unless the foreign material is discharged, and the usual treatment is therefore re-exploration of the wound and removal of the offending substance. In groin sinuses following aorto-femoral bypass grafts, removal of the graft would impair the arterial supply of the lower limb unless the infected graft can be replaced or bypassed.

IMPAIRED HEALING

FACTORS RETARDING WOUND HEALING

The vast majority of wounds heal without complication. It is a popular misconception that wounds heal slowly in the elderly; this is not so unless there are specific adverse factors or complications. Wound healing in general is retarded if blood supply is poor (as in arterial insufficiency of the lower limb) or if the wound is under excess suture tension. Other retarding factors are infection, long-term corticosteroid therapy, immunosuppressive therapy, previous radiotherapy, severe rheumatoid disease, malnutrition and vitamin and mineral deficiency, especially of vitamin C and possibly zinc.

WOUND DEHISCENCE ('BURST ABDOMEN')

Wound dehiscence, i.e. total wound breakdown, is an uncommon problem. It affects about 1% of abdominal wounds and usually occurs about 1 week after operation, preceded by profuse discharge of sero-sanguinous fluid from the wound. The sudden bursting open of the abdomen revealing coils of bowel is alarming to nurses and junior doctors but is remarkably pain-free for the patient. Infection and other factors already described may play a part but the usual cause is inadequate abdominal wall repair, often in the presence of infection. This may be compounded by mechanical disruption caused by coughing or abdominal distension.

The wound should initially be covered with sterile swabs soaked in saline and the patient returned to the operating theatre within a few hours for repair. This usually involves placement of **tension sutures** which incorporate large 'bites' of the whole thickness of the abdominal wall (see Fig. 12.3).

Fig. 12.3 Burst abdomen and repair with tension sutures

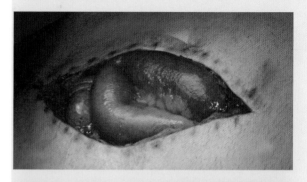

(a)

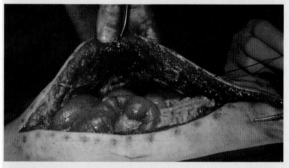

(b)

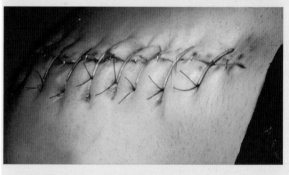

(c)

(a) Complete wound dehiscence 6 days after laparotomy for peritonitis. Note the exposed bowel spilling out of the wound. The patient had no particular risk factors so the cause was probably a poor technique of wound closure. **(b)** Operative photograph showing insertion of 'tension sutures' through the whole thickness of the abdominal wall. **(c)** The completed wound repair.

INCISIONAL HERNIA

Incisional hernia is a late complication of abdominal surgery. These hernias usually become apparent within the first postoperative year but sometimes develop as long as 15 years later; the overall incidence is about 10–15% of abdominal wounds. The hernia is caused by breakdown of the repair to the abdominal wall muscle and fascia. Predisposing factors are abdominal obesity, distension and poor muscle quality, poor choice of inci-

Fig. 12.4 Incisional hernia

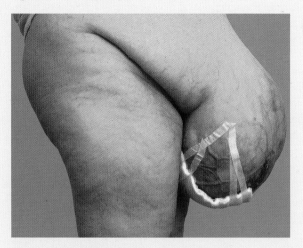

This 55-year-old woman presented with a massive incisional hernia through an old umbilical hernia repair scar. Her only complaint was of skin breakdown at its lowermost extent. Repair presented a huge challenge but was achieved using mesh.

sion, inadequate closure technique, postoperative wound infection and multiple operations through the same incision.

An incisional hernia usually presents as a bulge in the abdominal wall near a previous wound. The condition is usually asymptomatic but occasionally a narrow-necked hernia presents with pain or strangulation. Once an incisional hernia has appeared, it tends to enlarge progressively and may become a nuisance cosmetically or for dressing (see Fig. 12.4). Repair is indicated for strangulation, pain or inconvenience and usually involves placement of a synthetic mesh, either at open operation or laparoscopically.

COMPLICATIONS OF ANY SURGICAL CONDITION

RESPIRATORY COMPLICATIONS

Up to 15% of patients suffer from respiratory complications associated with general anaesthesia and major operations. The most common of these are **atelectasis and pneumonia**. Pre-existing lung disease greatly increases the risk of complications. Severely ill patients, including those with acute pancreatitis, and burns or trauma victims, are susceptible to the development of **acute respiratory distress syndrome**.

EFFECTS OF ANAESTHESIA AND SURGERY ON RESPIRATORY FUNCTION

Anaesthesia and surgery predispose to postoperative complications by altering lung function and compromising normal defence mechanisms as follows:

- **Lung tidal volume**—may be reduced by as much as 50%, depending on the incision site. Thoracic, upper abdominal and lower abdominal incisions (in decreasing order of effect) reduce lung volume
- **Lung expansion**—reduced by the **supine posture** during and after operation, pain, abdominal distension, abdominal constriction by bandages and the effects of sedative drugs
- **Ventilation rate**—usually increases and there is loss of normal periodic hyperinflation
- **Diminished ventilation and pulmonary perfusion**—result in reduced gaseous exchange

- **Airway defences**—compromised by loss of the cough reflex and diminished ciliary activity, which both lead to accumulation of secretions
- **Problems associated with laparoscopic abdominal surgery**—the pneumoperitoneum and head-down position lead to diaphragmatic splinting, a reduction in functional residual capacity and changes in intrathoracic blood volume. These lead to atelectasis, pulmonary shunting and hypoxaemia. Raised ventilatory airways pressure may lead to pulmonary barotrauma

ATELECTASIS

Pathophysiology and clinical features

Atelectasis or alveolar collapse occurs when airways become obstructed and air is absorbed from the air spaces distal to the obstruction. Bronchial secretions are the main cause of this obstruction. Predisposing factors include shallow ventilation, loss of periodic hyperinflation, inhibition of coughing and pooling of mucus. All of these are particular problems after thoracic and upper abdominal surgery. The resulting **ventilation/perfusion mismatch** produces a degree of right-to-left shunting of blood, and tends to cause a fall in PaO_2. If the obstructed airways are small, there is only minor segmental collapse, in which case localising signs are minimal and X-ray appearance is unremarkable. Despite this, the overall extent of collapse may be large and cause significant hypoxaemia.

Obstruction of a major airway causes collapse and consolidation of a whole lobe, resulting in the typical clinical signs of dullness to percussion and reduced breath sounds or **bronchial breathing**. Chest X-ray will show the lobe to be contracted and opacified with mediastinal shift and compensatory expansion of other lobes.

Most cases of atelectasis are relatively mild and pass undiagnosed, although the patient may be slow to recover from operation. The patient may be cyanosed, resulting from mild hypoxaemia, and have a mild tachypnoea, tachycardia and low-grade pyrexia, which all resolve spontaneously within a few days. Sputum culture (if any is produced) is usually negative but infection may complicate severe cases.

Prevention and treatment of atelectasis

Atelectasis is best prevented in patients undergoing major surgery by preoperative and postoperative physiotherapy. This includes deep breathing exercises, regular adjustments of posture and vigorous coughing. During physiotherapy, wounds should be supported by the patient's hand. Effective analgesia, e.g. infiltration of the wound with local anaesthetic or epidural analgesia, facilitates physiotherapy and mobility. Nebulised bronchodilators such as salbutamol may assist the patient to cough up secretions. Severe cases of diffuse atelectasis may require endotracheal intubation and positive-pressure ventilation. Lobar or whole lung collapse requires intensive physiotherapy and sometimes **flexible bronchoscopy** to aspirate occluding mucus plugs.

PNEUMONIAS

Bronchopneumonia is the usual form of chest infection seen in surgical patients. It occurs secondarily to chronic lung disease, chronic smoking or following atelectasis or aspiration of gastric contents. *Haemophilus* and *Streptococcus pyogenes* are the common infecting organisms but coliforms may be responsible in elderly, debilitated or seriously ill patients. *Pseudomonas* bronchopneumonia occurs in patients on ventilators or with bronchiectasis.

Infection is manifest by pyrexia, tachypnoea, tachycardia and a raised leucocyte count. The mucopurulent sputum is thick, copious and green. Antibiotics, usually amoxicillin or co-trimoxazole, are given on a 'best-guess' basis until sputum culture and sensitivities are available. Physiotherapy and encouragement to cough are equally important for recovery.

ASPIRATION PNEUMONITIS

Aspiration pneumonitis (Mendelson's syndrome) is a sterile, chemical inflammation of the lungs resulting from inhalation of acidic gastric contents. There is often a clear history of vomiting or regurgitation, followed by a rapid onset of breathlessness and wheezing. This may later become complicated by infection, i.e. bronchopneumonia, with its typical symptoms and signs. Chest X-ray shows characteristic 'fluffy' opacities, particularly in the lower lobes, which are most affected for anatomical and postural reasons.

Aspiration occurs when protective laryngeal reflexes are suppressed or when there is intestinal obstruction and regurgitation. Laryngeal suppression may be due to impairment of consciousness (e.g. during recovery from general anaesthesia or in alcoholic intoxication) or loss of consciousness after head injury.

Emergency anaesthesia in the non-starved patient poses special risks. Whenever possible, anaesthesia should be postponed for 4–6 hours after the last food or drink. In accident victims, it is important to note the time of last eating with respect to the time of the accident, and to remember that stress and anxiety may greatly delay gastric emptying. In pregnancy, gastric emptying is also much slower.

A patient with **intestinal obstruction** is at particular risk of inhalation of gastric contents. If possible, the stomach should be emptied by nasogastric tube. If general anaesthesia must be performed on the non-starved or otherwise at-risk patient, a **rapid sequence induction** technique is employed: as the patient loses consciousness, an assistant applies **cricoid pressure** to flatten the oesophagus against the cervical spine, preventing reflux of gastric contents. The airway is then secured with a cuffed endotracheal tube before the cricoid pressure is released. Oral antacids may be given beforehand to neutralise gastric acidity. Metoclopramide, given by injection, may also be used to hasten gastric emptying.

The mortality from aspiration pneumonitis approaches 50% and urgent treatment must be started should it occur. This involves thorough bronchial suction via an endotracheal tube (or bronchoscope if necessary), followed by positive-pressure ventilation and prophylactic antibiotics. Intravenous steroids are usually given to try to limit the inflammatory process, but their efficacy is unproven.

ASPIRATION PNEUMONIA

Aspiration pneumonia may complicate aspiration pneumonitis, but more often it develops insidiously, following chronic aspiration of infected food and oropharyngeal secretions. In the surgical context, debilitated, confused or elderly patients are the usual victims, but aspiration pneumonia is also seen in alcoholics, drug addicts and stroke patients. Achalasia of the oesophageal cardia and large hiatus hernias can lead to chronic aspiration, particularly occurring at night. The clinical features are of infection and lobar consolidation (usually of the lower lobe) progressing to **lung abscess** formation. The organisms are usually mixed oral anaerobes sensitive to penicillin, but prognosis depends more on the patient's general condition and is usually poor.

ACUTE RESPIRATORY DISTRESS SYNDROME

This syndrome of acute respiratory failure, formerly known as adult respiratory distress syndrome, is characterised by rapid, shallow breathing, severe hypoxaemia, stiff lungs and diffuse pulmonary opacification on X-ray. It can develop in response to a variety of systemic and direct insults to the pulmonary alveoli and microvasculature.

Acute respiratory failure has long been known to occur in many disparate conditions and has been given several different names such as shock lung, wet lung, post-traumatic respiratory insufficiency, Da Nang lung (Vietnam war) and white lung (after the typical X-ray appearance). In 1976, it was finally realised that the underlying pathological phenomena were similar, and were directly related to the well-recognised respiratory distress syndrome of newborn babies. The main conditions with which acute respiratory distress syndrome (ARDS) is associated are summarised in Box 12.3.

Pathophysiology of ARDS

The causative insults to the lung all have the effect of increasing the permeability of pulmonary capillaries leading to leakage of protein-rich fluid into the alveolar interstitium. This causes interstitial oedema which in turn **reduces lung compliance** and causes 'stiff lungs' and reduced alveolar ventilation.

Box 12.3 **Conditions associated with acute respiratory distress syndrome (ARDS)**

Direct insults to the lung

- Lung contusion
- Near-drowning
- Aspiration of gastric acid
- Inhalation of smoke and corrosive chemicals, e.g. chlorine, phosgene, nitrogen dioxide or ammonia
- Radiation pneumonitis

Systemic insults to the lung

- Multiple trauma with shock
- Systemic sepsis, e.g. after a colonic anastomotic leak
- Severe acute pancreatitis
- Major head injuries ('neurogenic pulmonary oedema')
- Fat, air and amniotic fluid embolism
- Major blood transfusion reaction or massive blood transfusion
- Disseminated intravascular coagulation
- Cardiopulmonary bypass
- Eclampsia
- Severe allergic reactions
- Drug overdose or sensitivity, e.g. heroin, barbiturates, paraquat, bleomycin

---

The alveolar lining cells (**type I pneumocytes**) are also damaged. This damage, combined with increased interstitial hydrostatic pressure, causes leakage of fluid into the alveolar spaces until they are filled. The result is disruption of the lung ventilation to perfusion ratio ($\dot{V}/\dot{Q}$ ratio), causing effective **right-to-left shunting** of blood. The intra-alveolar fluid later condenses to form a **hyaline membrane** which lines the alveoli. This is histologically similar to the neonatal form of the disease.

The full clinical syndrome often takes 24–48 hours to develop after the initial insult. If the patient eventually recovers, the interstitial damage may result in diffuse **interstitial fibrosis**. It is important to note that cardiac failure plays no part in the development of ARDS, although cardiac failure may later complicate the condition.

Clinical features of ARDS

The main clinical finding is rapid shallow respiration with only scattered crepitations heard on auscultation. There is usually no cough, chest pain or haemoptysis. Blood gas analysis reveals low PaO_2 but the $PaCO_2$ remains normal except in the most severe cases. Chest X-ray may be normal in the early stages, progressing rapidly through increased interstitial markings to complete or partial 'white-out' (see Fig. 12.5). ARDS may be difficult to distinguish from cardiac failure except that cardiac diameter is normal in ARDS, and cardiac failure usually responds to diuretic therapy.

Treatment of ARDS

The overall objective is to maintain respiratory function and cardiovascular stability while the underlying cause (e.g. sepsis) is brought under control. This should be carried out under intensive care conditions. The sooner the treatment is begun, the greater the chance of recovery.

Most patients require mechanical **ventilation** with **positive end-expiratory pressure (PEEP)** to achieve adequate oxygenation and to try to reverse alveolar oedema and collapse. Fluid balance is complex in these patients and requires monitoring of **right atrial pressure** using a central venous line. Cardiac output can be measured using trans-oesophageal ultrasound. One of the treatment aims is to produce a negative fluid balance and thus help minimise accumulation of fluid in the lung and interstitial tissue. Loop diuretic infusions or continuous veno-venous haemofiltration can be used to achieve this. Any associated renal failure can also be treated by this form of haemofiltration. In these patients, diuretics alone do not control pulmonary oedema but instead aggravate the hypovolaemia and shock associated with the underlying cause.

Renal failure is a common complication, sometimes prevented by early use of drugs such as dopamine. The

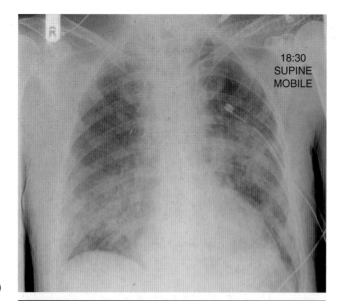

(a)

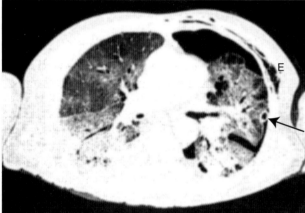

(b)

Fig. 12.5 Acute respiratory distress syndrome (ARDS)
(a) This middle-aged man underwent an oesophagectomy for carcinoma, with the proximal stomach anastomosed to the oesophageal remnant in the chest. He developed ARDS in the early postoperative period. The chest X-ray shows ill-defined alveolar opacification in the lung mid zones. Note the metallic vascular clips on the right side, the chest drain on the left side and the endotracheal tube and central venous line. **(b)** The CT scan shows bilateral consolidation in the dependent portion of both lungs with 'ground glass' opacification in the upper zones. There is a left pneumothorax with a chest drain in situ (arrowed); subcutaneous emphysema **E** resulting from the thoracotomy is also visible.

mortality rate for complicated cases of ARDS approaches 90%.

VENOUS THROMBOEMBOLISM (VTE)

PATHOPHYSIOLOGY

Venous thromboembolism is a major cause of complication and death after surgery or trauma and much of it is preventable. Venous blood is normally prevented from

- Previous venous thromboembolism
- Trauma and surgery (complex systemic effects)
- Increasing age
- Direct trauma to the pelvis and lower limbs, especially fractures
- Pre-existing lower limb venous disorders causing stasis
- Venous stasis during general or regional anaesthesia (loss of calf muscle pump and postural pressure on the calves)
- Malignant disease
- Immobility, e.g. bed-bound patients after operation or stroke
- Cardiac failure
- High-oestrogen oral contraceptive pill, oestrogen treatment, hormone replacement therapy
- Pregnancy
- Pelvic masses causing venous obstruction
- Groin masses obstructing femoral vein, e.g. femoral aneurysm, malignant lymph nodes
- Obesity
- Dehydration
- Blood disorders, e.g. polycythaemia, thrombocythaemia and pro-thrombotic disorders

clotting within the veins by a complex series of mechanisms which include local inhibition of the clotting cascade, prompt lysis of small clots that do form, and the flushing effect of a continuous flow of blood. In 1856, **Virchow** proposed in his 'triad' that venous thrombosis could be caused by abnormalities in the vein wall (trauma, inflammation); alterations in blood flow (stasis); and changes in the blood (hypercoagulability), and this explanation largely holds good today. The subtle balance within the veins can be disturbed by several local and systemic factors, many incompletely understood. Imbalance results in thrombus formation within the venous sinuses of the calf muscles and sometimes primarily in the pelvic veins. About 90% of deep vein thromboses (DVTs) start in the calf, and about a quarter propagate proximally to involve the femoral and pelvic veins, usually within a week of presentation. Calf vein thrombosis alone is rarely symptomatic yet it predisposes strongly to thrombosis propagating proximally. It has been shown that 80% of symptomatic DVTs involve proximal veins. Calf vein thrombi themselves rarely cause significant embolism but thrombi in the larger more proximal vessels are likely to become detached and migrate proximally to impact in the pulmonary arteries as pulmonary emboli.

The main **predisposing factors** to venous thromboembolism are summarised in Box 12.4, but thromboembolism can also occur in healthy individuals with no apparent predisposing factors. A proportion of these will

Age	Grade of surgery	Other risk factors	Risk of DVT (%)
20	Minor		1
40	Minor		3
60	Minor		10
60	Major		20
60	Major	Previous DVT	50
80	Major		40
80	Major	Previous DVT + infection or malignancy	96

Table 12.1 Factors affecting the risk of deep vein thrombosis after operation

have one or more **pro-thrombotic disorders** and investigation for these should be considered some time after the acute event. It should be remembered that patients may have been ill and dehydrated at home for some time before hospital admission and venous thrombosis may have been initiated before admission.

The risk of thromboembolism increases incrementally as the number and severity of local and systemic risk factors increase; this is neatly illustrated in Table 12.1. The impact of many of the predisposing factors can be minimised by **prophylactic measures against venous thromboembolism** in *all* hospitalised patients (see p. 184 below).

DEEP VEIN THROMBOSIS

Deep vein thrombosis (DVT) in the lower limbs is often silent, with the classic clinical features found in only a quarter of cases. These include swelling of the leg, tenderness of the calf muscles, increased warmth of the leg, and calf pain on passive dorsiflexion of the foot (**Homans' sign**). The presence of these features indicates that venous occlusion has extended at least as far as the popliteal veins.

Occlusion of the ilio-femoral veins tends to produce diffuse and sometimes massive swelling of the whole lower limb (see Fig. 12.6a). In addition, there is tenderness over the femoral vein in the groin. In severe cases (which are rare nowadays), the limb becomes painful and white, and boggy with oedema; this is known as **phlegmasia alba dolens** (painful white leg). In extreme cases, the limb becomes more painful and blue, with incipient venous infarction (**phlegmasia caerulea dolens**).

Asymptomatic DVTs have the same potential for causing both pulmonary embolism and long-term chronic venous insufficiency as symptomatic venous thromboses, thus emphasising the importance of prophylaxis for all patients at increased risk (see *Prevention of venous thromboembolism*, below). To complicate the problem, as many

as half of the patients who develop swelling and pain in the calf after operation do not have deep vein thrombosis.

Diagnostic tests for DVT

Colour duplex ultrasound is now the standard technique for investigation of cases where deep venous thrombosis is suspected. In surgical patients, scanning is likely to be the primary investigation as blood tests for D-dimers can be misleading after surgery (see *Diagnosis of pulmonary embolism* below). Colour duplex allows scanning of all the major lower limb deep veins for blood flow and contained thrombus, and can reliably exclude the diagnosis when the scan is normal. Previously, venography (phlebography) was the standard diagnostic technique. This involved cannulating a small vein in the foot and injecting contrast material. Duplex ultrasound is undoubtedly safer than venography and has a higher diagnostic reliability but both techniques are highly operator-dependent as regards making an accurate diagnosis. A typical venogram showing obstructed deep venous architecture is shown in Figure 12.7.

PULMONARY EMBOLISM

The classic picture of pulmonary embolism (PE) is sudden dyspnoea and cardiovascular collapse, followed by pleuritic chest pain, development of a pleural rub and haemoptysis. In hospital, this is often heralded by a collapse whilst seated on the toilet. Ten percent of PEs are estimated to be fatal within the first hour. The electrocardiogram (ECG) may show evidence of right heart strain (S wave in lead I, Q wave and inverted T wave in leads III—'S1, Q3, T3'). This clinical presentation, however, is uncommon and occurs only when 50% or more of the pulmonary arterial system is occluded. More extensive occlusion usually results in sudden death.

Smaller pulmonary emboli are more common and are often 'silent', presenting as non-specific episodes of general deterioration, confusion, breathlessness or chest

Fig. 12.6 Clinically obvious deep vein thrombosis

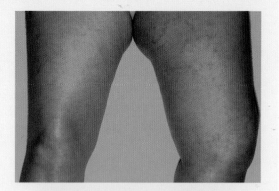

(a)

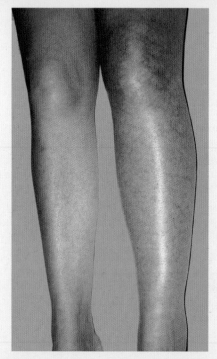

(b)

This woman of 45 underwent radical surgery for ovarian cancer. She suffered swelling and bursting pain in the whole of her left leg 5 days after operation. The left thigh **(a)** and leg **(b)** are both visibly swollen and blueish. On palpation, the limb felt warm. A massive ilio-femoral venous thrombosis was diagnosed on venography and the patient was anticoagulated. Luckily she did not suffer a pulmonary embolism and the limb returned to a normal diameter over 6 months. She will be at lifetime risk of post-thrombotic deep venous insufficiency.

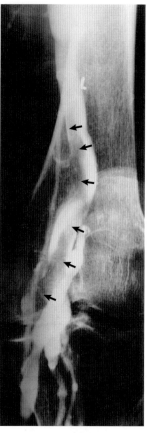

Fig. 12.7 Contrast venogram (phlebogram) of deep vein thrombosis
Venogram showing the popliteal veins in a patient who complained of calf pain 5 days after a laparotomy for obstructive jaundice. There is extensive thrombus in the deep veins (arrowed) which is only loosely attached to the vein wall and therefore in danger of embolisation to the lung. *Note:* this investigation has been largely superseded by colour duplex ultrasound scanning

pain. Note that the patient suffering small embolic events is heavily predisposed to a subsequent massive or fatal embolus; it is essential to recognise the condition and to treat it seriously. The patient often has a tachycardia and low-grade fever but there are no diagnostic changes on ECG. The condition may be attributed to chest infection, atelectasis or cardiac failure unless a diagnosis of pulmo-nary embolism is considered. There may be more specific diagnostic symptoms of small pulmonary emboli, includ-ing localised **pleuritic chest pain** and small **haemoptyses** in the form of blood-streaked sputum.

Venous thromboembolism is most common from about the fourth to the seventh postoperative day after major surgery but may present at any time during the postoperative month, sometimes after the patient has left hospital.

Diagnosis of pulmonary embolism (PE)

In suspected pulmonary embolism, chest X-ray and ECG are non-specific and of little value. The choice of investi-gation depends on the level of clinical probability. Several clinical scoring schemes can be used to consign patients to categories with low (~10%), intermediate (~25%) or high (~80%) risk of pulmonary embolism. These catego-ries are based on the sum of points allocated to **predis-posing factors** (past history of venous thromboembolism,

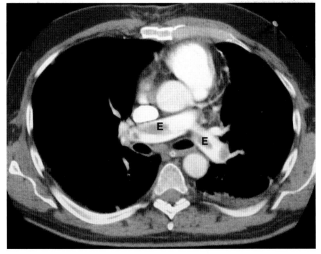

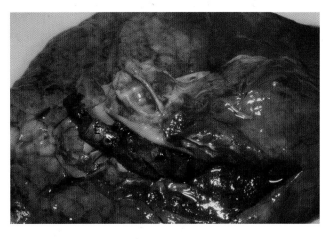

(a)

(b)

Fig. 12.8 Pulmonary embolism
(a) Thoracic CT pulmonary artery scan (CTPA) with intravenous contrast showing large emboli **E** in the pulmonary arteries. This is the investigation of choice where there is a high suspicion of PE. **(b)** Post-mortem specimen of lung from a patient who died of massive pulmonary embolism. Embolic material has been removed, but some remains in the pulmonary arteries **E**.

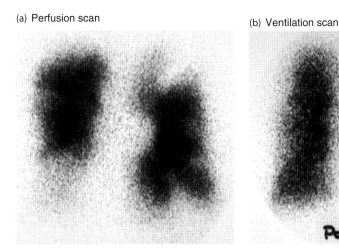

(a) Perfusion scan

(b) Ventilation scan

Fig. 12.9 Ventilation/perfusion (V̇/Q̇) scan in pulmonary embolism (posterior view)
This involves two separate radioisotope imaging procedures to demonstrate **ventilation/perfusion mismatch**. The patient inhales radioactive gas, and a gamma camera detects the distribution of radioactivity in the lung air spaces. An intravenous injection of radionuclide-labelled albumen microspheres is given before the **perfusion scan**. These lodge throughout the pulmonary artery bed except where occluded by thrombus. In pulmonary embolism, the ventilation scan is normal but areas of pulmonary under-perfusion (embolism) show as defects in the perfusion scan. In areas of infection or atelectasis (which are under-ventilated), the ventilation scan is deficient but the perfusion scan is normal. **(a)** Perfusion scan showing multiple filling defects typical of pulmonary embolism. **(b)** Ventilation scan from the same patient, which is normal. Impaired perfusion with normal ventilation is typical of pulmonary embolism.

immobility, malignancy) and the **presence of signs** of DVT, tachycardia or an alternative diagnosis. In the investigation of low probability cases, a diagnosis of PE can be excluded by negative results from tests with a high **negative predictive value**; in high probability cases, the test needs to have a high **positive predictive value**.

Blood tests for D-dimers have a high negative predictive value for pulmonary embolism (although levels are elevated after operation and therefore misleading). D-dimers are formed when cross-linked fibrin is lysed by

plasmin. When added to clinical suspicion, the result can be used to guide investigation; a low probability indicates that major investigations are unnecessary. In high probability cases, the quickest and most reliable method of confirming the diagnosis is by dynamic spiral or multi-slice computed tomographic pulmonary angiography (CTPA) using intravenous contrast (Fig. 12.8a). Where available, this has largely superseded radioisotope **ventilation/perfusion scanning** (V̇/Q̇ scanning), shown in Figure 12.9, and direct **pulmonary angiography**.

MANAGEMENT OF VENOUS THROMBOEMBOLISM

For most patients, removing or lysing lower limb thrombus or pulmonary embolus is impractical. The main objective, therefore, in managing deep vein thrombosis and pulmonary embolism is to halt the coagulation process by systemic anticoagulation, with the aim of preventing established thrombi from propagating and new thrombi from forming. Removal of thrombus is generally left to the normal body processes of lysis.

In the lower limbs, venous thrombi eventually become organised and firmly attached to the vessel wall, posing no further risk of embolisation. The thrombus is later invaded by granulation tissue and the veins eventually become recanalised, thus restoring venous flow. In the process, the valves are often destroyed, leading in the long term to **chronic venous insufficiency** (see Ch. 43), often many years later. After pulmonary embolism, if the patient survives the initial embolic episode, the emboli are efficiently removed by local thrombolysis, leaving little functional deficit.

Initially, anticoagulation is achieved with **intravenous heparin**. Local protocols vary but a typical one is to commence with a bolus dose of 5000 units (10 000 units in severe pulmonary embolism), followed by a continuous infusion of 15–25 units/hour/kg (24 000–48 000 units over each 24-hour period), with the dose adjusted to maintain the patient's **partial thromboplastin time** at 2–3 times normal. Heparin anticoagulation takes effect immediately and is continued for about 5 days, by which time acute symptoms have usually subsided. Often nowadays, full anticoagulation for DVT is effected and/or maintained using 12-hourly subcutaneous doses of unfractionated or low molecular weight heparin alone. After the initial dose (e.g. 15 000 units of unfractionated heparin), frequent laboratory monitoring is essential to ensure safe dosage. The subcutaneous route has the advantage that it can be employed on an ambulatory basis. In the mean time, oral **warfarin therapy** (which takes several days to become fully effective) is begun. Warfarin therapy is continued for 3–6 months, the period of highest risk of recurrent thromboembolism. Untreated, about 50% of patients with proximal DVT or PE will have a further thromboembolic event within 3 months. Patients who suffer repeated thromboembolic episodes when off anticoagulation may have to be maintained on warfarin for life. For these patients, in addition, a **filter** (e.g. a Greenfield filter) may be placed in the inferior vena cava via a percutaneous route to trap emboli migrating from leg and pelvic veins towards the pulmonary arteries.

In the rare case of sub-massive non-fatal pulmonary embolism with evidence of right ventricular dysfunction, surgical **embolectomy** may be appropriate. This is performed under cardiopulmonary bypass and is therefore no small undertaking. An alternative is **systemic thrombolytic therapy**, but this has an unacceptably high rate of serious bleeding and has largely been abandoned. However, the technique of manipulating a pulmonary artery catheter into the embolus and instilling high doses of **local thrombolytic drugs** or performing **clot suction** has occasionally been successfully employed.

PREVENTION OF VENOUS THROMBOEMBOLISM

The importance of **general measures** in preventing venous thrombosis needs to be emphasised. These include **early postoperative mobilisation**, **adequate hydration** and **avoiding pressure on the calves**. In addition, patients on oestrogen-containing oral contraceptives should ideally stop taking them (using replacement contraceptive methods) at least 6 weeks before major operations, as should patients on hormone replacement therapy (HRT). If these preparations are not to be stopped, consideration should be given to employing heparin prophylaxis for any operation.

For these and for patients at higher risk, as shown in Box 12.4 earlier, specific prophylactic measures should be taken to reduce the risk of deep venous thrombosis (and consequent pulmonary embolism). Prophylactic measures include the following:

- **Low-dose subcutaneous heparin**—this may be given as standard **unfractionated heparin** or as **low molecular weight heparin**. Both types are as effective for preventing deep venous thrombosis and pulmonary embolism but the chief advantage of low molecular weight heparin is that it is given only once a day instead of two or three times. Low-dose heparin is the most effective method of reducing venous thromboembolism in at-risk patients. It has been shown to reduce the rate of postoperative DVT by 70% in general surgical, urological, gynaecological, orthopaedic and trauma patients. Similar reductions are achieved in the rate of pulmonary embolism. The intravascular antithrombotic effect is not due to anticoagulation, but results from stimulation of platelet factor **antithrombin III**; there should be no detectable in vitro anticoagulant effect or any clinically significant effect on haemostasis during or after operation, although it is estimated that patients on low-dose heparin bleed about 10% more at major surgery
- **Calf compression devices**—several pneumatic and electrical devices are available for intraoperative calf compression to simulate normal muscle pump activity. These have the advantage of being non-invasive and easily applied to all patients, even those at low risk, but their effectiveness is less than low-dose heparin
- **Graduated compression 'anti-embolism' stockings**—the use of these stockings is simple and

widely practised. Provided they are correctly fitted, graduated compression stockings offer a suitable level of prophylaxis for patients at low or moderate risk. The stockings must be worn during operation as well as during the early postoperative period
- **Warfarin anticoagulation**—this is one of the best methods of prophylaxis for elective operations, and is widely used for major elective surgery in the Netherlands. It is considered impractical by many surgeons, not least because of the supposed risk of incidental and operative haemorrhage. In addition, the logistics of establishing preoperative anticoagulation and continuing dose monitoring afterwards require a great deal of resources

FLUID AND ELECTROLYTE DISTURBANCES

Fluid and electrolyte disturbances such as **dehydration** or **fluid overload**, **hyponatraemia**, **hypokalaemia** and **hyperkalaemia** frequently develop in the postoperative period. Fluid and electrolyte abnormalities are particularly common after major surgery of the bowel, especially if there have been massive fluid losses through vomiting, diarrhoea or sequestration in obstructed or adynamic bowel, or surgical complications. These problems are discussed in Chapter 2.

TRANSFUSION COMPLICATIONS

The management of blood transfusion and its complications is described in detail in Chapter 9.

URINARY RETENTION

Acute retention of urine is common in the early postoperative period. The usual problem is that the patient has been unable to pass urine following operation. The anuria is often drawn to the doctor's attention by a nurse several hours after operation but before the patient becomes distressed. **Acute retention** needs to be distinguished from true oliguria resulting from poor renal perfusion or acute renal failure; if this cannot be resolved clinically, ultrasonography will show whether the bladder is full of urine and the patient therefore in retention.

PATHOPHYSIOLOGY

Postoperative retention is much more common in men, particularly when there is a degree of prostatic hypertrophy. Patients with symptoms of bladder outflow obstruction ('prostatism') are at high risk of developing acute retention, although young male patients can also be affected.

Acute postoperative urinary retention seems to result from a combination of the following factors:

- Pre-existing bladder outlet obstruction
- Difficulty in passing urine in the supine position
- Embarrassment at passing urine without sufficient privacy
- Accumulation of a large volume of urine during the operation and recovery from anaesthesia, causing overfilling of the bladder
- Transient disturbance of the neurological control of voiding by general or spinal anaesthesia
- Pain from an abdominal or inguinal wound inhibiting normal contraction of the abdominal musculature and relaxation of the bladder neck
- Problems after certain operations which predispose to acute retention, e.g. abdomino-perineal resection of rectum or bilateral inguinal hernia repair
- Constipation—gross faecal loading is common in the elderly in hospital and is probably the most frequent cause of acute retention (and faecal incontinence)

MANAGEMENT OF POSTOPERATIVE URINARY RETENTION

Conservative measures

Most cases of postoperative acute retention can be managed conservatively, bearing in mind the precipitating factors mentioned above. If the problem is dealt with early, the patient is less likely to require catheterisation and this should be avoided if possible. However, if there is a history of symptoms of bladder outlet obstruction or previous prostatectomy, catheterisation is more likely to be needed. The first step is to ensure there is adequate **postoperative analgesia** and this may be all that is needed to enable the patient to pass urine. The next step is to help the patient out of bed in order to use a commode at the bedside or use a urine bottle standing at the bedside.

The patient will often need continuous support to stand if still unsteady from the anaesthetic or analgesia. For young male patients, a male assistant should be at hand if possible, as the presence of a young female can have a marked inhibitory effect!

If these measures fail, the patient should be wheeled into a bathroom for privacy and left alone for a while, if he (or she) is fit enough. The familiar sound of a tap left running often encourages micturition. If the patient still does not pass urine, it may be appropriate to encourage a bowel movement by means of a lubricant glycerine suppository. Defaecation is usually accompanied by bladder neck relaxation and micturition, so this may help.

Catheterisation

If conservative measures fail, catheterisation will usually be necessary. In females, bladder drainage and immediate removal of the catheter is often all that is required. In males, the catheter is usually left in situ until the following morning or until the patient is well. In patients with prostatic obstruction, a suprapubic catheter is a better option as it avoids urethral trauma and can easily be temporarily clamped to check if normal micturition has returned. Recurrent problems of retention are usually caused by bladder outlet obstruction and are managed as described in Chapter 35.

URINARY TRACT INFECTIONS

Urinary tract infections are common in the postoperative period, especially in women. The most obvious predisposing factor is urinary catheterisation. However, infections often occur without urethral instrumentation, in which case the cause is probably a combination of reduced urinary output which impairs 'flushing' of the bladder, incomplete bladder emptying in the supine posture, bacteraemia induced by operation or infection, and perhaps inadequate perineal hygiene.

Typical symptoms of dysuria and frequency may be absent or minimal and the diagnosis of urinary tract infection is often made on investigation of an unexplained pyrexia or septic episode. Treatment is by ensuring adequate fluid input and prescription of appropriate antibiotics such as trimethoprim.

ANTIBIOTIC-ASSOCIATED COLITIS

PATHOPHYSIOLOGY AND CLINICAL FEATURES

Colonic inflammation and other diarrhoeal disorders may be side effects of almost any antibiotic treatment. The conditions are largely due to selective overgrowth of intestinal organisms which then produce toxins that cause the damage. The clinical picture ranges from a mild attack of diarrhoea to profuse, life-threatening, haemorrhagic colitis.

Antibiotic-associated colitis may develop suddenly or gradually and occasionally becomes chronic or relapsing. Surgical patients are most likely to be affected in the postoperative period. *Clostridium difficile* is responsible for many of these cases, and in severe form the full picture of **pseudomembranous colitis** may develop. This can take a particularly virulent form. **Staphylococcal enterocolitis** is less common.

If a surgical patient on antibiotics develops diarrhoea and this is worse or more prolonged than might be expected after an operation, antibiotic-associated colitis should be suspected. Stool specimens should be examined by microscopy and culture and by measuring levels of *Clostridium difficile* toxin. Sigmoidoscopic inspection and biopsy of the rectum should also be performed. Treatment is based on the results of these tests. If *Clostridium difficile* infection is diagnosed, it is treated with oral met-ronidazole or, in resistant cases, with oral (non-absorbed) vancomycin.

ACUTE RENAL FAILURE

Acute renal failure is defined clinically as the abrupt onset of oliguria or anuria, associated with a steep rise in blood urea concentration. This is caused by failure to excrete nitrogenous waste products. The usual cause is **acute tubular necrosis**, but acute renal failure is sometimes caused by nephrotoxins. These include the **aminoglycoside antibiotics** gentamicin and tobramycin, myoglobin (released in the crush syndrome) and the 'hepatorenal syndrome' associated with obstructive jaundice (see Ch. 18). Acute renal failure is also a particular complication of surgery of the abdominal aorta, in which the renal arteries may become occluded by inadvertent damage or unrecognised embolism.

PATHOPHYSIOLOGY

The renal tubules are acutely sensitive to a variety of metabolic insults, particularly hypoxia and certain toxins. Hypoxia readily occurs if renal perfusion falls substantially; the usual surgical cause is an episode of severe or prolonged **hypotension**. This may be the result of hypovolaemic shock (haemorrhage or dehydration), cardiovascular collapse (postoperative cardiac failure or myocardial infarction) or septic shock. In the last, endotoxic and cytokine-initiated renal cell damage is also an important factor. Pre-existing **chronic renal disease** increases a patient's susceptibility to acute renal failure.

If the insult to the renal tubules is not overwhelming, the damage to the tubular cells is confined to disruption of cellular metabolism rather than tissue necrosis. This is potentially reversible, provided the patient can be maintained in good general condition while tubular recovery takes place. The usual sequence of recovery is that poor urine output continues for a period (**oliguric phase**), followed by **spontaneous diuresis** of large volumes of unconcentrated urine consisting of unmodified glomerular filtrate (**diuretic phase**). Urinary concentrating power then slowly improves as the tubules recover normal metabolic function. In contrast, when tubular damage is more extensive, the patient remains anuric or severely oliguric.

PREVENTION OF ACUTE RENAL FAILURE

Acute renal failure is largely preventable by careful attention to preoperative assessment, fluid balance, and prevention and prompt management of hypotension and sepsis, as well as dose monitoring of potentially nephrotoxic drugs. In high-risk patients (with pre-existing renal disease or obstructive jaundice and those undergoing cardiopulmonary bypass or aortic surgery), **intravenous renal dose dopamine** given during operation helps protect renal function.

DIAGNOSIS OF OLIGURIA

When urinary retention has been excluded and true **oliguria** or **anuria** is diagnosed, the problem is to differentiate between acute tubular necrosis and reduced renal perfusion. As a first step, a **urinary catheter** should be inserted to monitor the hourly rate of urine production, which should ideally be at least 30 ml/hour. *Note*: if a catheter is already in situ and stops draining, it may have become blocked.

Low urine output is most often caused by **reduced renal perfusion**, resulting from relative hypovolaemia or low cardiac output. This leads to diminished glomerular filtration and enhanced tubular reabsorption. The usual reason is inadequate replacement of a perioperative fluid deficit. To test this, an intravenous fluid challenge of 250 ml can be infused over a few minutes. If this restores urinary output, under-hydration is confirmed and the fluid balance must be corrected to prevent acute tubular necrosis. Potentially more serious causes of reduced renal perfusion include cardiac failure and acute myocardial infarction; these need to be considered in postoperative patients with a low urinary output. Only if poor renal perfusion (prerenal failure) can be excluded should acute renal failure be diagnosed.

MANAGEMENT OF ACUTE RENAL FAILURE

When acute renal failure is mild, simple conservation measures such as fluid restriction may sustain the patient until tubular function recovers. When complete (oliguric) renal failure occurs, serum urea, creatinine and potassium concentrations rise inexorably and the patient usually requires **haemofiltration** or **renal dialysis**. Fortunately, many of these patients recover renal function gradually over a few weeks or months and do not require permanent renal support.

PRESSURE SORES

PATHOPHYSIOLOGY

Elderly, debilitated and other bed-bound patients are extremely susceptible to pressure sores ('bed sores'), particularly over bony prominences such as the sacrum and heels (see Figs 12.10 and 12.11). Pressure sores occur because the frequent spontaneous adjustment of position that normally occurs in bed is lost through obtunded sensation and immobility. Diminished protective pain response plays an important part. Patients with diabetes may have a sensory neuropathy so they are unable to sense the damaging effects of prolonged pressure on a bony prominence. Tissue necrosis and the subsequent failure to heal result from a combination of factors including recurrent pressure ischaemia, poor tissue perfusion (from cardiac or peripheral vascular disease) and malnu-

Fig. 12.10 Typical heel pressure sore

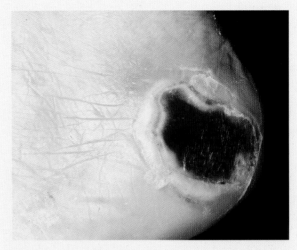

This elderly man presented with a ruptured abdominal aortic aneurysm and had a stormy postoperative course. At some stage, this heel was allowed to remain too long in one position, resulting in deep necrosis. He had no evidence of occlusive peripheral arterial disease.

Fig. 12.11 Osteomyelitis of the ischial tuberosity secondary to pressure ulceration

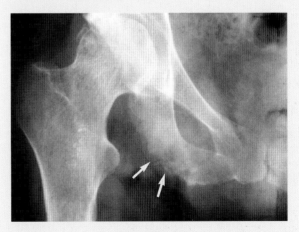

X-ray of the pelvis in an elderly bed-bound woman showing osteomyelitis of the ischial tuberosity (arrowed) underlying a deep long-standing sacral pressure ulcer.

trition. Note that patients who have experienced substantial weight loss and patients with relatively ischaemic lower limbs are at particular risk.

PREVENTION AND MANAGEMENT OF PRESSURE SORES

Once established, pressure sores are difficult to eradicate and prevention must be given high priority in patients at risk. Relatively hard surfaces such as accident and emergency department trolleys and operating tables may initiate pressure sores in susceptible patients in less than an hour. Likewise, pressure sores can develop in a remarkably short time in a hospital bed, particularly if the patient is incontinent of urine or faeces. Prevention of pressure sores on the ward is mainly a nursing responsibility; indeed, the incidence of pressure sores is a good indicator of the quality of nursing care.

Prevention of pressure sores involves the following procedures:

- **Special bed surfaces to spread the load**—these include (in ascending order of cost and complexity) pressure-relieving foam mattresses, electric ripple mattresses, water beds, suspended net beds and sophisticated low pressure continuous airflow beds
- **Relieving pressure on the heels**—use of ankle rests while on the operating table, use of heel pads, orthopaedic foam gutters and 'bean-bags' on return to the ward
- **Regular change of posture**—for most patients, this involves encouragement to get out of bed, at least into a bedside chair, and to mobilise beyond this as much as possible. A bed-bound patient requires regular turning so that the same skin area is not subjected to constant pressure
- Regular checking of pressure areas and local massage
- Management of incontinence

Treatment of established pressure sores is unsatisfactory unless the causative factors can be eliminated. This is often impossible in the permanently disabled patient. Avoiding pressure is the mainstay of treatment, supplemented by local cleansing and dressings designed to remove necrotic tissue and control secondary infection. For a deep sacral sore, major plastic surgery involving a rotational buttock flap is occasionally justified.

COMPLICATIONS OF OPERATIONS INVOLVING BOWEL

These include delayed return of bowel function, mechanical bowel obstruction, anastomotic failure, intra-abdominal abscesses, peritonitis, bowel fistula and acute bowel ischaemia.

DELAYED RETURN OF BOWEL FUNCTION

TEMPORARY INTERRUPTION OF PERISTALSIS

Any abdominal operation may temporarily disrupt peristalsis. This is particularly true where the operation is for peritonitis, an abscess or intestinal obstruction, or if the operation involves extensive handling of the bowel. Operations involving the retroperitoneal area such as aortic surgery may also disrupt peristalsis. The mechanism in this case is probably via a disturbance of parasympathetic activity. The problem is usually minor and mostly affects the small intestine. Patients may complain of nausea, anorexia and vomiting. This becomes obvious after oral fluids are reintroduced early in the postoperative period. This condition is often loosely described as **ileus** and is the reason for gradual reintroduction of fluids, followed by solids after abdominal operations. However, if ileus is prolonged, another cause such as an intraperitoneal collection of pus should be sought.

ADYNAMIC BOWEL DISORDER

Occasionally, a much more prolonged and extensive form of functional adynamic bowel disorder occurs. This presents with vomiting and protracted intolerance to oral intake. **Adynamic disorder** must be distinguished from true mechanical obstruction, which may require reoperation (see Ch. 19).

ACUTE GASTRIC DILATATION

Occasionally, adynamic disorder involves the stomach, causing acute gastric dilatation and accumulation of large volumes of gastric and duodenal reflux secretions. The warning feature is when the patient suddenly vomits a large volume of fluid which may, even on the first occasion, result in fatal bronchial aspiration. Preventing acute gastric dilatation is the main reason nasogastric tubes are used after upper gastrointestinal surgery or after relief of mechanical bowel obstruction. If acute gastric dilatation is suspected in any patient in whom recovery is unexpectedly slow, the abdomen should be examined daily for a **succussion splash**, and a nasogastric tube passed if the result is positive.

'PSEUDO-OBSTRUCTION'

Adynamic disorder involving the large bowel is conventionally but inaccurately described as **pseudo-obstruction**, as there is in fact no obstruction present. It may follow any abdominal operation, especially if the retroperitoneal area has been disturbed, as in nephrectomy or aortic surgery. Pseudo-obstruction is also a recognised complication of *non-abdominal operations* such as fractured neck of femur, especially in frail patients. Pseudo-obstruction may even occur without operation as a complication of severe hypokalaemia, trauma involving the lower spine and retroperitoneal area, or anti-Parkinsonian and other drugs. The diagnosis can rapidly be made on an 'instant' unprepared barium enema by excluding mechanical causes of obstruction. Treatment involves identification and treatment of the underlying cause, together with supportive measures such as an indwelling flatus tube until function returns.

MECHANICAL BOWEL OBSTRUCTION

EARLY POSTOPERATIVE MECHANICAL OBSTRUCTION

Postoperative mechanical obstruction of the bowel is uncommon. It may be caused by a loop of bowel becoming twisted or trapped in a peritoneal defect, unwittingly created at open operation or laparoscopy. **Fibrinous adhesions** may also cause obstruction, and these usually develop about 1 week after operation. In both cases, the obstruction may be transient and settle with conservative measures (nasogastric aspiration and intravenous fluids), or may progress to full-scale intestinal obstruction requiring laparotomy. If tenderness and systemic signs of toxicity appear, reoperation becomes urgent to exclude strangulation. Obstruction occurring after gastrectomy or gastroenterostomy may be due to oedema of the mucosa surrounding the anastomosis; this usually settles eventually with conservative measures although reoperation may be required.

LATE POSTOPERATIVE MECHANICAL OBSTRUCTION

Fibrinous adhesions may organise and persist as broad **fibrous adhesions** between adjacent loops of bowel or as isolated fibrous bands traversing the peritoneal cavity. These fibrous adhesions are a common cause of an isolated episode of small bowel obstruction or even infarction. Adhesions may also cause recurrent bouts of bowel obstruction months or years after abdominal operations. Most episodes will resolve spontaneously with conservative treatment, i.e. nasogastric aspiration and intravenous fluids, but failure of resolution or signs of strangulation (tenderness, toxaemia) will necessitate laparotomy.

Adhesive obstruction has become less common since talc powder on surgical gloves was discontinued in the 1970s and possibly even less common since the declining use of starch on surgical gloves. However, patients with recurrent intestinal obstruction due to adhesions present a serious surgical challenge. Each laparotomy becomes more difficult and hazardous for the patient. Therapeutic agents to prevent adhesions forming, often in the form of films, are currently under trial but conclusive evidence of their benefit is awaited.

ANASTOMOTIC FAILURE

Anastomotic leakage or breakdown is a major cause of postoperative morbidity after bowel surgery. Inadequate or delayed diagnosis and surgical intervention may lead to multiple and cumulative complications including sepsis, multi-organ dysfunction and failure, and fistulas.

Small anastomotic leaks are relatively common and lead to small **localised abscesses** which are walled off by surrounding gut and omentum. Small leaks manifest clinically by delayed recovery of bowel function resulting from local peristaltic dysfunction. Usually, the problem eventually settles with continued intravenous fluids and delayed reintroduction of oral intake. Reoperation, however, should be repeatedly considered if recovery is slow.

Major anastomotic breakdown results in generalised peritonitis, large abdominal abscesses, progressive sepsis and fistula formation. These are described below with the exception of systemic sepsis, which is described in Chapter 3.

INTRA-ABDOMINAL ABSCESSES

ABSCESS ASSOCIATED WITH BOWEL ANASTOMOSIS

An anastomotic leak from any part of the bowel may be walled off by small bowel and omentum in a vigorous intraperitoneal response (see Fig. 12.12). This results in formation of an abscess near the anastomosis. The patient will either be non-specifically unwell with delayed recovery, a swinging pyrexia and signs of local peritonitis, or more seriously ill with early signs of sepsis. A detailed description of the clinical features is given in Chapter 19. For systemic inflammatory response syndrome, see page 49.

Early reoperation is usually necessary to drain the abscess and prevent continued contamination of the peritoneal cavity. Where the anastomosis has broken down, both ends of the bowel should be brought out to form temporary stomas, since reanastomosis will almost certainly fail. The bowel can often be rejoined once the local infection and metabolic disruption have resolved.

OTHER INTRA-ABDOMINAL ABSCESSES

Intra-abdominal abscesses may also develop at sites remote from an anastomosis—for example, in the pelvis (**pelvic abscess**) or beneath the diaphragm (**subphrenic abscess**). These abscesses occur most often as a complication of treated peritonitis, particularly faecal peritonitis. They may also develop because of contamination of the operative site by faeces or other infected material, or by 'tracking' of an anastomotic abscess within the abdomen. Abscesses of this type usually produce a less severe illness than do those in direct communication with the bowel.

If an abscess is suspected, ultrasound or CT scanning may help to identify its location and guide needle aspiration or placement of a percutaneous drain, if appropriate. Surgical exploration may, however, be necessary.

Fig. 12.12 Intra-abdominal abscess following appendicectomy

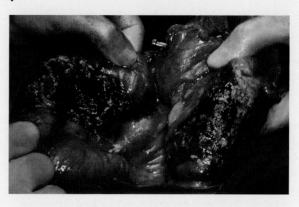

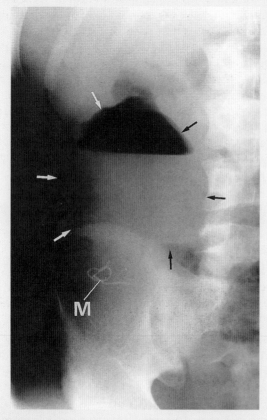

(a) This 16-year-old boy had an operation for removal of a perforated gangrenous appendix. He remained ill with anorexia and intermittent vomiting, general malaise and a swinging pyrexia. A large mass was palpable in the right side of the abdomen. Erect abdominal X-ray shows a huge abscess cavity (outline arrowed) with a gas bubble above a fluid (pus) level. Note the radiopaque marker **M** in a gauze swab packed into the open abdominal wound. **(b)** At operation, the abscess was surrounded by adherent small bowel, shown here.

PERITONITIS

Peritonitis in the postoperative period usually results from a major anastomotic breakdown causing widespread peritoneal contamination. Sometimes the cause of peritonitis is perforation of **obstructed or ischaemic bowel** or perforation of an incidental **peptic ulcer**. The clinical picture may develop rapidly over a few hours or, if infection spreads from an intraperitoneal abscess, more insidiously over a few days. The patient is systemically ill with severe, generalised abdominal pain; the abdomen is tender and rigid to palpation (see Ch. 19 for more details). *Note*: elderly patients with peritonitis may have surprisingly little tenderness. Generalised peritonitis progresses to sepsis and multiple organ failure unless promptly treated.

The patient is resuscitated and commenced on intravenous antibiotics and then returned to theatre for laparotomy. The abdomen is explored, the underlying cause is treated and peritoneal toilet is carried out. Early and vigorous treatment will usually save the patient's life.

BOWEL FISTULA

Fistula formation as a complication of surgery usually results from an anastomotic leak or infarction of a segment of bowel. A local abscess first develops then discharges to the surface via the wound or along the track of an abdominal drain. Anastomotic breakdown is more likely when there is obstruction of bowel beyond the anastomosis; the fistulous tract then provides a means of drainage for the obstructed bowel contents. With time, the drainage tract slowly becomes lined with epithelium from the bowel and the skin surface and the fistula becomes permanent. Occasionally a fistula develops in a patient after an operation for **bowel cancer**. In this case the fistula may be lined with malignant cells. Proximal small bowel fistulas result in the loss of large volumes of intestinal secretions containing digestive enzymes. This rapidly leads to dehydration and major electrolyte disturbances and usually causes gross intra-abdominal inflammation and skin destruction. The more proximal the origin of the fistula, the greater the volume of fluid and electrolyte loss and the more destructive its consequences.

The general state of the patient with a fistula depends on the extent of intra-abdominal infection. If this is minimal and there is no distal obstruction, the fistula usually closes spontaneously within weeks or months, provided the patient can be sustained in the interim. Proximal small bowel fistulas require **total bowel rest** (i.e. nil by mouth and a nasogastric tube) with full **parenteral fluid replacement and nutrition.** Somatostatin analogues may be given to substantially reduce the volume of secretion into the small bowel. Distal small bowel or large bowel fistulas may be managed with **enteral feeding** using low-residue elemental or semi-elemental fluid diets. These are often given via a fine-bore nasogastric tube.

When a fistula is associated with intra-abdominal infection, the patient is desperately ill, septic and hypercatabolic. These patients need intensive care management and reoperation. Laparotomy is required to bring the disrupted bowel ends to the surface as stomas and to drain the gross foci of infection; further laparotomies, even daily, may still be required before the intra-abdominal infection is brought under control. Mortality from these complicated fistulas is high.

ACUTE BOWEL ISCHAEMIA

Acute bowel ischaemia is an uncommon postoperative complication, usually occurring after abdominal aortic surgery. Infarction of the sigmoid colon follows inferior mesenteric artery ligation (usually a necessary part of the operation) if the collateral blood supply is compromised by obliterative atherosclerosis of the remaining mesenteric arteries. Fortunately, this problem is rare. The patient has usually progressed satisfactorily at first and then deteriorates unexpectedly several days after operation, often passing fresh blood per rectum. If untreated at this stage, the patient collapses with peritonitis due to colonic necrosis and perforation.

Clinical signs of acute bowel ischaemia are non-specific, but often the degree of collapse is out of proportion to the minimal abdominal signs. Plain abdominal X-ray may show 'thumb printing' of the affected bowel or the characteristic appearance of gas in the bowel wall. If acute bowel ischaemia is suspected, laparotomy must usually be performed urgently as perforation will soon occur and is nearly always fatal. Even with timely surgery, the prognosis is bleak.

13 Principles of cancer management

INTRODUCTION

In developed countries, people are living longer. This is mainly a result of public health measures which have improved infant mortality and reduced the burden of infectious diseases. Mortality from cardiovascular disease continues to dominate in late middle life, although in developed countries, smoking reduction, better control of blood pressure and the use of statins are substantially reducing deaths from atherosclerosis. Beyond late middle age, malignant disease begins to predominate. Huge strides have been made in recent years in understanding the molecular basis of cancer. Translating this into improved prevention, detection and treatment is a slow process but important progress has been made and the future for this approach is promising.

Malignant disease afflicts about a third of all people at some time in their lives and about one in four will die of it. Patients with malignant disease form a major part of the surgical workload and are responsible for as much as 40% of general surgical bed occupancy. Cancer patients impose disproportionate demands on services, since operations are often extensive and the patients are generally older, slower to recover and more prone to complications. At the same time, the total number of patients with malignant disease is rising because of increasing life expectancy and an increasing incidence of some cancers. In younger age groups, surgical workload from cancer is also expanding because of earlier detection, increased technical sophistication and increasing patient expectation. The incidence of common malignancies in Western countries is shown in Table 13.1.

Screening for malignant disease (see Ch. 6), notably cervical, breast and colorectal cancer, has had a significant but limited impact on mortality, partly because of lack of patient compliance (particularly in cervical and colorectal cancer) but also because of a relative inability to detect disease that is biologically early (in breast cancer).

Whether curative treatment can be offered depends on the location, the nature of the primary cancer (i.e. tissue type, metastatic potential) and the extent of spread, as well as other physiological factors such as the patient's hormonal status. Management of particular cancer types is becoming more protocol-driven as the outcomes of carefully conducted randomised trials have identified the most effective treatment regimens. Treatment increasingly involves a combination of surgical and other treatment modalities, particularly radiotherapy, chemotherapy, hormone manipulation and palliative symptom control.

Whilst the detection and treatment of various cancers is improving, dramatic press claims of 'breakthrough' cures are often premature and tend to raise false hopes. It is unlikely that a universal preventative or cure for cancer will appear. Instead, advances are likely to be incremental and specific to certain cancer types rather than covering the whole cancer spectrum.

NEOPLASIA

The main characteristic of all neoplasms is their uncontrolled growth that persists even after the initiating stimulus has been removed. Most neoplasms can readily be categorised as **benign** or **malignant** according to histological pattern and in most cases it is possible to predict the likelihood of invasion or of metastasis associated with a particular malignancy. Sometimes this is difficult; for example, distinguishing a leiomyoma from a leiomyosarcoma may only be achieved by following the long-term behaviour of the tumour. Neoplasms may also be difficult to distinguish clinically from other **tumour-like disorders** such as **hyperplasia** (e.g. parathyroid adenoma, a neoplasm, from parathyroid hyperplasia) or a **hamartoma** (a benign growth composed of a mixture of tissues normally found in that area of the body).

BENIGN NEOPLASMS

Benign neoplasms (tumours) usually grow slowly. They are typically well demarcated and often encapsulated, with a histological appearance closely reminiscent of the tissue of origin. Benign tumours present to the surgeon in a variety of ways as summarised in Box 13.1.

MALIGNANT NEOPLASMS

Malignant neoplasms or tumours are typically non-encapsulated with a poorly defined, irregular outline due to invasion into local tissues. They usually grow progressively and may grow rapidly. Histologically, the cells range from well differentiated to anaplastic, with the aggression of the neoplasm increasing as differentiation decreases. In **anaplastic tumours**, there is such loss of differentiation that little resemblance to the parent tissue remains.

The cells of malignant neoplasms and their nuclei often vary widely in shape and size. The extent of this **pleomorphism** also tends to correlate with the degree of malignancy and the future clinical behaviour of the tumour. The supporting tissue stroma of some malignancies may undergo fibrous hyperplasia, which accounts for some of the characteristic clinical features; these include hardness to palpation (induration), intestinal obstruction caused by annular carcinomas of the large bowel, and retraction and dimpling of skin overlying breast cancers. On the other hand, in highly aggressive tumours, the supporting tissue stroma may be inadequate for nutritional support, leading to necrosis and patchy haemorrhage within the tumour. This often presents as a sudden onset of pain and a mass.

Malignant tumours present in a variety of ways as summarised in Box 13.2.

CARCINOGENESIS

Multiple primary lesions and recurrences

Most cancers are probably caused by a combination of environmental factors and factors intrinsic to the patient. It has been estimated mathematically that about two-thirds of cancers can be attributed in some way to external environmental factors such as ionising radiation, virus infections and carcinogens in air, food and water. Many such factors are yet to be discovered but cigarette smoking is well recognised to be the most common carcinogen for lung, bladder and head and neck cancers. When cancer develops, it is likely that the whole of the affected organ or tissue has been altered in the same way

Table 13.1 Incidence of common malignancies in UK per year in men and women (from Cancer Research UK Scientific Yearbook 2005); figures have been rounded

Males		Females	
Prostate	30 000	Breast	41 000
Lung	23 000	Colorectal	16 000
Colorectal	18 500	Lung	15 000
Bladder	7500	Ovary	7000
Stomach	6000	Uterus	5000
Head and neck	5500	Lymphoma	4500
Lymphoma	5000	Melanoma	4000
Oesophagus	4500	Pancreas	3500
Kidney	4000	Stomach	3500
Leukaemia	4000	Bladder	3000

Box 13.1 Principal modes of presentation of benign tumours

- Lesion suspected by the patient to be malignant, e.g. breast lump
- Overt bleeding or occult blood loss causing anaemia, e.g. bowel polyps
- Local obstructive effects, e.g. leiomyoma of small intestine
- Pressure causing pain or dysfunction, e.g. neurofibroma
- Unacceptable cosmetic appearance, e.g. subcutaneous lipomas
- Production of excessive amounts of hormone by endocrine neoplasms, e.g. parathyroid adenoma, insulinoma, phaeochromocytoma

Box 13.2 Principal modes of presentation of malignant tumours

The primary lesion:

- Palpable or visible mass, e.g. breast or thyroid cancer
- Obstruction or other disruption of function of a hollow viscus, e.g. bowel obstruction by colorectal carcinoma, stridor in bronchial carcinoma
- Overt bleeding, e.g. bladder tumour or left-sided large bowel cancer
- Occult blood loss causing anaemia, e.g. carcinoma of stomach or caecum
- Obstructive jaundice, e.g. carcinoma of head of pancreas or extrahepatic bile ducts
- Skin lesion, often ulcerated, e.g. basal and squamous cell carcinomas, malignant melanoma, breast cancer
- Nerve invasion, e.g. facial nerve palsy from parotid carcinoma, recurrent laryngeal palsy from anaplastic carcinoma of thyroid

Note that pain is not a common presenting feature of primary malignancy except in the pancreas, lung and nasopharynx; pain is more often associated with metastatic disease

Metastatic deposits

- Enlarged lymph nodes (nodes tend to be hard, matted and non-tender). Intrathoracic nodes may cause superior vena caval obstruction
- Hepatomegaly, e.g. stomach, large bowel and pancreatic carcinomas
- Obstructive jaundice (usually due to lymph node mass in the porta hepatis compressing the bile ducts, but sometimes extensive liver deposits), e.g. stomach, large bowel and pancreatic carcinomas
- Abnormal masses distant from the primary lesion, e.g. abdomen, pelvis and skin
- Bone invasion causing bone pain or pathological fractures, e.g. prostatic and breast cancers

- Malignant effusions, e.g. pleural effusion in breast cancer, ascites with peritoneal deposits from intra-abdominal malignancies
- Pulmonary metastases—usually asymptomatic and found on chest X-ray
- Brain metastases—behavioural or personality changes, headache, fits, paresis, ataxias, etc.
- Neurological problems—spinal cord lesions caused by spinal fractures or by direct invasion

Generalised systemic manifestations (uncommon except for cachexia)

- Malignant cachexia (severe weight loss and wasting)—probably caused by the production of catabolic cytokines by the tumour
- Fever—characteristic of lymphomas and renal adenocarcinoma; also occurs when there is extensive tumour necrosis
- Migrating thrombophlebitis and chronic disseminated intravascular coagulation (DIC)
- Peripheral neuropathies, myopathies and rare autoimmune neuromuscular phenomena, e.g. myasthenic syndrome
- Other rare autoimmune phenomena, e.g. haemolysis
- Ectopic hormone production, e.g. antidiuretic hormone (ADH), adrenocorticotrophic hormone (ACTH), parathyroid hormone (PTH) and gonadotrophins (all rare in malignancies seen in general surgery)
- Production of fetal and embryonic proteins, e.g. carcino-embryonic antigen (CEA) produced by testicular tumours and colorectal and pancreatic carcinomas; alpha-fetoprotein (AFP) produced by testicular teratomas and hepatocellular carcinomas; prostate-specific antigen (PSA) in prostatic carcinoma—may be useful as **tumour markers** for diagnosis, monitoring treatment and long-term follow-up

---

by the carcinogen. Consequently, new primary tumours, as distinct from local recurrences, may develop later. This is a factor in deciding follow-up after treatment. However, clearly distinguishing between new primaries and recurrences is often impossible. Certain tissues, particularly those of the bladder, breast, skin, head and neck, and large bowel, are at particular risk of new primary carcinomas.

Growth and spread of malignant tumours

Malignant tumours spread by local **infiltration** and also by **distant metastasis** via lymphatics and the bloodstream and across coelomic cavities. Carcinogenesis, however, is not a single pathological event. Rather, the onset of uncontrolled proliferation and the capacity for distant spread evolve in a series of mutations over succes-

sive cell divisions. Many malignancies probably arise from a single cell line (i.e. are monoclonal) and the initial event is the acquisition of the capability of growing progressively in the native tissue. About 30 cell division cycles are probably needed to produce a clinically detectable lesion of 1 cm diameter containing 1000 million cells. Particular cellular properties enable a tumour to invade surrounding tissues and lymphatic or blood capillaries and then 'take root' in regional lymph nodes or other distant tissues. These properties are probably also products of multiple mutations that have given selective survival advantages. As time passes, the constituent cells of the tumour often become increasingly heterogeneous, both genetically and behaviourally.

These pathophysiological considerations have several important clinical consequences. Firstly, the earlier the primary tumour is detected and removed (i.e. the fewer cell division cycles), the greater the chance of complete cure. Unfortunately, mutations that permit metastasis may appear very early, i.e. by about 20 cell division cycles, when the primary lesion is too small to be detected (about 1 mm diameter).

There are two conflicting theories about the significance of regional lymph node involvement in carcinoma. Both views recognise that lymph node involvement implies a worse prognosis. **Halsted** believed that lymph nodes have an important function in halting spread, at least for a time, and that radical surgery to remove the nodes offers the best potential for a cure. In more than 50% of large bowel cancers, Halsted's view is probably correct and radical surgery remains the treatment of choice, offering a potential cure even in the presence of involved lymph nodes. In many other cancers, blood-borne (haematogenous) spread is often occult and probably occurs at an early stage, rendering the disease incurable by surgery. Unfortunately, identifying which patients have metastatic disease remains difficult, although better imaging, laparoscopy and biopsy techniques are improving pre-treatment diagnosis, whilst better understanding of lymph node drainage and wider excision of potentially involved nodes are leading to better prognostication and improved outcomes.

An alternative view about the significance of involved nodes, expressed by **Fisher**, is that metastases indicate failure of the host defences and are therefore a manifestation of systemic metastasis beyond the nodes. In the case of breast cancer, this has led to the increased use of systemic treatment with cytotoxic and hormonal therapy with the intention of eliminating or suppressing the growth of micrometastases. This has improved survival rates in a small proportion of patients. Nevertheless, radical local surgery remains important in controlling loco-regional disease in the breast, chest wall and axilla.

In practice, the probability of surgical cure when lymph node metastases are present depends on when the cancer develops the capacity for haematogenous spread. This is often about the same time as the capacity for lymph node metastasis appears. In these cases, surgical removal of metastases is ineffective because haematogenous metastases are usually multifocal by then. Occasionally blood-borne metastasis appears to be a solitary isolated event, and a cure can sometimes be achieved—for example, by partial hepatectomy in colorectal cancer metastases or pulmonary lobectomy for renal cell carcinoma, as well as in some paediatric malignancies. The liver, lungs, bone and brain are common target organs for haematogenous spread. Multiple metastases often respond temporarily to palliative chemotherapy, radiotherapy or hormone manipulation (e.g. carcinomas of breast, uterus, kidney and prostate) but complete cure is very rarely achieved.

This model of the development of metastatic potential means that future advances in cancer management need to focus on three factors: primary prevention, very early diagnosis, and research to find effective medical (i.e. non-surgical) approaches to treatment of metastases, e.g. radiotherapy, chemotherapy and hormonal manipulation.

TREATMENT OF MALIGNANT TUMOURS

BASIC PRINCIPLES OF CANCER MANAGEMENT

Two broad considerations determine the approach to treatment for any cancer patient. The first is whether an attempt can and should be made to achieve a **cure** or whether **palliation** is more appropriate; the choice depends on the nature of the tumour, the extent of local spread and whether distant metastases are believed to be present. The second consideration is the **prognosis**. This takes further factors into account, including the likely natural history of the type of cancer and the patient's age and comorbidity and his or her ability to withstand surgery. Systems of **staging** have been devised for each tumour type, many based on the **TNM system** which scores characteristics of the Tumour, the extent of regional lymph Node involvement and the presence of Metastases. Staging is used in planning treatment, as a guide to prognosis and as a standardised descriptive tool for comparing efficacy of treatment in different patients and in different centres.

Cancer often recurs some time after the primary treatment, and the success of treatment is often described in terms of patient survival after a given number of years rather than 'cure'. **Five-year survival** is often used as the yardstick and in many cases can be taken to imply cure. Nevertheless, some tumours, particularly breast cancer, may recur in a disseminated form as long as 30 years after apparently successful eradication. Conversely, colorectal cancer and testicular teratoma and seminoma rarely recur after the patient has survived 7 years.

TEAMWORKING IN CANCER MANAGEMENT

There is an increasing trend towards involving a range of specialists working in cooperative teams to manage patients with complex problems (Box 13.3). Structured multidisciplinary teams are an effective means of managing cancer cases where the diagnosis may need careful consideration and where the treatment package may involve radiotherapy, chemotherapy pre- or postoperatively, careful planning of an operation, prostheses or reconstructive surgery, stoma care and skilled specialist nursing or physiotherapy, as well as social and psychological support. Teams meet regularly to discuss individual cases and agree the whole course of management.

The benefits of working in this way stem from the battery of experience brought by experts in different disciplines, particularly in cases where diagnostic and therapeutic options are not clear. Cases can be discussed at any appropriate stage in the diagnostic and treatment process and an optimum treatment plan generated using the most current, evidence-based treatment tailored for the individual; the group has a joint responsibility for implementing the plan. A benefit for participants is that the discussion and cooperation with colleagues is an effective means of continuing professional development. Multidisciplinary teams have also been successfully introduced into other areas, for example managing neck lumps and rheumatoid disease. However, whilst this concept may seem ideal, having such a team is expensive and takes clinical staff away from other duties. It is clearly a luxury where health care is less developed and poorly funded.

TREATMENT OPTIONS

The main treatment options for malignant disease are **surgical excision**, **radiotherapy**, **chemotherapy** and **hormonal manipulation**, with two or more modalities of treatment often used in combination. The treatment offered to an individual patient will depend on tumour type and extent, the patient's overall fitness and, in particular, whether the aim is cure or palliation. A radical or aggressive approach to treatment using a combination of

---

therapies (e.g. surgery and pre- and/or postoperative radiotherapy and/or chemotherapy) may well be recommended where the aim is to cure, provided the scientific evidence supports this approach. In other patients where cure is not possible, or where disease has relapsed after radical treatment, the aim is to palliate, i.e. to alleviate the symptoms of disease.

Palliative care is a branch of medicine that focuses on quality of life rather than cure. All doctors practise palliative care at times when looking after patients who have potentially life-threatening illnesses. Palliation involves weighing up the benefits against the burdens of treatments, focusing on what is important to the patient and family. More complex cases may need the help of a specialist palliative care team, if available. This team can see patients before final diagnosis if there are difficult matters of symptom control, or psychological, social or spiritual problems. Some patients may need short admissions to specialist units (often called hospices) for symptom control or eventually for terminal care.

Most standard cancer treatments involve unpleasant **side effects** that are easily disregarded by both doctor and patient in their enthusiasm for treatment. The patient should be informed and then involved in reaching these decisions as much as he or she would like. The amount of information given varies between individuals—some patients may want the whole story, others may want less. Sometimes the information needs of the patient and family may differ but a doctor may speak to family members with the patient's consent. A diagnosis of cancer should rarely be concealed from a competent patient as suspicion and fear of the unknown often cause more distress than a frank explanation of the diagnosis and its ramifications. Time should be allowed for the patient to formulate further questions and a follow-up consultation arranged in a few days. It often helps the patient to have a friend or relative present. Patients are also helped by well-constructed printed information, by self-help groups and by specially trained cancer nurses who can spend the necessary time with the patient and act as an intermediary if necessary.

SURGERY FOR CANCER

GENERAL PRINCIPLES OF CANCER SURGERY (Box 13.4)

The ideal result of cancer surgery is the complete eradication of malignant disease without radically interfering with function. Nearly a third of cancer patients can be cured in this way; these are mainly patients with only primary disease (without nodal or metastatic disease). The decision about whether to embark on major elective surgery depends on careful assessment of the nature of the disease and its stage. Modern techniques of cross-sectional imaging, laparoscopy and intraoperative ultrasound greatly assist in this endeavour and may save

---

> **Box 13.3** **Contribution of members of the cancer multidisciplinary team**
>
> - **Surgeon**—specialises in the area in question, e.g. colorectal, upper gastrointestinal, breast
> - **Plastic surgeon**—if breast reconstruction is to be considered
> - **Oncologist**—considers whether adjuvant or neo-adjuvant radiotherapy/chemotherapy/hormonal therapy should be given
> - **Histopathologist**—determines tumour type, grade, markers for potential sensitivity to drugs or hormones, stage (e.g. TNM staging or Dukes' staging for rectal cancer)
> - **Radiologist**—assesses quality of imaging and staging by this method. Advises on further imaging in the light of discussion. Interpretation of findings to date
> - **Stoma care nurse/breast care nurse.** Stoma care nurse anticipates siting of stoma; prepares patient psychologically; marks site. Breast nurse assists with psychological and emotional support and may run specialist clinics
> - **Palliative care nurse/physician**—deals with quality of life, symptom control, and psychological, spiritual and social needs

---

Box 13.4 **The general principles of cancer management**

Note: detection of asymptomatic disease is covered in Chapter 6, including opportunistic screening, screening and surveillance of people with risk factors and population screening

1. **Pre-referral mechanisms**
- Patient education to recognise danger symptoms and signs
- Self examination by the patient. e.g. breast, testis
- Education, guidance and post-referral feedback for family practitioners in recognising danger symptoms and signs and reassuring the 'worried well'
- Appropriate referral to specialists helped by proformas containing indications to refer suspected skin, colorectal, breast, head and neck and upper gastrointestinal cancer
- Ready availability of early assessment and diagnostic tests

2. **Primary diagnosis after referral**—clinical assessment plus investigations, e.g. imaging, endoscopy, biopsy, fine needle aspiration cytology, laparoscopy

3. **Staging**—additional investigation to search for extent of spread:
- Local spread
- Lymph node spread
- Haematogenous spread (bone, lung, liver, brain)
- Peritoneal/pleural spread

4. **Multidisciplinary decision making**—to formulate the aims of treatment and to decide the optimum treatment:
- Treatment planning and timing of treatment, ideally based on randomised controlled trials (RCTs) but also on experience
- Treatment may involve a single entity, or combinations of surgery, neoadjuvant or adjuvant chemotherapy and/or radiotherapy, postoperative chemo- or radiotherapy, hormonal therapy
- Patients should be entered into clinical trials where best treatment is not established

Note that increasing specialisation and subspecialisation in the surgical treatment of rarer or more complex cancers produces better outcomes, e.g. sarcoma, oesophageal carcinoma

5. **The treatment**

6. **Repeat staging after operation or other treatment**—with knowledge of the operative findings and a review of the histology. This may change the postoperative plan for adjuvant therapy and provide information to calculate the statistical likelihood of survival/cure

7. **Post treatment surveillance**—for recurrence or appearance of new tumours in the field. Guidelines for different cancers are becoming available for the desirability, frequency and duration of clinical assessment, imaging and measuring tumour markers

8. **Audit** of local outcomes to improve quality of care. Participation in national audits

---

patients from fruitless radical surgery. Published critical reviews of the outcomes of different treatments for particular malignancies at different stages have also helped to guide the indications for surgery. The best information is Level 1 evidence coming from randomised controlled trials. For example, adenocarcinoma of the pancreas is treated by pancreatectomy nowadays only when there is a realistic chance of cure.

Where metastases appear confined to local lymph nodes, these nodes are usually excised along with the primary tumour or at a second operation. In gastric cancer, familiarity with the likely lymphatic drainage leads to targeted excision of particular lymph node groups; this, together with retrieval of increased numbers of lymph nodes, appears to be giving greater long-term cure rates. Even in the presence of incurable metastases, surgical excision of the primary lesion is sometimes required to relieve the local effects of the tumour, e.g. bleeding, pain or bowel obstruction, although similar results can often be obtained by radiotherapy, chemotherapy or physical means of destruction such as radiofrequency probes or lasers. Palliative surgery may also be required for locally advanced or metastatic disease to deal with specific dis-

tressing symptoms (e.g. dysphagia from oesophageal cancer, severe haemorrhage from a bladder tumour) or some emergency problem (e.g. acute bowel obstruction).

Sometimes surgery is used to **debulk** a tumour; this is combined with chemotherapy in an attempt either to improve the efficacy of chemotherapy (as in ovarian carcinoma) or to avoid leaving unstable tissue in abdominal lymph nodes (as in testicular teratoma). Increasingly, chemotherapy and/or radiotherapy is used to 'downsize' a malignant tumour to facilitate excisional surgery, e.g. rectal cancer. This is sometimes called 'downstaging', but since it has no effect on metastatic disease, this is an inaccurate use of the term.

RADIOTHERAPY

GENERAL PRINCIPLES OF RADIOTHERAPY

The value of ionising radiation in treating malignant tumours was recognised soon after the discovery of X-rays in 1895, and radiotherapy is now employed at some stage in managing about half of all patients with malignant disease. **Orthovoltage** X-rays (up to 250 kV) were the basis of conventional radiotherapy until the development of **megavoltage** irradiation in the late 1950s. Cobalt-60 machines provided more penetrating radiation initially, but these have been superseded by **linear accelerators** which provide photon beams with an energy of 5–20 MeV. With increased energy, the radiation dose peaks deep to the skin, thus avoiding the former severe skin reactions. Absorption of radiation by the target tissue causes highly reactive free radicals to appear which damage DNA and cause cell death at mitosis. With their high rate of proliferation, cancer cells are particularly sensitive, but normal tissues with a high rate of cell turnover (e.g. gut mucosa and bone marrow) are also vulnerable. The total dose administered depends on the aims of treatment, the site and volume of the tumour and its relationship to important normal tissues. Treatment is given in a variable number of sessions or **fractions** over a period of weeks to allow normal tissues to recover between treatments.

The larger the volume of tumour, the greater the dosage of irradiation required for its destruction. Since the dose is limited by the tolerance of normal tissues, radiotherapy is more effective for small lesions. Radiation dose is measured in **Gray** (Gy). A common daily dose is around 2 Gy, which is sufficient to destroy about 50% of viable cells in the average tumour; each subsequent dose destroys 50% of the remainder, causing a logarithmic decline in viable cell numbers as treatment proceeds. Planning radiotherapy for lesions deep within the body has improved markedly as a result of improved imaging using computerised tomography (CT scanning) and magnetic resonance imaging (MRI).

Radiation can be directed to a tumour in three ways:

- **External beam irradiation**—this is the method most commonly employed for skin lesions and deeply located tumours
- **Local application of radioisotopes (brachytherapy)**— this involves placing the radiation source upon or within the tissue to be irradiated. **Plaque** sources of radiation can be employed for skin malignancies, and radioactive **iridium wires or caesium needles** can be implanted in the oral cavity, prostate, skin and sometimes breast, giving high-dose local irradiation. Implantation is usually performed under general anaesthesia. For cancer of the uterus and cervix, the radioactive source is placed in a sealed container within the uterine or vaginal cavity; it can be inserted without risk to staff via a flexible tube from the radiation safe in which it is kept using computer control
- **Systemic radioisotope therapy**—radioactive iodine given by mouth or intravenously is a well-established treatment for thyrotoxicosis and can also be used for treating well-differentiated thyroid tumours provided the rest of the thyroid has been removed, even if extensive metastases are present. Attempts are still being made to direct radioisotopes precisely to cancer cells by attaching them to tumour-specific monoclonal antibodies, thus realising the dream of a 'magic bullet'; alas, this technique remains in the experimental stage

MAJOR APPLICATIONS OF RADIOTHERAPY

Radiotherapy has three major applications in cancer treatment: as a primary cure, as adjuvant treatment to surgery (and/or chemotherapy) or as palliation. The treatment objective must be clearly defined before treatment is begun.

Primary curative radiotherapy

Radiotherapy with curative intent is known as **radical radiotherapy**, and is widely used for basal cell and squamous cell carcinomas of the skin. It is also used for certain tumours which are technically difficult to remove or where surgery would be particularly mutilating, as in the head, neck and larynx. Radiotherapy can be directed at the primary lesion and regional lymph nodes if appropriate and rates of cure are comparable to those achieved by surgical excision. For example, in head and neck cancers without distant metastases, cure rates of 50–90% can be achieved with radiotherapy alone; similar results can be obtained in carcinoma of the cervix. Radiotherapy is employed in the treatment of most common solid tumours and in early cases of Hodgkin and non-Hodgkin lymphomas. The efficacy and application of radiotherapy for various tumour types is summarised in Table 13.2.

Radiotherapy can also achieve cure in up to 50% of bladder cancers, with salvage cystectomy reserved for recurrence.

Adjuvant radiotherapy

The principle underlying **adjuvant therapy**, whether radiological, chemical or hormonal, is that clinically undetectable micrometastases are often present in tissue surrounding a primary lesion, in regional nodes and in remote locations. These are believed to be responsible for local, regional and systemic recurrence after a primary lesion has apparently been completely removed.

Adjuvant radiotherapy can be applied to local tissue and regional nodes before surgery (known as **neoadjuvant therapy**, see below), after surgery or both, to try to eliminate micrometastases. Adjuvant radiotherapy is widely employed for cancer of the breast after removing the primary lesion locally or by mastectomy. If axillary nodes are involved, radiotherapy can be an alternative to radical lymph node clearance; survival rates are comparable to those achieved after surgery. However, the trend of opinion favours radical lymph node clearance for the improved diagnostic accuracy it provides and the prognostic value of knowing the number of nodes involved. The preference for surgery or radiotherapy remains one of local choice. Radiotherapy is also highly effective adjuvant therapy in seminoma of the testis.

Table 13.2 Applications of radiotherapy for treating malignant disease

Tumour type	Radiosensitivity	Indications
Head and neck	Moderate	Highly effective for localised lesions especially larynx
Lung Small cell Non-small cell	High (but largely palliative) Low to moderate	Enhances efficacy of chemotherapy but overall cure rate less than 10% Worth a trial in patients with inoperable disease for palliation
Breast	Moderate	Usually as adjuvant to surgery or to treat axillary nodal involvement or advanced local breast cancer
Thyroid Well differentiated Poorly differentiated (anaplastic)	High Low	High cure rate in combination with surgery (systemic radioiodine therapy) Rarely useful
Renal cell carcinoma	Low	Rarely appropriate
Transitional cell carcinoma of bladder	Moderate	Good cure rate for localised lesions
Testis	Moderate to high	Good (especially seminoma) but chemotherapy generally better (for teratoma)
Ovary	Very low	Rarely applicable
Uterus Cervix Body	Moderate Moderate	High cure rate for localised tumours; also as adjuvant therapy Adjuvant or palliative therapy
Gastrointestinal tract	Low to moderate	Increasingly used for adjuvant therapy in advanced rectal cancers. Definitive treatment for anal carcinomas
Lymphoma Hodgkin's Non-Hodgkin's	High High	Excellent cure rate for stage I and II disease High cure rate when used with chemotherapy
Multiple myeloma	High	Mainly used for palliation
Skin Basal or squamous cell carcinoma Melanoma	High Low	Highly curable Used to palliate metastases
Adult central nervous system	Low to moderate	Adjuvant therapy in well-differentiated gliomas Palliation of cerebral metastases
Paediatric malignancies	Variable	Often curative for brain tumours and effective for Wilms' tumour but limited by long-term effects on growth and development

Neoadjuvant radiotherapy

In certain cancers, treatment a short time before surgery with either radiotherapy or chemotherapy or both can bring benefits. This may enhance the cure rate for surgery or it may be used to 'downsize' a cancer to make surgery practicable, e.g. in locally advanced rectal cancer.

Palliative radiotherapy

Palliative radiotherapy is employed for local control of primary or metastatic lesions with the intention of treating symptoms and causing the minimum of side effects.

It is also employed to prevent impending complications, e.g. spinal cord compression. Much lower total doses are used for palliation than for attempts at cure; short courses or **single high-dose fractions** are usually adequate and are tolerable and convenient for the patient. Clearly, palliative radiotherapy can be justified only if expert assessment predicts that therapeutic benefit is likely.

Radiotherapy is particularly effective in controlling metastatic deposits in bone and brain. The pain of bone metastases can often be completely relieved by radiotherapy, as can some of the neurological manifestations of brain secondaries.

Radiotherapy is valuable in providing symptomatic relief in advanced disease. In ulcerating breast cancer, radiotherapy can shrink the primary lesion, controlling exudation and bleeding and permitting healing of overlying skin. Similarly, the distressing symptoms of cough, haemoptysis and pleuritic pain from advanced lung cancer can be eased by palliative radiotherapy. Symptoms associated with local tumour recurrence can often be controlled, e.g. haematuria from advanced bladder cancer or pain from rectal carcinoma. In abdominal malignancy, the main factor limiting the use of radiotherapy is incidental radiation injury to normal bowel. Late bowel damage can cause stricture formation, obstruction and continual bleeding, often years later. Indications for palliative radiotherapy are summarised in Box 13.5.

COMPLICATIONS OF RADIOTHERAPY

Despite the precise use of high-energy radiotherapy, side effects and complications still occur; the main early effects are outlined in Table 13.3.

Long-term side effects of radiotherapy

Modern radiotherapy using high-energy sources with meticulous treatment planning and delivery causes fewer side effects than the relatively empirical orthovoltage treatment used in the early days. Side effects such as **osteoradionecrosis** are rare (see Fig. 13.1), but **endarteritis obliterans** may be a long-term complication affecting any tissue subjected to radiotherapy. The effect is progressive impairment of blood supply, loss of special-

| **Box 13.5** | **Indications for palliative radiotherapy** |

Pain control
- Bone pain (especially breast, prostate and lung metastases)
- Nerve root and soft tissue infiltration (e.g. head and neck, brachial plexus)

Dyspnoea
- Shrinkage of tumour obstructing or compressing a large airway

Ulcerating and fungating lesions
- Breast, skin, head and neck tumours

Haemorrhage
- Haemoptysis
- Haematuria
- Rectal and cervical bleeding

Emergency complications
- Spinal cord compression
- Superior vena caval obstruction
- Raised intracranial pressure
- Obstruction of tubular viscera (e.g. oesophagus, upper gastrointestinal tract, ureters)

Space-occupying lesions caused by symptomatic brain metastases
- Brain metastasis causing hemiparesis

CASE STUDY

Fig. 13.1 Osteoradionecrosis after early orthovoltage radiotherapy for breast cancer

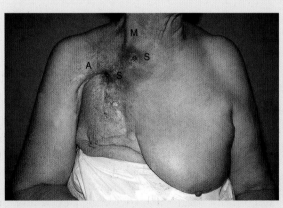
(a)

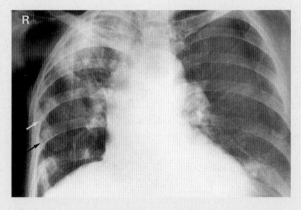
(b)

This 75-year-old woman had a radical mastectomy and orthovoltage irradiation for carcinoma of the right breast in 1949, 40 years before this photograph. She presented with two discharging skin sinuses below the clavicles, **S**. **(a)** Gross deformity of chest wall caused by excision of pectoral muscles at radical mastectomy (axilla **A**, sternomastoids **M**). Note sinus openings **S** leading down to sequestra, and widespread telangiectasia, a late result of radiotherapy. **(b)** Chest X-ray showing osteoradionecrosis of the ribs and scapula on the right side. There is typical patchy osteoporosis and osteosclerosis. Several healing pathological fractures are also evident (arrowed). Irradiation has induced lung fibrosis and pulmonary contraction resulting in a shift of the mediastinum towards the right.

Table 13.3 Early reactions and complications of radiotherapy

Reaction/complication	Management
Systemic side effects	
Malaise and fatigue—very common	These settle spontaneously with rest
Nausea, vomiting and anorexia	Anti-emetics
Effects occurring in irradiated tissues	
Skin (especially axilla, groin and perineum)	
Redness, itching and mild pain	Mild or moderate-strength topical steroids
Skin breakdown (in treatment of skin cancers, this heals after 3–4 weeks)	Moisture-retaining non-adherent dressings Silver–sulfasalazine cream
Abdomen and pelvis	
Nausea, vomiting, diarrhoea	Anti-emetics, antidiarrhoeals
Frequency, dysuria, haematuria (radiation cystitis)	Urinary alkalinising agents; exclude infection
Head and neck	
Dry mouth (xerostomia) due to salivary gland injury	Frequent oral fluids, moist oral swabs, careful attention to oral hygiene
Painful mouth, dysphagia and altered taste. This is due to inflammation and atrophy of oral mucosa (mucositis) and may also involve nasal mucosa	Topical steroids for ulcers, topical anaesthetic gels, antifungal agents for candidiasis, artificial saliva
Chest	
Painful dysphagia (radiation oesophagitis)	Local anaesthetic gel Compound antacid/alginate preparations, e.g. Gaviscon
Head	
Hair loss (alopecia)	Provision of wigs ('wig library')
Bone marrow	
Myelosuppression	Discontinue therapy, prophylactic antibiotics, platelet transfusion

ised tissues and replacement with fibrosis. In the chest, radiotherapy can cause pulmonary fibrosis and, in women treated for left-sided breast cancer, there is an increased long-term risk of cardiac events; treatment techniques have been modified as a result. In the gastrointestinal tract, the effects of radiation on bowel (**radiation enteritis**) can be particularly serious, with continued bleeding (in large bowel) and stricture formation (in small bowel). The same pathophysiological reaction probably accounts for delayed or incomplete healing after surgery with breakdown of intestinal anastomoses or formation of internal fistulae. **Radiation colitis** most commonly results from treatment of uterine cervical cancer.

CHEMOTHERAPY

GENERAL PRINCIPLES OF CHEMOTHERAPY

Success achieved with chemotherapeutic agents in curing many haematological and childhood malignancies encouraged the use of similar drugs to treat solid tumours previously treated only by surgery or radiotherapy.

Drugs destroy tumour cells in a variety of different ways, capitalising on their increased mitotic and meta-bolic rates. The main types of chemotherapeutic agent are as follows:

- **Antimetabolites**—analogues of normal cellular nutrients, e.g. methotrexate acts as a substitute for folinic acid
- **Alkylating agents**—these bind to DNA, e.g. nitrogen mustards
- **Drugs which cross-link DNA**, e.g. cisplatin
- **Drugs which disrupt the mitotic spindle**, e.g. vinca alkaloids, taxanes

These same cytotoxic mechanisms also affect normal tissues, though usually to a lesser extent, and are responsible for most of the side effects of chemotherapy. For many cancers, combinations of cytotoxic drugs obtain the best results. Particular combinations are chosen so the toxic effects of each drug impact on a different organ system; this means that each drug can be given in full tumour-toxic dose without excessive damage to normal tissues. The most effective drug combinations and doses for each tumour type have been established mainly by empirical trials. It has been difficult to find regimens that give better results than combinations developed in the 1970s and 1980s, e.g. CMF for breast cancer, CHOP for lymphoma and BEP for testicular cancer, although a

Box 13.6   Tumour sensitivity to cytotoxic chemotherapy

Highly sensitive tumours—reasonable prospect of cure

- Hodgkin's disease
- High-grade lymphomas
- Testicular tumours
- Choriocarcinoma
- Childhood leukaemias
- Wilms' tumour (nephroblastoma)
- Ewing's sarcoma
- Osteogenic sarcoma (lung metastases)

Moderately sensitive tumours—palliation is the main objective

- Breast cancer
- Ovarian malignancies
- Small-cell (oat-cell) carcinoma of lung
- Multiple myeloma
- Acute and chronic leukaemias in adults
- Low-grade lymphomas
- Colorectal cancer

Relatively insensitive tumours—cytotoxic therapy only indicated in special circumstances or with techniques of regional infusion

- Carcinoma of lung other than small-cell type
- Squamous carcinomas of the head and neck
- Carcinoma of uterus and cervix
- Melanoma
- Hepatocellular carcinoma
- Osteogenic sarcoma (primary lesions)
- Renal adenocarcinoma
- Bladder carcinoma

steadily increasing range of new chemotherapeutic drugs promise improvements. Drugs are usually given intravenously, often by infusion, in a series of four to six short courses separated by 3–4 weeks to allow recovery of normal tissues.

Experience has revealed a wide spectrum of sensitivities of different malignant tumours to cytotoxic therapy. These range from total destruction to no therapeutic effect. The sensitivities of different tumour types are summarised in Box 13.6.

MAJOR APPLICATIONS OF CHEMOTHERAPY

Primary curative treatment

This is mainly indicated for highly sensitive **germ cell tumours**, high-grade **lymphomas** and **solid tumours and leukaemias of childhood**. Chemotherapy may be used alone after obtaining a histological diagnosis (e.g.

Hodgkin's disease), or it may follow removal of the primary tumour (e.g. teratoma, Wilms' tumour), or it may be used first and then any residual tumour resected to achieve complete remission (e.g. abdominal para-aortic nodes in testicular teratoma).

Adjuvant chemotherapy

This involves systemic chemotherapy in addition to local treatment of the primary lesion in an attempt to destroy already disseminated but undetectable micrometastases. Adjuvant chemotherapy is often used for breast cancer where axillary lymph nodes are involved, particularly in premenopausal women. These patients are at high risk of developing widespread metastases later and adjuvant therapy is given in the hope of reducing the risk. In node-positive patients, both 5- and 10-year survival rates have been improved by between 5 and 15%. In recent years, adjuvant chemotherapy has become more widely employed as outcomes have improved (by a small amount), with fewer toxic side effects and better drugs to control nausea. As a result, treatment has become more acceptable to patients. In cancer of the colon and rectum, adjuvant chemotherapy, mainly using 5-fluorouracil (5FU), has a role in extending recurrence-free survival and life expectancy. Current information on this and other trials can be obtained from Cancer Research UK (www.cancerhelp.org.uk). For certain cancers including anal canal, cervix and some head and neck cancers, chemotherapy plus radiotherapy (**chemo-radiotherapy**) adds to the benefits of radiotherapy alone, often replacing the need for radical surgery.

General palliative treatment

General palliation is the rationale for using chemotherapy for disseminated malignancy in highly sensitive and moderately sensitive tumours. Cure is rarely achieved but quality of life may be greatly improved and, in some cases, life may be prolonged.

Palliation of distressing local symptoms

Cytotoxic therapy may sometimes be indicated for relatively insensitive tumours if local tumour effects are so distressing that even a small reduction in tumour mass might relieve them, e.g. breast cancer causing lymphatic obstruction. The objective is not to prolong life but to improve its quality.

SIDE EFFECTS OF CHEMOTHERAPY

Chemotherapy is toxic to tumour cells but also to normal body cells, especially those with rapid rates of turnover, e.g. bone marrow and gastrointestinal epithelium. Toxic effects are summarised in Box 13.7. Side effects are common but are rarely so severe that treatment is abandoned.

Toxic effects of chemotherapy

Bone marrow suppression

- Causes anaemia, thrombocytopenia and leucopenia (potentially fatal)

Immunosuppression

- Causes diminished resistance to opportunistic infections

Nausea and vomiting

- Tend to occur within an hour or two of chemotherapy
- Modern anti-emetics can usually control these symptoms but delayed nausea over the ensuing days remains a problem

Disruption of gastrointestinal epithelial turnover

- Causes diarrhoea and oral ulceration

Toxicity to hair follicles

- Particularly etoposide, cyclophosphamide and doxorubicin
- Causes hair loss (recovers 6 months after treatment)

Gonadal injury

- Loss of libido, sterility and possible mutagenesis

Long-term risk of inducing other malignancies

- 20–30 times the normal risk (but still low)

Rapid tumour destruction on a massive scale

- Leads to release of purines and pyrimidines (only a problem in leukaemias and lymphomas) which cause hyperuricaemia, presenting as obstructive uropathy and renal failure
- Hyperuricaemia can be prevented by giving prophylactic allopurinol

Chemotherapy offers substantial benefit and a chance of cure in some well-defined malignancies, as shown in Box 13.6. However, clinicians treating cancer need to be clear about their management objectives in advance of treatment, i.e. cure or palliation, based on the outcomes of published clinical trials wherever possible. Given the potential for side effects and the high cost, there is no place for speculative chemotherapy where scientific evidence shows no benefit.

HORMONAL MANIPULATION

GENERAL PRINCIPLES OF HORMONAL MANIPULATION

The growth of certain tumours, notably carcinoma of the prostate and some breast cancers, is partially dependent on sex hormones. Removal of the gonads or use of drugs which block or antagonise the appropriate hormone can have a valuable inhibitory effect on tumour growth.

MAJOR APPLICATIONS OF HORMONAL MANIPULATION

Prostatic cancer

Hormonal therapy is aimed at achieving testosterone suppression via surgical or medical castration. Surgical castration involves a bilateral orchidectomy, whereas medical castration involves the use of a **luteinising hormone releasing hormone (LHRH)** agonist. Castration can also be combined with an anti-androgen (combined androgen blockage) which blocks androgen receptor binding. LHRH analogues (gonadorelins) are as effective as orchidectomy for treating disseminated prostatic cancer. These drugs are given at intervals of 4 weeks or 3 months; initially they cause release of luteinising hormone from the anterior pituitary; this is followed by inhibition. **Anti-androgen drugs** alone (e.g. cyproterone, flutamide) have proved less effective and more toxic than gonadorelins but are usually administered initially to block the initial testosterone 'flare'. **Diethylstilbestrol (stilboestrol)** is a synthetic oestrogen which was used for many years before the synthetic LHRH agonists. It partly works by suppressing LHRH at hypothalamic level but may be cytotoxic to prostatic cancer cells in its own right. However, it is associated with a high risk of arterial and venous thrombosis and has fallen out of favour.

Breast cancer

Oral **tamoxifen**, an anti-oestrogen, has been shown to prolong survival after standard local treatment of oestrogen receptor ('ER') positive breast cancer. Its effect is beneficial at all ages but greatest in postmenopausal patients, and its use for 5 years post diagnosis has consistently given substantial survival benefits. Note that in postmenopausal women, oestrogens are produced by the peripheral conversion of androgens involving the enzyme **aromatase**. Aromatase inhibitor drugs reduce the action of aromatase, thereby lowering the quantity of oestrogen produced in the body. Emerging data suggest that drugs of this class may be superior to tamoxifen as adjuvant treatment, and they are frequently used in palliation. Tamoxifen can also give useful palliation in recurrent and metastatic breast cancer and it is worth considering a trial of treatment as the drug has few side effects. Advances in hormonal treatments now allow the use of second- and even third-line hormonal agents after relapse on tamoxifen. Duration of response to these treatments is often shorter than the initial treatment, but useful symptom relief may be obtained with minimal side effects.

In metastatic breast cancer, particularly with bony metastases, **oophorectomy** brings relief from pain in about 50% of cases. This may be achieved chemically with LHRH (gonadorelin) antagonists, producing a reversible menopausal state, surgically (usually laparoscopically) or by radiotherapy.

TARGETED THERAPIES

Oncologists have long dreamed of finding precise ways of delivering cancer-killing drugs so that they destroy cancer cells without damaging normal cells. Many refer to this idea as a 'magic bullet', and we are now entering an exciting era when this vision is becoming real. **Monoclonal antibodies** are now employed for this purpose. The antibody recognises certain protein configurations on the surface of particular types of cancer cells and 'locks' on to them. The intention is that this will cause the cells to destroy themselves or else trigger the body's immune system to recognise the marked cells as 'non-self' and attack them. So far, this has only limited application but much work is continuing in the field.

LYMPHOMA

The antigen CD20 is found on the surface of normal B-cell lymphocytes (but not their precursors) and is also present on the surface of nearly all the abnormal malignant B-cell lymphocytes found in 75% of non-Hodgkin lymphoma. The drug **rituximab** is a genetically engineered chimeric murine/human monoclonal IgG$_1$ antibody directed against the CD20 antigen and to which it 'locks'. Both normal and abnormal B-cells are destroyed but the body quickly replaces the normal cells, so any side effects from lack of B-cells are minimal. Rituximab combined with chemotherapy has increased response rates by 20% in B-cell lymphoma compared with chemotherapy alone and has become the desirable standard of care. However, the drug does cause infrequent serious adverse effects including muco-cutaneous reactions and the rare but fatal **infusion reaction complex** of organ failure.

BREAST CANCER

Human epidermal growth receptor 2 (HER2) is an antigenic protein of the human **epidermal growth factor receptor (EGFR)** family. HER2 is involved in transmitting growth signals from outside the cell to the nucleus and a strong signal causes the cell to divide. About 20% of breast cancers have excess HER2 (known as HER2-positive tumours), and in these a continuous growth signal causes accelerated cell division. **Trastuzumab** (trade name Herceptin) is a recombinant DNA-derived humanised monoclonal IgG$_1$ antibody which binds selectively with high affinity to the surface HER2 receptor. Its anti-cancer effects are brought about by blocking tumour cell growth and stimulating the immune system to destroy the tumour cells. It also acts in combination with chemotherapy to increase the cytotoxic cell destruction. Trastuzumab was used largely in clinical trials, particularly in recurrent and metastatic disease, but has been licensed in the UK by the National Institute for Health and Clinical Excellence (NICE) for use as part of primary therapy for HER2-positive breast cancers. As with all similar drugs, there are potential serious hazards including severe hypersensitivity reactions and adverse pulmonary events. There have been occasional infusion reaction complexes and rarely these have been fatal.

IMATINIB

In chronic myeloid leukaemia, the Philadelphia chromosome leads to production of an abnormal 'fusion protein' enzyme which continuously activates tyrosine kinase (TK) receptors. This causes uncontrolled cellular proliferation. A similar process occurs in **gastrointestinal stromal tumours (GIST)**, with activation of the **c-kit receptor**. Imatinib preferentially occupies the *TK* active receptor site, thereby decreasing the activity of several oncoprotein TK enzymes. As a result, the drug inhibits cellular proliferation and induces apoptosis (programmed cell death) in malignant cells.

THE FUTURE

Many other monoclonal antibodies and other small molecules that interfere with cellular receptors are under development or are already in clinical trials for a range of tumour types. It is likely that targeted therapies like this will improve the outcome for an increasing range of malignancies.

PALLIATIVE CARE

PRINCIPLES OF PALLIATIVE CARE

The principles of palliative care are outlined in Box 13.8. The diagnosis of cancer has immense significance to the patient and the patient's family. How it will affect them is governed by the type and spread of the cancer and by the treatment. Examples include:

- Psychological—adjustment reaction, anxiety, depression
- Social—loss of role: no longer able to care for family, no longer viewed as husband/wife/companion
- Financial—loss of job, expense of frequent hospital visits
- Spiritual—patient and family face up to mortality and ask questions about the meaning of life and their roles in the world
- Physical—pain, nausea, fatigue, dyspnoea

1. Palliative care is not just about dying people. Patients with cancer need to be helped to function as normally as they can for as long as they can. They often contemplate their own mortality and what is important to them

2. Ensure good communication by spending time with the patient and family (empathic listening and giving information according to the patient's needs are crucial). Some patients want more information than doctors give them; some want less. Find out about the patient in front of you. Explore the patient's concerns by asking open questions

3. Anticipate problems that might arise. Ensure that the patient/family know who to call if things go wrong. At an appropriate point, find out where a patient wants to die. Many choose home, some hospital. Hospices are another option. Terminal care at home needs coordinated planning. The family will often take most of the burden of care

4. Assess symptoms regularly. Medication may need to be changed frequently as the patient's condition changes

5. Be aware of different cultural practices and religious beliefs when caring for patients and families

6. Be aware of how looking after seriously ill patients can affect health care workers. Working as a team and discussing patients' care regularly helps professionals cope

In an effort to 'do all that is possible', there is a danger of concentrating on the primary disease while failing to treat the patient as a whole. Palliative care is concerned with addressing the problems listed above, but with the emphasis on the patient's own priorities, both during treatment and after treatment in those for whom cure is not possible.

Most patients with disseminated malignancy gradually deteriorate until they reach the terminal phase, when it becomes obvious that death will occur within the foreseeable future. A doctor's duty includes 'doing no harm' as well as trying to do some good, and there should be no ethical dilemma in withdrawing treatment that is unlikely to give benefit.

Increasingly, patients are living longer with an increased tumour load. Patients often experience complex symptoms with possible multiple aetiologies, resulting in treatment with multiple drugs. Diagnostic tests should be used judiciously to identify those causes that are remediable, but tests should be avoided that will not alter patient management. Proposed treatments should be negotiated with the patients and families, and time must be made available for clear and honest explanation. Palliative care focuses on **quality of life**, and addresses both physical and psychological needs of the patient and the family. Many clinicians, including family practitioners, are keen to look after their patients at the end of their lives and capable of doing so, ensuring a comfortable and dignified

demise. However, specialist palliative care physicians and nurses can support the primary care team and the patient and family in patients' homes and in specialist palliative care units (often called hospices).

APPROACH TO COMMON SYMPTOMS REQUIRING PALLIATION OTHER THAN PAIN

COMMUNICATION

Good communication is the foundation of palliative care. Giving patients and families time to talk about their thoughts and concerns will often in itself provide comfort. Patients may be concerned about their likely mode of death or how loved ones will cope when they are gone. Often, such worries can be allayed by these discussions.

Palliative pain relief is covered in the next section, and management of other common symptoms requiring palliation is detailed in Table 13.4. Effective management of the symptoms of advancing cancer requires frequent reassessment of the patient's condition, and frequent discussion with the patient to assess his or her own priorities. The doctor, patient and family need to work together to formulate a plan. Doctors must not hesitate to discuss complex situations with other colleagues and specialists to determine the best course of action.

Palliative care relies on a multidisciplinary team approach. Ideally, one health care worker (often in the primary care team) takes on the role of key worker and coordinates the patient's care and organises access to the specialist help needed.

Most patients will want to spend most of their time at home, away from hospital, supported by the primary care team, and many patients want to die at home. Terminal care at home is exhausting for families and they need support. The patient and family must know who they can contact, day or night, about problems if they arise. Handover between health professionals is increasingly important for care in the community. There should be immediate availability of specialist services and support, whether for admission or advice if needed. Family practitioners and community nurses often find palliative care a rewarding part of their jobs.

CANCER PAIN

About three-quarters of patients with advanced cancer have pain at some stage. How individuals perceive pain is influenced by the meaning of the pain to the patient (e.g. my cancer is getting worse), as well as other factors in the patient's life (social, spiritual and psychological), which, if deteriorating, can also worsen pain. Addressing these factors (in addition to appropriate analgesics) is an important way of helping these patients. Pain can be caused by:

Table 13.4 Common symptoms other than pain requiring palliation

Symptom	Causes	Management
Fatigue/asthenia (lack of energy)	Circulating factors released by tumour, chemotherapy, radiotherapy Pain, poor sleep, depression, anxiety	Open discussion with patient and family Encouraging gentle, regular exercise within limitations and a daily routine Address and treat remediable causes—check for anaemia Think of depression which often goes undiagnosed Think of a trial of corticosteroids
Loss of appetite (anorexia) and weight loss	Circulating factors released by tumour, chemotherapy, radiotherapy, chronic pain and nausea, fear, depression, anxiety, 'squashed stomach' syndrome, sore mouth, dysphagia	Explanation to patient and family of known causes Meticulous attention to oral hygiene Correct remediable factors Think of trial of corticosteroids or progestogen to stimulate appetite
Dysphagia	Tumours of pharynx, oesophagus and stomach Compression of oesophagus by extrinsic tumour (e.g. mediastinal lymph nodes) Oesophageal candidiasis	Options include insertion of stents, laser ablation, cryotherapy, brachytherapy (local radiotherapy) Radiotherapy, high-dose steroids Suspect in immunosuppressed patients or patients on steroids; diagnosis may require gastroscopy; may require prolonged treatment with oral antifungal agent
Nausea and vomiting	Drugs: opioids, NSAIDs and others Metabolic causes, e.g. hypercalcaemia, uraemia, liver failure Radiotherapy/chemotherapy Intracranial lesions causing raised intracranial pressure Gastric outlet obstruction Intestinal obstruction Constipation	Explanation to allay anxiety; review prescription Anti-emetic medication, e.g. haloperidol Anti-emetic drugs: cyclizine, short courses of $5HT_3$ antagonist and/or high-dose steroids High-dose steroids reducing to minimal maintenance dose, short course radiotherapy Prokinetic drugs, e.g. metoclopramide or domperidone If not candidate for surgery discuss with specialist. Needs honest discussion with patient—may not be able to stop patient being sick but should be able to reduce it If incomplete (e.g. no colic and passing wind) may benefit from prokinetic agents If complete, will need anti-secretory drugs (e.g. hyoscine butylbromide or octreotide) as well as anti-emetics (e.g. cyclizine or levomepromazine) Should be able to avoid nasogastric tube Prophylactic laxatives for all patients prescribed opioids; avoid bulk laxatives in preference to softening and stimulant agents
Breathlessness (dyspnoea), cough, choking	Pleural effusion, cardiac failure, infection, anaemia Laryngeal tumour, pulmonary tumour or major airway obstruction Lymphangitis carcinomatosa, multiple pulmonary metastases or infiltration Multifactorial: disease and debilitation Anxiety—common in breathlessness	Investigate and treat all reversible causes with regard to patient's overall condition May require stenting or local treatment, e.g. radiotherapy/laser/cryotherapy Trial of high-dose dexamethasone 16 mg daily; if beneficial reduce to maintenance dose, e.g. 2–4 mg daily Explanation to patient and family Trial of bronchodilator therapy Trial of intermittent oral morphine Trial of oxygen In terminal phase, continuous subcutaneous infusion of diamorphine and/or midazolam may be needed for sensation of breathlessness and associated anxiety Clear explanation, appropriate reassurance Anxiolytic drugs, e.g. small doses of lorazepam orally/sublingually or midazolam subcutaneously may help

Table 13.4 Common symptoms other than pain requiring palliation—cont'd

Symptom	Causes	Management
Constipation	There are many factors which make patients more likely to become constipated: immobility, weakness; general debility; poor oral intake; low dietary fibre; hypercalcaemia; hyperkalaemia Drugs, e.g. opioids and tricyclic antidepressants	Discuss nutritional options; encourage increased fluid intake; prescribe anti-emetic where nausea contributes to poor intake Laxatives: ● Bulking agents—should be reserved for moderately active patients with good fluid intake who are not on opioid medication ● Osmotic laxatives—lactulose (may cause flatulence and abdominal cramp); magnesium salts (sometimes unpalatable) ● Stimulants—senna, bisacodyl, danthron ● Lubricants—docusate (mainly a softener), liquid paraffin Often necessary to combine softening and stimulant agents Suppositories (glycerol and/or bisacodyl) Enemas sometimes necessary
Confusion	Unfamiliar stimuli Drugs, e.g. opioids, anticonvulsants, tricyclics Metabolic causes, e.g. uraemia, hypercalcaemia, hyponatraemia Cerebral metastases Infection Anxiety Cerebral hypoxia	Explanation and calming reassurance to patient and family Adequate lighting; familiar objects; minimise moving of patient within hospital Investigation and treatment of any reversible causes Medication if necessary: distressed patient may respond to oral or parenteral benzodiazepines, e.g. diazepam 5 mg b.d., or midazolam by continuous infusion; paranoid or hallucinating patients may require require haloperidol orally or subcutaneously, up to 20 mg/24 hours
Terminal restlessness (also known as terminal agitation/terminal anguish/terminal distress)	This is a diagnosis made by exclusion and can be distressing for the family	Explanation to family Rule out treatable causes: look for urinary retention; treat pain Sedation; often requires subcutaneous infusion, e.g. midazolam (benzodiazepine) 30–90 mg/24 hours ± levomepromazine 12.5–150 mg/24 h
'Death rattle' (i.e. distressing sounds of retained secretions in terminal stage of illness)	Accumulation of bronchial secretions and loss of control of muscles of larynx and pharynx	Explanation to family—more distressing to them than to the patient Positioning of patient often reduces sound and respiratory effort Early and continued use of antisecretory agent, e.g. glycopyrronium subcutaneously in divided doses or continuous infusion up to 1.2 mg/24 hours

- The cancer itself
- Treatment, e.g. oesophagitis following radiotherapy
- Debility leading to pressure sores
- Other illnesses, e.g. arthritis

ASSESSMENT OF PAIN

Patients frequently have more than one source of pain and each must be assessed carefully. Pain measurement tools (e.g. visual analogue or verbal rating scales) and charts can be helpful.

In assessing pain, it is most useful to use a classification that can help clinicians plan how to relieve it:

- Visceral pain—a constant 'tumour ache' caused by pressure of cancer or invasion of internal organs.

Although this can be severe, it is often sensitive to opioid medication
- Neuropathic pains—caused by pressure or destruction of nerves. Often patients find these pains difficult to describe, and that may be a clue to their aetiology. Sometimes words like 'tingling' or 'shooting' are used and the pain is in the distribution of a nerve root or peripheral nerve. Such pains are usually only partially responsive to opioids and require the use of adjuvant analgesics such as tricyclic antidepressants (e.g. amitriptyline), anti-epileptics (e.g. gabapentin) or corticosteroids to reduce oedema around tumours
- Bone pain—caused by infiltration of cancer into bones. Clinical features depend on the location of

the disease, e.g. bony spinal lesions may cause pressure on the spinal cord causing nerve pain, anaesthesia and weakness. Lesions of the skull base can lead to cranial nerve palsies

Often bony metastases lead to **incident pain** in which pain is tolerable at rest but becomes much worse with movement. This is often difficult to treat and requires the combination of local radiotherapy and bisphosphonate infusions (particularly in breast and prostate cancers and myeloma), together with analgesics. Note that incident pains are not usually responsive to opioids but that adjuvants (mentioned above) may help. It is often helpful to take extra medication before the activity that leads to pain.

PRINCIPLES OF CANCER PAIN MANAGEMENT

- The aim is to control pain as well as possible, with a balance between analgesia and the side effects of medication
- Analgesia should be given regularly not just as required ('p.r.n.')
- Analgesics should be titrated against the severity of pain using the three-step analgesic ladder developed by the World Health Organization (see Fig. 13.2). A patient who has reached the top of Step 2 but with pain believed to be opioid responsive should be given a strong opioid

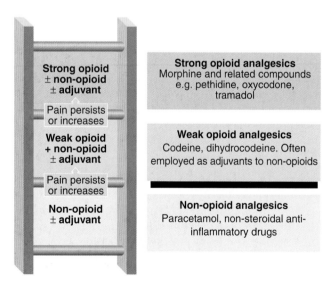

Fig. 13.2 Three-step analgesic ladder for cancer pain control (WHO 1986) (see Table 13.5 for adjuvants)
The World Health Organization has stated that pain relief should be:
(i) by the mouth—oral medication if possible
(ii) by the clock—regularly, not 'as required' (p.r.n.)
(iii) by the ladder—if, after reaching top dose on one rung of the ladder, pain is not controlled, go up the ladder

OPIOID ANALGESIA

Several strong opioids are listed on Step 3 of the WHO ladder but morphine is generally the one of choice. Most patients can be suitably managed for their pain relief with oral morphine, with the dose being titrated up or down according to analgesic requirements. Different pains vary in how sensitive they are to opioids, but for severe pain, no matter what the mechanism, an opioid trial is worth undertaking. Addiction is not a problem amongst cancer patients—they need the painkillers to treat their pain. If the pain abates in patients taking morphine, for example after radiotherapy, it is easy to reduce and sometimes to stop morphine. Nevertheless, this should be done gradually to prevent physical withdrawal symptoms.

Tolerance and diminishing effectiveness of morphine is uncommon, even among patients who take the drug for months. If a patient on a stable dose evidently requires an increase, this usually reflects disease progression.

Gradually increasing the dose of morphine according to the response avoids **respiratory depression**. This generally occurs only where the prescribed dose is excessive (greater than analgesic requirements), or where morphine metabolites accumulate because of reduced elimination, e.g. in renal impairment.

When considering starting morphine therapy, it is important to discuss the process with the patient and family to allay misconceptions. Some associate the need for morphine with imminent death, whilst others fear addiction or side effects.

Strong opioids are administered parenterally when patients cannot take oral medication because of dysphagia, persistent nausea, vomiting or profound fatigue. The intravenous route can be used in hospital but the **subcutaneous route** is preferred if the patient is managed at home. This route is suitable for single 'breakthrough' doses (less painful than intramuscularly) and for continuous infusion. Infusions are given via an indwelling 'butterfly' needle, usually controlled with a battery-operated syringe driver holding enough solution for 24 hours. In the UK, **diamorphine** is preferred to morphine because smaller volumes provide equianalgesic doses.

Establishing treatment

Once the use of morphine has been discussed and agreed with the patient, the preferred method for establishing dosage is by **titration**. The usual starting dose will be 5–10 mg of immediate-release morphine 4-hourly (or 2.5–5 mg for elderly patients). For those with renal or liver impairment or in the very elderly, a 6–8-hourly interval may be required. To accompany the regular 4-hourly dose, the same dose should be prescribed on an 'as required' basis for pain which 'breaks through' before the

Table 13.5 Adjuvant analgesics and other treatments for management of cancer pain

Treatment method	Indications
Non-steroidal anti-inflammatory agents—via oral/rectal/transdermal routes	Reduce inflammatory component in pain. Have a role for bony and other musculo-skeletal pains and may help neuropathic pains
Tricyclic antidepressants (usually as single evening dose)	Used in treatment of neuropathic pain. Also help patients to sleep. Can help mood as dose is increased
Anticonvulsants (e.g. gabapentin)	Valuable for neuropathic pain
Antispasmodics (e.g. hyoscine butylbromide—Buscopan)	Reduce visceral contractions in colicky visceral pain (intestinal, biliary, ureteric) and overt bowel obstruction
Muscle relaxants (e.g. diazepam)	Relieve muscle spasms
Antibiotics (e.g. metronidazole tablets or gel)	Help treat infected superficial lesions, e.g. ulcerated skin, breast or head and neck tumours (usually involve Gram-negative organisms)
Corticosteroids (e.g. dexamethasone 4–8 mg daily, prednisolone 30–60 mg daily) Dexamethasone causes less fluid retention	Shrink oedema associated with tumour to relieve pressure effects, e.g. cerebral tumours, spinal cord and peripheral nerve compression, liver capsule stretching, tumour swelling causing obstruction to bowel, biliary or urinary tracts
Topical anti-inflammatory agents	For oral and nasal mucositis, ulcerated skin lesions, radiation proctitis
Local palliative radiotherapy	For bone metastases, compressive lesions of brain and spinal cord, large airway and superior vena caval obstruction, fungating or bleeding superficial lesions
Bisphosphonates (e.g. pamidronate, clodronate)	Predominantly used for the relief of bone pain in metastatic breast cancer, and multiple myeloma. Can be given parenterally as bolus or continuously as oral therapy
Radioactive isotope therapy	Used for the relief of bone pain due to metastatic disease
Palliative chemotherapy	Sometimes relieves pain by shrinkage of chemosensitive tumours
Nerve blocks (often under radiological guidance)	Very helpful in treating pain in specific areas, e.g. intercostal blocks for chest wall pain, coeliac plexus blocks for pancreatic and other 'foregut' pain. Often reduce the overall requirement for systemic analgesia
Physiotherapy and associated physical modalities (e.g. massage, TENS, hot or cold packs)	Muscle spasm, inflammatory component of pains. Massage for muscle spasms and lymphoedema. TENS may help neuropathic pain
Skeletal immobilisation	Elective internal fixation of long bones for incipient or actual pathological fracture of long bones

next dose is due. If morphine helps the pain, the next day's regular dose (and p.r.n. dose) is $1/6$ of the total given in the previous 24 hours, or $1/2$ for slow-release morphine. If morphine does not help the pain, another analgesic approach is needed.

Successful treatment of cancer pain throughout the patient's life depends on carefully listening to the patient and carers to understand the changing situation, regular reassessment and detailed examination and documentation (using a pain chart wherever appropriate). A doctor working with a multidisciplinary team can achieve effective, acceptable pain relief for most patients. The patient can then concentrate on what to him or her constitutes a good quality of life.

A variety of other opioids are used less commonly in palliative care and usually for specific indications. These are summarised in Table 13.6.

Side effects of morphine and other opioids

The following should be remembered when commencing morphine:

- **Constipation** is common—prescribe a laxative and explain the need for regular use
- **Nausea** tends to occur at the onset of treatment and whenever the dose is increased but usually improves spontaneously. Prescribe an anti-emetic 'as required'

Table 13.6 Opioid drugs used in palliative care

Analgesic	Equianalgesic dose of oral morphine	Duration of action	Indications
Codeine 60 mg	6 mg	4–6 hours	Codeine or dihydrocodeine alone or in combination with paracetamol are used to treat mild to moderate pain May cause nausea or constipation
Tramadol 50 mg	5 mg	6 hours	Its effect on monoamine reuptake means that theoretically it may be useful for neuropathic pain
Diamorphine injection 10 mg	20–30 mg	4 hours	Where local regulations permit, it is preferred to morphine if parenteral route required as high solubility means smaller injection volume. Side effects as morphine
Fentanyl transdermal patch Lowest dose now 12 µg/hr	12 µg/hr equivalent to 30–60 mg of oral morphine in 24 hours	72 hours	Patch works by releasing depot drug into the skin. Takes 12 hours to reach analgesic levels so breakthrough treatment must be available when starting *Contraindicated* in unstable pain Often preferred to oral tablets by patients. Causes less constipation
Fentanyl lozenges Lowest dose 200 µg		1–4 hours	Can start to have its effect after 5– 10 minutes. May be useful for patients with incident pain who can take a lozenge before they want to move
Methadone 5 mg syrup	5–10 mg when given as single dose. Much more potent once drug has accumulated	4–5 hours single dose 6–12 hours after repeated doses	Used in specialist units; initial titration often complex owing to prolonged and variable half-life. Used in low dose, e.g. 2–5 mg nocte, for cough suppression
Oxycodone 5 mg—lowest strength capsule	10 mg	4–6 hours	May be better tolerated in some patients (e.g. elderly) as may cause fewer side effects, particularly confusion or hallucinations. Should be used only as second-line to morphine

N.B. There is no role for meptazinol or pethidine in the long-term treatment of cancer pain as they have limitations, e.g. analgesic ceiling, short duration of action, or accumulation of toxic metabolites, which render them unsuitable for regular long-term use

- **Drowsiness** resolves over 48–72 hours; if it does not, reduce dose or seek alternative strong opioid
- **Confusion, hallucinations**—especially in the elderly, if the starting dose is too high or the dose increased too rapidly. Look for renal impairment, hypercalcaemia or other causes. Reduce the dose if possible. Consider the use of an alternative strong opioid
- **Myoclonic spasms**, e.g. jerking—can occur if opioid dose is too high or if morphine metabolites build up because of renal impairment
- **Itch or bronchospasm**—occur occasionally and require a change to an alternative strong opioid

14

Principles of transplantation surgery

INTRODUCTION

Many patients face death because a single organ system such as kidney, liver, lungs or heart is failing, but could return to health if organ function could be restored. It is not surprising that physicians over the years have tried to achieve this directly, by transplanting a healthy organ from an animal or another human.

The scene for clinical organ transplantation was set early in the 20th century by Alexis Carrel. He was awarded the Nobel Prize for Physiology and Medicine in 1912 for his pioneering work in vascular surgery and transplantation with Charles Guthrie. Carrel, working with laboratory animals, found that **autografts** (organs removed and reimplanted into the same animal) could be expected to function indefinitely whereas **allografts** (organs transplanted between animals of the same species) rarely functioned for more than a few days. Early attempts at transplantation in man used **xenografts** (transplantation between different species) to transfer renal tissue from pigs, goats, rabbits and apes; these were uniformly unsuccessful.

The key to organ transplantation lay in the developing field of immunology, first with detection of the mechanisms involved in **graft rejection** and then the elaboration and application of techniques to minimise or prevent it. The first clinically useful transplant for humans involved pig heart valves. These consisted of simple avascular tissue, treated to render it non-immunogenic so as to avoid rejection. Porcine cardiac valve transplants have been used regularly in humans since the mid 1970s and have advantages over artificial valves in younger people and those in whom anticoagulation must be avoided.

Chemical immunosuppression designed to attenuate graft rejection has continued to advance, leading to improving success rates with transplantation of an expanding range of organs and tissues (see Table 14.1). Human cornea, kidney, liver, pancreas, heart, heart and lung, single or double lung and bone marrow transplantation are all now accepted as standard, although they are by no means free of rejection and other complications (see: http://www.ctstransplant.org/).

Promising results are latterly being achieved with small bowel transplantation for carefully selected patients with massive bowel loss. If recipient patients also have liver disease or extensive intra-abdominal desmoid formation (a rare tumour caused by proliferation of fibroblastic cells), **composite grafts** of more than one abdominal organ may be transplanted simultaneously. These are known as **cluster grafts** or **multivisceral transplants**, but are still uncommon outside a few highly specialised centres. The ultimate goal of transplant surgeons and immunologists is to be able to generate a state of **tolerance** between the graft and the recipient of a transplanted organ.

211

Table 14.1 Numbers of transplants performed during 1997 and 2003 in Europe and the USA

Organ	Europe		USA	
	1997	2003	1997	2003
Kidney Living donor	953	1 805	3386	6468
Cadaveric donor	11 193	12 119	7599	8389
Heart	2 402	1 998	2253	2022
Liver	4 018	4 961	3924	5039
Pancreas alone	98	156	194	460
Kidney + pancreas	285	450	841	846
Intestine	9	30	61	109

Organ transplantation already offers improved quality of life to renal transplant recipients and endows life itself to recipients of heart or liver grafts. This type of surgery is impossible without the generosity of carriers of donor cards and bereaved families in making organs available for transplantation. However, the UK donation rate of 12 donors per million population per year still lags behind the rate of 30–40 per million achieved in comparable European countries such as Austria, Spain and Northern Italy. This suggests that many more patients could benefit if the acceptability of these innovative procedures to the UK community could be enhanced. To achieve this, the results of this type of surgery and the ethical basis under which it is conducted need to be promoted more widely.

TRANSPLANT IMMUNOLOGY

MAJOR HISTOCOMPATIBILITY COMPLEX

Most tissue cells have a number of different surface **glycoproteins** which excite a response from the recipient's immune system if transplanted from one individual to another. These **histocompatibility antigens** are recognised by the recipient's immunocytes and the response generated involves both cell-mediated and humoral mechanisms. These responses cause destruction of the transplanted cells.

Each individual has several histocompatibility antigens but only one group is responsible for major graft rejection problems. These **major histocompatibility antigens** are coded for by a set of genes known as the **major histocompatibility complex (MHC)**. In humans, the MHC is located on a segment of the short arm of chromosome 6. It was first discovered in leucocytes and, although now shown to be present in all cells, it is still known as the **HLA complex** (human lymphocyte antigen system A). Within the human MHC, two major groups of antigens have been described known as class I and class II antigens, each with different structures and specificities. The principal class I loci are the **A and B antigens** and the principal class II loci are the **DR antigens**. Since each individual receives one set of genetic information from each parent, there are six principal loci (two each for A, B and DR) and any two individuals can differ at any or all of these loci. Certain HLA types are associated with particular autoimmune disorders, notably ankylosing spondylitis and coeliac disease, although the reason is unknown.

TISSUE TYPING AND TRANSPLANT SHARING SCHEMES

HLA typing of individuals is used to match the donor and recipient as closely as possible. In kidney transplantation, close HLA matching has been shown to give significantly improved graft survival, i.e. when donor and recipient are identical at all six loci or differ by only one A or B antigen. These grafts are known as **beneficial matches**. Tissue typing is usually performed serologically using specific antisera. More recently, increased accuracy has been obtained using new **DNA analysis based techniques** ('DNA fingerprinting').

Most developed countries have a national transplant sharing mechanism so that donors and recipients can be matched as closely and fairly as possible. Systems are designed to achieve an optimal balance between **utility** (the optimum use of a specific organ in terms of graft survival) and **equity** of access (the chance that an individual patient will receive a graft within a reasonable period). This typically combines the important matter of tissue matching with a range of other factors such as time on the waiting list.

The pattern of inheritance of tissue types within families shows that each child receives one set of genetic information (**haplotype**) from each parent. Siblings have a 1 in 4 chance of being **haplo-identical** and a 1 in 2 chance of having one haplotype in common. Fully HLA-matched sibling donors give the best chance of graft survival, followed by those with one haplotype in common. Other than the special case of monozygotic twins, there is still some rejection in HLA identical grafts between siblings owing to differences in minor histocompatibility antigens. ABO blood group compatibility is an obvious prerequisite for organ transplantation which must not be overlooked in the search for ever closer HLA matching.

IMMUNOSUPPRESSION

With all major organ transplants, the recipient's immune response must be suppressed, even if there is full HLA compatibility, so that rejection and graft loss can be minimised. Immunosuppressive therapy needs to be continued indefinitely, although dosage can usually be progressively reduced to maintenance levels after high-dose **induction therapy**. This is because a partly tolerant state is established by the diminution of the **host-versus-graft** response with time. Immunosuppressive drugs are employed in combination therapies, designed to allow lower doses of individual agents to minimise the side effects of each one, whilst optimising immunosuppression. The most widely used combination is **prednisolone**, **azathioprine** and **ciclosporin.**

In many cases, **polyclonal or monoclonal** antilymphocyte or antithymocyte globulins are added in the induction period. A recent significant alternative, now widely employed in induction for renal transplantation, has been the use of monoclonal antibodies directed at blocking the interleukin-2 (IL2) receptor.

Ciclosporin, a calcineurin inhibitor, represented a major advance over the earlier combination of azathioprine and corticosteroids, markedly improving graft survival after it was introduced in 1978. However, it has substantial side effects of its own in the form of nephrotoxicity, neurotoxicity, facial sebaceous hyperplasia causing coarsening of skin (most noticeable in young women) and a tendency to produce hirsutism.

In the search for better immunosuppressive drugs, ciclosporin has been modified to give more predictable gastrointestinal absorption, and new drugs continually appear. **Tacrolimus** is a macrolide; it is a potent immunosuppressive agent functioning as a calcineurin inhibitor, inhibiting the immune response in a manner similar to ciclosporin but with similar nephrotoxicity and neurotoxicity. Tacrolimus has largely replaced ciclosporin for liver transplantation, but both agents are still used in renal transplantation. Other newer agents include the antimetabolite **mycophenolate mofetil (MMF)**, which is now widely used in place of azathioprine. **Sirolimus (rapamycin)** is an alternative primary immunosuppressive agent to the calcineurin inhibitors and has the advantage that it does not have the nephrotoxic and hypertensive side effects of these agents. The abundance of new agents allows a tailored approach to immunosuppression for individual cases; this remains an exciting and important area of transplant research.

Complications of immunosuppression

All of these drugs, by their nature, suppress lymphocyte proliferation, antibody production and inflammation in varying degrees, and complications include impaired wound healing, peptic ulceration, vulnerability to infection, bone marrow suppression and occasionally development of malignancy (especially Epstein–Barr virus-related lymphoproliferative disorders). Each of the newer agents has its own unique side effect profile. In particular, mycophenolate mofetil may cause gastrointestinal disturbances, whilst sirolimus (rapamycin) is associated with hyperlipidaemias, mouth ulcers and occasionally pneumonitis. The long-term consequences of these hyperlipidaemias are unclear but it is interesting to note that sirolimus-coated coronary artery stents are associated with a reduced rate of reocclusion.

GRAFT REJECTION

Graft rejection continues to be a problem despite the increasing range of immunosuppressive agents. It can present in several ways:

HYPERACUTE REJECTION

This occurs within minutes or hours of transplantation and is caused by the presence of preformed antibodies resulting from previous transplantation, blood transfusion, pregnancy or ABO incompatibility. These antibodies can be detected if serum from the potential organ recipient is cross-matched with leucocytes from the lymph nodes or spleen of cadaveric donors or peripheral blood of living donors.

ACUTE REJECTION

This is a cell-mediated response and is common. Even with optimal immunosuppression, up to 30% of recipients are affected. Acute rejection usually occurs within 2 weeks in first-time grafts; it can usually be reversed by a temporary increase in immunosuppression, most often in the form of a short course of high-dose corticosteroid treatment or a brief course of antilymphocyte globulin.

CHRONIC REJECTION

This occurs months to years after transplantation and is probably the result of antibody-mediated rejection. It can occur even with effective long-term immunosuppression. It is often associated with gradual occlusion of arteries in the graft.

PRACTICAL PROBLEMS OF TRANSPLANTATION

SOURCES OF ORGANS FOR TRANSPLANTATION

Most tissues for transplantation are derived from cadaveric donors, with the organs being removed from the body as soon as possible after death has been confirmed. Any previously fit subject who becomes brain-dead as a consequence of a head injury, an intracranial vascular catastrophe or a primary intracerebral tumour can be a potential donor of intra-abdominal or intrathoracic organs; the last of these is acceptable because of the presence of an intact blood–brain barrier. Sufferers with these conditions have usually been resuscitated from the outset, with the circulation and respiration being maintained artificially. From such **'heart-beating'** donors, multi-organ donation procedures allow all appropriate organs to be removed and maintained in optimal condition for transplantation. Non-heart-beating donors can be used for bone, skin and corneal donation. Other organs such as kidneys and, more recently, livers can be transplanted from **controlled non-heart-beating donation**. These are donor patients with a hopeless prognosis where treatment is withdrawn in an intensive care setting. This allows the organs to be rapidly removed following cessation of the circulation.

Living-related and living-unrelated donation

In the case of kidney transplantation, donation from living family members gives excellent results. Initially, the UK was slow in accepting this option compared with the United States and Scandinavia, but this has now been reversed and a steadily increasing proportion of kidney grafts is now obtained in this manner.

Living unrelated donation (for example spousal donation) is also being practised more, again with remarkably good results despite the lack of tissue matching intrinsic to living-related cases. The risk to the donor is now small and laparoscopic live donor nephrectomy has improved the recovery time for donors and thus increased the acceptability of live donation. This procedure involves the kidney being mobilised laparoscopically before being removed via an incision substantially shorter than the conventional loin incision.

Living donation of livers is also becoming more common. It was introduced to allow donation of a small portion of the left liver from parent to child, but has now expanded to include right liver donation, which allows adult to adult transplantation. The risks for the donor are greater than in kidney donation. In countries such as Japan where the availability of cadaveric organs is limited for cultural reasons, these procedures are the mainstay of organ transplantation. The growing shortage of organs for transplantation has led to this technique being adopted even in countries where cadaveric liver transplantation is well established.

'BRAIN DEATH'

In many countries, criteria have been established to form a legal definition of brain death following irreversible brain stem injury, even in the presence of an intact circulatory system. Once the established criteria have been satisfied, and appropriate consent obtained from relatives, the subject becomes eligible for 'heart-beating' organ donation. The legal criteria for brain death in the UK are summarised in Box 14.1; similar criteria are used in other countries.

The diagnosis of brain death is made on the basis of purely clinical criteria in the UK. Electrocardiography, cerebral blood flow and other neurophysiological tests are not required. Appropriate clinical examination must, however, be performed by two senior doctors independent of the transplant team and must be repeated at least twice.

CONSENT

It is usual to seek the agreement of a potential donor's close relatives and to determine whether he or she had expressed any objection to donation during life. The matter is simplified if the potential donor carries a donor card, has placed his or her name on the national organ donor register or has left other written instructions for the family. The difficulty many doctors face in informing

---

Box 14.1 Legal criteria for diagnosis of brain death (UK)

Note this diagnosis is clinical and does not require special tests

1. There must be a positive diagnosis of severe structural brain damage
2. The condition causing brain damage must be irreversible
3. There must be complete loss of brain stem function— evidenced by fixed pupils, no spontaneous eye movements or response to caloric testing, absent corneal, eyelash and blink reflexes, absent laryngeal and cough reflexes, and no response to deep painful stimuli (note: some spinal reflexes may be retained despite brain death)
4. On removal of ventilatory support, there must be no spontaneous respiratory activity in the presence of a physiologically adequate increase in PCO_2
5. Any possible effects of hypothermia and drugs (e.g. muscle relaxants, respiratory depressants, alcohol) must be excluded

relatives of the death of a family member is compounded by having to request organ donation at the same time. However, this can be eased by knowing that the bereaved often gain consolation from knowing other lives will be saved by the donated organs and these gains can be set against their own loss. Awareness of the potential gains and benefits of transplantation can be increased by informed education and better availability of information for members of the public and for the medical profession.

ORGAN PRESERVATION AND TRANSPORT

Donors are often located in hospitals many miles from where the recipient operation is to be performed. There may also be delay in locating the recipient, and in getting the recipient into hospital and ready for operation. As a result, the organ to be transplanted is usually removed from the donor several hours before transplantation, driving the search for reliable techniques for organ preservation. **Hypothermia** alone reduces the metabolic demands of the organ and is the main method of organ preservation. The period of **warm ischaemia** is the time from circulatory arrest to effective cooling of the organ by perfusion with ice-cold preservation fluid. Warm ischaemia must be kept to a minimum to prevent irreversible damage to the organ. For kidneys, normal function will usually recover if warm ischaemia does not exceed 40–60 minutes. Longer periods of warm ischaemia result in markedly impaired function as a result of acute tubular necrosis but this can usually be overcome by continued haemodialysis until recovery of donor organ function. For the liver and heart, immediate function after transplantation is clearly essential and warm ischaemia must be avoided.

Two main methods are used for preserving organs between donation and transplantation:

- **Simple cold storage**. The organ is flushed with ice-cold preservation solution and stored at 0–4°C on ice. Using specially formulated solutions containing compounds designed to counter hypothermic cell swelling, it is now possible to store kidneys for 24–36 hours, livers for 12–18 hours and hearts for 4–6 hours
- **Continuous oxygenated hypothermic pulsatile perfusion** using special colloid-based (starch, plasma or albumin) solutions. This technique is more complicated and more expensive but enables kidneys to be stored for 2–3 days. The equipment is portable and can be used during transportation but the technique has not yet been extended to clinical preservation of other organs

SPECIFIC ORGAN TRANSPLANTS

KIDNEY TRANSPLANTS

Kidney transplantation is the longest established and most widely practised of solid organ transplants. It offers a substantial improvement in quality of life for patients with end-stage chronic renal failure who are otherwise faced with twice- or thrice-weekly haemodialysis or a regimen of continuous daily treatment with chronic ambulatory peritoneal dialysis. Donor organs can be obtained from any otherwise healthy donor up to 70 years of age or even older in certain cases.

The kidney is transplanted into an extraperitoneal location in the iliac fossa and the renal vessels are anastomosed to the iliac artery and vein (see Fig. 14.1). The ureter is implanted into the bladder using an intramural tunnel to prevent reflux. The non-functioning kidneys are usually left in situ unless infected or causing unmanageable hypertension.

The signs of **early acute rejection** of the kidney are oliguria, proteinuria, and pain and tenderness of the transplanted kidney. Luckily, this relatively common form of rejection can be easily reversed in most cases. Overall results of renal transplantation have steadily improved owing to more effective long-term immunosuppression and better-quality organs from 'heart-beating' brain-dead donors or living related donors. The survival rate of transplanted kidneys can be as high as 90–95% at 1 year. This falls by 5–10% each year thereafter, although there is evidence that the beneficial matching policy now in use may reduce the late graft attrition rate caused by chronic rejection.

HEART AND LUNG TRANSPLANTS

Cardiac transplantation has become a standard treatment for patients with ischaemic heart disease that is not amenable to coronary artery bypass grafting, and for patients with certain cardiomyopathies. A standard operative technique has been established employing **orthotopic** placement of the organ, i.e. replacing the diseased organ in the same anatomical location. The donor atria and graft vessels are sutured directly to those of the recipient. Monitoring for early rejection requires regular right-heart catheterisation and endomyocardial biopsy.

Using immunosuppressive protocols similar to those for kidney transplantation, the results of cardiac transplantation are now excellent, although the limited number of available donor organs means that cardiac transplantation is unlikely to ever be an option for all that could benefit. Novel techniques of **genetic engineering** have raised the possibility of breeding animals such as pigs with a specially engineered genetic make-up to allow

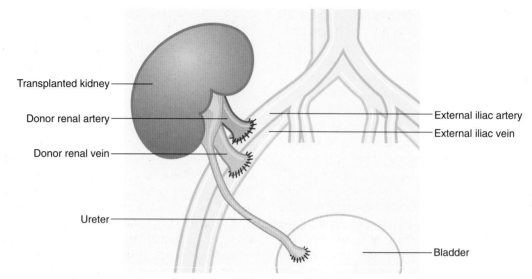

Fig. 14.1 Renal transplantation
The usual site for the transplanted kidney is in the pelvis, with anastomoses being constructed between the donor renal artery and vein, and the recipient iliac artery and vein, and between donor ureter and recipient bladder.

xenografts to be performed successfully. No such specially bred **transgenic** transplants have yet been performed in humans.

Combined heart and lung transplants are now also accepted as a standard treatment for patients with certain irreversible lung diseases such as cystic fibrosis, and good results are now obtained in specialist centres. Many cases have secondary heart disease and require a combined heart–lung transplant. In other cases the recipient's heart is healthy and can be transplanted into another patient; this is known as the **domino heart** procedure. Single or even double lung transplants are now also performed successfully in carefully selected patients with chronic respiratory failure.

LIVER TRANSPLANTS

The indications for liver transplantation in adults are end-stage non-malignant parenchymal liver disease, acute hepatic failure and certain inborn errors of hepatic metabolism. In children, liver-based inborn errors of metabolism and biliary atresia are the most common indications; the operation often needs to be performed during early infancy. Primary liver malignancies such as cholangiocarcinoma and hepatocellular carcinoma larger than 5 cm, and metastatic liver disease are no longer accepted as indications for liver transplantation as these malignancies inevitably recur early after transplantation in the immunosuppressed patient.

Rejection of the liver is less of problem than in kidney transplantation but the operation is more challenging. Most patients have advanced liver disease with disordered coagulation and often severe portal hypertension. A team

approach has evolved, with close cooperation between surgeons and specialist liver transplant anaesthetists. The diseased liver is removed and the new liver put in its place, the vena cava, portal vein and hepatic artery being reanastomosed in turn. Careful surgical technique combined with skilled anaesthetic monitoring and intraoperative replacement of clotting factors has transformed the procedure, and average blood loss during surgery is now only about 3 litres.

Results have improved greatly since the first liver transplant in 1963 and 1-year patient survival rates of 85–90% and 5-year survival figures of 70–75% are now standard (http://www.eltr.org/publi/index_rv.php3). For paediatric cases, the problem of an inadequate supply of donor organs has been solved by using reduced-size liver grafts. Either a lobe or a segment from a full-size adult organ can be transplanted, thus allowing disparities in size of up to 10 to 1 between donor and recipient. An adult liver can be divided into two parts to allow a child and an adult to receive grafts from a single donor organ. Techniques developed from living-related liver transplantation have more recently been extended to allow a liver graft to be divided for two adult recipients.

The late graft attrition rate for liver transplants appears to be much lower than for kidney grafts even though matching is by blood group only, without tissue typing. The 'Achilles heel' of liver grafting remains complications with the bile duct anastomosis. This can be performed using a direct duct-to-duct anastomosis or a Roux-en-Y loop but despite meticulous surgical technique, the complication rate from biliary strictures or leaks is still 10–15%. A further substantial problem is the increased risk of recurrent disease in the transplanted liver, particularly when the indication for transplantation is hepatitis C. Antiviral therapies are appearing but are not yet fully effective.

PANCREAS TRANSPLANTS

Pancreas transplantation offers the tantalising hope of a real cure for diabetes, thus avoiding its many late complications. These include myocardial ischaemia, peripheral vascular disease, peripheral neuropathy, nephropathy leading to renal failure and retinopathy leading to blindness. The pancreas presents a particular problem as the gland combines endocrine and exocrine function. The currently favoured technique involves transplanting the whole pancreas with a small segment of duodenum. The graft is placed in the pelvis and its vessels anastomosed to the iliac vessels in the same way as a kidney graft. In the initial technique for whole pancreas transplantation, the attached duodenal segment was anastomosed to the urinary bladder, allowing the exocrine secretions to drain into the urine. This technique has been largely replaced by one where the pancreas is anastomosed to a Roux-en-Y loop of bowel that gives enteric drainage of its enzymes. Graft survival rates of 70–80% are now being obtained and there is growing evidence that these grafts can arrest, and sometimes even partly reverse, the long-term complications of diabetes (http://www.iptr.umn.edu/). Currently, most pancreatic transplants are performed in diabetic patients with established renal failure and advanced complications of their disease. In these, the pancreatic transplant is combined with a renal transplant.

A different approach is transplantation of pancreatic endocrine tissue alone. This is achieved by transplanting **human islet cells** that have been extracted from pancreas by collagenase digestion. The islets are injected into the portal venous system and lodge in the liver sinusoids. The yield from extraction techniques has improved markedly, allowing a substantial percentage of the islets to be recovered from each pancreas. Technical developments have also improved the success rate but since it requires islet cells from more than one donor to achieve euglycaemia, it is less efficacious than whole pancreas transplantation whilst there remains a shortage of organ donors.

SMALL BOWEL TRANSPLANTS

A relatively recent advance in organ transplantation has been the development of small bowel transplantation. There is a growing number of patients who have lost all or most of their small bowel as a result of vascular problems, volvulus, necrotising enterocolitis, atresias or Crohn's disease, who are maintained on long-term parenteral nutrition. Specialist units can sustain such patients in good health for many years but the technique is expensive, inconvenient for the patients and leaves them at constant risk of infective complications from feeding lines as well as liver disease related to parenteral feeding. Small bowel may be transplanted alone or in combination with the liver in the case of coexisting irreversible liver disease. Experience is growing, with close to 1000 cases worldwide being recorded in the most recent international registry report (http://www.intestinaltransplant.org/). The indications for these techniques are still being considered, but results are expected to continue improving. In fact, it is beginning to rival long-term total parenteral nutrition in terms of survival, and already has clear advantages in quality of life.

POSTSCRIPT

Organ transplantation represents a stimulating fusion of complex surgical techniques with basic sciences that include immunology. Surgical techniques and basic sciences continue to improve year on year, gradually giving better technical results and hence better outcomes for patients. The success of transplantation generally has extended the range of potential transplant recipients into more technically demanding areas but the downside of this expansion is an exacerbation of the shortage of organ donors. As a result, innovations in the field of living organ donation are increasing the number of living kidney donors and driving other developments such as living liver donation. Transplantation is still evolving as a discipline, and its successes to date have increased the challenges rather than diminishing them.

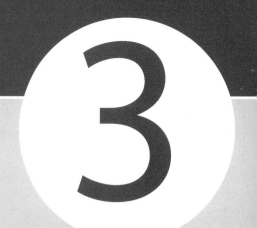

Principles of accident surgery

Major trauma

15

INTRODUCTION

Major trauma regularly captures the headlines but is statistically a relatively rare event in the UK and most of Europe. Major trauma is much more common in other parts of the world, some with much higher rates of road traffic collisions (e.g. Saudi Arabia) and yet others, higher levels of personal violence (e.g. South Africa, parts of the USA). Nevertheless, major trauma is the most common cause of death in young people almost everywhere.

For victims who survive the immediate trauma, there are two periods when there is a particularly high risk of death. The first occurs during the first or 'golden' hour after the accident (see next section) and the second occurs over the next few hours. Survival in the golden hour depends on the severity of injury, the competence of immediate care and the speed of transfer to an accident unit (in the UK, the average time to transport a non-trapped trauma victim to hospital is a surprising 57 minutes). Deaths after the first hour are for the most part avoidable, being largely caused by treatable conditions.

This chapter discusses the principles of management of serious and multiple injuries (including pre-hospital care, life support and resuscitation, assessment and triage, and prioritising urgent surgery), abdominal and thoracic injuries and major orthopaedic injuries.

PRE-HOSPITAL ASSESSMENT AND INTERVENTION

INTRODUCTION

The golden hour is a concept that comes from US war experience, popularised by Dr. R. Adams Cowley, a military surgeon. Severe injuries that cause substantial internal or external bleeding cause rapid circulatory decompensation for which the only effective treatment is likely to be expert management of shock and surgical arrest of bleeding. Thus, action to minimise the interval between injury and treatment gives the best chance of survival. Experience has shown that without treatment the survival rate in such patients falls off dramatically beyond 60 minutes. Rapid essential care at the accident scene and swift transport to a trauma centre is the key. This strategy is known as **scoop and run**, as opposed to **stay and play** that is best employed for less severe cases, in which the physiological derangement caused by transportation may be more detrimental than extending the period before hospital treatment.

ASSESSMENT AT THE SCENE OF THE ACCIDENT

'Reading the wreckage' could at one time give an idea of the likely patterns and severity of injury to passengers involved. However, modern cars have such sophisticated crumple zones that the visible damage gives little clue to the injuries. Major vehicle distortion may not cause severe injury, but such injuries can occur with apparently minor damage. The nature of damage to involved vehicles can provide some information, as the worst injuries tend to occur in head-on collisions or those affecting the front corners. Some estimate can also be obtained of whether there was a high- or low-velocity impact. If any passengers were killed or thrown out of vehicles, this indicates a high-velocity impact. Points to check include whether head restraints were in place, whether seatbelts were worn and whether airbags deployed. For motorcycle crashes it is best to assume that victims all have pelvic fractures until proved wrong. When a pedestrian is hit by a car, a 'bullseye' fracture of the car windscreen indicates a likely severe head injury.

Obvious injuries (e.g. traumatic amputations) are sought in the victims and their level of consciousness and mobility assessed. Trapped wounded need special treatment as they often have long extrication times and need analgesia, intravenous fluids and perhaps sedation to aid release. Trapped patients can quickly become hypothermic, and rapidly become hypovolaemic and acutely anaemic if major vessels are damaged (see Fig. 15.1). Note the problems of transfusing blood in the pre-hospital situation.

PREVENTION OF SECONDARY INJURIES AND DAMAGE

Primary injuries are those that result directly from the trauma. Secondary injuries occur as an indirect result of the trauma, e.g. secondary brain damage from hypoxia, fat embolism from long bone fractures, spinal cord damage due to an unstable spinal injury. Many of these are preventable with good immediate care, careful handling, rapid and appropriate resuscitation and elective ventilation if needed. Early stabilisation of long bone fractures minimises the risk of later multiple organ failure

and provides stable conditions in which a formal assessment of any less urgent head, chest or abdominal injuries can be made.

PRE-HOSPITAL CARE

Nowadays, much emphasis is placed on transporting the multiply injured patient rapidly to the most appropriate hospital or, in the case of serious head injuries, to a neurosurgical unit. The crucial need for rapid transfer is the guiding principle for the emergency field team and hence pre-hospital interventions are limited to the essentials. The need for endotracheal intubation is the main intervention that should delay transportation to hospital but occasionally anaesthetising the patient buys time for direct transfer to a specialised unit.

- **Airway and breathing.** The airway must be assessed and secured first, whilst ensuring that the **cervical spine** is immobilised (see next point). If the patient can speak, it can be assumed that the airway is patent, ventilation is intact and the brain adequately perfused. Note, however, that agitation may be a sign of hypoxia. In an unconscious or semi-conscious patient, the airway can usually be temporarily secured with a standard head tilt and chin lift or jaw thrust. If tolerated, the patient should then have two nasopharyngeal airways and a Guedel oropharyngeal airway placed to maintain airway patency. If the gag reflex is absent, **endotracheal intubation** is needed. If this proves unattainable, a useful rescue technique is to insert a laryngeal mask (LMA), as used in general anaesthesia; this may avoid the need for a surgical airway. As a last resort, a surgical airway can be achieved using a needle or surgical **cricothyroidotomy**. In all seriously injured patients, high-flow oxygen therapy (10–12 L/min) is mandatory.
- **Spine.** In an unconscious patient, particularly after a high-impact collision, a cervical spine fracture should be assumed until disproved. If the patient has

Clinical class of shock	Amount of blood lost		Blood pressure		Pulse rate	Respiratory rate	Extremities	Mental state
	Volume	Percentage	Systolic	Diastolic				
Class I	~750 ml	<15%	Normal	Normal	Normal	Normal	Normal	Alert
Class II	800 – 1500 ml	15–30%	Normal	↑	100 –120	Normal	Pale	Anxious or aggressive
Class III	1500 – 2000 ml	30–40%	↓	↓	~120+	↑~ 20/min	Pale	Anxious, aggressive or drowsy
Class IV	>2000 ml	>40%	↓↓	↓↓	120+ & thready	↑↑> 20/min	Ashen & cold	Drowsy, confused or unconscious

    Fig. 15.1 Clinical classification of hypovolaemic shock related to probable blood loss

Box 15.1 **Indications for immediate intubation and ventilation following a head injury or multiple injuries**

1. Glasgow Coma Score < 8 or falling score (see p. 246, Table 16.1)
2. Inability to maintain airway
3. Facial trauma or bleeding into the airway
4. Spontaneous hyperventilation causing hypocapnia
5. Inadequate ventilation causing hypoxia and/or hypercapnia
6. Seizures
7. Extreme agitation

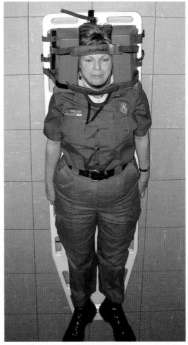

(a)

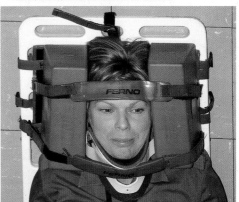

(b)

Fig. 15.2 Spine immobilised in a neutral position on a long spinal board

multiple injuries, the whole spine must be protected from secondary injury during transfer and assessment. After intubation if necessary, the spine is immobilised in a neutral position on a long spinal board. This usually requires a semi-rigid cervical collar, side head supports and strapping (see Fig. 15.2). Strapping is applied to head, shoulders and pelvis to prevent the body rotating independently of the neck

● **Circulation.** If the patient appears shocked by blood loss, one or more intravenous cannulae should be inserted in case fluid resuscitation is urgently needed. Venous filling is likely to be better in the early stages, so cannulation is easier and quicker than it would be in a collapsed patient in transit. However, it is a surprising fact that less than 10% of victims of blunt or penetrating trauma have early post-traumatic hypotension. One-third of these die of their wounds soon after injury (this **'non-survivable' proportion** recurs in every group studied since the Crimean War). This leaves two-thirds (2–3% of the trauma population) with post-traumatic hypotension due to blood loss. In all of these cases, it used to be thought that the blood pressure had to be rapidly restored. Recent research, however, has led to a different and more logical approach involving **permissive hypotension**, part of which is regular and careful **monitoring** to ensure that any deterioration is quickly recognised.

There are advantages in keeping the pressure low in trauma patients, provided organ perfusion can be maintained. It is now known that physiological compensation is effective at systolic pressures between 70 and 85 mmHg, and cerebral perfusion and urinary output are well maintained. Above this pressure, fresh clot is often dislodged ('**pop a clot**') and then bleeding recurs. A further disadvantage of unnecessary fluid resuscitation is that infusing only 750 ml of crystalloid activates cytokines and causes dilutional coagulopathy. Thus, in suitable patients, infused volumes can be reduced and clot disruption prevented by carefully managed permissive hypotension

—If a patient is **unconscious** without a palpable radial or pedal pulse, 250–500 ml fluid is given

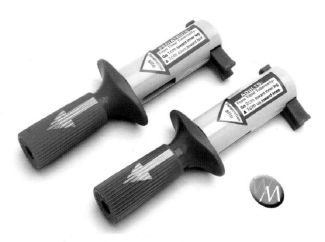

Fig. 15.3 Bone injection gun
Photographs courtesy of WaisMed Ltd.

immediately, followed by small boluses, repeated only until the point at which a pulse returns. This is known as **titration by pulse** and has been successfully employed in major trauma and in military campaigns. If intravenous access proves impossible, bone injection guns (Fig. 15.3) are a new and quick way of inserting an infusion cannula into the bone marrow

—If the patient is **unconscious** but has a palpable peripheral pulse, this indicates a systolic of above 80 mmHg and fluid resuscitation is not started

—If a patient is **conscious**, i.e. can speak and responds normally, systolic pressure can be assumed to be over 80 mmHg and, again, fluid resuscitation is not started

- **Wounds** should be covered with dressings to prevent contamination. Pressure dressings should be applied to bleeding wounds
- **Fractured limbs** should be realigned and splinted. This helps minimise blood loss, assists with pain control and may improve impaired peripheral perfusion

TRANSPORT TO HOSPITAL

Injured patients need to be transferred to an appropriate hospital as rapidly as is practicable. Most are taken in an ambulance by road, but transfer by helicopter can be quicker. If helicopter evacuation is available, it is important to consider whether the severity of injuries requires the facilities of a major trauma centre. If so, where is the nearest centre and how long would it take to transfer by road compared with helicopter (including time to call up the helicopter)? Overall, would there be any substantial time advantage?

Note that whilst helicopters can cover great distances quickly, they have important inherent disadvantages:

- When loading casualties, it is easy to displace endotracheal tubes, intravenous infusions and monitor cables. The utmost care is required in an anaesthetised patient to avoid disaster
- There is a greater potential for developing a pneumothorax when flying, particularly in a ventilated patient with chest injuries. It may be prudent to perform simple thoracostomies and leave them open in such cases. Tube drains are inappropriate
- The transport space in most helicopters is very restricted, so that access to the patient is poor and it is difficult to perform many commonly required resuscitation procedures. For this reason, patients must be relatively stable before they can be safely transferred by helicopter, and should have two intravenous access cannulae in situ, together with full monitoring

PRELIMINARY HOSPITAL MANAGEMENT OF MULTIPLE AND SERIOUS INJURIES

ORGANISATION OF THE ACCIDENT DEPARTMENT

The field team or ambulance service informs the trauma receiving unit as early as possible about the impending arrival of seriously injured patients, together with an assessment of numbers and the nature and severity of their injuries. This alerts the surgical and anaesthetic teams to be assembled, gowned and gloved, ready for when the patients arrive (see Box 15.2). Trauma units usually have a **resuscitation room** (see Fig. 15.4) where all necessary resuscitation equipment is located; this can now be made ready for immediate use, for example with infusion sets run through and drugs laid out.

Triage is the process of sorting patients into priority treatment groups on arrival to enable most efficient use of resources. The usual categories are shown in Table 15.1.

Success in managing individual patients with suspected life-threatening multiple injuries (or multiple patients with injuries) depends on good organisation. It involves concurrent activity between several professionals in the resuscitation room, but with one person, often the surgeon, designated **team leader**. The team leader must take overall medical responsibility as well as coordinate the activities of clinicians involved.

Box **15.2** **Major trauma team**

Members of the major trauma team

- Team leader
- Senior member of emergency department medical staff
- General surgeons—senior and junior
- Orthopaedic surgeons—senior and junior
- Anaesthetists—senior and junior
- Other specialist surgeons, e.g. cardiothoracic, neurosurgical as appropriate
- Senior nurses

(Note that one of the junior doctors needs to be nominated as 'scribe' to ensure accurate documentation of injuries and the sequence of events)

Departments to be notified of impending major trauma incident

- Radiology—on-call radiologist and radiographer
- Blood bank, haematology, biochemistry
- ITU
- Operating department
- Mortuary (in major disasters)

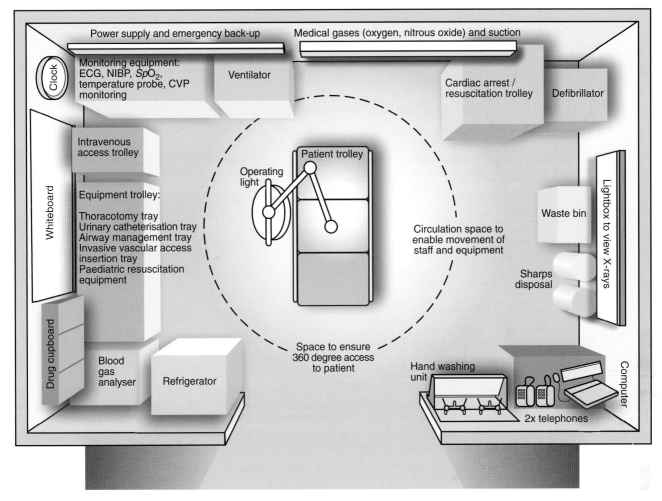

Fig. 15.4 'Bird's eye view' drawing of an ideal resuscitation room

Table 15.1 Triage priority groups

Category	Definition	Colour	Treatment
P1	Life-threatening	Red	Immediate
P2	Urgent	Yellow	Urgent
P3	Minor	Green	Delayed
P4	Dead	White	

INITIAL CARE IN THE ACCIDENT DEPARTMENT

By the time the seriously injured patient arrives in the resuscitation room, the first peak of deaths in the golden hour has passed and the main danger of death is from **hypovolaemia** (intrathoracic or intraperitoneal haemorrhage, blood loss from fractures) or from an expanding **intracranial haematoma**. (Note that most injured patients arrive at hospital with relatively trivial injuries and only a small minority require the extensive initial care described here.)

For the potentially seriously injured, the immediate priorities after arriving at hospital are:

- Rapid primary assessment combined with resuscitation
- Detailed secondary survey for all injuries
- Prioritisation and treatment of individual injuries

Training in this process has been standardised through **Advanced Trauma Life Support** (ATLS) courses, initiated by the American College of Surgeons and now run in many countries. These courses employ well-trained volunteers as 'patients' and participants are given training and assessment in real-life simulations using the 'ABCDE system' shown in Figure 15.5. The principle of ATLS is simple—the greatest threats to life should be treated first.

INITIAL ASSESSMENT OF THE SERIOUSLY INJURED PATIENT

Despite the urgency of the situation, primary assessment of the trauma patient must be performed in a systematic manner as soon as the patient arrives. The **primary survey**

1. PRIMARY SURVEY (ABCDE)

A. AIRWAY AND CERVICAL SPINE — is the airway obstructed?

Cervical spine
>   Cervical spine injury must be assumed in any seriously injured patient
>   **Immobilisation:** semi-rigid collar + sandbags or lateral head supports + strapping tape (see Fig.15.2)

Airway management
1. **Airway positioning:** head tilt + chin lift or jaw thrust ± look inside oropharynx if possible for foreign body (teeth, dentures) or other obstruction. Suction if blood/vomitus/secretions.
2. **Oropharyngeal/nasal airways:** Guedel airway + two nasopharyngeal airways or laryngeal mask airway (LMA)
3. **Definitive airway management:** endotracheal intubation if Glasgow Coma Score < 8 or other indication (see Box 15.1) CXR needed to check tube position
4. **Surgical airway management where tracheal intubation impossible, e.g. due to swelling, jaw fractures:** cricothyroidotomy (needle or surgical)

B. BREATHING AND VENTILATION — only assess breathing after airway is secure. Is patient breathing spontaneously and adequately ventilated?

Physical examination
>   Inspection, palpation, percussion and auscultation:
>   Observe specifically for injuries (**open wound, flail segment** of chest wall), distended neck veins (**cardiac tamponade**), tracheal deviation and asymmetrical expansion (**pneumothorax/tension pneumothorax**), dull percussion note (**haemothorax**)

Chest X-ray
>   Assess lungs, pleural spaces, chest wall and diaphragm

Treatment of life-threatening conditions
1. **Open chest wound:** seal with occlusive dressing to limit mediastinal 'flap' movement with each breath + tube thoracostomy
2. **Flail segment:** oxygen, monitoring, analgesia + endotracheal (ET) intubation + assisted ventilation if deterioration
3. **Cardiac tamponade:** pericardiocentesis
4. **Pneumothorax:** may need chest drain/tube thoracostomy if large pneumothorax
5. **Tension pneumothorax:** needle thoracocentesis + tube thoracostomy
6. **Haemothorax:** tube thoracostomy
7. **Diaphragmatic rupture:** repair surgically
8. **Serious head injury:** ET tube + assisted ventilation

C. CIRCULATION — assess circulation only when the patient's airway is secure and the above life-threatening conditions have been excluded, or identified and treatment under way

Physical examination
>   **Assess:** pallor, heart rate, blood pressure, temperature, capillary refill time, ECG and urine output. Is there any obvious external haemorrhage?

Management of shock and control of haemorrhage
1. Control external haemorrhage from bleeding open wounds by direct pressure on gauze pack
2. Insert two **wide-bore IV cannulae** into antecubital fossae (or other large veins)
3. If cannulation not possible, **venous cut-down** or **direct bone infusion** may be necessary
4. When venous access achieved, send blood for **urgent cross-matching**, and standard biochemical and haematological analysis
5. In the shocked patient, rapidly infuse two litres of **warmed crystalloid solution** through both peripheral intravenous lines; monitor response of pulse palpability, rate and BP and titrate rate of infusion (note permissive hypotension may be appropriate — see p.223)
6. If the patient fails to improve, consider transfusion of red cells. If the patient is rapidly deteriorating, O negative blood can be given
7. Consider likely causes of significant blood loss in the light of the history and clinical findings: e.g. thoracic trauma, abdominal injury, pelvic fracture, long bone fracture
8. **Catheterise** the bladder to monitor urine production and to provide a guide to renal perfusion
9. **Fracture management** — reduction of fractures may assist in haemostasis, especially femoral shaft fractures and sometimes pelvic fractures (also helps pain relief)
10. Relieve cardiac tamponade by **long needle aspiration**
11. Apply **external cardiac massage** in the case of cardiac arrest
Further management of circulation depends on likely source of blood loss, e.g. if abdominal injury is likely FAST ultrasound confirms and **laparotomy** may be required to control haemorrhage

D. DISABILITY of the central nervous system. Do not move on to assess 'D' until patient's circulatory state is stable

>   Basic **neurological assessment** is made using the **AVPU score**:
>   > **A** — Alert
>   > **V** — responding to Verbal stimuli
>   > **P** — responding to Painful stimuli
>   > **U** — Unresponsive
>   **Pupil size, inequality and reactivity to light** is also assessed
>   Estimate Glasgow Coma Scale if practicable and look for other neurological deficits

E. EXPOSURE of the whole patient, **ENVIRONMENT** and 'EXRAYS' (imaging)

The patient is **fully exposed**, including removal of all clothing, to allow rapid 'top to toe' assessment for external injury and for signs of injury which have not already been recognised and managed. The patient must be kept warm including warming intravenous fluids. Completion of the trauma series **X-rays, CT scans and FAST ultrasound** is performed

>   **Consider the following measures** to monitor the patient and aid further assessment, if not already done
>   > Urinary catheterisation
>   > Nasogastric or orogastric tube placement
>   > X-rays of cervical spine (lateral), chest and pelvis (trauma series)
>   > Focused abdominal Sonography for trauma (FAST)

Fig. 15.5 Primary survey and initial resuscitation
Management priorities for the patient with multiple injuries. In practice, anaesthetists usually deal with the airway and intravenous access and monitoring while surgeons evaluate the head and neck, chest, abdomen and pelvis for potential life-threatening injuries

Major disaster plan—receiving hospitals need a detailed (and rehearsed) plan for dealing with disasters from which many casualties are likely (e.g. train or air crashes). It can be summarised on action cards given to nominated staff when a major disaster is declared.

The plan defines precisely:

- How to recognise a major disaster and how to initiate the process
- The person responsible for each of the main functions (e.g. medical coordinator, field triage officer) and how to contact them
- Their precise duties
- Details of the responsibilities and actions required of all other team members

includes a rapid evaluation of the patient, resuscitation and crucial life-preserving treatment. A rapid history is taken whenever practicable, often as part of the secondary survey. A useful mnemonic for this essential history taking is **AMPLE**, as follows:

Allergies
Medicines and drugs
Past medical history
Last meal (including alcohol)
Events leading to accident

Other aspects of the history are usually obtainable from the field team's notes and include:

- Time of the incident
- Conscious level of patient when discovered and later changes in conscious level
- Details of drugs, fluids and other treatments administered at scene of accident

Conscious patients with suspected cervical spine injuries should be moved with extreme caution. Passive neck movements must not be attempted but the patient should be allowed to perform active movements unaided; spasm or pain will restrict movement if there is a significant injury. Patients should be 'log-rolled' by several people together in order to examine the back and to perform a rectal examination.

Primary survey and resuscitation is followed by a **secondary survey** designed to assess the potential for developing other life-threatening problems or complications. In the critically injured patient, the urgency of initial treatment may delay progress to the secondary survey. The primary survey and immediate resuscitation priorities for the multiply injured patient are summarised in Figure 15.5. The key clinical features sought in the secondary survey are given in Figure 15.6; individual systems are described later.

SECONDARY SURVEY

Head and neck

Look for bruising, soft tissue swelling; signs of basal skull fracture — Battle's sign (bruising over mastoid process), 'racoon eyes'
Lacerations
Depressed vault fractures
Facial and jaw fractures
Pupil size and responsiveness
Range of active neck movements

Chest (front and back)

Signs of respiratory distress — grunting/stridor
Bruising and skin imprinting
Penetrating injuries
Pattern and rate of respiration
Symmetry of chest movement
Gross mediastinal shift
Pattern of air entry throughout lung fields
Crepitus (subcutaneous air)

Abdomen and pelvis

External injuries as for chest (front and back)
Note: buttock injuries may penetrate abdominal cavity
Distension by gas or fluid (including blood)
Tenderness
Presence of palpable or percussible bladder
Pelvic fractures
Bleeding from urethral meatus
PR bruising, palpable pelvic haematoma or loss of anal tone (spinal injury)

Limbs

Neurovascular status of each limb
Lacerations
Deformities
Soft tissue swelling

Further definitive management of lesser injuries

Depends on findings from Primary and Secondary survey
May involve **further imaging ± surgery** or **ITU admission**
Before leaving the Emergency Department, **reassessment** is essential to ensure that the patient is safe to be transferred elsewhere

Fig. 15.6 Secondary survey
Special points to note in systematic examination of the seriously injured patient.

- Glasgow Coma Score
- Pulse rate, blood pressure, electrocardiogram (ECG)
- Respiratory rate
- Hourly urine output
- Oxygen saturation by pulse oximetry; blood gases
- Nasogastric aspiration

Note that the secondary survey must be **repeated**, often more than once, during hospitalisation as some major and many lesser injuries can be missed because of the urgency of the serious injuries. Up to 20% of multiple injury patients have injuries missed in the early stages.

RECORDING OF EVENTS

The time of examination and the clinical findings, together with details of investigations and treatments, must be carefully recorded in the patient's notes, not least for medico-legal purposes.

X-RAYS AND OTHER INVESTIGATIONS

In seriously injured patients, the chest, cervical spine and pelvis are X-rayed in the resuscitation room using portable equipment; this is known as a **trauma series**. The diagnostic quality of chest films must be good enough to exclude major chest wall, mediastinal and lung injuries and also to provide a baseline for comparison if the patient subsequently deteriorates. Cervical spine X-rays often fail to include C1, C7 and T1, and poor films must be interpreted with caution; if necessary they should be repeated or a CT scan of the area ordered. Generally, patients should not be moved to the CT scanner until they are stable—the machine is known as the 'donut of death' in ATLS parlance.

Portable skull X-rays are rarely performed nowadays if CT is available; CT scanning of the skull may be required urgently in head-injured patients. Focused abdominal sonography for trauma or FAST (see *Diagnosis of abdominal injuries*, below) is performed for suspected abdominal injuries and bleeding, but all other imaging is generally performed in the radiology department once the patient has been stabilised (see the following sections).

Initial **blood tests** should include haemoglobin estimation. Blood grouping and cross-matching or antibody screening should be performed and an appropriate number of units of blood ordered. In a desperate emergency, universal donor blood (group O, Rh negative) can be transfused without grouping or cross-matching, although plasma substitutes will usually suffice until compatible blood becomes available. Plasma electrolytes and glucose are usually measured, and arterial blood gases estimated if there is any suspicion of respiratory failure.

Further investigations are guided by the nature of the individual injuries, as detailed below and in the following chapters.

ABDOMINAL INJURIES

INTRODUCTION

Abdominal and thoracic injuries fairly often co-exist, and both penetrating and closed (blunt) injuries can affect both cavities at the same time. For this reason, it is logical to think in terms of **torso trauma**. Major injuries to the torso are a common cause of death at the scene of the trauma, for example from avulsion of the thoracic aorta, cardiac injury or massive liver injury. Immediate diagnosis and urgent laparotomy or thoracotomy offer almost the only hope of survival from these potentially fatal injuries, but often the injury is too extensive or time too short to intervene successfully. Less invasive techniques such as placement of a stent graft for aortic avulsion or continued transfusion until intra-abdominal pressure arrests haemorrhage in the case of massive liver injury have a place when the diagnosis is unambiguous.

The signs of external injury and their site provide clues as to the likely internal injuries. This is obvious with penetrating injuries but is also true of blunt injuries. For example, trauma to the left upper quadrant of the abdomen or left lower ribs is often associated with **splenic rupture** and similarly for the **liver** with right-sided injuries. Lower abdominal injuries may injure the **bladder**, and loin trauma damage the **kidney**. Central anterior chest trauma may damage the **heart** whilst injury to the clavicular area may traumatise the **brachial plexus or subclavian blood vessels**.

Abdominal injuries are uncommon compared with head and chest injuries and mortality can be low if they are managed promptly and appropriately. When death occurs, it is usually from massive haemorrhage. This usually arises from bursting injuries of the liver or spleen or from penetrating injuries to major arteries or veins, particularly in association with gunshot wounds. All of these represent major surgical challenges and the bleeding is sometimes uncontrollable. Note that **unrecognised injuries** are the principal **avoidable** cause of death.

It is important to remember that areas of the abdomen other than the main peritoneal cavity may be injured; **pelvic** viscera lie within a bony cage but extend low enough to be injured by wounds in the buttock or perineum. Similarly, the **retroperitoneal** viscera appear to be protected but are vulnerable to flank or back wounds, or to deep anterior stab wounds and any gunshot wounds. This area is not easily palpated and diagnosis requires cross-sectional imaging.

Overall, 20% of patients with closed abdominal trauma require operation. In penetrating injuries, 30% of those with stab wounds require operation and close to 100% of those with gunshot wounds.

DIAGNOSIS OF ABDOMINAL INJURIES

Clinical diagnosis is unreliable in blunt injuries because overt signs of bleeding or perforation of a hollow viscus may not develop until several hours after the injury. If early laparotomy is not indicated because the patient is stable, but the accident is judged to have been one involving high energy transfer, diagnostic investigations should be employed. Investigation is also desirable when an intra-abdominal injury is suspected in the following groups of patients (e.g. because of bruising or cloth printing on the skin):

- Those with impaired consciousness
- Those with thoracic, pelvic or abdominal wall injuries
- Those who need to be transferred to other units, e.g. by helicopter
- Those in whom prolonged investigation or treatment of other non-abdominal injuries is needed

Clinical observation

If surgical intervention is not judged necessary, nursing observations such as pulse and blood pressure are made at regular intervals and the patient re-examined frequently by a doctor for developing signs of peritonitis or intra-abdominal bleeding. Measurement of abdominal girth should not be used as it is unreliable and may give a false sense of security while the patient exsanguinates. Note that significant injuries will almost always become manifest within 24 hours.

Investigative techniques

Focused abdominal sonography for trauma (FAST)

Compared with clinical evaluation and diagnostic peritoneal lavage (see below), this has markedly improved diagnostic accuracy. It can even be applied in the pre-hospital setting. In pregnant patients it avoids the use of ionising radiation. The technique allows free intra-abdominal fluid to be reliably detected (an indication for urgent laparotomy in a haemodynamically unstable patient without other evident sites of blood loss), as well as the location and extent of solid organ haematomas and sometimes organ lacerations. A full torso ultrasound examination concentrates on five areas, the 'five Ps': Perihepatic, Perisplenic and Pelvic in the abdomen and Pleural and Pericardial in the chest. Ultrasound is less reliable than CT scanning for identifying specific injuries. Even in expert hands, ultrasound misses substantial injuries in about 10% of cases.

CT scanning

CT scanning should be performed only in stable patients. The main indications are abnormal abdominal signs at presentation or appearing later, or if ultrasound shows free intra-abdominal fluid.

CT can identify injuries to all solid abdominal and retroperitoneal organs (liver, spleen, pancreas, kidney), bowel perforations (indirectly by the presence of free gas and fluid), diaphragmatic rupture, retroperitoneal blood and pelvic and spinal fractures. It is very sensitive for showing free gas and can often identify the source of haemorrhage and the extent of injury in solid organ trauma, which may allow conservative management of less severe splenic and liver injuries. CT is also valuable for defining the extent and configuration of complex pelvic fractures.

Diagnostic peritoneal lavage (DPL)

This used to be widely employed to diagnose abdominal injury but the technique has been superseded by more accurate and less invasive investigations such as FAST or CT in units where the equipment is available. DPL involved instilling 0.5–1 L of normal saline into the abdominal cavity via a peritoneal dialysis catheter; the fluid was then allowed to run out. Blood or blood staining indicated intra-abdominal injury, but, importantly, a negative result did not exclude serious injury. Fluid recovered could be analysed for red and white blood cell counts, amylase and alkaline phosphatase, and examined for bile, bacteria or food fibres.

PENETRATING ABDOMINAL WOUNDS

STAB WOUNDS AND OTHER SHARP ABDOMINAL WOUNDS

Stab wounds may or may not penetrate the peritoneal cavity. They often cause little damage unless the blade penetrates the retroperitoneal area and injures the great vessels or pancreas. At one time, it was thought that all abdominal stab wounds required surgical exploration but current policy in most cases is towards more conservative management. A large series from Baragwanath Hospital, Soweto, South Africa, demonstrated that 70% or more patients could safely be managed by observation in hospital for 24 hours, with pulse and BP monitoring and serial abdominal palpation, and operated upon only if there were signs of deterioration. This is because many bowel perforations seal spontaneously without causing peritonitis, and bleeding from some internal wounds also stops by normal haemostasis. However, haemodynamically unstable patients and those with extensive or potentially contaminated penetrating wounds **must** be explored surgically without delay.

For most patients, the first step is to determine whether the peritoneum has been breached by exploring the wound under local anaesthesia. If it has, then laparoscopy should be employed to explore intra-abdominal viscera. If laparoscopy is unavailable, ultrasonography or CT scanning should be performed. If the peritoneum has not been breached and/or imaging is negative (as in most cases), conservative management with careful monitoring alone is appropriate. However, about one-third of those who later proved to have significant intra-abdominal injury were free of signs initially, emphasising the need for repeated clinical and ultrasonographic or radiographic reassessment.

BULLET AND OTHER MISSILE INJURIES

The severity of internal injury depends on the path and the mass of the missile and to a large extent on its velocity. Low-velocity missile wounds (e.g. hand-gun bullets) cause damage confined to the wound track, whereas high-velocity (i.e. rifle) bullet wounds injure widely and deeply. This is because the very much higher kinetic energy is dissipated in the tissues. In addition, **cavitation** is caused within the body tissues and debris is sucked into the wounds, causing contamination with clothing and soil. If the bullet hits bone, secondary missiles are created causing further injury. The size of the entry wound is no guide to the extent of injury, often being small because of the elastic recoil of the skin. Given the unpredictable extent of the injuries, **all** gunshot wounds must be surgically explored to check for visceral organ, intestinal and vascular damage. Buttock wounds should be treated in the same way.

CLOSED (BLUNT) ABDOMINAL INJURIES

Closed abdominal injuries usually result from road traffic collisions, falls, sporting contact injuries and accidents involving horses. Following substantial blunt injury, about 20% will require laparotomy. The **spleen** is the most vulnerable organ, especially in left-sided injuries to the lower chest or upper abdomen (see Fig. 15.7). **Liver injury** requires greater force of impact, usually from the front or right side. **Pancreatic and duodenal injuries** are uncommon and usually result from a heavy central abdominal impact, transecting the pancreas or retroperitoneal duodenum across the vertebral bodies. This most commonly occurs in children falling across the handlebars of their bicycles. The **kidneys** are vulnerable to punches or kicks in the loins.

Bowel is often damaged by rapid deceleration or crushing injuries, and is particularly vulnerable to tearing at sites where freely mobile bowel becomes attached to the retroperitoneum—at each end of the transverse colon, at the duodeno-jejunal flexure and in the ileocaecal area. A full **bladder**, common after a bout of heavy drinking, may rupture into the peritoneal cavity (or sometimes retroperitoneally) after abdominal impact. The **bladder** and **urethra** are also liable to be torn in association with displaced pelvic fractures. The clinical features and investigation of closed abdominal injuries are shown in Box 15.5.

PRINCIPLES OF MANAGEMENT OF CLOSED ABDOMINAL INJURIES

All patients with closed abdominal trauma should be admitted to hospital and closely observed. Compared with penetrating trauma, there is time for FAST ultrasound or CT scanning to diagnose the nature and extent of injury. As for penetrating injuries, urgent laparotomy is usually required in haemodynamically unstable patients and those with obvious peritonitis. A patient without evident visceral injury may be managed with permissive hypotension (see earlier) to minimise blood loss, once a head injury has been excluded, provided the pressure does not continue to fall. Less urgent laparotomy may be required if investigation reveals injuries requiring surgery or if clinical deterioration occurs. Indications include signs or investigations indicating gastrointestinal perforation (free gas on abdominal X-ray or scan, developing signs of peritonitis) and specific visceral injuries not amenable to conservative treatment, e.g. major splenic rupture.

INJURIES TO SPECIFIC SOLID ORGANS

Spleen (Fig. 15.7)

The spleen is the most commonly injured organ in blunt abdominal trauma. The organ should be preserved wherever possible because of the dangers of post-splenectomy sepsis. In one study, there was a 58-fold increase in the risk of sepsis; 2.4% of all post-splenectomy patients suffered sepsis and more than 50% of those were fatal.

CT scanning enables accurate assessment and classification of the extent of injury. Haematomas and capsular tears not extending deeply can often be managed conservatively. More severe injuries are treated by urgent laparotomy and splenic repair (splenorrhaphy) where possible. In a study including blunt and penetrating injuries, splenorrhaphy was found to be possible in 45% of cases, and there was a low risk of rebleeding. For repair, the spleen is mobilised and bleeding controlled with a vascular clamp at the splenic hilum; repair is performed by direct suture, fibrin glue or absorbable mesh bags. If this is insufficient, segmental resection or splenic artery ligation can be performed, but at least 50% of splenic substance must be preserved to maintain useful function. Removal of the whole spleen (splenectomy) is indicated for only the most severely injured spleens.

Liver

Isolated, relatively small liver injuries may be treated by surgical repair or local resection but major injuries are often best treated conservatively. This is because surgical control of bleeding from hepatic vessels deep within its substance may prove impossible, particularly if it is from the hepatic veins entering the inferior vena cava. Patients diagnosed with severe liver injuries should be discussed with specialists at a regional hepato-pancreatico-biliary (HPB) or liver unit. For conservative management, large-volume blood transfusions are sometimes given until abdominal tamponade stops the bleeding. If a major liver injury is encountered at surgical exploration and haemorrhage cannot be arrested, the liver should be packed with large pieces of surgical gauze, the abdomen closed and the patient stabilised. Ideally the patient should then be transferred to a major HPB centre because more extensive liver surgery may prove to be necessary when the packs are

1. History

- Substantial trauma to the abdomen or lower chest
- Seatbelt not worn in road traffic accident (especially driver impacting steering wheel)
- Abdominal pain after trauma
- Haematuria, particularly following trauma to the back or loin

2. Physical signs

- Skin bruising immediately after injury—suggests impact of sufficient force to cause internal damage
- Imprinting of cloth pattern on skin (cloth printing)—caused by compression of skin against vertebral bodies; implies a high energy transfer impact
- Unexplained hypotension—suggests concealed haemorrhage into the abdominal cavity or elsewhere
- Abdominal distension, i.e. increasing abdominal girth—from accumulating blood, urine or gas in the peritoneal cavity
- Increasing abdominal tenderness, guarding and rigidity (difficult to assess in the presence of abdominal wall bruising)—may indicate intestinal perforation or intra-abdominal bleeding
- Lateral lower rib fractures—may be associated with injury to spleen, liver or kidney
- Pelvic fractures, especially 'butterfly' fractures of all four pubic rami—often associated with bladder or urethral injury (especially in males) and pelvic vein injury
- Inability to pass urine and the findings of blood at the urethral meatus and/or perineal bruising—imply rupture of the urethra, usually at the pelvic diaphragm, i.e. post-membranous urethra (urethral catheterisation must not be performed and suprapubic employed instead); rectal examination may reveal a 'high-riding' prostate
- Damage to the anus or rectum may be palpable on rectal examination; the presence of blood suggests ano-rectal injury. If anal sphincter tone is low, this suggests neurological damage from a spinal injury

3. Investigation

- Plasma amylase level should be checked and, if raised, pancreatic injury investigated by CT scanning
- Chest and plain abdominal X-rays (supine and erect or lateral decubitus views) may show free intraperitoneal or retroperitoneal gas, rib or pelvic fractures associated with specific visceral injuries and radiopaque missiles such as bullets, shotgun pellets and glass
- Ultrasound and CT scanning—particularly useful in investigating solid organs, i.e. spleen (see Fig. 15.7), liver, kidneys, pancreas. Intravenous contrast CT is useful for large vessel injuries
- Urethrography—investigation of suspected urethral rupture
- Laparoscopy—increasingly important in investigation of closed abdominal trauma in stable patients. Can be performed under local anaesthesia

Fig. 15.7 Ruptured spleen

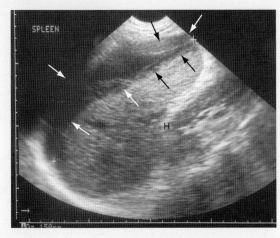

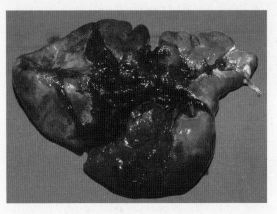

(a) (b)

(a) This 67-year-old woman sustained fractures of the left lower ribs in a fall. She was discharged from hospital the following day but presented again 6 weeks later with abdominal swelling, tenderness and anaemia. This ultrasound scan shows a large subcapsular splenic haematoma (arrowed), which had presumably developed slowly over the intervening period. The scan also shows intrasplenic haemorrhage **H**. She rapidly recovered after splenectomy. **(b)** This operative specimen comes from a 15-year-old girl who fell off her pony, which then trod on the left side of her chest. She was admitted to hospital with bruising over the lower ribs and tachycardia. At laparotomy, her spleen was found to be split completely in half, necessitating removal.

removed at an elective 'second look' laparotomy 48 hours later, although in most cases pack removal is uneventful.

Other organs

Pancreatic transection is treated by surgically removing the distal part of the pancreas and oversewing the stump. A crushing pancreatic injury may have to be treated with drainage alone. **Renal injuries** are usually managed conservatively unless nephrectomy is required for uncontrollable bleeding.

BOWEL INJURIES

Injuries to the small bowel are dealt with by simple suture or, if the mesenteric vascular supply is impaired, by resection and reanastomosis. Conventional treatment for right-sided large bowel injuries is resection and anastomosis of colon to ileum. Localised injuries to other parts of the colon without substantial intra-abdominal faecal contamination can usually be resected and joined end to end. After knife or gunshot wounds, simple repair gives good results provided there is minimal peritoneal contamination. Extensive injuries with contamination require **exteriorisation** of the damaged bowel ends to the abdominal wall, the proximal end as a colostomy and the distal end as a mucous fistula (see Ch. 27).

High-velocity penetrating injuries wreak havoc upon the gut, causing extensive devascularisation and multiple perforations; all necrotic or ischaemic tissue must be excised. The immediate dangers are peritonitis and systemic sepsis from gross contamination. Exteriorisation of viable bowel ends is mandatory for this type of injury.

LOWER URINARY TRACT INJURIES

Intraperitoneal rupture of the bladder is treated by laparotomy and suturing of the bladder, with a urethral catheter left in situ for 5–7 days until the defect has healed. **Extraperitoneal** bladder rupture is treated conservatively, with prolonged urethral or suprapubic catheterisation. Urethral tears require specialist urological management. If the urethral wall is partly intact (as shown on urethrography), it can be treated, at least initially, by catheterisation (usually suprapubic). Complete urethral avulsion injuries are usually treated by suprapubic catheterisation, with formal repair after local inflammation has settled. Formerly, attempts were made to 'railroad' a catheter through the disrupted urethra at operation, by passing instruments from the surgically opened bladder down the urethra and up the urethra from below. This treatment is no longer in vogue.

CHEST INJURIES

The types of chest injury, their clinical features and their treatment are summarised in Table 15.2.

GENERAL PRINCIPLES

Chest injuries are a common cause of death in patients with multiple injuries, although the death rate has fallen dramatically in countries where seatbelt wearing is compulsory. Seatbelts, however, often cause typical **sash pattern bruising** obliquely across the chest and minor rib and sternal fractures (Fig. 15.8). Sternal fractures are usually not of serious consequence but do carry a risk of causing myocardial injury. Ultrasound of the heart is desirable and cardiac function should be monitored with ECG until this can be excluded.

Serious chest injuries, particularly tearing injuries of the mediastinal contents (e.g. aorta, bronchi and oesophagus) may be present even without evidence of external injury. Diagnosis of serious chest injuries goes hand in hand with urgent resuscitative measures. Clinical signs may provide clues about the nature of the injury but the various diagnostic possibilities must all be considered so they are not missed. Good-quality chest X-rays (or CT scans) are essential and will usually reveal the diagnosis (see Fig. 15.9).

The main mechanisms of chest injury are penetrating trauma, blunt impact and crushing injuries, deceleration

Fig. 15.8 Seatbelt injury—case study

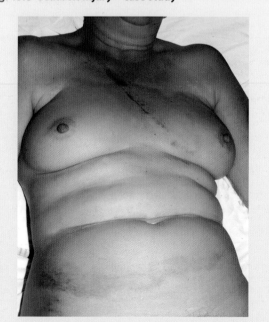

This 60-year-old woman was driving her car and suffered a severe frontal impact. The photograph shows the typical pattern of seatbelt bruising following this type of trauma. There was an undisplaced fracture of the body of the sternum but no major injuries; the seatbelt almost certainly saved the patient's life.

Table 15.2 Types of chest injury and their management

Nature of the injury	Clinical features	Treatment
Rib fractures	Localised pain on respiration or coughing; tenderness over fractures; usually visible on chest X-ray	Analgesia, intercostal blocks, physiotherapy, prophylactic antibiotics in chronic bronchitics
Flail chest, i.e. multiple rib fractures producing a mobile segment	Respiratory embarrassment; 'paradoxical' indrawing of the flail segment on inspiration	Intercostal block analgesia; endotracheal intubation and ventilation if hypoxic
Pneumothorax, i.e. air in pleural cavity causing lung collapse	Unilateral signs: loss of chest movement and breath sounds, percussion note resonant; sometimes chest wall emphysema; confirmed by chest X-ray	Intercostal drain with underwater seal
Sucking chest wound, i.e. open pneumothorax with mediastinum 'flapping' from side to side with each respiration	Gross respiratory embarrassment, audible sucking of air through chest wound	Sealing of chest wound with impermeable dressing; intercostal drainage
Tension pneumothorax, i.e. expanding pneumothorax causing progressive mediastinal shift to the opposite side and tracheal deviation	Signs of pneumothorax with disproportionate and increasing respiratory distress and hypoxaemia	Urgent chest drainage
Lung contusion	Deteriorating respiratory function; opacification of affected lung field on chest X-ray	Oxygenation, physiotherapy, mechanical ventilation in severe cases
Rupture of bronchus (uncommon)	Respiratory distress, surgical emphysema in the neck; suggested by air in mediastinum on chest X-ray (see Fig. 15.9a); confirmed by bronchoscopy	Operation by thoracic trained surgeon
Rupture of oesophagus (very rare)	May have surgical emphysema in the neck and pneumomediastinum on chest X-ray but diagnosis often missed until mediastinitis or empyema develops	Surgical repair if recognised early; surgical drainage and diversion for a late presentation
Haemothorax, i.e. blood in the pleural cavity. Usually arises from chest wall injury—rib fracture, lung parenchyma or minor venous injury. Most are self-limiting. Arterial injuries less common and more likely to need thoracotomy	Dull percussion note, breath sounds absent, tachycardia and hypotension due to blood loss	Most have stopped bleeding by the time of examination and only tube drainage is required. Dark, venous bleeding more likely to cease spontaneously than bright arterial bleeding. Tube must be large enough to drain without clotting, ideally 32–36 F; placed in sixth intercostal space in mid-axillary line. If patient haemodynamically stable, admit and observe. If continuing drainage of 200 ml+ per hour over 4 hours, should undergo thoracotomy
Cardiac tamponade, i.e. bleeding into pericardial cavity (usually penetrating trauma)	Hypotension, inaudible heart sounds, distended neck veins with systolic waves; enlarged, rounded heart shadow on chest X-ray; confirmed with ultrasound	Long needle aspiration via epigastric approach; operation if tamponade recurs
Cardiac contusion	May have arrhythmia or ECG changes similar to myocardial infarction	Conservative management
Rupture of aorta (usually results from deceleration injury)—fatal unless false aneurysm develops in mediastinum	Back pain, hypotension; systolic murmur or signs of tamponade in some cases; characteristic widening of mediastinum on chest X-ray; diagnosis confirmed by arteriography	Urgent thoracotomy and Dacron graft or minimal-access stent graft if available
Rupture of diaphragm, linear split usually in left diaphragm with herniation of gut into chest (penetrating or abdominal crush injury)	Respiratory distress, bowel sounds heard in the chest; diagnosis by chest X-ray and confirmed by barium meal; however, many cases are missed and only discovered much later; diagnosis may be made by laparoscopy or at laparotomy	Repair of diaphragm, usually via an abdominal approach

Fig. 15.9 Serious chest injuries

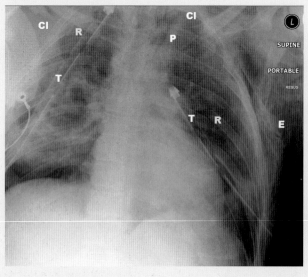
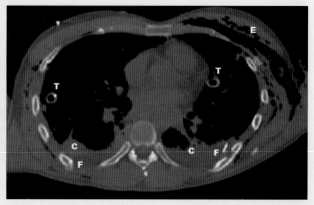

(a)   (b)

This 34-year-old male motorcyclist was hit by a car and then hit by another car whilst lying in the road. His GCS was 12–13 on arrival in the resuscitation room; brain, abdominal viscera and cervical spine were intact on CT. There were multiple fractures of ribs, scapula, clavicle, pelvis, humerus, femur and the chest injuries shown on CT **(b)**. His thoracic injuries were successfully managed conservatively. **(a)** Supine portable chest radiograph taken in the resuscitation room. It is not well centred, reflecting the difficulty in radiographing acutely unwell patients being resuscitated. The film shows bilateral clavicle **Cl, Cl** and rib fractures, pneumomediastinum **P**, surgical emphysema **E**, lung contusions and bilateral chest drains **T** inserted for pneumothorax. **(b)** CT scan of the patient on bone window settings showing surgical emphysema **E**, bilateral basal contusions of lungs **C, C**, chest drains **T, T**, and bilateral rib fractures **F, F**.

injuries and rupture of the diaphragm caused by abdominal compression. Less than 10% of chest injuries require thoracic surgical intervention but early recognition of those that do may be life saving.

Chest drains (tube thoracostomy)
Following trauma, chest drains are usually placed in the fourth or fifth intercostal space along the midaxillary line. The technique is shown in Figure 31.6, p. 462.

MAJOR ORTHOPAEDIC INJURIES

INTRODUCTION

This section contains a brief introduction to the main points of fracture management, followed by more detail on spinal and pelvic injuries.

- Pain—major orthopaedic injuries are extremely painful so good analgesia and early reduction is an important part of treatment, contributing to early mobilisation and reducing the potential for deep venous thrombosis (DVT)
- Blood loss—internal blood loss from fractures is often substantial (see Table 15.3), particularly if there are multiple fractures, and blood volume needs to be appropriately replaced. In pelvic fractures, external fixation may reduce blood loss
- Deformity—obvious deformity should be corrected as soon as possible using temporary splinting. This

treats pain and may assist vascular supply and limit blood loss
- Vascular and neurological integrity—where limbs are involved, this should be checked and appropriate investigation and intervention arranged
- Definitive fixation of fractures may be needed early or may have to be deferred until other life-threatening injuries have been dealt with

SPINAL FRACTURES

All patients suffering sufficient trauma should be considered to have a spinal injury until proved otherwise. Most attention is directed to the more vulnerable cervical spine, but the entire spinal column should be assessed for injury. The thoracolumbar spine is at risk in major trauma; in addition, 5% of patients with a spinal injury have a second

Table 15.3 Average blood loss from fractures

Site	Average loss (L)
Pelvis	1–4
Femur	1–2.5
Tibia	0.5–1.5
Humerus	0.5–1.5

fracture elsewhere in the spine. Definitive treatment of spinal injury requires specialist input.

CERVICAL SPINE

No patient without neck symptoms has ever been found to have an unstable cervical spine fracture, or has suffered neurological deterioration resulting from the injury. The cervical spine may be cleared clinically, without need for radiology, if the following conditions are met:

- Patient is alert and orientated
- No head injury
- No drugs or alcohol
- No neck pain
- No abnormal neurological signs
- No significant other injury that may distract the patient from complaining about a possible spinal injury
- **On examination:** no bruising or deformity around the neck, no tenderness and a normal pain-free range of active movement

Plain film radiology

The standard cervical spine series includes a lateral view (Fig. 15.10), an antero-posterior view and an open-mouth view to show the odontoid peg. Note that the lateral view alone will miss up to 15% of significant injuries. The lateral film **must** include both the base of the occiput and the upper part of the first thoracic vertebra. If the lower cervical spine is not seen, a CT scan of the region is indicated.

THORACIC AND LUMBAR SPINE INJURY

Thoracolumbar spine imaging is indicated if there is pain, bruising, swelling, deformity or abnormal neurological signs attributable to the thoracic or lumbar spinal regions. The presence of a fracture anywhere in the spine is an indication for full spinal imaging. Unconscious patients cannot be assessed clinically and require radiological clearance (i.e. exclusion of injuries) of the whole spine.

PELVIC FRACTURES

INTRODUCTION

The pelvis consists of a fused iliac bone, ischium and pubis on each side, forming an anatomical ring with the sacrum. Disruption of this ring requires at least two fractures or joint separations and requires substantial force. Hence pelvic fractures frequently involve injury to organs within the bony pelvis (bladder, urethra, rectum). In addition, the major iliac arteries and particularly veins that pass retroperitoneally through the pelvis are vulnerable to injury, sometimes causing massive haemorrhage.

The most common causes of pelvic fracture are motor vehicle collisions (50–60%), motorcycle crashes (10–20%) and pedestrians injured by cars (10–20%). The overall mortality rate from unstable pelvic fractures is about 10% in adults and 5% in children. Pelvic bleeding is the direct cause of death in about half, whilst infection of a retroperitoneal haematoma is responsible for most of the rest. If the patient with a substantial pelvic fracture is hypotensive on reaching the emergency department, the mortality rate approaches 50%; if pelvic fractures are open, mortality is about 30%.

CLINICAL EXAMINATION

On clinical examination, gentle bimanual compression and distortion of the iliac wings producing pain indicates likely fracture, as does palpable bony instability.

Other clinical indications of likely pelvic fracture include:

- Haematuria or signs of urethral injury in males, including high-riding prostate on rectal examination, scrotal haematoma or blood at urethral meatus
- Rectal bleeding, or a large haematoma or palpable fracture line on rectal examination
- Haematomas of the proximal thigh, above the inguinal ligament, over the perineum or in the flank
- Neurovascular deficits of the lower extremities

RADIOGRAPHY

Plain AP pelvic X-ray reveals 90% of pelvic injuries. If a fracture is present or suspected and the patient is stable, a pelvic CT scan should be performed. This is the best form of imaging for pelvic anatomy (including hip dislocation and acetabular fracture) and shows the extent of pelvic, retroperitoneal and intraperitoneal bleeding.

In a haemodynamically unstable patient without substantial intraperitoneal bleeding and an unstable pelvic fracture, initial management should include a simple wraparound pelvic splint. If this is unavailable, a version can be improvised using a bedsheet wrapped around the

Fig. 15.10 Cervical spine fractures

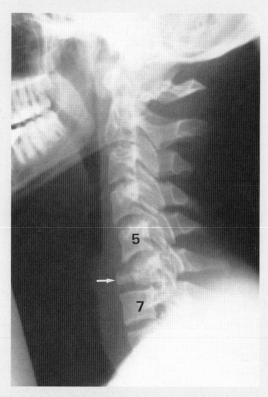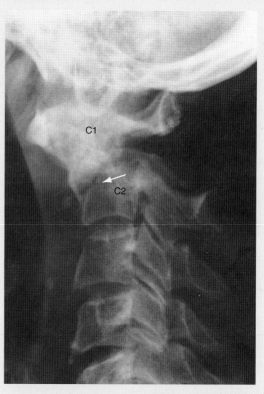

(a)

(b)

(a) This 17-year-old boy was admitted semi-conscious after crashing his motorcycle and landing head-first in a ditch. On examination he was tetraplegic and unable to move his upper or lower limbs although he could shrug his shoulders. This lateral cervical spine X-ray shows a burst fracture of the body of C6 (arrowed) with fragments in the spinal canal; there is also some posterior subluxation of C5. **(b)** Left lateral cervical spine X-ray from another unconscious young patient showing a fracture (arrowed) of the body of C2 and severe anterior subluxation of C1.

pelvis. Either should help control haemorrhage. Ideally, orthopaedic rigid external pelvic stabilisation should be applied but it is often difficult to organise rapidly. If blood pressure is still unstable, arteriography can determine the bleeding site; embolisation of the bleeding vessel may be possible as a means of control, or open surgery may have to be performed.

FURTHER TREATMENT

For unstable pelvic fractures, early stabilisation is important for pain control as well as for limiting bleeding. Patients need to be monitored over several days for signs of continuing blood loss, signs of infection or the development of neurovascular problems in the lower extremities.

Head and maxillofacial injuries

16

HEAD INJURIES

INTRODUCTION

Head injuries are a devastating problem with an enormous social and economic cost. Up to a million people attend emergency departments in the UK each year with head injury. Using the Glasgow Coma Scale (GCS, Table 16.1, p. 246) as a clinical indicator, 90% of these are classified as minor or mild with scores of 15 and 13 or 14 respectively, 5% as moderate (score 9–12) and 5% as severe (score 3–8). As many as 120 000 patients were admitted to hospital in England and Wales in 2004 for neurological observations following head injury, although this number should fall substantially with implementation of the 2003 NICE guidelines (Box 16.5, p. 247). Head injuries cause approximately 3500 deaths each year in the UK, amounting to about 0.6% of all deaths. Figure 16.1 shows how serious injuries represent only the tip of the iceberg of the impact of head injuries upon the health care system; the biggest problems are first, the acute management of the huge number of cases and second, coping with the chronic disability that the injuries cause.

Less than half the patients with head injuries attending emergency departments require CT scanning or hospital admission, and of these only a small proportion need specialist neurosurgical investigation and care. The difficulty is to recognise those at risk without over-investigating or admitting every single case to hospital. In order to streamline this process, various sets of guidelines have been produced, including the UK NICE guidelines (2003, http://www.nice.org.uk/page.aspx?o=CG004NICEguidel ine), which are summarised in Box 16.5. The main focus is detecting clinically important brain injuries (and injuries to the cervical spine—Box 16.1) and avoiding the need for admission of those with normal investigations. NICE guidelines depend, however, on ready access to CT scanning.

PATHOPHYSIOLOGY OF TRAUMATIC BRAIN INJURY

Traumatic brain injuries can be divided into **primary brain injuries**, which are the immediate result of the trauma, and **secondary brain injuries** which develop later as a result of complications. Treatment cannot reverse the primary brain injury but can deal with intracranial haematomas that would cause deterioration, and sustain the patient during the natural recovery period. Secondary brain injury is mostly caused by intracranial haematomas, ischaemia or hypoxia, and is largely preventable by prophylactic measures plus appropriate intervention. The death rate from head injuries could be greatly reduced by more widespread implementation of well-recognised management protocols, as discussed later. Prospects for improving care of head-injured patients depend on prompt triage, access to CT scanning, improved resuscitation, safe and rapid transfer to specialist units and expansion of neurosurgical critical care units.

At the cellular level, brain injury disrupts the neuronal cytoskeleton, which over a few hours leads to irreversible

237

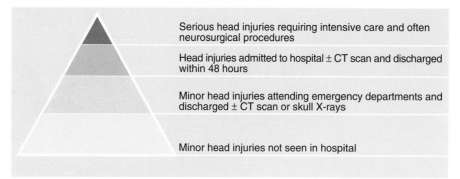

Fig. 16.1 **Workload caused by head injuries**

Box 16.1	'NICE'* guidelines for assessing cervical spine injuries

Indications for early imaging of cervical spine

- GCS less than 15 at time of assessment
- Paraesthesia/tingling/numbness in the extremities
- Focal neurological deficit
- Patient unable to actively rotate neck 45° to left and right
- Not possible to test range of movement in neck
- Patients with neck pain or tenderness aged 65 or more, or who have suffered a dangerous mechanism of injury

The investigation of choice is a 3 film series of good technical quality. CT is indicated as follows:

- Where X-ray is not possible or technically inadequate
- Where it is definitely abnormal or suspicious
- If clinical suspicion remains despite a normal study

CT should also be considered if other areas are being scanned for head injury/multi-region trauma, and a definitive diagnosis or exclusion of cervical spine injury is urgently needed.

* UK National Institute for Clinical Excellence

functional discontinuity of axons. Very high levels of extracellular glutamate accumulate, damaging neighbouring cells and causing a ripple effect of neuronal death and the release of further toxic molecules. Potential neuroprotective agents such as antagonists for glutamate and calcium have so far proved ineffective.

The brain has minimal capacity to functionally regenerate after injury but in general, the younger the patient, the better the prognosis. Young children can often recover full function after remarkably severe injuries because of the plasticity of the developing nervous system. With increasing age, the consequences of the primary injury are likely to be more severe; an important factor is that with advancing age, the brain shrinks, allowing greater mobility within the cranial vault under impact. This increases the risk of tearing intracranial veins that leads to subdural haemorrhage.

PRIMARY BRAIN INJURY

CONCUSSION

Concussion is a brain injury associated with brief loss of consciousness, usually for only a few minutes; it causes minor cognitive disturbances such as temporary confusion or amnesia. By definition there are no persistent abnormal neurological signs but there may be signs of neuronal injury on CT scanning.

DIFFUSE AXONAL INJURY

Axonal injury occurs in mild, moderate and severe head injuries, the number of axons damaged increasing with the severity of the injury. Axonal injury is visible on high-quality CT scans. Causative factors are similar to those that produce intracranial haematomas, but the trauma is usually initiated by contact with a broader object with less force and often with lateral movement. This condition does not cause raised intracranial pressure and treatment is supportive. Sequelae include organic and psychological dysfunction including loss of concentration, memory disturbances and personality changes such as depression or disinhibition. Higher cortical functions are affected most and take longest to recover. Many of these clinical features were formerly attributed to brain stem injury.

FOCAL BRAIN INJURIES

Focal injuries involve gross damage to localised areas of the brain and are readily visible on CT scanning. The main lesions are **cerebral contusion** or sometimes **laceration**, **haemorrhage** and **haematoma**, all of which may act as space-occupying lesions and are liable to result in secondary brain injury. The site and extent of the primary injury depend on the nature of the damaging force (see Fig. 16.2). Contusions may be small or large and occur beneath the area of impact (**coup**) or at the tips of the frontal or temporal lobes remote from the injury (**contrecoup**) caused by rebound of the brain within the skull at the time of impact (Fig. 16.3). With overt brain injury,

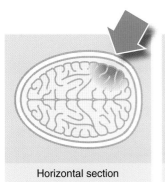
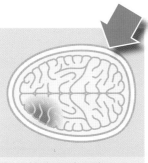
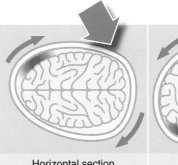
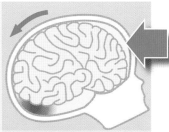

Horizontal section	Horizontal section	Horizontal section	Sagittal section

'Coup' or direct injury
Mechanism similar to deceleration injury
(a)

'Contre-coup' injury
Injury to side opposite blow because of rebound
(b)

Rotational injury
Inertia of brain suspended within cranium leads to tearing of surface vessels and subdural haemorrhage
(c)

Fig. 16.2 Mechanisms of brain injury
(a) The mechanism of 'coup' or direct injury is similar to a deceleration injury (shown in horizontal section). **(b)** A 'contre-coup' injury affects the side opposite to the blow because of rebound (horizontal section). **(c)** In rotational injury the inertia of the brain suspended within the cranium leads to the tearing of surface vessels and subdural haemorrhage (horizontal and sagittal sections).

CASE STUDY

Fig. 16.3 Focal brain injury

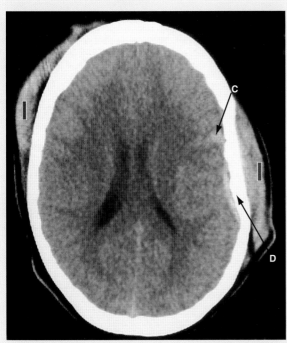

A cyclist was knocked off his bike by a car and suffered a head injury with loss of consciousness of 45 minutes. CT scan of head shows signs of soft tissue injury **I, I** in both left temporal ('coup') and right fronto-parietal regions ('contre-coup'). There is a depressed segment of skull bone in the left temporal region **D** and signs of intracerebral contusion **C** beneath both areas of injury. He gradually recovered without need for operation, but full cerebral functional recovery took several months.

there is usually a period of coma followed by a period of cognitive disturbance related to the extent of diffuse axonal injury or focal injury. Large contusions are associated with prolonged coma, small ones with lethargy and subtle focal deficits.

Brain injury is much more likely to have occurred if there is a skull fracture, but a skull fracture itself does not necessarily indicate brain injury.

SECONDARY BRAIN INJURY

Secondary brain injury may be caused by cerebral hypoxia, intracranial bleeding or infection. These are discussed in detail below.

CEREBRAL HYPOXIA

Oxygen deprivation to the brain after head injury is the most important and most easily preventable cause of secondary brain injury. It stems from ischaemia (lack of blood) or hypoxia (lack of oxygen in the blood). The damage is caused by **cellular hypoxia** or **raised intracranial pressure** due to cerebral oedema, or both. The most common cause is inadequate pulmonary oxygenation due to airway obstruction, alcohol or drug overdose, chest injury, inhalational pneumonitis, adult respiratory distress syndrome or central respiratory depression. Hypotension due to hypovolaemia may also contribute to cerebral hypoxia by reducing cerebral perfusion. Resuscitation is designed to prevent or treat both hypoxia and hypovolaemia.

INTRACRANIAL BLEEDING

Post-traumatic intracranial bleeding is traditionally classified into **extradural** (epidural), **subdural** or

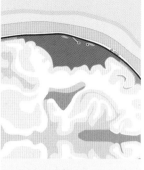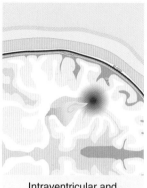

Extradural haemorrhage   Subdural haemorrhage   Intraventricular and
intracerebral haemorrhage

Fig. 16.4 Types of post-traumatic intracranial bleeding

intracerebral (see Fig. 16.4) but it has fairly recently become established that **subarachnoid** haemorrhage is also a common occurrence after moderate or severe head injury and carries a poor prognosis. With intracranial bleeding, local brain compression causes focal neurological effects as well as a general rise in intracranial pressure. The latter may cause **temporal lobe herniation** under the tentorium cerebelli or '**coning**' of the brain stem through the foramen magnum, or both, leading to neurological deterioration and often death.

An acute rise in intracranial pressure manifests with the following clinical signs:

- Deteriorating level of consciousness
- An enlarging, unresponsive pupil
- Central respiratory depression
- Falling pulse rate (late sign)
- Rising blood pressure (late sign)

Extradural (epidural) haemorrhage

About 10% of severe head injuries result in extradural haemorrhage and this is most common in children, adolescents and young adults. It is most likely to arise when there is a skull fracture in the temporal region (Fig. 16.5) but can occur without a fracture. It is usually caused by rupture of an artery, the middle meningeal or one of its branches; consequently the haematoma develops rapidly and needs urgent surgical intervention. Death will quickly follow unless the haematoma is evacuated rapidly. Emergency CT scanning is indicated to confirm the diagnosis and to show the position of the haematoma. With increased awareness of the problem and the more widespread availability of CT scanning, emergency 'blind' burr hole drainage of an extradural haemorrhage by a general surgeon is now rarely required. Urgent transfer to a neurosurgeon for consideration of craniotomy is usually the most appropriate course of action.

Pathologically, there is rapid accumulation of (arterial) blood between the skull vault and the tough dura mater with the extent of lateral spread limited by dural attachments (Fig. 16.4). The mass bulges into the underlying

Fig. 16.5 Temporo-parietal fracture with extradural haematoma

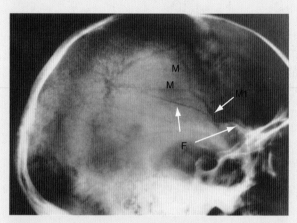

This 20-year-old man was admitted fully conscious after being knocked off a bicycle but deteriorated rapidly 2 hours later. Lateral skull X-ray showing a linear fracture (arrowed **F**) of the right temporo-parietal bones crossing the course of the anterior branch of the middle meningeal artery **M** on the temporal bone.

brain substance causing local compression and a rise in intracranial pressure.

The classic clinical picture in extradural haemorrhage is as follows:

- Loss of consciousness
- Rarely this is followed by a **lucid interval** but with severe headache and drowsiness
- Secondary decline in consciousness following any lucid interval
- Rapid development of a fixed, dilated pupil on the side of the injury and a hemiparesis on the opposite side

In many cases, unconsciousness is continuous from the outset. Extradural haematomas nearly always present within 24 hours of trauma.

Fig. 16.6 Subdural haematoma

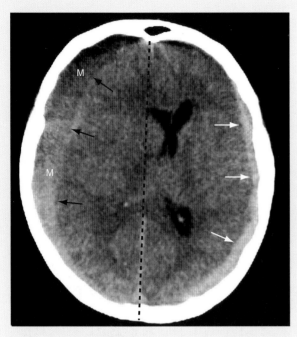

An elderly man suffered a head injury in a road traffic collision without loss of consciousness 48 hours previously. His conscious level gradually deteriorated and so this CT scan was performed. On the right side, there is a large subdural haematoma of mixed attenuation **M M** (black arrows define the edge of the brain). Such mixed attenuation suggests old liquefying thrombus and is consistent with its origin around the time of the accident. There is a smaller subdural haematoma on the left side (white arrows) of consistent attenuation suggesting that it arose more recently. Note the midline of the brain is shifted to the left by the mass effect of the larger haematoma and there is compression of the lateral ventricles. The patient required neurosurgical drainage.

Subdural haematoma

Subdural haematomas are more common than extradurals and occur in about 30% of severe head injuries (Fig. 16.6). Subdural haematoma usually results from the tearing of veins passing between the cerebral cortex and dura, or from laceration of the brain or cortical arteries. Blood accumulates relatively slowly in the large potential space between dura mater and arachnoid mater. The haematoma tends to spread laterally over a wide area. In contrast to extradural haemorrhage, there is usually underlying primary brain injury and the mortality is up to 50%. Subdural haematomas commonly occur in more than one site, either on the same side or on both sides (see Fig. 16.6).

In an acute subdural haemorrhage, there is usually clinical evidence of significant brain injury at the outset, with later deterioration. A lucid interval between initial loss of consciousness and later deterioration is rare. Acute subdural haemorrhage is more common in older adults because of increased brain mobility within the skull. Surgical evacuation of the clot may halt deterioration but recovery is often incomplete; many elderly patients die from this condition despite expeditious treatment. With increasing use of warfarin anticoagulation, acute subdural haematoma is seen more commonly after relatively trivial injury.

Chronic subdural haematoma

Subdural haematomas may develop gradually in the elderly following trivial, often unrecalled, head injury. This may become manifest weeks or months later as non-specific neurological deterioration, chronic headache or coma. Most patients do not present with a history of head injury and the diagnosis is made on investigation of neurological symptoms.

Intracerebral haemorrhage

Haemorrhage into the brain parenchyma is caused by primary brain injury. Small deep lesions are often associated with diffuse axonal injury and should be monitored for expansion using serial CT scans. A larger lesion or continuing haemorrhage produces an expanding mass lesion which should be evacuated early to prevent secondary brain damage.

INFECTION

Meningeal infection may cause secondary brain injury, with organisms entering via compound skull fractures. Fractures beneath scalp lacerations are easily diagnosed as being compound but others may be deceptive; for example, fractures of the skull base may communicate with the sphenoid or ethmoid sinuses, the nasal cavity or the external auditory canal. Similarly, fractures of the frontal bone often involve the frontal sinuses. Fractures of this type should always be assumed to be compound.

Early debridement of compound depressed fractures is important to minimise the risk of infection. There is no evidence to support the use of prophylactic antibiotics, which should be reserved for use when clinical infection is manifest; this usually becomes evident several days after injury.

SKULL FRACTURES

THE IMPORTANCE OF SKULL FRACTURES

A skull fracture indicates a severe impact. Consequently, patients with fractures are much more likely to sustain primary brain damage than those without. This became widely recognised after Teasdale's seminal paper in 1990 (see Table 16.2, p. 246). In addition, patients with skull fractures are 30 times more likely to suffer secondary brain damage by the mechanisms described earlier. Depressed fractures are often associated with some primary injury to the underlying brain but, paradoxically, the process of fracture may absorb some of the energy of impact and protect the brain.

If NICE guidelines are followed (Box 16.4), CT scans are performed on all patients with a reduced GCS and can virtually rule out fracture, intracranial haematoma and significant injury to the underlying brain. If CT scanning is not available, ordering plain X-rays for every patient with a head injury is expensive, time-consuming and inappropriate. Clinical criteria can identify most of those at significant risk of a skull fracture so that radiological resources can be employed cost-effectively (Box 16.2). Skull X-rays are less reliable than CT for detecting fractures. Note that even if no fracture is present, an intracranial haematoma may still be present, particularly in a child.

All patients diagnosed with skull fractures merit hospital admission for close observation (even if fully conscious).

TYPES OF SKULL FRACTURE

Linear or stellate fractures

These involve mainly the skull vault, often with little external sign of injury, although there may be some overlying scalp bruising or swelling. Linear fractures rarely exhibit displacement unless there are multiple fracture lines.

Depressed fractures

These fractures are usually caused by blunt injuries and the overlying scalp is usually lacerated or severely bruised; such fractures rarely produce serious primary brain injury unless they are depressed more than the thickness of the skull vault. Elevation of depressed fractures is usually performed for cosmetic reasons.

Compound (open) fractures

Either of the above types of skull fracture can be compound. If the dura is torn, there is a direct communication with the brain and a high risk of infection. Early debridement and dural closure are indicated. Compound fractures of the base of the skull are diagnosed clinically and with CT scanning.

Fractures of the base of the skull

These usually involve the anterior or middle cranial fossae. The characteristic clinical features are summarised in Box 16.3.

(a) AP, Towne's and lateral views of the skull

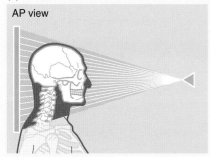

AP view

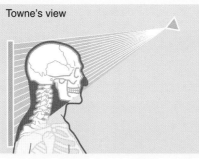

Towne's view

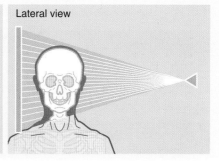

Lateral view

(b) 30° occipito-mental view of the facial bones

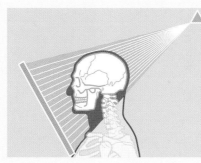

X-ray tube angled perpendicular to film

Fig. 16.7 A standard set of skull X-rays
(a) The standard set of skull X-rays includes three views: anterior-posterior (AP), Towne's view and lateral. For potential facial fractures, a 30° occipito-mental view may be added **(b)** The AP view is the standard frontal view of the skull. A calcified pineal may show a midline shift. The Towne's view shows the occipital bone, the zygomatic arch and the mandibular condyles if the mouth is open. The occipito-mental view of the facial bones shows the middle third of the face, fluid levels in the maxillary sinuses as well as the orbits and fractures of the orbital floor.

X-rays used for diagnosis of skull fractures

If CT is not available, a standard set of three X-ray films is taken: **lateral skull, AP skull and Towne's view** (see Figs 16.7 and 16.8). A careful and systematic search should be made for the presence of fractures as well as for lateral shift of the (calcified) pineal gland and fluid levels in the sphenoid and frontal sinuses. Fluid levels indicate a basal skull fracture. For suspected facial and orbital fractures, a 30° **occipito-mental** X-ray is the standard investigation.

MANAGEMENT OF HEAD INJURIES

ASSESSING ACTUAL OR POTENTIAL BRAIN DAMAGE

CLINICAL TRIAGE VERSUS CT DIAGNOSIS

Up to the end of the 1990s, triage of head-injured patients was intended to identify those likely to have an evolving intracranial haematoma. The process was based on clinical assessment, together with skull X-rays for patients with positive clinical indications (see Fig. 16.9). Large numbers of patients had to be admitted to hospital for observation because these methods were insufficiently reliable. The growing availability of CT at last made it practicable to use this investigation earlier and more often in the triage process, but there were theoretical risks of missing early evolving haematomas and concerns about the radiation dose involved, especially in children.

A UK National Institute for Health and Clinical Excellence (NICE) committee was charged with evaluating available evidence to construct new guidelines for head injury assessment, designed to reduce delay in detecting life-threatening complications and to ensure better outcomes. The committee concluded that early imaging rather than admission and 'head injury observation' would achieve their stated aims. The published NICE guidelines use head CT as the primary imaging modality, with **CT diagnosis** replacing **plain X-ray triage**. Skull X-rays (and regular head injury observations) are recommended to be restricted to infants at risk of intentional injury and situations where CT is unavailable. The potential benefits include early recognition of clinically significant intracranial haematomas and safely avoiding hospital admission where no lesion is found. However, the guidelines specify a tight timescale for obtaining CT and this

Fig. 16.8 Standard skull X-ray views and CT scan showing skull fractures

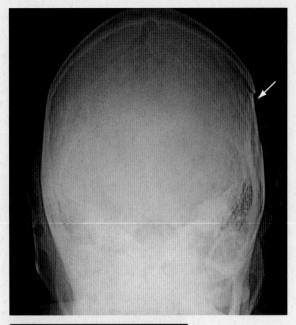

(a)

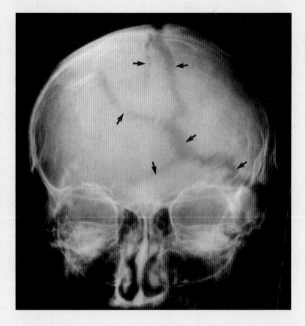

(b)

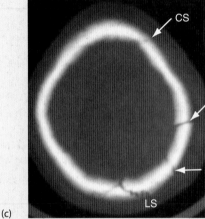

(c)

(a) Case study 1: Towne's view from a 19-year-old woman after a blunt blow to the side of the head; she was fully conscious. This shows a depressed fracture in the left parietal bone (arrowed) The segment of bone is depressed by more than the thickness of the skull and therefore needed surgically elevating. **(b) Case study 2:** this 24-year-old woman suffered a high impact speed road traffic accident (RTA) and was admitted to hospital deeply unconscious and with deep scalp lacerations. Her GCS was 5. This AP X-ray shows extensive fractures (arrowed) in the parietal, occipital and squamous temporal bones. Because of the lacerations, these fractures were considered compound. **(c)** CT scan of the upper part of the skull vault in a different patient after a road traffic collision showing a normal coronal suture **CS**. There are parietal fractures (arrowed) and **diastasis** (partial separation) of the lambdoid suture **LS**.

carries resource implications. Implementing NICE guidelines has been shown to increase the head scan rate two- to five-fold (from approximately 2% to 8%), reduce the rate of taking skull X-rays from about 40% to 4%, and reduce hospital admission rates from 10% to 4%. In published studies, the policy change has not resulted in any excess adverse events and there is a small overall cost saving.

CLINICAL ASSESSMENT

The most important factors in the history that indicate potential brain injury and a risk of future complications are **unconsciousness** and amnesia for events before the impact (**retrograde amnesia**). The duration of unconsciousness and amnesia are roughly proportional to the severity of brain injury. Witnesses should be questioned as to whether the patient was 'knocked out'. In practice,

however, the evidence is often unclear. If the patient was travelling in a car, the extent of injuries to other passengers may give an indication of the energy transfer in the accident. Careful questioning of the patient about events leading up to the accident usually reveals the duration of retrograde amnesia, if any.

On examination, particular attention should be paid to the level of consciousness, the pupil size and reactivity, and motor power in the limbs. The findings should be recorded periodically on a standard head injury proforma and the GCS calculated for each set of observations. A systematic neurological examination must also be performed, however trivial the head injury, in addition to a general examination.

If there is a deep scalp laceration or a history of penetrating injury, the scalp should be deeply probed with a gloved finger, which may reveal a small bony defect or step.

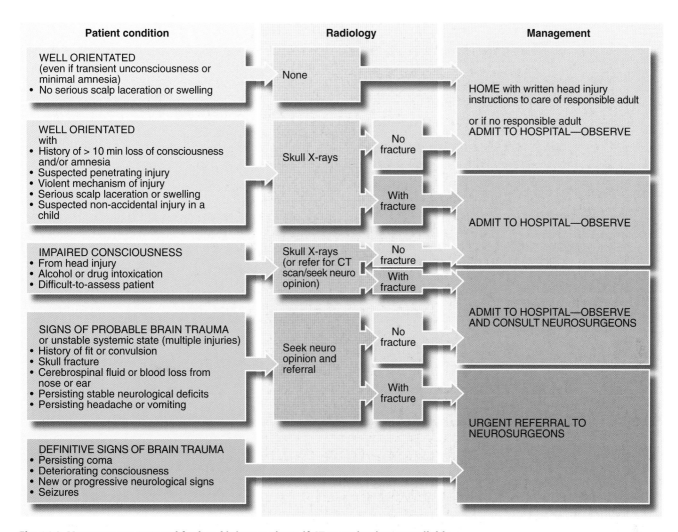

Fig. 16.9 Management protocol for head injury patients if CT scanning is not available

Level of consciousness

The level of consciousness is the most important single observation in head injury patients. However, unstructured clinical judgement is prone to error and lacks reproducibility. The GCS (see Table 16.1) overcomes these problems and is used world-wide for assessing severity of head injury and for monitoring progress. Level of consciousness can be categorised simply and reproducibly by this method. Formal assessment should take place after resuscitation and before intubation if possible, and should take into account any sedative drugs or alcohol taken and any direct orbital injuries. If eye opening and verbal responses cannot be used, the motor response is the most important observation; a patient unable to follow commands has a serious head injury. In patients with impaired consciousness, pressure over the supraorbital nerve at the orbital rim is usually employed to elicit pain. To be scored as being able to localise the pain, the patient's hand should rise above the clavicle. A **flexion response** to pain is manifest by a hand moving but not rising above the clavicle.

On the GCS, a score of 15 is normal. Reduced scores can sort patients into severity groups to help determine appropriate investigations and treatment. After a head injury, a score of 3–8 represents a *severe* head injury, 9–12 is *moderate*, 13–14 is regarded as *mild*, and 15 as *minor*. The probability of there being an intracranial haematoma likely to need surgery in these groups is shown in Table 16.2.

Aggressive behaviour in patients smelling of alcohol must **not** be assumed to result from intoxication (i.e. removal of social inhibition) because this behaviour also commonly arises from brain injury or hypoxia. A thorough examination and probably a CT scan should be performed with this in mind before employing sedation to quieten a disruptive patient. Comatose patients or those with multiple injuries are also often hypoxic. This causes cerebral swelling, thereby further depressing consciousness and damaging the brain. Accurate assessment of brain injury can therefore only be performed in a fully oxygenated patient.

Pupillary responses and eye movements

Pupillary size and response to light should be checked, along with the full range of eye movements and the visual fields if possible. Normal pupillary size and response to

Table 16.1 Glasgow Coma Scale

Clinical observation	Score*
Eye opening	
Spontaneous	4
To verbal command	3
To pain	2
None	1
Motor response	
Obeys commands	6
Localises pain	5
Flexion withdrawal to pain	4
Abnormal flexion (decorticate)	3
Extension to pain (decerebrate)	2
None	1
Verbal response	
Orientated	5
Confused conversation	4
Inappropriate words	3
Incomprehensible words	2
None	1

*On this scale, a patient's Glasgow coma score is the sum of the scores from the three sections. The worst total score is 3, the best is 15. After the initial score, the observations and scoring are repeated at intervals to look for deterioration

Table 16.2 Probability of intracranial haematoma requiring surgery according to the severity of head injury as assessed by GCS

Glasgow coma score	Severity of head injury	Probability of haematoma
3–8	Severe	1 in 7
9–12	Moderate	1 in 50
13–14	Mild	1 in 3500

light require the integrity of both the 2nd and 3rd cranial nerves, and pupillary changes are a fairly sensitive indicator of developing intracranial bleeding. However, benign pupil asymmetry is fairly common in the population at large and it is important to find out whether asymmetry was present beforehand if detected after a head injury. Unilateral changes to the pupil diameter or the light response after trauma are usually caused by 3rd nerve involvement. Pressure on one side of the brain forces the medial edge of the temporal lobe through the tentorial hiatus (herniation). This compresses the nerve in its long intracranial course on the same side. The result is pupillary dilatation and loss of the constrictor response to light on the same side as the lesion (ipsilateral). However, direct ocular trauma can also cause a mydriasis (dilatation of the pupil); in this case, there is usually a hyph-

aema (bleeding into the anterior chamber) or other obvious eye injury. Bilateral pupillary dilatation and loss of the light reflex are indications of potentially fatal brain stem injury, i.e. **'coning'**.

Limb movements and responses

In a fully conscious patient, tone, power and coordination can be readily assessed in the standard manner. If a subtle abnormality is suspected, the patient should be asked to close his or her eyes and hold the arms outstretched with palms upwards for 1 minute. Pronation or downward drift on one side is indicative of brain injury. For the semiconscious or unconscious patient, the pattern of limb response to painful stimuli provides a useful indication of the conscious level, as indicated in the Glasgow Coma scale (see Table 16.1).

PRACTICAL MANAGEMENT OF HEAD INJURIES

Patients with a GCS of 15 after a head injury can safely be discharged from hospital. Those with reduced scores will ideally have early CT scanning, following NICE guidelines (Box 16.4), and those with normal scans can also be discharged (unless other injuries make admission necessary) and the rest admitted for observation (Box 16.5). Patients admitted with uncomplicated minor head injuries who are fully alert can safely be allowed to go home after 24 hours even if there is a simple skull fracture. Patients should be advised to rest at home for at least a week as cognitive functions such as power of concentration are unlikely to recover rapidly (post-concussion syndrome, see later). Severely head-injured patients require urgent resuscitation and transfer to a neurosurgical unit.

If CT scanning is not available, a management scheme such as that shown in Figure 16.9 can be employed; the history is helpful in deciding whether apparently minor head injuries need skull X-rays (Box 16.2) or admission to hospital for observation (Box 16.6).

Head injury observations

The important observations for head injury patients admitted to hospital are shown in Table 16.3. These are sufficiently sensitive to provide early warning of developing complications. Observations are performed by nursing staff, the frequency depending on the state of the patient. If there is a skull fracture or any suggestion of reduced consciousness, confusion, disorientation, alcohol or drug effects, observations should be made at 30-minute intervals, at least for the first night, otherwise hourly. Observations are recorded or plotted on a special **head injury proforma** so that deterioration will be immediately obvious and can be reported to medical staff at once.

Box 16.4   'NICE' criteria for CT scan and consultation with a neurosurgical unit after head injury (GCS = Glasgow Coma Score)

General principles

- First stabilise airways, breathing and circulation (ABC)
- Clinically assess patients immediately with a GCS below 15
- If GCS is 8 or less, involve anaesthetist for airway management and resuscitation
- Perform early CT imaging where appropriate to detect brain and cervical spine injuries (skull X-rays + inpatient observation where CT unavailable)
- Exclude brain injury before attributing depressed conscious level to intoxication
- No systemic analgesia until assessed for conscious level and neurological deficit (local anaesthesia for fractured limbs/ other painful injuries)
- Record observations on a standard head injury proforma (a special one for under 16s)

Indications for head CT within 1 hour in adults or children

- GCS less than 13 at any time since injury
- GCS 13 or 14 at 2 hours after injury
- Suspected skull fracture, open or depressed, including signs of basal skull fracture (haemotympanum, 'panda' eyes, cerebrospinal fluid otorrhoea, Battle's sign)
- Post-traumatic seizure
- Focal neurological deficit
- More than one episode of vomiting

Indications for head CT within 8 hours in adults or children if the 1 hour criteria do not apply

- Antegrade amnesia (i.e. for events before impact) of more than 30 minutes
- Any loss of consciousness or amnesia plus:
  —Age 65 years or more
  —Coagulopathy (history of bleeding, clotting disorder, current warfarin treatment)
- Dangerous mechanism of injury (e.g. pedestrian struck by motor vehicle, occupant ejected from a motor vehicle or fall from more than 1 metre or five stairs).

Indications for prompt neurosurgical referral after head injury

The care of all patients with new, surgically significant abnormalities on imaging should be discussed with a neurosurgeon. Other criteria include:

- Persisting coma (GCS less than or equal to 8) after resuscitation
- Unexplained confusion for more than 4 hours
- Deterioration in GCS after admission (greater attention should be paid to motor response deterioration)
- Progressive focal neurological signs
- A seizure without full recovery
- Definite or suspected penetrating injury
- A cerebrospinal fluid leak

Note: A neurosurgical opinion should be sought based on clinical information; ideally, the CT images should also be transferred electronically to the neurosurgeon

Box 16.5   'NICE' criteria for admission to hospital following a head injury where CT is available and criteria have been followed

- New and clinically significant abnormalities found on imaging
- GCS has not returned to 15 after imaging, regardless of imaging results
- When CT scanning is indicated but cannot be done within the appropriate period
- Continuing worrying signs, e.g. persistent vomiting, severe headache
- Other sources of concern, e.g. drug or alcohol intoxication, other injuries, shock, suspected non-accidental injury, meningism or cerebrospinal fluid leak from nose or ear

Box 16.6   Criteria for admission to a general hospital after head injury when CT scan is not available*

Orientated patient

- Skull fracture or suture diastasis (separation)
- Persisting neurological symptoms or signs
- Difficulty in assessment, e.g. suspected drugs, alcohol, non-accidental injury, epilepsy, attempted suicide
- Lack of a responsible adult to supervise the patient
- Other medical condition, e.g. coagulation disorder

All patients with impaired consciousness

Notes:
1. Transient unconsciousness or amnesia with full recovery is not necessarily an indication for admission of an adult, but may be so in a child
2. Patients with head injuries may have other serious internal injuries which are easily overlooked
*Based on the report of the Working Party on Head Injuries, Society of British Neurological Surgeons, 1998

Observation	Sign of neurological deterioration
Conscious level (GCS)	Falling score
Pupil size and light response	Dilatation, loss of light reaction or developing asymmetry
Respiratory pattern and rate	Irregularity, slowing or reduced depth of breathing
Developing neurological signs	Focal signs point to localised intracranial damage
Pulse rate	Falling pulse rate (late sign)
Blood pressure	Rising blood pressure (late sign)

Table 16.3 Essential observations for head injury patients (findings should be recorded on a standard head injury proforma)

MANAGEMENT OF MODERATE AND SEVERE HEAD INJURIES

Most trauma deaths result from head injuries or from multiple injuries involving chest, abdomen and limbs. Some head injuries are so severe as to preclude survival, whilst others need urgent recognition and surgical decompression, e.g. extradural haemorrhage. For such cases, 4 hours is considered the maximum permitted delay between the injury and neurosurgical intervention for the condition to be potentially salvageable. Four hours easily passes given that at least an hour elapses before arrival at hospital plus the time spent in the resuscitation room, in the CT scanner, and the transfer to a neurosurgical unit.

Other deaths from head injuries occur unnecessarily, simply because ventilation (airway or breathing) has not been recognised as inadequate. This leads to hypoxaemia, hypercarbia and cerebral swelling, compounding the rising intracranial pressure. If patients are combative or severely agitated, there may be a need for general anaesthesia to enable control of PCO_2.

Initial management

Any patient who has focal neurological signs, whose conscious level is moderately depressed (GCS 14 or less) or who is unconscious, must be considered to have a significant head injury. The patient should be resuscitated and decisions made about the management of other injuries and the timing of CT scanning if other injuries need immediate treatment. If the receiving hospital does not have CT scanning facilities, the patient may need to be transferred to a regional centre after resuscitation. If the patient is deteriorating rapidly and an extradural haemorrhage is suspected, burr holes in the temporal region must be made immediately if the patient's life is to be saved.

Continuing care

The management of intracerebral haemorrhage and other major head injury complications is highly specialised. Many of these patients have other serious injuries and may need to be nursed and monitored in an intensive care or high-dependency unit with the assistance of anaesthetic staff.

The continuing care of the patient with a stable serious brain injury (usually in a neurological critical care unit) involves some or all of the following procedures:

- **Intensive monitoring** of vital signs and neurological status
- **Endotracheal intubation and artificial ventilation** if hypoxaemic
- **Nasogastric aspiration** for all unconscious patients to prevent inhalation of gastric contents
- **Monitoring of fluid and electrolyte balance** (hyponatraemia and hypoproteinaemia exacerbate cerebral oedema)
- **Monitoring of intracranial pressure** using a surgically implanted cerebral extradural catheter—75% of patients with severe head injuries in specialist units now have intracranial pressure monitored
- **Measures for the control of raised intracranial pressure**—successive protocols are employed for incremental rises, including controlled hyperventilation (reducing PCO_2 causes cerebral vasoconstriction, reduced cerebral oedema and hence reduced intracranial pressure), CSF drainage, mannitol infusion (for its osmotic effect in reducing cerebral oedema), hypothermia (although there is no solid evidence of benefit), barbiturates and decompressive craniotomy
- **Measures to maintain cerebral perfusion pressure**—may require intravenous infusion of fluids and perhaps inotropic cardiac support

REHABILITATION

Nearly all patients who have sustained a head injury experience long-term disability following discharge. This includes about half of those judged to have suffered a mild injury (GCS 13 or 14); even these so-called 'mildly' brain-injured patients have been shown to be moderately or severely disabled a year after injury. When MRI scanning is performed in 'mild' head injury patients, a surprisingly high incidence of parenchymal lesions is found, which perhaps explains the slow recovery. This disablement is termed **post-concussion syndrome**. Problems include headache, dizziness, mental deficits, slowness of thought, poor concentration, problems with communicating, inability to work, poor performance at school and difficulties with self-care.

Potential or actual disability needs to be recognised early, ideally before discharge from hospital. However, no reliable mechanism has been found to safely exclude patients from the need for follow-up. Ideally, all head injury patients should be followed up at least once, and expert and prolonged follow-up is mandatory following severe injuries and decompressive surgery. Long-term physical recovery after serious brain injury is helped by physiotherapy and occupational therapy, but recovery of intellectual powers is inevitably slow and cannot be speeded up. Patients can easily languish in the community unless the problems are recognised and supportive measures are put into place. This includes joining self-help groups such as Headway in the UK and other countries.

MAXILLOFACIAL INJURIES

GENERAL PRINCIPLES

Fractures of the facial skeleton are common, particularly after sporting injuries, road accidents and fights. The main fractures involve the mandible, the middle third of the face, the nasal bones, the orbit and the zygoma. Facial fractures rarely pose urgent management problems except for major middle third fractures (in which the upper jaw becomes detached from the base of the skull) and multiple mandibular fractures; both may result in upper airway obstruction, and these patients may require endotracheal intubation or cricothyroidotomy to safeguard the airway. Facial fractures are generally managed by maxillofacial surgeons, who may not be available in smaller hospitals. In most cases, delaying treatment for a few days does not adversely affect the outcome.

EXAMINATION FOR FACIAL FRACTURES

If there is any facial injury, the contour of the facial bones should be carefully palpated and the eyes examined before the oedema develops and obscures any underlying bony deformities. The extraocular muscle attachments may be disrupted by orbital wall fractures so the full range of eye movements must be formally examined and the patient questioned about diplopia in all positions. The patient should be asked if 'the teeth bite together normally', and the mouth should be examined both for missing or displaced teeth and for the state of the dental occlusion. Abnormalities of occlusion are a common and sensitive sign of a jaw fracture which might otherwise be missed. The full range of mandibular movements should also be checked to exclude fractures or dislocations involving the mandibular condyles.

RADIOLOGY

If facial fractures are suspected, X-rays should be taken of the facial bones with the particular views chosen according to the bones under suspicion. Interpretation of facial radiographs can be difficult for the non-specialist but most fractures can be identified if the main bony contours are carefully traced and compared with the opposite side.

Opacities or fluid levels in the maxillary sinuses (antra) usually represent haematoma. This commonly follows fractures of the bones surrounding the maxillary sinuses, e.g. zygoma or orbital floor.

MANDIBULAR FRACTURES

The common sites of mandibular fractures are shown in Figure 16.10. Because of the effects of oblique trauma, a fracture on one side is often accompanied by a fracture on the other side in a different position, e.g. body of mandible on one side and condylar neck on the other. Fracture lines tend to occur through points of weakness, e.g. mental foramina, unerupted third molar teeth or condylar necks. Most undisplaced mandibular fractures need no active intervention but displaced fractures require fixation. This can be achieved by wiring the lower teeth to the upper teeth, by direct wiring of the bones or by internal plate fixation (see Fig. 16.11). Any fracture passing through a tooth socket defines the fracture as 'compound' and prophylactic antibiotics should be administered.

FRACTURES OF THE MIDDLE THIRD OF THE FACE

Fractures of the middle third of the facial skeleton range from detachment of the palate and dental arch to complete separation of the middle third complex from the base of the skull. Diagnosis is based on clinical assessment. A simple test is to grasp the upper teeth or jaw between the fingers and attempt to move them independently of the skull. Treatment may involve disimpaction and usually requires sophisticated external fixation to the skull or internal plate fixation.

FRACTURES OF THE NASAL BONES

Trauma to the nose is extremely common and often results in nasal bone fracture. Less often, fracture dislocation of the septum occurs and may interfere with the nasal airway. Diagnosis is made on clinical grounds with the main features being flattening or lateral displacement

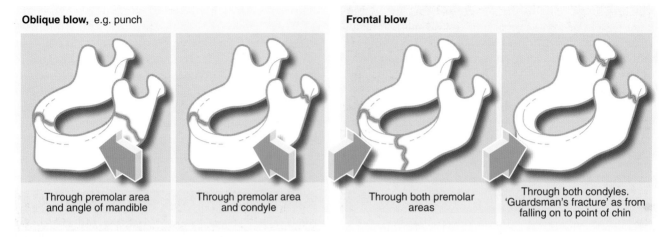

Oblique blow, e.g. punch

Through premolar area and angle of mandible

Through premolar area and condyle

Frontal blow

Through both premolar areas

Through both condyles. 'Guardsman's fracture' as from falling on to point of chin

Fig. 16.10 Common sites of mandibular fractures

Fig. 16.11 Oral pantomogram X-ray after plating of two mandibular fractures

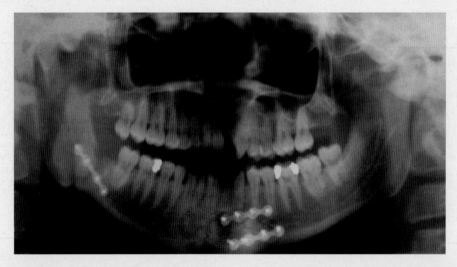

After a blow to the chin, fractures occurred at the angle of the mandible on the right and the anterior body on the left (see Fig. 16.10). Both fractures were immobilised by direct bone plating.

of the nasal bridge. Bleeding from the nose often indicates a nasal fracture. The fracture is usually reduced several days later by an ENT or maxillofacial surgeon.

FRACTURES OF THE ORBIT AND ZYGOMA

DEPRESSED FRACTURES OF THE ZYGOMA

A depressed fracture of the zygoma (see Fig. 16.12) is the most common fracture of the orbit and results from a blow to the cheek. The fracture line usually passes through the infraorbital foramen and causes a palpable step in the inferior orbital margin. The infraorbital nerve becomes compressed with any substantial degree of depression, causing paraesthesia or numbness in its area of sensory innervation, i.e. the upper lip, upper teeth and buccal mucosa on that side. Diagnosis may be suspected by flattening of the cheek contour; this is best seen from above and behind the patient. Overlying oedema may obscure a depressed fracture, and these patients warrant radiological examination. An associated fracture of the lateral orbital wall may produce enough bleeding for it to track forward under the conjunctiva. This type of subconjunctival haemorrhage has no visible posterior limit and is the characteristic sign of an orbital wall fracture (Fig. 16.13).

Treatment is indicated if there is inferior orbital nerve compression or a cosmetically unacceptable deformity. Reduction is usually accomplished via a temporal approach, sliding an elevator under the root of the zygoma, deep to the temporalis fascia.

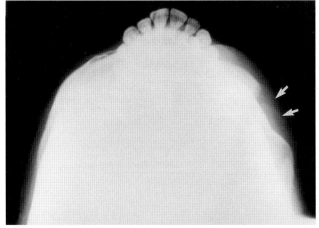

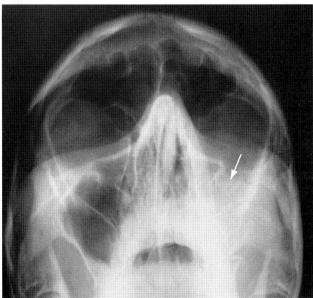

(a)

(b)

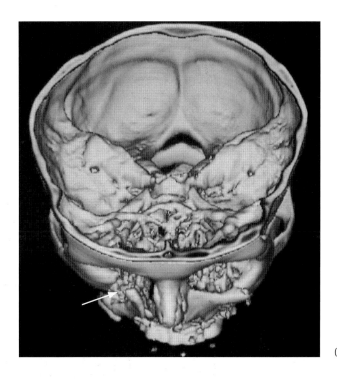

(c)

Fig. 16.12 Depressed zygomatic fractures
(a) Submento-vertical projection of a 43-year-old man who had been punched on the left cheek showing a depressed fracture of the zygomatic arch (arrowed). **(b)** 30° occipito-mental radiograph after a similar injury in a different patient. This patient had a depressed 'tripod' fracture of the zygoma manifest by discontinuity of the lower orbital margin (arrowed). Note that since the roof of the maxilla is involved, the maxillary sinus (the antrum) has typically filled with blood and is rendered radiopaque. **(c)** 3D reconstruction of CT scans showing a severely depressed fracture of right lower orbital rim involving maxilla and zygomatic body (arrowed). The left lower orbital rim is also fractured and displaced.

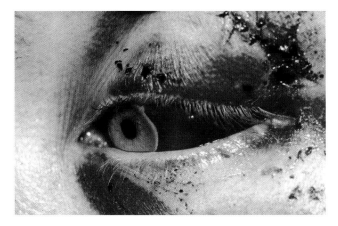

Fig. 16.13 Subconjunctival haematoma following a head injury
This 14-year-old boy fell off his bicycle and momentarily lost consciousness. This photograph shows a subconjunctival haematoma with no posterior limit indicating a fracture of the orbital wall, in this case the petrous temporal bone of the base of the skull.

BLOW-OUT FRACTURES OF THE ORBIT

A direct frontal blow to the orbit from an object about the size of a squash ball (3–4 cm) which may act like a plunger, causes a **'blow-out' fracture** of the orbital floor without damaging the orbital margin. Blow-out fractures can also occur after a blow to the inferior orbital rim which then causes a ripple effect, fracturing the floor of the orbit whilst the rim remains intact. The blow-out most commonly involves the floor of the orbit where the bony walls are thinnest. This causes herniation of peribulbar fat into the maxillary sinus and disrupts the function of the extraocular muscles, causing diplopia and restricted upward gaze (see Figs 16.14 and 16.15). Hence it is important to test eye movements in any patient with a facial injury. Diagnosis is suggested by finding an antral opacity (haematoma) on occipito-mental X-ray, but CT scanning of the orbit is required if the bony defect needs

251

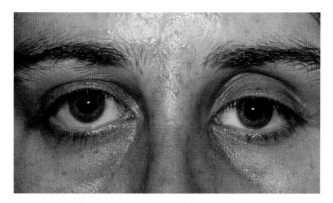

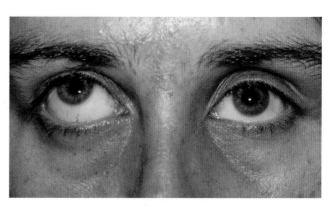

(a)

(b)

Fig. 16.14 Blow-out fracture of orbital floor
(a) This young man was punched in the left eye, causing a blow-out fracture of the orbital floor. **(b)** Note failure of upward gaze on the left due to trapping of the extraocular muscles in the fractured orbital floor.

Fig. 16.15 X-ray appearance of blow-out fracture of orbital floor

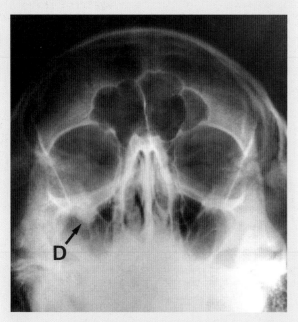

This 30-year-old man was hit on the right eye by a squash ball, causing a blow-out fracture of the orbital floor by hydraulic pressure. Orbital fat and extraocular muscles have been forced into the maxillary antrum and held there by the fractured bone edges. This causes the characteristic 'hanging drop' sign **D**. Upward gaze is restricted, resulting in vertical diplopia.

to be demonstrated. Treatment involves exploring the orbital floor and may require a bone graft or silicone implant.

INJURIES TO THE TEETH

Fractures and avulsions of the anterior teeth are common and may require immediate treatment in the emergency department. Correct first-aid treatment may preserve teeth which would otherwise be lost.

Fractures involving the loss of more than one-third of the crown should be seen urgently by a dental surgeon as the dental pulp may be exposed or endangered. Partially avulsed teeth need to be pushed back into position. This can usually be done with the fingers after local anaesthetic infiltration. Urgent dental referral for tooth splintage and root canal treatment is then required.

If a tooth is completely avulsed, it can often be successfully reimplanted by a dentist if it has been carefully cleaned and wrapped in a sterile, saline-soaked swab. Note that success with reimplantation diminishes proportionate to the time the tooth is out of the socket: under 30 minutes gives the best results. The discovery of missing or broken teeth in an unconscious patient should alert the examining doctor to the possibility of inhalation of tooth material into the bronchi or impaction in the lips or pharynx. Chest X-ray and examination of the perioral soft tissues should be performed in these cases.

COMMON ENT EMERGENCIES

The most common ear, nose and throat emergencies are illustrated in Figure 16.16.

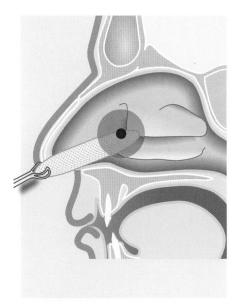

1. Active epistaxis

Management: apply topical local anaesthetic (e.g. Instagel). Pack gently with ribbon gauze or preformed sponge

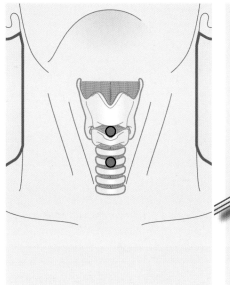

2. Acute upper airway obstruction

Management: sweep mouth with gloved finger for foreign body/denture; Heimlich manoeuvre to dislodge food inhaled into larynx. If these fail; stab laryngotomy (or rapid tracheostomy if trained and equipment to hand).
If in a restaurant, extend neck with rolled clothes under shoulders. Incise with steak knife and insert sheath from ball point pen

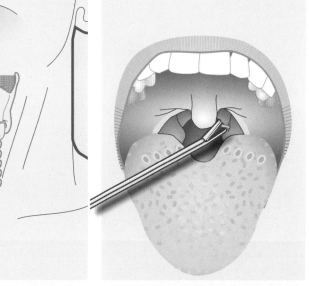

3. Fish bone in throat

Management: patient demonstrates position with finger tip, then apply lidocaine spray. Remove with forceps, using a headlight if available

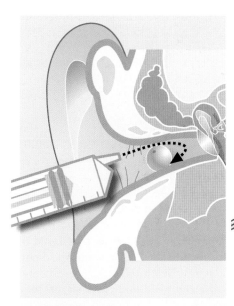

4. Foreign body in ear

Most commonly a bead in a child's ear. Management: remove using special sucker tip or gently syringe using a 20 ml syringe and water at body temperature.
No forceps!

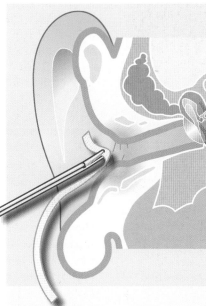

5. External otitis

Cause — usually *Staphylococcus* infecting hair follicles after swimming.
Management: Narrow ribbon gauze, soaked in antibiotic ointment + oral antibiotic against *Staphylococcus*, e.g. flucloxacillin

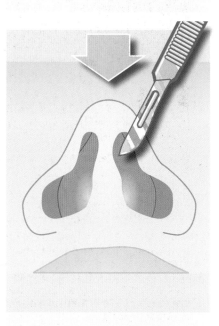

6. Septal haematoma following direct trauma

Note that the nose is blocked bilaterally. Management: incise and drain under local anaesthetic. If untreated likely to become a septal abscess leading to collapse of cartilage

Fig. 16.16 Common ENT emergencies

SOFT TISSUE INJURIES

Soft tissue injuries are defined here as cuts, lacerations, crushing injuries, missile injuries and impalements that do not involve bone or body cavities. The priority for treating soft tissue injuries depends on the primary survey as determined by the ABCDE system (Ch. 15).

Minor injuries are usually managed in primary care or emergency departments. These can be defined as superficial injuries not involving 'danger areas' such as the eye or hand, with no significant nerve or vascular injury and without heavy contamination. **Intermediate injuries** are defined as injuries that are not life threatening but require special attention, usually in hospital. **Major injuries** are those requiring more complex management in hospital, often with more than one specialty involved, e.g. general surgery, plastic and reconstructive surgery and orthopaedic surgery. Penetrating and other major **eye injuries** are a special case and need expert ophthalmic surgical care.

The detailed management of a soft tissue injury depends upon the following factors:

- The mechanism of injury (e.g. penetrating knife wounds, lacerations in road crashes, blast injuries, gunshot and missile injuries, burns, bites)
- The site of injury
- The extent and depth of wounds
- The types of tissue involved including nerves and blood vessels
- The extent of devitalisation of tissue
- Any contamination (e.g. with road dirt, soil or potential bacterial inoculation with animal or human bites)
- The possibility of retained foreign bodies

MINOR SOFT TISSUE INJURIES

Most minor wounds can be cleaned and sutured or closed with tissue glue immediately. Local anaesthesia is usually required. The danger of tetanus must be considered in any open wound that is more than purely superficial, and tetanus toxoid administered if previous immunisation is inadequate. Deep, soil-contaminated wounds (however small) in a non-immunised patient also warrant prophylactic penicillin. **Grazes** may need cleaning of road dirt but generally just require dressing with non-adherent dressings such as Mepitel.

INTERMEDIATE SOFT TISSUE INJURIES

Foreign bodies

The history of the injury can indicate the likelihood of foreign bodies being retained in the wound. The main types of foreign body are agricultural and road dirt and gravel, wood splinters, and glass and metal fragments. Plain radiology reveals metal and usually glass fragments (see Fig. 17.1) but the radiopacity of glass is variable and a negative X-ray does not exclude its presence. It is important to remember that a foreign body unrecognised at the time may result in litigation at a later date.

As a general principle, foreign bodies should be removed, especially if they are organic (e.g. wood) or likely to be contaminated. However, glass and metal fragments are often small, multiple and deeply embedded and may be difficult or impossible to locate at operation despite X-ray or ultrasound guidance. In such cases, it

Fig. 17.1 Glass in soft tissue wounds

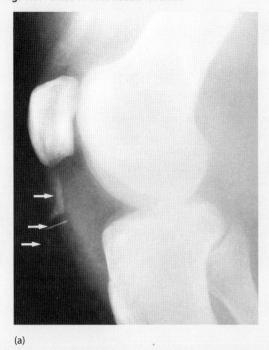
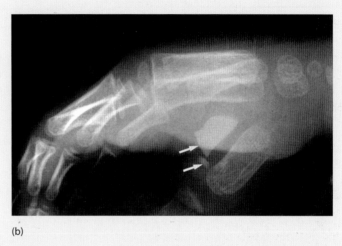

(a) (b)

(a) A 19-year-old woman with lacerations near the knee after falling on to broken glass. Note several fragments of glass (arrowed) in the infrapatellar soft tissues. **(b)** Fragments of glass (arrowed) in the palm of a 12-year-old boy after he fell through a glass door. In both these cases, the fragments were missed by casualty officers because X-rays were not requested despite a history of glass injury.

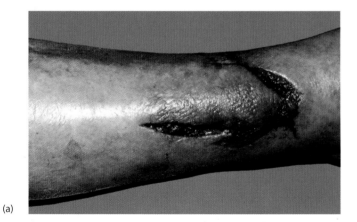
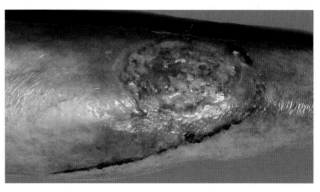

(a) (b)

Fig. 17.2 Flap laceration
(a) This wound was caused by a fall in which the patient's shin was scraped on a stone step. It is tempting to suture such a wound, but if this is done the flap will invariably undergo necrosis as in **(b)**. Most of these types of wound require split skin grafting.

is best not to embark on extensive exploratory surgery but to leave the fragments in situ where they rarely cause complications. The patient must be informed about what has been left and warned that superficial fragments often work their way to the surface and are shed spontaneously. The patient should be instructed to return if problems occur later. All of this information must be recorded in the patient's notes in case of future legal action.

Flap lacerations

Relatively minor trauma to the tibia commonly produces a V-shaped **flap laceration** (Fig. 17.2). This is most likely to occur in older patients or in patients on long-term corticosteroid therapy. If untreated, this injury habitually fails to heal because of poor blood supply to the flap and to the underlying tissue. Attempting to suture or tape a flap laceration into place increases tension in the flap, causing local ischaemia, tissue loss and ulceration. The most effective management is early excision of the flap and immediate split skin grafting. This can be performed under local anaesthesia and has been shown to take an average of two weeks to heal.

Facial lacerations

Minor facial lacerations generally heal well and can be primarily sutured in the accident department after careful cleaning. Infection is rare because of the excellent blood supply. Even ragged skin edges do not become devitalised and so trimming is rarely necessary. The main consideration is the expected cosmetic outcome, so great care should be taken with suturing technique, employing general anaesthesia if necessary. Complex lacerations, lacerations across the lip margin or eyelid and areas of substantial skin loss, especially on children and young people, should be managed by plastic surgeons (see next section).

Scalp lacerations

With scalp lacerations, the main considerations are to exclude brain injury and skull fracture and then determine whether the aponeurotic layer (galea) has been breached. In addition, haemostasis must be achieved; it is easy to underestimate the potential for blood loss from scalp lacerations, which may be sufficient to cause hypovolaemic shock, particularly in the elderly. Assessment and proper exploration is made easier by shaving the wound edges; large lacerations may need to be explored under general anaesthesia. If the aponeurosis has been breached, this should be repaired separately to prevent accumulation of a subaponeurotic haematoma that would be vulnerable to infection. Careful attention should be paid to achieving haemostasis from the major scalp blood vessels which lie in the superficial fascia between dermis and aponeurosis. Dense collagenous bands cross the superficial fascia and tend to prevent torn vessels contracting, thus hindering the spontaneous arrest of bleeding. Torn vessels need to be individually ligated or sutured.

MAJOR SOFT TISSUE INJURIES

Major injuries of soft tissues alone that require hospital treatment are uncommon; they can be classified as shown in Box 17.1. A primary survey (Ch. 15) determines the order in which injuries generally are managed, with life-threatening injuries being treated first. For other injuries, the urgency depends on the potential for deterioration (e.g. major blood loss, ischaemia or loss of an eye), the risk of infection and the availability of the necessary specialists. Contused or contaminated wounds need early cleansing and excision of all devitalised tissue (debridement), usually under general anaesthesia. If substantially contaminated, wounds are often left unsutured initially

---

| Box 17.1 | Classification of major soft tissue injuries |

- Vital part of the body, e.g. eye, hand, extensive facial lacerations
- Vascular injuries involving blood loss or ischaemia
- Nerve and tendon injuries requiring meticulous surgical repair
- Animal or human bites
- Gunshot, missile and stab wounds
- Traumatic amputation of digits or limbs
- Injuries involving substantial skin loss likely to need skin grafting, e.g. degloving injuries to limbs
- Contamination with soil, road dirt—requiring debridement and/or prophylactic immune serum or antibiotics
- Crush injuries
- Chemical injuries, e.g. acid, bleach, fertiliser
- Burns of more than 5% of body area or involving inhalation

---

to prevent wound infection and are then sutured a few days later by **delayed primary closure**. Less commonly, wounds are left open and are allowed to heal by **secondary intention** (see Ch. 3). Wounds involving skin loss may need early skin grafting.

INJURY TO A VITAL PART OF THE BODY

Eye

Injuries greater than 'sand in the eye' are best managed by ophthalmic specialists who are likely to require a slit-lamp and other instruments to fully assess the injury. Typical injuries include abrasions to the cornea, penetrating injuries (dart or pellets) and firework injuries.

Neck

Penetrating injuries to the neck must be treated with respect. Many vital structures are concentrated here and may be injured. These include major arteries and veins (carotid, jugular, subclavian, vertebral), the brachial plexus, some cranial nerves, the cervical sympathetic chain (see Fig. 17.3) and lung and pleura.

Lacerations to the limbs and hands (for traumatic amputation, see p. 262)

The main considerations with this type of injury are:

- **Possible nerve, tendon or vascular injury**— assessment includes testing sensation, movement, peripheral pulses and tissue perfusion (i.e. pulses, warmth, colour, capillary refilling after blanching). Tendon and nerve injuries are covered below
- **Tissue viability**—this is particularly important in the case of crush injuries and flap lacerations such as in the pretibial area (see above)

Fig. 17.3 Horner's syndrome caused by stab wound in the neck

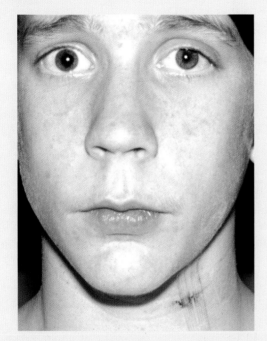

This 19-year-old was stabbed in the neck: the knife missed the great vessels but succeeded in damaging the cervical sympathetic chain, causing miosis (constriction) of the pupil as a result of unopposed parasympathetic activity.

- **Risk of infection**—the fingers and hands are vulnerable to infection of the pulp spaces and deep palmar space. Wounds need antibiotic prophylaxis against staphylococci and streptococci (e.g. flucloxacillin plus amoxicillin). They also need meticulous cleansing and exploration, if possible by a specialist hand or plastic surgeon. Injuries from bites (especially by dogs or humans) and bones (usually in meat workers) almost invariably become infected (see below).

Extensive facial lacerations

Facial injuries should be thoroughly cleaned and examined under local or general anaesthesia before repair to determine the extent of the damage; this should be performed within 12 hours of injury. Facial wound edges need minimal trimming because of the rich vascular supply. Important anatomical boundaries should be aligned first; these include the vermilion border of the lip, the rim of the eyelid and the eyebrow. Tissue layers should then be approximated individually—mucosa, muscle, cartilage and skin. Parotid duct injury should be considered in deep lacerations of the cheek and the duct repaired if possible. Photographic documentation is useful to help the patient appreciate the extent of injury and to provide an accurate record of progress.

Facial nerve integrity should be determined before anaesthesia is given. Nerve branches should be repaired if caused by a laceration posterior to a vertical line from the lateral canthus of the eye, but there is no point in doing so if the injury is anterior to this. Nerve repair should be performed no more than 72 hours after injury.

VASCULAR INJURIES INVOLVING BLOOD LOSS OR ISCHAEMIA

Where major **blood vessels** have been damaged, haemorrhage can usually be arrested, at least temporarily, by applying pressure on gauze swabs. If limb ischaemia is present, early vascular imaging and repair is needed. If substantial lengths of vessel have been lost, this involves vascular grafting. If revascularisation is delayed, **reperfusion injury** is probable and **compartment syndrome** is likely. Reperfusion injury occurs when blood flow is restored after a period of severe ischaemia. Much of the damage appears to be caused by free radicals formed as part of the inflammatory responses of damaged tissues and mediated by macrophages and inflammatory cytokines.

If a main artery and vein have both been severed, e.g. femoral artery and vein, the vein is always repaired first to allow venous drainage before repairing the artery. If nerves have also been cut, nerve repair is required using an operating microscope (microsurgery).

Compartment syndrome

The muscles of the leg below the knee and in the forearm lie within rigid fascial compartments. Restoring blood flow after a period of severe or total ischaemia leads to **reperfusion injury**, which in turn allows protein-rich fluid to leak from the damaged capillaries. This causes a rise in intracompartmental pressure (normally in the range of 0–10 mmHg) which compromises venous flow and later reduces capillary flow. This initiates a vicious circle that exacerbates the ischaemic insult and further increases the pressure. Arterial inflow is not usually impaired but compartment syndrome rapidly leads to irreversible nerve ischaemia and muscle necrosis.

The best form of management is pre-emptive **fasciotomy** at the time of revascularisation if the procedure follows a period of severe ischaemia or if there have been signs of ischaemic anaesthesia or paralysis before surgery. Fasciotomy involves incising the enclosing fascia of each compartment over a substantial length. The wound is left open and usually covered by split skin grafts a few days later. Fasciotomy can also be performed later if early postoperative signs suggest a developing compartment syndrome. Signs include altered sensation or paralysis in the distribution of nerves passing through the compartment (e.g. foot drop caused by ischaemia of the common peroneal nerve), muscle tenderness and excessive pain on passive movement. Note that peripheral pulses may still be present. Treatment of established compartment syndrome is often less satisfactory than pre-emptive treatment and may result in substantial disability.

PERIPHERAL NERVE INJURIES

Anatomy

In a peripheral nerve trunk, individual axons are sheathed in **endoneurium** and groups of axons are bundled in **fascicles**. Each fascicle is covered in tough **perineurium** composed of collagen and elastin and may contain both sensory and motor axons. A **peripheral nerve trunk** consists of a number of fascicles in a matrix of **epineurium** which also coats the nerve. Fascicles divide repeatedly along the course of a nerve, communicating with each other and intermixing rather than running neatly in parallel. This means that the arrangement and the type of axons and fascicles in one cross-section of the nerve may be very different from that in an adjoining cross-section. The difficulty of aligning the proximal arrangement with the distal arrangement is an important reason why functional recovery is poor if a segment of nerve is lost and has to be replaced with a nerve graft.

Types of injury

Nerve injuries were classified by Seddon in 1943:

- **Neuropraxia** is the mildest injury, in which nerve continuity is preserved and only transient functional loss occurs. Recovery takes place within 6–8 weeks on average, without Wallerian axonal degeneration. The lesion is probably biochemical and is caused by compression, blunt impact or nearby low-velocity missile injuries. Motor nerves are more sensitive to damage than sensory nerves and autonomic function is often retained
- **Axontmesis** occurs when there is interruption of the axon and its myelin but the perineurium and epineurium are preserved. Axontmesis results from more severe crush injury or contusion; axonal continuity is lost and complete denervation occurs but supporting structures remain intact. Electromyography (EMG) confirms muscle denervation distal to the injury. Recovery eventually takes place as a result of axon regeneration and is likely to be complete
- **Neurontmesis** involves complete functional disconnection of a nerve. Neurontmesis occurs with severe contusion, stretching or laceration of a nerve. Axons and their encapsulating connective tissue lose continuity and there is complete absence of motor, sensory and autonomic functions, which rarely recover without surgical intervention. In most cases, the nerve is not completely severed but suffers marked internal structural disruption. In this case, axonal regeneration causes a fusiform swelling of the

injured segment. If the nerve has been divided, fibroblast proliferation produces a dense fibrous scar which inhibits the ability of sprouting axons to enter distal tubules and seriously impairs nerve regeneration

Nerve regeneration

In **axontmesis**, calcium-mediated Wallerian (or antegrade) degeneration of the distal axon and myelin occurs early on. Within a few days, sprouting begins from the ends of the proximal axons. Regenerating fibres eventually cross the injury site and then progress distally at 1–2 mm a day through the undamaged tubules; these provide a precise path for reinnervation of target organs.

In **neurontmesis**, nerve lesions close to the parent cell often lead to death of the cell body. If cell death does not occur, axons sprout (as in axontmesis) but the first barriers are the scar and any intervening gap in the nerve. A neuroma forms on the proximal end of the nerve and functional distal recovery does not occur unless operative repair is performed. The most favourable injury for repair is a clean wound without segmental nerve loss.

Denervated muscle becomes irreversibly damaged after 18 months. Axons regenerate at about 2.5 cm per month provided they have an uninterrupted route, thus for any hope of functional recovery, the distance between the nerve injury and target muscle must be under 45 cm. As an example, if the ulnar nerve is injured in the brachial plexus, the wrist and finger flexors located in the forearm may recover, but the intrinsic muscles of the hand may not. The time taken for the axons to reach the end-organs depends on distance, provided the pathway is uninterrupted, but a further period is needed to achieve functional recovery. This is because the new axon needs to mature, the synapse has to be reconstituted, the end-organ must recover from trophic changes, and a critical number of axons must reach the target end-organs to accomplish neural control.

Clinical types of nerve injury

Compression

Compression affects the largest myelinated fibres most. Motor control is lost first and discrete sensation follows as compression continues. The underlying cause is probably nerve ischaemia; large myelinated fibres are more susceptible to this than smaller unmyelinated ones. In partial injuries, smaller pain-bearing and sympathetic fibres are often preserved, causing pain and hyperaesthesia in the nerve distribution. Compression injuries include so-called 'Saturday night palsy', where the radial nerve becomes compressed over the back of a seat in a patient who passes out under the influence of alcohol. Total loss of motor and sensory function is likely to occur. Adverse effects are spontaneously reversible unless ischaemia persists for more than 8 hours.

Traction

Traction, particularly stretching, is the most common mechanism of nerve injury and is often associated with fracture or dislocation. Nerves have little elasticity and can only stretch 4% without injury. Luckily, most traction injuries are self limiting and have a good prognosis; as many as 90% achieve good or fair recovery. The prognosis is worse when vascular trauma or open fractures are present, with only 65% recovering useful function.

Laceration

Lacerations such as those caused by a knife blade comprise up to 30% of serious nerve injuries. Exploration and repair is recommended in most cases of palsy following laceration.

Missile injury

Low-velocity gunshot missiles are less likely to sever nerves than sharp laceration injuries. However about 70% of missile wounds that require exploration for other reasons demonstrate complete or partial transsection of a nerve. In high-velocity missile injuries, cavitation of soft tissues caused by passage of the missile can produce nerve stretch injuries.

Repair of nerve injury

Direct repair

A clean sharp division of a nerve such as that caused by a knife wound should be repaired by primary anastomosis within 24 hours of injury. Simple **epineural repair** involves re-approximation of the nerve ends using a circumferential line of sutures. This type of repair is technically easier than **fascicular repair** which involves microsurgical anastomosis of fascicles or groups of fascicles.

Epineural repair is generally the method of choice for sharp nerve injuries. Results are often good if the fascicular patterns at the two cut ends are similar and where anatomic distortion is minimal. Even for proximal nerve trunk repair, where a plexiform layout of fibres is more likely, the chances of the correct type of axons passing down the proper fascicles appear to be as good as in fascicular repair. Epineural repair is also stronger and resists tension better. With compression, stretching or contusion injuries, repair should be undertaken between 8 weeks and 3 months of injury if there is no evidence of recovery.

Cable grafting

Autologous nerve grafting is needed if there is a large gap in a nerve. The most commonly used donor nerve is the **sural**, a large sensory nerve running down the posterior calf to the lateral dorsum of the foot. Several 'cables' are usually fashioned and attempts made to match proximal and distal fascicles. As indicated earlier, the plexiform and mixed nature of fascicles makes full recovery difficult to achieve.

Results of nerve repair

Assuming good technique, the following factors improve the prognosis for recovery after nerve repair:

- The repair involves purely sensory or motor nerves, e.g. the functional result of repair of a severed peroneal nerve (motor) is likely to be better than an equivalent median nerve repair (mixed)
- The lesion is distal rather than proximal because distal trunks have a more linear arrangement
- The patient is younger; children have better results than adults, and younger adults better than older adults
- The repair is undertaken soon after injury

TENDON INJURIES

Tendon injuries are common and are usually caused by trauma involving glass or knives (open injuries). Single or multiple tendons can be traumatised as well as neighbouring nerves, blood vessels and bone. Slicing injuries from knives and saws produce fairly predictable damage, but stabbing injuries (particularly from glass) can damage structures some distance from the site of entry. Tendons can also snap if overstressed. Such closed injuries commonly occur during sport, e.g. Achilles tendon rupture, or when there is abrupt muscle traction as in trying to prevent a fall, e.g. ruptured patellar tendon.

Complete division or detachment of a tendon causes immediate loss of its function, which is permanent unless repaired. Patients are usually immediately aware of difficulty in moving a finger, for example, but some injuries are less obvious if there is duplication in the function of muscles. Partial lacerations of tendons are not obvious but can be suspected if use of the tendon causes pain.

Assessment

Assessment of tendon injuries requires systematic testing of each and every tendon in the area, as well as adjacent nerves. The following signs should be noted when examining the limb. Examples are given for hand tendon injuries:

- **Position**—the exact site of the laceration will suggest which structures may have been injured
- **Posture**—when relaxed, the normal hand lies in a characteristic posture with the thumb tip held slightly flexed and fingers held in a cascade. Any change from this normal resting posture suggests tendon or nerve damage
- **Passive movement**—gentle pressure on each fingertip can reveal loss of tension or floppiness of a joint. Tendon function can be assessed by gentle pressure over the muscles in the forearm, which will normally cause movement of the relevant tendon
- **Active movement**—the best way of testing a tendon is to ask the patient to use the tendon by moving or tensing the relevant joint

Treatment

If a cut tendon is not repaired, its function is permanently lost, with resulting deformity, loss of movement and weakness. After an open injury, surgical exploration and repair should be performed early because late attempts at repair are technically more difficult. They are also less likely to succeed because unrepaired tendons retract, muscles shorten and atrophy, tunnels through which the tendons run shrink, and joints stiffen. Some closed ruptures of extensor tendons, however, are best managed by splinting, e.g. mallet finger.

Surgery

Exploration can be performed under regional or general anaesthesia, usually employing a tourniquet to prevent bleeding. The wound usually needs to be enlarged to allow thorough inspection of anatomical structures and to retrieve the tendon ends. The cut tendons are sutured together end-to-end and adjacent nerves repaired if necessary.

Rehabilitation

Skilled rehabilitation is essential as tendon repairs can break if overstressed and the repair can adhere to surrounding tissues. The key is **protected mobilisation** to allow early mobility without excessive stress on the repair. The repair needs to be splinted for 4 weeks or more, but it takes about 12 weeks to recover full strength.

Complications

- **Infection**—affects 5% and may cause failure of the repair. Contaminated wounds are at greatest risk
- **Tendon rupture**—affects 5–10% of repairs. Causes include technical failure, local and general factors delaying wound healing, and patient non-compliance
- **Tendon adhesion**—adhesion of the damaged tendon to the investing synovial sheath prevents the tendon from gliding freely. A small amount of adhesion is common, but sometimes further surgery is required to free the tendon (**tenolysis**)
- **Joint stiffness**—local joints can become stiff indirectly as a result of swelling, infection and immobility

ANIMAL-ASSOCIATED SOFT TISSUE INJURIES

Animals can cause human injury through bites, kicks, blunt trauma, goring with horns or lacerations from claws. Bite wounds in particular need prompt medical attention to reduce the risk of local infection. Tetanus is also a risk in puncture wounds or bites in a patient unprotected by tetanus immunisation.

Snakebite

Poisonous snakes are a hazard in many areas, although deaths from snakebite are rare. Snakebites are most common where dense human populations co-exist with large snake populations (e.g. South-East Asia, sub-Saharan Africa, and tropical America). Particularly dangerous venomous snakes include the Australian brown snake; Russell's viper and cobras in southern Asia; carpet vipers in the Middle East; and coral snakes and rattlesnakes in the Americas. The venom of a small or immature snake can be even more concentrated than that of larger ones; therefore all snakes should be left well alone. Less than half of all snakebite wounds actually contain venom, but travellers are advised to seek immediate medical attention whenever a bite wound breaks the skin. First-aid measures should include immobilising the affected limb and applying a pressure bandage that does not restrict limb perfusion (not a tourniquet), then moving the victim as quickly as possible to a medical treatment centre. Incision of the bite site is not recommended. Specific therapy for snakebites varies and should be left to the judgement of experienced local emergency medical personnel.

Arthropod bites and stings

The bites and stings of some arthropods (which include insects) can cause unpleasant reactions. Travellers should seek medical attention if a spider or insect bite or sting causes excessive redness, swelling, bruising or persistent pain. Patients who have a history of severe allergic reactions to bites or stings should consider carrying an adrenaline (epinephrine) autoinjector (EpiPen) in case of recurrence. Many insects and arthropods can transmit **communicable diseases**, even without the traveller being aware of a bite. This is particularly true when camping or staying in rural accommodation. Travellers to many parts of the world should be advised to use insect repellents containing DEET, protective clothing, and mosquito netting around beds at night. Stings from **scorpions** can be painful but are seldom dangerous except in infants and children. In general, exposure to scorpion stings can be avoided by sleeping under mosquito nets and by shaking clothing and shoes before putting them on.

Animal bites

Domestic pets cause more animal bites than wild animals, with dogs more likely to bite than cats; however, cat bites are more likely to become infected. The sharp pointed teeth of cats usually cause puncture wounds and lacerations that may inoculate bacteria into deep tissues. In Adelaide, Australia, about 6500 people are injured each year by dog attacks and 800 seek hospital treatment (7.3 per 10 000 population). Children up to 4 years required hospital treatment twice as often as adults, and men aged over 76 years twice as often as younger men; 90% of children suffered head and facial bites. In the USA, dog bites cause about 44 000 facial injuries requiring hospital treatment each year. This represents about 1% of all emergency room visits. Dog attacks kill 10–20 people each year in the USA, and in the UK there was an average of 2.3 fatalities a year between 1999 and 2004. Unfortunately, most of these fatalities are in young children where bites to the face, neck or head are extremely hazardous. Children are often bitten in these areas because of their small stature.

Dogs typically cause a crushing type of wound because of their rounded teeth and strong jaws. An adult dog can exert 200 pounds per square inch (psi) of pressure, and some large dogs are able to exert 450 psi. Such pressure may damage deep structures such as bones, vessels, tendons, muscle and nerves.

Bites of the **hand** generally have a high risk for infection because of the relatively poor blood supply. The complex anatomical structure also makes adequate cleansing of the wound difficult. In general, the better the vascular supply and the easier the wound is to clean (i.e. laceration vs. puncture), the lower the risk of infection.

The principles of treatment of bite wounds are inspection, debridement, irrigation and closure:

- Wounds should be carefully **inspected** to identify deep injury and devitalised tissue. Adequate inspection nearly always requires a general or regional anaesthetic. Care should be taken to visualise the deepest part of the wound and, if appropriate, to examine the wound through a range of motion
- **Debridement** is an effective means of minimising infection. Devitalised tissue, particulate matter and clots should be removed to prevent them from becoming a source of infection, as with any foreign body. Clean surgical wound edges result in smaller scars and promote faster healing
- **Irrigation** also helps prevent infection. A 19-gauge blunt needle and a 50 ml syringe provide adequate pressure and volume to clean most wounds. In general, 100–200 ml of irrigation solution per cm^3 of wound is required. Large, dirty wounds need to be irrigated in the operating theatre. Saline solution is an effective and inexpensive irrigating solution
- **Primary closure** can be considered in clean bite wounds or wounds that can be cleansed effectively. Others are best treated by **delayed primary closure**. Facial wounds are at low risk for infection because of the excellent blood supply, even if closed primarily. Bite wounds to the lower extremities, bites where there is a delay in presentation, or those in immunocompromised patients should generally be left open

Types of infection

Animal saliva is heavily contaminated with bacteria; over 130 disease-causing microorganisms have been isolated from dog and cat bite wounds, thus nearly all infections are mixed. In rabies areas, bites from non-immunised domestic animals and wild animals carry the risk of rabies and the need for prophylaxis should be considered, in addition to tetanus prophylaxis. While local infection and cellulitis are the leading causes of morbidity, sepsis is a potential complication of bite wounds. Meningitis, osteomyelitis and septic arthritis are additional concerns in bite wounds. Rabies is a generally fatal complication. However, the three infections mentioned below are probably the most significant:

Pasteurellosis

Pasteurella multocida is a bacterium carried naturally by most mammals in their mouths, including healthy cats, dogs and rabbits, and by some birds and fish. The organism is responsible for the most common bite-associated infection. The first signs of pasteurellosis usually occur within 2–12 hours of the bite and include pain, reddening and swelling of the area around the bite. Pasteurellosis can progress quickly, spreading centrally from the bitten area. The infection can spread and may cause flu-like symptoms such as fever, headaches, chills and swollen glands. If left untreated, it can cause pneumonia or systemic sepsis and, on rare occasions, death.

Streptococcal and staphylococcal infections

These bacteria can cause infections similar to those caused by *Pasteurella*. Redness and painful swelling occur at or near the site of the bite and progress proximally.

Human bites

Human bites can be as dangerous as animal bites because of the bacteria and viruses resident in the human mouth; the general principles of contaminated wound management apply. In a closed-fist injury, an opponent's tooth often inoculates the extensor tendon and its sheath. The resulting contamination cannot be removed readily through normal cleansing and irrigation. Patients may need to be admitted for intravenous antibiotic therapy, and surgical drainage may also be necessary.

When fingers are bitten, tendons and their sheaths lying close to the skin can become infected. The wound may appear to be trivial, but careful inspection is needed to exclude deeper injury. When a person is bitten on the head, wounds may appear innocuous, but subgaleal bacterial contamination can easily be missed. This is especially true in young children who have thin soft skin over the scalp and forehead. Such wounds are best cleaned, left open and closed secondarily. Use of antibiotics is debatable and has not been shown to reduce infection rates.

HIV transmission has occurred very rarely after a human bite. Exposure to saliva alone is not considered a risk factor for HIV (or hepatitis) transmission.

GUNSHOT, MISSILE AND STAB WOUNDS

Gunshot wounds and missile injuries need special attention. High-energy missiles may cause a small entry wound but produce havoc within (see Ch. 16). X-rays need to be taken and wounds explored under general anaesthesia.

TRAUMATIC AMPUTATION OF DIGITS OR LIMBS

Principles of digit and limb replantation surgery

Complete amputation of digits is common, especially in industrial accidents, but sometimes whole limbs are severed. With clean-cut injuries, it is possible to reattach the amputated part using microsurgical techniques to join the vessels and nerves. This cannot be done after crush or avulsion injuries or in grossly contaminated wounds. Even in ideal cases, recovery is slow and usually incomplete, necessitating many months away from work and much rehabilitation effort. Therefore, replantation should never be undertaken without carefully evaluating the likely benefits and ensuring the patient is fully involved in the decision. In digital amputation, the greatest disability results from loss of the thumb. There is no place for replantation of a single finger, even the index finger, because the remaining fingers rapidly adapt to the loss.

Replantation should only be considered if there has been no major crushing or degloving injury. Indications for replantation may include:

- Loss of whole upper limb or hand
- Loss of thumb alone
- Loss of all digits (replant thumb and one or two fingers)
- Loss of all fingers (replant one or possibly two fingers)

At the scene of the injury, the severed digit should be washed gently to remove obvious dirt and placed in a plastic bag which is then placed inside a second plastic bag containing ice or frozen peas. In this way it can be successfully preserved for up to 12 hours.

CONTAMINATION WITH SOIL AND ROAD DIRT

Superficial wounds such as grazes caused by motorcycle injuries and lack of protective clothing often become impregnated with road debris over wide areas. These need to be scrubbed clean, often under general anaesthesia. In the case of large contaminated and contused wounds involving muscle, the potential for **gas gangrene** must be considered. Dead tissue must be thoroughly excised, benzylpenicillin given prophylactically, and primary closure avoided in favour of delayed primary closure. Note that **hydrogen peroxide** must not be used in any wounds other than purely superficial ones because of the dangers of oxygen embolism causing brain damage.

CRUSH INJURIES

Crush injuries occur most commonly in earthquakes and during wars after buildings have collapsed on people. Rhabdomyolysis follows prolonged heavy continuous pressure on muscle and **crush syndrome** is caused by reperfusion injury when the damaged muscle is revascularised on removing compression. Damaged cells release potassium and potentially toxic substances such as myoglobin, phosphate and urate into the circulation. Water and extracellular electrolytes enter the damaged muscle. The net result is hypovolaemic shock with electrolyte disturbances leading to prerenal and toxic renal failure.

Following earthquakes, the incidence of crush syndrome has been estimated at 2–5% of those who are buried under rubble. About half of these develop acute renal failure, and half of those need dialysis. Crush syndrome is also seen following industrial incidents, particularly in mining, and in road traffic collisions.

Diagnostic criteria for crush syndrome include:

- A crushing injury to a large mass of skeletal muscle
- Sensory and motor disturbances in the compressed limb
- Swelling and tenseness of the limb a few hours later
- Myoglobinuria and/or haematuria
- Elevated serum creatine kinase (CK) with a peak greater than 1000 U/L
- Renal insufficiency hours or days later. This may manifest with oliguria (urine output less than 400 ml in 24 hours), decreased plasma calcium concentration and elevated plasma urea, creatinine, uric acid, potassium and phosphate

Presentation

Crush syndrome presents with profound shock. A limb trapped will be pulseless on release; later it will become red, swollen and blistered with loss of sensation and muscle power.

Reperfusion injury causes **compartment syndrome** to develop after release of compression. Once the compartment pressure exceeds capillary perfusion pressure (about 30 mmHg), tissues in the compartment become ischaemic.

Management

At the accident scene, if there has been a substantial crush injury, amputation of the limb on site will prevent crush syndrome. Clearly this takes fine judgement but a severely damaged limb may not be salvageable and crush syndrome causes substantial morbidity and can cause death. Venous access should be obtained early, and saline infused at 1000–1500 ml/h during extrication.

Once urine flow has been established, a mannitol-forced diuresis of up to 8 L/day should be maintained. Allopurinol may be given to reduce urate levels and protect the myocardium. If compartment syndrome seems likely, **fasciotomy** should be performed early to reduce muscle damage.

Hyperkalaemia and infection are common complications and may lead to the death of the patient. Intractable hyperkalaemia may benefit from dialysis. Disseminated intravascular coagulation can occur when there is massive tissue damage, and established acute renal failure requires appropriate management.

The earthquake in Marmara, Northern Turkey, in 1999 was well documented and had a mortality rate for crush syndrome of 15%. Peak levels of CK give useful prognostic information: levels greater than 100 000 U/L virtually always signify that haemodialysis will be needed or that the patient is likely to die. Children with extensive injuries do very poorly.

BURNS

INTRODUCTION

Burns affect everyone—young or old, rich or poor, in the developing or developed world—but the poor and underprivileged are more at risk and generally receive worse treatment. Burns cause devastating injuries. Initially there is severe pain and distress, but soon there is a massive assault on both physical and psychological aspects of those affected. There are visible physical scars and invisible psychological scars which together cause severe and long lasting disability.

EPIDEMIOLOGY

Thermal injury is common, with most burns being caused by flame injuries and many of the rest by scalds; electrocution and chemical injuries are uncommon. In the UK, about 250 000 people are burned each year; 112 000 attend accident departments for treatment and 13 000 are admitted to hospital. About 1000 have burns severe enough to need fluid resuscitation and, sadly, half of these are in children under 12. In an average year, burns cause 250 deaths in the UK. The incidence in the USA is higher, and in the developing world burns are an even more important problem with over 2 million burns a year thought to occur in India. Mortality in the developing world is also much higher, e.g. Nepal has 1700 burn deaths annually in a population of 20 million; the death rate there is 17 times higher than in the UK.

Two-thirds of burns occur in the home, of which 60% are associated with cooking. Half of all deaths in domestic fires occur between 10 p.m. and 8 a.m. and excess alcohol consumption often plays an important role. Fireworks and bonfires are frequent causes of domestic burns. The remaining third of burns largely occur in industrial accidents. **Most burns are preventable.** There is a male predominance except in the elderly. Young children and the elderly are at greatest risk from burns and also suffer disproportionate mortality from them. Twenty per cent of all burns occur in children up to the age of 4, 70% of these are scalds caused by spilling hot liquids or by exposure to hot bath water. Among the most common burns are those involving toddlers who pull containers of hot fluid over themselves from cookers and tables. These result in scalds to the outstretched arm, face, neck and front of the chest and these burns can cover a large area (see Fig. 17.4). Ten per cent of burns occur between the ages of 5 and 14.

Teenagers are often burned as a result of illicit activities, e.g. with petrol, explosives or high tension electricity. Overall, 60% of burns occur between the ages of 15 and 64, of which half are flame burns, often associated with inhalational injury; these tend to be deep dermal or full thickness burns (see Fig. 17.5). Ten per cent of those burned are over 65, often as a result of immobility, slowed reactions and decreased dexterity which place them at risk from scalds, contact burns and flame burns.

PATHOPHYSIOLOGY OF BURNS

In thermal burns of the skin, the depth of tissue destruction is an important determinant of local outcome. Skin burns are broadly divided into **partial** or **full thick-**

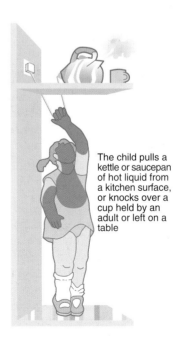

The child pulls a kettle or saucepan of hot liquid from a kitchen surface, or knocks over a cup held by an adult or left on a table

Fig. 17.4 Typical pattern of burns in a young child
The child pulls a teapot or cup of hot liquid from a table or when being held by a seated adult. The area shaded pink is typically burned.

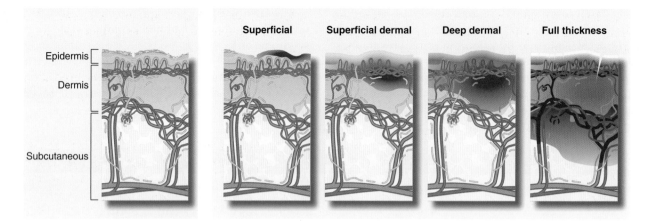

Fig. 17.5 Classification of depth of burns
- Erythema—red, dry skin that easily blanches then rapidly refills (not illustrated here)
- Superficial—red, moist wound that blanches and rapidly refills
- Superficial dermal—pale, dry, blanching wound that regains colour slowly
- Deep dermal—mottled cherry red and does not blanch (fixed capillary staining). The blood is thrombosed and fixed in damaged capillaries in the deep dermal plexus
- Full thickness—dry, leathery or waxy, hard wound that does not blanch. In extensive burns, full thickness burns can be mistaken for unburnt skin

ness. Partial thickness burns are those in which epidermal elements are spared, eventually allowing spontaneous healing without skin grafting. In deep partial thickness burns, the only epithelial remnants may be hair follicles and sweat glands which extend into the hypodermis, making regeneration slower. Full thickness burns are those in which all the epidermis has been destroyed. Skin grafting is usually necessary because epithelialisation from the margins is slow and prone to complications, in particular infection, fibrotic scarring and contractures.

The depth of damage caused by a thermal burn is not only a function of the temperature but also of the duration of exposure and the relative thickness of the skin (this is important in the very young and very old in whom the dermis is thinner). If applied for long enough, water at a temperature of only 45°C will cause full thickness destruction. This is often the mechanism of tragic burns in childhood. Note that the whole area of a major burn will not be uniformly deep.

Three zones of a major burn were described by Jackson in 1947. There is a central zone of **coagulation** in the area of maximum damage where skin cells are irreversibly damaged. This is surrounded by a zone of **stasis** characterised by decreased tissue perfusion. The importance of this zone is that injured cells can survive or die according to the effectiveness of treatment. Both of these zones extend deeply but the third zone, the outer zone of **erythema**, is superficial. The cells here are minimally injured and will recover in 7 days. It is important that this erythematous zone is not included in calculation of the burnt area.

| Box | 17.2 | Systemic changes occurring with large area burns (greater than 15% surface area in adults or 10% in children) |

- Surface and third space fluid losses lead to hypovolaemia
- Systemic inflammatory response syndrome occurs once burns affect 30% of body surface area
- Myocardial contractility becomes depressed
- In smoke inhalation, bronchoconstriction and ARDS occur
- Basal metabolic rate (BMR) increases up to 3-fold
- Function of the innate immune system becomes depressed
- General capillary permeability is increased
- Peripheral and splanchnic vasoconstriction occurs
- Red cells are destroyed by the burn
- Sepsis is likely if burns become infected, leading to organ failure and death

Systemic effects (Box 17.2)

Extensive burns cause substantial fluid losses. Destruction of the epidermis removes the normal barrier that prevents evaporation of body water. In addition, inflammatory exudation of protein-rich fluid into the extracellular space causes local oedema and blisters. The large volumes of fluid lost need to be replaced urgently (see Fig. 17.7). The amount lost depends on the area of the burn rather than the depth. Once 30% of the surface area is burnt, particularly if there is necrotic tissue, inflammatory mediators and cytokines released by the inflammatory response spill into the general circulation, causing a systemic inflammatory response. This provokes a generalised increase in capillary permeability, increasing the volume of plasma leaving the circulation into the 'third space'. Fluid losses are greatest in the first few hours but continue for at least 36 hours.

Extensive epidermal loss and the presence of necrotic tissue place the patient at high risk of infection. The main organisms are *Streptococcus pyogenes* during the first week and *Pseudomonas aeruginosa* thereafter. The risk of sepsis increases if burns become infected and this is responsible for organ failure and substantial mortality, even in this antibiotic era.

Electrocution burns

Electrical burns are caused by the conversion of electrical energy into heat, and electrocution is responsible for around 3% of admissions to burns units. The voltage is the key determinant of severity. Low domestic voltages just cause small deep contact burns at exit and entry sites. High-tension injuries occur at voltages over 1000 V and these cause large amounts of necrosis of bone and soft tissues and often limb loss. Muscle damage gives rise to rhabdomyolysis and renal failure. Contact with voltages greater than 70 000 V is invariably fatal.

The extent of burning is proportional to the electrical resistance of the tissue through which the current is transmitted. Bone offers the highest resistance; if current passes through a limb, the bones become heated and adjoining muscle is damaged in the process. Fasciotomy is likely to become necessary to decompress muscle compartments. Blood vessels also sustain intimal damage and thrombose. Deep tissue necrosis may not become clinically apparent until some days after an electrical burn and the extent of damage is often much greater than suspected.

Chemical burns

Chemical burns usually result from industrial accidents but may be caused by household chemical products. The severity depends on the agent, concentration and quantity, and duration of contact. Chemical burns tend to be deep because corrosives continue to act until fully removed. Alkalis such as cement tend to penetrate more deeply and cause worse burns than acids. **Hydrofluoric acid** is widely used in glass etching and circuit board construction and is a common cause of industrial chemical burns. It must be neutralised with topical or locally injected calcium gluconate to prevent the burning process continuing. The initial management of chemical burns is similar for all agents, i.e. remove all contaminated clothing and dilute or wash away the chemical by thoroughly irrigating the area, often by showering the patient.

Non-accidental injury (NAI)

Three to ten per cent of paediatric burns are due to non-accidental injury, i.e. deliberate harm to the child. Up to 30% of repeatedly abused children die. If non-accidental injury is suspected it is vital to follow the local NAI protocol.

ASSESSMENT OF THE BURNED PATIENT

HISTORY

The history should include information about the source of the burn, the temperature and the duration of contact and whether there was any inhalation of noxious gases.

CALCULATING THE BURNED AREA

Early assessment of the area of burns is important, not least because it helps determine the volume of fluid required for resuscitation. Area assessment is often badly done even by experts and is complicated by the fact that erythema needs to be excluded to avoid overestimating the extent. Preliminary assessment can be done immediately but definitive assessment should be deferred for a few hours until erythema settles.

All of the burned area needs to be exposed, ensuring the patient is kept warm by exposing areas sequentially. For adults, Wallace's rule of nines method of assessment (Fig. 17.6) is fairly reliable for medium to large areas and

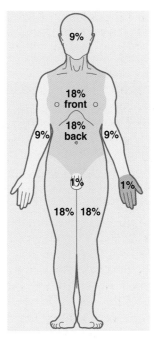

Fig. 17.6 Rule of nines
Wallace's rule for estimating the percentage of the skin surface area burned. A useful alternative estimate is that the area of the patient's own palm plus fingers is approximately 1% of the total skin area.

is quick to carry out; however, it is inaccurate for children. Another method is to use the area of the patient's palm and fingers to indicate roughly 1% of total body surface area. This is useful for estimating the area of small burns, and in very large burns where the **unburnt area** is counted. The most accurate method for all cases is to use **Lund and Browder charts** which compensate for variations in body shape that occur with age; the charts also give accurate assessment in children.

ASSESSING DEPTH OF BURN

Assessing the depth of burns at initial presentation is difficult, not least because most large burns are a mixture of different depths. Burns are dynamic wounds where the eventual depth can be influenced by the effectiveness of resuscitation and by inflammatory mediators as well as external factors such as bacterial proliferation, dehydration and cooling. For this reason it is important to review the burn regularly until it heals.

Depth assessment is not relevant for calculating fluid resuscitation but is important later for management of the burn. Figure 17.5 (p. 264) explains a widely used classification of the depth of burns, detailed below. In essence, partial thickness burns are capable of regenerating skin from preserved dermal adnexae whereas full thickness burns regenerate slowly from the edges and are likely to need surgical intervention and skin grafting. By way of preliminary assessment, if the burnt area is erythematous, blanches on pressure and retains pinprick sensation, it is partial thickness; charred skin or thrombosed skin vessels invariably indicate a full thickness burn.

Partial thickness burns may be classified as follows:

- **Superficial** burns—these affect the epidermis but not the dermis, e.g. sunburn
- **Superficial dermal** burns—these destroy the epidermis and upper layers of the dermis; blistering usually occurs. The burn may be covered with soot or dirt, which will need removing, and blisters should be deroofed so that the base can be checked. Capillary refill can be tested by pressure from a sterile cotton bud. A 21 g needle is used to test sensation and bleeding; pain is felt normally in superficial dermal burns and bleeding is brisk. Scalds tend to cause superficial to superficial dermal burns
- **Deep dermal** burns—these destroy all of the epidermis and most of the dermis, leaving only the deepest skin adnexae, sweat glands and some hair follicles, all of which are scanty. Accurate depth estimation here can be difficult. On needle testing, bleeding is delayed and only non-painful sensation is experienced

Full thickness burns are insensate and do not bleed on needling.

PRINCIPLES OF MANAGEMENT OF BURNS

Optimal treatment reduces the morbidity of burns as well as the mortality in large burns. Effective treatment shortens the period of healing, speeds return of function and reduces the need for secondary reconstruction.

First aid

At the scene of the burn, the first priority is to stop the burning process. The heat source must be removed and the flames doused. The patient's clothing is removed unless stuck to the burn, and **active cooling** employed to remove heat from the skin and arrest progression. Ideally this is achieved by immersing the burned area in tepid water (~15°C) for 15–20 minutes. This can cause hypothermia, especially in children.

Analgesia

Burns are very painful with pain being greatest in superficial burns. Pain relief is best achieved by cooling and covering burns in addition to giving analgesic drugs. In larger burns, opioids are given initially and NSAIDs later.

Dressings

Cling film (PVC film) is ideal as an initial burn dressing. It is essentially sterile and forms a pliable, non-adherent, impermeable barrier which is transparent to allow inspection. It should be laid on rather than wrapped around and covered with a blanket to keep the wound warm. Burned hands are enclosed in plastic bags. Prepacked cooling hydrogels, e.g. Burnshield, are available for applying at the scene of the burn.

Where should burns be managed?

Very small or erythema-only burns can be managed in primary care but all other patients should ideally be assessed and resuscitated (if necessary) in an emergency unit. Initial assessment will then determine whether treatment can be continued in a general hospital as an outpatient, whether hospital admission is required and whether transfer to a specialist burns unit is needed. Patients with extensive burns, i.e. involving more than 30% of body surface, should generally be transferred to a specialist burns unit as soon as initial treatment and resuscitation has been carried out. Facial burns should be referred to a specialist unit after covering with bland paraffin ointment (this is repeated every 1–4 hours to minimise crust). Other suggested referral criteria are summarised in Box 17.3.

OUTPATIENT MANAGEMENT OF MINOR BURNS

Patients suitable for outpatient management are adults without inhalation injury or significant comorbidity, with

Box 17.3   Criteria for referral to a burns centre

- Associated inhalational injury
- Partial thickness > 5% in a child or > 10% in an adult
- More than 1% full thickness
- Partial or full thickness burns to face, perineum, external genitalia, feet, hands and over joints
- Circumferential injury
- Chemical or electrical burns
- Extremes of age
- Non-accidental injury
- Comorbidity
- Non-healed burn 3 weeks after injury

partial thickness burns affecting less than 10% of body surface area. Children with less than 5% burns are also appropriately managed in this way. Patients with full thickness burns of up to 1% can also be managed as outpatients.

Immediate care involves analgesia and reassurance. Fluid resuscitation is not needed with this degree of burn. The main objective of local treatment is to prevent dehydration and infection of the burn site. Epithelialisation progresses faster in a moist environment. The burned area is cleaned of soot and debris with soap and water or weak chlorhexidine if necessary. Larger blisters are de-roofed and covered with a non-stick impregnated gauze dressing. Tulle gras (paraffin gauze) has long been used for this purpose but it soon dries out and adheres to the wound. A better alternative, although more expensive, is a soft silicone-coated net such as Mepitel. A generous layer of silver sulfadiazine cream (Flamazine) can be used instead; this antibacterial cream covers Gram-negative organisms including the common infecting organism, *Pseudomonas*. Either dressing is then covered by a thick absorbent layer of gauze and wool (Gamgee). Burns on the fingers and hands are best treated with a liberal coating of silver sulfadiazine cream and enclosing the hand in a plastic bag. The area should be checked at 24 hours and the dressing changed at 48 hours, by which time the depth should be evident and the treatment plan reviewed if necessary. Silver sulfadiazine cream can then be applied every 24–48 hours and skin slough should be excised as it separates. Partial thickness burns re-epithelialise within 14–21 days. If it has failed to heal within 3 weeks, the burn must be assumed to be full thickness and requires referral to a specialist unit.

Management of burns of specific depth

Superficial burns, typically sunburn, require only supportive therapy with regular analgesia and dressings for moist areas. Healing takes place within a week by regeneration from undamaged keratinocytes.

Superficial dermal burns. Blistering is common and exposed superficial nerves make these burns particularly painful. Progression to a deeper burn is unlikely. Healing is expected within two weeks from keratinocytes within sweat glands and hair follicles. The rate of regeneration depends on the density of adnexae, i.e. thin hairless skin on the inner arm or eyelid heals more slowly than thick or hairy skin of the back, scalp or face. Treatment is as described above although Hypafix is a special dressing that preserves mobility and allows washing with the dressing in place. It is applied directly to hand burns, for example. This dressing needs changing at least weekly by soaking in oil. Awkward facial burns are left open but liberally coated with antimicrobial creams or ointment. If the burns are still unhealed after 2 weeks, it can be assumed that the depth assessment was incorrect and the patient should be referred to a burns unit.

Deep dermal burns. These are the most difficult to assess. Superficial dermal burns may progress to deep dermal burns (with fixed capillary staining) within 48 hours. The density of skin adnexae is less at this depth and healing is slower and subject to contractures. Some of these burns heal spontaneously if kept warm, moist and free of infection, but if deep dermal burns are extensive or are in functionally or cosmetically sensitive areas they are better treated in a burns unit by excision to a viable depth and skin grafting within 5 days. This can reduce the morbidity and accelerate return to normal function.

Full thickness burns. All regenerative elements in the burned area have been destroyed; without grafting, wound contraction and distortion would be substantial. Ideally all full thickness burns need excision and grafting unless they are in an area where function would not be compromised and are less than 1 cm in diameter.

MANAGEMENT OF EXTENSIVE BURNS

Major burns are those affecting more than 20% of the body surface area. Managing them is a major challenge in which survival depends on accurate assessment, prompt and effective resuscitation, also the premorbid condition of the patient and whether there has been smoke inhalation. The main early aspects of management of serious burn victims are fluid replacement, assessment and treatment of inhalational respiratory problems and local management of the burns.

It is not easy to give an early prognosis. Clearly, aggressive treatment of someone who definitely will not survive is inhumane but victims of severe yet potentially survivable burns must be treated rapidly and effectively. The risk of dying from burns is greater with increasing area, with inhalational injury and in children under 3 and adults over about 60. High-voltage electrical burns are particularly lethal. Other medical conditions also increase the risk, e.g. alcoholism, epilepsy, diabetes, atherosclerosis and drug abuse.

> **Box 17.4   The Parkland formula for fluid resuscitation in the first 24 hours in major burns**
>
> - For adults, the total volume to be given over 24 hours is 3–4 ml Hartmann solution per kg body weight for each per cent surface area burnt
> - For children, the calculation is the same as for adults *plus* normal maintenance fluids
> - For all cases, half the estimated volume is given in the first 8 hours and the rest over the next 16 hours

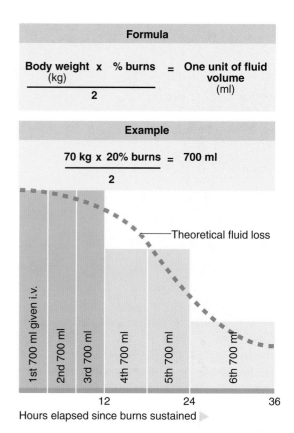

Fig. 17.7 Serious burns—a method for estimating fluid requirements over the first 36 hours (after Muir and Barclay)
The lower panel shows an example of a fluid replacement regimen for a 70 kg man with 20% burns. Each block represents one unit of fluid volume and is calculated as follows:

$$\text{Unit fluid volume} = \frac{70 \times 20}{2} = 700 \text{ ml}$$

Resuscitation and fluid management

As described earlier, adults with 15% and children with 10% body surface involvement lose sufficient fluid to be at risk of hypovolaemic shock. Fluid replacement depends on the extent of the burn and the weight of the patient. Hypovolaemia, particularly in the presence of myoglobinaemia, readily precipitates acute renal failure. Effective resuscitation maintains tissue perfusion in the **zone of stasis**, inhibiting depth progression. The greatest volume of fluid is lost in the first 8–12 hours, in which there is a general shift of fluid from intravascular to interstitial. Substantial fluid losses continue for at least another 36 hours. Rapid boluses of fluid should not be given early on as the raised intravascular hydrostatic pressure drives it rapidly out of the circulation.

Fluid requirements should be calculated from the time of injury, *not* the time of arrival in the emergency department. Colloids appear to offer no advantage over crystalloids and the volume required is estimated by referring to a well-tried formula such as that of Muir and Barclay shown in Figure 17.7, or the Parkland formula, Box 17.4. The Parkland formula has the advantage that it uses only crystalloids, it is easy to calculate and the rate can be adjusted by titrating against urine output.

These formulae are only a guide, however, and fluid balance must also be monitored according to pulse, blood pressure and urine output via a urinary catheter. Patients should also have 4–6-hourly estimations of packed cell volume, sodium, base excess and lactate. Note that patients with high-tension electrocution injuries need substantially more fluid than estimated by these formulae. In extensive full thickness burns, widespread red cell destruction occurs and blood transfusion may be needed.

MANAGEMENT OF THE BURNS

All wounds should achieve epithelial cover within 3 weeks to minimise scarring. Partial thickness burns usually re-epithelialise spontaneously given proper care, but full thickness burns require excision and skin grafting. Fingers, eyelids, limb flexures and genitalia nearly always require primary grafting soon after injury. For optimal care, grafting should be performed within 5 days of injury and patients needing transfer to a burns unit should reach there within a maximum of 10 days of injury.

The best covering for excised areas is autograft split skin from unburnt areas, ideally harvested near the recipient area to ensure best colour match. Sheets rather than postage stamp grafts should be used for hands and face. Wounds to be grafted must be free of infection; large areas of deep burns in particular need excising and grafting early to prevent infection and systemic sepsis. With extensive burns, skin grafting usually has to be performed in several stages because of a shortage of donor sites. Sites already used can be reused (**donor site rotation**) after 3 weeks or so; burned areas can be primarily excised and covered with temporary covering until donor sites become mature. Temporary coverings include cadaveric allograft skin, xenograft skin (e.g. pigskin), specially developed synthetic products or cultured epithelial autografts (sheets can be available in 3 weeks, skin cell suspensions in 1 week). Superficially burned areas can be treated with

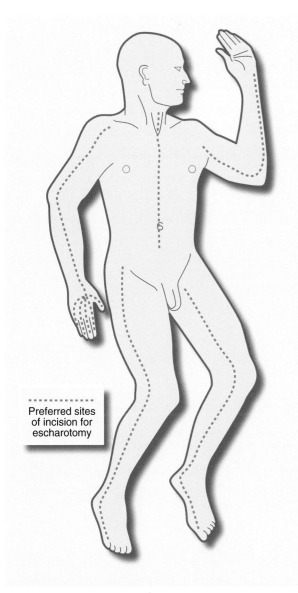

Preferred sites of incision for escharotomy

Fig. 17.8 Sites for performing escharotomy in deep circumferential burns

- A history of flame burns or burns in an enclosed space
- Stridor, tachypnoea or dyspnoea
- Singed nasal hair
- Full thickness or deep dermal burns to face, neck or upper torso
- Changes in the voice with hoarseness or a harsh cough
- Carbonaceous sputum or carbon particles visible in oropharynx
- Erythema or swelling of the oropharynx on direct inspection

The heat of inhaled gases is often sufficient to cause inflammatory oedema of the oral, nasal and laryngeal mucosa or even serious burns. Blackening by smoke or burnt skin around the nasal or oral cavities warns of inhalation injury. In addition, noxious gases can injure the lung parenchyma, resulting in pulmonary oedema, atelectasis and secondary pneumonias a day or two later.

Investigations include chest X-ray, blood gas and carbon monoxide estimations and upper respiratory tract examination with flexible pharyngoscopy and bronchoscopy.

Initial treatment involves administration of humidified air by mask and antibiotics to prevent chest infection. More severe cases require oxygen by mask, progressing to endotracheal intubation and intermittent positive pressure ventilation if blood gases deteriorate or pulmonary oedema develops.

FOLLOW-UP AND LATE TREATMENT

Burned areas should be protected from sun for 6–12 months by avoiding the sun or using sun block. Physiotherapy may be needed if mobility is impaired, and prolonged psychological support is necessary if deformity results from the burns or the treatment, particularly if it involves the face.

Local symptoms of severe **itching** and **dryness** are likely to occur. These can be helped by topical application of lanolin and specially made pressure garments. These also minimise skin contractures. If limitation of functional movement at joints or around facial orifices is not helped adequately by physiotherapy, operations to release scars may be needed, together with skin grafting.

Full thickness burns across joint flexures (including around the neck) may undergo severe fibrotic contraction even after grafting, seriously limiting movement. This difficult problem is likely to require plastic reconstructive operations.

dressings until healing occurs or graft sites become available.

Deep circumferential burns of the limbs and thorax begin to contract early and may restrict blood flow and respiratory movements. If excision and grafting is not done early, and if these signs develop, a procedure known as **escharotomy** is performed, involving incision of the eschar longitudinally down to bleeding tissue (Fig. 17.8).

INHALATIONAL INJURIES

Respiratory and systemic damage from inhalation of hot air, smoke and toxic gases (e.g. carbon monoxide or cyanides from burning upholstery) is a major cause of death and complications even if skin burns are slight (Box 17.5).

Symptoms, diagnosis and management

4

Non-acute abdominal pain and other abdominal symptoms and signs

INTRODUCTION

The diagnosis and management of non-acute abdominal complaints is an important part of the workload of a general surgical outpatient clinic. Most patients with abdominal complaints are investigated and treated as outpatients and only a proportion eventually need hospital admission or operation. The proportion of abdominal problems varies from one clinic to another depending on the availability of a medical gastroenterology service and of specialist gastroenterological surgical services.

The diagnoses made in patients seen in a surgical clinic are quite different from those made in emergency surgical admissions to hospital. Nevertheless, the surgeon in the clinic must remain alert to unfamiliar presentations of common conditions which more usually present acutely, e.g. an appendix mass.

The principal presenting symptoms of non-acute abdominal disorders are shown in Box 18.1. In addition, patients are often referred to a surgeon after discovery of an **abdominal mass**, **obstructive jaundice** or an **iron deficiency anaemia** caused by chronic blood loss.

The history can provide 70% or more of the clues to the diagnosis and so must be taken thoughtfully, accurately and with great care.

PAIN

CHARACTER, TIMING AND SITE OF THE PAIN

The key points to be covered in taking a history of abdominal pain are summarised in Box 18.2. Pain is a highly subjective phenomenon and the history will be coloured by the patient's own perception of the pain and its possible significance. Patients often use vague terms such as 'indigestion' and 'dyspepsia' to describe upper abdominal pain or discomfort associated with food. These terms should have little place in medical terminology, and what the patient actually means should be clarified by further questioning. In the history, the time-related features of the pain are highly significant in working towards a differential diagnosis and will only be elicited by diligent enquiry. It is important to establish when a pain first began. Sometimes, asking when the patient was last completely well will help pinpoint the real onset. When presenting a case history on a ward round, say 'the pain began six days ago' rather than, say, 'it began last Thursday'. Other details include whether the pain is continuous or periodic; there may be acute exacerbations on a continuous background pain, for example. If pain is periodic, enquire how frequently it occurs (minutes, hours, days, weeks or even constantly), and whether the frequency and severity vary.

Pain is described by patients in many different ways, although each pathological entity tends to have its own pain characteristics. The pattern will only come to light if all aspects of the pain history are enquired about.

The **site of origin** of the pain, particularly the site at which it first manifested, suggests the most likely anatomical structures to be involved. These are shown in Figure 18.1 (p. 277). The **distribution** and **radiation** of the pain provide further clues. Pain that extends through to the back suggests involvement of retroperitoneal structures, e.g. pancreas (carcinoma or chronic pancreatitis) or abdominal aorta (aneurysm). Gall bladder pain tends to radiate from the right hypochondrium around to the back on the right side. Renal pain tends to radiate from the loin down towards the groin and occasionally to the genitalia.

DISEASES CAUSING NON-ACUTE ABDOMINAL PAIN

The following conditions commonly cause non-acute abdominal pain. Each has certain characteristic features:

- **Gallstones and gall bladder dysfunction.** Biliary colic presents with irregularly recurrent bouts of severe pain which, though described as colic, characteristically last continuously for 1–12 hours. Some episodes are more severe and prolonged than others and often a particularly severe bout brings the patient into hospital. The pain is usually located in the upper abdomen—often on the right side, less often in the epigastrium—and may radiate to the back on the right. It is often precipitated by rich or fatty foods and may be associated with vomiting late in the attack

- **Peptic ulcer disease.** Typically there is intermittent 'boreing' epigastric pain which recurs several times a year and lasts for days or weeks at a time. It is not as severe as biliary colic unless there is perforation, which nearly always presents acutely. Retrosternal 'burning' occurs in peptic oesophagitis and tends to occur after large meals and on lying down. The association of pain with food varies according to the site of the ulcer disease: duodenal ulcer pain tends to be relieved by bland food and recurs 3–4 hours afterwards, typically in the early hours of the morning, whereas the pain of gastric ulcer and oesophagitis tends to be aggravated by food, especially if acidic or spicy. Peptic pain is generally relieved by antacids and virtually always by H$_2$-blocking drugs (e.g. ranitidine) or proton pump inhibitors (e.g. omeprazole), this 'trial of treatment' providing evidence towards a diagnosis

- **Chronic pancreatitis and carcinoma of pancreas.** These are typically associated with severe 'gnawing', persistent and poorly localised central pain which usually radiates through to the back and is often associated with anorexia and weight loss. The pain may be relieved by leaning forwards ('pancreatic position'). Early carcinoma of the pancreas, however, is often painless

- **Irritable bowel syndrome and constipation,** These conditions may produce a chronic symptom complex mimicking a partial obstruction of the bowel manifest by episodes of colicky pain. This is poorly localised, often 'bloating' pain, particularly post-prandially (after meals). It is of variable intensity and is often associated with transient disturbances of bowel function, particularly alternating diarrhoea and constipation. Passage of flatus or stool often temporarily relieves the symptoms

- **Diverticular disease and Crohn's disease**. Partial bowel obstruction can occur with diverticular disease of the sigmoid colon or with small bowel Crohn's disease. The symptoms are similar to those of complete bowel obstruction but more muted. In incomplete bowel obstruction, there is often some passage of flatus or even faeces but the patient otherwise appears obstructed. The term sub-acute obstruction is meaningless and should be abandoned

- **Chronic renal outflow obstruction (hydronephrosis) caused by stone, tumour or fibrosis**. There may be a 'dull', poorly defined, fairly constant loin pain which may be accompanied by typical urinary tract symptoms, e.g. haematuria and dysuria. It is often aggravated acutely by a high fluid intake

- **Gynaecological conditions**, particularly chronic pelvic inflammatory disease and ovarian tumours. These may reach the surgeon because of poorly defined lower abdominal pain. A gynaecological history should be taken in female patients; pelvic examination may reveal the cause

- **Non-surgical (i.e. 'medical') disorders causing abdominal pain**. These include liver congestion in heart failure (common), splenic infarcts or diabetes (both uncommon but important), acute intermittent porphyria, sickle-cell anaemia or tertiary syphilis (very rare). Patients sometimes present with abdominal pain for which no organic cause can be found despite extensive investigation. In these, irritable bowel syndrome or sensitivity to certain foods, e.g. gluten or wheat protein, need to be considered. Only as a last resort should the pain be attributed to psychological disturbances. Unnecessary operations may sometimes be performed on these patients

NON-ACUTE ABDOMINAL PAIN IN CHILDREN

This is common; the main organic causes are: 'infantile colic' (sometimes due to cow's milk allergy), irritable bowel syndrome in older children, chronic inflammatory bowel disease, recurrent streptococcal infections, and sometimes hydronephrosis caused by urinary tract obstruction. The so-called *periodic syndrome* is characterised by recurrent episodes of poorly defined and inconsistent abdominal pain and/or recurrent vomiting, sometimes sufficiently severe for the child to require admission and intravenous fluids. Abdominal migraine with or without nausea, pallor, photophobia abdominal lasting for up to three days is most common in the years before puberty. Psychosomatic abdominal pain may be the explanation if organic causes have been excluded and thus psychological and environmental factors, including the possibility of child neglect and abuse, should be explored (see Ch. 50).

APPROACH TO INVESTIGATION OF NON-ACUTE ABDOMINAL PAIN

A differential diagnosis must first be made on clinical grounds (Box 18.3 and Fig. 18.1). The choice (and order) of the numerous possible investigations should be efficient and economical, after considering how each one will support or help eliminate the most probable (and common) diagnoses and how it might influence management. Rarer diagnoses usually need more extensive and specialised investigation.

DYSPHAGIA

CLINICAL PRESENTATION

Dysphagia is the term used to describe difficulty in swallowing. The most common symptom is inability to swallow solid food, which the patient will describe as 'becoming stuck' or 'held up' before it either passes on into the stomach or is regurgitated. The patient usually reports that particular types of food are more difficult than others; fibrous foods, such as chunks of meat, usually cause the most trouble. The patient can usually indicate a precise level for the perceived obstruction. The true level of obstruction is usually some distance below that point.

Dysphagia is almost always caused by disease in or adjacent to the oesophagus but occasionally the lesion is in the pharynx or stomach. Oesophageal narrowing usually causes symptoms only when the lumen is unable to expand beyond a diameter of about 10 mm—the narrower the lumen, the more severe the symptoms. In many of the pathological conditions causing dysphagia, the lumen becomes progressively constricted and indistensible. Initially only fibrous solids cause difficulty but later the problem extends to all solids and later, even to fluids. Because narrowing is a gradual and insidious process, patients often compensate to a surprising degree (e.g. by liquidising all food) and may only present when they have difficulty in swallowing fluids or even their own saliva. By this time there is usually marked weight loss.

The common causes of dysphagia are outlined in Box 18.4, p. 279. **Pain** on swallowing or **odynophagia** (usually provoked by both food and drink, particularly if hot) is a distinctive symptom highly suspicious of carcinoma.

Achalasia is a major exception to the usual pattern of dysphagia in that swallowing of fluids tends to cause more difficulty than swallowing solids. In achalasia, there

Box 18.3 **Abdominal examination: 28 points to remember in examining a patient with abdominal symptoms**

General examination

1. Well-looking or ill (thin, emaciated, weak)?
2. Alert and responding normally or obtunded and slumped in bed?
3. Dehydrated (poor skin tone, sunken cheeks)?
4. Abnormal skin colour (pale, jaundiced, grey)
5. Signs of surgical wounds or dressings
6. End-of-bed charts—fever, tachycardia, fluid balance, trauma chart, pain chart, drug chart (e.g. strength and frequency of analgesia), modified early warning scores (MEWS)
7. 'Medical accessories'—i.v. infusion, urinary catheter, parenteral nutrition, monitoring equipment, oxygen mask

Peripheral stigmata of abdominal disease

1. Fingernails for koilonychia (spoon shaped nails in iron deficiency) and leuconychia (whiteness and opacity of nails, sometimes due to hypoalbuminaemia)
2. Hands for palmar erythema and Dupuytren's contracture (association with liver disease)
3. Eyes—yellow sclerae in jaundice, pale conjunctivae in anaemia
4. Mouth and tongue—for ulceration suggestive of Crohn's, angular stomatitis in anaemia, dehydration, telangiectasia in hereditary haemorrhagic telangiectasia
5. Supraclavicular fossa palpation for enlarged lymph nodes, particularly medial left-sided Virchow's node indicating upper GI malignancy (Troisier's sign)
6. Inspect abdominal skin for jaundice and scratch marks resulting from pruritus (itching), spider naevi (indicate likely liver disease)
7. Chest in males for gynaecomastia in liver disease

Abdominal inspection

1. Position the patient correctly (comfortable, near-flat, arms by sides) and expose the whole abdominal field ('nipples to knees', but not all at once)
2. Distended or scaphoid (sunken) abdominal shape?
3. Skin—wounds and scars, redness, purulent discharge or other signs of infection, erythema ab igne (see Fig. 18.2)
4. Bruising—umbilical or flank in acute pancreatitis; cloth printing (trauma cases)
5. Herniation (including usual primary sites and incisional hernias)

6. Caput medusae—enlarged veins radiating from umbilicus indicating portal venous obstruction
7. Visible peristalsis—usually indicating long-standing small bowel obstruction

Abdominal palpation (do not hurt the patient; watch the face for signs of discomfort)

1. Gentle overall palpation for obvious abnormalities
2. Overall firmer palpation at a deeper level provides detailed examination of abnormal masses—relationship to abdominal wall, size, shape, position, mobility, texture, hardness, fixation posteriorly or anteriorly, tenderness. Likely site or organ of origin?
3. Specific organ palpation—press in first, *then* ask the patient to breathe in deeply; gradually relax your pressure and seek the descending lower edge of the organ; repeat at 3 cm intervals moving upwards:
   - *Liver*—start as low as it might have reached, e.g. right iliac fossa, and work upwards as above. Map out palpable lower liver edge. If large, palpate surface for irregularities, e.g. metastases. The enlarging liver usually remains in contact with the anterior abdominal wall and is dull to percussion. Percuss also for upper border to gauge liver size; auscultate a large liver for vascular bruits
   - *Spleen*—tilt patient slightly towards right side, place left hand behind lower left ribs and gently lift. Start as low as enlargement might have reached, e.g. right iliac fossa, and palpate as for liver. Seek notch in lower edge. To be palpable, spleen needs to be enlarged 2–3 times normal. Percuss for overlying resonance due to gas in bowel superficial to it
   - *Kidneys*—as with the liver, a renal mass usually descends with inspiration since the kidneys lie just beneath the diaphragm. Bimanual palpation enables the posteriorly placed kidney to be felt by displacing it anteriorly (see Fig. 18.3). Place left hand in loin and attempt to push enlarged organ forwards on to examining hand
4. Examination for ascites (see Fig. 18.4)
5. Hernial orifices—inguinal and femoral for cough impulse; reducibility (see Ch. 32)
6. Rectal and/or vaginal examination if appropriate (see Table 18.1)
7. Percussion and auscultation if appropriate

is idiopathic destruction of the parasympathetic ganglia in Auerbach's (submucosal) plexus of the entire oesophagus, which results in functional narrowing of the lower oesophagus and peristaltic failure throughout its length. Thus the oesophagus becomes markedly distended and dilated, with solids settling towards the lower end and fluids spilling over into the airways causing **spluttering dysphagia**. This overspill and consequent symptoms tend to occur when the patient is lying flat at night. Achalasia often presents with chronic chest infection rather than dysphagia and the diagnosis is often reached late. Similar symptoms of overspill into the airways can be provoked by bulbar palsy, most commonly provoked by a stroke.

Bolus obstruction is an acute form of dysphagia, where a lump of food sticks at a narrowed part, completely obstructing the oesophagus.

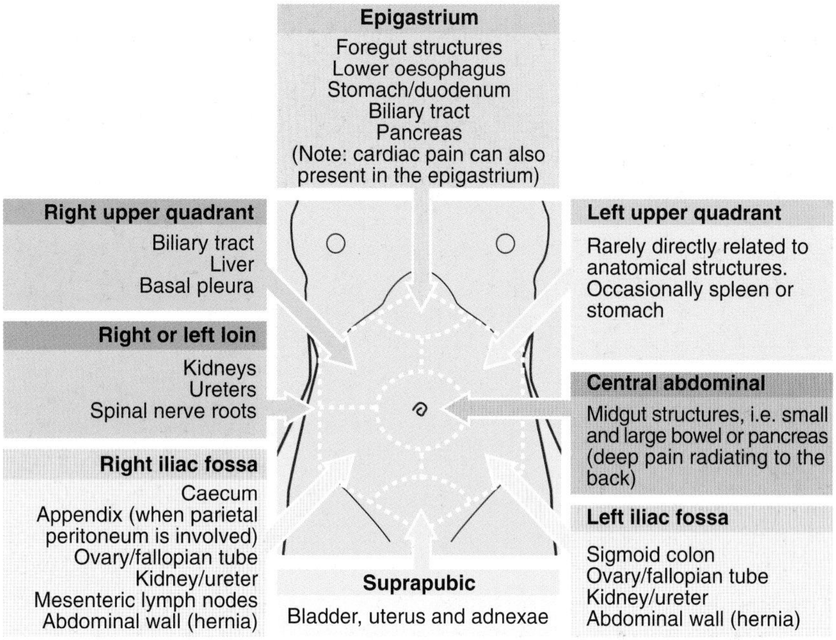

Epigastrium

Foregut structures
Lower oesophagus
Stomach/duodenum
Biliary tract
Pancreas
(Note: cardiac pain can also
present in the epigastrium)

Right upper quadrant

Biliary tract
Liver
Basal pleura

Left upper quadrant

Rarely directly related to
anatomical structures.
Occasionally spleen or
stomach

Right or left loin

Kidneys
Ureters
Spinal nerve roots

Central abdominal

Midgut structures, i.e. small
and large bowel or pancreas
(deep pain radiating to the
back)

Right iliac fossa

Caecum
Appendix (when parietal
peritoneum is involved)
Ovary/fallopian tube
Kidney/ureter
Mesenteric lymph nodes
Abdominal wall (hernia)

Left iliac fossa

Sigmoid colon
Ovary/fallopian tube
Kidney/ureter
Abdominal wall (hernia)

Suprapubic

Bladder, uterus and adnexae

Fig. 18.1 Anatomical significance of the site of abdominal pain

Fig. 18.2 Erythema ab igne

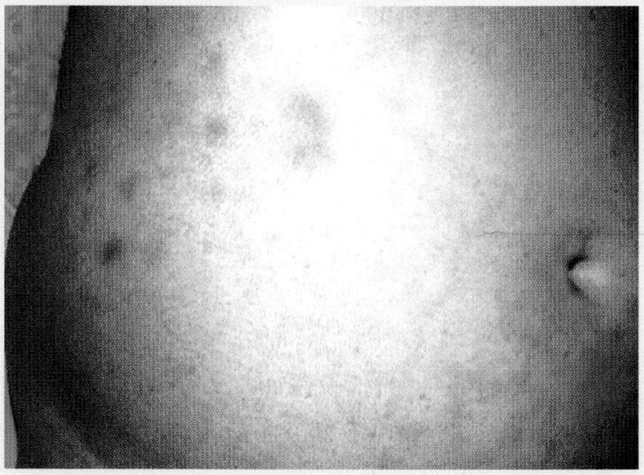

This woman of 45 suffered chronic pain in the right loin and had obtained some relief from regularly applying a hot water bottle to the area which resulted in typical skin damage. A staghorn calculus in the right kidney proved to be the cause.

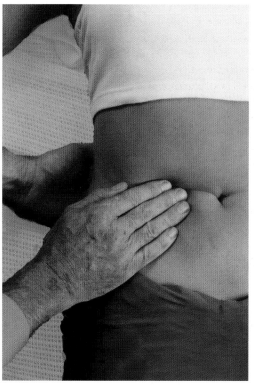

Fig. 18.3 Bimanual palpation of the abdomen
The posterior hand pushes forwards so that an enlarged viscus (usually retroperitoneal, e.g. kidney) or a mobile intra-abdominal mass is pushed onto the anterior examining hand. Note that this is not *ballottement*, which involves short sharp palpation anteriorly thus displacing ascites enabling a mass to bounce onto the examining hand.

APPROACH TO INVESTIGATION OF DYSPHAGIA

Dysphagia, particularly of recent onset, must be regarded seriously and fully investigated. A plain chest X-ray should be taken to exclude bronchial carcinoma; occasionally an oesophageal fluid level behind the heart is seen, resulting from an oesophageal stricture, hiatus hernia or achalasia. In high dysphagia, a flexible pharyngoscopy followed by

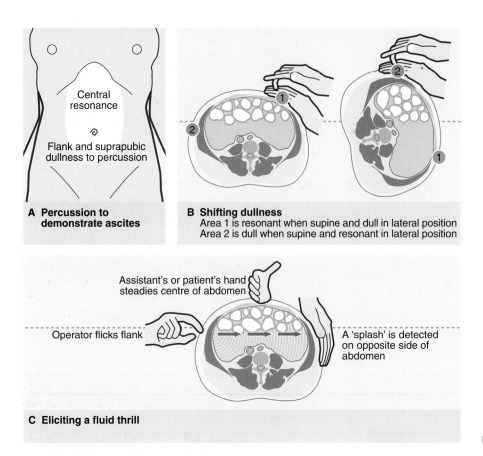

A **Percussion to demonstrate ascites**

B **Shifting dullness**
Area 1 is resonant when supine and dull in lateral position
Area 2 is dull when supine and resonant in lateral position

Central resonance

Flank and suprapubic dullness to percussion

Assistant's or patient's hand steadies centre of abdomen

Operator flicks flank

A 'splash' is detected on opposite side of abdomen

C **Eliciting a fluid thrill**

Fig. 18.4 Clinical signs of ascites

a barium swallow and meal is the usual sequence of investigation (note that oesophagogastroduodenoscopy—OGD—risks perforating a pharyngeal pouch). In lower dysphagia, flexible endoscopy (OGD) is usually performed, but both OGD and contrast radiography are often required. If a lesion has been demonstrated radiologically, OGD allows direct inspection and biopsy to confirm (or change) the diagnosis. In disorders of function, swallowing of barium-soaked bread or a video record of a barium swallow may be helpful in reaching a diagnosis. Oesophageal physiology measurements using manometry and pH monitoring are helpful in reaching a diagnosis of achalasia, especially in its early stages.

WEIGHT LOSS, ANOREXIA AND ASSOCIATED SYMPTOMS

Marked weight loss (**cachexia**) and loss of appetite (**anorexia**) are frequently manifestations of serious, insidious, often malignant abdominal disorders. They may be associated with a variety of other symptoms such as malaise, bloating, nausea, sporadic vomiting and regurgitation. These symptoms may have been unnoticed or dismissed as trivial by the patient and are only elicited by direct questioning.

The diseases which cause these symptoms may be grouped into four broad categories:

- **Intra-abdominal malignancies**, e.g. carcinoma of the stomach or pancreas, metastatic disease in the liver or widespread in the peritoneal cavity (arising particularly from stomach, large bowel, ovary, breast or bronchus), bowel lymphomas
- **'Medical' conditions**, e.g. alcoholism and cirrhosis, viral diseases (e.g. hepatitis or infectious mononucleosis), uncontrolled diabetes or thyrotoxicosis, malabsorption, renal failure, cardiac cachexia
- **Psychological disorders**, e.g. anxiety, depression, anorexia nervosa, bulimia
- **Chronic visceral ischaemia**, a very uncommon condition resulting from atherosclerotic narrowing of at least two of the three main visceral arteries—the coeliac axis and the superior mesenteric and the inferior mesenteric arteries—resulting in 'fear of food' and massive weight loss

APPROACH TO INVESTIGATION OF WEIGHT LOSS, ANOREXIA AND ASSOCIATED SYMPTOMS

In many patients, there may be other clinical clues to the main diagnosis or which suggest a line of investigation, e.g. pain, signs of anaemia or jaundice, or a palpable abdominal or rectal mass. More difficult are those cases where the symptoms occur alone. In this situation, basic

Obstruction arising in the oesophageal wall

Common

- Peptic oesophagitis (often associated with hiatus hernia)—sometimes causes fibrous stricture
- Carcinoma of oesophagus or cardia (uppermost part) of the stomach

Uncommon

- Candida oesophagitis, particularly after major surgery

Extremely rare

- Pharyngeal pouch
- Oesophageal web (Plummer–Vinson/Paterson–Kelly syndrome)
- 'Oesophageal apoplexy' due to haematoma in the wall
- Leiomyoma of the oesophageal muscle

Disorders of neuromuscular function

- Achalasia—uncommon
- Bulbar or pseudobulbar palsy—rare
- Myasthenia gravis—rare

External compression of the oesophagus

- Subcarinal lymph node secondaries from carcinoma of the bronchus—fairly common
- Left atrial dilatation in mitral stenosis—rare
- Dysphagia lusoria (compression from abnormally placed great arteries)—very rare

screening investigations (full blood count and erythrocyte sedimentation rate, urea and electrolytes, liver function tests and urinalysis) begin to differentiate 'medical' conditions from 'surgical' ones. If these screening tests fail to produce a lead, abdominal imaging using ultrasound or CT scanning may be indicated to exclude liver metastases or an occult intra-abdominal malignancy.

If investigations still reveal no cause, a psychological cause should be seriously considered. Before such a diagnosis can be accepted, there must be positive evidence of psychiatric disturbance. In practice, by this stage, previously concealed psychiatric features often become apparent; except for anorexia nervosa or bulimia, these are rare.

ANAL AND PERIANAL SYMPTOMS

Anal symptoms generate a large number of surgical outpatient referrals. Symptoms include bleeding and discharge, pain and itching, local swelling and a sensation of 'something coming down'. They often cause distress out of proportion to their pathological importance. The most common diagnoses are haemorrhoids, anal fissures and local abscesses, although the occasional infiltrating anal carcinoma or low rectal carcinoma or polyp must not be overlooked.

ANAL BLEEDING

This is an extremely common symptom. It is well tolerated by patients who usually believe that 'piles' (haemorrhoids) are responsible. Patients often present when the bleeding becomes excessive or when new and different symptoms develop. The characteristic feature of anal bleeding is fresh blood separate from the stool which may only be seen 'on the paper'. Fresh bleeding, however, may arise from malignancy in the rectum, sigmoid colon or anal canal and must be treated seriously. In addition to digital examination and proctoscopy, all patients require at least sigmoidoscopy; patients over 40 require colonoscopy, barium enema or contrast CT examination to exclude large bowel cancer, whether or not a benign anal cause, such as haemorrhoids, has already been found.

ANAL PAIN AND DISCOMFORT

The principal causes of chronic anal pain and discomfort are haemorrhoids and anal fissure. Haemorrhoids usually cause periodic anal discomfort and other anal symptoms rather than severe pain. Anal carcinoma is usually painless but may present with haemorrhoid-like pain. The difference is obvious on digital rectal examination.

Severe perianal pain which follows each episode of defaecation usually indicates a fissure in ano. This is a longitudinal tear typically in the posterior anal mucosa ending externally in a characteristic '**sentinel pile**', a small skin tag visible at the posterior anal margin. An anal fissure is often initiated by a bout of unaccustomed constipation. A perianal abscess may be responsible for anal pain even before the abscess is clinically detectable; the rare **intersphincteric abscess** may cause chronic pain and elude detection for weeks.

An acute onset of anal pain may be caused by a **perianal haematoma**, clearly visible at the anal margin, by strangulated or thrombosed haemorrhoids or by a perianal abscess.

Proctalgia fugax describes recurrent shooting pains in the anal area. Investigations should be performed to exclude local causes but usually no cause is found.

PERIANAL ITCHING AND IRRITATION

The most common cause of these symptoms is inadequate hygiene which results in local skin irritation. This is often exacerbated by scratching or application of various topical medications. The discharge associated with haemorrhoids, fistulae or tumours tends to keep the perianal skin moist, predisposing to low-grade fungal and bacterial infections. The longer these symptoms persist, the more difficult they are to eradicate and in fastidious patients a 'fixation' can develop. In children, threadworm infestation is a common cause of perianal itching; the itching is usually worse at night.

'SOMETHING COMING DOWN'

Haemorrhoids, skin tags ('memorials to past haemorrhoids') and occasionally mucosal or rectal prolapse cause this symptom. It is exacerbated by defaecation. Many patients tolerate the condition for some time before seeking medical advice and may have to push the lumps back manually after defaecation, presenting only when this becomes impossible. A pedunculated low rectal polyp may occasionally come through the anus and be confused with prolapsed haemorrhoids. Perianal warts are occasionally mistaken for lumps arising from within the anal canal.

PERIANAL DISCHARGE

A perianal discharge results from leakage of pus, inflammatory exudate or mucus from the anus or anal area. Pus may arise from a pilonidal sinus in the natal cleft or from an anal fistula. Inflammatory exudate or excess mucus may be produced by haemorrhoids, anorectal mucosal inflammation (proctitis), a villous adenoma or an ulcerating carcinoma.

APPROACH TO INVESTIGATION OF ANAL AND PERIANAL SYMPTOMS

Inspection of the anal area is followed by careful digital rectal examination (DRE) and proctoscopy. All three of these are mandatory (Table 18.1). Further examination follows the principles described earlier, but usually includes at least a rigid sigmoidoscopy. If pain makes these examinations impossible, a young patient can usually be assumed to have a fissure. In an older person, carcinoma of the anus must be excluded by examination under anaesthesia. Haemorrhoids appear as bulging bluish masses beneath the anal mucosa. They all arise above the squamocolumnar junction or dentate line ('internal piles') but may later extend beneath the perianal skin ('external piles') or prolapse through the anus ('intero-external piles').

A typical **anal fistula** appears as an inflammatory 'nipple' near the anal margin (see Fig. 18.6); it often exudes a discharge. In **proctitis**, the rectal mucosa is granular and reddened when seen on proctoscopy, and often bleeds to the touch (friability). An anal or low rectal carcinoma is a discrete ulcerated lesion with an indurated (firm, woody) base and a thickened margin. Diagnosis is confirmed by histological examination of a biopsy taken with special forceps.

The lymphatic drainage of the anal canal below the dentate line is to the inguinal lymph nodes and these should always be examined when a suspicious anal lesion is found.

CHANGE IN BOWEL HABIT, RECTAL BLEEDING AND RELATED SYMPTOMS

Normal bowel habit varies widely between different individuals in both frequency of defaecation and consistency

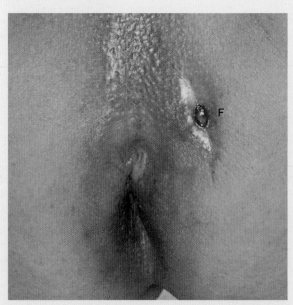

Fig. 18.6 Anal fistula

CASE STUDY

This man of 39 had presented with a perianal abscess 3 months previously that had been drained. He complained of persistent discharge which was found to be emanating from a fistulous opening **F** within the drainage scar. This proved to be a low fistula on further examination under anaesthesia.

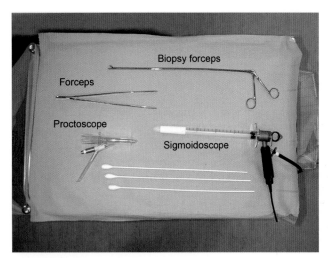

Fig. 18.5 Procto-sigmoidoscopy trolley
Typical layout of trolley prepared for proctoscopy and sigmoidoscopy in an outpatient clinic. Note the yellow waste bag on the left for contaminated swabs and waste and the paper bag on the right for waste wrapping from swabs, etc. Sigmoidoscopic biopsies are placed in a container of formol saline for fixation.

Table 18.1 Investigation of anal and colorectal symptoms

1. DIGITAL RECTAL EXAMINATION

Purpose	Inspection of the anal and perianal area for skin changes and lesions Palpation of the anal canal and lower rectum and surrounding tissues. Normally the firm walls of the anal sphincter are felt over the first 5 cm or so. Above that level, the rectal walls are soft and mobile
Preparation	Chaperone if necessary 'Consent'—written or implied Patient position to maintain dignity—usually left lateral with knees drawn up Equipment—good light, surgical gloves, gel lubricant, tissues
Technique ● **Inspection** ● **Palpation** Always minimise pain and discomfort—if pain/spasm prevents examination a fissure or anal carcinoma may be present Note that in the female, the uterine cervix is often felt anteriorly as a firm but localised mass. In the male, the normal prostate gland is felt near the tip of the finger anteriorly as a smooth, firm swelling about 2 cm in diameter with a midline groove between the lateral lobes	Sentinel pile; excoriation; ulceration, perianal haematoma; fistulous opening; scars; abscess; prolapsed mucosa or haemorrhoids; skin tags *In lumen*—faeces/blood/foreign body *In wall*—ulceration, polyp, thrombosed piles, internal opening of tract or fistula; Crohn's thickening; anal carcinoma; lack of normal softness *Outside wall*—prostatic enlargement (usually benign) can be palpated, as can irregularity or nodularity which may represent carcinoma; cervix; frozen pelvis; mass in pouch of Douglas Note: glove should be checked for blood/mucus/colour of stool

2. PROCTOSCOPY (Fig. 18.5; see also Ch. 30)

Purpose	Direct visualisation of mucosa of anal canal Must be done even if rigid sigmoidoscopy/barium enema/MRI to be done Therapy, e.g. sclerotherapy/ banding of haemorrhoids
Technique	The proctoscope with obturator in situ is lubricated and gently introduced into the anal canal to its greatest extent (10 cm). The obturator is removed and the instrument slowly withdrawn, ensuring that the mucosa of the entire anal canal is inspected
Findings in mucosa	Inflammation/granular surface Superficial ulceration Haemorrhoids—bleeding, degree of prolapse Anal carcinoma Solitary 'rectal' ulcer Pus Fistula Fibrous polyps Melanoma

3. RIGID SIGMOIDOSCOPY (for flexible sigmoidoscopy see text)

Purpose	**Visualisation** of the rectum up to recto-sigmoid junction—18–20 cm **Biopsy** of suspicious lesions or abnormal mucosa
Technique	As for proctoscopy for 10 cm or so. Obturator removed and proximal end closed with lens. Gentle inflation whilst inspecting lumen, manipulating and advancing' scope with least discomfort to patient Faecal loading may prevent visualisation; pain may limit examination to lower rectum only
Examples of pathology	Inflammation/granular surface Superficial ulceration Pus Polyps and adenomas Carcinoma Melanosis coli Strictures

---

| Box | 18.5 | Differential diagnosis of change in bowel habit |

- Carcinoma of colon, rectum or anus
- Diverticular disease
- Irritable bowel syndrome
- Crohn's disease of small or large bowel
- Ulcerative colitis
- Drug effects, e.g. codeine phosphate, iron, laxative abuse
- Reduction in fibre content of diet
- Parasitic infestations, e.g. giardiasis
- Following acute bacterial or parasitic colitis
- Changes in resident bacterial flora, e.g. antibiotic-associated diarrhoea
- Malabsorption syndromes
- Thyrotoxicosis

Note: in many cases, no cause is found

---

of stool. For an individual, transient changes in bowel habit are usually insignificant but persistent change often leads to the patient seeking medical advice. Departure from the norm may have several different aspects, occurring in various combinations. The differential diagnosis of a change in bowel habit is summarised in Box 18.5.

FREQUENCY OF DEFAECATION AND STOOL CONSISTENCY

Chronic constipation or diarrhoea marks the extremes of change, although some patients develop an erratic pattern of bowel action. Changes all may signify serious disease and deserve investigation. The index of suspicion is further raised if there is rectal bleeding or tenesmus (for definition, see p. 284). Waking from sleep to evacuate the bowels should be treated seriously, especially if it occurs frequently.

Stool consistency varies according to diet but the stool is usually 'formed'. Persistently unformed stools, i.e. 'looseness', is only abnormal if it represents a change from the patient's usual habit.

Constipation

Constipation arises for four main reasons:

- Incomplete bowel obstruction, e.g. faecal impaction, an obstructing carcinoma or stricture in the bowel wall, or occasionally an extrinsic lesion such as ovarian cancer
- Loss of peristalsis, e.g. acutely due to drugs such as narcotics, antidepressants or iron, chronic diverticular disease, chronic laxative abuse
- Inadequate fibre intake or poor fluid intake, which decrease faecal volume and prolong intestinal transit time

- In bed-bound patients, multiple factors including immobility, diet, inadequate fluid intake, drug effects

Diarrhoea

Chronic diarrhoea is most often caused by irritation or inflammation of the small or large bowel. The inflammatory bowel diseases (ulcerative colitis and Crohn's disease) are important diagnoses. Chronic parasitic infestations of the large bowel with amoebae or of the small bowel with *Giardia lamblia* are easily overlooked. In areas where these diseases are not endemic, patients may give a history of foreign travel. Chronic diarrhoea may follow an acute attack of *Salmonella* or other coliform infection. Less commonly, a blind loop of small bowel remaining after bypass surgery becomes colonised with gut flora, causing changes in intraluminal metabolism (**blind loop syndrome**). The most common diagnosis in diarrhoea after intestinal infection is irritable bowel syndrome.

Bile salts irritate the bowel. Therefore if the enterohepatic circulation is disrupted, e.g. after distal small bowel resection, defective reabsorption of bile salts may cause diarrhoea. A less common cause of diarrhoea is the increased volume of bowel contents in various malabsorption syndromes. Finally, when no physical cause can be found, concealed laxative abuse or an anxiety state should be considered. Early morning diarrhoea on its own rarely indicates serious disease.

Erratic bowel habit

Some patients develop an erratic bowel habit with bouts of constipation interspersed with episodes of frequency and looseness of stool. The most common cause is **irritable bowel syndrome**, which can be attributed to a heightened pain response in conjunction with a possible over-production or change in production of normal enteric gas. In particular the symptoms include a marked gastrocolic reflex, i.e. a call to stool immediately after eating. In **diverticular disease**, constipation and 'rabbit-pellet' faeces are the dominant characteristics but there may be episodic diarrhoea, often during periods of inflammation. This may be caused by intermittent release of proximal liquefied stool past the partially obstructed solid faeces (**spurious diarrhoea**). Incomplete bowel obstruction of this type may also occur in carcinoma of the left colon, Crohn's disease or faecal impaction.

Patients treated with broad-spectrum antibiotics, particularly the cephalosporins, may develop **antibiotic-associated diarrhoea**. If caused by *Clostridium difficile*, this is known as **pseudomembranous colitis**; the symptoms are due to changes in colonic bacterial flora (see Ch. 12).

CHANGES IN THE NATURE OF THE STOOL

Stools are normally brown owing to the presence of urobilin, a breakdown product of bile. In biliary obstruction, bilirubin does not reach the gut and the stools become pale. Stools in obvious jaundice are often described as 'putty-coloured' or 'clay-coloured'.

Stools may also be pale when they contain excess fat as in various malabsorption syndromes. In coeliac disease (gluten enteropathy) the stool is often loose and offensive. In fat malabsorption, the stools tend to float because of the excessive fat content and the patient has difficulty flushing them away. This is known as **steatorrhoea**.

Undigested food in the stool indicates failure of digestion and absorption. This can be normal when the diet is extremely high in fibre. It may, however, indicate malabsorption or a 'short-circuit' in the bowel due to previous bowel resection or a fistula between bowel loops.

PRESENCE OF FRANK BLOOD, ALTERED BLOOD OR MUCUS IN THE STOOL

Note: acute gastrointestinal haemorrhage is covered in Chapter 19.

Frank rectal bleeding

When a patient has seen blood in the stool, a careful history should be taken regarding the colour, i.e. fresh or altered blood, and also the relationship of the blood to the stool. Blood alone may be passed, or it may appear before or after the stool. There may be blood mixed with the stool or coating it. The only evidence may be blood-staining of the stool after defaecation.

Bright red blood usually indicates a lesion in the rectum or anus. When blood is clearly separate from the stool it suggests an anal lesion, most commonly haemorrhoids but occasionally proctitis or a carcinoma. If the blood is on the surface of the stool it suggests a lesion such as a polyp (see Fig. 18.7) or carcinoma further proximally, either in the rectum or descending colon. These observations have little diagnostic reliability. As a general rule, rectal bleeding should be assumed to be caused by tumour until proven otherwise!

When blood is mixed with the stool, it usually indicates even more proximal disease. This is usually in the left side of the colon or occasionally in the transverse colon. Carcinoma or inflammatory ulceration is often the cause. In such cases the blood, being 'older', is darker.

When the blood originates further proximally in the gastrointestinal tract, e.g. peptic ulcer, it is so altered by 'digestion' that it may not be recognised as blood by the patient. The stool is typically shiny black or plum-coloured. In rapid bleeding from stomach or duodenum, the stools become fluid and are described as 'tarry'. This is known as **melaena** and has a characteristic odour. Patients on iron therapy have greenish-black or charcoal-coloured, formed stools which should not be mistaken for altered blood. In this case, faecal occult blood testing should be negative.

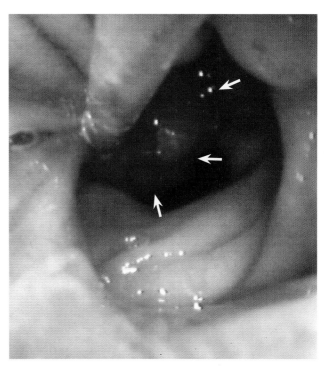

Fig. 18.7 Colonoscopic appearance of a polyp in the sigmoid colon
This 2 cm polyp (arrowed) was found to be the cause of rectal bleeding. It was easily removed with a colonoscopic snare soon after this photograph was taken.

Occult faecal blood loss

A persistent trickle of blood from the gastrointestinal tract may not alter the appearance of the stool. This 'occult' blood may be detectable only by chemical tests. Despite the small daily quantities involved, this hidden blood loss can cause serious iron deficiency anaemia. This test can be done either at the bedside or in the laboratory, but it is sensible to perform three tests to prevent false negatives.

Rectal passage of mucus or pus

Mucus ('slime') or pus may be passed alone or with the stool. Patients rarely volunteer this information but will report it when asked. The most common cause is irritable bowel syndrome. **Villous adenomas** typically secrete copious mucus, but this may also occur with frank carcinoma of the rectum. Mucus and pus may be noted in the inflammatory bowel disorders and occasionally in diverticular disease. An anal leak of mucus may be a feature of haemorrhoids and causes itching (**pruritus ani**). A patient sometimes reports passing a mass of purulent material. This usually represents spontaneous discharge of a perianal or pararectal abscess, and will often have been preceded by anal or perineal pain.

TENESMUS

Tenesmus is an unpleasant sensation of incomplete evacuation of the rectum. The sensation causes the patient to attempt defaecation (often with straining) at frequent intervals. The most common cause is probably irritable bowel syndrome. Another common cause is an abnormal mass in the rectum or anal canal. This may be a carcinoma, polyp or thrombosed haemorrhoid. Occasionally a prostatic carcinoma invades around the lower rectum producing tenesmus. In some cases, despite extensive investigation, no organic cause is found for tenesmus.

APPROACH TO INVESTIGATION OF CHANGE IN BOWEL HABIT

In the case of chronic diarrhoea, stool specimens should be examined for ova and parasites and cultured for *Shigella* and *Salmonella* species. After rectal palpation and proctoscopy as described earlier, the next step in investigation is sigmoidoscopy, either rigid or flexible. **Rigid sigmoidoscopy** (rectoscopy) permits direct visual examination and biopsy of the mucosa up to the rectosigmoid junction; the term sigmoidoscopy is misleading in this case as it does not include the sigmoid colon proper. **Flexible sigmoidoscopy**, on the other hand, allows examination as far as the splenic flexure. The majority of large bowel lesions responsible for altered bowel habit occur in this region. Biopsies of the rectal wall should also be taken both for histology (e.g. for Crohn's disease) and for microbiological examination.

Further investigation is based on the differential diagnosis assembled during clinical examination. Barium enema X-ray, contrast CT scanning or colonoscopy is indicated in the majority of cases. Note that low rectal lesions cannot reliably be demonstrated on barium enema, and preliminary sigmoidoscopy is mandatory. If Crohn's disease is suspected, barium studies of the small bowel may also be required.

Flexible fibreoptic endoscopes can be used to directly examine the colon above the rectosigmoid junction. The shortest, the **flexible sigmoidoscope**, may be employed with no preparation or following a simple enema and can thus be used in the outpatient clinic. An excellent view can be obtained as far as the splenic flexure, allowing examination of the area in which over 50% of large bowel cancers occur. Since colonoscopy is a time-consuming and rather uncomfortable procedure, patients usually require intravenous sedation and analgesia, and occasionally general anaesthesia. Therefore colonoscopy is usually performed in hospital or dedicated units as short-stay day cases. Remember that more than one colonic adenoma or carcinoma can occur at the same time (synchronous lesions), so a full colonic examination is needed if one of these lesions is found.

IRON DEFICIENCY ANAEMIA

A common reason for surgical referral is persistent or severe anaemia believed to be caused by chronic intestinal blood loss. The patient may have presented initially with symptoms of chronic anaemia, namely lethargy, generalised weakness, breathlessness or even angina. Just as often, the anaemia has been recognised during general physical examination or on a blood count.

Chronic anaemia has many causes. Iron deficiency is the most common and is the only one with a cause likely to need surgical treatment. In blood films, iron deficiency anaemia is characterised by hypochromic, microcytic red blood cells. Serum iron level is low and transferrin elevated. Iron deficiency anaemia can be caused by chronic low-grade blood loss (which is often occult), inadequate dietary iron intake or absorption, or a combination of both. In some patients, the pattern of iron deficiency may be complicated by a coexisting anaemia from another cause, particularly the 'anaemia of chronic illness'. For example, an elderly patient with rheumatoid arthritis may have a chronic normochromic, normocytic anaemia due to chronic disease, as well as an iron deficiency anaemia caused by gastric bleeding provoked by non-steroidal anti-inflammatory drugs. Pernicious anaemia or folate deficiency anaemia may also underlie an iron deficiency anaemia.

APPROACH TO INVESTIGATION OF ANAEMIA

Investigation of a patient with suspected iron deficiency anaemia has five main components:

- History—seeking sources of blood loss from the various tracts (see Box 18.6) and excluding inadequate dietary iron intake. Previous gastrectomy may cause vitamin B_{12} deficiency and also diminished acid output, which may prevent adequate iron absorption. Drug history—aspirin, other NSAIDs and corticosteroids may be the cause of chronic gastroduodenal blood loss. A history of drug treatment for peptic ulcer or antacids for 'indigestion' may also indicate a source of blood loss
- Physical examination—seeking an abdominal mass, an enlarged Virchow's node in the left supraclavicular area (indicative of intra-abdominal malignancy), a rectal lesion or signs of a 'medical' cause
- Confirmation of iron deficiency anaemia and exclusion of common 'medical' causes of anaemia such as rheumatoid arthritis or chronic leukaemias— examine blood film, measure ESR, serum iron and transferrin, B_{12} and folate. When there is a 'mixed' anaemia, measuring iron stores in a bone marrow biopsy is the definitive method of diagnosing iron deficiency. Small bowel biopsies may demonstrate coeliac disease in a proportion of patients with simple anaemia without bowel symptoms

Lesions in the gastrointestinal tract

- Ulcerating tumours or polyps of the following (in order of frequency): caecum, stomach, the rest of the large bowel, and (rarely) stromal tumours of small bowel, e.g. leiomyosarcoma (GIST)
- Chronic peptic ulceration, i.e. hiatus hernia with reflux oesophagitis, gastric and duodenal ulcers or stomal ulceration following gastric surgery. All may be induced or aggravated by ingestion of aspirin and other non-steroidal anti-inflammatory drugs. These drugs can also cause chronic gastric haemorrhage from superficial erosions
- Other 'ulcerating' lesions of the bowel, e.g. haemorrhoids, angiodysplasias of colon or small bowel
- Chronic parasitic infestations, e.g. hookworm (extremely common in some developing countries)

Lesions in the female genital tract

- Heavy menstrual loss (menorrhagia is an extremely common but easily overlooked cause)
- Carcinoma of uterus or cervix (usually presents as abnormal vaginal bleeding rather than anaemia)

Lesions in the urinary tract (rarely sufficient to cause anaemia)

- Transitional cell carcinoma of bladder, pelvicalyceal systems or ureters
- Renal cell carcinoma (may cause haematuria but rarely anaemia)
- Chronic parasitic infestations, e.g. schistosomiasis (common in some developing countries)

- Testing of specimens of stool for occult blood (at least three specimens should be tested)
- Pursuing clues that suggest the origin of bleeding by using special investigations such as endoscopy and contrast radiology. When occult blood is found in the faeces and there are no digestive symptoms, colonoscopy is usually performed first, looking for tumours, polyps, inflammatory bowel disease or angiodysplasias. If negative, this is followed by gastroscopy. Both may be performed in the one session. If both are negative, it may be appropriate to proceed to small bowel contrast radiography. More recently, **capsule endoscopy** has become available. A free capsule containing a miniature video imaging device is swallowed, transmitting views of the entire gastrointestinal tract as it passes distally (see Ch. 5)

Occasionally, gastrointestinal bleeding continues, even though all investigations appear normal. The next step is often to repeat the appropriate investigations. If bleeding is rapid and serious enough to merit operation and no obvious lesion is found, the whole small bowel may be examined by operative endoscopy (enteroscopy). The small bowel is opened and a colonoscope threaded along its full length, transilluminating the bowel in the process. Small bowel angiodysplasias can only be reliably located by this method or by capsule endoscopy.

OBSTRUCTIVE JAUNDICE

THE NORMAL ENTEROHEPATIC CIRCULATION (Fig. 18.8)

The **haem** component of spent red cells is normally broken down to bilirubin (mainly in the spleen and bone marrow), bound to albumin and transported to the liver. This relatively stable protein–pigment complex is insoluble in water and is not excreted in the urine. In the liver, the complex is split and the bilirubin conjugated with glucuronic acid which makes it water-soluble, before it is excreted into the bile canaliculi. The normal concentration of both conjugated and unconjugated bilirubin in the blood is very low. Bacterial action in the bowel converts conjugated bilirubin into colourless **urobilinogen** and pigmented **urobilin** which imparts the brown colour to normal faeces. Some urobilinogen is reabsorbed, passing to the liver in the portal blood, and is then re-excreted in the bile. The entire process is called an **enterohepatic circulation** (see Fig. 18.8). A small amount of urobilinogen escapes into the systemic circulation and is excreted in the urine, colouring it yellow.

Bile acids (salts) are synthesised in the liver from cholesterol-based precursors. These are excreted in bile to the duodenum and facilitate lipid digestion and absorption in the small intestine. About 95% of the bile acids are reabsorbed in the distal ileum and returned to the liver via the portal vein, only to be re-excreted in the bile. Thus both bilirubin and bile acids are involved in enterohepatic circulations.

PATHOPHYSIOLOGY OF OBSTRUCTIVE JAUNDICE

If biliary outflow becomes obstructed, conjugated bilirubin is dammed back in the liver from where it enters the bloodstream and causes a gradual rise in plasma bilirubin. Once the plasma bilirubin level exceeds about 30 μmol/L, jaundice should be clinically detectable. Above 60 μmol/L, jaundice is obvious. Conjugated bilirubin, being water-soluble, is excreted in the urine, turning it dark.

In obstructive jaundice there is diminished or absent excretion of bile into the bowel, causing changes in the faeces. There is less urobilin to darken the stool and fewer bile acids, resulting in defective fat absorption. The two combine to give the stool a characteristic 'putty' colour.

A particular consequence of poor dietary fat absorption is malabsorption of vitamin K. This leads to decreased hepatic synthesis of clotting factors, notably prothrom-

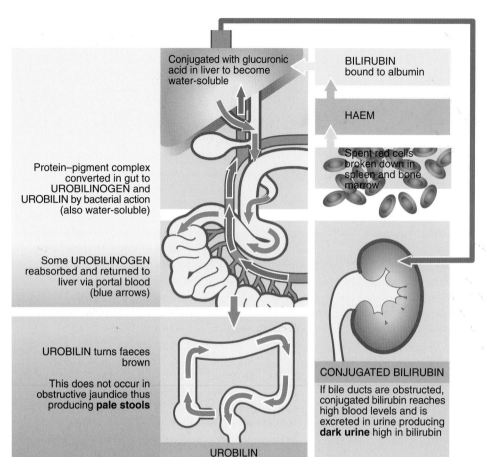

Conjugated with glucuronic acid in liver to become water-soluble

BILIRUBIN bound to albumin

HAEM

Spent red cells broken down in spleen and bone marrow

Protein–pigment complex converted in gut to UROBILINOGEN and UROBILIN by bacterial action (also water-soluble)

Some UROBILINOGEN reabsorbed and returned to liver via portal blood (blue arrows)

UROBILIN turns faeces brown

This does not occur in obstructive jaundice thus producing **pale stools**

CONJUGATED BILIRUBIN

If bile ducts are obstructed, conjugated bilirubin reaches high blood levels and is excreted in urine producing **dark urine** high in bilirubin

UROBILIN

Fig. 18.8 Normal dynamics of bilirubin excretion and the effects of obstructive jaundice Note that urobilinogen will appear in substantial quantities in the urine if large amounts are produced because of haemolytic anaemia, or if there is liver cell damage.

bin. Impairment of blood clotting is not so great as to cause spontaneous haemorrhage or bruising but there is a significant risk of haemorrhage during surgery or after liver biopsy. Thus the patient's coagulation profile must be checked before any invasive procedure. The coagulopathy is corrected with parenteral vitamin K or, in the case of an urgent procedure, fresh frozen plasma. Biliary obstruction also dams back bile acids, which raises their blood concentration leading to deposition in the skin; this sometimes causes intense itching.

HISTORY AND EXAMINATION OF PATIENTS WITH OBSTRUCTIVE JAUNDICE

History-taking

This should include enquiry about episodes of pain typical of gallstone disease, previous episodes of obstructive jaundice which resolved spontaneously, or previous biliary tract surgery. Previous attacks of acute pancreatitis also suggest gallstone disease. Other important aspects of the history include:

- Change in colour of urine and stools, i.e. dark urine and pale stools
- Drug history, e.g. oral contraceptive pill—potential for intrahepatic cholestasis

- Risk factors for viral hepatitis—blood product transfusion, intravenous drug abuse, tattoos, shellfish ingestion, sexual exposure
- Alcohol intake—if excessive, predisposes to pancreatitis and cirrhosis
- Symptoms associated with malignancy—anorexia, weight loss and non-specific upper gastrointestinal disturbance is common in carcinoma of the pancreas, a disease more common in the elderly
- A history of inflammatory bowel disease predisposes to **sclerosing cholangitis** although this is relatively rare

Examination

Early jaundice is a subtle physical sign and will be missed unless the patient is examined in a good light, preferably daylight. Jaundice is first detectable in the sclera of the eye and soon afterwards in the skin of the abdominal wall. In some cases of obstructive jaundice, the patient develops generalised itching (pruritus) and scratch marks may be apparent. The general stigmata of liver disease, such as spider naevi and liver 'flap', are only found when jaundice is caused by primary liver disease rather than extrinsic obstruction.

The abdomen should be examined, particularly for ascites, an enlarged liver or spleen, abnormal masses or a palpable gall bladder. An enlarged liver may be caused

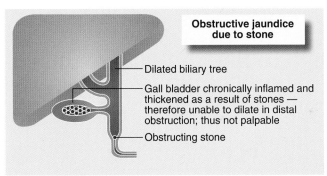

Fig. 18.9 Courvoisier's law

Labels for left figure (Obstructive jaundice due to stone):
- Dilated biliary tree
- Gall bladder chronically inflamed and thickened as a result of stones — therefore unable to dilate in distal obstruction; thus not palpable
- Obstructing stone

Labels for right figure (Obstructive jaundice due to carcinoma):
- Dilated biliary tree
- Thin-walled gall bladder dilates in distal obstruction; thus becomes palpable
- Carcinoma of pancreas or periampullary region obstructing common bile duct

by primary or secondary malignancy. In a jaundiced patient, splenomegaly with hepatomegaly is an important sign of chronic parenchymal liver disease (usually cirrhosis) and indicates portal hypertension. Ascites in a patient with obstructive jaundice is almost always due to disseminated intra-abdominal malignancy.

Courvoisier's 'law' (see Fig. 18.9) was formulated in 1890 and states that obstructive jaundice in the presence of a palpable gall bladder is not due to stone (and is therefore likely to be caused by tumour). The argument is that gallstones cause chronic inflammation leading to fibrosis of the gall bladder, which prevents its distension. An alternative explanation is that intermittent stone obstruction leads to thickening of the gall bladder wall, which prevents distension. In malignancy, progressive obstruction occurs over a short period and the gall bladder distends easily.

Particular attention is paid to the colour of the stool found on rectal examination, as a pale stool is characteristic of obstructive jaundice. The urine should also be inspected. In obstructive jaundice, it is usually dark yellow or orange from the presence of conjugated bilirubin, and froths when shaken due to the detergent effect of bile acids.

Conditions causing obstructive jaundice are illustrated in Figure 18.10.

APPROACH TO INVESTIGATION OF JAUNDICE

A patient with clinical signs of obstructive jaundice is usually investigated step by step as follows:

Urine tests

The presence of bilirubin in the urine, together with an indication of its concentration, is easily established by clinic or ward bedside dipstick urine tests. Substantial quantities usually mean biliary obstruction.

Blood tests

- Infective hepatitis should be excluded by serological screening for hepatitis B and C. Other antigen and antibody tests may be carried out if suspicion of infective hepatitis is high. A history of transfusion, intravenous drug abuse or travel to developing countries may increase the likelihood of an infection
- Confirm that the jaundice is obstructive by means of liver function tests, although these are not completely reliable in this respect. Obstructive jaundice is characterised by an elevated level of plasma bilirubin, predominantly in the conjugated form. There is also marked elevation of plasma alkaline phosphatase (liver isoenzyme) which is derived from bile canaliculi. The transaminases, derived from hepatocytes, are usually only mildly elevated
- When biliary obstruction is intrahepatic (e.g. cholangiocarcinoma obstructing only one duct) there may be a mixed biochemical picture with evidence of hepatocyte damage as well as duct obstruction. Liver function tests are, however, an unreliable guide and ultrasonography of the liver is mandatory
- Mild jaundice is commonly found in patients with Gilbert's syndrome, caused by a mild congenital abnormality of haemoglobin metabolism without serious significance
- Coagulation studies should be performed because of likely defects in clotting
- Tumour markers should be tested for in patients with a previous history of gastrointestinal malignancy

Imaging

Hepatobiliary ultrasonography

This is the simplest means of demonstrating dilated intrahepatic ducts (see Fig. 18.11), liver secondaries, a dilated extrahepatic biliary system or gall bladder abnormalities including stones. Ultrasound may reveal the cause of obstructive jaundice to be a tumour in the head of the pancreas or enlarged lymph nodes in the porta hepatis. Ultrasound, however, is unreliable for demonstrating pathology in the lower portion of the biliary tree; although it may show gallstones, it is unreliable for excluding them. In particular it may not visualise common bile duct stones or lesions in the head of the pancreas.

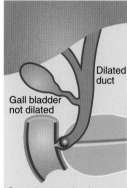

Gall bladder not dilated

Dilated duct

Stone impacted at lower end of CBD

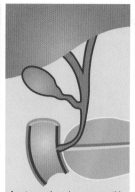

Gall bladder may dilate and become palpable (Courvoisier's sign)

CBD compressed by carcinoma as it passes through the head of pancreas

May also invade or compress 2nd part of duodenum

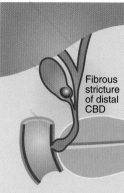

Acute or chronic pancreatitis may compress CBD in a similar way by inflammation or scarring

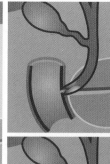
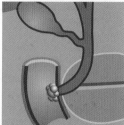

Fibrous stricture of distal CBD

| **1** | **Stones in common bile duct very common** | **2** | **Carcinoma of head of pancreas common** | **3** | **Pancreatitis uncommon** | **4** | **Mirizzi's syndrome rare** | **5** | **Periampullary malignant tumours uncommon** |

Suggested by a history of pain typical of biliary colic. Jaundice may be progressive (If stone is firmly impacted), fluctuant without ever disappearing altogether (if a stone alternately impacts and disimpacts), or intermittent (if multiple small stones successively impact then pass through the lower end of the common bile duct)

Typically causes painless jaundice which is persistent or progressive. The gall bladder may become palpable (see Courvoisier's law, Fig. 18.9)

Common bile duct is obstructed by inflammatory swelling in acute pancreatitis or by scarring in chronic pancreatitis

Found in about 1% of cholecystectomy patients. Gallstones impacted in Hartmann's pouch cause inflammation of the gall bladder which then fuses with the CHD causing secondary stenosis.
Large impacted stones sometimes cause pressure necrosis of the adjoining duct walls leading to chole–choledochal fistula

Include carcinomas of the ampulla, distal bile duct or duodenum (uncommon). Obstructive features are similar to carcinoma of head of pancreas

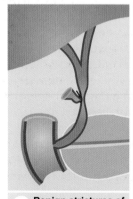

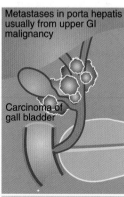

Metastases in porta hepatis usually from upper GI malignancy

Carcinoma of gall bladder

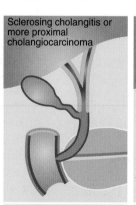

Sclerosing cholangitis or more proximal cholangiocarcinoma

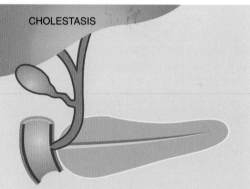

CHOLESTASIS

| **6** | **Benign strictures of the common bile duct uncommon** | **7** | **Other malignant tumours rare** | **8** | **Intrahepatic or hilar bile duct obstruction rare** | **9** | **Intrahepatic cholestasis common** |

May be due to surgical damage (fairly common) or inflammation caused by previous stone. Obstructive features are similar to carcinoma of head of pancreas

May cause bile duct obstruction above the ampulla. Examples include lymph node metastases in the porta hepatis (fairly common), primary cholangiocarcinoma (uncommon) and carcinoma of the gall bladder

Primary cholangiocarcinoma; sclerosing cholangitis (rare)

Note: hepatic metastases rarely cause obstructive jaundice

Viral hepatitis is a common cause

Systemic sepsis often causes low grade jaundice (due to liver dysfunction)

Idiosyncrasy to certain drugs (including chlorpromazine, oral contraceptives and chlorpropamide) interferes with bile excretion from hepatocytes, presumably by affecting membrane transport

Widespread hepatic lymphoma is a classical but rare cause

Fig. 18.10 Causes of obstructive jaundice

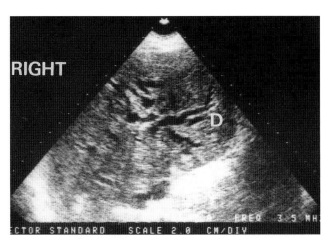

Fig. 18.11 Ultrasonogram showing dilated intrahepatic ducts
An ultrasound scan in an 80-year-old man with obstructive jaundice. This transverse section through the liver shows the characteristic 'double-barrel shotgun sign' **D**, with two parallel tubular structures representing major branches of the bile duct and portal vein. Normally, the portal vein is four times wider than the corresponding bile duct. Here they are the same diameter.

CT scanning

This may be the next stage if ultrasound findings are equivocal. CT is particularly useful for demonstrating primary or secondary tumours but may miss a small carcinoma at the lower end of the common bile duct.

Endoscopy—diagnostic and therapeutic

If ultrasound demonstrates dilated ducts, endoscopic retrograde cholangiopancreatography (ERCP) is frequently the next investigation (see Fig. 18.12). It is now usual practice to drain an obstructed bile duct at the same procedure if practicable, either by sphincterotomy and stone removal or by placing an intraluminal **stent**. This may be the definitive treatment for duct stones or inoperable carcinomas; for patients requiring operation, stenting is sometimes used to allow the jaundice to settle and liver function to improve. The role of diagnostic ERCP in jaundice is gradually being supplanted by magnetic resonance cholangiopancreatography (MRCP) described in Chapter 5.

Laparoscopy and liver biopsy

If bile ducts are not dilated, liver biopsy or biopsy of demonstrated secondaries may be performed (with ultrasound or CT guidance). Because clotting is frequently abnormal, clotting studies must be performed before any invasive procedure. Abnormalities are corrected by giving daily vitamin K injections and, if a clotting defect remains, infusing fresh-frozen plasma before and during any invasive procedure.

In patients unsuitable for percutaneous biopsy, or those who require visualisation of other organs, laparoscopy may be used to visualise the liver directly and to obtain biopsy specimens from suspicious areas. Occasionally, a firm diagnosis cannot be made before operation; abdominal exploration and frozen section histology may provide the answer. Laparotomy provides an opportunity for treatment at the same time.

PRINCIPLES OF MANAGEMENT OF OBSTRUCTIVE JAUNDICE

The primary aim of treatment is to relieve the obstruction of the biliary tract. Obstructed bile is often infected and a fulminant **acute cholangitis** can develop at any time. Back-pressure interferes with other liver functions such as synthesis of albumin and clotting factors. Eventually structural liver damage ensues.

Three categories of obstruction may be defined according to surgical treatment options:

- Potentially curable obstructions
- Obstruction due to incurable tumour
- Terminal disease

Potentially curable obstructions

These include bile duct stones and strictures as well as small tumours of the lower bile ducts, duodenum or ampullary region (*periampullary tumours*) (see Fig. 18.10, p. 288).

The number, size and position of **bile duct stones** may have been identified before operation by ERCP or MRCP. Stones may be removed at ERCP by dividing the ampullary sphincter using a 'bow-string' diathermy wire via the duodenal endoscope. Sometimes, if the stone is very large or impacted, the obstructed bile may be drained by endoscopic placement of a tube alongside it within the bile duct without stone removal. These tubes are known as **stents**, named after the inventor of earlier devices. Current large-bore duodenal endoscopes allow peroral placement of biliary stents up to about 4 mm in diameter.

When available, endoscopic sphincterotomy or stent placement is the initial treatment of choice for virtually all patients with common bile duct stones causing obstructive jaundice but particularly so for the following groups:

- Acute cholangitis, where it may be required urgently
- Patients who have previously had a cholecystectomy
- If laparoscopic cholecystectomy is planned
- Debilitated elderly patients where laparotomy would be specially hazardous

If cholecystectomy is the chosen treatment, bile duct stones can be identified by X-ray cholangiography performed during the operation (**peroperative cholangiography**) and removed surgically. Operative **choledochoscopy** is one technique where a flexible or rigid 'scope allows a visual check for completeness of stone removal.

Many surgeons undertaking laparoscopic cholecystectomy routinely perform operative cholangiography but

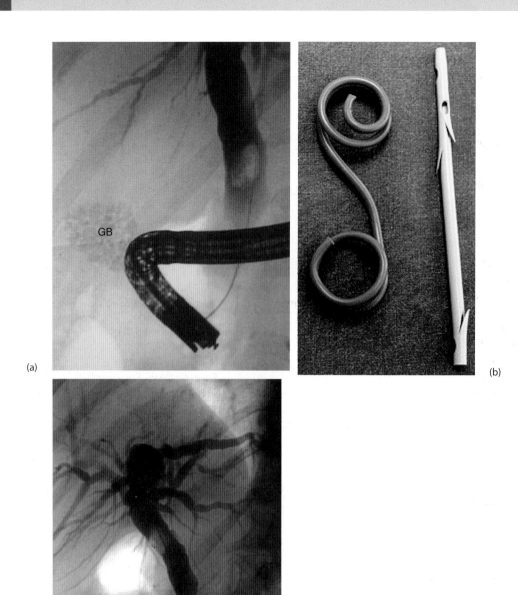

Fig. 18.12 Endoscopic stenting
(a) Diagnostic endoscopic retrograde cholangiogram (ERC) showing an enlarged common bile duct containing a single large stone. A collection of radiopaque gallstones is seen in the gall bladder **(GB)**. **(b)** Two types of biliary stent: the pigtail type on the left and the notched variety on the right, as used in this patient. **(c)** Despite endoscopic sphincterotomy, the bile duct stone could not be retrieved so a tubular self-retaining stent has been placed to relieve the obstructive jaundice. The stone was successfully removed endoscopically on a later occasion.

only a small proportion undertake laparoscopic exploration of the common bile duct as this is a difficult and time-consuming procedure.

Bile duct strictures can be treated by long-term stenting. Strictures are usually due to post-surgical fibrotic scarring but occasionally result from inflammatory scarring due to cholecystitis with jaundice (**Mirizzi's syndrome**). The 'gold standard' for more severe strictures or for iatrogenic division or ligation of the common bile duct is surgical reconstruction of the bile ducts.

Small **tumours in the periampullary region** may be amenable to complete excision, thereby relieving biliary obstruction. A complete cure is often achieved. **Adenocarcinoma of the head of the pancreas** is a common cause of obstructive jaundice but the long-term prognosis is poor even after a successful radical pancreatico-duodenectomy (which itself can have a high mortality rate). This may get better as specialist surgical centres improve preoperative staging and achieve better surgical outcomes. If an operation for potentially curable malignant disease is planned, it is now considered better not to stent beforehand to relieve the jaundice because of the risk of introducing infection. Note, however, that the precautions in Table 18.2 must be observed in such cases.

Obstruction due to incurable tumour

Such obstructions are commonly caused by carcinoma of the head of the pancreas, less often with lymph node metastases in the porta hepatis and rarely from carcinoma of the gall bladder. At present, the trend is towards palliative treatment because few cases have potential for curative surgery. Stenting is the palliative treatment of choice with bile duct and, if necessary, duodenal stenting. The alternative is bypass surgery; various operations can bypass the biliary obstruction by joining small bowel to the gall bladder or bile duct proximal to the obstruction or to dilated ducts within the liver. If the duodenum becomes obstructed by invading tumour, a surgical gastro-jejunostomy can be performed. For carcinoma of the head of the pancreas, **triple bypass** (see Ch. 24) is the classic palliative operation.

All these techniques merely overcome the problem of obstructive jaundice and have no influence on the course of the disease. Eventually and often within a few months, the patient succumbs to other manifestations of the cancer. Percutaneous **coeliac ganglion blockade** provides effective palliation for intractable pain.

Terminal disease

By the time obstructive jaundice has developed, some patients have reached a terminal stage of their cancer. In these cases, stenting may still be indicated but surgical interference may be difficult to justify; the aim should be to relieve distress and allow a dignified death. Some patients experience severe itching which may be lessened by drugs such as antihistamines or chlorpromazine. Oral cholestyramine is not indicated because it only removes bile salts which are able to reach the bowel.

SPECIAL RISKS OF SURGERY IN THE JAUNDICED PATIENT

Despite the fact that most obstructive jaundice can now be relieved preoperatively by stone removal or stenting,

Table 18.2 Special precautions to be taken when operating on a patient with obstructive jaundice

Potential complication	Pathophysiology	Prophylaxis
Infection	Obstructed bile is usually infected with aerobic gut organisms, and is under pressure. Instrumentation may precipitate ascending cholangitis, leading to sepsis and multiple organ dysfunction Spillage of infected bile during operation causes peritoneal contamination and risks intraperitoneal or wound infection	Preoperative drainage of bile into the bowel by endoscopic sphincterotomy or stenting is sometimes used Prophylactic antibiotics against gut flora should be given
Endotoxaemia and renal failure	Endotoxins appear in the systemic circulation. These predispose to multiple organ dysfunction syndrome (MODS) by activating components of the inflammatory cascade and may precipitate a systemic inflammatory response. Renal function is particularly vulnerable if renal perfusion is already impaired Postoperative 'hepatorenal syndrome' (i.e. acute renal failure) which manifests as oliguria and hyponatraemia	Prophylactic antibiotics Ensure adequate hydration during any period of restriction of oral fluid throughout—preoperative intravenous fluids and osmotic diuretics during operation Insert urinary catheter to monitor output
Hepatic impairment	Biliary back-pressure on the liver causes defective clotting factor synthesis (even if vitamin K given) and defective hepatic metabolism of certain drugs Patients with chronic parenchymal liver disease withstand the stresses of major abdominal surgery and anaesthesia poorly	Avoid drugs excreted by the liver. Give antibiotics to minimise endogenous endotoxin production
Fat malabsorption	Biliary obstruction causes diminished absorption of fats including fat-soluble vitamins such as vitamin K (a co-factor for prothrombin synthesis). This results in defective clotting	Monitor clotting Give parenteral vitamin K to improve prothrombin ratio, 24 hours preoperatively if possible; if necessary, fresh-frozen plasma perioperatively
Thromboembolism	Paradoxically, considering the clotting deficiency, postoperative deep vein thrombosis is common	Prophylactic subcutaneous low-dose heparin injections

surgery must still sometimes be performed in a jaundiced patient. This poses a greater risk from preoperative and postoperative surgical complications, as shown in Table 18.2.

ABDOMINAL MASS OR DISTENSION

An abdominal mass is sometimes discovered by the patient but more often by medical examination. An older patient with a definite palpable mass is likely to have a malignant tumour, but benign cysts, inflammatory masses, aneurysms or atypical hernias may be responsible. Occasionally masses have a 'medical' cause, e.g. hepatosplenomegaly of chronic lymphocytic leukaemia. Commonly, one of the 'five Fs'—fetus, faeces, flatus, fat or fluid—may masquerade as a 'surgical' mass or distension. These are common causes of embarrassment! An abdominal mass may be discovered without any related clinical features; usually, however, the patient has gastrointestinal symptoms, anaemia or jaundice in addition. A careful history will often reveal useful clues as to the cause of the mass.

CLINICAL ASSESSMENT OF AN ABDOMINAL MASS (see Table 18.3)

History

A thorough history will probably provide clues to the specific organ system involved. Important features include: how long has it been there; how did the patient come to notice it; is it always present or does it sometimes disappear (e.g. a hernia may reduce); is it getting bigger or smaller? A history of intra-abdominal malignancy years before should be regarded with grave suspicion: the disease may have recurred or a related new primary developed. This is especially common in large bowel cancer but uncommon once 7 years have elapsed since treatment.

General examination

General examination should seek systemic signs of disease (e.g. cachexia, anaemia and jaundice) or signs of malignant dissemination (e.g. supraclavicular lymphadenopathy in suspected stomach cancer). Abdominal and pelvic examination must be thorough and, if appropriate, proctoscopy and sigmoidoscopy should be performed.

EXAMINATION OF AN ABDOMINAL MASS

The location of the mass, its relations to other structures, its mobility and its physical characteristics, such as size, shape, consistency and pulsatility give valuable information about the organ of origin and the likely pathology. **Hernias**, e.g. incisional, umbilical and sometimes interstitial (Spigelian) hernias (see Ch. 32), may present as localised swellings but they usually shrink or reduce completely when the patient is supine or under anaesthesia. Unless the diagnosis of a hernia is considered, it may be overlooked. An incarcerated (irreducible but not obstructed) hernia is more appropriately considered a true 'mass'.

EXAMINATION OF MASSES IN SPECIFIC REGIONS OF THE ABDOMEN (see Fig. 18.1)

Mass in the right hypochondrium (right upper quadrant or RUQ)

A right hypochondrial mass is usually of hepatobiliary origin. If so, it will be continuous with the main bulk of the liver both to palpation and percussion. When the liver is diffusely enlarged, the inferior margin is regular and well defined and the consistency is usually normal. When infiltrated with primary or secondary cancer, the palpable liver may be hard and irregular or the liver may appear diffusely enlarged. Carcinoma of the gall bladder is indistinguishable from hepatic cancer on palpation. Rarely, a Riedel's lobe—a congenitally enlarged part of the right lobe—is mistaken for a pathological mass. Less commonly, a right hypochondrial mass is a diseased gall bladder. When a liver mass is suspected, other signs of liver disease should be sought. A mass continuous with the liver above and with a typical pear-shaped rounded outline is likely to be a mucocoele of the gall bladder. A more diffuse, tender mass may be an empyema of the gall bladder.

Epigastric mass

A mass in the epigastrium is usually due to a cancer of the stomach or transverse colon or sometimes omental secondaries from ovarian carcinoma. Cancer involving the left lobe of the liver may also present in this way (Fig. 18.13). These masses are usually hard and irregular and

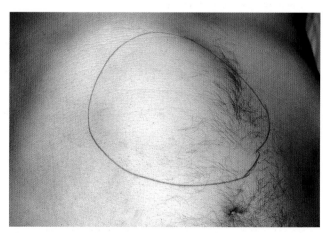

Fig. 18.13 Epigastric mass
This man of 44 presented having discovered an epigastric mass. It was asymptomatic. The margins of the mass are outlined on the skin. The mass moved downwards with respiration and proved to be a massive liver metastasis from a tiny pancreatic primary adenocarcinoma.

Table 18.3 **Causes of hepato-splenomegaly**

Hepatomegaly	Splenomegaly	Hepato-splenomegaly
Physiological Riedel's lobe		
Malignant tumours Hepatocellular carcinoma Secondary carcinoma		
Infective **Viral** Hepatitis, Epstein–Barr virus, cytomegalovirus **Bacterial** Tuberculosis, leptospirosis, liver abscess **Protozoal** Malaria, schistosomiasis, amoebiasis, histoplasmosis, hydatid disease	Hepatitis, Epstein–Barr virus, cytomegalovirus Subacute bacterial endocarditis, typhoid, tuberculosis, leptospirosis Malaria, toxoplasmosis, brucellosis, schistosomiasis, leishmaniasis (kala-azar)	Hepatitis, cytomegalovirus Tuberculosis, leptospirosis Malaria, toxoplasmosis, brucellosis, schistosomiasis, leishmaniasis (kala-azar)
Alcoholic liver disease Fatty liver Early cirrhosis		
Systemic diseases Wilson's disease Haemochromatosis Cellular infiltration, e.g. amyloid, sarcoid	Sarcoidosis Amyloidosis Rheumatoid arthritis (Felty's syndrome) Storage diseases (e.g. Gaucher's)	Amyloidosis Storage diseases (e.g. Gaucher's)
Benign tumours Hepatic adenoma		
Congestive cardiac disease Right heart failure Tricuspid regurgitation (pulsatile liver) Budd–Chiari syndrome	**Congestive splenomegaly** Hepatic vein thrombosis Portal vein thrombosis Splenic vein thrombosis Cirrhosis with portal hypertension	**Congestive hepatosplenomegaly** Hepatic vein thrombosis Portal vein thrombosis Splenic vein thrombosis Cirrhosis with portal hypertension Budd–Chiari syndrome
Haematological disease **Lymphoproliferative disorders** Lymphoma Leukaemias	Lymphoma Leukaemias	Lymphoma Leukaemias
Myeloproliferative disorders	Chronic myeloid leukaemia Myelofibrosis Polycythaemia rubra vera Essential thrombocythaemia	Chronic myeloid leukaemia Myelofibrosis Polycythaemia rubra vera Essential thrombocythaemia
Anaemia	Haemolytic anaemia Megaloblastic anaemia	Megaloblastic anaemia
Miscellaneous Primary biliary cirrhosis Polycystic liver disease	Thyrotoxicosis	Infantile polycystic disease

are mobile or fixed according to the degree of invasion. Occasionally an epigastric mass is an isolated enlargement of the left lobe of the liver or massive para-aortic lymph nodes due to lymphoma or testicular secondaries. A pulsatile epigastric mass is likely to be an abdominal aortic aneurysm.

Mass in the left hypochondrium (left upper quadrant or LUQ)

A cancer of the stomach or splenic flexure of the colon may present as a mass in the left hypochondrium. Tumour masses can usually be distinguished clinically from an enlarged spleen as the latter often has a discrete 'edge' and lies more posteriorly. Note that a normal-sized spleen is not palpable.

Mass in the loin or flank

A mass in the loin or flank is likely to be of renal origin and can best be felt on **bimanual palpation** (see Fig 18.3). Very rarely, a hernia occurs in the lumbar region; this reduces spontaneously as the patient rolls over.

Mass in the left iliac fossa

Masses in the left iliac fossa usually arise from the sigmoid colon. A hard faecal mass may be mistaken for a cancer but it can often be indented like putty. A solid sigmoid mass is usually due to tumour or a complex diverticular inflammatory mass. Ovarian masses and sometimes eccentric bladder lesions may be palpable in either iliac fossa. These lesions, however, arise from out of the pelvis and can often be pushed up on to the abdominal examining hand by digital pressure in the rectum or vagina (bimanual palpation—most effectively performed under general anaesthesia). Note that a rectal examination is mandatory in a complete abdominal examination.

Hernias in the groin are common (see Ch. 32) and may be chronically irreducible (incarcerated). Occasionally, an interstitial (Spigelian) hernia develops above the groin in either iliac fossa. This presents a somewhat confusing picture on examination by virtue of its site and because the peritoneal sac herniates between the layers of the abdominal wall.

Suprapubic mass

Suprapubic masses usually arise from pelvic organs such as the bladder or uterus and its adnexae. A palpable bladder is most commonly due to chronic urinary retention and the patient should be catheterised and then examined again. A distended bladder is dull to percussion and disappears on catheterisation. Bladder enlargement is usually symmetrical and may extend above the umbilicus. The margins may be difficult to define accurately because of the bladder's soft consistency. Only massive bladder tumours are palpable and would be accompanied by urinary tract symptoms and urine abnormalities. Sometimes large bladder stones are palpable abdominally.

A uterus may be palpable abdominally when enlarged by pregnancy or fibroids. Bimanual examination involves digital examination of the vagina at the same time as palpation of the lower abdomen with the other hand. Ovarian tumours, particularly cysts, may become enormous and extend well up into the abdomen; again, bimanual examination (under general anaesthesia if necessary) helps to distinguish the origin.

Mass in the right iliac fossa

The right iliac fossa is a common site for an asymptomatic mass. It may be due to unresolved inflammation of the appendix which becomes surrounded by a mass of omentum and small bowel, giving rise to an **'appendix mass'** (see Ch. 26). There is usually a recent history of right iliac fossa pain and fever. A carcinoma of the caecum may become very large without causing symptoms of obstruction because the caecum is large and distensible, and the faecal stream at this point is quite liquid. Thus, a caecal carcinoma often presents as an asymptomatic right iliac fossa mass; iron deficiency anaemia is often evident by this stage. Crohn's disease of the terminal ileum often presents with a tender mass, usually with typical symptoms of pain and diarrhoea.

Central abdominal mass

A central abdominal mass may originate in large or small bowel, as a result of malignant infiltration of the great omentum or from retroperitoneal structures such as lymph nodes, pancreas, connective tissues or the aorta. Retroperitoneal masses are only palpable if they are large. One of the most common central abdominal masses is an aneurysm of the abdominal aorta. Aneurysms usually arise just above the aortic bifurcation (at the umbilical level) which explains their central location in the upper part of the abdomen. The characteristic feature of an aneurysm is its **expansile pulsation**; other solid masses may transmit pulsation from large vessels nearby, but these masses are not expansile.

Several different types of hernia may present near the centre of the abdomen. Most common is an **incisional hernia** which protrudes through part or the whole of an abdominal wall incision. This may occur at any time after operation, from days to years later. It usually results from poor closure technique or postoperative infection. **Paraumbilical** or **umbilical hernias**, common in the obese, occur centrally and diagnosis is usually straightforward. **Divarication of the recti** (rectus abdominis muscles, not a true hernia) involves the recti being splayed apart, often as a result of pregnancy or obesity, leaving the central anterior abdominal wall devoid of muscular support. This condition is easily recognised because of its typical 'keel' shape and its symptomless nature; treatment is rarely necessary. Divarication and midline hernias can best be demonstrated when the abdominal muscles are contracted, e.g. the supine patient raises both heels from the bed.

Rectal mass and findings on pelvic examination

An abdominal or pelvic mass may be palpable solely on rectal (or vaginal) examination. The mass may be a rectal cancer or a cancer in the loop of sigmoid colon lying in the pelvic cavity; the latter is unlikely to be visible on sigmoidoscopy. Sometimes, secondary deposits from an impalpable tumour in the upper abdomen may seed the pelvic cavity. This may produce a hard anterior lump or even a solid mass filling the pelvic cavity. The latter condition is known as a **frozen pelvis**. Frozen pelvis can also occur with endometriosis or local spread of a carcinoma of cervix or, rarely, prostate.

INTERPRETATION OF A FINDING OF ASCITES

Ascites is defined as a chronic accumulation of fluid within the abdominal cavity and has many causes, some malignant and some non-malignant. Ascites can usually be recognised clinically only when the volume exceeds 2 litres, but even then it is easily overlooked. Dullness to percussion in the flanks and suprapubic region with central resonance is suspicious of ascites and should be followed by an attempt to elicit a fluid thrill or 'shifting dullness' (see Fig. 18.4).

Malignant ascites

In ovarian or colonic cancer, the peritoneum is sometimes seeded with tumour deposits which secrete a protein-rich fluid containing malignant cells. This **malignant ascites** may reach a volume of several litres. The peritoneum may be peppered with thousands of minute seedlings without a palpable mass or there may be several large masses hidden by the ascitic fluid. Such widespread peritoneal involvement may cause abdominal distension which is often difficult to recognise on abdominal examination. It should be suspected if a patient with a past history of gastrointestinal or ovarian carcinoma has other symptoms suggestive of malignancy such as anorexia or marked weight loss.

Lymphatic obstruction

A rare cause of ascites is massive obstruction of abdominal lymphatic drainage. This is usually caused by malignant involvement of para-aortic lymph nodes with lymphoma or metastatic testicular malignancy. **Chylous ascites**, in which the ascitic fluid is milky-white, is rare and is due to proximal lymphatic obstruction and the presence of chylomicrons in the fluid originating from mesenteric lymphatics.

Tuberculosis

Abdominal **tuberculosis** is an uncommon cause in developed countries but is common in the developing world. Tuberculosis can occasionally present as ascites; this form is characterised by multiple tiny peritoneal tubercles, clinically indistinguishable from tumour secondaries. If discovered at operation, biopsies must be taken because the condition is usually curable, unlike its malignant counterpart.

Non-surgical causes

Ascites is commonly caused by gross congestive cardiac failure, constrictive pericarditis, severe hypoalbuminaemia or portal venous obstruction, the last occurring in cirrhosis and occasionally with liver metastases.

DIFFUSE ABDOMINAL DISTENSION

In diffuse distension without a palpable abdominal mass, sinister causes need to be excluded. Gas within the bowel is a common cause for long-standing and often intermittent abdominal pain and distension. It usually occurs in healthy young adults, particularly women, in association with irritable bowel syndrome or air swallowing during hyperventilation. Chronic gaseous abdominal distension may also be found in elderly patients with partial volvulus of the sigmoid colon. Clinical assessment will usually diagnose these problems and avoid unnecessary investigation.

Gross faecal loading may also be responsible for abdominal distension. This is often seen in children with abdominal pain and sometimes in young adults with irritable bowel syndrome. Asymptomatic chronic constipation is common in the elderly, and a faecal mass palpable through a thin abdominal wall can give the impression of a sinister mass.

APPROACH TO INVESTIGATION OF AN ABDOMINAL MASS OR DISTENSION

Laboratory tests

Blood, urine and stool investigations will be performed as suggested by the history and examination, e.g. full blood count, function tests, dipstick urinalysis and faecal occult bloods.

Radiology

A chest X-ray should be performed if malignancy is suspected. Ultrasonography or CT scanning (see Fig. 18.14) is useful for demonstrating the size and origin of a mass and one or other is often the first choice if pathology is suspected in the liver, biliary tree, pancreas, aorta or pelvic organs, or to confirm ascites. For pelvic masses, transvaginal or transrectal ultrasound is usually the

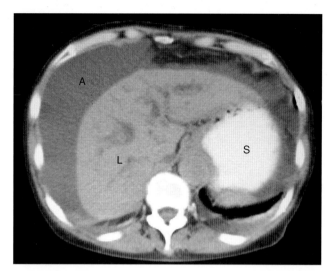

(a)

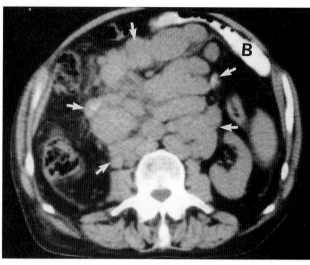

(b)

Fig. 18.14 CT scans showing gross ascites and enlarged lymph nodes
In **(a)** note the darker grey homogeneous shadow of fluid **A** around the liver **L** and the contrast in the stomach **S**. **(b)** Retroperitoneal mass of lymph nodes due to lymphoma. This CT scan was taken to assess the stage of spread of a known lymphoma. This 40-year-old woman presented with a large rubbery lymph node mass in her neck and was also found to have a large central abdominal mass. Abdominal CT scanning showed an enormous mass of lymph nodes (arrowed). Small bowel **B** is seen anteriorly, enhanced by orally administered contrast material.

investigation of first choice. CT scanning is most valuable in defining masses in the retroperitoneal area, e.g. pancreas, aorta or kidneys, but may be the investigation of choice for suspected large bowel cancer in frail patients. Ultrasound or CT scanning can be used to guide needle biopsy or aspiration cytology precisely. Contrast studies, e.g. barium meal, barium enema or intravenous urography, may be indicated by the clinical findings.

Endoscopy

Flexible endoscopic techniques such as gastroscopy or colonoscopy enable direct examination and biopsy of many gastrointestinal lesions. Gastro-duodenoscopy is indicated if symptoms are suggestive of oesophago-gastro-duodenal pathology, flexible sigmoidoscopy or colonoscopy if the findings suggest large bowel pathology, and ERCP may be used to outline the biliary and pancreatic duct systems if appropriate.

Other methods of tissue diagnosis

A tissue diagnosis should be obtained even if disseminated malignancy seems obvious. It can influence palliative and supportive treatment and, occasionally, an apparently hopeless case proves on histology to be treatable or even curable. Examples are tuberculosis, lymphoma or a germ cell tumour such as teratoma. Techniques of obtaining tissue for histology include needle or excision biopsy of enlarged cervical lymph nodes, and percutaneous biopsy of liver or an intra-abdominal mass (which may be guided by ultrasound or CT). Paracentesis abdominis (i.e. needle aspiration of ascitic fluid) is a safe and

simple way of obtaining a specimen for cytology and microbiology. Finally, when less invasive methods have failed to provide the necessary information, direct biopsy of tumour at diagnostic laparoscopy or open operation usually provides the definitive diagnosis.

Examination under anaesthesia, laparoscopy and exploratory laparotomy

Examination under anaesthesia (EUA) is sometimes necessary for estimating the mobility and spread of pelvic tumours. General anaesthesia with a muscle relaxant allows thorough abdominal palpation and bimanual examination of the pelvis via rectum and vagina and the taking of biopsies. This may not be possible without anaesthesia because of tenderness or abdominal wall muscle tone. EUA is often combined with cystoscopy or other rigid endoscopies. Laparoscopy, widely used in gynaecology, is now a widely available diagnostic and therapeutic tool in general surgery. It allows direct inspection and biopsy of masses and visualisation of the extent of local spread governing resectability, as well as allowing a search for intra-abdominal metastases. Samples can be taken for cytology to demonstrate intraperitoneal spread. Special ultrasound probes may be applied directly to the liver and other organs where lesions are suspected which are too small to be detected by standard non-invasive ultrasonography. Diagnostic laparotomy, often necessary before the advent of modern imaging techniques, is now required only when less invasive procedures have failed to provide a clear diagnosis or when treatment to relieve symptoms such as bowel obstruction is urgently required.

The acute abdomen and acute gastrointestinal haemorrhage

19

INTRODUCTION

The term **acute abdomen** is widely understood but is difficult to define precisely. Typically, the symptoms are of acute onset and strongly suggest an abdominal cause; abdominal pain is almost always a prominent feature. The illness is of such severity that admission to hospital appears essential and operative surgery is a likely outcome. Many of the disorders causing an 'acute abdomen' are serious and potentially life-threatening unless treated promptly. On the other hand, simple and relatively trivial conditions such as constipation can produce acute and severe symptoms mimicking the early stages of an acute abdomen. These lesser diagnoses may only become apparent after a period of observation or after special investigations.

Major gastrointestinal haemorrhage is also a common reason for acute surgical referral, and is manifest by vomiting of blood (**haematemesis**) or profuse rectal bleeding or the passage of **melaena** (altered blood). Many such patients are initially referred to a general (internal) physician or gastroenterologist, especially if the presumptive diagnosis is bleeding from a peptic ulcer or oesophageal varices. Management is usually conservative, at least initially, and may be undertaken in an internal medicine unit, or occasionally in a combined gastroenterology and surgery unit.

Acute surgical emergencies constitute about 50% of all general surgical admissions (see Table 19.1). About half of these are for abdominal symptoms, predominantly pain, and half of those in this group resolve without operation. The rest undergo emergency surgery (e.g. for ruptured abdominal aortic aneurysm) or a scheduled surgical procedure during the same admission (e.g. cholecystectomy on the next available operating list), or arrangements are made to have an operation later (e.g. interval appendicectomy for resolving appendix mass).

The common abdominal causes for emergency admission are summarised in Figure 19.1. The list is not meant to be exhaustive and excludes obscure medical causes like acute intermittent porphyria or tabes dorsalis, as well as conditions mainly confined to infants and children (see Ch. 50).

BASIC PRINCIPLES OF MANAGING THE ACUTE ABDOMEN

In managing the acute abdomen, the first goal is to resuscitate the patient. For practical purposes this means intravenous fluids where indicated and, usually, administration of analgesia. The next goal is to make a broad diagnosis on the basis of history, examination and laboratory tests and imaging if indicated. Most patients undergo plain radiology of chest and abdomen (Box 19.1).

If peritonitis is suspected, a chest X-ray in the erect position is performed. All of this will help to decide whether an operation is necessary and if so, how urgently it is required. It will also clarify if non-surgical treatment is necessary, e.g. antibiotics for diverticulitis or cystitis (lower urinary tract infection, UTI) or conservative measures for acute pancreatitis. Sometimes it is evident that the patient has an acute abdomen, i.e. peritonitis, that demands urgent surgery. Often, the precise diagnosis and the procedure required cannot be known until the abdomen is opened.

The broad diagnosis is based on the likely pathophysiological phenomena responsible for the patient's clinical state. Does the clinical picture suggest intestinal obstruction, bowel strangulation, peritonitis, intra-abdominal abscess, intra-abdominal bleeding or acute bowel ischaemia, or is there obvious gastrointestinal haemorrhage? More than one of these phenomena may occur at once. For example, strangulation is usually associated with signs of obstruction. Each of the main phenomena is described in detail in the following sections.

DISORDERS AND DISEASES CAUSING THE ACUTE ABDOMEN

INTESTINAL OBSTRUCTION

PATHOPHYSIOLOGY OF INTESTINAL OBSTRUCTION

Any part of the gastrointestinal tract may become obstructed and present as an acute abdomen. Gastric outlet obstruction, however, presents differently and is described in Chapter 21. The causes of intestinal obstruction are many and varied, as outlined in Figure 19.2.

Obstruction leads to dilatation of bowel proximally and disrupts peristalsis. The manner of presentation depends on the level of obstruction within the gastrointestinal tract (i.e. stomach, proximal or distal small bowel or large bowel) and on the completeness of obstruction. The most acute presentation is upper small bowel obstruction which manifests within hours of onset. This is because the large volume of gastric and pancreaticobiliary secretions is prevented from moving onwards, so it regurgitates into the stomach and is vomited. In contrast, distal large bowel obstruction is often much more chronic and may be present for days or weeks before the patient seeks treatment.

SYMPTOMS OF INTESTINAL OBSTRUCTION

Symptoms and physical signs are summarised in Box 19.2 (see p. 305).

Table 19.1 Composition of acute general surgical admissions in a typical district general hospital without a separate head injury or urological emergency service (gastrointestinal causes are shown in bold type)

Reason for admission	Percentage of admissions
Non-specific abdominal pain, resolving without surgery	**25%**
Head injuries	20%
Acute appendicitis	**12%**
Acute abdomen due to other causes	**12%**
Abscesses	10%
Arterial emergencies	5%
Urological emergencies	5%
Hernia/scrotal emergencies	5%
Gastrointestinal haemorrhage	**3%**
Soft tissue wounds	2%
Burns	1%

Box 19.1 Plain radiology in the acute abdomen—what to look for

Five main image densities are detectable on radiographs:

- White—metallic objects
- Off white—calcified structures
- Medium shades of grey—most soft tissues
- Dark grey—fat
- Black—gas

How to review an abdominal X-ray:

1. Check **name** is correct and **date** is current
2. Note **type of X-ray**, i.e. plain or contrast, erect or supine
3. Is the image of adequate **diagnostic quality**, i.e. appropriate density. Does it show the whole abdomen?
4. **Bowel gas and bowel wall**—note distribution and dilatation (small bowel diameter less than 3 cm, most large bowel less than 5 cm, caecum less than 9 cm). Absence of gas may indicate a displacing mass, ascites (central) or acute pancreatitis (ground glass appearance). Faeces appear mottled; 'faecal loading' may mean constipation or obstruction. Rigler's sign is strongly suggestive of bowel perforation
5. **Non-bowel gas**—free intraperitoneal gas, e.g. subphrenic gas in perforation of bowel, gas within bowel wall in necrosis, gas in biliary tree after sphincterotomy or fistula into bowel
6. **Calcification**—aortic wall in aneurysm, pancreas, renal and ureteric stones, gallstones, pelvic phleboliths (calcified old venous thrombi), teratomas, fetus. Bones of spine and pelvis—osteoarthritis, metastases (lytic or sclerotic), Paget's disease, fractures
7. **Soft tissues**. Thickened bowel wall. Check outline of kidneys (are both present?; length equal to 3 or more vertebral bodies) and psoas muscles (obscured in retroperitoneal inflammation)
8. **Artefacts**—artificial objects placed by medical personnel (central venous line, nasogastric tube, metal vessel or Fallopian tube clips, biliary, vascular or bowel stents, inferior vena caval filter, intrauterine contraceptive device
   —foreign bodies—embedded bullets, glass fragments, objects inserted rectally
   —projection of buttons, safety pins, rings on hand, coins, body piercing

In patients with an acute abdomen, always review chest X-ray for the following:

- Hiatus hernia
- Heart size
- Lung fields
- Pneumothorax
- Diaphragms: relative height; gas under
- Bony changes
- CVP line position

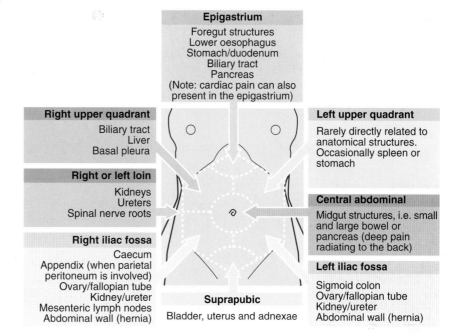

Fig. 19.1 Common causes of acute abdominal pain
Note: Non-specific abdominal pain which resolves without operation is relatively common. A watch and wait policy may be wise in the absence of critical signs.

Vomiting

Obstruction of the bowel eventually leads to vomiting; the more proximal the obstruction, the earlier vomiting develops. Vomiting can occur even if nothing is taken by mouth because saliva and other gastrointestinal secretions continue to be produced and enter the stomach. Remember that at least 10 litres of fluid are secreted into the gastrointestinal tract each day. The nature of the vomitus gives important clues about the level of obstruction. For example, vomiting of semi-digested food eaten a day or two earlier strongly suggests gastric outlet obstruction, particularly if there is no bile present in the vomitus. Copious vomiting of **bile-stained fluid** suggests upper small bowel obstruction. If the vomitus is thicker and foul-smelling (**faeculent**), a more distal obstruction is likely. This change to faeculent vomiting usually takes place gradually after about 24 hours of complete obstruction and is often an indication for urgent operation. The term faeculent vomiting is something of a misnomer as it contains putrefying and altered small bowel contents rather than faeces.

Pain

Fluid and swallowed air proximal to an obstruction together with continuing peristalsis cause pain. The general area of the pain gives clues as to the embryological origin of the affected bowel: upper, middle or lower abdominal pain originates in foregut, midgut or hindgut respectively. In obstruction, pain is not usually the most prominent symptom. It is of variable intensity, often quite mild, and usually colicky and occurring in short-lived bouts as peristalsis attempts to overcome the obstruction. In the small

bowel, peristaltic action often increases for 24–48 hours after the onset of obstruction and then fades after that.

Constipation

Distal to the obstruction, bowel gas is absorbed and the propulsion of bowel contents is arrested. The resulting **absolute constipation**, i.e. no faeces or flatus is passed rectally, is pathognomonic of bowel obstruction. The longer the duration of absolute constipation, the more significant it becomes in the diagnosis of obstruction.

Effects of the competence of the ileocaecal valve

Symptoms develop more gradually in large bowel obstruction because of the large capacity of the colon and caecum and their absorptive activity. If the ileocaecal valve remains competent however, retrograde flow of accumulating bowel contents is prevented and the thin-walled caecum progressively distends with swallowed air and eventually ruptures. In about half the cases of large bowel obstructions, the ileocaecal valve becomes incompetent and allows the small bowel to distend, delaying the onset and perhaps acuteness of obstructive symptoms. Operation is clearly more urgent if the ileocaecal valve does remain competent.

Incomplete obstruction

If the bowel is only partially obstructed, the clinical features are less clearly defined. Vomiting may be intermittent and the bowel habit erratic. Chronic incomplete obstruction leads to gradual hypertrophy of the muscle of the bowel wall proximally. Peristaltic activity in this hypertrophic muscle is responsible for the bouts of colicky

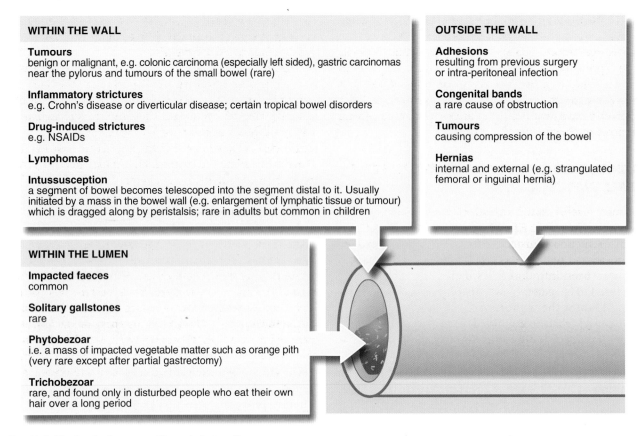

WITHIN THE WALL

Tumours
benign or malignant, e.g. colonic carcinoma (especially left sided), gastric carcinomas near the pylorus and tumours of the small bowel (rare)

Inflammatory strictures
e.g. Crohn's disease or diverticular disease; certain tropical bowel disorders

Drug-induced strictures
e.g. NSAIDs

Lymphomas

Intussusception
a segment of bowel becomes telescoped into the segment distal to it. Usually initiated by a mass in the bowel wall (e.g. enlargement of lymphatic tissue or tumour) which is dragged along by peristalsis; rare in adults but common in children

OUTSIDE THE WALL

Adhesions
resulting from previous surgery or intra-peritoneal infection

Congenital bands
a rare cause of obstruction

Tumours
causing compression of the bowel

Hernias
internal and external (e.g. strangulated femoral or inguinal hernia)

WITHIN THE LUMEN

Impacted faeces
common

Solitary gallstones
rare

Phytobezoar
i.e. a mass of impacted vegetable matter such as orange pith (very rare except after partial gastrectomy)

Trichobezoar
rare, and found only in disturbed people who eat their own hair over a long period

Fig. 19.2 Mechanical causes of bowel obstruction

pain, which may be more prominent than those found in complete obstruction. The pain is often accompanied by **visible peristalsis**, which is the hallmark of incomplete obstruction, although it can only be seen in thin patients. The most common cause is a slowly progressively obstructing colonic cancer. Note that incomplete obstruction should *not* be called subacute obstruction as the term is inaccurate and misleading.

PHYSICAL SIGNS OF INTESTINAL OBSTRUCTION

General examination

Vomiting, diminished fluid intake and sequestration of fluid in the small bowel commonly lead to **dehydration**. This is clinically manifest by extreme dryness of the mouth and characteristic loss of skin turgor and elasticity. Gas-filled loops of bowel proximal to the obstruction produce gaseous **abdominal distension**; the more distal the obstruction, the greater the distension. General examination may also reveal signs of anaemia or lymphadenopathy attributable to the primary disorder.

Groin examination

It is essential that the groins are examined for hernias. An obstructed femoral hernia is usually very small and rarely causes local symptoms. Instead it produces symptoms and

signs of small bowel obstruction. Similarly, a strangulated femoral hernia is often no bigger than a large grape and is rarely red or tender; consequently, it is easily missed if not specifically sought. This is a clinical point of particular importance—an obstruction due to an irreducible hernia will not settle with the usual conservative treatment.

Abdominal examination

On abdominal inspection, scars of previous operations may be important, both from the nature of the disease and the surgery as well as the possibility of adhesive obstruction. Rarely, episodes of **visible peristalsis** may be observed in thin patients where the obstruction is incomplete and of long duration.

On palpation, the most striking feature is the lack of abdominal tenderness; the exception is when strangulation has occurred. Obstruction with tenderness *must* be diagnosed as strangulation, necessitating urgent operation after fluid resuscitation. Note that a large abdominal mass causing obstruction may be palpable.

On **percussion**, the centre of the abdomen tends to be resonant and the periphery dull because bowel gas rises to the most elevated point; this may be difficult to distinguish from ascites.

On **auscultation**, bowel sounds in obstruction are traditionally described as being loud and frequent, high-pitched and tinkling; nevertheless, in practice, obstructed bowel sounds may or may not be increased. They have an echoing, cavernous quality or else can sound like the gentle lapping of water against a boat. This is due to fluid sloshing about in distended, gas-filled loops of bowel. A **succussion splash**, heard on gently shaking the patient's abdomen from side to side, may add weight to the clinical diagnosis of obstruction.

RADIOLOGICAL INVESTIGATION OF SUSPECTED BOWEL OBSTRUCTION

The most useful initial investigation is a plain supine abdominal X-ray (see Figs 19.3 to 19.5). Bowel proximal to an obstruction is distended by gas, but gas is virtually absent beyond the obstruction although some rectal gas may have been introduced if a digital examination was performed. The pattern and distribution of bowel gas often indicates the approximate site of obstruction. In small bowel obstruction, fluid levels are likely to be visible if an erect or decubitus X-ray has been taken. The degree of distension is determined by measuring bowel diameter on the X-ray, but ensure that the image is not magnified or reduced. If it is, there may be a measurement scale on the image with which to compare the bowel (see Box 19.1 for normal dimensions).

The ileocaecal valve may or may not remain competent when large bowel obstruction occurs and this is a key determinant of the rate of likely deterioration of the patient's clinical condition. The caecum and ascending colon are less muscular than the rest of the colon, so obstruction at any point distal to the caecum means that these areas dilate the most and are most likely to perforate. Once the radiological diameter of the caecum reaches 10 cm, it is in imminent danger of rupture and an operation is needed urgently.

In large bowel obstruction of less acute onset, where the patient does not require urgent surgery, an unprepared radiological contrast enema is helpful to demonstrate the site and nature of the obstruction (including sigmoid volvulus) and to distinguish mechanical obstruction from pseudo-obstruction (see below). A computerised tomography (CT) scan can also help to elucidate the underlying diagnosis. CT scanning gives an indication of the level of obstruction but may not give the precise diagnosis. Other useful information such as the presence of

Fig. 19.3 Radiological appearances of obstructed bowel

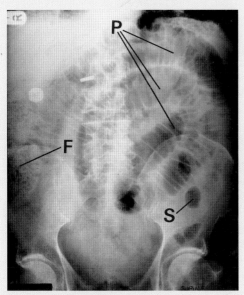

(a) Supine abdominal film in a man of 67 presenting with vomiting and abdominal distension. The film shows mid small bowel obstruction. Dilated small bowel fills the upper left quadrant and centre of the abdomen, and can be identified by the valvulae conniventes (plicae circulaies **P**) which extend across the whole width of the lumen. The small bowel distal to the obstruction is collapsed and is not visible on this film. The large bowel is also collapsed, with faecal loading of the ascending colon (**F**) and only a small amount of gas in the sigmoid colon (**S**). Note also the metallic tip of the nasogastric (NG) tube and the incidental radiopaque gallstone.

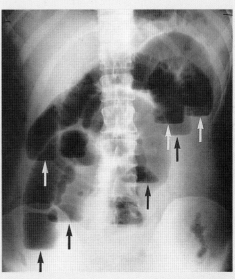

(b) Erect film showing multiple loops of dilated small bowel and multiple fluid levels. The obstruction was caused by a small carcinoma of the medial wall of the caecum encroaching upon the ileal opening. Note: erect abdominal films are rarely taken nowadays.

CASE STUDY

Fig. 19.4 Radiological appearances of obstructed bowel

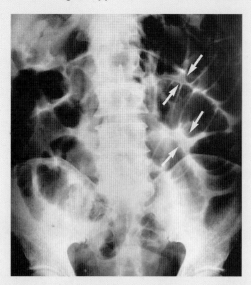

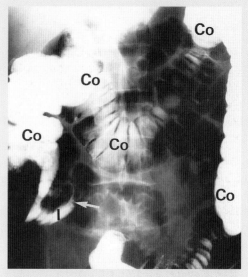

(a) Supine abdominal X-ray in a middle-aged man with several days of symptoms of small bowel obstruction. The abdomen is filled with grossly dilated small bowel loops. In addition, the small bowel wall is thickened, as shown by the apparent space between loops of bowel (arrowed); this is a characteristic feature of prolonged obstruction.

(b) 'Instant' contrast enema showing contrast filling the normal colon **Co** and distal ileum **I** which abruptly terminates at the obstruction (arrow). The obstruction proved at laparotomy to be caused by a band adhesion resulting from an operation for appendicitis 25 years previously.

hepatic metastases may radically influence management, for example using a bowel stent to relieve the obstruction rather than operating.

THE ADYNAMIC BOWEL

Temporary disruption of normal peristaltic activity without mechanical blockage causes the symptoms of **adynamic bowel disorder**. It occurs most commonly after abdominal surgery in which the bowel has been handled, and small bowel is particularly susceptible. The condition is known as **ileus** or **paralytic ileus**. Normal **postoperative ileus** should not persist for more than about 4 days. It is one of the reasons why fluids and solids are usually introduced gradually after abdominal surgery. Persisting postoperative 'ileus' is a cause for careful clinical management as it is usually due to a complication of surgery such as anastomotic leakage or an intra-abdominal abscess. Both of these have adverse local effects upon bowel wall function, and often require timely reoperation.

Occasionally electrolyte disturbances, such as hypokalaemia, or anti-Parkinsonian drugs are responsible for adynamic bowel disorder. The condition is also common in patients admitted to intensive care, particularly the multiply injured.

Pseudo-obstruction of the colon

A form of adynamic bowel disorder peculiar to the large bowel is called **pseudo-obstruction**. The term, however, is a misnomer as no mechanical obstruction is present. It can be caused by a wide range of apparently unrelated conditions that compromise bowel peristalsis. These include retroperitoneal inflammation or haemorrhage, neurological conditions, certain drugs (e.g. anticholinergics), pregnancy, orthopaedic injuries or surgery (particularly in the elderly) and prolonged recumbency.

Physical signs are similar to those of mechanical obstruction except that bowel sounds are not of the obstructed type or may be inaudible. The diagnosis of pseudo-obstruction is based on the clinical findings and confirmed if no mechanical obstruction is found on 'instant', i.e. unprepared, contrast enema.

Pseudo-obstruction eventually resolves with conservative measures in most cases. It is important to identify and treat any obvious precipitating cause. Neostigmine is sometimes used for those failing to respond to conservative measures but close cardiac monitoring is required. Surgery is rarely necessary but is sometimes indicated if mechanical obstruction cannot be excluded or if no recovery is evident after prolonged conservative management.

PRINCIPLES OF MANAGEMENT OF INTESTINAL OBSTRUCTION

Once intestinal obstruction has been recognised and the approximate level of obstruction identified, management proceeds as follows:

Fig. 19.5 Radiological appearances of obstructed bowel

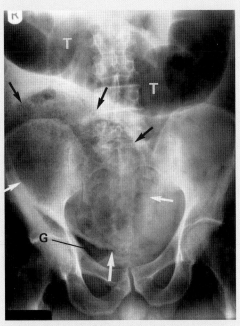

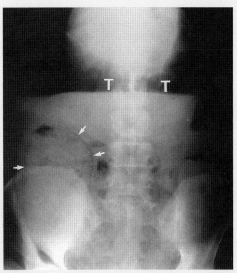

(b) Erect film showing gas in the caecal wall which indicates necrosis and is caused by the extreme distension. Note also the long fluid level in the transverse colon **T, T**.

(a) Supine film of an elderly man showing gross caecal dilatation with loss of haustration (surface folds). In large bowel obstruction, this typically occurs if the ileocaecal valve remains competent—a condition that carries a high risk of perforation. In this case, the transverse colon **T** is dilated with gas and there is complete absence of colonic gas on the left side of the abdomen where the descending and sigmoid colon lies. From this, it can be deduced that the colon is obstructed near the splenic flexure. In fact, this patient had an obstructing carcinoma at the splenic flexure and the caecum had perforated, as shown by the presence of gas **G** in the extra-peritoneal tissues.

- Resuscitation is an essential first step (see Ch. 4). Oral intake is discontinued and intravenous fluids are given, the volume and type of fluid determined by the state of hydration, the duration of the obstruction and plasma electrolyte abnormalities. Note that after prolonged vomiting, patients may be seriously depleted of fluid and electrolytes
- If the patient is vomiting or there is marked small bowel dilatation, a nasogastric tube is passed and the gastric contents aspirated. This will control nausea and vomiting, remove swallowed air and reduce gaseous distension. Most importantly, it will minimise the risk of inhalation of gastric contents, particularly during induction of general anaesthesia
- At least two-thirds of uncomplicated cases of obstruction are due to adhesions and will usually resolve with conservative measures employed for a maximum of 4 days. Those that resolve do not usually require operation during this episode
- Large bowel obstruction due to faecal impaction can be relieved by enemas or manual removal of faeces

- Operation may be required to relieve the obstruction. Provided strangulation can be excluded and the caecum is not dangerously distended, operation can safely be deferred for a day or two. Nevertheless, few obstructions that have not begun to settle with 48 hours of adequate conservative treatment will resolve without intervention. This interval gives time for the patient to be resuscitated and for any desirable investigations. The obstruction may settle during this period, particularly if caused by adhesions following previous surgery
- **Bowel stenting.** In some cases of left-sided colonic obstruction found to be due to malignancy, the obstruction can be relieved with an endoscopically placed expanding metal stent. Surgery can then be deferred until the patient's condition has been optimised. If incurable metastatic disease has been identified, resectional surgery may be avoided
- At operation the cause of the obstruction is confirmed and dealt with appropriately (see Fig. 19.6)

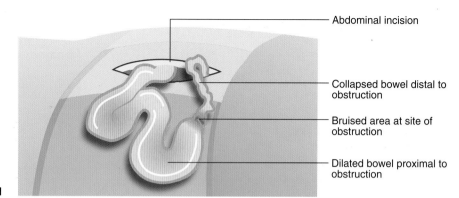

Fig. 19.6 Findings at operation for simple band obstruction of small bowel

— Abdominal incision

— Collapsed bowel distal to obstruction

— Bruised area at site of obstruction

— Dilated bowel proximal to obstruction

BOWEL STRANGULATION

PATHOPHYSIOLOGY OF BOWEL STRANGULATION

Strangulation occurs when a segment of bowel becomes trapped so that its lumen becomes obstructed and its blood supply compromised. If unrelieved, this progresses to **infarction** and eventually perforation. Strangulation can occur when there is an external hernia, when loops of bowel become trapped within the abdominal cavity or when there is mass rotation of bowel, twisting and compressing the mesentery (**volvulus**).

The process of strangulation begins with partial obstruction of the bowel due to external pressure or twisting. Venous return is initially obstructed and the combined effect is to cause oedema of the bowel wall which further aggravates the obstruction. The closed loop of bowel becomes progressively dilated by gas produced by fermentation. The combination of gas pressure and venous back pressure progressively inhibits arterial inflow, causing ischaemia and then infarction.

Strangulation most commonly occurs when small bowel is caught within a hernia (inguinal, femoral, umbilical or incisional). The bowel undergoes necrosis and soon perforates within the hernial sac. The perforation may be contained initially but generalised peritonitis usually ensues. Clinically, the patient first develops symptoms and signs of small bowel obstruction. A newly irreducible hernia can usually be found and this is likely to be tender and inflamed. However, a strangulated femoral hernia is a trap for the unwary. As indicated earlier, these are often deceptively small and non-tender and will be missed unless the groins are carefully examined.

Bowel may also become strangulated within the abdominal cavity if a loop becomes trapped by fibrous bands or adhesions (congenital or resulting from previous surgery) or passes through an omental or mesenteric defect. Similarly, strangulation occurs if a large loop of bowel becomes twisted several times on its mesentery, a condition known as volvulus. Small bowel volvulus is rare and occurs only when its mesentery has an unusually small base. Recognition is vital because the entire small bowel may be lost if treatment is delayed. The sigmoid colon (or occasionally the caecum) is particularly susceptible to volvulus if it becomes excessively distended; this is most commonly seen in elderly patients with chronic constipation and in countries where the staple diet is extremely high in fibre.

SYMPTOMS AND SIGNS OF BOWEL STRANGULATION

Intra-abdominal strangulation causes the usual symptoms and signs of bowel obstruction (see Box 19.2) but these are accompanied by **abdominal tenderness** which should be an alerting signal as it is not a feature of uncomplicated bowel obstruction. The tenderness is probably due to pressure on the already distended closed loop. When compared with those with uncomplicated obstruction, patients with strangulation are systemically more unwell, with a tachycardia and a leucocytosis. Pain increases progressively and the pulse rate rises further. Once these signs are evident, or earlier if tenderness is also present, strangulation is diagnosed and conservative treatment must be abandoned.

PRINCIPLES OF MANAGEMENT OF SUSPECTED BOWEL STRANGULATION

When strangulation is diagnosed or even suspected, operation must be performed urgently (after rapid fluid resuscitation) to try to prevent infarction and perforation (see Fig. 19.7). The patient is otherwise managed as for uncomplicated obstruction. There are no specific investigations to help diagnose bowel strangulation, which is a clinical diagnosis best confirmed at laparotomy.

PERITONITIS

PATHOPHYSIOLOGY AND CLINICAL FEATURES OF PERITONITIS

Peritonitis is defined as inflammation of the peritoneal cavity and may be localised or generalised. This includes

Symptoms

- Vomiting—time of onset and nature of the vomitus suggest the level of obstruction
- Absolute constipation (i.e. no flatus or faeces passed rectally)—pathognomonic of complete obstruction (but not present in partial obstruction)
- Abdominal pain—usually colicky in character, often mild in uncomplicated obstruction and more severe in strangulation

Physical signs

- Dehydration—caused by vomiting, lack of fluid intake and fluid sequestration in obstructed bowel
- Abdominal distension—due to gas-filled loops of bowel. The more distal the obstruction, the greater the distension
- Visible peristalsis—uncommon finding; usually encountered in a very thin patient with prolonged but incomplete distal small bowel obstruction
- Abdominal tenderness—important feature distinguishing bowel strangulation from uncomplicated obstruction
- Central resonance to percussion with dullness in the flanks—gas within dilated bowel loops rising to the uppermost point in the abdomen
- Abnormal bowel sounds—exaggerated, lapping, sloshing, perhaps high-pitched or tinkling. Bowel sounds are absent or normal in adynamic obstruction

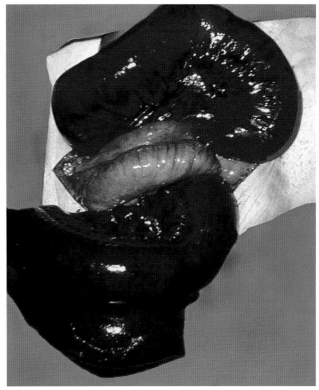

Fig. 19.7 Necrotic bowel after strangulation
This photograph, taken at operation for bowel obstruction, shows a dilated necrotic loop of small bowel which has strangulated after passing through a congenital defect in the sigmoid mesocolon. The bowel was on the point of perforation.

the serosal coverings of the bowel and mesentery, the omentum and the lining of the abdominal cavity. At the outset, peritoneal inflammation is often **localised** and the affected area contained by a wrapping of omentum, adjacent bowel and fibrinous adhesions. This may, however, be insufficient to prevent spread, and **generalised peritonitis** results. Sudden perforation of any viscus almost invariably leads to life-threatening generalised peritonitis.

Localised peritonitis occurs in the vicinity of any primary intra-abdominal inflammatory process. Acute appendicitis is a typical example. Once the parietal peritoneum becomes involved, pain becomes localised to the affected area and is exacerbated by movement of the abdominal musculature. The area is tender to palpation and the overlying abdominal wall muscles contract when examination is attempted. This sign is known as **guarding**. If the palpating hand is quickly removed, the sudden movement of the peritoneum causes intense pain which is described as **rebound tenderness**. However, this test is unkind and its diagnostic value overstated. Rebound tenderness is better elicited by gentle percussion and can often be inferred from the history. Hospital 'speed bumps' thus may perform an important diagnostic role! Rectal

examination should be performed as anterior tenderness can be a sign of pelvic peritonitis but note that the examining finger does not reach the appendix itself. Localised peritonitis is usually accompanied by mild systemic 'toxicity', i.e. low-grade fever, malaise, tachycardia and leucocytosis.

With **generalised peritonitis**, the patient becomes seriously ill, sometimes extremely rapidly after the precipitating event, e.g. perforation. There is massive exudation of inflammatory fluid into the peritoneal cavity causing hypovolaemia. This is often compounded by toxaemia from absorbed products and systemic sepsis if infection is present. The severity of the systemic illness depends on the cause of the peritonitis and is most severe when there is widespread contamination by faeces, pus or infected bile. Peritonitis is less severe when infection is absent (e.g. perforated duodenal ulcer in its early stages).

On examination in generalised peritonitis, the abdomen is rigid and tender (although this may not be evident in the very elderly or mentally obtunded) and bowel sounds are absent because of peristaltic paralysis. As mentioned, rectal examination provides a means of direct palpation of the pelvic peritoneum and will usually reveal anterior tenderness. This is a most important sign and is strong evidence of peritonitis.

Box	19.3	Causes of peritonitis

Localised peritonitis

- Transmural inflammation of bowel, e.g. appendicitis, Crohn's disease, diverticulitis
- Transmural inflammation of other viscera, e.g. cholecystitis, salpingitis

Generalised peritonitis

- Chemical peritonitis: irritation of the peritoneum by noxious materials, e.g. bile, stomach or small bowel contents (due to perforation), enzyme-containing exudates of acute pancreatitis or blood
- Bacterial peritonitis: spreading intraperitoneal infection, e.g. rupture of intra-abdominal abscess or faecal contamination due to bowel perforation, trauma, surgical spillage or anastomotic leak after recent bowel surgery

Generalised peritonitis is an indication for early laparotomy. The only exception to this is acute pancreatitis, which can be usually be excluded by serum amylase estimation. CT scans are often performed in patients with peritonitis but they rarely change management and may delay definitive treatment.

The causes of peritonitis are summarised in Box 19.3.

INTRA-ABDOMINAL HAEMORRHAGE

Blood may enter the abdominal cavity from a variety of sources including ruptured ectopic pregnancy, leaking aortic aneurysm or blunt trauma, especially to the liver and spleen. Blood in the abdominal cavity causes moderate peritoneal irritation and symptoms similar to peritonitis, but often more muted. Distinguishing between the two is usually not difficult because the history and other symptoms and signs give enough clues. In an unstable patient with obvious intraperitoneal bleeding, this is best diagnosed and managed at laparotomy. In the less urgent situation, suspected intra-abdominal bleeding may be confirmed by CT or ultrasound scan, which may give clues as to the cause and help the sometimes difficult decision of whether to manage conservatively or by operation.

PRINCIPLES OF MANAGEMENT OF PERITONITIS

Local peritonitis is treated according to the diagnosis. For example, appendicitis requires appendicectomy whilst acute diverticulitis and salpingitis are usually managed with antibiotics.

With generalised peritonitis, the patient is at risk of death from systemic sepsis. As soon as the diagnosis is made, high doses of antibiotics are given intravenously. With the exception of acute pancreatitis, generalised peritonitis requires urgent laparotomy to discover the cause,

to clear the contaminating material (**peritoneal toilet**) and to undertake definitive treatment.

INTRA-ABDOMINAL ABSCESS

PATHOPHYSIOLOGY AND CLINICAL FEATURES OF INTRA-ABDOMINAL ABSCESS

There are two common causes of intra-abdominal abscess. The first occurs after bowel perforation, when omentum and adjacent bowel attempt to wall off the defect. The second is a complication of bowel surgery where there has been localised faecal contamination during operation or an anastomotic leak later. Appendiceal perforation may cause a local abscess or one which tracks down into the pelvis. Diverticular disease often causes a **pericolic abscess** or **complex inflammatory mass**, particularly in the rectosigmoid area or pelvis. Less commonly, perforation of a colonic carcinoma results in a pericolic abscess. Gall bladder perforation is rare but occasionally results in a right-sided **subphrenic abscess**. Finally, perforation of an ulcer in the posterior wall of the stomach may produce a **lesser sac abscess**.

With intra-abdominal abscesses, abdominal pain is usually continuous rather than colicky and tends to increase relentlessly. Local bowel irritation may cause diarrhoea or adynamic bowel disorder. A swinging pyrexia is an important sign which points to the diagnosis of an abscess and there is usually a marked leucocytosis. The patient is otherwise relatively well, except with a postoperative abscess where there is a degree of systemic inflammatory response or even of multi-organ dysfunction (see Ch. 3). There may be a palpable abdominal inflammatory mass. These most commonly originate with acute appendicitis or acute diverticular disease. Rectal examination may reveal a hot, tender mass (a **pelvic abscess**), displacing the rectum backwards—a classic finding in the febrile post-appendicectomy patient. These patients usually complain of diarrhoea caused by inflammation close to the rectum.

Ultrasound or CT of the abdomen and pelvis is most useful in demonstrating the site and size of an abscess, and drainage may be possible under imaging control. When an abscess is suspected but cannot be demonstrated, radioisotope scanning using the patient's own radionuclide-labelled white cells may be helpful (see Fig. 19.8).

PRINCIPLES OF MANAGEMENT OF AN INTRA-ABDOMINAL ABSCESS

With a pelvic abscess in an otherwise well patient, there is usually no advantage in giving antibiotic treatment or attempting to drain the abscess because, given time, the abscess will usually drain spontaneously and safely into the rectum. Discharge of the abscess is recognised when the patient passes pus and blood per rectum; this is followed by resolution of the fever and healing.

Fig. 19.8 Radioisotope scan showing a large pelvic abscess

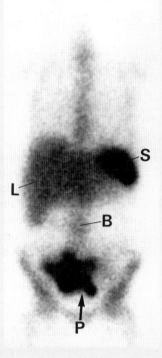

(a)

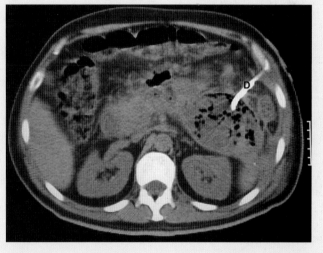

(b)

(a) Radionuclide scan of a 47-year-old woman who presented with lower abdominal tenderness and a swinging pyrexia. The patient's own leucocytes were labelled with a radionuclide. This image shows a large pelvic abscess (**P**), shown later to be due to diverticular perforation. Note also the radioisotope uptake by the spleen (**S**), liver (**L**) and bone marrow (**B**), which is a normal feature of such scans.

(b) CT-guided percutaneous placement of a drain **D** into an abscess of the pancreatic tail following an attack of acute pancreatitis. Note the pancreas remains generally swollen.

Small subphrenic abscesses may also resolve without intervention but larger ones can usually be drained percutaneously under ultrasound control. Many intra-abdominal abscesses can be successfully treated using percutaneous drainage but be aware that these methods deal only with the abscess and not the underlying cause. Laparotomy may be required to deal with an intra-abdominal abscess, particularly if the underlying cause needs treatment or if it is technically unsuitable for percutaneous drainage.

PERFORATION OF AN ABDOMINAL VISCUS

PATHOPHYSIOLOGY AND CLINICAL FEATURES OF PERFORATION

Disease in any hollow abdominal viscus may be complicated by perforation into the peritoneal cavity. The common sites of perforation are stomach and duodenum (from peptic ulcer), sigmoid colon (from diverticular disease or carcinoma) and the appendix (from acute appendicitis). The symptoms and signs of a perforated viscus depend on the nature of its contents, the volume of spillage and the effectiveness of the local defences.

A small perforation may be immediately walled off by omentum and nearby bowel but a local abscess will then develop. In this case, symptoms and signs are often grumbling and rather non-specific at first but develop into those typical of an intra-abdominal abscess (see previous section). A common example of this is appendicitis in adults. A small diverticular perforation without faecal spillage may cause localised peritonitis which may even resolve spontaneously. At the opposite extreme, a large colonic perforation due to a stercoral tear from severe constipation causes sudden overwhelming faecal peritonitis, which is often fatal despite treatment. A perforated peptic ulcer causes marked abdominal signs of peritonitis, typically 'board-like' rigidity, but little initial systemic upset. This is because the fluid spilled is usually sterile. Acute cholecystitis occasionally perforates if the inflammation is severe enough to cause necrosis.

Perforation is essentially a clinical diagnosis but can usually be confirmed by the presence of free gas in the

307

Fig. 19.9 Free perforation of abdominal viscus shown on plain chest X-rays

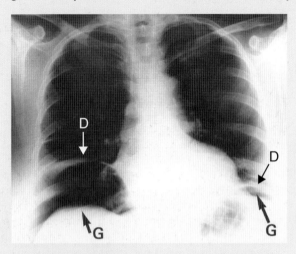

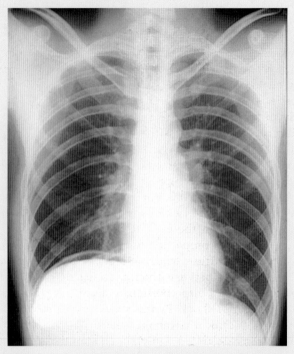

(a) Erect chest X-ray from a man of 60 with a perforated sigmoid diverticulum who presented with a sudden onset of severe abdominal pain. The film shows large radiolucent gas shadows **G, G** under each hemidiaphragm **D, D**. Fortunately in this case, no faeces entered the peritoneum and the patient did not suffer shock or peritonitis.

(b) Free gas under the diaphragm. This 22-year-old man presented with a 48-hour history of abdominal pain, initially central but latterly it had moved to the right iliac fossa (RIF). Clinically he had tenderness and rebound in the RIF. This erect chest X-ray shows free gas beneath both sides of the diaphragm indicating perforated bowel. Unusually, in this case it was due to a perforated appendicitis.

peritoneal cavity on plain radiography. This can be seen as a radiolucent line beneath one or both hemidiaphragms on an erect chest film (see Fig. 19.9) or on a lateral decubitus film of the abdomen. Note that plain radiographs do not always demonstrate free gas when there is a perforation but that CT scanning is very sensitive for detecting even small quantities of free gas. Free gas is rare in the case of perforated appendicitis, but very large amounts of gas are typically seen with perforated duodenal ulcers and colonoscopic perforations. If imaging fails to support the clinical findings, action should be based on the clinical diagnosis.

PRINCIPLES OF MANAGEMENT OF PERFORATION

Perforation is a surgical emergency. Most cases require urgent operation to repair the defect or resect the segment of diseased bowel. Duodenal ulcer perforations can be plugged with omentum or closed by suture and this may be accomplished at open surgery or laparoscopically. In large bowel perforations, a Hartmann's procedure, which leaves a temporary colostomy (see Ch. 27), is frequently required because healing of an anastomosis may be

impaired if there has been peritoneal contamination. There is, however, a trend in specialist units towards performing primary anastomosis even in these cases. Very rarely, in perforation following colonoscopy for example, conservative management is appropriate provided there are few clinical signs. This is because faecal contamination is minimal as the bowel is already clean. In the elderly or unfit, perforated duodenal ulcers may also be managed conservatively using restriction of oral fluids, nasogastric aspiration, acid suppression and antibiotics; however, the outcome is unpredictable and the approach should be reserved only for patients unsuitable for general anaesthesia or surgery.

ACUTE BOWEL ISCHAEMIA

PATHOPHYSIOLOGY AND CLINICAL FEATURES OF INTESTINAL ISCHAEMIA

Acute occlusion of the **superior mesenteric artery** may lead to acute ischaemia of the primitive midgut-derived structures, i.e. jejunum, ileum and right colon (see Fig. 19.10). This causes massive infarction of the right side of the colon and most of the small bowel and later, fatal perforation. There are two fairly distinct types of acute superior mesenteric occlusion. The first is **embolism**, which usually originates from left atrial thrombus in atrial fibrillation or from left ventricular wall thrombus after recent myocardial infarction. Secondly, **thrombosis** of the artery may occur. This is usually a terminal event in gross low output cardiac failure or is secondary to atherosclerotic stenosis; thrombosis takes place more readily if the mesenteric vessels are already diseased. The vulnerability of the superior mesenteric artery territory is poorly understood, as is the sparing of the coeliac and inferior mesenteric territories, but it probably relates to the nature of the collateral blood supply.

Acute bowel ischaemia can be a difficult diagnosis to make because of the lack of specific clinical features or diagnostic tests. In the early stages, pain is often very severe and out of proportion to the clinical signs. There may be mild diffuse tenderness but the abdomen is usually soft to palpation without guarding. As the process evolves, there is a disproportionate degree of cardiovascular collapse or shock. By this stage, arterial blood gas analysis will show a metabolic acidosis and the plasma lactate may be elevated. On plain abdominal X-ray, gas may be visible within the bowel wall. By this time, surgery

is unlikely to be successful. Diagnosis depends therefore on clinical suspicion but for most cases the outlook is grim no matter how early the diagnosis is made.

Some cases of intestinal infarction are due to **mesenteric vein thrombosis**. The cause may be a prothrombotic disorder but is often idiopathic. In these patients, the infarction is often patchy and localised resections may allow some patients to survive.

PRINCIPLES OF MANAGEMENT OF INTESTINAL ISCHAEMIA

If intestinal ischaemia is suspected, laparotomy must be performed urgently unless it is clearly going to be fruitless. Very occasionally, it is possible to restore the mesenteric arterial supply by embolectomy or vascular bypass before the bowel becomes necrotic. If the infarcted segment is not too extensive and the rest of the bowel looks healthy, resection gives a reasonable chance of recovery and an adequate amount of bowel to sustain nutrition. Even with short segments of residual small bowel, supplementary nutrition may allow prolonged survival; however, in nearly half the cases, the extent of necrosis is so great that resection is unrealistic and the patient should be allowed to die with as little interference as possible. In a few patients with arterial or venous infarction, massive resection and subsequent small bowel transplantation may be appropriate.

Examination and investigation of the acute abdomen are summarised in Boxes 19.4 and 19.5.

Fig. 19.10 Intestinal ischaemia

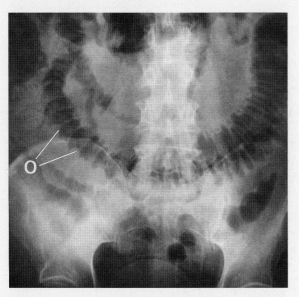

This 68-year-old woman with atrial fibrillation presented with collapse but only moderate abdominal pain. The patient had embolised her superior mesenteric artery (acute SMA occlusion) which supplies the embryological midgut-derived structures. The whole of her small bowel and the right half of her colon were necrotic but the left half of the colon was intact. This film shows the typical gross thickening of small bowel folds caused by swelling from oedema and intramural haemorrhage **O**.

Box	19.4	**Special points to note in examining a patient with an acute abdomen**

General examination

See Box 18.3 (p. 276)

Abdominal examination

- Inspection
  —distension, visible peristalsis, previous operation scars, obvious hernias, range of abdominal movement with respiration
  —always inspect the loins and back
- Palpation and percussion
  —tenderness, guarding, rigidity, rebound tenderness, pain on percussion
  —free fluid, succussion splash
  —groins for hernias and their reducibility, external genitalia
  —abdominal masses (including a full bladder)
  —abnormal pulsation (?aneurysm)
- Auscultation
  —bowel sounds, mesenteric arterial bruits

Box 19.5   Investigation of the acute abdomen

Blood tests

Haematology

- Haemoglobin
  - —may be normal immediately after an acute bleed
  - —low haemoglobin concentration may represent chronic anaemia due to occult blood loss rather than acute haemorrhage
- White blood count—leucocytosis is non-specific and rarely of much diagnostic value unless greater than about 14×10^3/L
- Blood group and ordering of blood for transfusion—for severely anaemic patients, in major haemorrhage or when major surgery is contemplated

Biochemistry

- C-reactive protein
  - —non-specific indicator of inflammatory activation
  - —confirms organic illness if substantially elevated
- Plasma amylase—whenever pancreatitis cannot be excluded
- Urea and electrolytes—indicated in vomiting and diarrhoea, dehydration, poor urine output, diuretic therapy, urinary tract disease, known or suspected renal failure, pancreatitis and sepsis
- Glucose—for diabetics or those with glycosuria (beware of hyperglycaemia due to acute stress or steroid therapy)
- Liver function tests and calcium estimation—for pancreatitis and acute biliary disease
- Clotting studies—for acute pancreatitis and septicaemia (disseminated intravascular coagulation), severe bleeding (consumption coagulopathy) or those with a history of bleeding disorders

Urine tests

- Ward ('stick') testing—for blood, protein, bile, glucose, nitrites and white cells
- Microscopy—for red and white blood cells, organisms
- Culture and sensitivity—in suspected urinary tract infections
- Strain urine for stones—in ureteric colic
- Pregnancy test in females if appropriate

Imaging (see Box 19.1)

Plain radiography

- Erect chest X-ray
  - —cardiovascular disease or abnormality, e.g. cardiomegaly, thoracic aneurysm, aortic dissection, cardiac failure

- —respiratory disease
  - —suspected visceral perforation (gas under diaphragm)
- Supine abdominal X-ray (erect or decubitus if necessary)
  - —bowel (gas pattern and dilatation, fluid levels, gas in the wall, faeces and faecoliths)
  - —urinary tract ('KUB' = kidneys, ureters and bladder) shows kidney size and position, calculi
  - —biliary tract (gallstones, gas in biliary tree in gallstone ileus)
  - —aortic calcification (aneurysm)
  - —psoas shadows (obscured by retroperitoneal inflammation or haemorrhage)

Ultrasound

- Gallstones
- Pelvic abnormalities in obstetric and gynaecological practice
- 'Chronic' enlargement of the spleen
- Abdominal aortic aneurysm (AAA)
- Free abdominal fluid and gas indicating perforated bowel
- Other stones
- Dilated ducts; air in biliary tree
- Hydatid, teratomas and other cysts
- Intra-abdominal abscesses and masses

Contrast radiology

- 'Instant' barium enema in colonic obstruction or acute colitis
- Emergency intravenous urography in ureteric colic

CT scanning

CT can give rapid, cost-effective evaluation of acute abdominal pain but should not supplant clinical examination nor unreasonably delay surgical exploration in the deteriorating patient. Diagnostic value of CT is better if timing, contrast (i.v. and/or oral) and other variables are tailored to the working diagnosis.

- Assessment of abdominal trauma—severity and grading of solid organ injury, free intra-abdominal fluid and gas; retroperitoneal injuries including pancreatic and duodenal rupture and vascular injury
- Often first choice for ureteric colic, suspected aortic aneurysm or aortic dissection
- Useful where diagnosis remains in doubt, e.g. suspected bowel perforation (detects small amount of free gas), acute diverticulitis
- Investigation of postoperative complications—abscesses, fluid collections
- Severe acute pancreatitis, especially if necrosis suspected

MAJOR GASTROINTESTINAL HAEMORRHAGE

PATHOPHYSIOLOGY AND CLINICAL FEATURES OF GASTROINTESTINAL HAEMORRHAGE

Major gastrointestinal haemorrhage presents either as vomiting of blood or passage of frank or altered blood rectally. Vomited blood (**haematemesis**) may be fresh or partly digested. In the latter case, it is dark and may have the typical appearance of 'coffee grounds'. Haematemesis usually indicates bleeding from the oesophagus, stomach or duodenum.

Blood loss beyond the duodenum is usually passed rectally. The extent to which it is altered by digestion and the degree of mixing with the stool are useful indicators of its level of origin. Upper gastrointestinal bleeding is often manifest by **melaena**. This is the passage of loose, reddish-black, tarry stools with a characteristic foul smell. With upper gastrointestinal bleeding proximal to the duodeno-jejunal (DJ) flexure at the ligament of Treitz, haematemesis or melaena or both can occur. Haematemesis is more likely if the bleeding is rapid. The main causes of major gastrointestinal haemorrhage are summarised in Figure 19.11.

COMMON CAUSES OF GASTROINTESTINAL BLEEDING

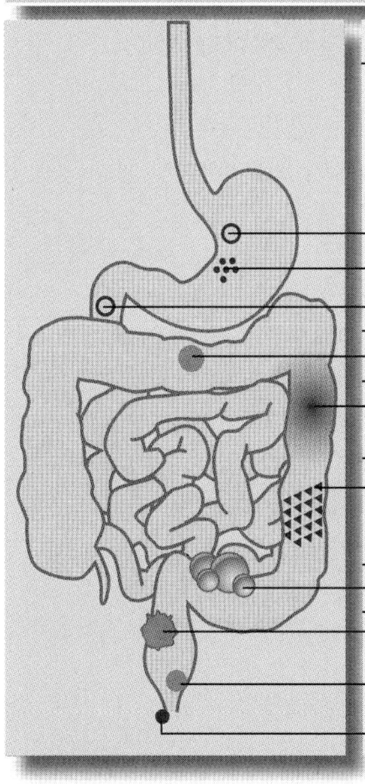

Pathology	Clinical features	Frequency
Acute and chronic gastric ulcers Gastric erosions Chronic duodenal ulcer	Haematemesis and/or melaena	Very common
Polyps or carcinoma of colon	Altered blood per rectum	Common
Ischaemic colitis	Abdominal pain then fairly fresh rectal bleeding	Fairly common
Angiodysplasias of colon	Pattern of bleeding depends on location within colon; increasingly recognised with the rise in colonoscopy	Fairly common
Diverticular disease	Fresh rectal bleeding	Common
Carcinoma of rectum	Fresh rectal bleeding but rarely in large quantities	Common
Rectal polyps		
Haemorrhoids		

UNCOMMON CAUSES OF GASTROINTESTINAL BLEEDING

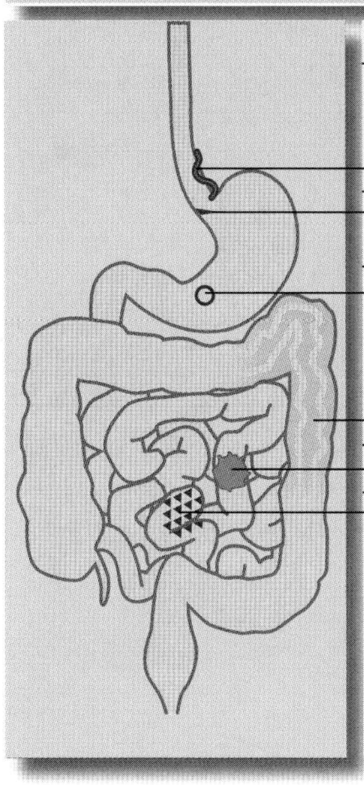

Pathology	Clinical features	Frequency
Oesophageal varices	Haematemesis and/or melaena	Uncommon
Mallory–Weiss oesophageal tears	Haematemesis or altered blood per rectum	Uncommon
Stress ulcers	Haematemesis and/or melaena	Uncommon
Acute or fulminant ulcerative colitis	Bloody diarrhoea	Uncommon
Malignant small bowel tumours	Altered blood per rectum	Rare
Angiodysplasias of small bowel	Altered blood per rectum	Rare

Fig. 19.11 Causes of gastrointestinal haemorrhage

MANAGEMENT OF UPPER GASTROINTESTINAL HAEMORRHAGE

Initial management and resuscitation

Any patient presenting with severe upper gastrointestinal haemorrhage is at risk of dying from hypovolaemic shock. This may occur with the initial event or as a result of rebleeding. There is a very real danger of rebleeding in the high-risk patients (see Fig. 19.12) during a hospital stay (about 50%) and a combined management policy has been shown to reduce mortality for all cases of upper gastrointestinal haemorrhage from 10% to about 2%. Hospitals should have clearly written and agreed protocols for combined medical and surgical management of upper gastrointestinal haemorrhage so that patients do not 'slip through the net' and perish by default (Fig. 19.12).

Clinical history, examination and investigation

More than two-thirds of patients presenting in Western countries with upper gastrointestinal haemorrhage nowadays are over 60 years of age and one-third of these have a history of taking aspirin or other non-steroidal anti-inflammatory drugs. Other specific details of the history may be relevant. These include alcohol consumption, previous peptic ulceration or gastric surgery, or a history of cirrhosis and variceal haemorrhage. In earlier times, the mean age of presentation was much younger, probably because of poorer living conditions, higher alcohol and tobacco intake and perhaps greater *Helicobacter pylori* infection rates.

Abdominal examination is usually unremarkable but general examination may show signs of chronic liver disease suggesting possible gastro-oesophageal varices. Rectal examination may reveal melaena stool or altered blood and this can be helpful if the history of haematemesis has not been substantiated, e.g. 'coffee-ground' vomiting not seen by a doctor.

The volume of blood said to have been vomited or passed per rectum is unreliable as a measure of blood loss because a great deal may remain in the bowel. It is therefore essential to obtain good venous access as a first step and then to perform a full blood count, urea and electrolytes and prothrombin ratio and liver function tests, to send blood for grouping and antibody screen (or crossmatching), and to order blood for transfusion in high-risk cases (see Fig. 19.12 and below). ECG and chest X-rays are useful in patients over 65 years or with cardiorespiratory disease. The patient should be made ready to go to the operating theatre at a moment's notice, rather than having

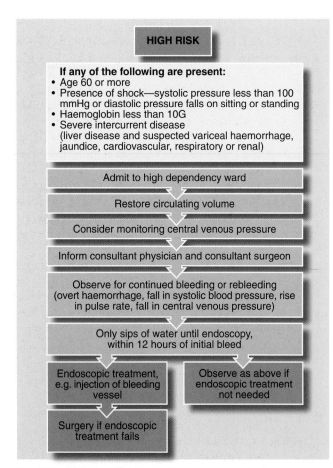

HIGH RISK

If any of the following are present:
- Age 60 or more
- Presence of shock—systolic pressure less than 100 mmHg or diastolic pressure falls on sitting or standing
- Haemoglobin less than 10G
- Severe intercurrent disease (liver disease and suspected variceal haemorrhage, jaundice, cardiovascular, respiratory or renal)

Admit to high dependency ward

Restore circulating volume

Consider monitoring central venous pressure

Inform consultant physician and consultant surgeon

Observe for continued bleeding or rebleeding (overt haemorrhage, fall in systolic blood pressure, rise in pulse rate, fall in central venous pressure)

Only sips of water until endoscopy, within 12 hours of initial bleed

Endoscopic treatment, e.g. injection of bleeding vessel | Observe as above if endoscopic treatment not needed

Surgery if endoscopic treatment fails

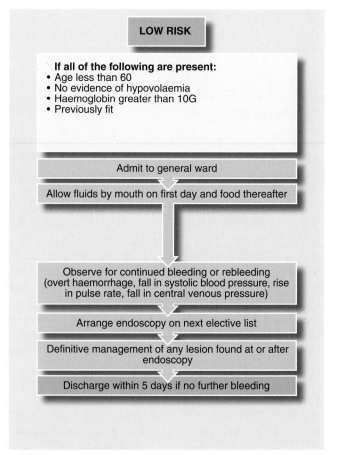

LOW RISK

If all of the following are present:
- Age less than 60
- No evidence of hypovolaemia
- Haemoglobin greater than 10G
- Previously fit

Admit to general ward

Allow fluids by mouth on first day and food thereafter

Observe for continued bleeding or rebleeding (overt haemorrhage, fall in systolic blood pressure, rise in pulse rate, fall in central venous pressure)

Arrange endoscopy on next elective list

Definitive management of any lesion found at or after endoscopy

Discharge within 5 days if no further bleeding

Fig. 19.12 Risk stratification in the management of acute upper gastrointestinal haemorrhage

to chase laboratories for results or blood for transfusion when the patient suddenly deteriorates!

Stratification of risk

Patients with acute upper gastrointestinal haemorrhage should be stratified clinically into a **low-risk group** (non-life-threatening) and a **high-risk group** (where continued bleeding or likely rebleeding is potentially life-threatening). This stratification is based on age, the presence of shock, the haemoglobin concentration and the presence of complicating disease (see Fig. 19.12). Stratification determines the priorities of management and enables concentration of resources on those who really need it. Further risk factors may be found at endoscopy (see next section).

It is vital that patients with signs of shock are monitored and resuscitated thoroughly; the rate and volume of intravenous fluid replacement (whether plasma expanders or blood) is adjusted against the responses of pulse rate, blood pressure, central venous pressure and hourly urine output.

Endoscopic management of acute upper gastrointestinal haemorrhage

Patients clinically at high risk should be assessed early by a surgical team, even if admitted under the care of a gastroenterologist or (internal) physician. Ideally, the same surgical team should remain responsible for that patient until recovery. This continuity of surgical care ensures that a decision to operate can be made without procrastination if conservative management fails.

All patients with upper gastrointestinal haemorrhage require endoscopy to determine the site and activity of bleeding, to diagnose oesophageal varices and to determine suitability for endoscopic treatment. Endoscopy also assists the surgeon in locating the source if surgery becomes necessary. Urgent endoscopy, within 12 hours of the first bleed, should be performed in clinically high-risk patients; all others should be endoscoped on the next available list, but ideally within 24 hours. Even in the most acute upper gastrointestinal haemorrhage, gastroscopy can usually be performed on the operating table before operation. Duodenal or gastric ulceration should be easily identifiable (although these should be found at operation without this assistance), but the real value of endoscopy is the ability to diagnose unusual sources of bleeding, most of which present particular operative problems. Thus, oesophageal ulceration or a Mallory–Weiss tear (see Ch. 22) may be discovered, and the surgeon can avoid operating on unsuspected variceal haemorrhage. Even in patients with known varices, endoscopy is essential, as in 50% of cases blood loss will be from a completely different lesion, e.g. peptic ulcer, gastric erosions.

Unexpected endoscopic features may also place apparently low-risk patients into a high-risk category. These are:

- **Active spurting from an artery in an ulcer bed**. Endotherapy by gastroscopic injection of adrenaline (epinephrine) or an adrenaline (epinephrine)/ sclerosant mixture should be attempted; there is a 25–40% rebleed rate even in expert hands and the patient must be closely monitored as these patients often need surgery
- **A visible elevated vessel or protruding adherent clot (Dieulafoy lesion)**. These lesions double the above risk of rebleeding to 50–80%. If the patient is hypotensive as a result of blood loss, the risk of rebleeding is 80%
- **Bleeding gastro-oesophageal varices**. Mortality is 30%. Immediate treatment is required with endoluminal rubber band ligation or injection sclerotherapy. Tamponade with special balloon catheters may also be necessary prior to endotherapy

Low-risk patients usually stop bleeding with conservative management after the initial haemorrhage that precipitated admission to hospital and are unlikely to rebleed. They may be given sips of water and acid suppression therapy (although there is little scientific evidence to support this practice), monitored by observation for rebleeding, pulse rate and blood pressure, and endoscoped on the next available list.

Surgical management

A policy of early surgery for patients over 60 has been shown to reduce mortality. Urgent surgery is also required for patients defined clinically or endoscopically as being at high risk and who suffer one rebleed, or for any patient who suffers two rebleeds. Immediate surgery is required for patients with exsanguinating haemorrhage or those unable to be stabilised during initial resuscitation. Occasionally blood loss is so rapid that an unguided laparotomy must be performed immediately to staunch the flow.

The choice of surgical procedure depends on the source of haemorrhage but there is a trend towards less radical procedures now that postoperative medical management of peptic ulcer disease has improved. Bleeding is arrested with under-running sutures after gastrotomy or duodenotomy and attempts are made to preserve the pyloric ring. Gastric and duodenal ulcers should be biopsied for *Helicobacter* testing and in case of malignancy in gastric ulcers. Gastrectomy or vagotomy and pyloroplasty are rarely necessary (see Ch. 21). Anti-*Helicobacter* therapy is given later if peroperative or postoperative testing is *H. pylori* positive.

MORE DISTAL GASTROINTESTINAL HAEMORRHAGE

More distal gastrointestinal bleeding is not usually investigated immediately to find the site but is managed conservatively, anticipating spontaneous cessation. Around

Fig. 19.13 Angiogram showing angiodysplasia of caecum

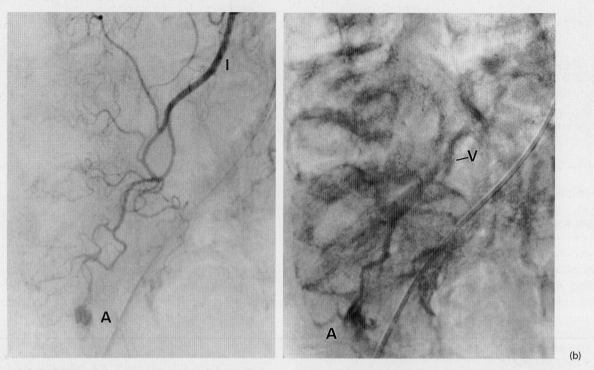

(a)

(b)

This man of 70 had been admitted to hospital on 12 occasions for rectal bleeding and chronic anaemia and had received 55 units of blood transfusion in all. On the last admission, this superior mesenteric arteriogram was performed, revealing the source of blood loss. **(a)** Subtraction film showing the arterial phase; the ileocolic artery **I** feeds a knot of abnormal blood vessels, an angiodysplasia **A**, at the lower pole of the caecum was responsible for the bleeding. **(b)** Subtraction film of the venous phase; the angiodysplasia **A** is still visible and there is early filling of a large draining vein **V**. These appearances are typical of angiodysplasia; the caecum is the most common site of occurrence. The lesion was resected by right hemicolectomy.

80% settle without transfusion, and the majority of the remaining 20% settle with transfusion alone. If bleeding continues, it is an important principle that the source of bleeding should be localised by investigation so that appropriate treatment can be accurately targeted. 'Blind' laparotomy is often unsatisfactory because the cause may need non-surgical treatment or the source of bleeding may be difficult or impossible to find.

Blood loss from diverticular disease and ischaemic colitis is usually self-limiting. Several small bleeds may occur over a few days but the volume lost is usually small and hypovolaemia is rare. Typically the presentation is late and the bleeding has often stopped, with blood per rectum the only evidence.

Investigation involves colonoscopy once the bleeding has stopped; the procedure can be dangerous whilst luminal blood limits vision. Sigmoidoscopy and barium enema are alternatives, but bleeding usually arises from the mucosa and this is not well demonstrated radiologically. Occasionally an unsuspected carcinoma or polyp is discovered.

In ulcerative colitis, the diagnosis is evident from the other symptoms and signs, and management depends on the success of medical treatment (see Ch. 28). Persisting large bowel haemorrhage which is less rapid but recurrent is usually due to **angiodysplasias** (see Ch. 29). Colonoscopy can be both diagnostic and therapeutic for bleeding angiodysplasia. If colonoscopy is negative, impossible or unsatisfactory, radioisotope scanning using the patient's own labelled red cells or highly selective arteriography may be used to localise the source of bleeding at least to a general area of bowel (see Fig. 19.13). At laparotomy the whole bowel can be examined and any suspect area resected if appropriate. However, purely mucosal lesions are undetectable at operation so, as a last resort, a colonoscope inserted through an incision in the bowel wall can be used to examine the whole colon and small bowel for bleeding sites. This may be the only operative means of diagnosing small bowel angiodysplasia. Occasionally, therapeutic embolisation of localised bleeding lesions using selective angiography is employed.

Gallstone diseases and related disorders

20

INTRODUCTION

Gallstones and related disorders account for all but a small proportion of biliary tract disease in most countries. Liver flukes are an important cause of bile duct inflammation and obstruction in the Far East and South East Asia; the fluke *Fasciola hepatica* can also infect people in Western Europe, usually via infested watercress. The most important of the remaining diseases, cholangiocarcinoma and sclerosing cholangitis, are discussed in Chapter 24. Gallstone disease is also known as **cholelithiasis**. When stones are present in the bile ducts, this is known as **choledocholithiasis**.

Most gallstone-related disease presents with pain, typically located in the epigastrium or right hypochondrium (right upper quadrant or RUQ). The character of the pain varies with the diagnosis; in most cases, it is acute and intermittent rather than chronic. The severity ranges from very severe and requiring hospital admission to moderately severe and able to be managed at home. For the less severe group, gallstone disease tends to be investigated in the outpatient clinic. Less commonly, gallstone disease presents as pain and **jaundice** caused by a stone passing into and obstructing the common bile duct.

Non-acute upper abdominal pain is a common cause of surgical referral, accounting for up to 7% of outpatient referrals in a typical district general hospital. Of these, about half will be diagnosed as having gallstone disease. Furthermore, about 25% of elective abdominal operations on adults in district general hospitals are performed for gall bladder disease. There is thus considerable scope for the future development of effective preventative measures and better non-surgical methods of managing gallstone disease.

STRUCTURE AND FUNCTION OF THE BILIARY SYSTEM

Bile collects in the canaliculi between hepatocytes and drains via collecting ducts within the portal triads into a system of ducts within the liver. These progressively increase in diameter until they become the **right** and **left hepatic ducts** which fuse to form the **common hepatic duct** 3–4 cm outside the liver. This is joined further distally by the **cystic duct** to become the **common bile duct** (see Fig. 20.1). The common bile duct is 4–5 cm long and passes down behind the duodenum then through the head of the pancreas to drain via the **ampulla of Vater** into the medial wall of the second part of the duodenum. The **sphincter of Oddi** within the ampulla prevents reflux of duodenal contents. In most cases, the **main pancreatic duct** joins the common bile duct at the ampulla although it may enter the duodenum independently.

The **gall bladder** is a muscular sac lined by a mucosa characterised by a single, highly folded layer of tall columnar epithelial cells. The lining epithelium is supported by loose connective tissue which contains numerous blood vessels and lymphatics. Mucus-secreting glands are found at the neck of the gall bladder but are absent from the body and fundus. The proximal part of the duct is disposed into a spiral arrangement called the **spiral valve**, the function of which is not well understood. The gall

315

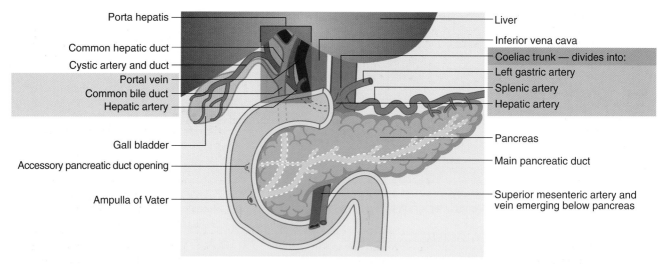

Fig. 20.1 Surgical anatomy of the gall bladder, biliary tract and pancreas
The coeliac trunk (the foregut artery) arises from the aorta and divides into the hepatic, splenic and left gastric arteries. The hepatic artery divides into right and left branches, mirrored by the extrahepatic right and left hepatic ducts. These join caudally to form the common hepatic duct; this in turn is joined by the cystic duct to form the common bile duct (CBD). The **porta hepatis** consists of the hepatic arteries, the extrahepatic bile ducts and the portal vein

bladder lies in a variable depression in the undersurface of the right hepatic lobe and is covered by the peritoneal envelope of the liver. The common bile duct is a fibrous tissue tube lined by a simple, tall columnar epithelium. It is normally up to 0.6 cm in diameter and this can be measured on ultrasound scanning.

Bile is made continuously by the liver and passes along the biliary tract to the gall bladder where it is stored. Bile is concentrated by as much as 10 times in the gall bladder by a process of active mucosal reabsorption of water. Lipid-rich food passing from stomach to duodenum promotes secretion of the hormone **cholecystoki-nin-pancreozymin** (CCK) by endocrine cells of the duodenal mucosa. This hormone stimulates contraction of the gall bladder, squeezing bile into the duodenum. Bile salts (acids) act as emulsifying agents and facilitate hydrolysis of dietary lipids by pancreatic lipases. If bile fails to reach the duodenum because of biliary tract obstruction, lipids are neither digested nor absorbed, resulting in the passage of loose pale foul-smelling fatty stools (**steatorrhoea**). Furthermore, the fat-soluble vitamins (A, D, E and K) are not absorbed. The lack of vitamin K soon leads to inadequate prothrombin synthesis and hence defective clotting. This may pose problems of haemostasis if surgery is necessary in a patient with obstructive jaundice.

PATHOPHYSIOLOGY OF THE BILIARY SYSTEM

GALLSTONE COMPOSITION

In developed countries, most gallstones are **mixed** and contain a predominance of cholesterol; this is mixed with some **bile pigment** (calcium bilirubinate) and other **calcium salts**. A small proportion are virtually 'pure' cholesterol stones ('**cholesterol solitaire**'). In Asia, most gallstones are composed of bile pigment alone. The composition and pathogenesis of the various types of gallstone are summarised in Table 20.1, and some examples are illustrated in Figure 20.3.

The physical structure of mixed gallstones gives an insight into the historical sequence of their formation. There is usually a small core of organic material, which often contains bacteria. The main part of the stone is made up of concentric layers, demonstrating that stones do not form in a single episode but by a series of discrete precipitation events. Furthermore, in the same gall bladder, there are often several 'families' of gallstones, each of a different size. This suggests that each generation began at a different time, presumably due to a transient change in local conditions. All families then build up at the same rate by lamination, leading to the range of different sizes. Radioisotope dating studies have shown that the average gallstone is 11 years old when removed!

The full story of how the common variety of cholesterol-predominant (mixed) stones is formed has not yet been elucidated but several clues are available. The main factors are: (a) changes in concentration of the different constituents of bile, (b) biliary stasis and (c) infection. It is likely that several subtle abnormalities combine synergistically to bring about precipitation of bile constituents.

Bile salts and lecithin are responsible for maintaining cholesterol in a stable **micelle** formation. The normal

Table 20.1 Composition and pathogenesis of gallstones

Chemical composition	Pathogenesis	Characteristics
Mixed stones (75–90% of all stones) Cholesterol is the predominant constituent Heterogeneous mixture of cholesterol, bile pigments and calcium salts in a laminated structure around a 'core' (Fig. 20.2)	Combination of: • Abnormalities of bile constituents • Bile stasis • Infection	Multiple stones with several generations of different sizes often found together Stones may be hard and faceted (where they have developed in contact) or irregular, 'mulberry'-shaped, and softer Colours range from near-white through yellow and green to black Most are radiolucent but 10% are radiopaque
Cholesterol stones (up to 10% of all stones)	As for mixed stones	Large, smooth, egg- or barrel-shaped and usually solitary ('cholesterol solitaire') Yellowish. Up to 4 cm diameter and may fill the gall bladder. Radiolucent
Pigment stones Calcium bilirubinate (uncommon in developed countries, common in Asia)	Excess bilirubin excretion due to haemolytic disorders, e.g. haemolytic anaemias, infections, malaria, leukaemias	Multiple, jet-black, shiny 'jack' stones; 0.5–1 cm diameter. Usually of uniform size and often friable
Calcium carbonate stones (rare)	Excess calcium excretion in bile	Greyish faceted stones Radiopaque

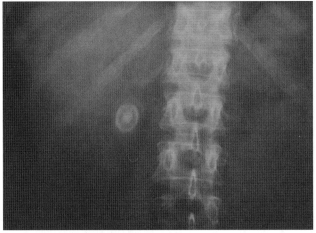

Fig. 20.2 X-ray of radiopaque gallstone
Plain abdominal X-ray showing large radiopaque gallstone in the right upper quadrant. Note that the stone is obviously laminated, having built up in layers over many years. Note also that only 10% of mixed stones are radiopaque.

micellar structure of bile supports a greater concentration of cholesterol than could otherwise be held in solution and it is therefore inherently unstable. An excess of cholesterol in proportion to bile salts and lecithin is probably one of the main factors in cholesterol stone formation. This is supported by the fact that patients in whom the terminal ileum has been resected or who have chronic distal ileal disease have a threefold risk of developing cholesterol-rich stones. The mechanism is likely to be as follows: the terminal ileum is the main site for reabsorption of bile salts and when it is diseased or has been removed, reabsorption declines, leading to bile salt loss via the bowel and, eventually, a decline in the bile salt pool. The remaining bile salts are then insufficient to maintain the micellar structure of cholesterol in suspension leading to precipitation.

Precipitation from bile is enhanced by **biliary stasis**. This occurs if the gall bladder becomes obstructed or its contractility becomes defective. It is not known whether obstruction of the gall bladder outlet is a primary event in the formation of stones but it is believed to play a part in their continued accretion. Obstruction could be caused by dysfunction of the spiral valve in the cystic duct, by reflux of duodenal contents (which may be infected) or by small stones already formed. The muscular gall bladder wall is damaged by long-standing inflammation or infection which interferes with its ability to empty. Pregnancy is also a predisposing factor.

THE ROLE OF INFLAMMATION AND INFECTION

The relative roles of inflammation and infection in gallstone formation are still in doubt, but probably both play a part. Abnormalities of bile composition may cause **chemical inflammation** of the gall bladder, resulting in inflammatory exudation and perhaps accumulation of inflammatory debris. **Bacteria** usually form the organic nidus upon which gallstones are built; they enter the gall bladder intermittently by reflux from the duodenum or via the bloodstream. This process is probably normal in itself but becomes pathological if the bacteria are not flushed out, as occurs when the gall bladder does not adequately empty. Once stones are formed, episodic bacterial ingress could be responsible for periods of precipitation in which layers of the laminated structure are built up. Indeed, some gallstones continue to harbour bacteria

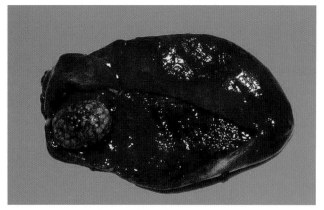

(a) Thick-walled chronically inflamed gall bladder found to be obstructed at its neck by a single stone. Note the stone is an aggregate of many smaller stones.

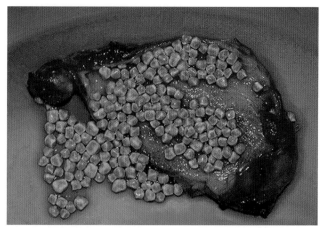

(b) Multiple small gallstones in the gall bladder, all of much the same 'generation'.

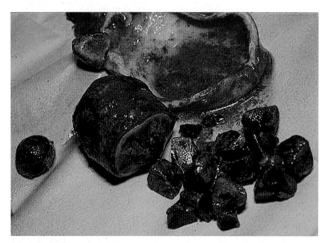

(c) Gallbladder containing one huge stone and multiple smaller stones. These stones all fitted together with adjoining facets.

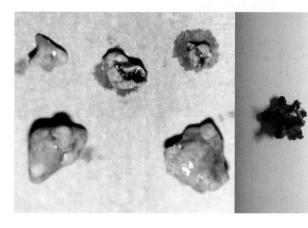

(d) Different types of gallstones—pale irregular stones of different ages on the left and a pigment 'jack' stone on the right.

Fig. 20.3 Types of gallstone

and so the process becomes self-perpetuating. In support of this is the fact that faecal organisms can be cultured from at least 25% of cholecystectomy specimens.

THE ROLE OF CHRONIC OBSTRUCTION

Transient obstruction of the gall bladder by stone may cause episodes of acute pain (**biliary colic**). If the obstruction persists, the gall bladder becomes chemically inflamed causing **acute cholecystitis**. If obstruction does not resolve by itself and the contents do not become infected, the gall bladder becomes distended with mucus; this is known as a **mucocoele**, and is often palpable and tender. If the contents become infected, an abscess develops within the gall bladder and this is known as an **empyema of the gall bladder**.

The majority of gall bladders removed for chronic pain show a range of histological features more in keeping with a **chronic obstructive aetiology** than an infective one. These features include intact but often atrophic mucosa,

submucosal and subserosal fibrosis, hypertrophy of the muscular wall, and mucosal diverticula extending into the muscular layer (known as **Rokitansky–Aschoff sinuses**). Evidence of active or previous infection is uncommon. Inflammatory infiltrates are mainly associated with traumatic gallstone erosion of the mucosa or intrusion of inspissated bile into the gall bladder wall, particularly around the mucosal diverticula. In some cases the gall bladder is so grossly scarred, distorted or contracted that its absorptive and contractile functions have been completely destroyed.

OTHER PATHOLOGICAL MECHANISMS

In about 10% of patients with typical symptoms of gall bladder disease, no stone can be demonstrated during investigation or at operation. In some of these cases, a stone may have passed out of the duct system into the bowel. In other cases, chronic inflammation occurs independently of stones, the so-called '**cholecystitis sans** stones'; again, chronic obstruction may be the aetiology. Finally, the terms '**biliary dyskinesia**' and '**cystic duct syndrome**' may sometimes explain the condition where patients have typical symptoms of gall bladder disease but standard investigations are essentially normal. When biliary manometry is used, some of these patients are shown to have an abnormally high pressure in the sphincter of Oddi. Confirming this diagnosis is difficult but a fair proportion of patients suspected of this are cured by endoscopic sphincterotomy or surgical sphincteroplasty.

EPIDEMIOLOGY OF GALLSTONES

In developed countries, at least 10% of the adult population probably develop gallstones during their lifetime, although most remain asymptomatic. Gallstones are rare before adulthood and increase in prevalence with age. Women are affected four times as often as men and it appears that pregnancy is a very important predisposing factor; obesity and diabetes may also play a part. The typical patient is said to be a 'fair fat fertile female of forty', but many gallstone patients do not fit this description. Gallstone disease is rare in the rural communities of developing countries but is increasing with urbanisation. Western-style processed foods, high in fats and refined carbohydrates but poor in fibre, may be responsible. Their contribution to gall bladder disease would be compatible with the theory that changes in the composition of bile are an important factor in stone pathogenesis.

INVESTIGATION OF GALL BLADDER PATHOLOGY

When gallstone disease is suspected, investigation has the following objectives:

- Exclude haematological and liver abnormalities and other metabolic disorders
- Establish whether gallstones are present in the gall bladder and/or common duct and whether the gall bladder wall is abnormally thickened
- Assess the integrity and patency of the bile duct system and the pancreatic duct (if there is any suggestion of obstruction)

BLOOD TESTS FOR HAEMATOLOGICAL AND LIVER ABNORMALITIES

In many straightforward cases, no blood tests are necessary except to exclude anaemia in susceptible groups such as women of childbearing age. **Haemolytic disorders** such as hereditary spherocytosis, thalassaemia and sickle-cell trait should be considered as they may predispose to pigment stones. Liver function tests are indicated if there is any suggestion of jaundice or other liver abnormality. Finally, blood cultures to exclude systemic infection may be appropriate in seriously ill patients.

IMAGING IN THE INVESTIGATION OF GALL BLADDER PATHOLOGY

Investigation for gall bladder disease aims to demonstrate the presence of stones and signs of chronic gall bladder inflammation. Ultrasonography is the mainstay of investigation but other investigations are occasionally employed.

Ultrasonography

Ultrasonography (see Fig. 20.4) is reliable for identifying stones in the gall bladder and any increase in thickness of the gall bladder wall (caused by inflammation or fibrosis). Ultrasound provides a simple and accurate means of demonstrating **dilatation of the common duct** system, which often indicates distal duct obstruction. Unfortunately, it is unreliable for identifying bile duct stones directly, particularly at the lower end, because the image tends to be obscured by overlying duodenal gas. Ultrasound has the great advantage of being suitable for use in the seriously ill or jaundiced patient.

INVESTIGATION OF THE BILIARY DUCT SYSTEM

See Figure 20.5.

The non-jaundiced patient

Patients with gallstones but no history of obstructive jaundice do not require preoperative investigation for duct stones. If cholecystectomy is performed, **intra-operative** (also known as per-operative) **cholangiography** may be carried out. A cannula is passed through the cystic duct into the common bile duct and radiopaque contrast material injected to fill the biliary tree; contrast should flow into the duodenum. X-rays or fluoroscopic imaging are then used to demonstrate the duct morphology and any abnormalities such as duct dilatation, filling defects caused by stone or distortion of the tapering lower end of the common duct, as well as obstruction of flow into the duodenum. If cholangiography shows a stone or stones, the duct may be explored at the time or else dealt with later by endoscopic retrograde cholangio-pancreatography (ERCP).

A different problem is the patient with a history of **transient jaundice** possibly attributable to stones. Most cases will have either operative cholangiography at cholecystectomy or preoperative ERCP.

The jaundiced patient

When obstructive jaundice has been diagnosed, it is important to distinguish between stone and tumour in order to plan appropriate management.

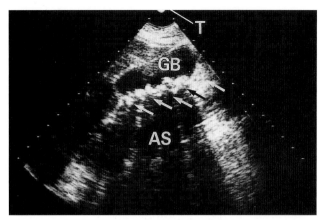

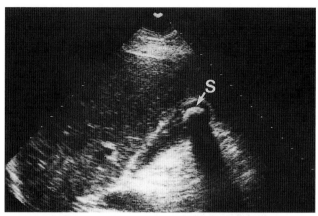

(a) Longitudinal scan of gall bladder in a 46-year-old woman who complained of intermittent attacks of right upper quadrant pain. The scan shows the outline of the gall bladder **GB** and a layer of gallstones (arrowed) along its posterior wall. The stones each cast a clear acoustic shadow **AS** beyond them. Note that these shadows can be projected back to the transducer **T**.

(b) Longitudinal scan of the gall bladder in a 37-year-old woman showing a single large stone **S** in the fundus. Note that only the anterior surface of the stone is seen (as an arc) because all sound waves are reflected from it, casting a dense acoustic shadow beyond. Note that ultrasound is a poor method of demonstrating stones at the lower end of the common bile duct.

Fig. 20.4 Biliary ultrasound scans

Ultrasonography is usually the initial investigation. This shows the extent of dilatation of both intrahepatic and extrahepatic ducts and may even show a stone lodged at the lower end of the duct. If stones are demonstrated in the gall bladder, this adds weight to the impression that stones are blocking the duct rather than tumour, but the two can coexist. The ultrasound scan will usually demonstrate the presence of a carcinoma of the pancreatic head or enlarged lymph nodes in the porta hepatis; either may cause extrahepatic biliary obstruction.

Ultrasound may make the diagnosis, but if more detailed information is required, biliary tract morphology can be outlined using magnetic resonance cholangio-pancreatography (MRCP). This produces images of the biliary tree and pancreatic ducts. Adjustment of the settings at the time of the scan can produce different images of the anatomy, for example to show the pancreatic head. If MRCP does not yield the necessary information, the ducts can be visualised by direct injection of contrast. There are two methods: ERCP and, more rarely, percutaneous transhepatic cholangiography. ERCP is the more useful investigation; it also allows the ampullary region

to be inspected for tumour. Furthermore, the pancreatic duct may be outlined if required. If stones are found in the common bile duct, it is often possible to perform immediate **endoscopic sphincterotomy**, releasing the stones, thus diagnosing and relieving the jaundice in one procedure. This may be life-saving for the patient with ascending cholangitis and is the treatment of choice on its own for the patient who is a poor risk for laparotomy or laparoscopy.

Percutaneous transhepatic cholangiography is used in exceptional circumstances, for example if ERCP is unsuccessful because of previous gastric surgery. It involves inserting a long, fine (22 gauge) needle through the skin into one of the dilated intrahepatic ducts under radiological control. Contrast medium is then injected. An obstructing stone produces a characteristic rounded filling defect as opposed to the tapering stricture typical of tumour.

Ultrasound scanning via the endoscope is a useful technique to show greater detail at the lower end of the common bile duct or to examine lesions in the ampulla or head of the pancreas with greater clarity.

CLINICAL PRESENTATIONS OF GALLSTONE DISEASE

The names attached to the various clinical syndromes associated with gallstones are somewhat confusing and at best imprecise. This is partly because more than one pathological process may occur at once; hence the true diagnosis can often be made only in the histopathology laboratory.

Gallstones may cause chronic, low-grade symptoms, often labelled **chronic cholecystitis**. However, many of

these symptoms may be due to irritable bowel syndrome or chronic aerophagia (air swallowing).

Severe bouts of pain occur if the gall bladder becomes acutely obstructed, even transiently; this is known as **biliary colic**. Acute inflammation of the gall bladder is known as **acute cholecystitis**. It may be complicated by a **mucocoele of the gall bladder**, abscess formation (**empyema**) or, uncommonly, free **perforation**. Rarely,

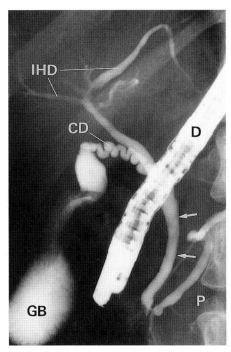

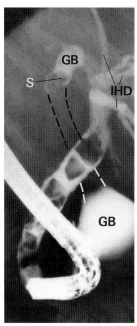

(a) Normal ERCP showing duodenoscope **D** in the second part of the duodenum. Contrast has been injected first into the pancreatic duct **P** and then into the common bile duct (arrowed). Note also the cystic duct **CD**, gall bladder **GB** and intrahepatic bile ducts **IHD**.

(b) Endoscopic retrograde cholangiogram in a woman of 77 who presented with mild epigastric pain and obstructive jaundice. The film shows multiple large stones in the common bile duct, represented by filling defects. The common bile duct is moderately dilated, but the intrahepatic ducts **IHD** are not. The fundus and neck of the gall bladder **GB** are shown, but the body is empty of contrast (dotted lines). There is a stone **S** near the neck of the gall bladder.

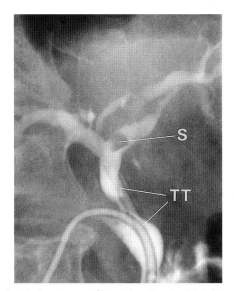

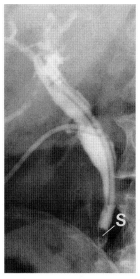

(c) and (d) Postoperative T-tube cholangiogram films taken (routinely) 7 days after open cholecystectomy and removal of stones from the common bile duct (two different patients). The films show the T-tube **TT** in situ. In (c), a stone **S** can be seen in the left hepatic duct, and in (d), another stone **S** can be seen at the lower end of the common bile duct. Both stones were successfully retrieved percutaneously 6 weeks later. The T-tube was removed and steerable grasping forceps passed into the biliary system through the skin defect. Each stone was then grasped and drawn to the surface along the track.

Fig. 20.5 Investigation of the biliary duct system

large stones in the common bile duct ulcerate directly into the duodenum causing **fistula** formation. If they pass down the small bowel and impact in the terminal ileum and cause obstruction, this is called **gallstone ileus**. Finally, gallstones probably predispose to **carcinoma** of the gall bladder in the very long term. The spectrum of clinical disorders associated with gallstones is summarised in Figure 20.6.

CHRONIC SYMPTOMS SUGGESTIVE OF GALL BLADDER DISEASE

CLINICAL FEATURES

Many patients are referred with a long history of almost daily pain which is poorly localised in the right upper quadrant or epigastrium. It is often accompanied by nausea or even vomiting. The pain may be exacerbated by large or fatty meals and may radiate around towards the back. The symptoms are often rather vague and ill defined; this probably explains why patients often delay consulting a doctor. Examination rarely reveals more than vague upper abdominal tenderness.

MANAGEMENT

Most of these patients turn out not to have gallstones on ultrasonography. The most frequent diagnosis is probably irritable bowel syndrome but the differential diagnosis includes peptic ulcer disease, urinary tract infection and chronic constipation. Note that even if a patient has upper abdominal symptoms and demonstrable gallstones, this does not prove the one is caused by the other. Asymptomatic gallstones are a common incidental finding and it sometimes takes fine clinical judgement to decide whether cholecystectomy is likely to cure the symptoms.

When symptoms are characteristic of gall bladder disease, no special investigations other than ultrasonography are required. When the symptoms are less clear-cut, a more extensive search is necessary, perhaps including upper gastrointestinal endoscopy, plasma amylase and ECG as well as bowel investigations.

BILIARY COLIC

CLINICAL FEATURES

Intermittent cystic duct obstruction by stone is probably the most common reason for symptoms from gallstones. Typically, patients are female and chiefly fall into two groups: the young or middle-aged, often overweight woman, where there is likely to be little histological evidence of inflammation in the gall bladder, and the elderly woman in whom the gall bladder is grossly thickened, chronically inflamed and shrunken. The same conditions arise less frequently in males.

Biliary colic describes the symptom complex that arises from sudden and complete obstruction of the cystic duct or the common bile duct by stone. The pain produced is severe; it typically rises to a plateau over a few minutes then continues unrelentingly. Note that this pain does not have the strikingly intermittent brief peaks of other forms of colic. These patients writhe in agony until the pain resolves spontaneously after several hours or after opiate analgesia. A bout of vomiting often heralds the end of the attack and the patient feels exhausted and sore for the next day or so. There is commonly a history of previous similar episodes. There are few positive findings on examination: the patient is afebrile but there may be some local tenderness due to gall bladder distension. If the attack does not settle within 24 hours, acute cholecystitis is a more likely diagnosis (see below).

MANAGEMENT

Most cases of biliary colic can safely be managed at home if the diagnosis is recognised. Relief of pain usually requires only one injection of an opiate and the attack then passes. Severe attacks of biliary colic usually lead to emergency hospital admission since the differential diagnosis includes other conditions that may require urgent operation, e.g. perforated peptic ulcer. A presumptive diagnosis can be made on clinical grounds but ultrasound is important in making a definitive diagnosis. Ultrasound examination should be performed as soon as possible since early diagnosis may save several unnecessary days in hospital. In acute gallstone disease, cholecystectomy scheduled for the next available list is preferred by many surgeons but others perform the operation electively at a later date. Early operation appears to be the better option, reducing the risk of the complications of gallstones.

If a mucocoele of the gall bladder is found on ultrasonography, the attack is likely to persist and there is a high risk of an **empyema of the gall bladder** developing. In this case, cholecystectomy often becomes obligatory during the current admission.

Cholecystectomy is the definitive treatment for attacks of biliary colic. Patients are frequently put on a low-fat diet initially or whilst awaiting operation and this often relieves symptoms, presumably by removing a stimulus to gall bladder contraction. It also facilitates weight loss, if appropriate.

In younger patients, cholecystectomy is usually straightforward. The gall bladder is usually found to contain stones or thick dark biliary sludge and its wall is often thin, although it may sometimes be inflamed. In a few patients, the gall bladder is thickened and scarred and technically more difficult to remove. Techniques of cholecystectomy are discussed on pages 326–8.

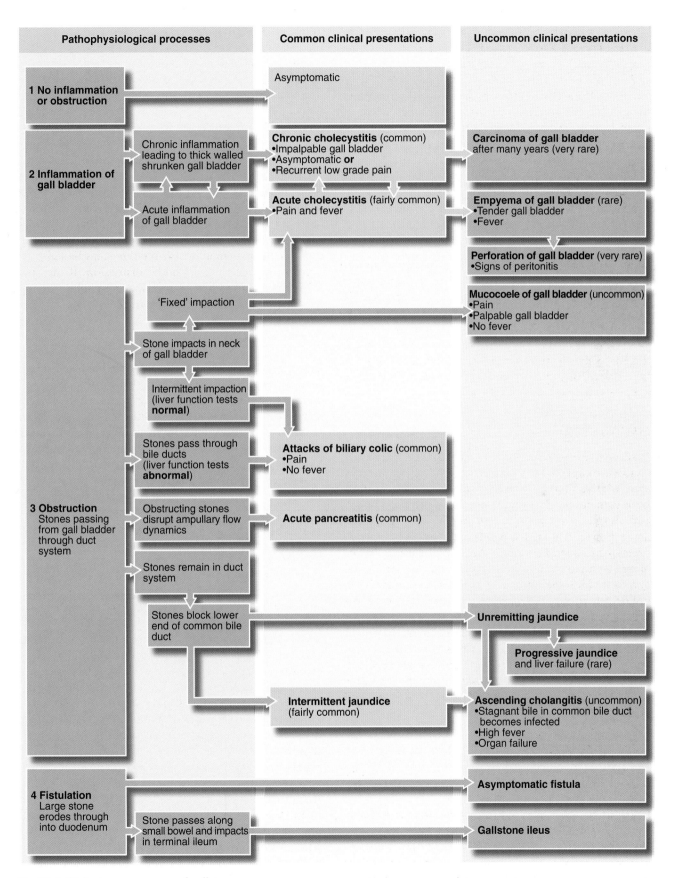

Fig. 20.6 Clinical consequences of gallstones

ACUTE CHOLECYSTITIS

PATHOPHYSIOLOGY AND CLINICAL FEATURES

Several factors contribute in varying degrees to cause acute inflammation in an obstructed gall bladder. These include physical and chemical irritation and, later in the episode, bacterial infection. The clinical result is acute cholecystitis, which often presents as a surgical emergency. In contrast to biliary colic, the patient is usually systemically unwell with a fever and tachycardia. On examination there is tenderness in the right upper quadrant, more marked on inspiration, and a tender inflammatory gall bladder mass may be palpable. The term 'Murphy's sign' is often misused in this context; it was originally used to describe tenderness at the tip of the ninth rib. Being inflammatory in origin, the clinical course of acute cholecystitis is more prolonged than biliary colic, usually lasting several days before settling or else precipitating urgent surgery.

MANAGEMENT

As with biliary colic, a presumptive clinical diagnosis may be made but it is worthwhile obtaining an early definitive diagnosis. Ultrasonography is usually sufficient to support the diagnosis by revealing stones and a thickened gall bladder wall.

As previously described, most patients with acute cholecystitis have a chemical inflammation and therefore do not require antibiotics. Oral intake should be restricted to fluids, and an intravenous infusion should be set up if necessary. When acute cholecystitis is accompanied by gall bladder infection, symptoms and signs are more marked and antibiotics should then be given.

Acute cholecystectomy

The patient with acute cholecystitis will need a cholecystectomy at some stage. Early cholecystectomy, performed within a few days of the onset of the attack, is becoming more popular. The procedure is as safe as elective surgery, convenient for the patient and an efficient usage of hospital beds. The alternative policy of conservative management involves discharging the patient after the acute attack resolves with readmission for elective cholecystectomy after about 6 weeks, by which time the inflammation has usually settled. However, in the mean time, there is a risk of further acute attacks or some other manifestation of gallstone disease such as acute pancreatitis. Even if delayed cholecystectomy is preferred, the acute attack may not settle, necessitating cholecystectomy on the same admission.

When operation is performed during the acute illness, the gall bladder is found to be obstructed and tense. The serosal surface is oedematous and inflamed with petechial haemorrhages or even purulent exudate and there are fibrinous adhesions to nearby structures. The gall bladder neck or cystic duct is blocked by an impacted stone and the gall bladder is usually found to contain further stones or sludge mixed with inflammatory exudate. Bowel organisms can be cultured from the contents in about 70% of cases.

In older patients and in males, the operation may be much more difficult; the gall bladder may be grossly inflamed, thickened and scarred and has to be patiently dissected out of the liver bed. Great care must be taken to avoid damaging the bile ducts. The gall bladder often contains several stones and may be filled with pus. A bacterial culture swab should be taken from within the gall bladder at operation as any postoperative infective complications are likely to involve the same organisms.

Empyema of the gall bladder

In a more extreme clinical variant, the gall bladder becomes distended with pus. The condition, known as an empyema, represents an abscess of the gall bladder. As with abscesses elsewhere, a swinging pyrexia is often found. Sometimes part of the gall bladder wall becomes necrotic, leading to perforation. This may be walled off by adjacent omentum, resulting in localised abscess formation and a palpable gall bladder mass. Occasionally, perforation leads to a subphrenic abscess or generalised peritonitis. These patients require surgery without delay. **Gangrenous cholecystitis** and perforation are rare because the gall bladder has a rich blood supply from its hepatic bed as well as from the cystic artery.

CHOLECYSTO-DUODENAL FISTULA AND GALLSTONE ILEUS

These uncommon complications of gallstones result from the inflamed gall bladder becoming adherent to the adjacent duodenum and a stone ulcerating through the wall to form a cholecysto-duodenal fistula. The fistula decompresses the obstructed gall bladder and allows stones to pass into the bowel and gas to enter the biliary tree. As such, the condition is usually harmless and unsuspected. It may be diagnosed on plain abdominal X-ray by the presence of gas outlining the biliary tree (see Fig. 20.7). Sometimes a fistula is discovered at operation.

Occasionally, a solitary cholesterol stone passing into the bowel is so large that after traversing the small bowel it impacts in the narrowest part, the distal ileum, causing small bowel obstruction or **gallstone ileus** (see Fig. 20.7). This occurs in the elderly and presents as an unexplained intermittent and sometimes incomplete small bowel obstruction. Unfortunately, the diagnosis is often difficult to make as the stone is usually radiolucent and delayed diagnosis is detrimental to the patient. In an elderly patient with distal small bowel obstruction, the diagnosis needs to be considered and can be confidently made if gas is recognised in the biliary tree on a plain abdominal X-ray.

Fig. 20.7 Gallstone ileus—case study

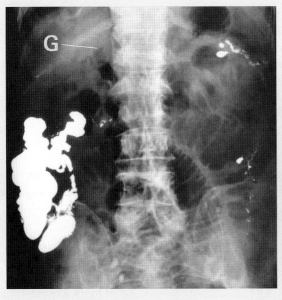
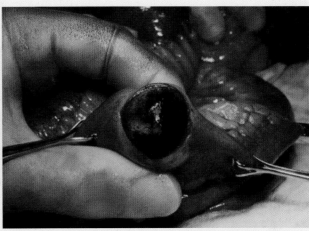

(a)   (b)

This 78-year-old woman presented with a gradual onset of small bowel obstruction. A large cholesterol solitaire stone had ulcerated from the gall bladder into the duodenum, travelled down the small bowel and finally impacted in the distal ileum causing complete obstruction. **(a)** This plain supine abdominal X-ray shows widespread small bowel dilatation. The diagnostic feature is the presence of gas **G** in the biliary tree (in this case, the common bile duct and cystic duct). **(b)** Photograph showing 'cholesterol solitaire' stone being removed from the distal ileum at operation. This had caused **gallstone ileus** by obstructing the terminal ileum. The gall bladder and fistula did not require surgery

CARCINOMA OF THE GALL BLADDER

Chronic irritation by stone over a long period is believed to predispose to adenocarcinoma of the gall bladder. This condition is rare and only found in the elderly. The presenting symptoms are similar to chronic inflammatory gall bladder disease. Jaundice may develop if the tumour obstructs the bile ducts. Carcinoma of the gall bladder is usually an unexpected finding at cholecystectomy for stones and is usually incurable by the time of detection.

BILE DUCT STONES

PATHOPHYSIOLOGY

Bile duct stones nearly always originate in the gall bladder and pass through the cystic duct. Most stones are small enough to pass out of the biliary system into the duodenum but may cause biliary colic or mild jaundice during transit. This explains many of the symptoms of recurrent gallstone-related disease.

Initially, stones in the bile ducts are small and enlarge progressively in situ. This is evident from the occasional finding of multiple faceted gallstones fitting neatly together in the common duct which could only have formed within the duct. The common bile duct is narrowest at its lower end and stones too large to pass out tend to lodge at this point. A stone here either becomes impacted, causing **progressive jaundice**, or acts as a ball-valve, causing **intermittent jaundice**. Obstruction results in gradual dilatation of the biliary tree; if dilatation is long-standing it does not regress even after the obstruction is removed and may lead to stagnation of bile and further stone formation. Note that the gall bladder rarely distends in this condition even when the common bile duct is completely obstructed. This is because of the inflammatory fibrosis or mural hypertrophy caused by gallstones (Courvoisier's law—see Ch. 18, p. 287).

CLINICAL PRESENTATIONS OF STONES IN THE BILIARY TRACT

Obstructive jaundice

Stones in the common bile duct, as stated earlier, are a common cause of obstructive jaundice and must be considered in the differential diagnosis; details are given in Chapter 18.

Asymptomatic duct stones

Any patient with gallstones may have duct stones although asymptomatic duct stones are rare. Standard practice used to be to perform operative cholangiography at every operation. However, most surgeons now perform selective cholangiography in patients with any signs, symptoms or investigations suggesting passage of stones.

Acute pancreatitis

Stones passing through or lying near the ampulla of Vater may interfere with drainage of pancreatic enzymes into the duodenum. Bile reflux into the main pancreatic duct may then cause acute pancreatitis (see Ch. 25).

Ascending cholangitis

Bile stasis in the common duct occurs with chronic obstruction and dilatation and predisposes to bacterial infection. The infection then extends proximally to involve the intrahepatic duct system. The condition is known as ascending cholangitis and is a potent cause of systemic sepsis. It is characterised by intermittent attacks of pain, swinging pyrexia and jaundice. This triad is also referred to as **Charcot's intermittent hepatic fever** and is often accompanied by marked weight loss. Ascending cholangitis is a serious condition and may culminate in life-threatening **acute suppurative cholangitis**. The bile duct must be drained urgently, either by surgical operation or preferably by endoscopic sphincterotomy.

MANAGEMENT OF GALLSTONE DISEASE

NON-SURGICAL TREATMENT OF GALLSTONES

Whatever the clinical manifestation of gallstone-related disease, most cases are treated surgically. A small proportion, however, are suitable for oral drug therapy. **Chenodeoxycholic acid** (a bile acid) and related drugs increase the bile salt pool and inhibit hepatic cholesterol secretion. When administered over a long period, these drugs cause slow dissolution of cholesterol stones. Unfortunately, the drugs have several disadvantages:

- Very slow action
- Only small, cholesterol-predominant stones can be dissolved
- High rate of stone recurrence after successful treatment
- Frequent drug-related side effects, e.g. severe diarrhoea and hepatic damage

For these reasons, drug therapy has largely gone out of favour and should only be considered in patients unfit for general anaesthesia with small radiolucent stones in a gall bladder which concentrates contrast and contracts in response to a fatty meal.

SURGICAL MANAGEMENT OF GALLSTONES

INDICATIONS FOR SURGERY AND PREPARATION OF THE PATIENT

There are two main indications for cholecystectomy:

- Symptomatic gallstone disease
- Asymptomatic gallstones when there is a reasonable likelihood of future symptoms or complications

In most cases high-quality biliary ultrasound is the only imaging study required. This demonstrates gall bladder disease and gallstones and the diameter of the intrahepatic and extrahepatic bile ducts. Information from ultrasound about gall bladder wall thickness or the number and size of stones has not proved useful in predicting the feasibility of laparoscopic surgery. If there are stones in the duct system, common duct exploration is added to cholecystectomy or else stones are extracted at ERCP.

Any jaundiced patient is at particular risk during surgery because of infection, hepatic impairment, defective clotting, acute renal failure and venous thrombosis (see Table 18.2, p. 291). It is often preferable to relieve obstructive jaundice prior to surgery by endoscopic sphincterotomy and stone extraction or bile duct stenting to minimise some of these complications. In patients presenting with jaundice caused by operable carcinoma of pancreas; however, the obstruction is often deliberately not relieved preoperatively because the duct dilatation simplifies its anastomosis to bowel. It also minimises the risk of introducing infection into a stagnant biliary tree.

CHOLECYSTECTOMY—OPEN VERSUS LAPAROSCOPIC SURGERY

The traditional method of cholecystectomy was by open operation at laparotomy. Laparoscopic cholecystectomy has rapidly increased in popularity in recent years and is already the gold standard method of treating gallstones. All surgeons performing this operation must, however, also be able to competently perform a difficult open operation in order to cope with the occasional conversion to open operation necessitated by unexpected complications or particular difficulties arising during a laparoscopic operation.

LAPAROSCOPIC MANAGEMENT OF GALL BLADDER DISEASE

Absolute contraindications to laparoscopic cholecystectomy include generalised abdominal infection, the late stages of pregnancy and major bleeding disorders. Relative contraindications for less experienced surgical teams include morbid obesity, acute cholecystitis, untreated bile duct stones including obstructive jaundice, previous

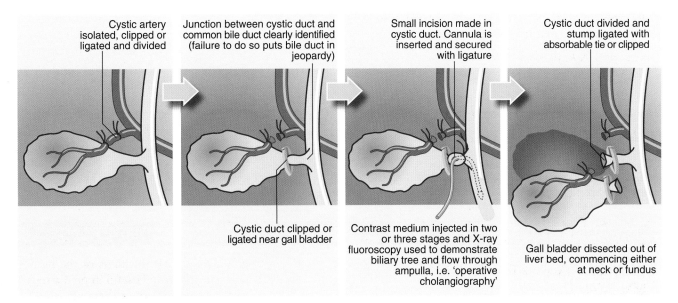

Cystic artery isolated, clipped or ligated and divided

Junction between cystic duct and common bile duct clearly identified (failure to do so puts bile duct in jeopardy)

Small incision made in cystic duct. Cannula is inserted and secured with ligature

Cystic duct divided and stump ligated with absorbable tie or clipped

Cystic duct clipped or ligated near gall bladder

Contrast medium injected in two or three stages and X-ray fluoroscopy used to demonstrate biliary tree and flow through ampulla, i.e. 'operative cholangiography'

Gall bladder dissected out of liver bed, commencing either at neck or fundus

Fig. 20.8 Principal steps in cholecystectomy

abdominal surgery (adhesions) and intra-abdominal malignancy.

Patients undergoing laparoscopic surgery should be prepared for and have consented to open surgery in case conversion proves necessary. In most centres, 1–5% of elective patients require conversion. If bile duct stones are suspected, preoperative ERCP (or equivalent magnetic resonance investigation) is advisable and stone extraction may be carried out if necessary. With experience, at least 95% of stones can be successfully extracted by this method of endotherapy. Some surgeons favour operative cholangiography in every case to give a 'road map' of the duct anatomy, to exclude bile duct stones and to provide experience for when cholangiography is essential. However, many surgeons practise 'selective' cholangiography for only those patients who have had abnormal liver function tests at any time or a dilated duct on ultrasound scanning, or in patients with clinical evidence of earlier passage of stone, for example previous acute pancreatitis or jaundice.

Operative technique

The main steps in cholecystectomy are shown in Figure 20.8 and a common operating theatre set-up for laparoscopic cholecystectomy is shown in Figure 20.9. The patient is anaesthetised and a pneumoperitoneum established via an open Hassan procedure using an automatic gas insufflator. The open method is very safe and is gradually superseding the blind Veress needle technique. A 10 mm cannula is then placed into the abdomen to accommodate a video laparoscope. The abdominal cavity is inspected for other pathology. Three additional abdominal punctures are usually made to introduce operating instruments. The cystic duct and artery are identified and

an operative cholangiogram performed (if desired) percutaneously across the abdominal wall. It is extremely important to be certain of the ductal anatomy before cutting anything because of the distortion introduced by retraction of the gall bladder and the limitations of the two-dimensional imaging system. If in doubt, perform a cholangiogram.

The cystic duct is doubly secured with metal or plastic clips, the gall bladder is dissected from the liver bed using diathermy or ultrasonic coagulation probes, and haemostasis is secured. The now free gall bladder is usually removed via the umbilical port. To achieve this, the laparoscope is moved to the upper midline port and forceps inserted through the umbilical cannula. The neck of the gall bladder is grasped and pulled into the cannula and the entire cannula and gall bladder neck withdrawn through the abdominal wall. If large stones prevent its passage, the incision is enlarged. The umbilical fascial defect should be sutured to prevent herniation but the upper midline puncture and the lateral punctures are usually left unsutured.

Results of laparoscopic cholecystectomy

Most patients are able to walk and tolerate food within 6 hours of operation and up to 80% can be discharged within 24 hours. The intervals before return to work and other normal activities are significantly reduced compared with open cholecystectomy.

Bile duct injuries occur in approximately 0.5% of patients. The risk of bile duct injuries is undoubtedly related to the experience of the operating team but has been reported to be twice as high in laparoscopic surgery as open surgery. The consequences of bile duct injury can be catastrophic; patients have died with multi-organ failure

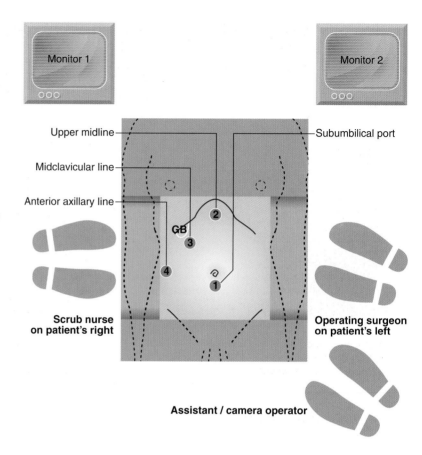

Fig. 20.9 Operating theatre arrangement for laparoscopic cholecystectomy
A common arrangement of the various operating ports (numbered 1–4) is shown. The subumbilical port **(1)** is usually placed with the Hassan open technique to take a 10 mm video laparoscope. A Veress needle is still sometimes used for initial gas insufflation. At the upper midline port **(2)** a 10 mm trocar is placed 5 cm below the xiphoid under video vision to the right of the falciform ligament. This is used to introduce operating instrument—curved dissectors, clip applier, and suction and irrigation tubes. At the midclavicular **(3)** and anterior axillary **(4)** lines, 5 mm trocars give access for grasping forceps, which are used to retract the gall bladder, and liver retractors.

Table 20.2 Potential complications of laparoscopic cholecystectomy

Stage of procedure	Complication
Placement of insufflation needle, trocar or other instruments	
During operation	Injuries to bowel Injuries to blood vessels, e.g. iliac artery Diaphragmatic injury with tension pneumothorax
Postoperative	Bleeding from trocar insertion sites Subcutaneous emphysema
Late	Herniation through trocar entry points and bowel strangulation
Trauma to biliary system	
During operation	Injuries to common bile ducts and hepatic ducts Bleeding from cystic or right hepatic artery Gall bladder perforation with spillage of bile and stones
Postoperative	Bleeding and bile leakage from liver bed Bile leakage from cystic duct remnant Retained bile duct stones
Other complications	Bowel damage by diathermy or laser

resulting from unrecognised biliary peritonitis whilst others have required open operations to repair bile ducts and have risked the consequences of long-term bile duct strictures. Other potential complications are listed in Table 20.2.

OPEN CHOLECYSTECTOMY

The choice of incisions for open biliary surgery includes upper midline, right paramedian, oblique subcostal (Kocher's) and transverse. The operative steps are the same as in laparoscopic surgery.

OPERATIONS ON THE COMMON BILE DUCT

Exploration of the common bile duct

If stones are known to be present in the bile ducts, the common duct may be explored, either laparoscopically or at open surgery. The duct is opened through a longitudinal incision and stones retrieved, often with some difficulty, by a combination of manipulation, irrigation, grasping with stone forceps and use of a balloon catheter. **Operative choledochoscopy** is often used to check for residual stones and to remove difficult stones. The flexible fibreoptic choledochoscope gives good visibility and manoeuvrability and can also be used in laparoscopic surgery by deploying it via one of the 5 mm ports. After exploration, a latex T-tube is usually inserted to drain bile

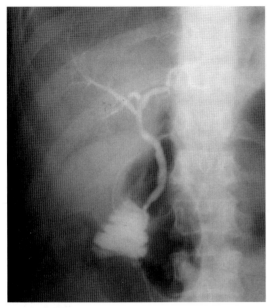

(a) Normal operative cholangiogram. The bile ducts are not dilated, the hepatic ducts fill, and contrast flows easily into the duodenum. There are no filling defects in the duct and the duct tapers normally at its lower end.

Fig. 20.10 Operative cholangiograms

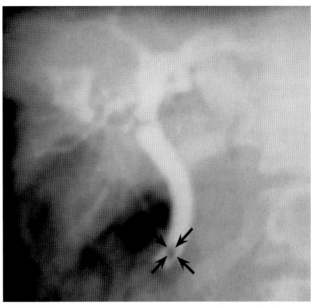

(b) Operative cholangiogram showing dilated bile ducts with a stone at lower end. This poorer quality image was seen better on the screen of the image intensifier used in the operating theatre. A filling defect (arrowed) is seen towards the lower end of the common bile duct representing a stone. This was removed at operation via a choledochotomy.

to the exterior, with the transverse limb placed within the common bile duct. The main purpose of a T-tube is to provide access to the biliary tree for a further cholangiogram about 1 week after operation (**T-tube cholangiography**, see Fig. 20.10). This is to ensure that no stones remain and to allow any oedema at the ampulla to settle.

Procedures to facilitate bile duct drainage

When the common bile duct is grossly dilated and contains multiple stones, it may be difficult to ensure complete stone clearance at exploration. This is because fragments of stone adhere to the wall. Furthermore, such a duct is usually stretched and baggy and remains so postoperatively, predisposing to stasis and further stone formation. It is therefore a useful precaution at open operation to make an anastomosis between the bile duct and adjacent duodenum known as a **choledocho-duodenostomy**. This ensures bile drainage even if stones or debris have been left behind. The anastomosis must be wide or it will predispose to ascending cholangitis.

An alternative operation, **transduodenal sphincteroplasty**, involves opening the second part of the duodenum and splitting the sphincter of Oddi by a large longitudinal incision. The mucosal edges are then sutured in apposition to minimise stricture formation. This operation may also be used to remove a firmly impacted stone from the lower end of the common duct. After any opera-

tion in which bile ducts are opened, an abdominal drain should be placed nearby to minimise the hazards of any biliary leakage. Few of these operations are performed nowadays as these patients are often better and more safely managed by endoscopic sphincterotomy.

ENDOSCOPIC MANAGEMENT OF BILE DUCT STONES

With the widespread availability of ERCP and endoscopic sphincterotomy, stones in the common duct can often be retrieved without an open operation. This technique represents a real advance in the management of duct stones over the earlier need for open surgery. **Endoscopic sphincterotomy** may be employed in the following circumstances:

- Urgent drainage of the bile duct in obstructive jaundice complicated by cholangitis. Definitive surgery can thus be deferred until the risks of infection have been minimised
- Retrieval of stones missed at operation. This avoids a difficult and hazardous operation to explore or re-explore the duct
- Removal of duct stones in patients unfit for operation (gallbladder left in situ)
- Some cases of acute pancreatitis due to gallstones
- Preparation of a jaundiced patient for elective gall bladder surgery

COMPLICATIONS OF BILIARY SURGERY

The procedure-specific complications of laparoscopic cholecystectomy are listed in Table 20.2. General complications of cholecystectomy are described below.

The retained stone

Despite considerable care at exploration of the common duct at open surgery, stones occasionally remain in the duct system after operation and are revealed by postoperative T-tube cholangiography. Until the 1970s, there were only two courses of remedial action. The first, attempting to flush the stone into the duodenum by irrigating the T-tube with heparin, saline or bile acids, was rarely successful. The second choice was a further laparotomy. Reoperation was technically difficult and carried a greatly increased risk of morbidity and mortality. Retained stones are now usually retrieved by ERCP and sphincterotomy, although it is still possible to retrieve retained stones percutaneously via a mature T-tube track using steerable grasping forceps or a Dormia basket.

Retained stones sometimes make themselves known many years later, when, having enlarged, they cause pain or obstructive jaundice. This possibility should be considered if a patient with previous biliary tract surgery develops typical pain or obstructive jaundice.

Biliary peritonitis

Bile leaking into the peritoneal cavity is irritant and causes a chemical peritonitis. If the bile is infected, it causes generalised peritonitis and sepsis with a high risk of fatality. Bile tends to leak through suture lines because of its detergent action. Therefore, whenever the duct system has been opened, a drain should be left in the vicinity for at least 5 days. Small leaks after biliary operations usually settle spontaneously but if biliary peritonitis develops, the area must be urgently drained percutaneously or, more often, re-explored surgically and drained, with intravenous antibiotic cover.

Bile duct damage

The bile ducts can easily be damaged at cholecystectomy or common duct exploration unless their anatomy, which is commonly aberrant, is carefully displayed. The most serious error is unrecognised transsection or ligation of the common duct. This presents as a major biliary leak or increasing jaundice; urgent re-exploration and reconstruction is mandatory. Lesser degrees of bile duct damage from crushing, overuse of diathermy or a careless ligature will heal but eventually result in a fibrotic stricture. This presents much later with obstruction. Regardless of how the bile ducts are damaged, complex reconstructive surgery is usually required, although endoscopic placement of a long-term stent allows rescue of some strictured ducts without operation. In the medium term, however, stents inevitably become blocked and have to be replaced every 3–6 months.

Haemorrhage

The cystic and hepatic arteries and the vascular liver bed are vulnerable to operative trauma and bleed profusely. Removing a grossly inflamed or fibrotic gall bladder is particularly hazardous. Manoeuvres to control haemorrhage may damage other structures, passing unnoticed at the time; this is a common cause of bile duct trauma.

Hazards of pre-existing jaundice

These are discussed under *Obstructive jaundice* in Chapter 18 (p. 285).

Ascending cholangitis and other infections

Ascending cholangitis can be a late complication of biliary surgery where an anastomosis has been formed between bile ducts and bowel. Reflux of intestinal contents and organisms takes place continually in such cases but active infection only occurs when bile stagnates in the duct system because of inadequate drainage. Usually the diameter of the anastomosis has shrunk to a point when it no longer drains adequately. Ascending cholangitis may also occur early after common duct exploration for jaundice, since bile in this situation is nearly always infected. Prophylactic antibiotics should always be used when operating on jaundiced patients with duct obstruction to minimise this complication.

An early complication of biliary surgery is a **subphrenic abscess**. This must be considered if the patient develops an unexplained swinging fever a few days after operation. Diagnosis may be elusive and is best made by ultrasound. Treatment is by percutaneous needle drainage under ultrasound guidance or occasionally by open operation.

Peptic ulceration and related disorders

21

INTRODUCTION

Peptic ulcer disease encompasses disorders of the oesophagus, stomach and duodenum. The conditions share the symptom of epigastric pain and all have the common aetiology of mucosal inflammation that is associated, to a greater or lesser extent, with gastric acid–pepsin secretions. Recent work has demonstrated that the most important aetiological factor in gastric and duodenal ulcer disease is chronic mucosal infection with the bacterium *Helicobacter pylori*. Peptic disorders, together with gallstone disease, are the most common causes of organic upper abdominal pain.

With the advent of highly effective pharmacological agents to block acid secretion and more reliable diagnostic and treatment monitoring techniques such as flexible

endoscopy, the use of surgery in peptic ulcer disease has declined by over 90% in the last 30 years. Recent antibiotic and other treatments against *H. pylori* promise even greater reductions and perhaps permanent cure for many peptic ulcer disorders. Most patients with suspected peptic ulcer disease are treated empirically by family practitioners; the rest are largely managed by gastroenterologists. Only a minority present to surgeons because of failed medical treatment. Rates of emergency complications such as perforation and haemorrhage have remained relatively static but peptic pyloric stenosis has markedly declined as chronic ulceration has become less common. Nevertheless, because of the diagnostic difficulties posed by upper abdominal symptoms, surgeons still manage many patients who turn out to have peptic disorders.

PATHOPHYSIOLOGY AND EPIDEMIOLOGY OF PEPTIC DISORDERS

PATHOPHYSIOLOGY OF PEPTIC ULCERATION

Inflammation, probably initiated by *H. pylori* infection and sustained by the combined effect of gastric acid and pepsin upon the mucosa, is probably the cause of all peptic disorders of the upper gastrointestinal tract other than reflux oesophagitis. *H. pylori* is a Gram-negative microaerophilic spiral bacterium which has the ability to colonise the gastric mucosa over a very long period. In many cases, infection appears to have been acquired in

childhood and there is often an association with poor living conditions in early life. Normally, a dynamic balance is maintained between the inherent protective characteristics of the mucosa (the mucosal barrier) and the irritant effects of acid–pepsin secretions. The delicate balance between secretion and protection may be disrupted by diminution of mucosal resistance or excessive acid–pepsin secretion or a combination of both. In some cases, the mucosal surface may become eroded by the direct action of some external agent, e.g. strong alcohol. Whatever the aetiology, the range of pathological

331

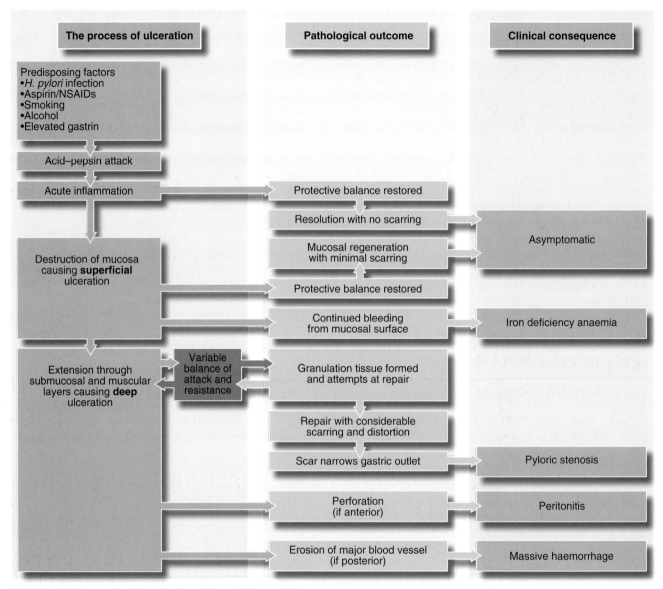

Fig. 21.1 Pathogenesis of peptic ulceration and its possible outcomes
Note that pain is a common factor in any active ulceration.

outcomes is similar and is summarised in Figure 21.1. If, at any stage, the balance of resistance over attack is restored, the process is halted and the tissue repaired. This explains the chronic and remittent nature of peptic ulcer disease.

OUTCOMES OF BREACHES OF THE MUCOSAL BARRIER

When the protective mucosal barrier is breached, the delicate underlying connective tissue is exposed to acid–pepsin attack, exciting an acute inflammatory response. If the protective balance is restored at this early stage, the inflammation will resolve and the epithelium regenerates. Little if any residual damage will result. If, however, the healing balance is not restored, continued acid–pepsin attack on the unprotected submucosa leads to an **acute**

peptic ulcer. This tends to become progressively larger and deeper.

From here, there are several possible outcomes. Sometimes the ulcerative process continues virtually unchecked through the full thickness of the gut wall. The ulcer perforates and intestinal contents escape into the peritoneal cavity resulting in peritonitis. More often, the layer of necrotic slough and acutely inflamed underlying tissue in the ulcer base temporarily resist acid–pepsin attack. This allows granulation tissue to form which initiates the process of fibrous repair. If, for example, acid-reducing drugs are used, the ulcer may heal, leaving a small scar with normal overlying mucosa. Usually, however, a tenuous balance is established between resistance and attack, matched by an unstable equilibrium between the rate of repair and the rate of tissue destruction. A chronic peptic ulcer then results which may persist for many years, its size and symptoms varying as mucosal resistance and exacerbating factors fluctuate.

If local or systemic factors change and swing the balance in favour of repair, the lesion may heal completely. On the mucosal surface, the healed ulcer site is usually puckered by scar contraction in the muscular wall. Externally, the serosa is thickened and may adhere to adjacent structures. If scarring occurs in a narrow part of the tract, i.e. the lower oesophagus or pyloric region, the lumen may become even narrower to produce a stricture, and subsequent acute mucosal inflammation and swelling may then precipitate obstruction. If healing does not occur at all, a chronic ulcer may slowly enlarge and deepen. Continual bleeding from the ulcer may cause chronic anaemia. Ulceration may erode into a large blood vessel causing acute major haemorrhage, particularly if the ulcer lies on the posterior wall of the duodenum; if it lies on the anterior wall, it may perforate into the peritoneal cavity.

EPIDEMIOLOGY AND AETIOLOGY OF PEPTIC ULCER DISEASE

THE SIZE OF THE PROBLEM

Chronic peptic ulcer disease is very common in developed countries, affecting around 10% of the population

at some time in their lives. The incidence of **duodenal ulcer** has been falling over the last 30 years, probably because of improved living conditions, reduced smoking and good medical therapy. The incidence of **gastric ulcer** is probably constant, although increasing numbers of cases are revealed as a result of NSAID-provoked haemorrhage.

Untreated duodenal ulcer seems to have a natural history characterised by recurrent attacks over 5–10 years then a gradual spontaneous remission. About 15% of patients have severe symptoms and aggressive disease. In many sufferers, symptoms are trivial or sporadic and settle spontaneously or with the help of antacids, and medical advice may never be sought.

Peptic ulceration is relatively rare in developing rural communities, despite a high incidence of *H. pylori* gastroduodenal infection. This implies that environmental factors associated with Western life are additional aetiological factors in the disease.

SITES OF PEPTIC ULCERATION (see Fig. 21.2)

Stomach and duodenum

Around 98% of all chronic peptic ulcers occur in the duodenum or stomach, and sometimes both at the same time. The most common sites are in the **first part of the duodenum** (known endoscopically as the duodenal bulb)

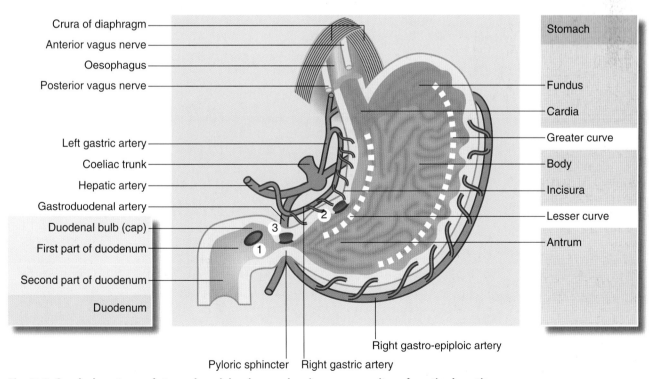

Fig. 21.2 Surgical anatomy of stomach and duodenum showing common sites of peptic ulceration
Acid secretion by the gastric mucosa is controlled by two mechanisms: **(a)** the vagus nerve stimulates acid secretion by the parietal cells (cholinergic stimulation) and **(b)** gastrin (produced by the APUD cells in the antrum) promotes secretion of acid and pepsin by the parietal and peptic cells of the fundus and body. The second is mediated via H_2 receptors. **(1)** Marks the common site for duodenal ulcers which may be anterior or posterior; **(2)** the site of pyloric channel ulcers; and **(3)** the common site of lesser curve gastric ulcers.

or the **gastric antrum**, particularly along the lesser curve. A chronic **stomal ulcer** may also appear at the margin of a surgically created communication between stomach and intestine (gastroenterostomy).

In the rare **Zollinger–Ellison syndrome**, a gastrin-secreting tumour of pancreatic origin overstimulates acid–pepsin production and causes severe and widespread peptic ulceration. The ulcers commonly involve stomach and duodenum and extend into the second part of the duodenum or even further distally.

Oesophagus

Peptic inflammation and superficial ulceration may involve the lower oesophagus. It is almost always secondary to acid–pepsin reflux, which itself is often associated with hiatus hernia. *H. pylori* infection (see below) is probably not an important factor here. Reflux causes intermittent destruction of the lower oesophageal mucosa by acid or bile (or both), causing **linear ulceration** and prompting vigorous attempts at healing. One outcome is replacement of the normal squamous epithelium with metaplastic columnar mucosa. This is known as **Barrett's oesophagus** and is one of the few known predisposing factors for adenocarcinoma of the lower oesophagus, a condition that has increased by 70% over the last 25 years (see Ch. 22). Chronic peptic ulcers, similar to gastroduodenal ulcers, may also develop at the lower end of the oesophagus.

AETIOLOGICAL FACTORS IN PEPTIC DISEASE

H. pylori infection

Despite extensive research, the precise aetiology of peptic ulcers was obscure until fairly recently. The importance of *H. pylori* infection as the main initiating factor has finally been universally accepted following the pioneering work of Dr Barry J. Marshall and Dr J. Robin Warren in Perth, Australia in the early 1980s. In a dramatic demonstration of Koch's postulates, Marshall produced a duodenal ulcer in himself a few days after ingesting cultured *H. pylori*. The ulcer proved to be *H. pylori*-positive on biopsy and was cured by anti-*Helicobacter* antibiotic therapy. The pair won the Nobel Prize in Physiology or Medicine for 2005 for their discovery of the bacterium *H. pylori* and its role in gastritis and peptic ulcer disease. Prior to their work, it had always been believed that microorganisms could not live in the highly acid environment of the normal stomach. However, gastric biopsies had frequently shown intramucosal bacteria, which they were eventually able to culture in vitro. These spiral-shaped organisms appear able to penetrate protective surface mucus and then accumulate in the region of intercellular junctions. There they may excite inflammation, stimulating excess acid–pepsin production or compromising normal protective mechanisms.

The jigsaw began to fit together when it was found that peptic ulcers could regularly be successfully treated with a combination of bismuth and antibiotics. Later work showed that *H. pylori* infection in duodenal ulcer patients was associated with a six-fold increase in gastric acid production which remitted when the infection was eliminated. There is now evidence that *H. pylori* is carcinogenic, initiating certain types of gastric lymphoma and some cases of gastric cancer. The broad picture is now evident: *H. pylori* causes a chronic infection with complications that include gastric and duodenal ulcer, gastric mucosa-associated lymphoma and gastric cancer. Only a tiny percentage of patients with duodenal or gastric ulcers are *H. pylori*-negative. Tests for *H. pylori* infection include serum **anti-*H. pylori* IgG**, direct tests on gastric biopsies for urease produced by the organism, hydrogen breath tests and histological examination of biopsy specimens.

Further details of this fascinating story remain to be worked out; for example, why not all patients with *H. pylori* infection develop upper gastrointestinal lesions, and why not all patients with certain gastric cancers have been exposed to *H. pylori*. There is even speculation that elimination of *H. pylori* may predispose some patients to gastric cancer.

Acid–pepsin production

Parietal cells secrete acid in direct or indirect response to acetylcholine, gastrin and histamine. It is likely that the common mediator is histamine. The final common pathway for hydrogen ion secretion is via activation of a specific enzyme, H^+/K^+ ATPase, which exchanges hydrogen ions generated in the parietal cell for potassium ions in the gastric lumen. In **duodenal ulceration**, the fundamental abnormality appears to be excessive production of acid–pepsin by the stomach, both basal (i.e. overnight) and stimulated. This may be a defensive response to *H. pylori* infection mediated via a de-inhibition of APUD endocrine cells of the gastric antrum. These cells normally secrete **gastrin** in response to gastric distension and protein ingestion and are an important factor in controlling acid–pepsin secretion. In duodenal ulcer patients, resting gastrin levels are not elevated but there appears to be an exaggerated gastrin response to intake of food.

In patients with **gastric ulcers**, measured acid secretion is either normal or low, and the essential problem seems to be diminished resistance to acid–pepsin attack, probably related to the quantity or quality of mucus produced. Nevertheless, reduction of acid production by medical or surgical means is effective in healing gastric ulcers.

Mucosal resistance

There are several mechanisms which protect the upper gastrointestinal mucosa against autodigestion. Somatostatin and prostaglandins are inhibitors of parietal cell secretion and the latter have other cytoprotective properties. Two forms of mucus, soluble and insoluble, are secreted continuously by gastric and duodenal mucosa; they contain bicarbonate and together maintain the cell surface pH at neutrality. Mucosal blood flow probably plays an important part by removing hydrogen ions that back-diffuse into the cells.

With increasing age, there is reduced turnover of surface cells and generalised mild mucosal atrophy, which might explain why the incidence of gastric ulcers rises with age. Non-steroidal anti-inflammatory drugs (NSAIDs) prescribed for arthritic disorders are commonly and increasingly identified as the causative factor for acute presentations of peptic ulceration, particularly in later life. NSAIDs probably have their greatest effect systemically rather than locally, via their blocking effects on prostaglandin production. Indeed, in elderly patients presenting with upper gastrointestinal bleeding or perforation, ulceration may occur after only a few NSAID tablets have been taken, or at any stage during a long period of medication. This risk is not diminished by enteric-coated preparations, nor by administration by routes other than orally, e.g. as suppositories. The risk of NSAID-induced ulceration increases steeply in later life. All of these drugs have been incriminated and their power to provoke peptic ulceration is in direct proportion to their effectiveness at relieving arthritic symptoms. A history of 'indigestion' in patients taking NSAIDs must be taken seriously.

Other mucosal irritants

Alcohol, aspirin and other NSAIDs are all known to induce acute mucosal inflammation directly (**acute gastritis**). In a susceptible individual, the inflammation may persist, resulting in chronic ulceration. Prolonged heavy alcohol intake is also a recognised risk factor. Reflux of pancreatic digestive enzymes back through the pylorus may also play a part, and is probably caused by defective pyloric closure. Another possible factor is antral stasis (perhaps also caused by abnormal pyloric function), leading to increased gastrin secretion. The area of the junction between parietal and antral cells on the lesser curvature of the stomach has been noted to be particularly vulnerable to gastric ulceration, although the reason is not understood.

Smoking

Cigarette smoking is twice as common in patients with chronic peptic ulcer disease as in the general population. Its pathogenic role is attributed to increased vagal activity, and its effect on producing relative gastric mucosal ischaemia. Cessation of smoking, however, greatly assists in the healing of peptic ulcers.

INVESTIGATION AND CLINICAL FEATURES OF PEPTIC DISORDERS

INVESTIGATION OF SUSPECTED PEPTIC ULCER DISEASE

The diagnosis and management of peptic disorders relies mainly on flexible endoscopy, which revolutionised the process after its introduction in the late 1960s. Barium meal contrast radiography has largely been superseded by endoscopy.

ENDOSCOPY

Oesophago-gastro-duodenoscopy, also known as OGD or gastroscopy, involves visual examination of the mucosa using a steerable, flexible endoscope. Gastroscopy enables direct and comprehensive examination of the whole area of the upper gastrointestinal tract that is prone to peptic ulcer disease.

In peptic ulcer disease, gastroscopy has definite advantages over contrast radiography, which by its nature can only demonstrate substantial structural abnormalities and then only as two-dimensional images. Shallow mucosal abnormalities such as superficial ulceration or vascular malformations are invisible on barium meal but can be directly inspected and diagnosed from their endoscopic appearance. Distortion resulting from previous disease or surgery often interferes with radiological interpretation. This too can usually be overcome by endoscopic inspection.

Benign gastric or oesophageal ulceration can be reliably distinguished from malignancy if endoscopic biopsies are taken from several places around the ulcer edge. In patients with peptic disorders, biopsies of distal gastric mucosa are now taken routinely to investigate *H. pylori* infection.

In acute upper gastrointestinal haemorrhage, gastroscopy is almost mandatory, as described in Chapter 19. Gastroscopy can identify the site of the bleeding and is particularly useful if gastro-oesophageal varices are suspected to be the source of bleeding. Gastroscopy also allows recognition of features which can help stratify patients into low or high risk of rebleeding and it provides an important means of treating bleeding sites by injection of vasoconstrictors or sclerosants.

CONTRAST RADIOLOGY

Contrast radiography of the upper gastrointestinal tract is nowadays used largely to determine swallowing function and to give an idea of the effectiveness of gastric emptying. It involves the patient swallowing barium suspension (**barium meal**). Its passage is followed through the upper gastrointestinal tract by fluoroscopic imaging, with points of special diagnostic importance recorded on film or electronically. During the investigation, the patient is tilted and rolled in various directions to demonstrate the whole region of interest. Effervescent tablets are given to produce gaseous distension of the stomach and duodenum and spread the contrast in a thin, even layer over the mucosal surface. This standard **double contrast technique** improves the imaging of mucosal detail, particularly when the duodenum is relaxed by giving

intravenous anticholinergic drugs such as hyoscine butylbromide.

PRESENTING FEATURES OF PEPTIC ULCER DISEASE

The various ways in which peptic inflammation affects the oesophagus, stomach and duodenum are summarised in Table 21.1.

Table 21.1 Clinical consequences of peptic ulcer disease in different anatomical sites

Pathological process	Clinical lesion	Symptoms
Oesophagus		
Transient acid–pepsin reflux	Mild reversible acute inflammation, i.e. transient oesophagitis	Burning retrosternal pain (i.e. 'heartburn')
Recurrent acid–pepsin reflux or failure of oesophagus to expel acid by peristalsis (often found in hiatus hernia)	Episodes of acute inflammation, i.e. reflux oesophagitis—probably reversible with no scarring	Recurrent epigastric and retrosternal pain. Chronic iron deficiency anaemia may occur
Persistent severe reflux	Chronic low-grade blood loss Continuous severe inflammation with superficial ulceration. May lead to chronic ulceration and/or stricture	Severe retrosternal pain, dysphagia and sometimes recurrent small haematemeses
Stomach		
Acute gastric irritation, e.g. by NSAIDs or alcohol	Acute (reversible) mucosal inflammation, i.e. acute gastritis or erosive/ haemorrhagic gastritis	Epigastric pain, vomiting, acute upper gastrointestinal bleeding
Acute reduction in mucosal resistance provoked by visceral ischaemia or the systemic inflammatory response syndrome (usually in intensive therapy unit patients or after burns)	Widespread superficial gastric ulceration (gastric erosions)	May bleed uncontrollably or perforate
Chronic *H. pylori* infection, probably with longstanding diminished resistance to acid–pepsin attack, with or without extrinsic irritation	Chronic or recurrent gastric ulceration	Epigastric pain—characteristically exacerbated by food (especially if acid or spicy), anorexia and weight loss Symptoms of chronic anaemia
Duodenum		
Episodic acid–pepsin attack	Acute (reversible) mucosal inflammation, i.e. duodenitis	Episodic epigastric pain
Chronic *H. pylori* infection, probably with persistent acid–pepsin attack	Duodenal ulceration (may involve pyloric canal)	Epigastric pain—typically relieved by food and occurring several hours after food, especially at night
Pre-existing duodenal scarring causing pyloric stenosis with superadded acute inflammation and mucosal swelling	Complete pyloric obstruction	Symptoms of chronic anaemia Severe vomiting, dehydration, shock, gross electrolyte disturbance (hypochloraemic alkalosis)
Both stomach and duodenum		
Periodic loss of protective equilibrium	Recurrent ulceration	Intermittent symptomatic episodes
Erosion of a major vessel in ulcer floor	Severe haemorrhage	Massive haematemesis or melaena
Unchecked ulceration	Perforation and peritonitis	Acute severe abdominal pain and shock

Epigastric pain (usually described as 'boreing', 'gnawing' or 'burning') is the principal presenting symptom and is common to peptic disorders whatever the site. Pain is often accompanied by other forms of discomfort, often described by the patient as 'indigestion' or 'dyspepsia'. A more specific description may suggest particular diagnostic entities. Retrosternal pain ('heartburn') suggests reflux oesophagitis, whereas bitter regurgitation ('waterbrash') is characteristic of both oesophageal reflux and duodenal ulceration. Nausea or vomiting, anorexia (loss of appetite) and abdominal fullness or bloating are common in gastric ulcer and pyloric stenosis, but may also occur in a variety of other upper gastrointestinal disorders, e.g. gallstone disease and irritable bowel syndrome.

The relationship of symptoms to food intake may help to distinguish gastric from duodenal ulceration; gastric ulcer pain is typically exacerbated by food and duodenal ulcer pain relieved by it.

Untreated peptic disorders are by nature protracted, with exacerbations and remissions over weeks or months. Symptoms tend to follow the disease activity and often wax and wane over many years before finally remitting.

Peptic ulcers may be virtually asymptomatic, particularly those caused by NSAIDs. Recognition then depends on acute presentation with bleeding or perforation or on investigation of iron deficiency anaemia. Asymptomatic peptic ulceration should always be suspected if there is no obvious cause for anaemia.

NON-ACUTE CLINICAL PRESENTATIONS OF PEPTIC ULCER DISEASE

PEPTIC DISORDERS OF THE OESOPHAGUS

All peptic disorders of the oesophagus are associated with reflux of gastric contents. These disorders range from mild reversible inflammation, through moderate acute inflammation with superficial ulceration (**reflux oesophagitis**), to severe persistent inflammation. The latter may lead to **fibrotic scarring and stenosis** (see Fig. 21.3) and sometimes **chronic peptic ulceration**. In many patients, reflux is associated with hiatus hernia (see Ch. 22); in the remainder the mechanism of the damaging reflux is poorly understood but is probably related to faulty neuromuscular coordination of the functional sphincter at the gastro-oesophageal junction.

In conjunction with gastroscopy, barium meal examination is often useful for demonstrating strictures, hiatus hernia or the existence of gross reflux and the relationship of abnormalities to the level of the diaphragm; both investigations are usually necessary.

On gastroscopy, reflux oesophagitis is characterised by mucosal reddening and, in more severe cases, by typical linear superficial ulceration (see Fig. 21.4). Peptic strictures occur only in the last few centimetres of the distal oesophagus and are recognised if the lumen is found to be too narrow to allow the endoscope to pass. The stricture is usually located just above the oesophago-gastric junction, which itself often lies above the diaphragm because of inflammatory shortening of the oesophagus. The normal oesophago-gastric junction is about 40 cm from the incisor teeth when seen on endoscopy (endoscopes have distances marked on them). The mucosa near the stricture varies in the amount of inflammation and ulceration present. Specialised intestinal metaplasia, dysplasia and carcinoma must be excluded by biopsies because the visual appearances may not be characteristic. Occasionally, a deep chronic ulcer occurs in the lower oesophagus; this looks and behaves like a gastric or duodenal ulcer. When squamous oesophageal epithelium is repeatedly damaged by reflux, it may be replaced by metaplastic columnar epithelium. This is known as **Barrett's oesophagus** and there is strong evidence that it predisposes to malignant change. If found, it should be biopsied to exclude dysplasia. When dysplasia is severe, there is about a 1% annual risk of malignant change and continued surveillance or surgery is highly desirable. Standard protocols are usually employed for surveillance of Barrett's oesophagus.

PEPTIC DISORDERS OF THE STOMACH

Peptic disorders of the stomach range from mild inflammation (**gastritis**) to **chronic gastric ulcers**, and most often occur in the antral region and along the lesser curve beyond the incisura.

Chronic gastric ulcers must be distinguished from malignant ulcers. The site of occurrence may aid recognition of a benign ulcer, but carcinoma may occur in any part of the stomach, with the region of the gastro-oesophageal junction now being the most common. Malignancy can only be excluded by histological examination of multiple representative biopsies taken from around the ulcer circumference (not the base) or by examining the whole ulcer in a resection specimen. In most cases, carcinoma probably arises de novo but occasionally a benign ulcer may undergo malignant transformation.

GASTRITIS

Gastritis can only be proved by endoscopy and appears as widespread reddening of the mucosa. If biliary reflux from the duodenum into the stomach is evident, the condition is sometimes referred to as '**biliary gastritis**' on the assumption that it is caused by the irritant effect of biliary and pancreatic secretions. Acute gastritis, often caused by alcohol (chronic alcoholism or single alcoholic

Fig. 21.3 Peptic stricture of the oesophagus

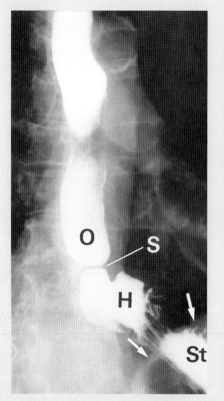
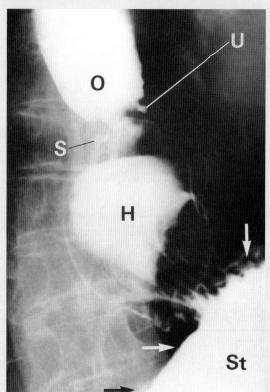

(a)

(b)

(a) A barium swallow in a 60-year-old woman who complained of burning retrosternal pain when lying flat (present for several years) and the recent onset of pain and difficulty when swallowing solid foods. The X-rays show the lower end of the oesophagus **O** and stomach **St**, part of which lies above the level of the diaphragm (position arrowed), forming a sliding hiatus hernia **H**. There is a tight stenosis in the last 2 cm of the oesophagus due to a peptic stricture **S**. **(b)** At greater magnification, barium can be seen filling the crater of a chronic peptic ulcer **U** immediately above the stricture.

Fig. 21.4 Reflux oesophagitis

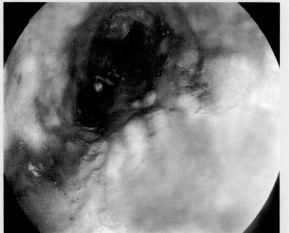

Gastroscopic view of the lower end of the oesophagus in a woman of 62 with a long history of reflux. Note the patchy ulceration **U** and the irregular fibrotic cardia caused by recurrent ulceration and attempts at healing. Further scarring may cause stricture formation.

binges) or aspirin/NSAID ingestion, can cause symptoms of sufficient severity to warrant gastroscopy. The mucosa often exhibits patchy shallow ulceration (**erosive gastritis**) and is friable and easily traumatised, causing bleeding.

STRESS ULCERS

Acute 'stress' ulcers are single or multiple small discrete superficial lesions that may develop rapidly in seriously ill patients, often in intensive care units. This condition may be a complication of extensive burns, systemic sepsis (possibly via visceral hypoperfusion), multiple trauma, major head injuries, uraemia or terminal illness. Stress ulcers typically present with haemorrhage (**haemorrhagic gastritis**), which is sometimes catastrophic, and occasionally with perforation. There is minimal mucosal inflammation around the ulcers and the aetiology may be primarily mucosal ischaemia rather than peptic. The risk of this life-threatening complication can be minimised in vulnerable patients by prophylactic treatment with proton pump inhibitors.

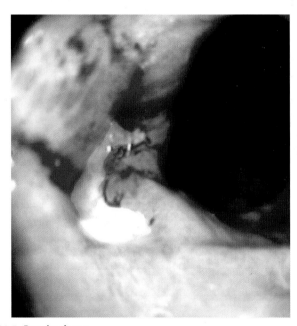
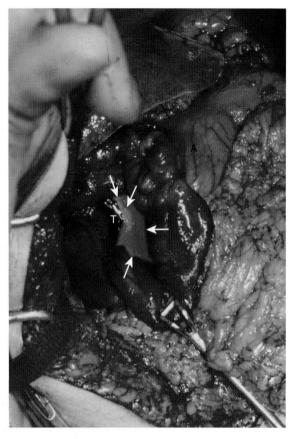

(a)   (b)

Fig. 21.5 Peptic ulcers
(a) Lesser curve benign gastric ulcer as seen through a gastroscope. At the original examination, the ulcer could be viewed from several directions and biopsies taken of the edge to exclude malignancy. **(b)** Photograph taken at emergency laparotomy for bleeding duodenal ulcer. The pylorus has been opened longitudinally and a deep chronic posterior ulcer crater is identified (arrowed). Thrombus **T** overlying an eroded artery is visible. A bleeding artery in the ulcer crater was under-run with sutures to arrest the haemorrhage.

CHRONIC GASTRIC ULCERATION

Chronic gastric ulcers vary greatly in size but the majority are small (less than 2 cm in diameter). **Giant ulcers** (up to 10 cm) are occasionally seen in the elderly; if posteriorly situated, they may erode through the stomach wall, obliterating the lesser sac and adhering to the surface of the pancreas. In these cases, the ulcer base or floor is composed of pancreatic tissue and erosion may cause catastrophic haemorrhage. Often symptoms are minimal before the acute event.

Benign gastric ulcers are typically regular in outline with a base consisting of white fibrinous slough. The ulcer gives the impression of having been punched out of the gastric wall, and there is no heaping-up of the mucosal margin as seen in malignant ulcers. The surrounding mucosa is surprisingly normal, although there may be radiating folds resulting from chronic fibrotic contractures. The typical endoscopic appearance of a gastric ulcer is shown in Figure 21.5a and the barium meal appearance in Figure 21.6.

Peptic disorders of the stomach typically cause severe, often disabling, epigastric pain which tends to be exacer-

bated by food, especially if acidic or spicy. The pain may be so severe that patients lose weight and develop a fear of food. Symptoms tend to persist for weeks or months, fluctuating in intensity and then disappearing completely, only to recur weeks or months later. Symptoms are a poor guide to disease activity or response to treatment. Indeed, major ulcers may be silent. Both can be monitored only by repeated gastroscopy until healing. A rare complication of peptic disease is perforation of a gastric ulcer into the transverse colon. The resulting gastro-colic fistula causes true faecal vomiting.

PEPTIC DISORDERS OF THE DUODENUM

DUODENITIS

Duodenitis, a non-ulcerative form of duodenal inflammation, has a similar endoscopic appearance to gastritis. It is commonly discovered in patients suspected of having duodenal ulceration, and probably represents a mild form of peptic disease.

Fig. 21.6 Chronic gastric ulcer

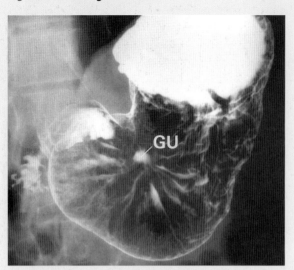

Double contrast barium meal in a 54-year-old man with a 6-month history of epigastric pain after meals. A gastric ulcer crater **GU** containing barium is seen on the lesser curve. Abnormal folds of gastric mucosa radiate out from the ulcer. Endoscopy and biopsy are indicated to exclude malignancy.

CHRONIC DUODENAL ULCERATION

Chronic duodenal ulcers almost exclusively occur in the pyloric channel and the first part of the duodenum. The latter area is known endoscopically as the 'duodenal bulb' and radiologically as the 'duodenal cap'. On endoscopy, duodenal ulcers have a range of appearances similar to chronic gastric ulcers. There is usually a single ulcer but two or more ulcers at one time are common ('kissing ulcers' occur on opposing walls of the duodenum). Malignancy is very rare in the duodenal bulb, so biopsy of the ulcer for this purpose is seldom necessary; biopsy of the gastric antrum for confirmation of *H. pylori* infections is, however, indicated. The radiological characteristics of duodenal ulcers are shown in Figure 21.7.

Duodenal ulcer symptoms follow the same general pattern as for gastric ulcer but with important exceptions. The pain tends to appear several hours after a meal ('hunger pain') and is relieved by eating. A typical history includes episodic early morning waking (often around 2 a.m.) with epigastric pain; this pain is relieved by drinking milk and eating bland foods. Consequently, undiagnosed patients tend to gain weight from the increased intake of food and milk. This is in contrast to the weight loss often associated with gastric ulcer. Symptoms in duodenal ulcer are more useful as a guide to disease activity and response to treatment than in gastric ulcer; this, and the extreme rarity of duodenal malignancy, removes the

Fig. 21.7 Chronic duodenal ulceration

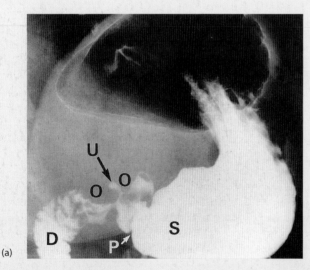

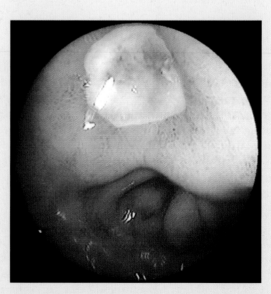

(a)

(b)

(a) A 35-year-old man complaining of epigastric pain at night and before meals. Barium meal examination: stomach marked **S**, and part of duodenum **D** and pylorus **P**. The X-ray shows a deep chronic duodenal ulcer **U** with contrast filling the ulcer crater; on either side are large areas free of contrast **O** caused by a ring of oedematous duodenal mucosa surrounding the ulcer.
(b) Endoscopic view of lesser curve gastric ulcer. This ulcer has probably only been present for about 4 months. It does not show surrounding scarring and distortion of the gastric wall that would be characteristic of longstanding ulcers.

need for regular gastroscopic follow-up in most cases of duodenal ulcer.

NON-ULCER DYSPEPSIA

In many patients presenting with upper abdominal pain, no evidence can be found of peptic ulcer or other organic disease despite competent assessment and investigation often including gastroscopy. In such cases, particularly those of long standing and in which symptoms are atypical, the diagnostic label of non-ulcer dyspepsia may be applied. There is probably no single cause of non-ulcer dyspepsia but a range of mechanisms, from 'excess acid' to irritable bowel syndrome. Some patients respond to mild antacids, others to dietary modification and yet others to changes to their life to reduce stress. If the patient proves to be *H. pylori* positive on biopsy or other test, eradication is probably indicated, but there is a poor correlation between elimination of infection and relief of symptoms.

MANAGEMENT OF CHRONIC PEPTIC ULCER DISEASE

Both the nature and the management of peptic ulcer disease have undergone extraordinary changes over the past four decades. The aim of treatment has always been to heal the ulcer with the minimum harm or inconvenience to the patient and with the lowest risk of recurrence. Several decades ago, medical management was relatively ineffective and was largely confined to antacid drugs, bland diets and bed rest. The only definitive treatment was major surgery and it was widely employed, often after a long period of chronic symptoms. Surgery was deferred as long as possible in the hope of spontaneous remission, and patients often had to 'earn' their operations by years of suffering! Partial gastrectomy offered the best cure rate and was thus the most common operation despite its mortality of 2–10% and its serious long-term complication rate. Later, various versions of vagotomy were shown to be almost equally effective, but with fewer complications.

The principles of modern management of peptic disorders are summarised in Box 21.1.

CONTROL OF PREDISPOSING OR AGGRAVATING CAUSES

The patient's history may reveal adverse factors which can be easily eliminated. These are summarised at the start of Box 21.1. Radical dietary modification is unnecessary; patients should merely be advised to avoid food which they find aggravates the symptoms. Spicy or acidic foods are often blamed.

Aspirin and other NSAIDs should be avoided, although this is often difficult in patients with arthritic disorders;

| Box | **21.1** | **Principles of management of peptic disorders** |

Control of predisposing or aggravating causes
- Modify diet, reduce alcohol intake, cease smoking, avoid irritant and ulcer-provoking drugs (aspirin and other NSAIDs), avoid stress, reduce oesophageal reflux by losing weight and attention to posture

Elimination of proven *H. pylori* infection
- Combined therapy with anti-acid and antibiotic combinations

Diminishing of irritant effects of acid–pepsin
- Simple antacid drugs, alginate preparations, liquorice derivatives, bismuth preparations

Administration of mucosal protective agents
- Sucralfate

Reduction of acid secretion
- H_2-receptor-blocking drugs (cimetidine, ranitidine), proton pump inhibitors (PPIs, e.g. omeprazole), surgical vagotomy (rarely employed nowadays)

Surgical removal of intractable ulcers and gastrin-secreting tissue
- Partial gastrectomy

Correction of secondary anatomical problems
- Dilatation of oesophageal strictures, operations for pyloric stenosis and hiatus hernia

---

the detrimental effect of these drugs is greatest in the elderly, the main sufferers from arthritis. The ulcerogenic effect of these drugs is directly proportional to their effectiveness and relates largely to their systemic anti-cyclo-oxygenase activity. There is therefore little to be gained from changing drugs within the group or by using them in enteric-coated or suppository form. If NSAIDs cannot be avoided in patients with a predisposition to peptic ulceration, concurrent use of cytoprotective drugs may be indicated.

Specific **cyclo-oxygenase 2 (COX-2) inhibitors** once held out a promise of minimising adverse NSAID effects on the upper gastrointestinal tract, but the recognition of increased cardiac mortality has limited their application. COX-1 is an enzyme present throughout the body that initiates the production of prostaglandins, key mediators in both health and disease. COX-2, on the other hand, is an inducible form of the enzyme present at very low levels in normal tissues; in disease, it stimulates production of prostaglandins that mediate inflammation and pain.

Patients with oesophageal reflux, especially if associated with hiatus hernia, can minimise the damage by

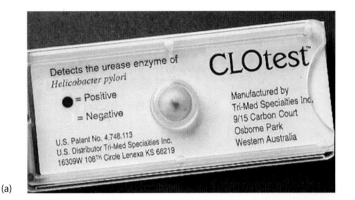

(a)

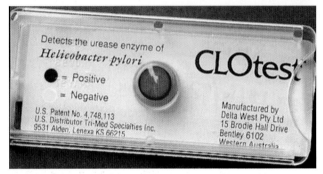

(b)

Fig. 21.8 Proprietary urease testing kit for _H. pylori_
Biopsies of gastric or duodenal mucosa are placed in the well and the result read after a set period. A positive result is indicated by the colour change seen here in **(b)**.

simple mechanical measures such as losing weight, elevating the head end of the bed and avoiding stooping.

ELIMINATION OF PROVEN _H. PYLORI_ INFECTION

Once _H. pylori_ has been confirmed, treatment involves a short course of acid inhibition combined with antibiotic treatment. Eradication usually produces long-term ulcer remission, and reinfection with _H. pylori_ is rare. A triple regimen including a proton pump inhibitor (e.g. omeprazole) and two antibiotics (clarithromycin plus either amoxicillin or metronidazole) given for 1 week eliminates _Helicobacter_ in over 90% of cases. Longer courses give potentially higher elimination rates but produce more side effects and lower compliance. Confirmation of eradication can be achieved by re-endoscopy and rapid urease testing, or by breath testing.

DIMINISHING OF IRRITANT EFFECTS OF ACID–PEPSIN

An array of proprietary antacid preparations is available over the counter and on prescription. When used assiduously, they promote ulcer healing almost as effectively as any other drug, although more slowly. The main active ingredients are few. **Sodium bicarbonate** offers rapid but temporary relief of symptoms, while **magnesium trisilicate** or **aluminium hydroxide** promotes ulcer healing.

Some of these agents, however, interfere with proton pump inhibitors. **Colloidal bismuth compounds** have been in use for many years. They have an antacid action and have been found to be active against _H. pylori_.

Alginate preparations form a foamy layer on the surface of gastric contents, coating the upper stomach and lower oesophagus and protecting it from oesophageal reflux.

ADMINISTRATION OF MUCOSAL PROTECTIVE AGENTS

Sucralfate is a complex of aluminium hydroxide and sulphated sucrose that is minimally absorbed from the gastrointestinal tract. It is believed to act by binding to denuded areas of mucosa and protecting them from acid–pepsin attack. It has been shown to be as effective as H_2-blockers in providing symptom relief and healing when given in the dose of 2 g twice daily. It does not interfere with other drugs and is safe in pregnancy. It is also effective for preventing stress ulcers in seriously ill patients.

REDUCTION OF ACID SECRETION

Acid secretion by the gastric mucosa is normally controlled by two mechanisms:

- Direct cholinergic stimulation of parietal cells mediated via the **vagus nerve**. This is under reflex control originating in the cerebral cortex triggered by the sight and taste of food
- Gastrin is secreted by APUD cells in the gastric antrum and promotes acid secretion via histamine released from mast cells in the vicinity of the parietal cells. The histamine receptors on the parietal cells are distinct from those elsewhere in the body and are designated as **type 2 (H_2) receptors**; these receptors are not blocked by standard 'antihistamine' drugs such as chlorphenamine. Gastrin secretion is partly controlled by the vagus and partly by local (vagally independent) reflexes initiated by gastric distension and the presence of food or alcohol in the stomach

From this, two practical methods have been found to reduce acid secretion: drugs which selectively block H_2-receptors or the proton pump mechanism (described earlier), and surgical division of the vagus nerve.

H_2-receptor blockade and proton pump antagonists

H_2-receptor blocking drugs were developed in the 1970s and were the first 'medical' revolution in the management of peptic disorders. **Cimetidine** was alone in the market for several years but was joined by **ranitidine**, which has a few minor advantages but is no more effective for healing ulcers. H_2-receptor antagonists are highly effective in

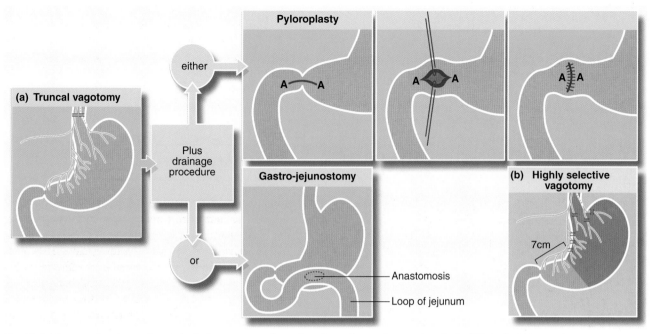

Fig. 21.9 The vagotomies and gastric drainage procedures (rarely performed nowadays but of historical interest)
(a) Truncal vagotomy is followed by a drainage procedure, either pyloroplasty (Heinecke–Mikulicz is illustrated) or gastro-jejunostomy. In gastro-jejunostomy an anastomosis is created to the most dependent part of the stomach; a short efferent loop of jejunum is brought up either in front of the transverse colon and sutured to the anterior wall of the stomach (antecolic), or behind the transverse colon via an incision in the mesocolon and sutured to the posterior wall of the stomach (retrocolic). **(b)** Highly selective vagotomy does not require a drainage procedure. Only the parietal cell mass is denervated, preserving the innervation of the pylorus and antrum plus the rest of the abdominal viscera.

reducing gastric acid secretion. Symptomatic response is rapid, usually within a day or two, and healing follows within a few weeks in 70–90% of cases. Recurrence rates, however, are high even with maintenance therapy, with 50–75% of patients developing further symptoms within 2 years.

A newer group of drugs, the substituted **benzimidazoles**, are extremely potent and reduce acid production to near zero by direct inhibition of the proton pump. **Omeprazole** and other variants are often employed for oesophagitis, recurrent ulcers and Zollinger–Ellison syndrome. Where *H. pylori* infection is present, the use of these drugs alone is not recommended as the recurrence rate is unacceptably high.

Vagotomy

Vagotomy was first performed in the 1920s and popularised by Dragstedt from 1943. It gradually superseded classic partial gastrectomy as the surgical treatment of choice for chronic duodenal ulcer. The various vagotomy operations illustrated in Figure 21.9 are now only of historical interest. The simplest involved dividing the anterior and posterior vagal trunks close to the abdominal oesophagus just below the diaphragm (**truncal vagotomy**). The operation is effective in promoting ulcer healing but paralyses gastric motility and slows pyloric emptying. A surgical **drainage procedure**, usually pylo-

roplasty ('V & P'), less commonly **gastro-jejunostomy**, was therefore a necessary part of the operation.

Attempts to reduce the gastric emptying complications of truncal vagotomy led to operations designed to preserve the innervation of the distal antrum and pylorus whilst denervating the proximal acid-secreting portion of the stomach. **Highly selective vagotomy** preserved the nerves of Latarjet and avoided the need for a gastric drainage procedure. Early postoperative side effects were fewer but ulcer recurrence rates were higher than for truncal vagotomy.

All surgical treatments for duodenal ulcer were eclipsed by the introduction of the H_2-blockers and the operation rate is now only 1% of that of four decades ago. The vagotomies are now occasionally employed for chronic symptomatic duodenal ulceration that recurs after effective elimination therapy; most are performed laparoscopically.

Surgical removal of intractable ulcers and gastrin-secreting tissue

Partial gastrectomy was occasionally used for patients where medical management had failed to heal a benign gastric ulcer or to treat repeated recurrences. The operation had the dual role of removing the ulcer and the gastrin-secreting mucosa. The classic gastrectomy for chronic gastric ulcer was known as the **Billroth I** type

343

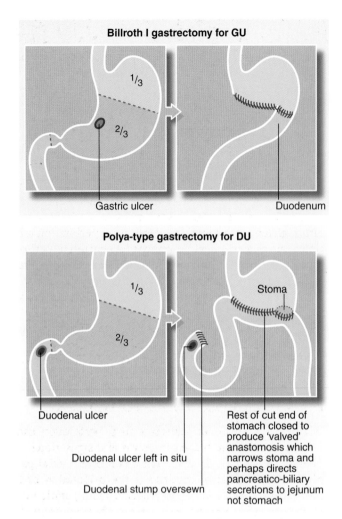

Billroth I gastrectomy for GU

Gastric ulcer

Duodenum

Polya-type gastrectomy for DU

Stoma

Duodenal ulcer

Duodenal ulcer left in situ

Duodenal stump oversewn

Rest of cut end of stomach closed to produce 'valved' anastomosis which narrows stoma and perhaps directs pancreatico-biliary secretions to jejunum not stomach

Fig. 21.10 Types of partial gastrectomy formerly performed for peptic ulcer disease

---

Box 21.2 Side effects of partial gastrectomy

- Inability to eat normal-sized meals due to reduced gastric capacity
- 'Dumping' due to rapid emptying of stomach contents—common but most patients adapt with time
- Episodic bilious vomiting due to reflux of bile into stomach via the anastomosis
- Tendency to bolus obstruction of the gastric outlet stoma
- Weight loss due to a combination of above factors and malabsorption—especially common in women
- Vitamin B_{12} deficiency due to loss of gastric intrinsic factor; may present as macrocytic anaemia or subacute combined degeneration of the spinal cord—potentially catastrophic, occurring many years after operation and preventable by regular vitamin B_{12} (hydroxycobalamin) injections
- Iron deficiency anaemia due to reduced iron absorption—common but easily prevented by taking iron tablets, e.g. once weekly
- Malignant change in gastric remnant possibly due to bacterial production of carcinogens—rare

---

(Billroth, 1881) and involved removing the distal two-thirds of the stomach. The gastric remnant was then anastomosed to the first part of the duodenum (see Fig. 21.10).

The standard partial gastrectomy for duodenal ulcers was a **Polya-type gastrectomy**, also involving resection of the distal two-thirds of the stomach but anastomosing the cut end of the stomach to the side of a loop of proximal jejunum (gastro-jejunostomy). The cut end of the duodenum (duodenal stump) was closed and the ulcer left in situ to heal (see Fig. 21.10). Numerous variations on gastrectomy have been described over the years and many still carry their authors' names, e.g. Polya (1911), Finsterer (1909), Billroth II (1881), Hofmeister (1908), Balfour (1934). The use of eponymous titles to describe particular operations has become somewhat confused, but the essential difference is whether the gastric remnant is anastomosed to the duodenum (Billroth I-type) or to a jejunal loop (Polya-type).

In general, partial gastrectomy was highly effective in relieving symptoms and preventing recurrence of peptic disease, but long-term side effects were a serious problem affecting 30–40% of patients.

Complications and side effects of partial gastrectomy

Partial gastrectomy is a major operative procedure yet recovery tends to be surprisingly straightforward. A small proportion of patients develop serious complications such as duodenal stump leakage and anastomotic breakdown. However, the main complications of partial gastrectomy occur in the long term and may not become manifest for years (see Box 21.2). Recurrent ulceration after partial gastrectomy was rare and occurred in the gastric remnant or at the stomal margin. The usual reason was that insufficient stomach had been removed, but occasionally malignant change was responsible (3% risk over 15 years). Abnormally high acid production was another cause, sometimes due to Zollinger–Ellison syndrome or hyperparathyroidism.

Correction of secondary anatomical problems

The main anatomical problems secondary to peptic disease are oesophageal stricture and pyloric stenosis.

Oesophageal strictures can usually be managed by periodic dilatation and medical or surgical treatment of the underlying cause. With the patient intravenously sedated, a guide-wire is inserted across the stricture endoscopically, and then metal or plastic dilators are inserted over it. Occasionally, reflux continues to cause damage and stricturing; it may then become necessary to perform anti-reflux surgery.

EMERGENCY PRESENTATIONS OF PEPTIC ULCER DISEASE

The emergency presentations of peptic ulcer disease are acute haemorrhage, perforation and, much less commonly, pyloric stenosis. Peptic ulcer disease was responsible for much major emergency abdominal surgery until the early 1970s. Since then there has been a remarkable reduction in emergency presentations of peptic ulcer, and emergency surgery is now a rarity except in elderly patients taking NSAIDs for arthritic symptoms. This change was well under way before the introduction of effective modern drug therapy and can probably be attributed to the progressive improvement in living standards after World War II.

HAEMORRHAGE FROM A PEPTIC ULCER

Acute bleeding from a peptic ulcer presents with haematemesis or melaena or both. Management is discussed in detail in Chapter 19.

PERFORATION OF A PEPTIC ULCER

Perforation of a gastric or duodenal ulcer into the peritoneal cavity causes peritonitis. Until about 25 years ago, these perforations were a common cause of an acute abdomen but the incidence has fallen in parallel with the general decline in peptic ulcer disease. Nowadays, as with haemorrhage, perforations of peptic ulcers occur most commonly in elderly patients taking NSAIDs. Occasionally, a younger patient presents with a perforated duodenal ulcer without an obvious predisposing cause.

Duodenal ulcer perforations are two or three times more common than gastric ulcer perforations. The perforation typically occurs on the anterior surface of the duodenal bulb just beyond the pylorus. There is often a short history of NSAID ingestion, but a long history of taking such drugs does not rule them out as an aetiological factor. About half the patients with a peptic ulcer perforation have had recent ulcer symptoms but the other half are asymptomatic.

Gastric ulcer perforations are uncommon and occur virtually always in the elderly. About a third of these are due to perforation of a gastric carcinoma but present in the same way as a perforated peptic ulcer. This explains why standard surgical treatments for gastric perforation include excision or extensive biopsy of the ulcer. Oesophageal peptic ulcers occur much less commonly and perforate even more rarely.

CLINICAL PRESENTATION OF PERFORATED PEPTIC ULCER

Perforation of a gastric or duodenal ulcer usually presents as a sudden onset of epigastric pain, rapidly spreading to the whole abdomen. The pain is continuous and is aggravated by moving about. Paradoxically, there may be vomiting of brownish or even blood-stained fluid. On examination, the patient is in obvious pain but is not shocked or toxic.

There is generalised involuntary abdominal guarding, which in younger patients is so tense as to be described as '**board-like rigidity**', although this may be absent in the elderly. There is also generalised abdominal tenderness but this may only be detectable on firm palpation because of muscle spasm of the abdominal wall. After several hours, abdominal wall rigidity tends to relax although tenderness remains. Peptic ulcer perforation initially causes a chemical, as opposed to bacterial, peritonitis, unlike more distal bowel perforations. This explains the lack of general toxicity in the early stages. If untreated for more than 24 hours, secondary infection may take place and systemic signs appear.

If posterior wall gastric ulcers perforate, they leak gastric contents into the lesser sac, which tends to confine the peritonitis. These patients thus present with less marked symptoms.

DIAGNOSIS OF PERFORATED PEPTIC ULCER

Diagnosis of an upper gastrointestinal perforation can usually be made from the symptoms and signs alone. A plain erect radiograph of the chest will often reveal gas under the diaphragm, confirming the perforation of a hollow viscus but not its origin. This radiographic evidence of perforation, however, is not always present. If perforation is suspected but the signs are equivocal, an abdominal radiograph may be taken after the patient has swallowed 25 ml of water-soluble contrast; this may confirm the leakage. Diagnostic gastroscopy is contraindicated because the stomach must be inflated during this examination and air and gastric contents would erupt into the peritoneal cavity.

SURGICAL MANAGEMENT OF PEPTIC PERFORATION

Emergency surgery is indicated in nearly all cases of upper gastrointestinal perforation. The patient is first resuscitated and a nasogastric tube inserted. The operation is most commonly performed at laparotomy, but laparoscopic management of perforated duodenal ulcers is now well established with equally good results. The principles are similar in either case. At surgery, the abdomen is inspected and the diagnosis confirmed. 'Peritoneal toilet' is performed to remove fluid and food contaminating the peritoneal cavity. A perforated duodenal ulcer is usually obvious as a punched-out hole near the pylorus. An anterior gastric perforation is also obvious, but a posterior gastric ulcer is not visible unless the lesser sac is opened, usually along the greater curve.

Fig. 21.11 Gastric outlet obstruction

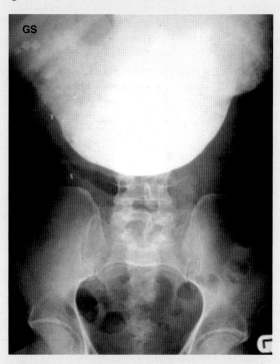

GS

Barium meal examination in a woman of 78 who presented with a 2-week history of vomiting. She was grossly dehydrated with a hypochloraemic alkalosis. She was resuscitated and a nasogastric tube passed. This film shows huge gastric dilatation and no flow of barium beyond the pylorus. She also has incidental gallstones (**GS**). The obstruction proved to be due to chronic duodenal ulceration, but a diagnosis of carcinoma of the gastric antrum must be considered in such a patient.

In duodenal perforation, simple closure of the perforation by suturing a vascularised flap of omentum over the defect is the treatment of choice, accompanied by the taking of biopsies for *H. pylori* testing. This should be followed later by *Helicobacter* eradication therapy if positive.

In perforated gastric ulcer, the classic operation was Billroth I gastrectomy, including the whole ulcer in the resection. However, local excision of the ulcer and simple closure are increasingly employed, provided the ulcer is believed to be benign. In any case, the ulcer edge must be biopsied in several places to be certain.

CONSERVATIVE MANAGEMENT OF PERFORATED DUODENAL ULCER

If an elderly, unfit patient presents late with a perforated duodenal ulcer, many surgeons treat this conservatively. This involves nasogastric aspiration, intravenous fluids, gastric acid suppression and antibiotics. Many of these patients who might otherwise have succumbed with major surgery recover satisfactorily.

PYLORIC STENOSIS

The pyloric canal and the immediate pre-pyloric area are common sites of chronic ulceration. Ulcers in this area are probably aetiologically related more closely to duodenal than gastric ulcers and should be managed accordingly. There may be typical symptoms of chronic duodenal ulcer or the presentation may be with pyloric stenosis and a minimal history of ulcer pain. Chronic ulceration near the pylorus causes fibrosis, which may progress to stricture formation. In the early stages, this leads to partial gastric outlet obstruction. An acute exacerbation of the ulcer leads to mucosal swelling and pyloric sphincter spasm, which then precipitates complete luminal obstruction.

CLINICAL FEATURES OF PYLORIC STENOSIS

These patients rarely give any recent history of peptic ulcer pain but tend to present with a short history (a few weeks at most) of episodic and sometimes projectile vomiting. This is unrelated to eating, and the vomitus typically contains foul-smelling semi-digested food eaten a day or more previously. It does not contain green bile. Often patients do not seek medical advice until they have become severely dehydrated with gross electrolyte disturbance.

On clinical examination, undernourishment, dehydration, constipation, weakness and weight loss may dominate the picture. Because the stomach is full of residual fluid and food, shaking the patient's abdomen from side to side produces an audible **succussion splash**. Gastric peristalsis may be visible in longstanding cases and a dilated stomach full of residual food may be palpable. On plain abdominal X-ray, it may be possible to see the grossly dilated stomach filled with mottled food material.

Several gastric washouts using a large-bore oral tube will be necessary to clear the gastric residue before endoscopy or barium meal is attempted.

Nowadays, distal gastric cancer is a more common cause of gastric outlet obstruction. With cancer, the obstruction does not resolve with conservative treatment whereas benign stenoses often do.

The differential diagnosis of gastric outflow obstruction also includes carcinoma of the head of the pancreas (with or without obstructive jaundice) and, rarely, chronic pancreatitis.

BIOCHEMICAL ABNORMALITIES IN PYLORIC STENOSIS

The biochemical disturbances in these patients are complex and depend on the volume and composition of fluid lost by vomiting and on the body's compensatory mechanisms. Hydrogen and chloride are the principal ions lost in the vomitus. In response, the kidney conserves hydrogen ions by exchanging them for sodium ions (and some potassium ions), which are necessarily lost in the urine. The kidney also conserves chloride ions by exchanging them for bicarbonate ions. The net result may be a profound depletion of total body sodium (which is not accurately reflected in the plasma sodium level), profound hypochloraemia and profound metabolic alkalosis (**hypochloraemic alkalosis**). The plasma urea level is often high as a result of dehydration. Finally, the proportion of ionised calcium in the serum may fall as a result of the alkalosis, inducing tetany.

MANAGEMENT OF PYLORIC STENOSIS

The first management priority in gastric outlet obstruction is resuscitation. Fluid and electrolyte deficiencies are corrected by infusion of physiological saline with added potassium chloride. The volume required often amounts to 10 litres or more. Rehydration will usually return the blood urea level to normal but may unmask an anaemia serious enough to require blood transfusion.

Often the obstruction has a significant inflammatory element, and acid suppression and *Helicobacter* eradication will produce a significant clinical response. If these fail, or malignancy is suspected, endoscopy should be repeated. Operative treatment may then become necessary.

22

Disorders of the oesophagus

INTRODUCTION

Diseases of the oesophagus form a small but significant part of the workload of some general surgeons but the majority of oesophageal surgery is performed in specialised units. Most cases are managed by medical gastroenterologists except those likely to require surgery, when close collaboration between medical and surgical specialists is needed.

Difficulty in swallowing, known as **dysphagia**, is the most common presenting symptom. **Reflux oesophagitis** and other peptic disorders of the lower oesophagus (often associated with hiatus hernia) and **oesophageal carcinomas** are the main conditions encountered. **Achalasia** and **pharyngeal pouch** are occasionally seen; **oesophageal web** (as in Plummer–Vinson syndrome) and **leiomyoma** are extremely rare.

Oesophageal varices secondary to cirrhosis usually present as massive haematemesis. Surgical treatment is seldom required as most acute cases are now managed with non-surgical therapy.

CARCINOMA OF THE OESOPHAGUS

PATHOLOGY AND CLINICAL FEATURES OF OESOPHAGEAL CARCINOMA

The oesophagus is lined by stratified squamous epithelium. Historically the majority of oesophageal malignancies were **squamous carcinomas**. The minority were **adenocarcinomas** occurring in the lower third of the oesophagus, probably derived from metaplastic intestinal mucosa, i.e. Barrett's oesophageal changes. However, over the last three decades there has been a slow but steady reversal in the proportions of patients presenting with these histological subtypes; currently adenocarcinoma makes up 60–70% of new cases. Squamous and adenocarcinomatous forms are both only moderately differentiated in general and behave aggressively.

Tumours at the gastro-oesophageal junction originate from three areas: the distal oesophagus ('type 1'), the cardia of the stomach ('type 2') or the subcardial gastric wall ('type 3'). Oesophageal cancers may fungate into the lumen but more often infiltrate diffusely along and around the oesophageal wall. Once through the wall, the tumour invades adjoining mediastinal organs.

Difficulty in swallowing (dysphagia) is the classic symptom, but it tends to develop insidiously. Patients initially have trouble with solids but they tend to compensate (liquidising their food, for example) before seeking medical advice. Later they have trouble swallowing liquids. By the time a patient presents with dysphagia, the tumour is often incurable and lymphatic spread to mediastinal nodes has already occurred. Sometimes, involvement of other mediastinal organs, e.g. recurrent laryngeal nerve invasion or an oesophago-tracheal fistula, produces the first symptoms. Low oesophageal lesions tend to metastasise to upper abdominal nodes and the liver.

EPIDEMIOLOGY AND AETIOLOGY OF OESOPHAGEAL CARCINOMA

The incidence of oesophageal cancer in Western countries is relatively low compared with carcinoma of the colon and stomach. It accounts for about 5% of all deaths from cancer, with males and females equally at risk. The disease is usually advanced by the time of presentation, hence the mortality rate is appalling, with 75% dying within a year of presentation and only 6% surviving 5 years (see Fig. 22.1).

Oesophageal carcinoma is uncommon before the age of 50 years. At least 50% of tumours occur in the lower third of the oesophagus and only about 15% in the upper third. Heavy alcohol intake is associated with at least a 20 times greater risk and smokers have at least five times the risk of non-smokers; however, these risk factors classically predispose only to squamous cell carcinoma.

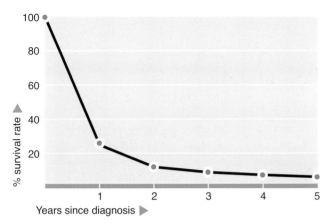

Fig. 22.1 **Survival after diagnosis of oesophageal carcinoma**

Since 1980 there has been a 70% increase in the proportion of oesophageal adenocarcinomas relative to squamous cell carcinomas in many Western countries. The reason is not clear, but may be related to the widespread use of acid-suppressing medication and possibly to alterations in diet. There appears to be no familial predisposition but people with structural and functional disorders, such as peptic oesophagitis and stricture, achalasia, oesophageal web or pharyngeal pouch, are all at considerably greater risk of the disease. Most women who develop upper third lesions have a pre-existing oesophageal web or pharyngeal pouch, both in themselves very rare.

Areas of exceptionally high incidence have been reported in China, elsewhere in the Far East, and around the Caspian Sea. There is some evidence that a fungus which grows on food grain may be responsible. This epidemiological pattern suggests that chronic local tissue irritation is an important aetiological factor, with different factors perhaps predisposing to the two main histological types. One common finding in dietary studies is an association with low intake of fruit and vegetables, and attention is particularly focused on lack of dietary antioxidants which may allow unopposed free radicals to cause excessive tissue damage.

INVESTIGATION OF SUSPECTED OESOPHAGEAL CARCINOMA

Dysphagia or pain on swallowing (**odynophagia**) in a middle-aged or elderly patient demands urgent investigation in order to exclude carcinoma (see Box 22.1). General physical examination is usually unrewarding except in very advanced disease. In these cases, there may be signs of **wasting**, **hepatomegaly** due to metastases, a **Virchow's node** in the left supraclavicular fossa or sometimes **hoarseness** as a result of recurrent laryngeal nerve involvement. Direct inspection of the oesophagus using a flexible endoscope is necessary and biopsies are taken of any suspicious areas.

Staging the tumour

Once carcinoma of the oesophagus is diagnosed, it is important to establish the extent of local invasion and discover whether metastasis to thoracic or abdominal lymph nodes or the liver has occurred; this will determine whether potentially curative treatment is appropriate or just palliative treatment. CT scanning is the principal investigation but it frequently understages the disease. **Staging laparoscopy** can show peritoneal or visceral metastases not seen on CT scan; some units employ staging **thoracoscopy** to assess the pleural cavity for the same reasons. **Endoscopic ultrasound (EUS)** demonstrates very clearly the different layers of the gut wall and thus helps to delineate the tumour more accurately both in length and, more importantly, depth of invasion (T stage). It has a high sensitivity and specificity for locally involved lymph nodes. It can also be used to biopsy suspicious nodes in otherwise inaccessible locations (**EUS-guided biopsy**), thus enhancing the staging process and in some cases preventing unnecessary surgery. Once more

Fig. 22.2 Barrett's oesophagus and oesophageal carcinoma

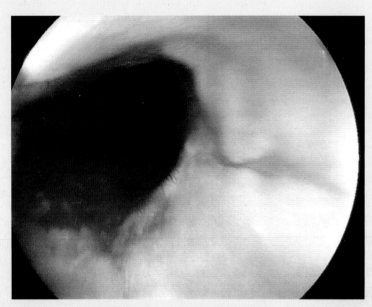

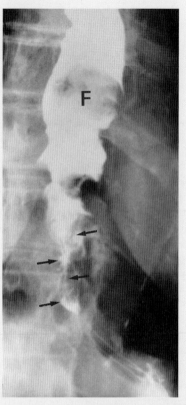

(a)

(b)

(a) Endoscopic view of Barrett's oesophagus demonstrating linear ulceration and deeper red mucosa with chronic ulceration at the oesophago-gastric junction. Diagnosis is confirmed on biopsy. This condition is potentially premalignant. **(b)** Barium swallow in an elderly man who presented with almost complete dysphagia. The film shows the lower end of the oesophagus which has an irregular narrowing of the lumen (arrowed). This appearance did not alter in several views of the same area and is characteristic of malignancy. Nevertheless, endoscopy is usually performed to obtain histological confirmation by means of biopsies. The oesophagus above is moderately dilated and contains a bolus of food **F** which cannot pass onwards.

than four lymph nodes are involved, the greater the number of involved nodes, the lower the chances of surgical cure.

MANAGEMENT OF CARCINOMA OF THE OESOPHAGUS

The ideal treatment would be to eliminate the cancer. In practice, this can rarely be achieved because of overt or occult spread. Even if cure is impossible, oesophageal obstruction must be relieved to allow the patient to eat and to prevent the appalling consequence of complete obstruction, i.e. inability to swallow even saliva.

Surgical resection of the tumour is mainly employed only when the aim is cure. For incurable patients with dysphagia, palliative procedures to restore swallowing such as argon plasma tissue coagulation, laser treatment or stent insertion can be effective and are certainly preferable to major surgery, particularly if life expectancy is short.

Adjuvant therapy in addition to surgery has a role in some patients with carcinoma of the oesophagus, although clinical trials are still continuing to determine the precise indications. Most often, radiotherapy is given alone or in combination with chemotherapy (chemoradiotherapy) before surgery (**neoadjuvant therapy**) in an attempt to shrink or downsize the tumour.

Historically, radiotherapy has been given as the sole form of treatment for squamous carcinoma. Intubation of the tumour was often needed before radiotherapy to avoid total obstruction as a result of swelling in the short term. Results of this form of radiotherapy were often disappointing because of adverse local effects. Radiotherapy nowadays tends to be reserved for palliation.

The choice of treatment depends on the patient's fitness and the stage of the disease. Comorbidity due to the adverse effects of alcohol and cigarettes, for example chronic lung disease or cirrhosis, may influence the decision. Cardiac fitness is assessed clinically and by electrocardiography (ECG) and sometimes echocardiography. In addition, spirometry and blood gases should be performed to assess the patient's fitness for thoracotomy. If the FEV$_1$ is less than 2 L, single lung ventilation used during thoracotomy is unlikely to be tolerated. A preoperative staging workup usually includes CT scanning of chest and abdomen and endoscopic ultrasound. Diagnostic laparoscopy may be undertaken for tumours at the gastro-oesophageal junction to assess serosal involvement and peritoneal spread.

Surgery

Once a decision has been made to undertake surgery, the choice of operation depends on the level of the lesion. In general, the aim is to remove the tumour with an appropriate safety margin, to perform a two-field lymphadenectomy (removing mediastinal and abdominal lymph nodes) and to achieve a leak-free anastomosis.

Lesions above the carina (the tracheal bifurcation) are usually dealt with by a three-stage **oesophagectomy** known as the **McKeown operation**, with all stages performed at the same operation. The first stage is to mobilise the tumour and the oesophagus via a right thoracotomy with the patient in the left lateral position. The second stage involves rolling the patient into a supine position and performing a laparotomy to allow the stomach to be mobilised and fashioned into a conduit. A third incision is then made in the neck through which oesophagus and tumour are delivered and the gastric conduit is anastomosed to the cervical oesophagus. A cervical anastomosis is safer than an intrathoracic one, as the consequences of anastomotic leakage would be less devastating.

If the tumour arises lower in the oesophagus, a two-stage **Ivor Lewis operation** is usually performed. The abdomen is opened first, and the stomach mobilised and fashioned into a conduit. The patient is then turned into a left lateral position and the right chest opened, the oesophagus mobilised and the tumour and lymph nodes excised. Finally the gastric conduit is drawn up into the chest and anastomosed to the proximal oesophageal remnant. If this is impossible, a loop of jejunum or a single end of jejunum (Roux-en-Y) is drawn up and used to make the connection (see Fig. 22.3). Controversy exists

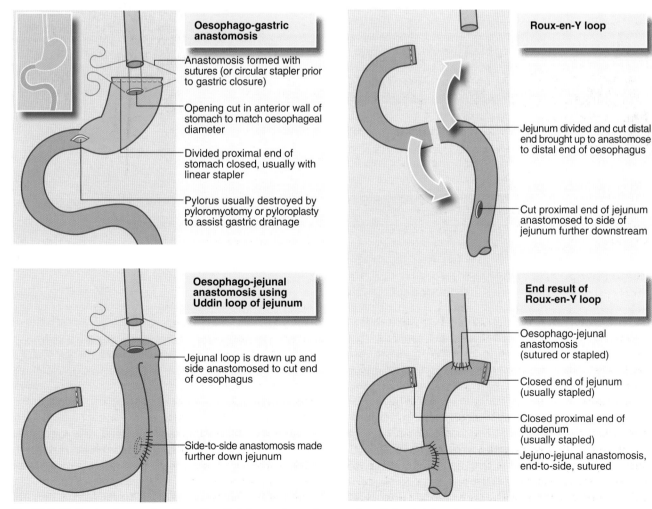

Oesophago-gastric anastomosis

- Anastomosis formed with sutures (or circular stapler prior to gastric closure)
- Opening cut in anterior wall of stomach to match oesophageal diameter
- Divided proximal end of stomach closed, usually with linear stapler
- Pylorus usually destroyed by pyloromyotomy or pyloroplasty to assist gastric drainage

Oesophago-jejunal anastomosis using Uddin loop of jejunum

- Jejunal loop is drawn up and side anastomosed to cut end of oesophagus
- Side-to-side anastomosis made further down jejunum

Roux-en-Y loop

- Jejunum divided and cut distal end brought up to anastomose to distal end of oesophagus
- Cut proximal end of jejunum anastomosed to side of jejunum further downstream

End result of Roux-en-Y loop

- Oesophago-jejunal anastomosis (sutured or stapled)
- Closed end of jejunum (usually stapled)
- Closed proximal end of duodenum (usually stapled)
- Jejuno-jejunal anastomosis, end-to-side, sutured

Fig. 22.3 Methods of reconstruction after distal oesophagectomy and partial or total gastrectomy

about whether extending lymphadenectomy into the neck, so-called 'three-field lymphadenectomy', is beneficial. The procedure increases the operative risks and only appears to benefit a subgroup with proximal tumours and fewer than five nodes involved.

An operation that gained some popularity is **transhiatal oesophagectomy**. A thoracotomy is avoided by mobilising the oesophagus and the cancer by blunt dissection from the abdomen via the diaphragmatic hiatus and via a neck incision, performing the anastomosis in the neck after resection. However, interest is waning, chiefly because of concerns that the safety margins of excision may be insufficient for potential cure and adequate lymphadenectomy is impossible in the chest. There is also an increased risk of damaging veins in the chest during dissection (particularly the azygos vein) and causing catastrophic haemorrhage.

There is increasing interest in laparoscopic approaches to these cancers, and many units in Europe, Australia and America are now regularly performing laparoscopic oesophagectomies and gastrectomies. Techniques involve combined laparoscopic and thoracoscopic approaches. Perioperative morbidity and mortality and cancer recurrence rates appear to be at least comparable with open surgery, and there are the additional benefits of minimal access surgery. In the UK, most centres still largely undertake open surgery but several leading centres are beginning to produce satisfactory results with this approach.

Oesophagectomy is always a major undertaking and carries the potentially fatal risk of anastomotic breakdown. This may lead to mediastinitis, lung abscess or oesophago-pleural fistula. Patients need to be made aware of the risks in relation to the benefits, as well as the likely prolonged convalescent period and the long-term morbidity. Postoperative problems include dysphagia, small capacity for food (early satiety), and reflux.

Inoperable lesions

If operation is inappropriate, oesophageal patency can often be restored by palliative ablation of the tumour with absolute alcohol injections or by cutting a pathway through the tumour with laser therapy via a gastroscope. Both of these treatments can be repeated as the tumour regrows. Alternatively, the oesophagus can be intubated by inserting a cloth-covered metal stent (see Fig. 22.4) through the lesion. This is usually done under intravenous sedation, using the endoscopic technique of **pulsion intubation.** First the oesophageal lesion is dilated then the stent inserted using X-ray guidance. These tubes relieve symptoms, but food has to be liquidised and the tube kept 'clean' by taking fizzy drinks after eating. If the lesion is situated in the lower oesophagus, stent insertion effectively bypasses the tumour but also counteracts any residual function of the lower oesophageal sphincter. This renders the patient more susceptible to acid reflux, for which antacid medication may need to be prescribed.

Fig. 22.4 Intubation of oesophageal cancer: cloth-covered metal stent in situ

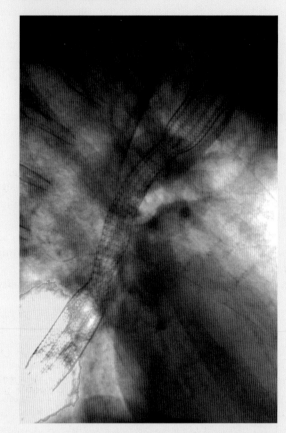

This 70-year-old man presented with inoperable carcinoma of the middle third of the oesophagus. The malignant stricture was dilated via a flexible gastroscope and a Dacron-covered metal stent inserted to keep the stricture open as a palliative measure. This lateral chest X-ray shows the stent in situ.

HIATUS HERNIA AND REFLUX OESOPHAGITIS

PATHOPHYSIOLOGY

The oesophagus is essentially a tube of smooth muscle conveying food to the stomach by peristalsis. At the lower end of the oesophagus there is a tonically active sphincter mechanism. Its contraction coordinates with oesophageal peristalsis, relaxing to allow food to enter the stomach. The purpose of the sphincter mechanism is to prevent reflux of stomach contents into the oesophagus. After passing through the diaphragm, the oesophagus continues for about 2 cm within the abdomen before joining the stomach. The sphincter mechanism is not completely understood but it probably involves several components: a functional (but not anatomical) sphincter of the oesophageal wall immediately above the diaphragm and the smooth muscle at the gastric cardia. This is reinforced by

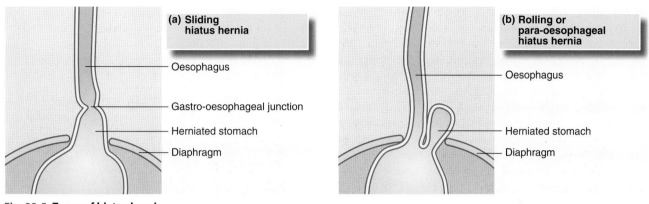

Fig. 22.5 Types of hiatus hernia
(a) Sliding hiatus hernia, which is common. This type disrupts the physiological anti-reflux mechanism. (b) Rolling or para-oesophageal hiatus hernia, which is rare. The anti-reflux mechanism is usually left intact.

contraction of the diaphragmatic crura, by the acute angle at which the oesophagus enters the stomach and by the 'flutter valve' effect of intra-abdominal pressure on the abdominal portion of the oesophagus causing collapse of the lumen.

Hiatus hernia is an abnormality which occurs when the proximal part of the stomach passes through the diaphragmatic hiatus proximally into the chest (see Fig. 22.5). Around 90% of hiatus hernias are of the **sliding type**, in which the gastro-oesophageal junction is drawn up into the chest and a segment of stomach becomes constricted at the diaphragmatic hiatus. The hernia tends to slide up into the chest with each peristaltic contraction. These hernias may become huge and, rarely, may contain the whole stomach including the pylorus and first part of the duodenum, sometimes with part of the colon as well. In the 10% of non-sliding cases, the gastro-oesophageal junction remains below the diaphragm and a bulge of stomach herniates through the hiatus beside the oesophagus. These are described as **para-oesophageal** or **rolling hiatus hernias**.

In sliding hiatus hernia, the lower oesophageal sphincter mechanism often becomes defective, causing reflux of acid–peptic stomach contents into the oesophagus. This is not a problem with rolling hiatus hernias which more usually present with pain, possibly due to torsion of the stomach within the hernial sac.

Hiatus hernia in adults is commonly associated with smoking and obesity. The pressure of intra-abdominal fat may be contributory. Hiatus hernia can also be a congenital abnormality presenting in early infancy.

CLINICAL FEATURES OF REFLUX OESOPHAGITIS

Hiatus hernia is common, especially in women, and becomes more common with advancing years. Only a small proportion of patients with a hiatus hernia actually experience symptoms of **acid–peptic reflux**, i.e. 'heartburn'; moreover, reflux can occur without a hiatus hernia.

Research has shown that the adverse effects of reflux are more likely to affect patients with impaired peristaltic 'clearing' of gastric contents from the lower oesophagus. Reflux causes acute inflammation (**oesophagitis**). This is experienced as burning retrosternal pain (**heartburn**), bitter-tasting regurgitation or other forms of 'indigestion'. Symptoms are typically worse at night when the patient lies flat in bed or on bending forward during the day.

If reflux is severe and persistent, mucosal destruction is recurrent and inflammation becomes chronic. Progressive scarring leads to fibrosis of the wall and this may lead to narrowing (stricture) of the lumen and the symptom of dysphagia. Longstanding oesophageal reflux predisposes to the development of **Barrett's oesophagus** with normal squamous oesophageal epithelium being replaced by metaplastic columnar mucosa. Barrett's oesophagus is the only known predisposing factor for adenocarcinoma of the lower oesophagus, which, as mentioned earlier, has increased by 70% in developed countries since 1980. Histological examination of biopsies may reveal **specialised intestinal metaplasia** (SIM) or **severe dysplasia**, both of which are markers for malignant change, supporting the metaplasia/dysplasia/carcinoma model for the evolution of lower oesophageal cancer.

Occasionally, oesophageal reflux symptoms are severe and acute, causing chest pain which may easily be mistaken for angina or even myocardial infarction. There is often an element of **oesophageal spasm** which, like angina, is relieved by glyceryl trinitrate and similar drugs. This may confuse the diagnosis.

In general, hiatus hernias can be assessed with endoscopy, with biopsy if necessary. The latter is important to exclude carcinoma, especially if dysphagia is experienced. In specialised units, **oesophageal manometry studies** are used to assess the muscular function of the oesophagus and **oesophageal pH studies** are performed to assess the extent and severity of reflux. These studies are often used to help determine which patients are likely to benefit from surgery. Rarely barium swallow examination (see

Fig. 22.6 Sliding hiatus hernia

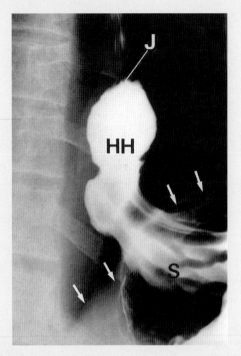

Sliding hiatus hernia in a 63-year-old woman. The hiatus hernia is marked **HH**, the stomach **S** and the oesophago-gastric junction **J**; the position of the diaphragm is arrowed.

Figs 22.6 and 22.7) may be necessary to delineate complicated anatomy.

MANAGEMENT OF HIATUS HERNIA AND REFLUX OESOPHAGITIS

Nearly all patients can be managed conservatively, with surgery reserved for intractable cases. Treatment is aimed at reducing acid–pepsin activity and preventing reflux.

Reducing reflux

Weight reduction, where appropriate, is the most effective long-term anti-reflux measure. Changes in the diet will often of themselves improve symptoms of reflux. For example, **alcohol** causes the sphincter to relax and many medical students can personally vouch for the combined effect of beer and spicy food! Other foods known to precipitate reflux are coffee, tea and chocolate. Reflux can be reduced substantially by taking smaller, more frequent and drier meals, by using blocks to elevate the head of the bed at night and by sleeping on more pillows in an upright position. **Smoking** induces sphincter relaxation, and quitting often reduces reflux dramatically. Patients should also be advised to wear loose-fitting clothing, and avoid bending or straining soon after meals. **Alginate drugs**, available in liquid or chewable tablet form, produce a foamy surface layer on the stomach contents and are said to coat the lower oesophagus, protecting it from the effects of reflux. These drugs are most effective if taken soon after food.

Prokinetic agents

Drugs that stimulate motility can have a useful effect in reflux. **Metoclopramide** is a dopamine antagonist that stimulates gastric emptying and increases small bowel transit as well as enhancing contraction of the oesophageal sphincter. **Cisapride** is a prokinetic drug without dopamine antagonist action; it is thought to stimulate motility by releasing acetylcholine in the intestinal wall. This drug is helpful in oesophageal reflux, gastric stasis and some cases of non-ulcer dyspepsia. Unfortunately it has been linked with cardiac complications and its licence has been withdrawn for widespread prescription. It can, however, still be prescribed on a named-patient basis.

Reducing acid–pepsin production

Reducing acid–pepsin attack is probably the mainstay of treatment for reflux disease. It is accomplished as for chronic peptic ulcer disease (see Ch. 21). Simple antacid drugs and H_2-receptor antagonists are sometimes effective but in severe cases **omeprazole** or another proton pump inhibitor (PPI) is the drug of choice. Drugs and food that irritate the lower oesophagus should be avoided.

Management of strictures

Inflammatory fibrous strictures used to be regularly dilated with gum-elastic **bougies** of progressively increasing size under general anaesthesia via a rigid oesophagoscope. Nowadays, dilatation is usually performed under intravenous sedation using flexible gastroscopy under X-ray control. A flexible guide-wire is first positioned across the stricture via the endoscope and graded metal or plastic dilators passed over the wire to dilate the stricture. If the stricture recurs and causes dysphagia despite suitable conservative treatment for reflux, an anti-reflux operation may be indicated. This usually allows healing of mucosal damage and may prevent further stricture formation.

Surgery for hiatus hernia and reflux oesophagitis

Surgery is reserved for intractable symptoms, recurrent stricture and chronic peptic ulceration which fail to respond to PPI therapy. This particularly includes patients with Barrett's oesophagus (having excluded those with a high risk of malignancy by biopsy). Surgery may also be indicated for the young or middle-aged patient in whom PPIs produce a partial or complete response but who do not wish to take long-term medication. The traditional operations for formal repair of hiatus hernia, performed via chest or abdomen (e.g. Belsey Mark IV), have largely been superseded by **Nissen fundoplication**. This abdominal (or thoracic) operation involves dissection of the

Fig. 22.7 Sliding hiatus hernia

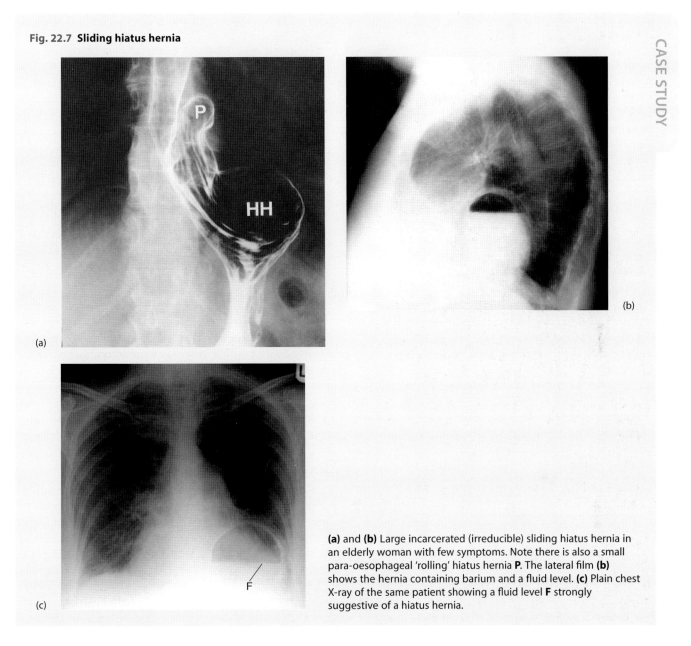

(a)

(b)

(c)

(a) and (b) Large incarcerated (irreducible) sliding hiatus hernia in an elderly woman with few symptoms. Note there is also a small para-oesophageal 'rolling' hiatus hernia **P**. The lateral film **(b)** shows the hernia containing barium and a fluid level. **(c)** Plain chest X-ray of the same patient showing a fluid level **F** strongly suggestive of a hiatus hernia.

gastro-oesophageal junction at the hiatus, tightening up the crura (which may have become lax, thus allowing the hiatus hernia to develop) and wrapping the gastric fundus around the intra-abdominal portion of the oesophagus to recreate a flutter valve.

In experienced hands, laparoscopic Nissen fundoplication is the operation of choice and allows the patient a rapid return to normal levels of activity. Clinical trials have shown that the laparoscopic approach gives results comparable to open fundoplication. Typical side effects of any Nissen operation include temporary dysphagia, gas-bloat syndrome (due to retained air and a decreased ability to belch) and consequently increased flatus. These problems usually settle in time, but must be clearly explained to the patient before obtaining consent for operation. The most significant (but fortunately rare)

postoperative complication is that of a **slipped wrap**. In this case, the fundal wrap slips down onto the stomach, or up through the hiatus into the chest (usually after a bout of excessive vomiting). In either case, the patient usually presents with acute onset chest and/or upper abdominal pain and dysphagia. This complication should be managed as a surgical emergency with diagnostic confirmation followed by early reoperation.

ACHALASIA

PATHOPHYSIOLOGY AND CLINICAL PRESENTATION OF ACHALASIA

Achalasia is an uncommon disorder of oesophageal motility. Normal peristalsis is disrupted throughout the oesophagus, causing uncoordinated and inadequate relaxation of the lower oesophageal sphincter.

In pathological terms, there is a poorly understood neurological defect involving Auerbach's myenteric (parasympathetic) plexus. As mentioned, the entire oesophagus is affected rather than just the cardia, as the obsolete term 'achalasia of the cardia' would imply. The condition presents in two main age groups, young adults and the elderly. In the latter, the cause may be a central rather than a local neurological defect. Achalasia, as with any structural abnormality of the oesophagus, predisposes to carcinoma.

Clinically, the cardiac sphincter becomes constricted and the proximal oesophagus dilates with accumulated fluid and solids. Difficulty in swallowing fluids is the usual presenting symptom. Solids tend to sink to the lower end of the dilated oesophagus, whereas fluids spill over into the trachea causing **spluttering dysphagia** (see Ch. 18) and coughing, particularly at night. Vomiting and retrosternal pain may occur in more severe cases. The degree of dysphagia tends to vary and probably depends on the amount of food residue in the oesophagus at the time.

INVESTIGATION OF SUSPECTED ACHALASIA

Chest X-ray may demonstrate that the mediastinal shadow is widened by a dilated oesophagus; sometimes a fluid level is visible in the oesophagus behind the heart. At endoscopy there is the typical appearance of a capacious distal oesophagus, usually with food and fluid residue, and a tight lower oesophageal sphincter that may or may not admit the tip of the gastroscope. It is important to visualise the oesophago-gastric junction in order to exclude an occult neoplasm masquerading as achalasia (**pseudoachalasia**). Barium swallow examination reveals gross dilatation of the oesophagus with a tapering constriction at the lower end. The constriction barely allows contrast to pass into the stomach (see Fig. 22.8). Under fluoroscopic screening, uncoordinated purposeless peristaltic waves can often be seen; these are described as **tertiary contractions** and are distinct from the normal coordinated pattern of primary and secondary contractions. Oesophageal manometry is the cardinal test for achalasia, demonstrating excessive lower oesophageal sphincter pressure that fails to relax on swallowing and abnormal peristalsis in patients with a more chronic history.

Fig. 22.8 Late-stage achalasia in a 60-year-old man

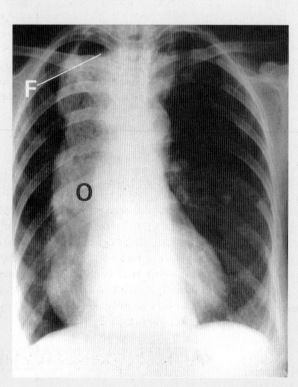
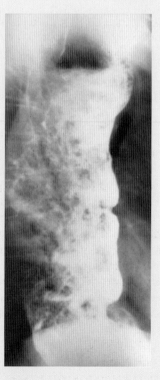

(a)   (b)

(a) The chest X-ray shows gross mediastinal widening caused by a massively dilated oesophagus **O** filled with food debris. Note the mottled appearance of the oesophagus and the fluid level **F** at its upper end. Note also the absence of a gastric air bubble below the diaphragm. This is characteristic of achalasia. **(b)** Barium swallow in the same patient. This confirms the findings on the chest X-ray.

Fig. 22.9 Oesophageal carcinoma secondary to achalasia

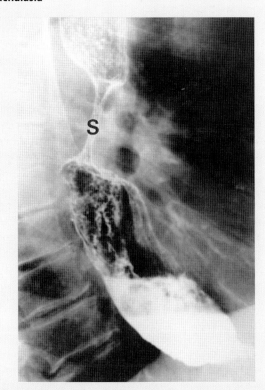

Malignant stricture **S** in the middle third of the oesophagus in a 60-year-old woman with achalasia of long standing. She had a Heller's myotomy at the age of 26. Note that this surgery does not reduce the inherent predisposition to carcinoma.

Fig. 22.10 Pharyngeal pouch

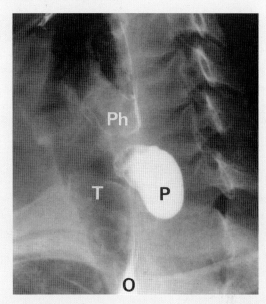

Lateral view during barium swallow examination in a 41-year-old man complaining of mild dysphagia; the X-ray shows a contrast-filled pouch **P** extending from the pharynx **Ph**. Note the gas-filled trachea **T** lying anteriorly. **O** = oesophagus.

MANAGEMENT OF ACHALASIA

The condition is by its nature incurable, and treatment is directed at relieving the distal obstruction. The standard operation is via the abdomen, and involves a longitudinal incision of the lower oesophageal and upper gastric muscle wall until the mucosa bulges through (**Heller's cardiomyotomy**); this is best combined with a partial fundoplication to overcome the almost inevitable reflux it will cause. The operation can be performed open or laparoscopically. Balloon dilatation is sometimes used as an alternative to operation and results appear to be virtually as good in experienced hands. Patients with achalasia should be followed up and periodically endoscoped to exclude developing carcinoma (see Fig. 22.9).

PHARYNGEAL POUCH

Pharyngeal pouch is a rare cause of dysphagia. It arises at the junction of pharynx and oesophagus, and probably results from lack of coordination between the inferior constrictor muscle and cricopharyngeus during swallowing. At this point, there is an area of relative weakness known as **Killian's dehiscence**. The result is a progressive mucosal outpouching between the two muscles. The condition is best diagnosed by barium swallow (see Fig. 22.10). Pharyngeal pouch is easily perforated during endoscopy, and therefore if endoscopy is performed to investigate 'high' dysphagia this diagnosis should be considered and the procedure performed by an experienced endoscopist. Treatment of pharyngeal pouch is by surgical excision from the side of the neck, or via a completely endoluminal approach.

OESOPHAGEAL WEB

Circumferential mucosal folds (or webs) may occur in the oesophagus producing annular narrowing of the lumen and causing dysphagia. They also predispose to carcinoma in the long term. In the upper oesophagus, they are found in association with severe iron deficiency anaemia, particularly in women. The triad of dysphagia, anaemia and atrophic glossitis is known as **Plummer–Vinson** or **Paterson–Brown-Kelly syndrome**.

GASTRO-OESOPHAGEAL VARICES

PATHOPHYSIOLOGY OF GASTRO-OESOPHAGEAL VARICES

Gastro-oesophageal varices result from **portal venous hypertension**. The most common cause is cirrhosis

Fig. 22.11 Endoscopic view of oesophageal varices

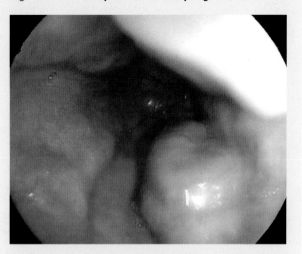

This man of 63 was known to have alcoholic cirrhosis and had suffered one acute gastrointestinal haemorrhage, treated successfully by injection of bleeding varices. The bulging blue masses can be seen protruding into the oesophageal lumen.

of the liver, usually associated with alcohol abuse. Less common causes include portal vein thrombosis, hepatic vein thrombosis (**Budd–Chiari syndrome**) and schistosomiasis.

As resistance to flow and pressure rises in the portal venous system, abnormal venous communications develop between the peripheral part of the portal system and the systemic venous circulation. This is known as **portal-systemic shunting**. Multiple large veins appear in the peritoneal cavity and retroperitoneal area, making any form of abdominal surgery hazardous. Large submucosal veins also appear at the lower end of the oesophagus and gastric fundus, and these are known as **gastro-oesophageal varices** (see Fig. 22.11). These varices can produce massive gastrointestinal haemorrhage, possibly related to rises in intravariceal pressure. Up to 40% of cirrhotic patients suffer variceal haemorrhage at some stage.

A further result of portal hypertension is splenic enlargement. This may produce the effects of **hypersplenism**, namely anaemia, thrombocytopenia and leucopenia. Patients in the late stages of cirrhosis also develop **ascites**.

If massive portal-systemic shunting of blood occurs either spontaneously or as a result of a surgically created shunt to treat portal hypertension, **portal-systemic encephalopathy** may develop. This is due to toxic substances such as ammonia being absorbed from the intestine and passing directly into the systemic circulation without first traversing the liver where they would normally be detoxified.

ELECTIVE MANAGEMENT OF GASTRO-OESOPHAGEAL VARICES

Gastro-oesophageal varices are not usually treated unless they have bled. Occasionally, elective treatment is carried out in cases where haemorrhage is considered highly likely; with the improving efficacy of banding and sclerotherapy, some clinicians believe that lower-risk asymptomatic varices should be treated electively. After recovery from an acute bleed, varices should be treated at planned intervals by banding or injection sclerotherapy until they are eliminated.

MANAGEMENT OF BLEEDING GASTRO-OESOPHAGEAL VARICES

Diagnosis and resuscitation

When a patient with known cirrhosis or varices presents with massive upper gastrointestinal haemorrhage, the first priority is resuscitation. Following this, the source of haemorrhage is sought by endoscopy. In fact only about half of these patients will be bleeding from oesophageal varices. The rest have bleeding gastric varices, gastric erosions or Mallory–Weiss tears of the lower oesophagus. In this last condition, arterial bleeding is the cause and it does not respond to measures designed to treat bleeding varices, but is usually self-limiting. Occasionally, bleeding duodenal or gastric ulcers are found. The management of the patient varies according to the diagnosis. Whatever treatment is undertaken, it must be remembered that cirrhotic patients often have defective clotting which may be further exacerbated by massive haemorrhage. It is prudent to perform clotting studies and give specific corrective factors.

Treatment

If bleeding is from varices, an attempt may be made at endoscopy to band or inject them with a sclerosant (e.g. ethanolamine or sodium tetradecyl sulphate (STD)). The mainstay of initial treatment is an **octreotide infusion**. More than 75% of patients initially respond to this therapy. Meanwhile, resuscitation continues with blood volume replacement, fresh-frozen plasma and platelets. Excess water and sodium should be avoided as this rapidly migrates into the peritoneal cavity as ascites. Hepatic encephalopathy should be anticipated as a result of the protein load of blood in the bowel and oral neomycin or lactulose administered. Delirium tremens may also require treatment if the patient is an alcoholic.

In patients not responding to octreotide, an attempt is made to apply tamponade. After endotracheal intubation to protect the airway, a special tube is passed through the mouth into the stomach and a balloon inflated. Traction is exerted on the upper end for up to 4 hours to arrest the haemorrhage. Several varieties of tube are in use: the

Sengstaken–Blakemore tube has separate intra-gastric and oesophageal balloons and depends for its action upon physiological arrest of bleeding. Most cases cease bleeding with inflation of the gastric balloon alone and traction. The **Linton balloon** is an alternative comprising a single large intra-gastric balloon (300–600 ml) which allows simultaneous endoscopy and rubber banding or injection sclerotherapy of varices.

Operative surgery for oesophageal varices has dwindled in recent years because of the effectiveness of injection sclerotherapy. Now that the problem of variceal haemorrhage can be overcome, the mortality in these patients is related to the progression of the underlying cirrhosis.

If variceal haemorrhage continues despite effective conservative therapy, transjugular intrahepatic portal-systemic stenting (**TIPS**) is sometimes used. This involves cannulating the internal jugular vein and placing an angiography catheter within the intra-hepatic vena cava. Using combined fluoroscopy and ultrasound, the catheter is guided into the portal system within the liver. Then an expanding metal stent is placed to connect the intra-hepatic portal system to the vena cava.

As a last resort, emergency surgical treatment is performed, but all operations carry a high mortality in such seriously ill patients. The simplest operation is **transgastric oesophageal stapling**. A circular stapler is passed into the oesophagus via a gastrotomy, a ligature tied around the oesophagus between the staple cartridge and the anvil, and the gun fired. This places two rows of staples through the full thickness of the oesophageal wall, disconnecting the longitudinal veins. However, this is not effective for bleeding gastric varices.

Emergency **portal-systemic shunting** operations are occasionally used but carry a risk of portal-systemic encephalopathy, although they reliably arrest haemorrhage. Shunting operations are still sometimes used fol-

Table 22.1 Child's criteria for assessing operative risk in portal hypertension

Risk factor	Score points		
	1	2	3
Encephalopathy	None	Minimal	Marked
Ascites	None	Slight	Moderate
Bilirubin (μmol/L)	< 35	36–50	> 50
Albumin (g/L)	> 35	28–35	< 28
Prothrombin ratio	< 1.4	1.4–2.0	> 2.0

Each criterion is scored and the total added:
Child's grade A (good risk) scores 5–6
Grade B (moderate risk) scores 7–9
Grade C (bad risk) scores 10–15

lowing recovery from acute haemorrhage but many doctors believe that repeated rubber banding or injection sclerotherapy via a flexible endoscope is the best prophylaxis against further haemorrhage.

All types of surgical portal-systemic shunts carry a risk of **encephalopathy**, although shunt design has been modified to minimise this risk. The original operation was **portacaval shunting**, in which the main portal vein was anastomosed to the inferior vena cava. Later variations include **mesocaval shunting** in which the superior mesenteric vein is connected to the inferior vena cava via an interposition graft, and **lienorenal shunting** (the **Warren shunt**) in which the splenic vein is anastomosed to the left renal vein. The last is said to cause the lowest incidence of encephalopathy but is also the least effective for decompressing the portal venous pressure.

Operative risk in these patients has been calculated using **Child's criteria**, shown in Table 22.1.

23 Tumours of the stomach and small intestine

INTRODUCTION

Benign tumours occasionally occur in the stomach but unfortunately most gastric tumours are malignant. Nearly all of these are adenocarcinomas, whilst the rest are lymphomas or the occasional carcinoid tumour or sarcoma. True adenomatous **gastric polyps** are rare; most gastric polypoid lesions are small benign hyperplastic nodules.

Tumours of the small bowel are rare. Of the malignant tumours, lymphomas and stromal tumours (GIST) are much more common than adenocarcinomas. **Peutz–Jeghers syndrome** is a rare inherited disorder characterised by multiple benign polyps in the small bowel and perioral pigmentation. It is fairly commonly encountered at student examinations (see Ch. 27)!

CARCINOMA OF STOMACH

PATHOLOGY OF GASTRIC CARCINOMA

Gastric carcinomas are almost exclusively adenocarcinomas. Two distinct histopathological groups are recognised, each with its own epidemiological associations.

The **intestinal type** of carcinoma has histological features similar to intestinal epithelium. Cells grow in clumps and there is a marked inflammatory infiltrate. The second variety is the **diffuse type**. Here the cells are singular, often arranged in single file and surrounded by a marked stromal reaction. The tumour cells have large intracellular **mucin** droplets which displace the nucleus to the cell periphery, giving the characteristic **signet ring appearance** (Fig. 23.1).

Gastric carcinomas develop in three morphological forms; the intestinal type largely produces fungating tumours and malignant ulcers and the diffuse type causes infiltrating carcinomas. The first two have a better prognosis than the last.

- **Fungating tumours**—these polypoid lesions may grow to a huge size
- **Malignant ulcers**—these probably result from necrosis in the centre of broad-based solid tumours. Malignant ulcers are often larger than peptic ulcers (except for the giant benign ulcer of the elderly) with a heaped-up indurated (hardened) margin. There is no surrounding mucosal puckering as occurs in inflammatory scarring
- **Infiltrating carcinomas**—this form spreads widely beneath the mucosa, and diffusely and extensively invades the muscle wall. This causes marked thickening and rigidity and the entire stomach contracts to a very small capacity. The condition is known as **linitis plastica** and its appearance is likened to a 'leather bottle'. Linitis plastica affects a slightly younger age group than intestinal-type cancer and has a very poor prognosis. Diagnosis may be delayed because the endoscopic changes are often subtle and standard biopsies of the mucosa may not show malignancy

'**Early gastric cancer**' is defined as cancer limited to the mucosa and submucosa. This is rarely detected in patients who present with symptoms but is found most often as a result of endoscopic screening or else fortuitously whilst investigating possible peptic ulcer. Results of surgery in this group are excellent, with a cure rate of about 90%.

EPIDEMIOLOGY OF GASTRIC CARCINOMA

Gastric cancer is the second most common cancer in the world and also the second most frequent cause of cancer deaths; it is surpassed only by lung cancer. The disease is rare before the age of 50 and increases in frequency thereafter. Males have one and a half times the risk of females, and the disease is more common in lower socio-economic

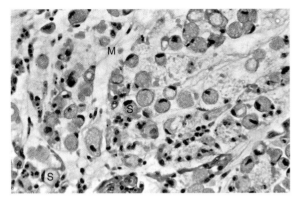

Fig. 23.1 Carcinoma of the stomach—histopathology
High-power view of typical infiltrating type of gastric carcinoma showing numerous signet ring cells **S**. This appearance is due to the presence of intracellular mucin **M**.

groups. Japan has the highest annual incidence with a crude rate of 124 per 100 000 per year in men and 60 in women. In the UK, equivalent rates are 21 for men and 12 for women, and in the USA 10 for men and 6 for women. The offspring of Japanese immigrants to America carry no higher risk than other Americans, providing evidence that environmental rather than racial factors are central in the aetiology. In much of the Western world, both the incidence and death rates of gastric cancer have steadily decreased over recent years, and this results almost exclusively from a decline in the intestinal type. In Japan, the age standardised mortality rate for men has fallen from 63 per 100 000 per annum in 1970 to 29 in 1997; in the USA equivalent rates were 8.4 in 1970 falling to 4.1 in 1997.

The epidemiology of gastric carcinoma gives enticing clues as to the causes of the disease. There are marked regional variations in incidence which are largely explained by disparities in the rate of intestinal-type carcinomas. This, and the fact that this type is more prevalent in lower socio-economic groups, strongly suggests that environmental factors play an important part in the genesis of this histological type. However, there is probably no single common aetiological factor but rather a combination of co-factors that bring about malignant change. Japan with its very high incidence of this disease continues to play a leading role in research into early detection and management.

AETIOLOGY OF GASTRIC CARCINOMA AND PREMALIGNANT CONDITIONS

Atrophic gastritis

Multifocal atrophic gastritis (type B) has been identified as a condition that precedes intestinal-type gastric cancer. It probably represents one step of a sequence running from superficial gastritis, via atrophic gastritis, to intestinal and colonic metaplasia, dysplasia and even-

tually to cancer. Multifocal atrophic gastritis is the result of **chronic inflammation** and appears first on the lesser curve of the stomach. Risk factors for type B gastritis include *Helicobacter pylori* infection and certain items of diet (see below). Either may initiate the process and thereafter act along the same sequence towards malignancy. The **diffuse corporeal type of gastritis (type A)** that occurs in pernicious anaemia is a much weaker aetiological factor for cancer. Patients with this have a three-fold to six-fold increase in risk of developing gastric cancer, but the absolute risk remains low.

Helicobacter pylori infection

H. pylori is known to initiate peptic ulceration, and in recent years chronic *H. pylori* infection has become a prime suspect for initiating intestinal-type gastric cancer. The organism has the ability to colonise gastric mucosa over long periods and cause chronic gastritis which, in some cases, eventually progresses to type B multifocal atrophic gastritis. In one biopsy study of gastric cancers, *H. pylori* was found in 90% of intestinal-type cancers, whilst only 30% of the diffuse type were infected. Levels of IgG antibody to *H. pylori* were elevated in gastric cancer patients compared with controls, with odds ratios of between 4 and 6 in favour of a causative association; the risk progressively increased with rising antibody levels. However, more than 60% of controls without gastric cancer had elevated antibodies, so the picture is not simple. The carcinogenic mechanism of *H. pylori* may involve alterations to the gastric acid–pepsin environment, with increased cell turnover and possibly enhanced mucosal susceptibility to ingested carcinogens. *H. pylori* eradication does not reverse the gastric atrophy but does improve the enzymic and hormonal secretory capacity. As mentioned on page 365, *H. pylori* also appears likely to be involved in **gastric lymphoma** of the **mucosa-associated lymphoid tissue (MALT)** type.

Dietary factors

Dietary factors shown to influence the incidence of gastric cancer include excess intake of salt and nitroso compounds and a low intake of ascorbic acid. In this respect, diets high in dried and salted fish and salt-cured and smoke-cured meats appear to create a particular risk. Lettuce grown in temperate climates appears to offer a protective effect.

CLINICAL FEATURES OF GASTRIC CARCINOMA

Symptoms are often minimal until late in the course of the disease so that 70% of patients present with advanced local and/or metastatic disease. Lesions at the inlet or outlet of the stomach cause **obstructive symptoms** earlier than those in the body of the stomach where the diameter allows for substantial growth before encroaching on the

Box 23.1	Presenting features of gastric carcinoma

- Often asymptomatic until a late stage
- Non-specific epigastric pain and dyspepsia
- Iron deficiency anaemia
- Nausea and vomiting
- Anorexia and early satiety
- Feeling of abdominal fullness or discomfort
- Marked weight loss (cachexia)—late stage
- Epigastric mass (late stage)
- Left supraclavicular mass (metastasis in Virchow's node)
- Obstructive jaundice (metastases in the porta hepatis)
- Pelvic mass (metastases to ovaries)

forward progress of food. Vomiting occurs if the gastric outlet becomes obstructed, typically by tumours of the antrum, and dysphagia occurs with gastro-oesophageal tumours. Such cancers are not necessarily early in pathological terms, however. In patients proved to have true early gastric cancer, retrospective appraisal has shown that a high proportion had pre-existing upper gastrointestinal symptoms, most often dyspepsia and epigastric pain with food, although these were not necessarily caused by the cancer.

In **advanced disease**, up to half of patients are asymptomatic and the rest have pain, nausea, vomiting, anorexia or a feeling of fullness after small meals (**early satiety**). Sometimes these symptoms have been present for many months before the patient presents. **Anaemia** resulting from chronic occult blood loss is common and one-third have positive stool tests for occult blood. Overall, one-third have **cachexia** (severe weight loss and wasting). This usually indicates the presence of metastatic disease and may be the only manifestation of cancer; indeed, dramatic weight loss in the absence of other symptoms should alert the clinician to possible gastric carcinoma. This, or the presence of an epigastric mass, indicates that the possibility of surgical cure is remote. Of the 70% who present with advanced local disease (stage T_3), more than half have extensive abdominal nodal spread and half have distant metastases.

Fortunately, patients are now tending to present earlier, perhaps because persistent indigestion and upper gastrointestinal symptoms are more likely to prompt investigation than previously.

The presenting features of gastric carcinoma are summarised in Box 23.1.

Spread of gastric cancer

Invasive gastric cancer progresses to involve submucosal lymphatics, and the depth of penetration through the gastric wall correlates closely with the likelihood of nodal metastases. The tumour, node, metastasis (TNM) system is now the standard staging structure agreed internationally, with additional Japanese nomenclature designating particular groups of lymph nodes draining the stomach as **stations**, numbered 1–16. Lymphatic metastatic spread initially involves nodes in the coeliac axis and periduodenal area; these are known as perigastric stations 1–6. Involvement of these stations is considered N_1 in the TNM system. Positive nodes in the para-aortic area, splenic hilum and porta hepatis indicate a more advanced stage, with porta hepatis nodes sometimes causing obstructive jaundice. Involvement of these 'secondary' stations signals N_2, N_3 or even M_1. Clearance of these more distant lymph node stations is achieved by the radical R2 gastrectomy (pioneered in Japan). Histology of the nodes enhances the accuracy of TNM staging and improves the ability to predict long-term survival after surgery.

Direct spread and metastasis

- **Direct spread** into the transverse colon is not unusual in neglected cases and sometimes results in **gastro-colic fistula** formation, with true faecal vomiting
- **Transperitoneal spread** may involve the surface of the ovaries (**Krukenberg tumour**) or form masses in the pouch of Douglas; in either case a mass is often palpable on rectal examination
- **Remote lymph node spread**—the left supraclavicular (**Virchow's**) lymph node classically becomes invaded via the thoracic duct, giving a palpable mass (**Troisier's sign**) sometimes found at initial presentation
- **Haematogenous spread** to involve liver, lungs, brain and bone is common, and symptoms or signs of these may be the reason a doctor is consulted

Investigation of suspected gastric carcinoma

Initial diagnosis

Early detection radically increases the chances of surgery curing the condition. Hence the aim of investigation is to detect gastric cancer as early as possible. A high index of suspicion and early endoscopy for non-specific symptoms improve the chances of early detection. In one American series for example, where early endoscopy is the rule, only 15% of gastric cancers were unsuitable for operation at initial diagnosis, and half the operations were performed with the aim of cure.

In areas with a high incidence of gastric cancer, **endoscopic screening** is an effective and popular method of detecting early disease. It is widely employed in Japan, with the result that over 40% of cancers operated upon after screening have been in a pre-symptomatic stage and can truly be defined histologically as 'early gastric cancer'. About 90% of these patients undergo potentially curative operations.

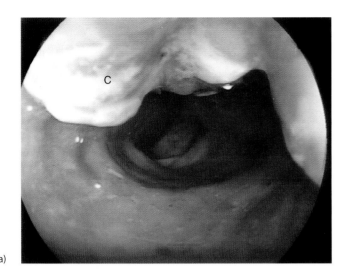
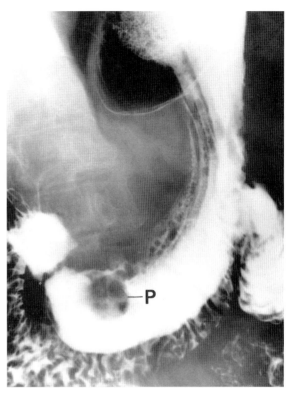

(a)

(b)

Fig. 23.2 Endoscopy and barium meal showing carcinoma of the stomach
(a) Gastroscopic view of large fungating intestinal-type carcinoma of stomach in the prepyloric region **C**. This corresponds to the barium meal examination in **(b)**. Diagnosis was confirmed by endoscopic biopsy.

Barium meal was the standard investigation for many years but it was often difficult to differentiate between benign gastric ulcer and carcinoma, even on double contrast studies. The radiological appearances of typical gastric malignancies are shown in Figures 23.2 and 23.3. **Endoscopy**, which allows visual inspection and biopsy, is now the favoured investigation for suspected carcinoma of the stomach. The site of a lesion may be important as benign ulcers are usually found on the lesser curve or in the prepyloric area whereas carcinomas arise in any part of the stomach, including the lesser curve. The initial endoscopy in a patient with carcinoma gives an accurate diagnosis in 90% of those with **exophytic** lesions (where the tumour grows into the lumen from one area of the gastric wall) but only 50% for **infiltrating** lesions. Multiple biopsies improve these rates, as do repeat endoscopy and re-biopsy of suspicious lesions.

Staging
Once cancer is diagnosed, knowing the stage helps determine the most appropriate treatment and whether surgery is likely to benefit the patient. **CT scanning** is most widely employed and gives an idea of the extent of local tumour invasion, lymph node involvement and hepatic metastases. **Laparoscopy** after CT improves the accuracy of staging, with disseminated disease sometimes being discovered, thus saving the patient an inappropriate laparotomy. **Endoscopic ultrasonography** (EUS) via a flexible endoscope is increasingly utilised in staging and gives an image with high resolution. It is highly accurate for deter-

Fig. 23.3 Barium meal showing linitis plastica

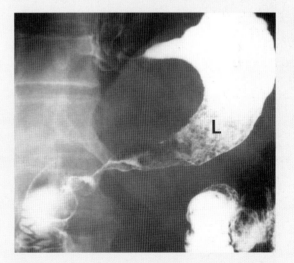

Linitis plastica-type infiltrating carcinoma of the stomach **L**. Note the shrunken appearance of the whole stomach caused by widespread submucosal invasion of the tumour. Endoscopic biopsy may not give the correct diagnosis because the mucosa is often intact. This 60-year-old woman presented with anorexia. She had a total gastrectomy but died 5 months later of widespread metastases.

mining the depth of penetration of small gastric cancers, and hence the 'T' (tumour) stage. Local spread (e.g. into pancreas), nodal involvement, left hepatic lobe metastases and ascites are also demonstrable by this method.

MANAGEMENT OF GASTRIC CARCINOMA

Like oesophageal cancer, gastric cancer is increasingly managed in specialist upper gastrointestinal centres. This consolidates surgical, radiological and oncological expertise and ensures that other professionals such as anaesthetists, theatre staff, ITU/HDU staff, dieticians and physiotherapists become experienced in managing these cases and can all contribute to the multidisciplinary team (MDT). In many places, multidisciplinary meetings are held regularly to discuss and agree the treatment plan, allow regular reviews of progress and conduct clinical audit. In the UK, most chemotherapy and radiotherapy is undertaken only within clinical trials and only after MDT plans have been formulated.

Radical surgery

As described, metastasis from gastric cancer is often early, widespread and occult. For this reason, **radical surgery** offers the only prospect of cure even when the tumour appears small. Radical gastrectomies are very major and time-consuming operations and careful staging needs to be performed before surgery to ensure that there is a realistic chance of cure. Note that the decision to attempt surgical removal also depends on the general fitness of the patient.

Japanese surgeons have developed radical R1 and R2 gastrectomies for patients where cure is the intention. Both involve total or subtotal gastrectomy; R1 also removes local nodal stations whilst R2 removes local and secondary nodal stations. In Japan, these procedures have greatly improved 5-year survival rates and have almost eliminated local recurrences. If the gastric cancer proves to be confined to the mucosa and submucosa, 5-year survival approaches 90%; with local nodal involvement survival is about 50%. With more distant spread, survival falls dramatically to 5%. Western results have not yet matched these, largely because of higher surgical complication rates.

Chemotherapy and radiotherapy

Gastric cancers are known to respond to both chemotherapy and radiotherapy but there is little evidence for much real benefit of adjuvant treatment. Postoperative chemotherapy alone is ineffective but combined pre- and post-operative treatment has shown promising outcomes in recent studies. The epirubicin–cisplatin–5 FU (ECF) regimen is effective against gastric cancer and the recent MAGIC trial improved 5-year survival from 23% for surgery alone to 36% for chemotherapy and surgery.

Radiotherapy has not been regularly used in gastric cancer but may have a place in palliation, particularly for local recurrence.

Palliative procedures

For patients with advanced cancer, it is wrong to perform heroic but ultimately ineffective surgery. Even patients with obviously incurable tumours may have few symptoms, and for them major surgery is likely to prejudice the quality of their remaining life. Palliative surgical bypass procedures or local resections should be reserved for relieving symptoms that cannot be treated in other ways. If tumour bleeding, necrosis or encroachment on the gastric lumen results in distressing symptoms such as nausea, anorexia, vomiting (gastric outlet obstruction may be complete) or symptoms of anaemia, palliative gastrectomy may be required. After palliative gastrectomy, patients survive an average of 12 months, compared with about 3 months without operation. Gastric outlet obstruction may sometimes be relieved by placing a self-expanding intraluminal stent, and this may circumvent the need for surgery.

GASTRIC POLYPS

Most gastric polyps are benign **hyperplastic nodules** of the gastric mucosa. They may be single or multiple and can occur anywhere in the stomach. They are all less than 1.5 cm in diameter and can confidently be observed by 'watchful waiting' as they almost never become malignant.

Genuine **adenomatous polyps** are rare. These are true neoplasms, with histological and morphological forms similar to adenomatous polyps of the large intestine (see Ch. 27). Adenomas are usually single, large and asymptomatic. Most are found incidentally on radiological or endoscopic examination. Up to 40% show histological features of malignancy. Treatment is by endoscopic excision biopsy (**submucosal resection**). Regular surveillance endoscopy needs to be arranged afterwards to monitor for recurrences or new lesions.

GASTROINTESTINAL STROMAL TUMOURS (GIST)

Gastrointestinal stromal tumours are very rare mesenchymal tumours that can arise anywhere in the gastrointestinal tract. They were once thought to be leiomyomas because of the histological similarity, i.e. loose bundles of spindle cells closely resembling muscle layers. However, immunocytochemical markers can now distinguish the mesenchymal tissue types and differentiate them from muscle and nerve tumours. GISTs have now been identified as originating from the **interstitial cells of Cajal**, the so-called 'pace-makers' of gut motility; these display CD34 and CD117 ('kit') proteins. GISTs are most frequently found in the stomach and can range from less than 1 cm to more than 20 cm. The risk of malignancy is determined partly by the tumour location but mostly by size and histological mitotic index (see Table 23.1). Most gastric GISTs are small (< 5 cm) and have a low mitotic index.

GISTs are often diagnosed incidentally at endoscopy. They can be sessile (domed) or pedunculated lesions (on a stalk; Fig. 23.4b), covered by normal mucosa. Small lesions may be asymptomatic; large lesions produce the symptoms or signs of any abdominal mass. Tumours over 5 cm in the gastric antrum may cause intermittent gastric outlet obstruction by impacting in or passing through the pylorus (Fig. 23.4b). Furthermore, they are prone to haemorrhage via a central 'umbilicated' ulcer (Fig. 23.4a);

these typically present after an acute episode of haematemesis. Following diagnosis and before surgery, the patient may need to be staged by CT to confirm the size and exclude metastases (local, nodal or hepatic). Suitable biopsies allow immunocytochemical analysis, but it can be difficult to obtain sufficiently deep samples. Local resection is appropriate if the lesion has low malignant potential; malignant lesions require full oncological clearance as for other gastric cancers.

Small bowel gastrointestinal stromal tumour

GISTs of small bowel are histologically similar to gastric tumours but may present by obstructing the lumen or growing outwards from the outer wall of the bowel (Fig. 23.5). Primary resection and anastomosis is the usual treatment and survival is influenced by the size and mitotic counts.

Table 23.1 Risk of aggressive behaviour of gastrointestinal stromal tumours

Risk of aggressive behaviour (malignant potential)	Greatest dimension (cm)	Mitoses per 50 microscope high-power fields
Very low	< 2	< 5
Low	2–5	< 5
Intermediate	< 5 5–10	6–10 < 5
High	> 5 > 10 Any size	> 5 Any number > 10

GASTRIC AND SMALL BOWEL LYMPHOMAS

PATHOLOGY AND CLINICAL FEATURES OF LYMPHOMAS

Primary lymphomas sometimes arise in the stomach or small bowel. They constitute about 10% of gastric malignancies. As with peptic ulcer and gastric adenocarcinoma, *H. pylori* infection is an important initiating factor. In non-Hodgkin lymphoma, the small bowel lymphoid tissue may become involved.

CASE STUDY

Fig. 23.4 Gastrointestinal stromal tumour

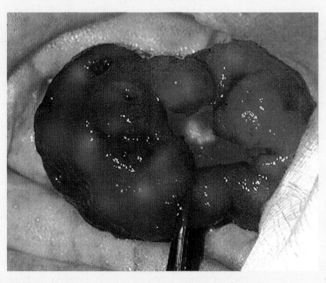
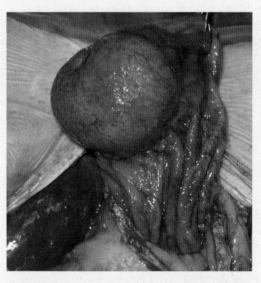

(a)   (b)

(a) This 64-year-old woman presented with recurrent iron deficiency anaemia. A large ulcerated polyp had been seen at endoscopy. Here, the stomach has been opened at laparotomy and the polyp is held up in the surgeon's hand. Deep peptic ulcers can be seen on its surface. Histologically, it proved to be a gastrointestinal stromal tumour (GIST), previously called a leiomyoma. **(b)** Another gastrointestinal stromal tumour which had become impacted in the pylorus causing gastric outlet obstruction. It was delivered through the gastrotomy, excised and the defect closed with sutures.

Fig. 23.5 Malignant gastrointestinal stromal tumour (leiomyosarcoma) of the jejunum

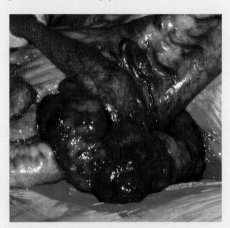

This operative specimen shows a large fleshy lesion on the outer surface of the upper jejunum. The patient was a 33-year-old woman who presented with iron deficiency anaemia refractory to oral iron. An abnormality was finally seen on a barium small bowel study after many fruitless investigations. This tumour was histologically well differentiated and amenable to resection; after 5 years, there was no recurrence.

Fig. 23.6 Intussuscepting tumour of small bowel

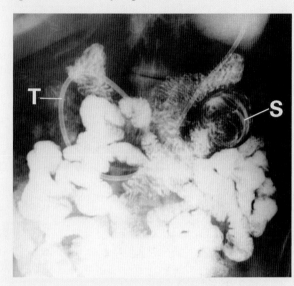

This 35-year-old woman suffered several self-limiting episodes of small bowel obstruction. During one of those episodes this small bowel barium enema was performed by placing the tip of a naso-jejunal tube **T** just distal to the duodeno-jejunal flexure and instilling barium. A small bowel intussusception is demonstrated by the 'coiled spring' sign **S**, due to the presence of barium between the telescoping layers of bowel. At surgery, a gastrointestinal stromal tumour was found to be responsible.

In the stomach, lymphomas become extensive, diffusely infiltrating the stomach wall or, less often, projecting into the lumen as bulky ulcerating masses. The symptoms (if any) and endoscopic appearances closely resemble gastric adenocarcinoma but recognising lymphoma is important because the prognosis after treatment is much better. Note that good quality biopsies are the only reliable means of diagnosis. Unlike gastric carcinoma, lymphomas tend to occur in children and young adults. Some cases of low-grade lymphoma have been reported to resolve following *Helicobacter* eradication, but this is only successful if the disease is detected early.

In the small intestine, lymphomas also produce bulky lesions which may obstruct, ulcerate, bleed or even perforate. Occasionally, a lymphoma provides the focus for an intussusception (see Figs 23.6 and 23.7 and also Fig. 50.14, p. 742). Small bowel lymphoma may be a complication of coeliac disease but the risk is only about 6 times higher than for the general population.

MANAGEMENT OF LYMPHOMAS

Investigation of both stomach and small intestine involves barium studies and endoscopic biopsy, but histological examination is essential to distinguish lymphomas from primary or secondary carcinoma. Tissue is obtained by laparotomy or laparoscopy. Primary **small bowel** lymphomas are often localised lesions, amenable to surgical excision. Postoperative radiotherapy or chemotherapy or both may be necessary. Treatment gives a 5-year survival rate of

around 50%. Radiotherapy alone effectively treats some primary **gastric** lymphomas, emphasising the importance of a tissue diagnosis before surgery is embarked upon.

CARCINOID TUMOURS

PATHOLOGY OF CARCINOID TUMOURS

Carcinoid tumours probably arise from APUD cells of the gastrointestinal endocrine system. Thus, they can arise anywhere in the gastrointestinal tract or in tissues embryologically derived from it including the pancreas and biliary system. More than 50% of carcinoid tumours are found in the appendix, and most of the remainder occur in the small intestine.

CLINICAL PRESENTATION OF CARCINOID TUMOURS

Appendiceal carcinoid tumours are usually discovered incidentally in appendicectomy specimens and virtually always remain small and benign. In contrast, carcinoid tumours elsewhere in the bowel spread locally in the bowel and mesentery, later becoming disseminated to the liver and other sites. The bowel lesions usually present with symptoms of partial or complete obstruction.

Fig. 23.7 Intussuscepting tumour of small bowel

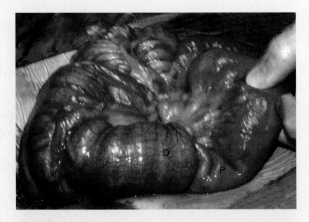

(a)

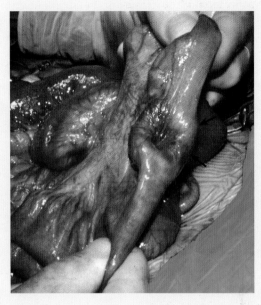

(b)

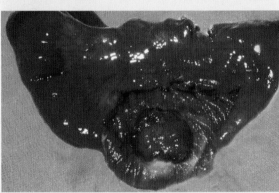

(c)

This 22-year-old man presented with small bowel obstruction. At laparotomy, the obstruction was found to be caused by an ileo-ileal intussusception. This set of operative photographs **(a)** shows how the proximal ileum **P** had intussuscepted into the distal ileum **D**. When this was reduced **(b)**, an abnormality of the bowel wall could be seen to have formed the apex of the intussuscipiens (arrowed). In **(c)**, a polypoid tumour **P** can be seen on the luminal surface, which proved histologically to be a lymphoma.

Carcinoid tumours secrete a variety of catecholamines, including **serotonin**. When there is a large volume of tumour, usually in the form of liver metastases, enough catecholamines are secreted to cause the **carcinoid syndrome**. This is characterised by an array of clinical phenomena including transient 'hot flushes', hypotension, asthma and diarrhoea. A metabolite of serotonin, **5-hydroxy-indoleacetic acid** (5-HIAA), can be measured in the urine as a diagnostic marker.

MANAGEMENT OF CARCINOID TUMOURS

Treatment usually involves resection of the primary lesion along with the local lymph nodes. An appendiceal carcinoid present at the tip only and less than 2 cm in diameter can be treated by simple appendicectomy. In patients with metastatic disease, the condition progresses very slowly. It responds well to surgery, and in the typical young patient a more radical approach can be recommended than for other intra-abdominal malignancies. Metastatic carcinoid is not curable by radiotherapy or chemotherapy.

The full carcinoid syndrome is usually associated with large volume hepatic metastases which are not amenable to surgical or other cure. It is uncommon and symptoms can be controlled with the help of drugs such as **octreotide**, a somatostatin analogue. Radiotherapy is useful if pain is caused by massive liver enlargement and it may induce some shrinkage.

OTHER TUMOURS OF THE SMALL INTESTINE

Small bowel tumours include **solitary benign angiomas**. These are usually found incidentally at operation or autopsy but sometimes present with intussusception or chronic haemorrhage.

Adenocarcinomas do occur in the small intestine, especially in the duodenum, but are rare compared with stomach and large bowel. Small bowel adenocarcinomas present with bowel obstruction, biliary obstruction when in the periampullary region, bleeding or symptoms of metastases. Barium follow-through examination for chronic symptoms may demonstrate the lesion, but more commonly it is found and resected at a laparotomy for acute obstruction, only being recognised later on histological examination. Unfortunately, metastasis to regional lymph nodes or the liver has already occurred in many patients by the time of presentation.

Peutz–Jeghers syndrome is described in Chapter 27 (p. 404).

Tumours of the pancreas and hepatobiliary system

24

INTRODUCTION

Adenocarcinomas derived from ductal cells of the exocrine pancreas make up more than 90% of pancreatic cancers. These have the worst survival of all gastrointestinal malignancies, with only about 12% of patients surviving 1 year and only 2% surviving 5 years. Much less commonly, malignancy arises from **exocrine acinar (secretory) cells** (2% of pancreatic cancers) or from **endocrine islet cells** (8% of pancreatic cancers). Most endocrine tumours manifest because of the effects of excess hormone secretion, e.g. insulin, glucagon, gastrin. Around 90% of insulinomas are benign but most of the other endocrine tumours are malignant, although survival is often prolonged.

The typical presenting features of non-endocrine pancreatic adenocarcinoma are severe and intractable abdominal pain, marked weight loss and obstructive jaundice caused by compression of the common bile duct. Jaundice is often the first presentation, but pain usually develops at a later stage. Obstructive jaundice is also a frequent presentation of the less common **periampullary carcinomas.** These include primary cholangiocarcinomas of the biliary tree and adenocarcinomas of the ampulla of Vater and duodenum.

Sclerosing cholangitis is a rare non-malignant condition which has similar modes of presentation to pancreatic cancer and is therefore included in this chapter. In contrast, the uncommon **carcinoma of the gall bladder** often presents with symptoms suggestive of cholecystitis, although jaundice develops later in many cases.

Primary liver tumours are rare in developed countries but relatively common in some developing countries, where hepatitis B and C are the main predisposing factors. **Secondary liver tumours** are common in all countries as a result of haematogenous spread of many types of malignant tumour.

CARCINOMA OF THE PANCREAS

PATHOLOGY

Carcinoma of the pancreas is usually an adenocarcinoma arising from cells lining the duct system. About 70% of tumours arise in the head of the gland (the largest part) and the remaining 30% in the body or tail. The tumours tend to form a well-differentiated ductular pattern but the sheets of cells between the ducts often appear more anaplastic. Despite the organised histological pattern, this is a highly malignant tumour. It metastasises early to local lymph nodes (including nodes in the porta hepatis), to the peritoneum and to the liver via the portal vein (see Fig. 24.1). By the time of presentation, the malignancy has already disseminated in nearly all cases and the prognosis is dire.

Carcinoma of the pancreas presents at a mean age of 65 and is extremely rare under the age of 50. In the Western world, the incidence is similar in males and females and the disease ranks third equal with oesophageal cancer among gastrointestinal carcinomas after large bowel and stomach. Nevertheless, it is relatively uncommon in absolute numbers, being responsible for about 7000 deaths each year in the UK, although the numbers in developed countries continue to rise. Its incidence is three-quarters that of gastric carcinoma, and overall it represents only 3% of all malignancies. Risk factors include cigarette smoking (2–3 times the risk and presenting 15 years earlier) and previous resectional gastric surgery (2–5 times the risk). The action of ingested nitrosamines and *N*-nitroso compounds is probably the common factor.

CLINICAL FEATURES OF PANCREATIC CARCINOMA

There are no suitable screening tests for the disease and so pancreatic cancer nearly always presents with

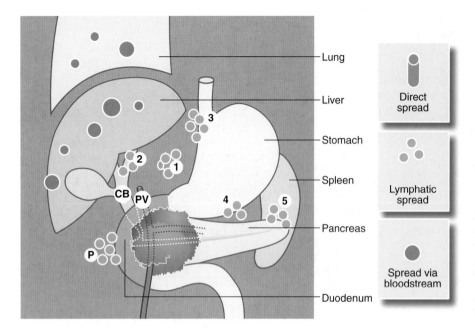

Fig. 24.1 Spread of carcinoma of the pancreas
Direct spread may involve the common bile duct **CB** where it traverses the pancreas, the duodenum and the portal vein **PV**. Lymphatic spread may reach the paraduodenal peritoneum **P** and the nodes of the coeliac axis **1**, the porta hepatis **2**, the lesser and greater curves of the stomach **3, 4** and the hilum of the spleen **5**. Spread may also occur via the bloodstream to the liver, lungs, etc.

Box 24.1   Presenting features of pancreatic carcinoma

Common presenting features

- Substantial weight loss (about 80% of cases)
- Abdominal pain (about 60%)
- Obstructive jaundice, often without pain (about 50%)

Less common presenting features

- Acute pancreatitis (rare)
- Diabetes mellitus (preceding or following diagnosis)
- Gastric outlet obstruction (due to external compression)
- Thrombophlebitis migrans (recurrent superficial venous thromboses)
- Pancreatic steatorrhoea (due to pancreatic duct obstruction)

---

symptoms and signs. The main presenting features are substantial weight loss (80%), abdominal pain (60%) and obstructive jaundice (50%). Ascites and an abdominal mass are uncommon. The presenting features of pancreatic carcinoma are shown in Box 24.1.

Pain and other abdominal symptoms and signs

The **pain** of pancreatic carcinoma is severe and continuous and is typically described as 'deep' and 'gnawing'; it may drive patients to suicide. The pain tends to be nocturnal and poorly relieved by analgesics but may be alleviated somewhat by leaning forwards from a sitting position ('the pancreatic position'). This severe pain usually represents locally advanced disease with extension of tumour beyond the pancreas and involvement of retroperitoneal nerves, particularly around the coeliac axis. There are often ill-defined **dyspeptic symptoms** like anorexia, nausea or sporadic vomiting. **Weight loss** is often dramatic even without liver metastases, and is much greater than can be explained by anorexia alone.

OBSTRUCTIVE JAUNDICE

Jaundice, often without pain, develops insidiously over several weeks, and is associated with pale stools and dark urine. During this time, the patient or his/her relatives first notice yellow discoloration of the sclerae; as the condition progresses the skin gradually assumes a deep greenish-yellow hue. Pruritus (itching) develops in the later stages but surprisingly it is less common early on. This form of obstructive jaundice is caused by compression of the common bile duct in its course through the head of the pancreas. As a result, the proximal bile duct system, including the gall bladder, becomes dilated. The gall bladder often dilates and becomes palpable (**Courvoisier's law**, see Ch. 18, p. 287). Obstruction of the bile duct may also be caused by metastasis to lymph nodes in the porta hepatis. Liver metastases alone rarely cause jaundice.

Note that carcinoma of the pancreas and other obstructing tumours of the biliary tree typically produce an unremitting, painless and progressively deepening jaundice. In contrast, the jaundice of gallstone disease tends not to be so profound and tends to fluctuate in intensity and there is usually a history of typical biliary pain.

APPROACH TO INVESTIGATION OF SUSPECTED PANCREATIC CARCINOMA (Box 24.2)

A patient presenting with obstructive jaundice should be initially investigated as described in Chapter 18.

Fig. 24.2 Carcinoma of the head of the pancreas

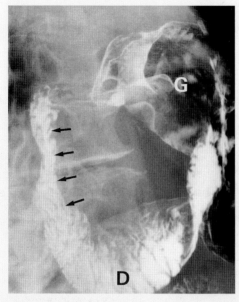

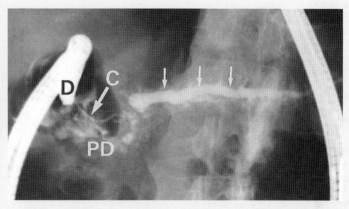

(a)   (b)

(a) This 77-year-old man presented with 4 weeks of painless obstructive jaundice. This barium meal shows the gastric antrum **G** and duodenum. The duodenal loop **D** is grossly expanded by the obstructing effect of the head of the pancreas. The medial wall of the second part of the duodenum (arrowed) is compressed and distorted by the tumour. **(b)** Endoscopic retrograde pancreatogram in a jaundiced patient with carcinoma of the head of the pancreas. The tip of the duodenoscope **D** lies opposite the ampulla of Vater, into which a catheter **C** has been passed. The distal pancreatic duct is dilated (arrowed) and the proximal duct **PD** is compressed and distorted by the tumour.

Box 24.2 Investigation of suspected pancreatic carcinoma

If patient jaundiced—suspect diagnosis from age, typical history, signs, liver function tests

If patient not jaundiced—suspect diagnosis on ultrasound or CT (differential diagnosis is often pancreatitis)

- **Primary imaging**—usually CT scan
- **Confirm histology**—CT-guided biopsy, endoscopic ultrasound-guided needle aspiration cytology
- **Assess primary tumour in detail**—site, size, local invasion especially of blood vessels using ultrasound, high-definition CT
- **Assess metastatic spread**—liver, nodes, peritoneum using CT, laparoscopy, ± laparoscopic ultrasound

When investigations are complete, the multidisciplinary team considers whether curative treatment is feasible and how to plan and implement it. If curative treatment is not appropriate, consider what palliative treatment is necessary

If pancreatic cancer proves to be the likely diagnosis, the optimum patient management is via a streamlined diagnostic pathway carried out in a specialised, high-volume pancreatic centre serving a population of perhaps 2–5 million. This enables prompt diagnosis, palliative procedures where appropriate, and timely and expert resectional surgery without stenting for the 10–15% of cases where cure can be attempted.

CT and ultrasound imaging

Ultrasound is used to look for masses in the pancreas and liver, and for dilated bile ducts and stones in the gall bladder. (Note that conventional transabdominal ultrasound is unreliable for detecting stones in the common bile duct.) Further diagnostic information about pancreatic masses can be obtained from high-resolution CT scans, which should be performed before endoscopic retrograde cholangio-pancreatography (ERCP) to ensure a virgin field that is free of artefact. CT can show the extent of the tumour and the presence and volume of liver metastases. It can also demonstrate **vascular tumour invasion** of the superior mesenteric and portal veins, and the superior mesenteric artery and coeliac axis, any of which would diminish the feasibility of surgical resection. The extent of primary and/or metastatic disease shown on imaging may be such that the tumour is pronounced **inoperable** (i.e. not resectable with the intention of cure), in which case

371

Fig. 24.3 Carcinoma of the head of the pancreas

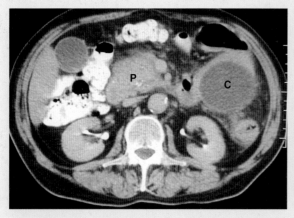
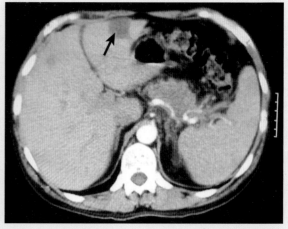

(a)   (b)

(a) CT scan showing enlargement of the head of the pancreas **P** most suspicious of carcinoma. The dark circular lesion within the tail of the pancreas is a secondary cyst or pseudocyst **C**. **(b)** CT scan further cephalad (towards the head) of the same patient showing one obvious low-attenuation lesion in the liver consistent with a metastasis (arrowed). The diagnosis of carcinoma of the pancreas was confirmed on percutaneous biopsy of the pancreatic lesion. Thus this 54-year-old man had inoperable disease. Unfortunately, this is all too common a presentation.

palliative measures are instituted and the patient is saved a fruitless attempt at resection.

Endoscopic ultrasound (EUS) and needle aspiration cytology

In patients with jaundice where ultrasound and CT suggest that a carcinoma of the pancreatic head may be resectable, further detail can be acquired by **endoscopic ultrasound**. In this, an ultrasound probe is positioned in the second part of the duodenum via an upper gastrointestinal endoscope. This allows precise visual ultrasound examination of the pancreatic head and its associated vessels as well as the duodenum and ampullary region. In addition, ultrasound-guided **needle aspiration** sampling of suspicious lesions can be performed for cytological examination, to establish a diagnosis before surgery or to guide oncological management. Endoscopic ultrasound is currently accepted as the gold standard for assessing primary tumour size, site and vascular involvement and thus its potential operability. However, its accuracy is severely impaired if a stent has been placed to relieve jaundice; this is an argument for specialised investigation and treatment so stenting can be avoided if resection is feasible.

Magnetic resonance cholangio-pancreatography (MRCP)

MRCP produces images that are similar to ERCP in diagnostic usefulness but it is particularly useful in biliary obstruction to confirm choledocholithiasis (bile duct stones) or to investigate obstructive lesions of the bile duct itself such as cholangiocarcinoma or primary sclerosing cholangitis.

Endoscopic retrograde cholangio-pancreatography and therapeutic intervention

ERCP (see Fig. 24.2b) is no longer the primary diagnostic tool but is employed mainly for therapeutic intervention. For obstructive jaundice due to stone, ERCP is the main mechanism for removing duct stones. For inoperable carcinoma of the pancreatic head, placing a tubular stent across the obstruction allows palliation of jaundice by draining the biliary tree. The same strategy is used if a stone proves irremovable at the first attempt. If left in place long enough, plastic stents eventually become encrusted and occluded but, sadly, patients with inoperable pancreatic cancer rarely survive long enough for stent occlusion to become a problem. Wider bore expanding metallic stents are now available but indications for their use are yet to be defined.

Lesions in the body and tail of the pancreas

When pancreatic cancer is suspected in a non-jaundiced patient and no alternative diagnosis has yet been made, abdominal CT scanning can be more reliable for confirming the diagnosis than ultrasound, although small tumours may still be missed (see Fig. 24.3a and b). Endoscopic ultrasound can be useful for examining the body and tail of the pancreas via the stomach, and again ultrasound-guided aspiration cytology can be employed. CT scanning also gives an idea of the extent of local invasion into the retroperitoneal area and the portal vein and shows metastatic deposits in the liver parenchyma and lymph nodes; this can help the surgeon decide whether the lesion is resectable. CT-guided needle biopsy can obtain specimens for histopathology. However carcinomas involving the body and tail do not cause the early warning sign of jaundice and thus tend to present late in the natural history of the disease; this means that operability is highly unlikely. It is worth noting that CT scanning can understage the disease, chiefly because it does not detect small-volume peritoneal deposits.

Accurate staging of pancreatic cancer enables resection to be offered to those most likely to profit, whilst avoiding unnecessary surgery in those for whom it would provide no benefit. Staging laparoscopy is often the final evaluation before resection, allowing inspection and biopsy of the peritoneum for small metastases; it can be combined with ultrasound via the laparoscope, although this latter technique has been largely superseded by high-quality CT and endoscopic ultrasound.

Cystic neoplasms

Cystic neoplasms of the pancreas are sometimes discovered incidentally on CT scanning or ultrasonography. Often the investigation has been prompted by non-specific upper abdominal symptoms. Cystic neoplasms can be difficult to differentiate from pancreatic pseudocysts, but CT and endoluminal ultrasound (EUS) can help define the morphology and allow aspiration of material for cytology and biochemical analysis (CEA, CA19.9 and amylase). Once a pseudocyst has been excluded, the differential diagnosis of the cystic neoplasm includes **serous and mucinous cystadenomas** and **cystadenocarcinomas**. Radical resection is the treatment of choice for most of these since all cystic neoplasms may have a malignant potential and are largely curable if treated early enough. However, if EUS-guided aspiration reveals a serous lesion and it has no adverse radiological or biochemical features, observation by 'watchful waiting' may be a management option. The presence of mucus, however, identifies a mucinous pancreatic lesion that has a greater potential for malignancy and should be resected.

MANAGEMENT OF PANCREATIC CARCINOMA

It is an unfortunate truth that most patients with pancreatic cancer present at an incurable stage because of local invasion or metastases. Only about 15% have apparently localised disease with a potential for cure by resection. Where resection of the pancreatic head is indicated, **Whipple's operation** (pancreatico-duodenectomy, see Fig. 24.6, p. 376) is the standard type of procedure. It is a major undertaking with high operative morbidity and mortality; even in high-volume specialist centres, opera-

tive mortality is 1–2% with a 15–20% morbidity (pancreatic leaks, delayed gastric emptying, wound infections) and a 5-year survival of only 15–20%.

Postoperative adjuvant chemotherapy confers a modest survival advantage, and the large-scale clinical trial ESPAC 3 is continuing. This aims to determine the merits of 5-fluorouracil (5FU) regimens versus gemcitabine, but early success has meant that an initial study arm with no treatment has been dropped.

Palliation of pancreatic cancer

When there is obvious widespread disease, the patient should be allowed to die with minimal surgical interference but with careful attention to symptom control. Adequate analgesia is fundamental; severe pain can often be substantially relieved by permanent **blockade of the coeliac ganglion**, which is performed percutaneously under radiological control or endoscopically under ultrasound guidance using EUS. If **obstructive jaundice** is the dominant feature, this can usually be relieved by inserting a plastic or metal biliary stent (**endoprosthesis**) into the compressed bile duct at ERCP. In difficult cases where ERCP is unsuccessful, a percutaneous transhepatic route (percutaneous transhepatic cholangiogram, PTC) can be valuable, either to pass a guide-wire to the duodenum and facilitate the ERCP procedure or to place a stent directly; techniques are illustrated in Figure 24.4. Bypass can be achieved surgically at laparotomy (usually a '**triple bypass**' procedure, consisting of choledocho- or cholecysto-jejunostomy, gastroenterostomy and jejuno-jejunostomy, see Fig. 24.4). This procedure is now uncommon but is undergoing a resurgence as it often provides longer-lasting relief than palliative stenting of the bile duct and/or duodenum. Note that duodenal obstruction can also be bypassed by laparoscopic gastroenterostomy.

BILIARY AND PERIAMPULLARY TUMOURS

Adenocarcinomas originating from the epithelium lining the biliary duct system are known as **cholangiocarcinomas**. They may develop anywhere in the intrahepatic or extrahepatic duct system but are more common in the upper third of the extrahepatic bile duct, near the confluence of the right and left hepatic ducts ('Klatskin' tumour). The less common **intrahepatic cholangiocarcinomas** present in a manner similar to primary hepatocellular carcinomas. Since most of the biliary system remains patent in these cases, jaundice is rare. In contrast, **extrahepatic cholangiocarcinomas** tend to obstruct bile drainage. They present with painless progressive jaundice in the same way as carcinoma of the pancreatic head. Additionally cholangiocarcinomas are more likely to occur in patients with **primary sclerosing cholangitis**. Distinguishing cholangiocarcinoma from the multiple

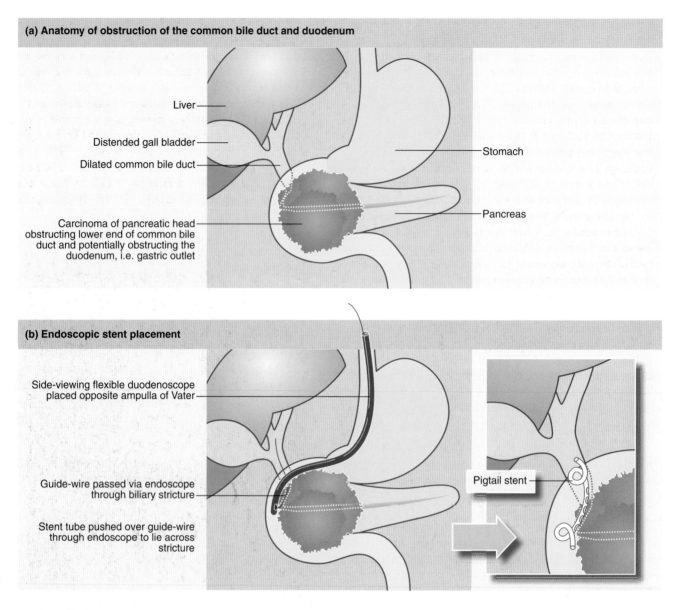

(a) Anatomy of obstruction of the common bile duct and duodenum

Liver

Distended gall bladder

Dilated common bile duct

Stomach

Pancreas

Carcinoma of pancreatic head obstructing lower end of common bile duct and potentially obstructing the duodenum, i.e. gastric outlet

(b) Endoscopic stent placement

Side-viewing flexible duodenoscope placed opposite ampulla of Vater

Guide-wire passed via endoscope through biliary stricture

Stent tube pushed over guide-wire through endoscope to lie across stricture

Pigtail stent

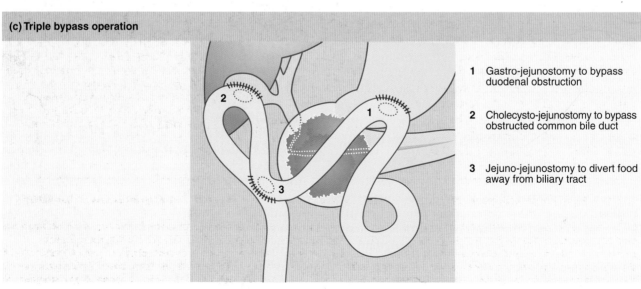

(c) Triple bypass operation

1   Gastro-jejunostomy to bypass duodenal obstruction

2   Cholecysto-jejunostomy to bypass obstructed common bile duct

3   Jejuno-jejunostomy to divert food away from biliary tract

strictures that are the hallmark of sclerosing cholangitis can be challenging.

Cholangiocarcinomas have a dense fibrous stroma and tend to grow along the duct system rather than producing focal proliferative lesions. The resulting smooth elongated stricture can be demonstrated by ERCP, MRCP or transhepatic cholangiography (see Fig. 24.5). Histological proof of malignancy may be difficult to obtain owing to the fibrous nature of the tumour. Unlike pancreatic cancer, cholangiocarcinomas are often slow-growing and metastasise late. Despite this, lymph node involvement at presentation is common, and extension along bile ducts and involvement of the nearby portal vein and hepatic arterial branches results in a low operability rate and an even lower long-term survival. Radical procedures combining partial hepatectomy with excision of the involved biliary tree and 'en bloc' portal vein resection and reconstruction may offer better clearance and improved survival for selected patients.

An unusual part of the spectrum of periampullary lesions is adenocarcinoma arising at the ampulla of Vater. Here it forms a polypoid lesion projecting into the duodenum and obstructing biliary drainage causing jaundice. These tumours are friable and tend to bleed persistently, giving a positive result on faecal occult blood testing. An association with intestinal polyposis syndromes has been described. Diagnosis is made at endoscopy at which the tumour is visible and accessible to biopsy. Very rarely, adenocarcinoma arises in the duodenal mucosa itself and causes obstructive jaundice if situated close to the ampulla. Again, the lesion is readily diagnosed at ERCP and biopsy.

MANAGEMENT OF EXTRAHEPATIC CHOLANGIOCARCINOMA AND PERIAMPULLARY CARCINOMA

Extrahepatic and periampullary cancers can often be treated by curative resection by Whipple's pancreaticoduodenectomy. This extensive procedure involves resection of most of the extrahepatic biliary system as well as the whole duodenum, the head of the pancreas and usually the distal stomach, as illustrated in Figure 24.6. Operative morbidity and mortality are similar to the operation for pancreatic cancer, but the prognosis is often better because the obstructing tumour is usually still small, with less extensive local and regional spread.

CARCINOMA OF THE GALL BLADDER

Carcinoma of the gall bladder is a disease of old age and is nearly always associated with longstanding stone disease. Chronic inflammation is likely to be the carcinogenic factor. Diagnosis of early gall bladder cancer is usually made incidentally at cholecystectomy and in this special case wide excision of the gall bladder bed plus hilar lymphadenectomy may be possible, offering the chance of cure. In most cases, the diagnosis is late and the patient presents with advanced disease and jaundice. Direct invasion of the liver together with lymphatic spread

Fig. 24.5 Cholangiocarcinoma

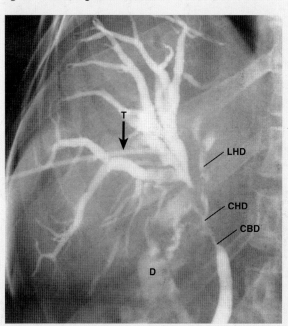

Percutaneous transhepatic cholangiogram in a 66-year-old man with painless progressive jaundice from an inoperable cholangiocarcinoma; this X-ray shows a long stricture of the common bile duct **CBD**, common hepatic duct **CHD** and left hepatic duct **LHD**. Some contrast has flowed through into the duodenum. The cystic duct is obliterated, preventing filling of the gall bladder. A percutaneous drainage tube **T** has been inserted into the right hepatic duct system prior to an attempt to place a stent across the stricture by the same route. Some contrast has flowed through into the duodenum **(D)**. Nowadays, most stents are placed endoscopically (see Fig. 24.4).

Fig. 24.4 Palliative procedures for obstructive jaundice caused by carcinoma of the head of the pancreas or a periampullary tumour
(a) Obstruction of the common bile duct and duodenum. Carcinoma of the pancreatic head obstructs the lower end of the common bile duct and potentially the duodenum, i.e. the gastric outlet. **(b)** Endoscopic stent placement. The sphincter of Oddi may require a preliminary endoscopic sphincterotomy prior to intubation. A self-retaining plastic stent, placed endoscopically or percutaneously, lies in situ across the biliary stricture. Note the 'pig-tail' ends of this type of stent which curl up when the wire is removed, retaining the stent in the correct position. **(c)** Triple bypass operation, less commonly performed nowadays because of the efficacy of endoscopic stenting and the short life expectancy of patients with pancreatic cancer.

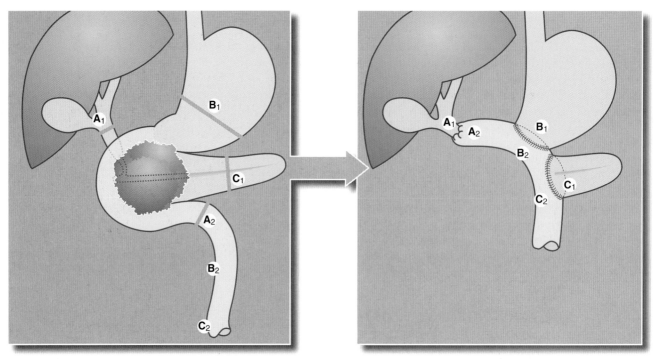

Fig. 24.6 Whipple's operation (pancreatico-duodenectomy)
(a) Structures are divided at the lines A_1, A_2, B_1, C_1. **(b)** The distal half of the stomach, the entire duodenal loop, the head and body of the pancreas and the lower end of the common bile duct are all removed, then reconstruction is performed with anastomoses between A_1 and A_2, B_1 and B_2 and C_1 and C_2.

make resection impracticable at this stage and survival is usually brief.

PRIMARY SCLEROSING CHOLANGITIS

Primary sclerosing cholangitis (PSC) is a rare condition, probably of autoimmune origin, which results in progressive fibrosis that causes multiple strictures of the biliary system. This luminal narrowing causes gradual and progressive obstructive jaundice and, later, secondary cirrhosis. The condition may arise sporadically but often occurs in association with longstanding ulcerative colitis. The bile duct stenosis is usually diffuse with a characteristic appearance on ERCP (see Fig. 24.7), but just occasionally the condition is localised to the extrahepatic biliary system. Here it gives a radiological appearance indistinguishable from cholangiocarcinoma, thereby providing a diagnostic dilemma. Management is by endoscopic dilatation of clinically significant strictures and prescribing choleretic drugs to improve bile flow. In advanced cases, liver transplantation is an option. Interestingly, up to 10% of these have demonstrated cholangiocarcinoma in the excised native liver.

ENDOCRINE TUMOURS OF THE PANCREAS

The neuroendocrine cells of the islets of Langerhans give rise to a variety of uncommon tumours. These often produce excess hormone secretions that are responsible for the usual presenting features. The islet cells make up only 2% of the pancreatic mass and comprise cells of four types: **alpha cells** secrete glucagon, **beta cells** secrete insulin, **delta cells** secrete somatostatin and F or **PP cells** secrete pancreatic polypeptide.

INSULINOMAS AND GLUCAGONOMAS

The most common endocrine tumours of the pancreas are **insulinomas** derived from beta cells. Nevertheless these occur in only 1.7 per million people per annum. The main symptoms are cerebral disturbances caused by attacks of hypoglycaemia, particularly when fasting or exercising. The attacks are relieved by oral or intravenous glucose. About 90% of insulinomas are single and 90% are benign and amenable to curative resection. They occur with equal frequency in the head, body and tail of the pancreas. Histologically, insulinomas are almost always benign; malignancy is only diagnosed on the appearance of metastases.

The diagnosis of insulinoma is usually made late, often after the manifestations of hypoglycaemia have resulted in accusations of alcoholism or referrals for psychiatric or neurological advice for abnormal behaviour or epilepsy. When inappropriate hyperinsulinaemia causing hypoglycaemia has been confirmed, CT scanning and selective pancreatic arteriography (see Fig. 24.8) can identify the site of the lesion. When this is unsuccessful, venous sam-

Fig. 24.7 Sclerosing cholangitis

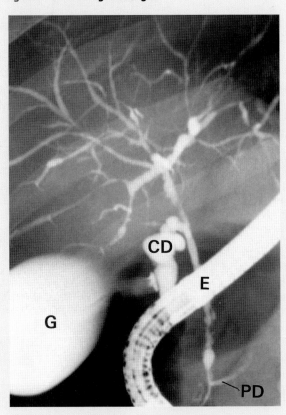

ERCP in a 52-year-old man with longstanding ulcerative colitis who developed painless jaundice. There is widespread irregular narrowing of both the intrahepatic and extrahepatic bile ducts typical of sclerosing cholangitis. Note the endoscope **E**, the normal gall bladder **G** and the cystic duct **CD** filling with contrast. The proximal part of the pancreatic duct **PD** also contains contrast.

Fig. 24.8 Insulinoma as seen on a selective arteriogram (subtraction film)

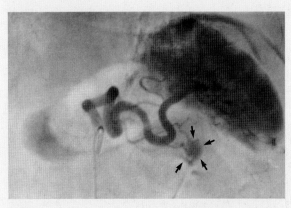

This 31-year-old woman suffered from bouts of faintness which proved to be caused by intermittent hypoglycaemia. Selective splenic arteriography demonstrated an abnormal mass of blood vessels about 1.5 cm in diameter (arrowed) in the tail of the pancreas representing an insulinoma. The tail of the pancreas was excised and the patient's symptoms disappeared.

pling may help and intraoperative ultrasound can usually locate lesions unable to be visualised by any other technique. Insulinomas are usually small and can be dealt with by simple enucleation although larger lesions or those placed deep in the head of the pancreas may entail formal pancreatic resection.

Alpha cells may give rise to **glucagonomas**; these are very rare and present with diabetes mellitus and a characteristic skin rash known as **migratory necrolytic erythema**.

ZOLLINGER–ELLISON SYNDROME

Gastrin-secreting tumours (**gastrinomas**) are rare, occurring at the rate of only 1 per million per annum. They arise in the pancreatic islets or from ectopic cells in the duodenal wall. About 25% develop in patients with multiple endocrine neoplasia type 1 (MEN 1), described briefly below. Gastrinomas cause severe and intractable

peptic ulceration and diarrhoea, and this is known as Zollinger–Ellison syndrome.

The diagnosis is made by demonstrating persistently high serum gastrin levels. The tumour is localised by CT scanning and selective pancreatic angiography. Many of the lesions are too small to be demonstrated by either method and their location can only be established using intraoperative ultrasonography at laparotomy. About 60% of gastrinomas are classified as malignant but they grow slowly and metastasise late. Thus, excision is often curative. In patients where the primary tumour is inoperable, palliation with high-dose **proton pump inhibitors (PPIs)** often prevents peptic ulcer symptoms and complications.

MULTIPLE ENDOCRINE NEOPLASIA SYNDROMES (MEN)

Pancreatic neuroendocrine cell tumours sometimes form part of a multiple endocrine neoplasia syndrome (MEN), of which two types are recognised, MEN 1 and MEN 2, as follows:

- MEN 1—islet cell tumours, pituitary adenomas and parathyroid hyperplasia
- MEN 2—medullary carcinoma of the thyroid (often in childhood), phaeochromocytoma and parathyroid adenoma

PRIMARY TUMOURS OF THE LIVER

Primary malignant tumours of the liver are uncommon in developed countries. Of those that do occur, the majority are **hepatocellular carcinomas** derived from hepatocytes. Even less commonly, other elements in the liver give rise to tumours such as **angiosarcoma**. Also an increasing number of benign liver lesions are found incidentally during ultrasound examinations for gallstones. The most frequently found are benign cysts and haemangiomas which do not need treatment.

More rarely, benign solid areas of **focal nodular hyperplasia (FNH)** are discovered. These are more prevalent in women and tend to be associated with use of the oral contraceptive pill. Other benign solid lesions include **hepatic adenomas**. Focal nodular hyperplasia is much more common than adenoma (in a ratio of 9 : 1) but adenoma may lead on to hepatoma and hence most liver surgeons recommend resection of these whilst hyperplasia can safely be left. These two conditions are similar radiologically, but focal nodular hyperplasia may have a characteristic central scar seen on imaging.

HEPATOCELLULAR CARCINOMA

Hepatocellular carcinomas (also known as **hepatomas**) are malignant, slow-growing tumours which often arise multicentrically and synchronously throughout the liver. Unusually for malignancy, an aetiological factor can be identified in nearly all cases; factors include pre-existing infection with hepatitis B and especially hepatitis C, alcoholic cirrhosis, haemochromatosis and chronic active hepatitis. Eighty percent have some form of pre-existing cirrhosis. In developed countries, **alcoholic cirrhosis** is the most common aetiological factor; indeed, hepatoma occurs in about 25% of patients with cirrhosis of more than 5 years' standing. The risk in patients with **haemochromatosis** and **chronic active hepatitis** is even higher. Hepatocellular carcinoma is one of the most common cancers in parts of Africa and the Far East. Here the usual cause is hepatitis B induced cirrhosis, but other environmental carcinogens have also been implicated; these include **aflatoxin**, produced by a species of *Aspergillus* growing on stored grains and peanuts. Various **parasitic infestations**, e.g. schistosomiasis, *Echinococcus* (tapeworm) and *Clonorchis sinensis* (liver fluke), also predispose to hepatocellular carcinoma. In developed countries, the peak incidence is between the ages of 40 and 60, but in those developing countries where the disease is common, most cases occur between 20 and 40.

Clinical features and management of hepatocellular carcinoma

The presenting features of hepatocellular carcinoma are anorexia, weight loss, abdominal pain and distension, often with jaundice and ascites. These are often associated with non-abdominal stigmata of cirrhosis. On examination, a liver mass may be palpable. Ultrasound or CT scanning can establish the size and position of the liver mass or masses and guide needle biopsy. However, a very high alpha-fetoprotein blood level is sufficient to establish the diagnosis.

By the time of initial diagnosis, hepatocellular carcinoma is usually widespread in the liver, rendering curative resection impossible. Occasionally, small lesions are resectable but only in those rare instances where co-existing cirrhosis is minimal. At one time, liver transplantation appeared to offer the necessary radical resection and replacement of the diseased liver, but results with large tumours proved unsatisfactory, recurrence being the rule. Transplantation is more promising, however, when there are fewer than 3 tumours and they are smaller than 5 cm (i.e. meeting the 'Milan' criteria). In such cases the outcomes are comparable to those for liver transplantation for the underlying liver disease alone, with 5-year survival in the region of 70%. In patients with known cirrhosis, it is important to identify developing tumours early; UK hepatology units carry out regular ultrasound surveillance and alpha-fetoprotein estimations in patients who would potentially be candidates for liver transplantation.

By way of palliation, local administration of cytotoxic drugs by 'chemo-embolisation' via an intra-arterial cannula is sometimes undertaken and radiofrequency ablation can be used for small lesions arising in cirrhotic livers where transplantation is not an option due to advanced age, comorbidities or patient choice.

SECONDARY LIVER TUMOURS

Secondary tumours in the liver are extremely common. They arise from a wide variety of primary sources, especially the stomach, pancreas, large bowel, breast and bronchus. Liver metastases are initially asymptomatic but the patient begins to feel ill with anorexia and weight loss as the liver parenchyma is progressively destroyed. Jaundice is unusual and tends to appear only at a terminal stage. Jaundice then results from a combination of compressive obstruction of the intrahepatic biliary system and gross parenchymal loss so that bile pigments cannot be excreted. Consequently, the biochemical picture tends to be a mixed hepatitic and obstructive pattern.

A substantial proportion of colorectal cancer patients are cured by primary surgery, but those that eventually die of colorectal cancer almost universally have metastatic liver disease. There is no benefit to be gained by resecting metastatic disease in most other sites, but colorectal liver metastases represent a special case where there may be a real chance of cure. In fact, 10–20% of colorectal cancer patients who develop liver metastases may be suitable for curative resection. As a result of recent optimistic reports, increasing numbers of patients are considered for liver resection.

The liver has a large reserve capacity and a remarkable regenerative capacity. This means that up to 70% of the volume of liver tissue can be surgically resected, provided there is no other liver disease. More and more patients are being considered for resection because of advances in surgical technique and a willingness to undertake extensive or multiple resections. Resection is sometimes combined with chemotherapy and/or radiofrequency ablation to 'downsize' the tumour. Surgery of this type is a major undertaking, best practised in specialised units. It can be performed with an operative mortality of around 2% and a 5-year survival of 30–40%. If further metastases appear in the hypertrophied regenerating liver, further resection can sometimes be carried out and even isolated lung metastases can be excised. In some series, this aggressive policy is pushing the 5-year survival close to 50%.

In other primary cancers such as breast and bronchus, liver metastases usually indicate surgically incurable disease, reflecting the systemic nature of the malignancy. Occasionally, however, metastases from renal cell carcinoma or neuroendocrine tumours have been successfully resected. If liver metastases are painful, palliation by systemic chemotherapy may retard their growth and suppress symptoms. Multiple inoperable metastases can be controlled by a range of physical methods including local cryotherapy, radiofrequency ablation, laser destruction and percutaneous alcohol injection. Such treatments are unlikely to extend survival, however, and controlled clinical trials of benefit are notably lacking.

25 Pancreatitis

INTRODUCTION

Pancreatitis is a common inflammatory disorder of the pancreas that is characterised by abdominal pain. Most cases present in an acute form known as **acute pancreatitis** and attacks range in severity from mild to severe. Severe attacks are particularly life-threatening, with a mortality of around 20%.

Some patients suffer recurrent acute attacks (**acute relapsing pancreatitis**) and a small proportion suffer a persistent form known as **chronic pancreatitis**; this is much more common in men and is often associated with high alcohol intake.

ACUTE PANCREATITIS

AETIOLOGY AND EPIDEMIOLOGY OF ACUTE PANCREATITIS

Gallstones and alcoholism together account for about 80% of acute pancreatitis world-wide. These and the other main causes of acute pancreatitis are listed in Table 25.1. **Opie** first pointed out the relationship between gallstones and pancreatitis in 1901 based on autopsy evidence. Later it became clear that stone obstruction of the ampulla of Vater allowed bile to reflux into the pancreatic duct, thus activating enzymes within the gland. Small gallstones may cause transient obstruction as they pass through the ampulla via the bile ducts, or larger stones may impact at the lower end of the common bile duct. Beyond this, the precise mechanism of gallstone pancreatitis remains obscure even today.

The proportion of acute pancreatitis caused by alcoholism varies from country to country; for example, about two-thirds of patients in the UK have a gallstone aetiology whereas in parts of the USA and continental Europe about two-thirds have an alcoholic aetiology. Longstanding high alcohol intake for at least 2 years is usually required to cause alcoholic pancreatitis; the mean daily alcohol intake in the subjects of one study was 140 g compared with 40 g in controls. Occasionally acute pancreatitis can result from a single session of heavy drinking—students finishing exams beware! The mechanism of alcoholic pancreatitis is unknown but is believed to be a direct toxic effect of alcohol on the pancreas in genetically predisposed individuals. In most cases of acute pancreatitis the initiating factor is some form of **pancreatic duct obstruction**. This is most often due to gallstones, but chronic alcoholic pancreatitis may also contain an obstructive element caused by inflammatory swelling and scarring.

In developed countries, the annual incidence of acute pancreatitis requiring hospital admission is about 1 : 2000 population and the mortality is about 2%. About 15% fall into the defined clinical category of **severe pancreatitis**. Women are affected more than men, but men are more likely to suffer recurrent attacks. Most patients are over 45 years of age and the peak incidence is between 50 and 60 years. The reported incidence appears to have risen by a factor of 10 over the last 40 years, with only part of this increase being attributable to improved diagnosis. The other factors are unknown.

PATHOPHYSIOLOGY OF ACUTE PANCREATITIS

Acute pancreatitis is characterised by the sudden onset of diffuse inflammation of the pancreas. A range of diverse factors initiate disturbances of cellular metabolism, chiefly concerned with membrane stability. This leads to

Table 25.1 Aetiology of acute pancreatitis

Condition	Frequency
Obstruction	
Gallstones	30–70% of cases
Congenital abnormalities: pancreas divisum with accessory duct obstruction; choledochocoele; duodenal diverticula	5% of cases
Ampullary or pancreatic tumours	3% of cases
Abnormally high pressure in the sphincter of Oddi (over 40 mmHg)	1–2% of cases
Ascariasis (second most common cause in endemic areas, e.g. Kashmir)	Depends on locality
Drugs and toxins	
Alcohol excess	30–70% of cases
Drugs: ('**SAND**'—**S**teroids and sulphonamides, **A**zathioprine (and 6-mercaptopurine), **N**SAIDs, **D**iuretics such as furosemide and thiazides, and didanosine); also antibacterials such as metronidazole and tetracycline, H$_2$ blockers and many other classes of drug	1–2%
Scorpion venom	Very rare
Snake bites	Very rare
Iatrogenic and traumatic causes	
Following endoscopic retrograde cholangio-pancreatography (ERCP) or endoscopic sphincterotomy	2–6% of patients having the procedure
Following cardiopulmonary bypass	0.5–5% of patients having bypass
Blunt pancreatic trauma, usually due to motor vehicle accidents	Very rare
Repeated marathon running	Very rare
Metabolic causes	
Hypertriglyceridaemia (> 11 mmol/L)	2% of cases
Hypercalcaemia	Rare
Hypothermia	Rare
Pregnancy	Rare
Infection	
AIDS: secondary infection with cytomegalovirus and others	About 10% in patients with AIDS
Other viruses: mumps, chickenpox, Coxsackie viruses, hepatitis A, B and C	Very rare
Idiopathic pancreatitis	
No definable cause after thorough diagnostic evaluation including ERCP; research studies show about two-thirds of 'idiopathic' cases have gallstone microlithiasis	10–12% of cases

inappropriate activation of zymogens (pre-enzymes) within the pancreas. Activation of **trypsin** is probably the key initiating event and this overwhelms intrinsic anti-trypsin activity, leading to **interstitial oedematous pancreatitis**. Fortunately, the extent and severity of inflammation remain mild and self-limiting in most patients and any systemic effects are mild. In the least severe cases there is minimal peritoneal exudation, and no pancreatic changes are detectable on contrast-enhanced CT scanning. In more severe disease, the pancreas becomes swollen and oedematous but remains viable. If laparotomy is inadvertently performed at this stage, clear,

---

Box 25.1   Mnemonic for the causes of acute pancreatitis: 'I get smashed'

I   Idiopathic
G   Gallstones
E   Ethanol
T   Trauma
S   Steroids
M   Mumps
A   Autoimmune
S   Scorpion/snakes
H   Hyperlipidaemia/hypercalcaemia
E   ERCP
D   Drugs

Box 25.2   History and investigations helpful in determining the cause of acute pancreatitis*

History

- Previous gallstones
- Alcohol intake
- Family history
- Drug intake
- Exposure to known viral causes or prodromal symptoms

Initial investigations (acute phase)

- Pancreatic enzymes in plasma
- Liver function tests
- Ultrasound of gall bladder

Follow-up investigations (recovery phase)

- Fasting plasma lipids
- Fasting plasma calcium
- Viral antibody titres
- Repeat biliary ultrasound
- MRCP
- CT (helical or multislice with pancreas protocol)

* Adapted from UK guidelines for the management of acute pancreatitis. Gut 2005; 54: 1–9.

---

non-infected peritoneal fluid can be seen, with whitish patches on the great omentum and mesentery representing areas of **fat saponification** ('fat necrosis'). If saponification is extensive, calcium becomes sequestered in areas of fat necrosis and this is incriminated in the fall of blood calcium level characteristic of severe acute pancreatitis.

As severity increases, trypsin and other enzymes cause increasingly extensive local damage as well as activation of complement and cytokine systems that lead to the development of systemic inflammatory response syndrome (SIRS) leading to organ failure. Manifestations include shock, acute respiratory distress syndrome (ARDS), renal failure and disseminated intravascular coagulation (see Ch. 2). At this stage, **acute peripancreatic fluid collections** become detectable on CT scanning. The most severe pancreatitis is associated with **pancreatic necrosis**. An element of ischaemia within the gland, together with an associated reperfusion injury, has been incriminated in transforming acute oedematous pancreatitis into this necrotising disease. Complications are common and mortality in this group (even without infection) is up to 10%.

A substantial proportion of patients with pancreatic necrosis develop **infection** of the necrotic pancreas, usually with Gram-negative organisms translocated from the bowel. This occurs within 2 weeks of the onset and greatly increases mortality. Diagnosis of this crucial development can be difficult to make. **Pancreatic abscess formation** is a different phenomenon, developing later and having a somewhat better prognosis.

In patients dying of acute necrotising pancreatitis, autopsy reveals the peritoneal cavity to be filled with a dark, blood-stained inflammatory exudate containing fine lipid droplets. This gives the condition its name of **acute haemorrhagic pancreatitis**. The peritoneal surface is grossly inflamed and semi-digested and all that is left of the pancreas is a necrotic mass.

Box 25.3   Clinical features of acute pancreatitis

Mild attack

- Acute abdominal pain
- Minimal or rapidly resolving abdominal signs, e.g. abdominal distension, some abdominal tenderness and guarding, absent bowel sounds
- Minimal systemic illness
- Moderate tachycardia

Severe attack

- Severe acute abdominal pain
- Severe toxaemia and shock
- Generalised peritonitis (diffuse abdominal tenderness, guarding, rigidity, absent bowel sounds)
- Acute respiratory distress syndrome (may develop during the first few days)

CLINICAL FEATURES OF ACUTE PANCREATITIS (see Box 25.3)

Acute pancreatitis presents as a patient with an acute abdomen. Pain begins suddenly and is severe and continuous from the outset. Initially it is poorly localised in the central and upper abdomen and is often described by the patient as 'going through to the back'. As the peritoneal cavity becomes involved over the next few hours, the pain spreads throughout the abdomen and, if the diaphragmatic peritoneum becomes inflamed, may be referred to the **shoulder tips**. Unrelenting vomiting may be an early feature. In the early stages, the patient is restless and constantly changes posture in the search for a comfortable position. Pain is most often relieved by leaning forward in the so-called '**pancreatic position**'. With the onset of chemical peritonitis, movement becomes increasingly painful and the patient tends to lie very still. The clinical signs depend on the severity of the inflammatory process and the stage to which it has progressed.

INVESTIGATION OF SUSPECTED PANCREATITIS

Acute pancreatitis must be excluded in any adult presenting with acute abdominal pain, and in any child with peritonitis not readily attributable to appendicitis. The British Society of Gastroenterology and other similar organisations have produced comprehensive guidelines on the management of acute pancreatitis (http://www. bsg.org.uk/pdf_word_docs/pancreatic.pdf).

Plasma amylase

Amylase is one of the enzymes absorbed into the circulation in pancreatitis; **plasma amylase** measurement is simple to perform in the laboratory and provides a generally reliable diagnostic test. A plasma amylase level above 1000 i.u./ml is usually regarded as diagnostic of acute pancreatitis but amylase levels are often lower in alcoholic pancreatitis, particularly during recurrent attacks. Any upper abdominal inflammatory condition near the pancreas (e.g. cholecystitis, perforated peptic ulcer or strangulated bowel) may cause a moderate rise in plasma amylase, although this rarely reaches 1000 i.u./ml. Plasma amylase levels rise rapidly at the outset of an attack of pancreatitis, and levels of 10 000 i.u./ml or more may be recorded on admission to hospital. However, the levels fall as the patient recovers and the diagnosis of pancreatitis should not rely on an arbitrary threshold; rather the amylase level at any particular time should be interpreted in relation to the time elapsed since the onset of abdominal pain. Most other enzyme estimations have not proved more sensitive or specific than amylase although **serum lipase** estimation may be useful in difficult or late-presenting cases. In addition, elevated alanine amino-transferase (ALT) levels are highly specific for gallstone pancreatitis.

The peak amylase level is not an indicator of the severity of the pancreatitis or of the likelihood of subsequent complications. However, persistently raised levels over several days warn of developing complications. Note that false negative amylase results may occur in lipaemic serum. In this case, true results can be obtained on diluted specimens.

On rare occasions, the serum amylase may be normal in acute pancreatitis. This occurs where most of the gland has been destroyed by severe pancreatitis. It may also occur if a patient presents several days into an attack, by which time the amylase may no longer be elevated. If pancreatitis is strongly suspected but the serum amylase is normal, the diagnosis may be confirmed by appropriate radiological imaging (see next section).

Once the patient is in the recovery phase of the illness, fasting bloods should be taken for calcium levels and for plasma lipids, particularly triglycerides. Viral antibody titres may be useful in cases of idiopathic pancreatitis.

Imaging

Plain X-rays of both chest (erect) to look for free gas under the diaphragm, and abdomen (supine) are usually performed during the initial investigation. Abdominal X-ray may show a featureless 'ground-glass' appearance if peritoneal exudate is present. Bowel gas tends to be absent except perhaps for a '**sentinel loop**' of dilated adynamic small bowel in the centre of the abdomen. Note, however, that these signs are not specific for pancreatitis and are often absent. Rarely, radiopaque gallstones are visible.

An **ultrasound scan** of the biliary tree is essential but good images are not always obtained; a delay of 48–72 hours may allow an improved image quality. The goal is to look for small calculi in the gall bladder or bile ducts which are typically responsible for gallstone pancreatitis. If no definite cause for the pancreatitis is found, a repeat ultrasound examination should be performed following recovery from the attack.

CT scanning has a limited role in acute pancreatitis. In terms of initial diagnosis, it is indicated only when the clinical and biochemical findings are equivocal, particularly if the amylase is normal and other intra-abdominal pathology such as perforation or infarction needs to be excluded. In **severe pancreatitis**, contrast-enhanced CT scanning is also valuable in demonstrating the presence of necrosis, however necrosis cannot be identified until at least 4 days after the onset of symptoms. CT scans performed too early in the course of the disease cannot predict the final severity of the disease and are unlikely to influence management of the patient during the first week.

Endoscopy

In patients where a cause for pancreatitis is not evident from the history or initial imaging studies, endoscopic retrograde cholangio-pancreatography (**ERCP**) may have an important diagnostic role. In this group of patients, a cause can be found in about 50%, e.g. small pancreatic or periampullary tumours, pancreatic duct stricture, gallstones, congenital pancreas divisum or a high-pressure sphincter of Oddi. Early sphincterotomy also has an important role in management.

Table 25.2 A mnemonic ('PANCREAS') for remembering the modified Glasgow scoring system of severity prediction in acute pancreatitis

Mnemonic letter	Criterion	Positive when
P	PaO_2	< 8 kPA or 60 mmHg
A	Age	> 55 years
N	Neutrophil count	> 15 × 10⁹/L
C	Calcium (blood)	< 2 mmol/L
R	Raised plasma urea	> 16 mmol/L
E	Enzyme (plasma lactate dehydrogenase, LDH)	> 600 i.u./L
A	Albumin (plasma)	< 32 g/L
S	Sugar (plasma glucose)	> 10 mmol/L

After E M Moore, with permission

Box 25.4 Criteria for early identification of severe pancreatitis (after Ranson)

Severe pancreatitis, with a high risk of major complications or death, is defined by the presence of three or more of the following features:

On admission

- Age over 55 years (non-gallstone pancreatitis) or 70 years (gallstone pancreatitis)
- Leucocyte count greater than 16 000 × 10⁹/L
- Blood glucose greater than 10 mmol/L in a patient who is not diabetic
- Lactate dehydrogenase (LDH) greater than 350 i.u./L
- Serum glutamic oxaloacetic transaminase (SGOT) > 100 u/L

During the next 48 hours

- Haematocrit increase of more than 10%
- Serum urea increase of more than 10 mmol/L despite adequate i.v. therapy
- Hypocalcaemia (corrected serum Ca < 2.0 mmol/L)
- Low arterial PO_2 (< 8 kPa or 60 mmHg)
- Metabolic acidosis (base deficit more than 4 mEq/L)
- Estimated fluid sequestration more than 6 L

CLINICAL CLASSIFICATION

The initial clinical picture cannot be relied upon to predict which patients are likely to deteriorate. Only a small proportion eventually suffer necrotising pancreatitis but a case of mild pancreatitis can rapidly deteriorate to 'death's door'. To provide **early warning** of severity, each patient with acute pancreatitis is placed into one of two categories, **mild** or **severe**. This provides an indicator of prognosis within the first 48 hours and is central to the formulation of a management strategy. Categorisation is based on carefully tested scoring systems originally developed by **Ranson** in USA (see Box 25.4) and modified by **Imrie** (Glasgow criteria—see Table 25.2). If three or more of the factors listed are present, the patient is diagnosed as having severe pancreatitis and should be admitted to an intensive care or high-dependency unit for careful monitoring. The more adverse factors present, the worse the prognosis. Even if a patient is initially placed in the mild group, continued observation is essential as a swing to severe pancreatitis can occur at any time.

Mild acute pancreatitis

Mild attacks are common. The patient looks generally well with minimal systemic features. Nevertheless, there is often considerable pain. The abdomen is usually distended and diffusely tender but with little guarding. Bowel sounds are absent as a result of inflammatory ileus and rectal examination is normal. The patient may be mildly jaundiced as a result of periampullary oedema. The differential diagnosis in this situation includes biliary colic, acute cholecystitis, an acute exacerbation of a peptic ulcer or even a small perforation of a peptic ulcer. Lower lobe pneumonia or an inferior myocardial infarction may sometimes present in this way. Sometimes the diagnosis is made after the serum amylase is unexpectedly found to be elevated.

Severe acute pancreatitis

In a severe attack the patient looks apathetic, grey and shocked and there are typical abdominal signs of generalised peritonitis, i.e. extreme tenderness, guarding and rigidity. In this case, the differential diagnosis includes other major abdominal catastrophes, especially faecal peritonitis from perforated large bowel and concealed haemorrhage from a leaking aortic aneurysm or ruptured ectopic pregnancy. Massive bowel infarction due to arterial occlusion may present in this way but the abdominal signs are often less marked. An important early and dangerous complication of severe acute pancreatitis is acute respiratory distress syndrome (**ARDS**). The clinical features of acute pancreatitis are summarised in Box 25.3.

MANAGEMENT OF ACUTE PANCREATITIS

Mild attacks

The management of acute pancreatitis has been the subject of international debate and there are now numerous guidelines available, including those from the World Association of Gastroenterology and the International Association of Pancreatology. In the UK, the guidelines most used are those published by the British Society of Gastroenterology, updated in 2005.

Mild attacks require no further emergency investigation once diagnosed, and are managed by fluid resuscitation and analgesia. There is no evidence to support the use of antibiotics in mild cases and recovery is usually rapid. At one time oral intake was often withheld, intending to 'rest' the pancreas, but there is no evidence of benefit and these patients need no dietary restriction. Later management is aimed at treating predisposing factors. Gallstones should be sought by ultrasonography; if present, cholecystectomy is the definitive treatment and is performed 2–4 weeks after recovery, preferably on the same admission. Ductal stones should be removed endoscopically before discharge from hospital. Alcohol abuse must be discouraged.

Severe attacks

A severe attack is defined by reference to a list of criteria which should be evaluated on admission and over the next 48 hours (see Table 25.2 and Box 25.4, p. 384). Patients with severe pancreatitis may die early in the attack because of profound systemic toxaemia (SIRS), shock and multiple organ dysfunction syndrome (MODS); see Chapter 2. ARDS develops rapidly with little warning but a deteriorating arterial PO_2 may herald its onset. This is an indication for urgent ventilatory support before the condition becomes established.

Even when pancreatitis is severe, supportive measures are still the mainstay of treatment. These include **oxygen supplementation** and careful intravenous **fluid resuscitation**. A nasogastric tube is passed to aspirate the stomach if gastroparesis causes troublesome vomiting. Enteral nasogastric or naso-jejunal feeding has been reported in some series to significantly decrease morbidity. If starvation is prolonged and enteral feeding is not tolerated because of ileus, then total parenteral nutrition may be necessary.

Gross fluid and electrolyte disturbances as well as hypocalcaemia are also likely to occur. Fluid balance in the shocked patient is complicated by massive losses of protein-rich fluid into the peritoneal cavity and interstitially ('third space'). This sequestration of fluid needs to be countered by large amounts of colloid and crystalloid solutions, carefully monitored by measuring central venous pressure and hourly urine output. Any patient recognised to have severe pancreatitis or anyone with acute pancreatitis, however mild, who develops signs of serious deterioration should be admitted to an intensive care unit without delay for close monitoring and vigorous treatment of cardiovascular, pulmonary, renal and septic complications. Box 25.5 lists recommended investigations to guide management.

Plasma amylase may be measured daily to chart the progress of the disease; as the inflammation begins to resolve, the amylase levels fall accordingly. However, C-reactive protein (CRP) is a better indicator of systemic inflammation and hence developing necrosis and other

---

> **Box 25.5** **Recommended frequent investigations in severe acute pancreatitis**
>
> - Haemoglobin estimation and white cell count
> - Arterial blood gas estimations
> - Blood sugar
> - Plasma electrolytes, creatinine and urea
> - 'Liver function tests' (i.e. bilirubin, alkaline phosphatase, lactate dehydrogenase (LDH), transaminases, serum proteins)
> - Plasma calcium and phosphate
> - C-reactive protein on Day 1 and 5

---

complications. If the CRP is elevated at > 100 on Day 5, complications such as pancreatic infection, abscess or pseudocyst are likely to be responsible. Biochemical estimations, particularly liver transaminases and bilirubin, are charted regularly, looking chiefly for evidence of biliary obstruction; renal function tests are performed for evidence of acute renal failure.

Prophylactic parenteral antibiotics (e.g. a cephalosporin or imipenem) should be administered to minimise the risk of any pancreatic necrosis becoming infected, even though the evidence for benefit is not strong.

Endoscopy and surgery in severe acute pancreatitis

All patients suspected of having or proven to have a gallstone aetiology should undergo urgent therapeutic ERCP, and this should take place within 72 hours of the onset of pain. This applies whether severe pancreatitis is predicted from diagnostic criteria or has been confirmed. All of these patients require **sphincterotomy** of the sphincter of Oddi whether or not stones are found in the common bile duct. If stones are seen or if cholangitis or jaundice is present, biliary stenting is also usually required.

There is no role for surgery during the acute attack but in patients with stones laparoscopic cholecystectomy with operative cholangiography should be performed before discharge from hospital. This is because deferring cholecystectomy until months after the acute attack increases the risk of another attack. In the small group of critically ill patients with infected necrotic tissue and infected peripancreatic fluid collections, surgical debridement with or without continuous peritoneal irrigation is unavoidable, but mortality remains high.

The principles of management of acute pancreatitis are summarised in Box 25.6.

COMPLICATIONS OF ACUTE PANCREATITIS

Mortality

About 15% of patients admitted to hospital with acute pancreatitis have severe disease, which carries a high risk

Box	25.6	Principles of management of severe acute pancreatitis

(Treatments added according to severity of attack)

- Resuscitation with intravenous fluids and early oxygen supplementation
- 'Nil by mouth'
- Nasogastric tube and gastric aspiration
- Intravenous antibiotics
- Intensive care:
    —fluid and electrolyte management
    —treatment of hypocalcaemia
    —ventilatory support
- Laparotomy and pancreatic necrosectomy

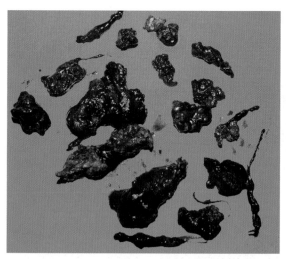

Fig. 25.1 Pancreatic necrosis
Necrotic pancreas removed 16 days after a severe attack of pancreatitis complicated by peripancreatic infection. The patient made a slow recovery but became diabetic in the convalescent period.

of potential complications. It is important to be aware, however, that about 10% of patients initially diagnosed with mild pancreatitis will deteriorate markedly during admission and become severe. In severe pancreatitis, mortality is 8–10%, i.e. 2% of all cases, and obese patients have a much higher mortality. About half of those that die do so within the first week, usually of ARDS and pulmonary failure. The other early life-threatening complications are associated with **multiple organ dysfunction (MODS)** as a result of systemic inflammatory activation. Manifestations include cardiovascular collapse aggravated by fluid shifts, renal failure made worse by hypotension, and disseminated intravascular coagulopathy. If death occurs after the first week, infective complications on top of existing organ failure are the usual cause.

Pancreatic necrosis and infection

In cases of severe pancreatitis, **pancreatic and peripancreatic necrosis** may manifest during the first 2 weeks of the attack (see Fig. 25.1). Necrosis is identified using intravenous contrast-enhanced CT scanning in which the necrotic pancreas does not opacify, having lost its blood supply. Infection of devitalised pancreatic and peripancreatic tissues occurs in about one-third of patients with severe pancreatitis despite prophylactic antibiotics, and is often lethal. With infection, the pancreatitis fails to resolve and signs of systemic inflammation appear. Infection may be suspected by the appearance of gas bubbles within pancreatic fluid collections but can be confirmed only by percutaneous aspiration (with microscopy and culture of the aspirate), usually performed under CT guidance. In proven infected cases, operative debridement, drainage and sometimes continuous peritoneal irrigation may be necessary, along with aggressive organ support.

Fluid collections around the pancreas

During the initial attack, **acute fluid collections** may develop around the gland. Most of these resolve sponta-

neously, but for those that do not, CT-guided percutaneous drainage is valuable. Fluid collections persisting for longer than 6 weeks are termed **pancreatic pseudocysts** (see below). Late in the course of the disease, a **pancreatic abscess** may develop. This is a well-localised collection of pus within the gland, and contrasts with **infected necrotising pancreatitis** which appears earlier and is not localised.

Pancreatic pseudocyst

A pancreatic pseudocyst is a collection of pancreatic enzymes, inflammatory fluid and necrotic debris, usually encapsulated within the lesser sac. Pseudocysts appear in 1–8% of cases of acute pancreatitis and are less likely to resolve spontaneously than the early acute fluid collections. A pseudocyst is not a true cyst (i.e. there is no epithelial lining) although the surrounding tissues become thickened by the inflammatory response. Pseudocysts may occur after even a moderate attack of pancreatitis and sometimes reach the size of a football! An upper abdominal mass may be palpable. If a pseudocyst is suspected, CT scanning is the investigation of choice (see Fig. 25.2).

Management varies according to the size of the cyst. Larger cysts, especially those larger than 10 cm, are unlikely to resolve. Those around 6 cm can be safely observed for up to 6 months, provided they have a typical appearance on CT scanning and are asymptomatic. If the cyst has failed to resolve by then, operative intervention should be considered. Operation, either by laparoscopy or an open approach, involves 'marsupialising' the pseudocyst into the posterior wall of the stomach. This can be performed after about 6 weeks, when the wall of the pseudocyst has 'matured' enough to hold sutures.

Fig. 25.2 Pancreatic pseudocyst

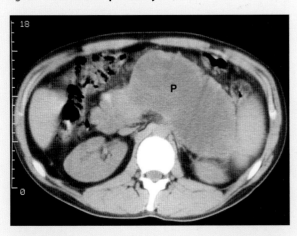

This 57-year-old man was admitted to hospital with an acute abdomen 3 weeks before this scan. He was found to have acute pancreatitis due to gallstones. The symptoms and signs of pancreatitis smouldered on and the CRP and plasma amylase failed to return to normal. This CT scan of his upper abdomen shows the cause of the persistent pancreatitis, a pseudocyst arising from the tail of the pancreas **P**.

Pancreatic abscess

Pancreatic abscesses occur in 1–4% of cases of acute pancreatitis. Certain patients remain systemically well despite pancreatic necrosis, with an illness that may grumble on for several weeks. There is a recurrent high swinging fever indicating the presence of an abscess. By that time, the necrotic pancreas is likely to have formed a discrete red-grey mass lying free within the pancreatic bed and bathed in pus; the pus may extend widely in the retroperitoneal tissues. Operation is then required to remove the necrotic tissue and drain the abscesses.

Complications of severe pancreatitis

Severe acute pancreatitis can cause wide-ranging complications in almost every system of the body:

- Multi-organ failure may lead to renal failure, respiratory failure, cardiac failure, and haematological and coagulation disorders
- Direct local pressure effects, inflammation and hypotension may cause portal vein thrombosis
- Local pressure plus hypotension may cause bowel ischaemia—the transverse colon is commonly affected because of the position of the middle colic artery
- Pseudoaneurysms may form in vessels such as the splenic artery because of inflammatory damage to the arterial wall and fluid collections around them
- Internal pancreatic fistulae may form, particularly if necrosis causes disruption of the pancreatic duct or the wall of a pseudocyst. The result may be pancreatic ascites, mediastinal pseudocysts, enzymatic mediastinitis or pancreatic pleural effusions

Late complications of acute pancreatitis

Diabetes mellitus, and intestinal malabsorption due to loss of pancreatic secretions sometimes occur after severe attacks, but it is surprising how uncommon these are considering the extent of pancreatic damage that occurs.

RECURRENT, RELAPSING AND CHRONIC PANCREATITIS

RECURRENT ACUTE PANCREATITIS

Some patients suffer recurrent attacks of acute pancreatitis, usually resulting from alcohol abuse or gallstone disease. The first and second attacks may be severe, but attacks after that almost never produce lethal complications. The patient is entirely well between attacks. In different patients, the attacks vary in severity but are rarely extreme. This condition is often described as 'chronic relapsing pancreatitis' but both types are better described as recurrent acute pancreatitis.

CHRONIC PANCREATITIS

Other patients suffer persistent and severe upper abdominal pain, similar in character to a prolonged attack of acute pancreatitis. This condition is known as chronic pancreatitis. These patients do not develop the other clinical features of acute pancreatitis and may not develop elevated amylase levels (hyperamylasaemia). The pain is so severe and so persistent as to drive some patients to suicide. Carcinoma of the pancreas and chronic pancreatic inflammation should both be considered in patients with this pattern of pain. Inflammatory swelling of the pancreatic head occasionally causes obstructive jaundice but carcinoma in this position is a far more common cause of jaundice.

Despite the pain, there are usually no abnormal abdominal signs. The plasma amylase may be moderately elevated on occasions; the diagnosis of chronic pancreatitis may, however, be missed if raised amylase levels are not detected. This may be because tests are not done at an appropriate time or the patient is unfortunate enough never to have elevated levels. There is a danger that these patients may be dismissed as suffering from psychosomatic pain.

Ultrasound or CT scans may show glandular swelling (sometimes difficult to differentiate from pancreatic carcinoma) and a dilated pancreatic duct. If ERCP is performed, the pancreatic duct system may look normal or else may be distorted and irregular in calibre, confirming chronic inflammation and fibrosis (see Fig. 25.3). Sometimes pancreatic duct stones are demonstrated.

Fig. 25.3 Retrograde pancreatography

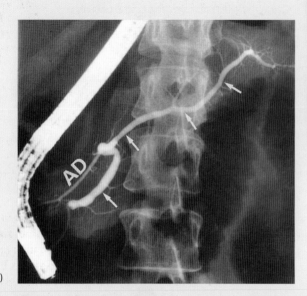

(a)

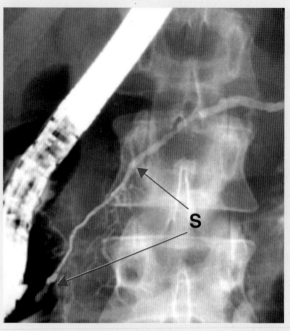

(b)

These films were both obtained by injecting contrast into the pancreatic duct using a flexible duodenoscope. **(a)** This pancreatogram is normal. The main duct (arrowed) narrows regularly towards the tail of the pancreas and there are no strictures or dilatations along its length. The accessory pancreatic duct **AD** also fills in this patient. **(b)** This pancreatogram is from a man of 26 with a history of severe upper abdominal pain. There is a long stricture of the main duct between the red arrows **S** of unknown origin. Typical changes of chronic pancreatitis, i.e. irregularity of the wall with dilatations and poor filling of small ducts, are seen in the duct distal to the stricture.

Chronic pancreatitis may cause years of misery, perhaps eventually 'burning out' as the gland atrophies completely. It is important to make the diagnosis in good time so that pain can be relieved. In the long term, malabsorption or diabetes is more likely to develop than after acute pancreatitis.

Pancreatic calcification seen on abdominal X-rays is diagnostic of chronic pancreatitis but is a rare finding and is sometimes found in asymptomatic patients (see Fig. 25.4). X-rays are therefore of little clinical value.

Treatment of chronic pancreatitis is far from satisfactory. Surgery is only useful if structural abnormalities can be found. Surgical procedures include removal of pancreatic duct stones, partial pancreatectomy of the body and tail for duct stenosis, sphincteroplasty of the pancreatic duct opening, or occasionally total pancreatectomy. Chemical coeliac ganglion blockade provides useful (and often permanent) pain relief, but does nothing to prevent inflammation. If there are multiple duct strictures, the pancreatic duct can be surgically split along its whole length and the side of a loop of jejunum sutured to the gland to allow unrestricted drainage. Interventional endoscopy can be employed for dilatation and stenting of isolated pancreatic duct strictures.

Fig. 25.4 Pancreatic calcification in chronic pancreatitis

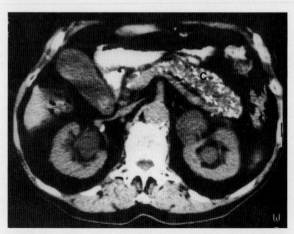

This obese 55-year-old man had a long history of severe abdominal pain and alcohol abuse. Pancreatic calcification was not visible on a plain abdominal X-ray but extensive calcification is clearly seen on this CT scan.

Appendicitis

INTRODUCTION

Acute appendicitis is the most common cause of intra-abdominal infection in developed countries and appendicectomy is the most common emergency surgical operation. In the UK, 1.9 females per thousand have the operation each year compared with 1.5 males, and about 1 in 7 people eventually undergo the operation. Surprisingly, the incidence of appendicitis fell by about 30% between the 1960s and the 1980s, for reasons unknown.

Appendicitis can occur at any age but is most common below 40 years, especially between the ages of 10 and 20. It is rare below the age of 10 and very rare below 2 years. Appendicitis is rare in rural parts of developing countries, but in the cities the incidence approaches that of the West. This different susceptibility in people of similar ethnic origin is probably related to a much reduced intake of dietary fibre in city-dwellers.

Acute appendicitis should be included in the differential diagnosis of all patients presenting to hospital with acute abdominal pain. Even previous appendicectomy does not absolutely rule out the diagnosis. Despite lay impressions, a positive diagnosis is often difficult to make and this is partly because of the wide range of differential diagnoses and the lack of specific diagnostic tests for the confirmation or exclusion of appendicitis. Sometimes a non-inflamed appendix is found at operation but a good proportion of these 'unnecessary' appendicectomy operations is unavoidable. Diagnostic laparoscopy can improve diagnostic accuracy, particularly in young women, and can also be used therapeutically to remove an inflamed appendix.

ANATOMY OF THE APPENDIX

The appendix is a blind-ending tube arising from the caecum at the meeting point of the three taeniae coli, just distal to the ileo-caecal junction. The base of the appendix thus lies in the right iliac fossa, close to **McBurney's point**. This is two-thirds of the way along a line drawn from the umbilicus to the anterior superior iliac spine (see Fig. 26.6, p. 397). In most cases, the appendix is mobile within the peritoneal cavity, suspended by its mesentery (**meso-appendix**) with the appendicular artery in its free edge. This is effectively an end-artery, with anastomotic connections only proximally.

The appendix has been described as lying in several 'classic' sites, but apart from the true retrocaecal appendix, the organ probably floats in a broad arc about its base (see Fig. 26.1). Only inflammation will fix it in a particular place. Its position will then determine the clinical presentation of the disease. In about 30% of appendicectomies, the appendix lies over the brim of the pelvis ('**pelvic appendix**'). In some cases, the appendix lies retroperitoneally behind the caecum and is often plastered to it by fibrous bands. Thus, an inflamed retrocaecal appendix may irritate the right ureter and psoas muscle, and may even lie high enough to simulate gall bladder pain.

Histologically, the appendix has the same basic structure as the large intestine. Its glandular mucosa is separated from a loose vascular submucosa by the delicate muscularis mucosa. External to the submucosa is the main muscular wall. The appendix is covered by a serosal layer (the visceral layer of peritoneum) which contains the large blood vessels and becomes continuous with the serosa of the meso-appendix. When the appendix lies retroperitoneally, there is no serosal covering. A prominent feature of the appendix is its collections of lymphoid tissue in the lamina propria. This lymphoid tissue often has germinal centres and is prominent in childhood but diminishes with increasing age.

The mucosa contains a large number of cells of the gastrointestinal endocrine amine precursor uptake and decarboxylation (APUD) system. These secrete mainly serotonin and were formerly known as **argentaffin cells**.

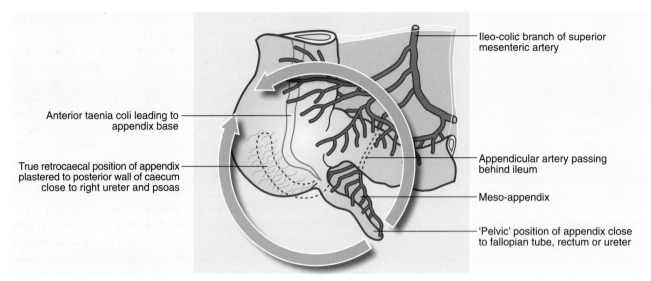

Fig. 26.1 Surgical anatomy of the appendix
The appendix can be positioned anywhere on the circumference shown by the arrowed arc.

Carcinoid tumours commonly occur in the appendix and arise from these cells.

PATHOPHYSIOLOGY OF APPENDICITIS

Appendicitis is probably initiated by obstruction of the lumen caused by impacted faeces or a faecolith. This explanation fits with the epidemiological observation that appendicitis is associated with a low dietary fibre intake.

In the early stages of appendicitis, the mucosa becomes inflamed first. This inflammation eventually extends through the submucosa to involve the muscular and serosal (peritoneal) layers. A fibrinopurulent exudate forms on the serosal surface and extends to any adjacent peritoneal surface, e.g. bowel or abdominal wall, causing a localised peritonitis.

By this stage the necrotic glandular mucosa sloughs into the lumen, which becomes distended with pus. Finally, the end-arteries supplying the appendix become thrombosed and the infarcted appendix becomes necrotic or **gangrenous**. This usually occurs at the distal end and the appendix begins to disintegrate. Perforation soon follows and faecally contaminated appendiceal contents spread into the peritoneal cavity. If the spilled contents are enveloped by omentum or adherent small bowel, a localised **abscess** results; otherwise spreading peritonitis develops. The evolution of acute appendicitis is illustrated histologically in Figure 26.2.

CLINICAL FEATURES OF APPENDICITIS

The pathophysiological evolution of appendicitis and the corresponding symptoms and signs are illustrated in Figure 26.3.

CLASSIC APPENDICITIS

Acute appendicitis classically begins with poorly localised, colicky central abdominal **visceral pain**; this results from smooth muscle spasm as a reaction to appendiceal obstruction. Anorexia and vomiting often accompany the pain at this stage.

As inflammation advances over the ensuing 12–24 hours, it progresses through the appendiceal wall to involve the parietal peritoneum (which is innervated somatically). At this stage the pain typically becomes **localised** to the right iliac fossa. Signs of local peritonitis can be elicited at this stage, i.e. tenderness, guarding and rebound tenderness. This classic picture is seen in less than half of all cases, largely because the localising symptoms and signs vary with the anatomical relations of the inflamed appendix and the vigorousness of the body's defences.

OTHER PRESENTATIONS OF ACUTE APPENDICITIS

If the appendix lies in the pelvis near the rectum, it may cause local irritation and diarrhoea. If it lies near the bladder or ureter, inflammation may cause urinary symptoms of frequency, dysuria and (microscopic) pyuria, i.e. leucocytes in the urine. These findings may be mistakenly interpreted as urinary tract infection. An inflamed retrocaecal appendix produces none of the usual localising symptoms or signs, but may irritate the psoas muscle causing involuntary right hip flexion and pain on extension. A high retrocaecal appendix may cause pain and tenderness below the right costal margin. An inflamed appendix near the Fallopian tube causes pelvic pain sug-

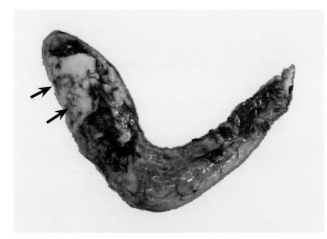

(a) Macroscopic photograph showing acutely inflamed appendix. The distended tip shows a purulent exudate on the serosal surface (arrowed).

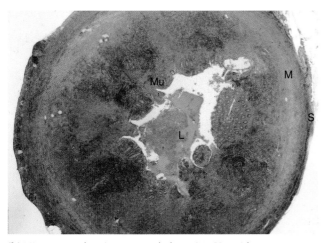

(b) Microscopy showing mucosal ulceration **Mu** with acute inflammatory cells within the lumen **L**. Inflammation extends through the muscle wall **M** to the serosal surface **S**.

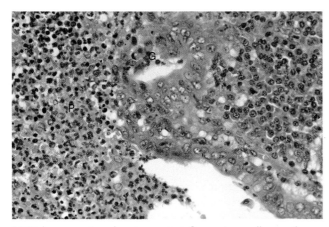

(c) High-power view showing acute inflammatory cells, mostly polymorphs **P**, destroying glands **G**.

Fig. 26.2 Acute appendicitis

gestive of an acute gynaecological disorder such as salpingitis or torsion of an ovarian cyst.

The early phase of poorly localised pain typically lasts for a few hours until peritoneal inflammation produces localising signs. If untreated, the inflamed appendix may become gangrenous after 12–24 hours and perforate, causing spreading peritonitis unless it is sealed off by omentum. The whole abdomen becomes rigid and tender and there is marked systemic toxicity. Perforation is particularly common in young children. Sometimes, the pathological sequence is extremely rapid and the patient presents with sudden peritonitis.

In older patients, a gangrenous or perforated appendix is more likely to be contained by the greater omentum or loops of small bowel. This results in a palpable **appendix mass**. This may contain free pus and is then known as an **appendiceal abscess**. As with any significant abscess, there is a tachycardia and swinging pyrexia. An appendix mass usually resolves spontaneously over 2–6 weeks. In the elderly, a delayed diagnosis may produce an appendix abscess, walled off by loops of small bowel. There may be no palpable mass and the symptoms and signs may not be recognisable as appendicitis. These include nonspecific abdominal pain and features of small bowel obstruction due to localised paralytic ileus. Occasionally, appendicitis may present in a most unusual way. Examples include discharge of an appendix abscess into the Fallopian tube presenting as a purulent vaginal discharge, and inflammation of an appendix lying in an inguinal hernia presenting as an abscess in the groin.

MAKING THE DIAGNOSIS OF APPENDICITIS

Acute appendicitis is a clinical diagnosis, relying almost entirely on the history and physical examination. Investigations are only useful in excluding other differential diagnoses. Ideally, the diagnosis should be made and the appendix removed before it becomes gangrenous and perforates. This markedly reduces the risk of infective complications. On the other hand, unnecessary appendicectomies must be kept to a minimum.

Diagnosis of acute appendicitis poses little difficulty if the patient exhibits the classic symptoms and signs summarised in Box 26.1. The problem occurs when the symptoms and signs are not typical. The patient may present at a very early stage, or the signs may have some other pathological cause. At least two out of every three children admitted to hospital with suspected appendicitis do not have the condition.

If the evidence for acute appendicitis is insufficient and no other diagnosis can be made, the patient should be kept under observation, admitted to hospital if necessary and re-examined periodically. Eventually, the symptoms settle or the diagnosis becomes clear.

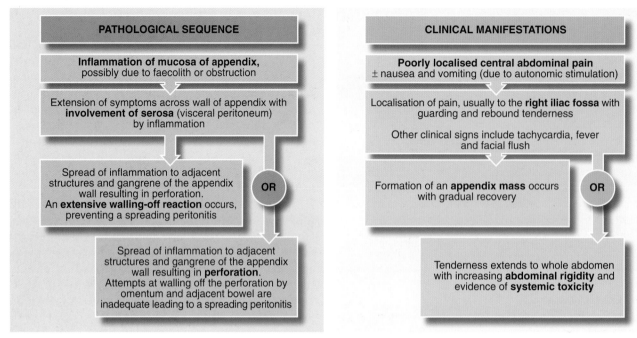

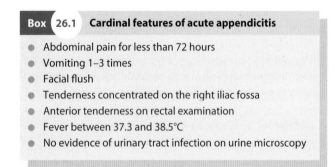

Fig. 26.3 Pathophysiology and clinical manifestations of acute appendicitis

| Box | 26.1 | **Cardinal features of acute appendicitis** |

- Abdominal pain for less than 72 hours
- Vomiting 1–3 times
- Facial flush
- Tenderness concentrated on the right iliac fossa
- Anterior tenderness on rectal examination
- Fever between 37.3 and 38.5°C
- No evidence of urinary tract infection on urine microscopy

SPECIAL POINTS IN THE HISTORY AND EXAMINATION

Acute appendicitis typically runs a short course, between a few hours and about 3 days. If symptoms have been present for longer, appendicitis is unlikely unless an 'appendix mass' has developed. A recent or current sore throat or viral-type illness, particularly in children, favours the diagnosis of **mesenteric adenitis** (inflammation of the mesenteric lymph nodes analogous to viral tonsillitis). Urinary symptoms suggest **urinary tract infection** but may also occur with pelvic appendicitis.

The patient with appendicitis is typically quiet, apathetic and flushed; the lively child doing jigsaw puzzles almost never has appendicitis! Oral foetor may be present but is not a reliable sign of appendicitis. Cervical lymphadenopathy tends to suggest a viral origin for the abdominal pain. Mild tachycardia and pyrexia are typical of appendicitis but a temperature much over 38°C makes the diagnosis of acute viral illness or urinary tract infection more likely.

Signs of peritoneal inflammation in the right iliac fossa are often absent in the early stages of the illness. The patient should be asked to cough, blow the abdominal wall out and draw it in; all of these cause pain if the parietal peritoneum is inflamed. In children, it may be difficult to interpret apparent tenderness, especially if the child cries and refuses to cooperate. This can usually be overcome by distracting the child's attention whilst palpating the abdomen through the bedclothes or even with the child's own hand under the examiner's hand. Several signs (e.g. Rovsing's sign—pressure in the left iliac fossa causing pain in the right iliac fossa) have been described that are said to point to the diagnosis of appendicitis but these are all unreliable. One useful test is to ask the child to stand, then to hop on the right leg. If this can be achieved, there is unlikely to be any significant peritoneal inflammation.

Rebound tenderness was traditionally demonstrated by palpating deeply, then releasing the hand suddenly. However, this can cause excessive and unexpected pain. A kinder and more precise way method is to perform gentle percussion in the right iliac fossa. This displaces and irritates inflamed peritoneum in a controlled way; if this is painful, then rebound is present. Anterior peritoneal tenderness on rectal examination (i.e. pelvic peritonitis) supports the diagnosis of appendicitis, provided other signs are consistent, but note that the appendix itself cannot be palpated rectally. In pelvic appendicitis, rectal tenderness may be the only abdominal sign. Lack of this sign does not, however, exclude appendicitis.

Box 26.2 Main differential diagnoses of acute appendicitis

Urinary tract infection (cystitis or pyelonephritis)

- Unlikely if nitrites are absent from dipstick testing of the urine and can be excluded if there are not significant numbers of white blood cells or bacteria on urine microscopy

Mesenteric adenitis

- Common in children and often associated with an upper respiratory infection or sore throat
- Inflammation and enlargement of the abdominal lymph nodes, probably viral in origin
- Fever is typically higher than in appendicitis (i.e. greater than 38.5°C) and settles rapidly
- A firm diagnosis can only be made at laparotomy or laparoscopy, but gradual resolution favours this diagnosis

Large bowel disorders

- Constipation may cause colicky abdominal pain and iliac fossa tenderness. There is no fever and the rectum is loaded with faeces
- Diverticulitis affecting the caecum or the sigmoid colon (when lying in the right iliac fossa) is usually diagnosed only at operation

Gynaecological disorders

- The pain of ovulation about 14 days after the last menstrual period (mittelschmerz) may cause right iliac fossa pain. There is often a history of similar pain in the past. There are no signs of infection and the pain settles quickly
- Salpingitis (most commonly chlamydial) causes lower abdominal pain, often with a vaginal discharge. Digital vaginal examination typically reveals adnexal tenderness, and moving the cervix from side to side induces pain ('cervical excitation')
- Torsion of, or haemorrhage into a right ovarian cyst may produce symptoms like appendicitis, but there is no fever. A tender mobile mass may be palpable in the right suprapubic region or on vaginal examination. This diagnosis can be confirmed with ultrasound
- Ectopic pregnancy. May present with anaemia and/or hypotension. A pregnancy test is mandatory

Small bowel pathology

- An inflamed or perforated Meckel's diverticulum (see Fig. 26.4) may present exactly like appendicitis
- Terminal ileitis due to Crohn's disease (or, more rarely, *Yersinia pseudotuberculosis*)
- Necrotic small bowel from strangulation usually presents with intestinal obstruction

Acute pancreatitis

- Pain is predominantly central
- If there is tenderness in the right iliac fossa, it will also be present in the epigastrium
- If in doubt, the serum amylase should be measured

Gastroenteritis

- Vague abdominal pain and tenderness which may be associated with vomiting and diarrhoea
- Usually improves steadily during a period of observation

DIFFERENTIAL DIAGNOSIS

The differential diagnosis of acute appendicitis theoretically includes all the causes of an acute abdomen shown earlier in Box 12.1 However, the main conditions of practical importance are summarised in Box 26.2, along with the main features distinguishing them from acute appendicitis. These other conditions rarely need operation. Certain uncommon conditions such as *Yersinia* ileitis and inflamed Meckel's diverticulum (Fig. 26.4) are included in the list but they can only be distinguished from appendicitis at operation.

THE EQUIVOCAL DIAGNOSIS

If acute appendicitis can be diagnosed confidently on clinical grounds, no further investigations other than those dictated by potential comorbidity are required unless there are secondary problems such as anaemia or dehydration. It is worth emphasising that there are no diagnostic tests specific for appendicitis; where the diagnosis is in doubt, the patient **must** be re-examined every few hours to identify changes in the clinical picture to ensure that deterioration is detected early. Missing an evident clinical diagnosis and sending the patient home causes unnecessary pain and suffering and is likely to prompt a claim for medical negligence

Certain investigations may be useful where the diagnosis is in doubt. The white blood count is usually unhelpful, as a modest rise occurs in many conditions. If there is a great rise (say to over 16×10^3), the clinical diagnosis of appendicitis is usually already clinically obvious, but it helps to exclude non-suppurative gynaecological pathology. Urinalysis must be performed if there is any suggestion of a urinary tract infection. A **pregnancy test** should be performed in females of child-bearing age.

Various **scoring systems** have been devised to try to improve the accuracy of clinical diagnosis in suspected appendicitis. The most well known of these is the Alvarado score (see Table 26.1) but the results are too variable for it to be of universal clinical benefit.

Abdominal X-rays are not needed unless there is confusing evidence of abdominal pathology after a period of

Fig. 26.4 Perforated Meckel's diverticulum

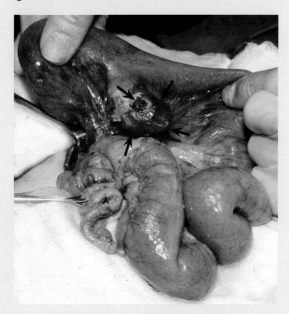

This man of 28 presented with a typical history and clinical findings of acute appendicitis. However, at operation he was found to have a normal appendix but a perforated Meckel's diverticulum (arrowed). The diverticulum was resected and the appendix also removed to prevent future confusion and the patient made a good recovery. On histological examination, the Meckel's was found to contain gastric mucosa.

Table 26.1 Scoring system for the diagnosis of acute appendicitis based on the Alvarado score

	Score
Migration of pain from central abdomen to right iliac fossa	1
Anorexia	1
Nausea or vomiting	1
Tenderness in right iliac fossa	2
Rebound tenderness	1
Raised temperature ($\geq$ 37.5°C)	1
Raised leucocyte count $\geq 10 \times 10^9$/L	2
Neutrophilia of $\geq$ 75%	1
Total	**10**

The Alvarado scoring system is an objective, structured means of assessing patients with right iliac fossa pain, but has proved unreliable in diagnosing acute appendicitis. However, patients with an initial score of 4 or less are very unlikely to have appendicitis and do not need hospital admission unless symptoms worsen. In patients with appendicitis, 40% have rising scores, confirming this is a progressive disorder in which symptoms and signs evolve with time.

observation. The presence of a single fluid level in the right iliac fossa or even widespread small bowel dilatation suggests local adynamic bowel disorder due to appendicitis causing functional obstruction, but this is an uncommon finding. Even less commonly, a perforated appendix may allow sufficient free gas to escape to be revealed on plain X-rays. In adults with an equivocal diagnosis of appendicitis, the plasma amylase should be measured because the early features of appendicitis and pancreatitis can be similar. Abdominal ultrasound can be helpful to detect an abscess or mass, or non-appendiceal pathology, but cannot be relied upon to show uncomplicated appendicitis. CT scanning is claimed to be accurate but submits the patient to a high radiation dose and greatly increases the cost of investigation. Laparoscopy is increasingly used in women of menstruating age in whom gynaecological pathologies are common. However, this is an invasive investigation requiring a general anaesthetic and is best employed when an operation is clearly indicated but the diagnosis is still ambiguous.

PROBLEMS IN THE DIAGNOSIS OF APPENDICITIS

THE VERY YOUNG

Appendicitis is rarely seen below 2 years of age, but when it does occur, the 'typical' abdominal symptoms and signs are obscure or absent. An infant or toddler may display signs of infection without revealing the abdominal origin. Abdominal X-rays may demonstrate dilated loops of bowel and fluid levels. Generalised peritonitis supervenes all too rapidly in this age group because the abdominal defence mechanisms are rudimentary, in particular the 'wrapping' effect of the greater omentum. Laparotomy is usually indicated in an ill infant with abdominal signs.

THE ELDERLY

Appendicitis tends to develop more slowly in the elderly. The appendix wall becomes fibrotic with age and the area is more readily walled off by omentum and adherent small bowel. Indeed, many cases probably resolve spontaneously. In those who reach hospital, the history is often as long as one week. Symptoms and signs of obstruction may be present, including vomiting, colicky abdominal pain and obstructed bowel sounds. A mass may be palpable if the patient is relaxed and not too tender but often it can be palpated only under general anaesthesia. Abdominal X-rays may reveal fluid levels in the right iliac fossa.

PREGNANCY

Appendicitis occurs at least as often during pregnancy as at other times but the diagnosis can be difficult. The

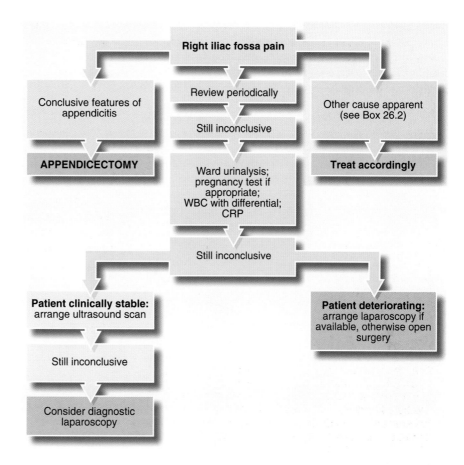

Fig. 26.5 Summary—management of suspected appendicitis

appendix is displaced upwards by the enlarging uterus so that abdominal pain and tenderness are in a much higher position than usual. The diagnosis and management of the pregnant patient must be shared with an obstetrician. Laparoscopy may be indicated if the diagnosis is in doubt but this becomes technically difficult beyond 26 weeks. Mortality from appendicitis for both mother and fetus rises as the pregnancy progresses and can be as high as 9% for the mother and 20% for the fetus in the third trimester.

THE 'GRUMBLING' APPENDIX

Recurrent bouts of right iliac fossa pain occur in some children and are often labelled as 'grumbling appendix'. Appendicular pathology is probably not the cause in most of these cases. Persistent chronic inflammation of the appendix probably does not occur, but recurrent bouts of appendicular colic or low-grade acute appendicitis undoubtedly do. These children may have several abortive admissions for abdominal pain and it may eventually be justifiable to remove the appendix to allay parental anxiety. A non-inflamed appendix containing a faecolith or threadworms (assumed to have caused the pain) is often found. The pain will be cured in no more than half.

The management of suspected appendicitis is summarised in Figure 26.5.

APPENDICECTOMY

The annual death rate from appendicitis has fallen dramatically since 1960. In 1934 there were 3193 deaths from appendicitis in the UK, whereas by 1982 this had fallen to 110. The improvement results from several factors including better general nutrition, earlier presentation, better preoperative preparation and better anaesthesia. Deaths that now occur are usually due to dehydration and electrolyte changes which are unrecognised or ineffectively treated before surgery, often as a result of a late or missed diagnosis. Infective complications of appendicitis have fallen dramatically since the 1970s because of the widespread use of prophylactic antibacterial agents.

ANTIBIOTIC PROPHYLAXIS

In appendicitis, most intra-abdominal infective complications and wound infections occur in perforated or gangrenous appendicitis. The majority of the infecting organisms are anaerobic and the infections can largely be prevented by prophylactic metronidazole. Rectal suppositories are just as effective as intravenous metronidazole and are cheaper but are best given 2 hours before operation. Aerobic organisms are involved in a smaller number of cases and some surgeons therefore advocate additional prophylaxis with an antibiotic such as a cephalosporin.

TECHNIQUE OF APPENDICECTOMY

The principal steps in appendicectomy are illustrated in Figure 26.6 and should be understood by any doctor called upon to assist in the operation. Increasingly, laparotomy is being replaced by laparoscopic diagnosis and surgery, but the principles are similar.

Open appendicectomy

A low skin crease incision (**Lanz**) rather than the higher and more oblique one centred on McBurney's point is now favoured as it gives a better cosmetic result. The superficial (Scarpa's) fascia (well marked in children) is then incised and the three musculo-aponeurotic layers of the abdominal wall are split along the line of their fibres. This produces the '**gridiron**' **incision**, described as such because the fibres of external oblique and internal oblique run at right angles to each other. The peritoneum is then lifted and opened and may reveal pus or mucopurulent watery fluid; a swab of this is taken for microscopy and culture. The appendix is located digitally and delivered into the wound; further exploration may be needed if it does not lie in the immediate vicinity. A retrocaecal appendix will require mobilisation of the caecum by dividing the peritoneum along its lateral side.

Once the appendix has been delivered into the wound, its blood supply in the meso-appendix is divided between clips and ligated. The appendix base is crushed with a haemostat which is then reapplied more distally. An absorbable ligature is then tied around the crushed area. After this preparation, the appendix is then excised. A 'purse-string' suture may be placed in the caecum near the appendix base, the appendix inverted and the suture tied, although this practice has fallen out of favour generally as it is not used in laparoscopic surgery and patients have not suffered adverse consequences from its omission. If the appendix was found to be perforated or gangrenous, or if pus was found, thorough peritoneal toilet is performed. A sump sucker is guided down into the pelvis with a finger to suck out any fluid, and the area is then gently swabbed out with gauze to remove any adherent infected material. Any pus or a faecolith left in the pelvis predisposes to subsequent pelvic abscess.

The peritoneum, internal oblique and external oblique are each closed with two or three absorbable sutures. Drainage is not usually recommended unless there is a thick-walled abscess cavity which will not collapse. If the appendix is perforated or gangrenous, delayed primary closure of the skin is advisable as this reduces the rela-

---

Box 26.3 Complications of appendicitis (see also p. 394)

Intraperitoneal complications

Early

- Appendix stump blowout—spillage of colonic contents into the peritoneal cavity
- Generalised peritonitis—perforated or gangrenous appendix, virulent organisms, late presentation or diagnosis
- Abscesses—local, pelvic, subhepatic, subphrenic
- Retained faecolith causing chronic local infection
- Haematoma due to slippage of a vascular ligature or a mesenteric or omental tear

Early or late (even many years later)

- Intestinal obstruction due to adhesions

Late

- Infertility due to tubal occlusion following pelvic infection

Abdominal wall complications

Early

- Superficial wound infection
- Deep wound infection
- Dehiscence

Late

- Incisional hernia

Notes:
1. Gangrenous or perforated appendix has higher risk of infective complications
2. Undiagnosed appendicitis or a late diagnosis is likely to lead to a higher incidence of complications, particular infective ones such as generalised peritonitis and systemic sepsis

---

tively high risk of wound infection. The superficial layers are left open initially and closed after 48 hours if the wound is clean.

After operation, oral fluids, followed by solids, are gradually increased unless vomiting or other complications occur, and most patients are able to be discharged on the second or third postoperative day.

Laparoscopic appendicectomy

Laparoscopy is a valuable technique that allows the appendix to be found wherever it may lie. It also permits visualisation of the rest of the abdominal cavity and the pelvis, thus improving diagnostic accuracy over open operation and minimising negative appendicectomies. It is strongly indicated in patients who are clearly unwell and in need of an operation but in whom the diagnosis is not clear. It is particularly useful in women of menstruating age and in any patient with pelvic symptoms. If the appendix is abnormal or if there is free fluid in the peri-

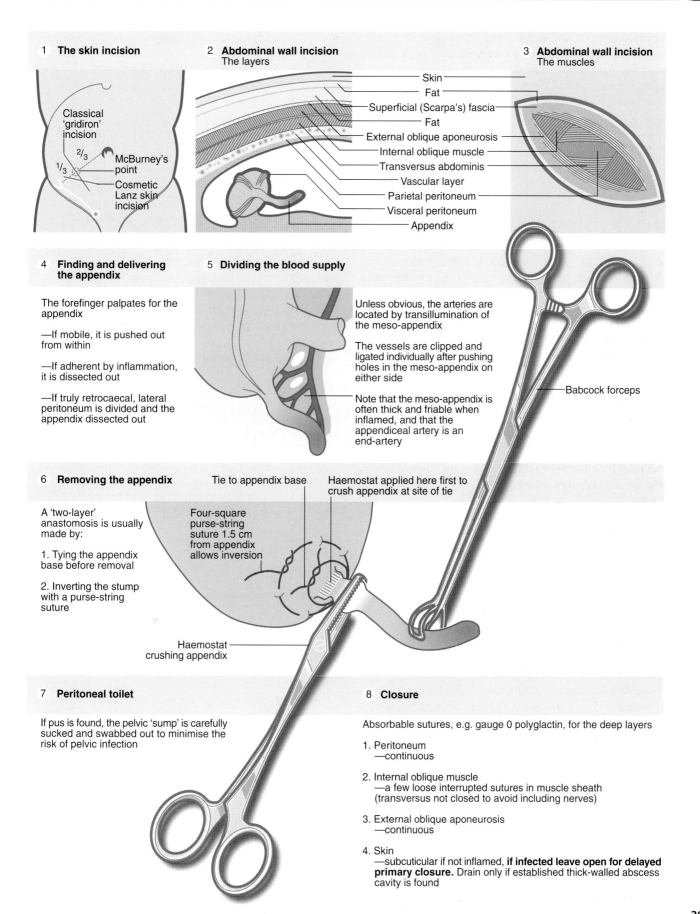

1 The skin incision

Classical 'gridiron' incision

2/3
1/3

McBurney's point

Cosmetic Lanz skin incision

2 Abdominal wall incision
The layers

Skin
Fat
Superficial (Scarpa's) fascia
Fat
External oblique aponeurosis
Internal oblique muscle
Transversus abdominis
Vascular layer
Parietal peritoneum
Visceral peritoneum
Appendix

3 Abdominal wall incision
The muscles

4 Finding and delivering the appendix

The forefinger palpates for the appendix

—If mobile, it is pushed out from within

—If adherent by inflammation, it is dissected out

—If truly retrocaecal, lateral peritoneum is divided and the appendix dissected out

5 Dividing the blood supply

Unless obvious, the arteries are located by transillumination of the meso-appendix

The vessels are clipped and ligated individually after pushing holes in the meso-appendix on either side

Note that the meso-appendix is often thick and friable when inflamed, and that the appendiceal artery is an end-artery

Babcock forceps

6 Removing the appendix

A 'two-layer' anastomosis is usually made by:

1. Tying the appendix base before removal

2. Inverting the stump with a purse-string suture

Tie to appendix base

Haemostat applied here first to crush appendix at site of tie

Four-square purse-string suture 1.5 cm from appendix allows inversion

Haemostat crushing appendix

7 Peritoneal toilet

If pus is found, the pelvic 'sump' is carefully sucked and swabbed out to minimise the risk of pelvic infection

8 Closure

Absorbable sutures, e.g. gauge 0 polyglactin, for the deep layers

1. Peritoneum
   —continuous

2. Internal oblique muscle
   —a few loose interrupted sutures in muscle sheath (transversus not closed to avoid including nerves)

3. External oblique aponeurosis
   —continuous

4. Skin
   —subcuticular if not inflamed, **if infected leave open for delayed primary closure.** Drain only if established thick-walled abscess cavity is found

Fig. 26.6 Appendicectomy—operative technique

toneal cavity for which no other cause can be found, appendicectomy is performed. Laparoscopic appendicectomy is a particularly useful tool in the obese, obviating the need for a large incision and the high risk of wound infection. Some surgeons use laparoscopy as a diagnostic tool and then convert to an open operation but laparoscopic appendicectomy may be performed if the appropriate skills and instruments are available.

The principles and techniques are similar to the open operation but laparoscopy is more technically demanding. The meso-appendix may be clipped or divided by diathermy and the appendix base is ligated using preformed 'endo-loop' sutures. The base of the appendix is rarely buried and must never be diathermied. Superior visualisation and good access allow a thorough washout to be performed. Laparoscopic removal of the appendix has a lower wound infection rate and may allow an earlier return to normal activities.

THE 'LILY-WHITE' APPENDIX

If the appendix is found not to be inflamed at open operation (colloquially termed 'lily-white'), it should always be removed because an appendicectomy scar would lead doctors in future to assume that the appendix has been removed. The abdomen is explored as allowed by the incision to search for a cause for the symptoms:

- **Mesenteric lymph nodes** in children may be grossly enlarged by mesenteric adenitis—this is probably viral in origin

- **The terminal ileum** may be thickened and reddened by Crohn's disease or, more rarely, by *Yersinia* ileitis. The latter is a self-limiting condition caused by the organism *Yersinia pseudotuberculosis* and requires no specific treatment. The appendix is removed but the bowel left untouched. If possible, an enlarged mesenteric node is removed for histological examination
- **A Meckel's diverticulum** may be found within 60 cm of the ileocaecal valve—if inflamed, this is removed but a wide-mouthed non-inflamed diverticulum is usually left alone
- **Both ovaries can usually be palpated**—ovaries may be twisted, inflamed or enlarged or an inflamed Fallopian tube may be seen
- **Cholecystitis, sigmoid diverticulitis** (with the sigmoid displaced to the right), **inflammation of a caecal diverticulum, hydronephrosis** or a **leaking aneurysm** are rarely found

THE APPENDIX MASS

A vigorous response to appendicitis may result in a mass in the right iliac fossa, often with fever. Usually the patient has few systemic symptoms or signs of ill health. A conservative regimen followed by interval appendicectomy 6 weeks later (**Ochsner–Sherren regimen**) was advocated in pre-antibiotic days but is now less favoured. Early operation under antibiotic cover is now performed more frequently.

Colorectal polyps and carcinoma

27

INTRODUCTION

Carcinoma of the colon and rectum is the third most common malignancy in both men and women in Western countries. In the UK, the lifetime risk of colorectal cancer is 5%, although the condition is less common in the developing world. Colorectal cancer is not only extremely common, it is also potentially preventable by screening the colon for premalignant lesions, namely **adenomatous polyps**. Surgery for large bowel cancer is generally rewarding, with high rates of cure achieved by timely resection.

Most cancers arise as a result of a complex interaction between genetic and environmental factors. The Western diet in particular has been incriminated in much of the geographical variation in incidence. About 5% of colorectal cancer is strongly genetically linked. It is important to recognise patients in this small group of **inherited colorectal cancer syndromes** as there are effective guidelines available for the screening and treatment of patients with these high-risk syndromes.

Most colorectal cancers originate in the glandular mucosa and are therefore histologically **adenocarcinomas**. Other forms of malignancy in the large bowel such as **carcinoid tumour** or **lymphoma** are rare. Squamous carcinomas occur at the anus or in anal canal skin but these have an entirely different aetiology and different methods of management; they are discussed in Chapter 30.

Surgery is the mainstay of treatment for colorectal cancer. The common procedures and the complications of large bowel surgery are outlined in this chapter and the different types of intestinal stomas and their indications are described.

COLORECTAL POLYPS

The term **polyp** can cause more confusion than understanding. The term is simply a morphological description and is used to describe any localised lesion protruding from the bowel wall into the lumen; it does *not* imply any specific pathology. This conforms to the use of the term elsewhere in the body, e.g. allergic nasal polyps or endometrial polyps. A simple pathological classification of large bowel polyps is shown in Box 27.1, emphasising the range of polyp types that can occur there.

ADENOMATOUS POLYPS AND ADENOMAS

Polyps are a common finding in the large bowel. Most colorectal polyps are **adenomas** (i.e. benign neoplasms) and all of these adenomatous polyps have the potential for **malignant change**. In general, it takes about 5–10 years for an adenomatous polyp to progress to invasive cancer. Early removal prevents progression from benign adenoma to adenocarcinoma. The process by which the epithelial cells acquire increasingly severe genetic mutations is termed the **adenoma–carcinoma sequence**. Thus if polyps are found at endoscopy, all of them should be meticulously removed (Fig. 27.1c) and subjected to histological examination to establish their nature.

Most adenomas are typically polypoid and **pedunculated** or dome-shaped and **sessile** (stalkless), allowing easy recognition and removal by diathermy snare. The much less common **flat adenomas** occur in developed countries but are particularly found in the Far East. These can be small and are most often seen at colonoscopy

Neoplasms

- Adenomas—very common, all potentially premalignant; these include villous, tubular and tubulo-villous types
- Early carcinomas—common
- Lymphomas—rare
- Leiomyomas and leiomyosarcomas—rare
- Lipomas and liposarcomas—rare
- Carcinoid tumours—rare

Hyperplasias

- Metaplastic mucosal polyps—very common
- Lymphoid aggregations—common in young children

Hamartomas

- Angiomas—uncommon
- 'Juvenile polyps'—uncommon; small malignant potential
- Peutz–Jeghers polyps—uncommon; small malignant potential

Inflammatory polyps

- 'Pseudopolyps' of severe ulcerative colitis

---

displaying a minimally elevated rim and depressed centre. Recognition at colonoscopy requires special dye-spray techniques. Flat adenomas can be removed by injecting saline into the submucosa to 'lift' the flat lesion before excising the abnormal mucosa with diathermy, sometimes in several pieces.

Adenomatous lesions examined histologically display a range of epithelial abnormalities ranging from mild to severe dysplasia, through carcinoma in situ, to early invasive cancer. In invasive cancer, the cellular abnormality has breached the basement membrane, from where extension eventually occurs through the muscularis mucosa and into the submucosa. As a general rule, the larger the lesion, the more likely it is to be malignant: only 1% of polyps smaller than 1 cm are malignant whereas about half of those larger than 2.5 cm are malignant.

Even in apparently benign lesions, there may be discrete areas of frank malignancy; thorough histological examination is needed if these are not to be overlooked. With pedunculated lesions removed by colonoscopic snaring, it is crucial to establish whether there is invasion of the stalk: if the stalk is clear of cancer, further treatment is not usually required.

Patterns of colonic adenoma

Three patterns of lesion are recognised histologically: tubular adenomas, villous adenomas and tubulo-villous adenomas (Fig. 27.1d).

Tubular adenomas

These are small pedunculated or sessile lesions in which the adenoma cells retain a tubular form similar to normal colonic mucosa. Tubular adenomas have the least potential for malignant transformation.

Villous adenomas

Villous adenomas are usually sessile (no stalk) and frond-like (papilliferous) lesions which tend to secrete mucus. The epithelial component of villous adenoma is more dysplastic than that of tubular adenomas and there is a correspondingly greater potential for malignant change; as with tubulo-villous adenomas, the malignant potential is proportional to the size.

Tubulo-villous adenomas

Histologically, these lesions are intermediate between tubular and villous adenomas and they comprise the majority of colonic polyps. Most are pedunculated, and the stalk is covered with normal colonic epithelium. The stalk probably develops by the action of peristalsis dragging the tumour mass distally and can range from about 0.5 to 10 cm long.

Distribution of colorectal adenomatous polyps

Adenomatous polyps can occur in any part of the large bowel, although three-quarters of them arise in the rectum and sigmoid colon. (This exactly parallels the distribution of carcinomas and provides strong corroboration that most cancers develop from polyps.)

Adenomas often arise singly (particularly villous adenomas) but more than 20% of patients with colonic polyps have **multiple polyps** and these are most often tubulo-villous. Patients with frank carcinoma are often found to have coexisting benign adenomas (**synchronous**) and these are likely to become malignant later if not removed (see Fig. 27.2). This explains why the whole colon should be examined before colectomy wherever possible, preferably by colonoscopy, and why long-term follow-up after treatment of large bowel cancer should include regular colonoscopy.

Symptoms and signs of colorectal polyps

Many polyps cause no symptoms, at least in their early stages, and remain undiagnosed or are found incidentally on colonoscopy or barium enema examination. Symptomatic polyps present typically with **rectal bleeding** and sometimes **iron deficiency anaemia** due to occult blood loss. **Mucus production**, especially from villous adenomas, may be so copious as to be the main presenting complaint. Very occasionally, symptomatic **hypokalaemia** may develop because so much potassium-containing mucus is lost. Distal lesions may occasionally produce **tenesmus** (a painful urge to defaecate) or they may **prolapse** through the anus. Rarely, large polyps can cause obstructive symptoms or intussusception.

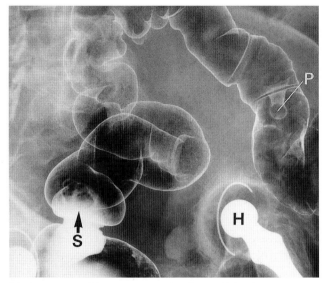

(a)

(a) This 65-year-old man presented with rectal bleeding. On sigmoidoscopy, a large polypoid lesion was seen in the upper rectum. The X-ray shows the rectum and sigmoid colon during a barium enema (note the hip prosthesis **H**), demonstrating two polyps: a sessile rectal lesion **S**, visible at sigmoidoscopy, and a pedunculated polyp **P** in the sigmoid colon. No other polyps were demonstrated in the large bowel. Sigmoidoscopic biopsies showed no malignancy, but the lesions looked suspicious and were removed by surgically resecting the upper rectum and sigmoid colon. Histology showed the rectal lesion was an adenoma, but it was found to have early invasive carcinoma in one area. The sigmoid polyp proved to be a benign tubulo-villous adenoma.

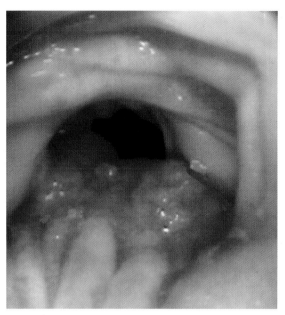

(b)

(b) A 2 cm polyp on a long stalk in the sigmoid colon.

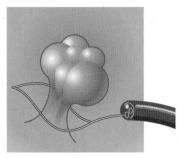

(c)

(c) The snare loop is tightened around the stalk of the polyp before applying diathermy current to remove it and coagulate the blood vessels in the stalk.

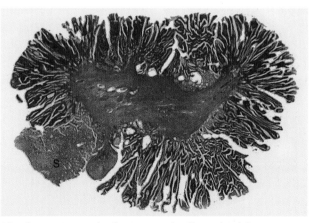

(d)

(d) Adenomatous polyp having mainly villous glandular architecture. The example shown has a well-defined stalk **S**, although this is more typical of tubular or tubulo-villous polyps, villous adenomas often having a broad base.

Fig. 27.1 Colorectal polyps

Diagnosis and management of colorectal polyps

For symptomatic patients, visualisation of the colon is needed. All colorectal investigation is to some degree invasive and uncomfortable and the benefits have to be made clear to patients, whilst their dignity and privacy is respected as far as possible. In the outpatient clinic, **rigid sigmoidoscopy** (which actually visualises the rectum) is most often performed initially, as nearly half of all polyps lie within reach of the 25 cm rigid instrument. **Flexible sigmoidoscopy**, usually performed without bowel preparation or after a simple phosphate enema, reaches past the sigmoid and ascending colon to the splenic flexure, covering 75% of the area at risk, but to view the remainder of the bowel requires **colonoscopy**. Colonoscopy is the 'gold standard' investigation: it allows direct visualisation of the entire large bowel, and polyps may be removed at the same time. For this reason, it is the first-line investigation in many centres. However, there are disadvantages: it requires a full day's bowel preparation and the procedure

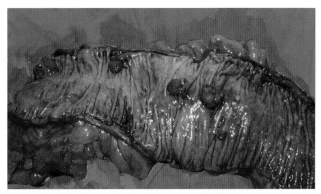

Fig. 27.2 Multiple colonic adenomatous polyps
This length of opened descending colon is from a 64-year-old man who presented with an invasive carcinoma of the rectum (not shown here). Several adenomatous polyps of various sizes can be seen in this part of the bowel; the larger polyps have greater malignant potential.

often requires sedation because of the discomfort. Furthermore, colonoscopy carries a 1 : 1000 risk of major haemorrhage or perforation. Sessile, small or flat adenomas in any location can be difficult to recognise even at colonoscopy and these potentially malignant lesions can be missed, especially if bowel preparation has been poor.

In elderly or infirm patients, **a CT pneumocolon** examination may be performed instead of an endoscopic procedure, although it is less sensitive for detecting polyps. It is less invasive and does not require sedation but bowel preparation is needed, and if polyps are found, colonoscopy is still required. Other alternative investigations include double contrast barium enema examination or unprepared CT scan.

Once an adenomatous polyp is found or a colorectal cancer has been treated, that patient is known to be at risk of forming further polyps elsewhere in the large bowel and requires follow-up colonoscopies. Intervals between colonoscopies are set according to guidelines determined by the number, size and pathology of polyps at each investigation and vary between 1 and 5 years.

Ideally, people at risk would be **screened** to detect asymptomatic polyps (as well as invasive cancers) so they can be removed before undergoing malignant change. Pilot projects have proved reasonably successful in reducing the numbers presenting with late colorectal cancer and are likely to be rolled out on an increasing scale. In England and Wales, a national bowel cancer screening programme will employ faecal occult blood testing every 2 years for people between 60 and 69 years of age. This test has been shown to aid detection of about 50% of asymptomatic cancers and is predicted to reduce mortality from colorectal cancer by 15%. Greater reductions could undoubtedly be achieved if patient compliance could be improved or if colonoscopy for screening on a large scale could be successfully implemented.

ADENOCARCINOMA OF COLON AND RECTUM

EPIDEMIOLOGY OF COLORECTAL CARCINOMA

As shown in Table 27.1, colorectal cancer is the third most common cause of death from cancer in the developed world; it is responsible for about 16 150 deaths in the UK every year. Almost a third of these cancers arise in the rectum. The disease is rare before the age of 50 (except in inherited colorectal cancer syndromes, see later) but common after the age of 60. There is little difference in incidence between the sexes.

Apart from increasing age, **diet** seems to be an important factor. Colorectal cancer is a more common disease in developed countries, with the lowest rates found in developing areas of Asia and Africa. However, sporadic cases are seen in younger males in the Indian subcontinent. The discrepancy was first highlighted by Denis Burkitt in the early 1970s and led to the belief that the Western low-fibre, high-fat diet may be in some way responsible. Studies of migrants from areas of low incidence to those of high incidence have shown that they rapidly achieve the cancer incidence of their new homeland. Daily intake of red or processed **meat** has been shown in the large European EPIC study to increase the risk by 30%; conversely, twice weekly intake of **fish** reduces it by 30%. It is likely that excess dietary fats also act as carcinogens. As regards **alcohol**, excess beer appears to increase the risk of colorectal cancer, whereas wine does not. However, any type of alcohol in excess appears to hasten malignant change in adenomas. In addition, the typical low-**fibre** Western diet results in a much slower whole-gut transit time and it may be that carcinogens in the stool thereby maintain contact with the bowel mucosa for longer. Low-fibre diets are usually low in fruit and raw vegetables and consequently low in **antioxidants**, which are thought to have a protective role.

Epidemiological studies have shown a reduction in colorectal cancer in people taking a small dose of **aspirin** daily (75–150 mg) as prophylaxis against cardiovascular disease. Furthermore, recent evidence has shown that type 2 **diabetic patients** have a 50% increase in risk, particularly if control of glycated haemoglobin is poor. There is some evidence that long-term usage of insulin increases colorectal cancer risk but the risk is small when compared with the absolute benefits of good glycaemic control.

Ulcerative colitis, a chronic inflammatory condition of the large bowel (discussed in Ch. 28), carries an inde-

Table 27.1 Death rates from colorectal cancer compared with other malignancies (UK 2004). Cancers are listed in order of frequency

Males (UK)	Number of deaths in 2004	Rate per million population	% of all male cancer deaths in 2004
1. Lung	19 500	667	24.4
2. Prostate	10 200	349	12.7
3. Colon and rectum	8650	296	10.8
4. Stomach and oesophagus	8270	283	10.3
5. Kidney and bladder	5350	183	6.7
6. Leukaemias, lymphomas and myelomas	5180	206	6.4
7. Pancreas	3400	116	4.2
8. Brain and CNS	2050	70	2.6
9. Liver (including secondaries with unknown primary)	1590	54	2
10. Malignant melanoma	1000	34	1.2
All others	14 800		18.5
All male cancers	**80 000**		

Females (UK)	Number of deaths in 2004	Rate per million population	% of all female cancer deaths in 2004
1. Lung	13 550	444	18.5
2. Breast	12 350	404	16.8
3. Colon and rectum	7500	246	10.2
4. Leukaemias, lymphomas and myelomas	5320	175	7.2
5. Stomach and oesophagus	4850	159	6.6
6. Ovary	4435	145	6
7. Pancreas	3645	119	5
8. Kidney and bladder	3075	101	4.2
9. Uterus and cervix	2730	90	3.7
10. Brain and CNS	1400	46	1.9
All others	14 500		19.8
All female cancers	**73 350**		

Since 1997, there have been marked changes in death rates from some cancers: colorectal cancer deaths have fallen by 12% in females, but by only by 4% in males. Lung cancer deaths have *risen* by 6% in females, but *fallen* by 13% in males, no doubt due to changes in cigarette consumption. As a result, lung cancer has now overtaken breast cancer as the prime cause of cancer deaths in females. Deaths from breast cancer have fallen by only 8%, despite huge investments in national screening, and there has been a fall of 15% in female stomach and oesophageal deaths for reasons unknown.

pendent risk of bowel neoplasia. After 10 years of active disease, the cancer risk rises by 1% each year.

Finally, **inherited genetic conditions** may give rise to colorectal cancer. They are discussed below. This is the main explanation for the higher risk of cancer developing in first-degree relatives of patients with early-onset cancers. For this reason, it is important to ask about a family history of bowel or other potentially inherited cancers in patients presenting with bowel symptoms.

INHERITED CONDITIONS CAUSING BOWEL CANCER

A small proportion of bowel cancers result from inherited conditions but they account for a disproportionate number of those patients presenting when young. Identifying these 'at risk' families allows counselling, surveillance and cancer prevention, often through referral to specialist Familial Colorectal Cancer clinics. These inherited conditions may be divided into the **polyposis syndromes**, in which sufferers develop large numbers of polyps early in life likely to undergo malignant change, and **hereditary non-polyposis colorectal cancer (HNPCC)**, in which sufferers have 'normal' or low numbers of adenomatous polyps which tend to progress to cancer. The latter is the most common condition predisposing to bowel cancer.

Polyposis syndromes

The most important polyposis syndrome is **familial adenomatous polyposis (FAP)**, both because it occurs reasonably commonly (1 : 30 000 people) and because of the inevitability of large bowel cancer developing if untreated. An autosomal dominant defect in the APC gene causes a hundred or more adenomatous polyps to develop in the large bowel by the mid teen years. Affected patients usually have one parent with the condition. Each affected individual is certain to develop colorectal cancer, at an average age of 40, unless preventative measures are taken. Ideally, prophylactic surgery to remove the area at risk should be performed in early adulthood. One option is subtotal colectomy and ileorectal anastomosis which removes nearly all the large bowel but has the disadvantage that the retained rectum requires careful long-term surveillance. The alternative is to remove the rectum as well (**panproctocolectomy**) and then perform an ileostomy or an **ileal pouch** restorative procedure.

Another important polyposis syndrome is **Peutz–Jeghers** syndrome, which causes hamartomatous polyps throughout the gastrointestinal tract. Patients often have freckles around the mouth and on the hands, feet and genitalia. Half of these patients are likely to die by the age of 50 because of polyp-related emergencies such as bowel intussusception or cancer. These patients are prone to develop cancers of small and large bowel, stomach, pancreas, testis and breast.

Hereditary non-polyposis colorectal cancer (HNPCC)

Hereditary non-polyposis colorectal cancer syndrome (also known as **Lynch syndrome**) results from defects in mismatch repair genes which mend damaged DNA. The condition carries a 70% lifetime risk of colorectal cancer, but also a substantially increased risk of other 'indicator' cancers such as those of endometrium, ovary, urothelium, small bowel and brain, and sometimes several of these. Families can be difficult to identify because of the diversity of cancers and incomplete genetic penetrance (i.e. not everyone carrying the genetic defect will develop cancer). When patients under 45 develop indicator cancers, they can be tested for markers which suggest the genetic condition. If positive, formal genetic tests are then undertaken. Those at risk should be offered colonoscopy every 2 years from the age of 25 if practicable.

PATHOPHYSIOLOGY OF COLORECTAL CARCINOMA

Colorectal carcinomas exhibit a wide range of differentiation which broadly correlates with their clinical behaviour and prognosis (Fig. 27.3). Most carcinomas are initially **exophytic** (i.e. protruding into the lumen) and later ulcerate and progressively invade the muscular bowel wall. Eventually, the tumour involves the serosa and surrounding structures. Stromal fibrosis may cause luminal narrowing, which is responsible for the common acute presentation of **large bowel obstruction**.

Large bowel carcinomas metastasise via lymphatics and the bloodstream, and by the time of diagnosis as many as 25% of patients already have widespread metastases (Fig. 27.4). Lymphatic spread is sequential, first to mesenteric nodes and then onward to para-aortic nodes. Occasionally lymph node involvement is directly responsible for the clinical presentation. For example, para-aortic nodes may present as a palpable mass or cause **duodenal obstruction**. Other enlarged nodes may compress the bile ducts in the porta hepatis causing **jaundice**.

Haematogenous spread is predominantly to the liver and usually occurs later than lymphatic spread; therefore a patient with early lymph node involvement at the time of presentation has a better chance of avoiding liver metastases. Despite this, hepatic involvement does occur without evidence of lymphatic spread. Haematogenous spread to other sites such as lung or bone is uncommon but can occur, as may systemic manifestations.

PRESENTATION OF LARGE BOWEL CARCINOMA

Late presentations as a result of metastases have been discussed in the last section. For local disease, the mode

Fig. 27.3 Cancers of the colon and rectum

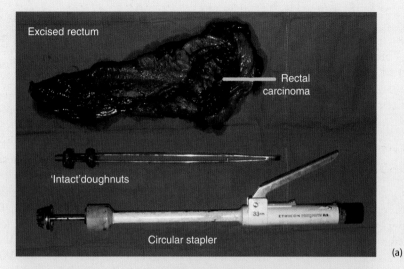

Excised rectum

Rectal carcinoma

'Intact'doughnuts

Circular stapler

(a)

(a) Annular carcinoma of rectum in a 68-year-old woman who presented with large bowel obstruction. A low anterior resection was performed with a covering loop ileostomy. The bowel was rejoined using the circular stapler. Two complete 'doughnuts' of tissue indicate successful firing of the stapler. **(b)** Synchronous cancers of the transverse colon. This elderly man presented with a change in bowel habit, with constipation and overflow diarrhoea. Preoperative barium enema examination revealed two cancers that were resected at operation and the ends anastomosed.

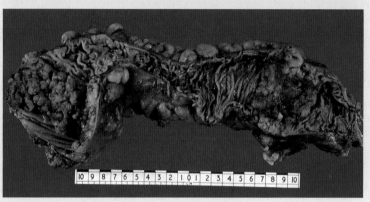

(b)

of growth and clinical presentation of large bowel cancer depend to some extent on the site of the lesion.

Blood loss and anaemia

Carcinomas of the caecum and ascending colon rarely cause obstruction unless the ileo-caecal valve is involved. This is because the right colon has a larger diameter than the left colon and the faecal stream is more fluid. However, occult **bleeding** from the tumour surface commonly causes iron deficiency **anaemia**, and these patients typically present with anaemia and a palpable mass in the right iliac fossa

Change of bowel habit and large bowel obstruction

Colorectal cancers usually give out blood and mucus into the lumen. This tends to alter the bowel habit towards a looser stool. Thus a recent history of loose stool is more likely to predict cancer than increasing constipation,

especially since constipation is so common in the elderly population. Faeces in the left colon are more solid and the intraluminal pressure is higher, thus cancers here are more likely to obstruct. The more distal the tumour, the more likely it is to cause obstruction. Colonic cancers tend to progressively encircle the bowel wall, encroaching on the lumen and producing an **annular stenosis**. It has been estimated that it takes a year to involve each quarter of the bowel circumference.

Large bowel obstruction may be partial or complete. **Partial obstruction** may present as a change in bowel habit, often noticed as constipation with intermittent 'overflow' diarrhoea. **Complete obstruction** will precipitate emergency hospital admission (see Ch. 19).

Rectal bleeding

Carcinomas distal to the splenic flexure often cause visible blood to be passed per rectum. The character of the blood and the nature of its mixing with stool depend on how far proximally the lesion is from the anus.

Fig. 27.4 Hepatic and other metastases from colonic carcinoma

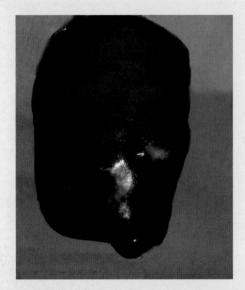

This 49-year-old man presented with a 9-month history of rectal bleeding, found to be due to a sigmoid colon carcinoma which was resected. Two years later he was found on ultrasound screening to have a single metastasis in the right lobe of the liver. No other metastases were found so he underwent a resection of the right lobe of the liver; the resected specimen is seen here. Unfortunately, he returned 3 years later with a malignant paraduodenal mass and widespread peritoneal metastases, from which he died.

Tenesmus

Lesions (carcinomas or polyps) in the lower two-thirds of the rectum may be perceived as masses of faeces. This stimulates a persistent defaecation response, causing an unpleasant sensation of incomplete evacuation known as tenesmus.

Perforation

A cancer invading through the bowel wall may stimulate a vigorous local inflammatory process resulting in a **pericolic abscess** which contains the perforation, at least for a while. This occurs most often in the rectosigmoid area and usually presents with left iliac fossa pain and tenderness and a swinging fever. The differential diagnosis is acute diverticulitis or a diverticular abscess.

A carcinoma anywhere in the colon (but rarely in the rectum) may perforate and present as an acute abdomen with **peritonitis**. Occasionally a carcinoma may erode into a nearby organ creating a malignant **fistula**. Fistulation can occur into stomach, bladder, uterus or vagina, or direct to the skin.

CLINICAL SIGNS IN SUSPECTED COLORECTAL CARCINOMA

The symptoms and signs of colorectal cancer are illustrated in Figure 27.5. General examination may show features suggesting disseminated malignant disease, e.g. obvious cachexia and weight loss or supraclavicular node enlargement. Abdominal examination is normal in most patients but may reveal a mass in the colon, enlargement of the liver (hepatomegaly) due to metastases, or ascitic fluid. Unfortunately, all of these signs represent late and often incurable disease.

Rectal examination is mandatory in all suspected cases as a high proportion of carcinomas occur in the lowest 12 cm of the large bowel and can be reached with an examining finger. In addition, intraperitoneal tumour spread into the pouch of Douglas may be palpable anteriorly through the rectal wall. The degree of **fixation** of a rectal tumour to surrounding structures can also be evaluated digitally and this gives some indication of potential operative difficulty. Finally, the glove should be inspected for blood and mucus as well as stool colour and consistency.

Investigation of suspected colorectal carcinoma

Proctoscopy and rigid or flexible sigmoidoscopy are usually performed at the initial consultation for all patients complaining of bowel symptoms. About 50% of colorectal cancers lie within reach of a rigid sigmoidoscope and 75% within reach of a flexible sigmoidoscope. Lesions can be biopsied through either instrument.

A history of rectal bleeding should be fully investigated in patients over about 45 years and in any patient if the symptoms or signs suggest malignancy. This applies even if a local cause such as haemorrhoids is found, since these are so common that they will often be found coincidentally. **Flexible sigmoidoscopy** is the investigation of choice for rectal bleeding as the causative lesion has a high probability of being found in the left side of the colon. If a tumour is found, the rest of the bowel must still be examined for synchronous tumours or further polyps.

In patients complaining of a change in bowel habit (particularly looser stools) or unexplained anaemia, a bowel lesion could be left or right sided, and thus the entire colon must be examined by colonoscopy or barium enema examination (Fig. 27.6).

Blood tests

Anaemia often results from a bowel neoplasm, and abnormal liver function tests suggest substantial liver metastases. Raised blood urea can result from rectal lesions compressing the ureters, whilst hypokalaemia occasionally results from lesions producing excess mucin. Tumour markers are neither sensitive nor specific for a primary

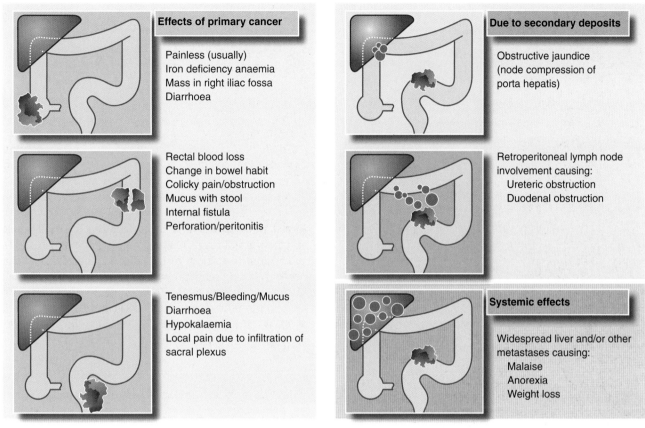

Effects of primary cancer

Painless (usually)
Iron deficiency anaemia
Mass in right iliac fossa
Diarrhoea

Rectal blood loss
Change in bowel habit
Colicky pain/obstruction
Mucus with stool
Internal fistula
Perforation/peritonitis

Tenesmus/Bleeding/Mucus
Diarrhoea
Hypokalaemia
Local pain due to infiltration of
sacral plexus

Due to secondary deposits

Obstructive jaundice
(node compression of
porta hepatis)

Retroperitoneal lymph node
involvement causing:
    Ureteric obstruction
    Duodenal obstruction

Systemic effects

Widespread liver and/or other
metastases causing:
    Malaise
    Anorexia
    Weight loss

Fig. 27.5 Symptoms and signs of colorectal cancer

diagnosis of colorectal cancer but **carcino-embryonic antigen** (CEA) is used to monitor for cancer recurrence.

Imaging for staging

When colorectal malignancy is diagnosed and irrespective of distant spread, surgery is likely to be necessary to relieve symptoms. **Staging** is performed to guide oncological planning and counselling of the patient. Liver and lung metastases are sought, along with any other evidence of spread within the abdomen or to bone. CT scanning is the most useful investigation for all of these but liver ultrasound scanning may be more sensitive for detecting small liver metastases. If CT is not available, chest X-ray will reveal whether there are lung metastases. MRI scanning can add important information about the extent of local spread of rectal cancer to aid treatment planning.

In a patient presenting as an emergency with complete large bowel obstruction, plain abdominal X rays often show large bowel dilated by gas down to the level of obstruction and empty of gas beyond it. The level is often at the sigmoid colon or recto-sigmoid junction. CT scan or sigmoidoscopy may confirm the likely diagnosis of carcinoma. Similarly, an 'instant' Gastrografin enema (i.e. without bowel preparation) can confirm the diagnosis and at the same time exclude **pseudo-obstruction**.

MANAGEMENT OF COLORECTAL CARCINOMA

Surgical resection is the main treatment for colorectal carcinoma. For tumours localised to the bowel wall, resection offers an excellent chance of complete cure; for tumours at a more advanced stage, chemotherapy and radiotherapy may be required to increase the chances of cure. For rectal cancers, chemoradiotherapy may be given preoperatively (known as **neoadjuvant therapy**) to shrink the tumour to improve the chances of successful surgical removal. There is a trend for patients with cancers to be referred for multidisciplinary team discussion, where surgeons, oncologists, radiologists, palliative care doctors and colorectal specialist nurses discuss all aspects of the case and formulate a plan of management.

For advanced disease, even with very extensive tumours, palliative resection is usually worthwhile to relieve obstruction or to prevent continuing blood loss. In frail patients with metastatic disease in whom any surgery is too risky, a **stent** can often be placed endoscopically to hold open the bowel and relieve obstruction.

STAGING OF COLORECTAL CARCINOMA

Staging of colorectal carcinoma influences the need for further treatment by chemotherapy or radiotherapy. It

Fig. 27.6 Caecal and colonic carcinomas: barium enema examinations

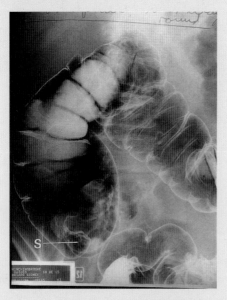

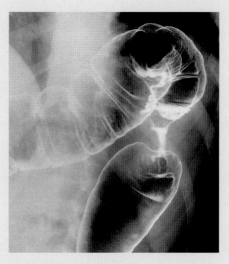

(a)

(b)

(a) Polypoid carcinoma arising on the medial wall of the caecum in a 73-year-old man with an iron deficiency anaemia and a mass in the right iliac fossa. Note the lesion is growing out into the lumen; it is recognised by the overlapping double shadows **S**.
(b) Typical 'apple-core' lesion just distal to the splenic flexure of a man of 39 who complained of rectal bleeding. With this degree of stenosis, it was surprising that he had had no change in bowel habit. Acute obstruction would probably soon have occurred if the tumour had not been recognised and resected. The patient is unusually young for colorectal carcinoma in the Western world.

also gives an estimate of the statistical probability of surviving 5 years and the likelihood of cure. Final staging of colorectal cancer depends on information from several sources: the findings at laparotomy, histological examination of the resected specimen and the radiological and other imaging for distant organ spread. The two most widely used staging systems are the tumour/node/metastasis (**TNM**) and **Dukes' classification**. Dukes was a pathologist and staged tumours based on the specimens he received. His classification was first described for rectal carcinomas and later for colonic carcinomas; it is outlined in Table 27.2.

Approximately a quarter of all patients with colorectal cancer are incurable at presentation; all of these die within 5 years. Of the others that undergo radical surgery with the aim of cure, 50% are alive and well 5 years later. Very few patients surviving 5 years die later of recurrent disease.

OPERATIONS FOR COLORECTAL CANCER

The principles of colorectal tumour resection are as follows:

- Operative access is achieved by laparotomy, usually via a long midline incision. In specialist units, laparoscopic or laparoscopic-assisted surgery is sometimes employed

- The affected segment of bowel is removed with a margin of normal bowel. A minimum of 5 cm clear each side of the tumour removes local lymphatics likely to be involved. In practice, the precise lines of resection are determined by the distribution of mesenteric blood vessels (see Fig. 27.7). For example, lesions in the ascending colon are treated by removal of the whole right colon (right hemicolectomy), as the right colic artery has to be ligated in order to remove a section of the right colon. There must be a good blood supply to the cut ends of bowel to ensure healing

- A wedge-shaped section of colonic mesentery is removed with the bowel. This contains the primary field of lymph node drainage. If there are other obvious lymph node metastases, these are usually included in the resection specimen

- **Rectal cancers** are a special case and an outline of standard operations is given in Figure 27.8. The preferred operation is a sphincter-saving **anterior resection of rectum**; provided the lower edge of the tumour is 1–2 cm above the anal sphincters, the sphincter can be preserved in most patients. This operation involves excising the tumour with an appropriate length of bowel plus an intact envelope of fat around it (the **mesorectum** containing local lymph nodes). Ideally this is to a distance of 5 cm below the primary tumour, although a margin of

Table 27.2 Staging and survival rates from treated colorectal carcinoma

UICC stage	TNM stage	Modified Dukes' stage	Approximate 5-year survival
Stage 0	Carcinoma in situ Tumour confined to the bowel wall with no extension into the extrarectal or extracolic tissues.		
Stage I	Tumour invades submucosa (T1) Tumour invades muscularis propria (T2) No lymph node metastases	**A**	85–95%
Stage II	Tumour invades beyond muscularis propria (T3) Tumour invades into other organs (T4) No lymph node metastases	**B**	60–80%
Stage III	1–3 regional lymph nodes involved—any T (N1) 4 or more regional lymph nodes involved—any T (N2) No distant metastases	**C** C1: apical node not involved (node furthest from tumour) C2: apical node involved	30–60%
Stage IV	Distant metastasis (M1) Any T stage, any N stage	**D**	< 10%

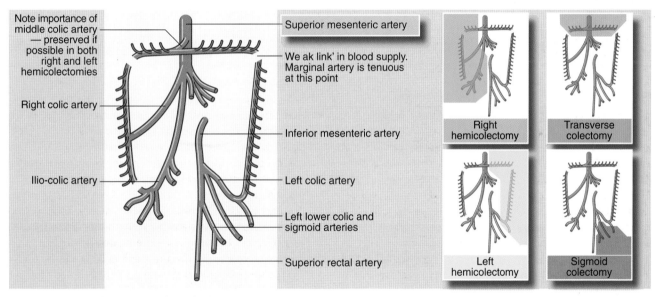

Fig. 27.7 Standard operations for colonic cancer

1 cm is acceptable when the tumour is very low. The proximal end of bowel is then anastomosed to the distal stump. Alternatively, a pelvic reservoir is created using a **J-pouch** technique (Fig. 27.8). This has been shown to reduce the frequency and urgency of defaecation without increasing surgical complications. A temporary ileostomy or colostomy is sometimes used to aid healing of a low anastomosis. If the sphincter is involved, the entire rectum and anus has to be removed via an **abdomino-perineal resection (APR)**, with the proximal end of bowel brought out as a colostomy

- In most cases, the two cut ends of bowel can be joined (anastomosed) without the need for a

temporary or permanent colostomy. (The indications for stomas and their types and management are described on pp. 412–415.) The method used to rejoin the bowel depends on the site of the anastomosis, the preference of the surgeon and whether there is much disparity in diameter between the ends to be joined. Methods of large bowel anastomosis are shown in Figures 27.9 and 27.10.

BOWEL CLEANSING TECHNIQUES PRIOR TO SURGERY

It was commonly believed that preoperative bowel preparation decreased the risk of anastomotic leaks and hence

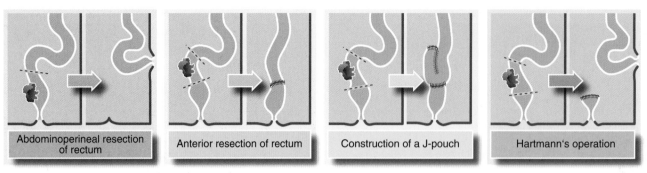

Fig. 27.8 Standard operations for rectal cancer
Hartmann's procedure is described on pages 413–415.

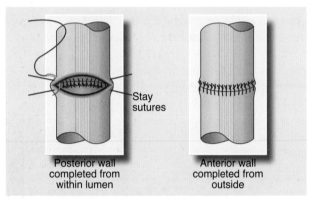

Fig. 27.9 Single-layer method of bowel anastomosis
A single-layer anastomosis using interrupted absorbable sutures is the safest and most commonly used method of anastomosis for nearly all types of bowel. If the bowel cannot be rotated, the posterior layer sutures are placed from inside the bowel and knotted within the lumen. Sutures usually incorporate the muscle wall and submucosa but not the mucosa.

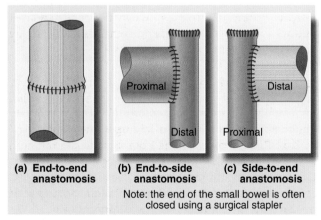

Fig. 27.10 Methods of matching the diameter of the bowel ends to effect a safe anastomosis
(a) An end-to-end anastomosis is used when bowel ends are of similar diameter. **(b)** An end-to-side anastomosis is used where the proximal end is greater in diameter than the distal end, e.g. in small bowel obstruction. **(c)** A side-to-end anastomosis is used where the distal end is greater in diameter than the proximal end, e.g. in right hemicolectomy.

infective complications. Despite meta-analysis studies showing that this is not the case, a recent study with better methodology confirmed that bowel preparation reduced anastomotic leak rate. Most surgeons prefer bowel to be prepared whenever possible because an empty bowel makes the surgery more convenient. In order to clear the bowel of faecal material, a combination of the following procedures is employed:

- **Withdrawal of solid foods**. The patient may be limited to fluids or a low-fibre diet for a few days before operation
- **Purgation**. This is usually with oral stimulant laxatives (e.g. sodium picosulfate). Note that the diarrhoea caused by this method may easily dehydrate elderly patients. In addition, oral purgatives should not be given to patients with partial bowel obstruction since they may precipitate complete obstruction with pain and a risk of perforation
- **Enemas and distal bowel washouts**. When there is bowel obstruction, only distal washouts and enemas can safely be given preoperatively. In these cases, it is possible to clear the proximal colon of faeces by an 'on-table washout' during the operation, once the tumour has been resected. This involves inserting a Foley catheter through the wall of the caecum (usually through the appendix stump) and irrigating 2–3 L of warm saline into the colon. This is drained into a bucket via a large-bore tube placed in the distal end of the colon

PERIOPERATIVE PROPHYLACTIC ANTIBIOTICS

A variety of faecal commensals and other organisms cause abdominal infections after large bowel surgery. These include *Escherichia coli* and other Enterobacteriaceae (Gram-negative aerobes), *Bacteroides* and related organisms (Gram-negative anaerobic rods), *Staph. aureus* (Gram-positive aerobic cocci), *Enterococcus faecalis* (Gram-positive anaerobic cocci) and the Clostridia (Gram-positive anaerobic rods). For prophylaxis, an antibiotic combination is chosen to cover the main organisms. Popular regimens are shown in Box 27.2. It is important to achieve high circulating blood levels by the time of operation, so the first dose is usually given at anaesthetic induction or with the premedication.

THE ROLE OF ADJUVANT RADIOTHERAPY AND CHEMOTHERAPY

Adjuvant radiotherapy and chemotherapy is usually offered to patients with Dukes' C cancers to increase the chance of prolonged survival. There is also a marginal benefit for those with Dukes' B but the potential advantages have to be weighed against the unpleasant side effects of treatment. As mentioned earlier, neoadjuvant chemoradiotherapy (given before surgery) is particularly relevant for rectal tumours tethered in the pelvis, where shrinking a large tumour can make it operable. Such therapy may enable the anal sphincter to be preserved by **downstaging** the tumour. Where rectal tumours extend through the bowel wall, particularly anteriorly, a course of radiotherapy directly before surgery has been shown to reduce local pelvic recurrence. Radiotherapy after surgery is probably less effective and risks radiation damage to small bowel now lying in the pelvis.

For chemotherapy in large bowel cancer, **5-fluorouracil (5-FU)** is the chief adjuvant agent; it is often given in combination with its biomodulator, **folinic acid**. Newer drugs such as oxaliplatin and irinotecan are being investigated in clinical trials and may give greater benefit.

MANAGEMENT OF ADVANCED DISEASE AND RECURRENCE

The primary tumour is usually resected to relieve its local effects even when distant metastases have been diagnosed. Most of these patients die within 1 or 2 years and only about 1 in 10 survives 3 years; none survives 5 years. The exception is metastasis confined to the liver (see below), where partial liver resection is enabling prolonged survival in about 40% of patients.

The **liver** is the most common site of distant metastasis. Liver metastases may be discovered at imaging for staging before operation, at operation or later as a result of surveillance with ultrasound, CT or blood tumour marker (CEA) estimation. Occasionally there may be only one or two metastases confined to a resectable anatomical lobe. These may be excised locally or the affected segment of liver removed by partial hepatectomy. Given the relatively good outcome, liver resections for metastases are increasingly performed. PET scanning can be used to look for occult metastases elsewhere before attempting liver resection.

Patients with liver metastases seldom become jaundiced until the disease is very advanced, since jaundice only occurs when the parenchyma is almost completely destroyed or major bile ducts are compressed at the porta hepatis. Specific treatment for this late event is rarely effective, although oral dexamethasone may temporarily reduce metastatic tissue oedema and relieve symptoms. Colorectal tumours sometimes metastasise to **bone**, particularly the lumbar spine, and painful lesions may be palliated by radiotherapy.

Metastatic colorectal carcinomas are most often treated with 5FU, with oxaliplatin as a second-line agent. This can substantially prolong survival and improve quality of life. Colorectal carcinomas also respond to radiotherapy but its use is restricted because the radiation beam cannot be directed at the tumour without damaging normal bowel nearby.

'Recurrences' within the colon usually represent new cancers arising metachronously from pre-existing or new adenomas. Careful examination of the entire colon before the first operation is likely to reduce such recurrent disease. In **rectal cancer**, local recurrence is now seen in 5–20% but this was a more common problem before the importance of mesorectal excision was realised. Such recurrences often cause intractable perineal pain; occasionally a fungating mass grows in the anal region or buttocks. These very distressing complications may be palliated to a degree with radiotherapy.

COMPLICATIONS OF LARGE BOWEL SURGERY

The complications of large bowel surgery are summarised in Box 27.3. Infection arising from faecal contamination is the main early complication of large bowel surgery. Contamination may result from perforation prior to operation, inadvertent faecal spillage during the operation or postoperative anastomotic leakage or breakdown.

Three main types of infection occur: wound infection and dehiscence, intraperitoneal abscesses, and generalised peritonitis. Intra-abdominal infection carries a high risk of systemic sepsis and multi-organ dysfunction, particularly after emergency operations. All of these infective complications are radically reduced by appropriate use of prophylactic antibiotics.

Box 27.3	Complications of large bowel surgery

Early complications

Local

- Inadvertent damage to other organs, e.g. ureter, bladder, duodenum or spleen—usually recognised at operation
- Haemorrhage, e.g. slipped ligature
- Wound infection—cellulitis, abscess or wound edge necrosis
- Intra-abdominal abscess—at site of surgery, pelvic or subphrenic

Regional

- Anastomotic leak or breakdown—local or general peritonitis
- Stoma problems—sloughing or retraction
- Compartment syndrome in legs due to prolonged elevation during surgery (rare)

Systemic

- New onset atrial fibrillation or flutter—often indicates anastomotic breakdown
- Systemic sepsis leading to multi-organ dysfunction syndrome

Later complications

- Diarrhoea—due to short bowel
- Division of pelvic parasympathetic nerves—causes sexual/bladder dysfunction
- Small bowel obstruction—due to pelvic peritoneal adhesions or tangling of small bowel with colostomy or ileostomy, or later as a complication of radiotherapy causing small bowel damage

STOMAS

INDICATIONS AND GENERAL PRINCIPLES

It is often necessary to divert the faecal stream to the anterior abdominal wall via a stoma. The effluent is collected in a removable plastic bag attached by adhesive to the abdominal skin. Stomas are named according to the part of the bowel opening on to the abdominal wall, i.e. **ileostomy** or **colostomy**. (The term **urostomy** is used for the ileal conduit that connects ureters to the skin surface in patients whose bladder has been removed.)

Stomas may be permanent or temporary. Wherever possible, the need for a stoma should be anticipated before operation and discussed with the patient. This is done to ensure that informed consent is obtained and to prepare the patient for what is often perceived as a 'fate worse than death'. Specialised **stoma nurses** assist in planning and aftercare. Before the operation they counsel the patient, who is encouraged to try out a dummy appliance and talk to other stoma patients. The stoma nurse also identifies and marks the most suitable and comfortable site for the stoma appliance. This takes into account the patient's occupation and leisure activities, clothing and ability for self-care.

Permanent stomas

These are necessary when there is no distal bowel segment remaining after resection or when for some reason the bowel is not to be rejoined. A **colostomy** is required after **abdomino-perineal resection** of a low rectal or anal canal tumour. An **ileostomy** (see Fig. 27.12) is employed after excision of the whole colon and rectum (pan-proctocolectomy) unless a pouch reconstruction is performed. Sometimes in patients with severe and permanent incontinence, a colostomy may make a better life possible. Permanent stomas must be carefully sited to facilitate

long-term management, usually below the belt line. Colostomies are usually fashioned in the left iliac fossa and ileostomies in the right iliac fossa.

Temporary stomas

Emergency procedures

A temporary stoma may be created (even by an inexperienced surgeon) as an emergency measure to relieve complete distal large bowel obstruction causing proximal bowel dilatation. If the ileo-caecal valve remains competent in complete obstruction, the caecum can rupture and cause death by peritonitis. Thus if a patient with large bowel obstruction has a dilated caecum but no small bowel dilatation on plain abdominal X-ray, the ileo-caecal valve is likely to be competent. If the patient develops right iliac fossa pain, perforation is imminent. Perforation can be prevented by a timely diverting stoma; the obstructing lesion may be removed at the same operation or later.

Defunctioning stomas

A 'defunctioning' stoma (ileostomy or colostomy) may be used to protect a more distal anastomosis at particular risk of leakage or breakdown by preventing intraluminal pressure rises and by diverting the faecal stream. Common examples are a technically difficult low rectal anastomosis (flatus and faeces may leak from the anastomosis), an anastomosis performed after resection of an obstructing lesion (distension may compromise the blood supply), or emergency resection involving unprepared bowel (solid faeces may remain impacted in the lumen). Reversing the temporary stoma to restore bowel continuity is often a relatively simple procedure, usually performed after 3–4 months. Some surgeons like to perform a limited contrast enema to demonstrate anastomotic integrity before closing the stoma.

Bowel rest

A temporary colostomy may be used to 'rest' a more distal segment of bowel or a perineum involved in an inflammatory process, by diverting the faecal stream. Examples include pericolic abscess, complex anorectal fistulae and major surgical perineal wounds.

TYPES OF STOMA

The way in which a stoma is fashioned depends on its purpose. The main types of stoma are described below and illustrated in Figure 27.11. Colonic stomas are designed with the bowel mucosa lying flush with the skin. Small bowel stomas are fashioned with a 'spout' of bowel protruding about 3 cm, to ensure that the irritant small bowel contents enter the ileostomy appliance directly rather than flowing on to the skin (Fig. 27.12).

Loop stoma

This type of stoma is designed so that both the proximal and distal segments of bowel drain on to the skin surface (see Fig. 27.11a). This deflects proximal effluent to the skin surface and provides a 'blow-off' valve for the distal loop. Loop stomas are used mainly for temporary defunctioning. It is straightforward to reanastomose the ends at reversal; the loop is then dropped back into the abdomen. The most common form of loop stoma is the **loop ileostomy**; occasionally a **loop transverse colostomy** is used.

Split or 'spectacle' stoma

This is the ultimate form of defunctioning stoma although it is rarely used, having been largely superseded by the loop stoma. After resection, both proximal and distal bowel ends are brought separately to the skin surface. The proximal end stoma passes stool into a stoma appliance; the distal stoma (or **mucous fistula**) defunctions the bowel beyond it and produces just a little mucus.

End stoma

This type of stoma is usually permanent. An end **colostomy** is most commonly used to 'resite the anus' on to the abdominal wall after removal of the rectum and anal sphincter (i.e. abdomino-perineal resection). An **ileostomy** may be employed after subtotal or pan-proctocolectomy, particularly in fulminant colitis. Later, some form of reconstruction may be considered, involving the creation in the pelvis of a pouch or reservoir of several loops of ileum sutured side-to-side which is connected to the anus. The anal sphincter mechanism is preserved so that the patient is usually continent and can control evacuation.

Hartmann's procedure: end colostomy and rectal stump

Hartmann's procedure is a relatively safe technique, particularly for less experienced surgeons, and carries less overall risk than primary anastomosis. It is employed

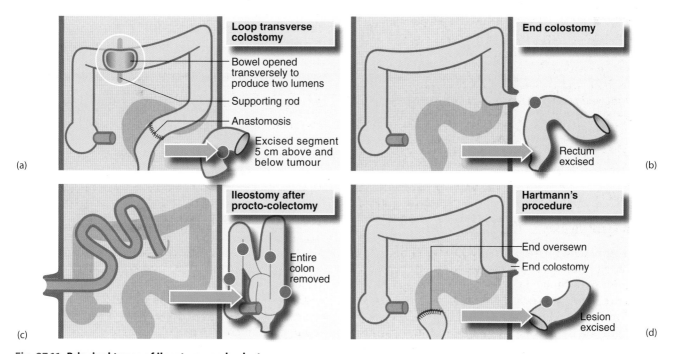

(a)

Loop transverse colostomy
— Bowel opened transversely to produce two lumens
— Supporting rod
— Anastomosis
Excised segment 5 cm above and below tumour

(b)

End colostomy
Rectum excised

(c)

Ileostomy after procto-colectomy
Entire colon removed

(d)

Hartmann's procedure
— End oversewn
— End colostomy
Lesion excised

Fig. 27.11 Principal types of ileostomy and colostomy
(a) Loop transverse colostomy is usually temporary, and is used to defunction the distal bowel. **(b)** End colostomy is usually permanent. **(c)** Ileostomy after procto-colectomy is permanent. Note the protruding 'spout' produced by everting the ileum. **(d)** End colostomy in Hartmann's procedure sometimes becomes permanent.

Fig. 27.12 End ileostomy

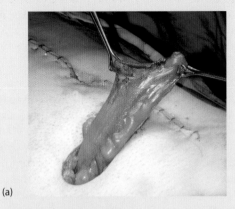
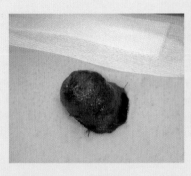
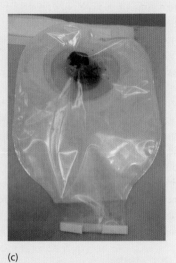

(a)   (b)   (c)

This man of 45 had suffered remittent ulcerative colitis for 12 years which could only be managed with high doses of steroids. He underwent subtotal colectomy and formation of this end ileostomy. Later, he will be considered for a pouch reconstruction. **(a)** Formation of ileostomy. The end of the ileum is brought to the surface via an opening made in the right iliac fossa at a point predetermined by the stoma therapist. **(b)** The end of the ileum has been turned back on itself like a cuff to form a spout or Brook ileostomy. **(c)** The stoma bag placed in the operating theatre.

Table 27.3 Complications of ileostomy and colostomy

Complication	Treatment
Early complications	
Mucosal sloughing or necrosis of the terminal bowel due to ischaemia	Reoperation and refashioning of the stoma
Obstruction of stoma due to oedema or faecal impaction	Exploration with a gloved finger and sometimes glycerol suppositories or softening enemas
Persistent leakage between skin and appliance causing skin erosion and patient distress, often due to inappropriate location of stoma (e.g. over skin crease)	May respond to stoma nursing care or require a resiting operation
Late complications	
Parastomal hernia due to abdominal wall weakness	Resiting of stoma
Prolapse of bowel	Refashioning of stoma
Parastomal fistula	Refashioning of stoma
Retraction of 'spout' ileostomy	Reoperation and refashioning of a new ileostomy
Stenosis of stomal orifice	Refashioning of stoma
Perforation after colonic irrigation	Emergency operation
Psychological and psychosexual dysfunction	May require counselling or measures to reverse stoma

after emergency resection of rectosigmoid lesions where primary anastomosis is inadvisable because of obstruction, inflammation or faecal contamination, or surgical inexperience. It may be the choice of treatment for frail or debilitated patients. At Hartmann's operation, the lesion is resected, the proximal bowel is made into an end colostomy (the same as that employed after an abdomino-perineal resection) and the cut end of the distal remnant closed with sutures or staples (see Fig. 27.11d). Secretions from the residual rectum still pass through the anus. Several months later when local inflammation has resolved, a decision may be made to reconnect the bowel, depending on the fitness and the preference of the patient. However, the colostomy is so well tolerated that some patients prefer to keep it permanently rather than undergo another major operation.

Irrigation technique for managing a colostomy

An ileostomy tends to work continuously during the day whereas a colostomy is intermittent. Some patients with a colostomy prefer to dispense with a stoma bag by using a technique of colonic irrigation. Once every few days the patient passes a litre or more of water into the colostomy via a special spout, then the water is allowed to drain out, with the aim of emptying the entire colon. After this, the stoma is covered with a dry dressing as a stoma bag is not needed until the next irrigation.

Complications of colostomy and ileostomy

These are summarised in Table 27.3.

28 Chronic inflammatory disorders of the bowel

INTRODUCTION

Substantial inflammation in any part of the small or large bowel usually presents with diarrhoea (i.e. frequent passage of loose stools). When inflammation affects the large bowel, the diarrhoea often contains blood. **Chronic diarrhoea** is defined as lasting for longer than 6 weeks. Chronic diarrhoea is to be distinguished from the acute diarrhoea of gastroenteritis which is usually of viral origin or related to food poisoning and is thus self limiting.

A chronic change of bowel habit to looser and more frequent stools, whether containing blood or not, raises the possibility of three categories of diagnosis: **infective causes** (bacillary or amoebic), **inflammatory bowel diseases** (ulcerative colitis, Crohn's disease or rarer forms of non-infective colitis) and **neoplasms** (covered in the previous chapter).

The term **inflammatory bowel disease** is usually employed to describe the two chronic remittent bowel disorders, **ulcerative colitis** and **Crohn's disease**, and these make up the bulk of this chapter. They share many pathophysiological and clinical features, for example both conditions present most often with chronic diarrhoea. However, Crohn's disease can involve small or large bowel or both, whilst ulcerative colitis is confined to the large bowel. When large bowel alone is inflamed, it is important to differentiate between the two conditions because their management and the spectrum of complications differ substantially (see Table 28.1).

These inflammatory bowel diseases are chronic and relapsing in nature. They have variable responses to treatments, with a potential for complications after major surgery. Thus the long-term care needs to be carefully managed, with well thought out decisions about investigation, drug treatment, managing social factors and the timing of surgery, which sometimes involves a stoma. The most effective management and the best outcomes result from close cooperation between medical and surgical gastroenterologists and associated practitioners such as stoma nurses. For the most part, patients can be managed on an outpatient basis but acute exacerbations or complications may require hospital admission. Surgery is usually indicated when medical management has failed or when complications such as fulminant colitis, obstruction, toxic dilatation of the colon or perforation occur. In addition, ulcerative colitis is a long-term risk factor for developing **colorectal cancer**.

Ulcerative colitis and Crohn's disease are relatively common causes of bowel inflammation in developed countries, but in developing countries **infections** that cause chronic inflammation of the large bowel are more common. These may also be contracted by travellers. **Amoebiasis** in particular may mimic ulcerative colitis, and **tuberculosis** may mimic Crohn's disease. **Pseudomembranous** and other forms of **antibiotic-related colitis** are increasingly common in hospitalised patients after antibiotic treatment; they are discussed in Chapter 12. Pseudomembranous colitis is of increasing importance in hospital practice. Whilst typical cases can be readily diagnosed and treated, severe forms of the condition may require emergency colectomy and have also been incriminated as a cause of fatality in elderly patients. Symptoms may occur as long as 6 months after antibiotic use.

Infective causes must be excluded where possible before a diagnosis of inflammatory bowel disease is made because life-threatening complications can result from treating infective conditions with the immunosuppressive drugs used for inflammatory bowel disease.

EPIDEMIOLOGY AND AETIOLOGY OF INFLAMMATORY BOWEL DISEASE

Ulcerative colitis and Crohn's disease are considered to be separate entities but in 10–15% of cases no clear distinction can be made; this is termed **indeterminate colitis**. Little is known about their aetiologies but it is possible

Table 28.1 Comparative features of ulcerative colitis and Crohn's disease

	Ulcerative colitis	Crohn's disease
Pathology		
Inflammation	Recurrent acute inflammation with intervening quiescent phases	Chronic relapsing inflammation
General distribution	Continuous involvement of affected part of colon	Skip lesions in any part of gastrointestinal tract
Rectal involvement	Always	About 25%
Ileal involvement	Backwash ileitis only	Involved in 80% of cases; exclusive to ileum in 50% of cases
Depth of wall involved	Mucosa only	Transmural, including serosa
Mucosal changes	Widespread irregular superficial ulceration with or without pseudopolyps	Fissured ulceration causing 'cobblestone' appearance
Granuloma formation	Absent	Characteristic but not always present
Mesenteric adenopathy	Reactive hyperplasia only	Lymph nodes often enlarged; granulomas may be present
Fibrosis of wall	Minimal	Marked
Main clinical features		
Diarrhoea	Severe during acute attacks, often causing incontinence	Less prominent
Rectal bleeding	Very common	Less common
Abdominal pain	Mild cramping 'pre-defaecation' pain with diarrhoeal attacks	Dominant feature—persistent or grumbling pain with severe acute attacks
Abdominal mass	No	Relatively common
General debility	Less marked	Characteristic
Complications		
Strictures	Rare	Common and often multiple
Fistulae	Rare	Common
Anal and perianal lesions	Uncommon	Common
Massive haemorrhage	Occurs in fulminant disease	Rare
Intestinal obstruction	Rare	Incomplete obstruction is common
Perforation	Complication of toxic megacolon	Free perforation rare but perforation causing local abscess formation or internal fistula common
Toxic megacolon	May occur in fulminant attacks	Rare
Malignant change	High risk with severe/longstanding disease	Low risk
Management		
Local 5-ASA/steroids	Left-sided active disease	Less effective
Systemic steroids	Severe exacerbations	Severe exacerbations
Oral 5-ASA	To treat mild attacks Long-term maintenance	Less effective
Immunosuppressives	In severe cases unresponsive to steroids As steroid-sparing agent	'Steroid sparing' in intractable cases
Surgery	Less common —in longstanding disease with evidence of dysplasia or malignancy —in fulminant colitis —in uncontrolled chronic disease	Commonly required

that the diseases may share some aetiological factors or even represent different facets of the same disease.

Epidemiological studies indicate that ulcerative colitis and Crohn's disease are relatively common in the developed communities of Western Europe, North America, Australasia and South Africa. The incidence appears to be much lower in Southern and Eastern Europe and Japan. The diseases are rare in most of Africa, Asia and South America. In the West, the incidence of Crohn's disease appears to have increased over the past 50 years (to 100 per 100 000 people per year), whilst ulcerative colitis (200 per 100 000) has remained static or has even declined.

Most cases of inflammatory bowel disease develop in the late teen years and twenties, with little difference between males and females. Social class seems to be irrelevant as does urban versus rural living. In the USA, white people are three times more susceptible to ulcerative colitis than black people and five times more susceptible to Crohn's disease.

The aetiology of the inflammatory bowel diseases remains obscure despite extensive epidemiological, clinical and laboratory research. There is a familial incidence: 6–8% of patients with ulcerative colitis and about 20% of those with Crohn's disease have first-degree relatives with the same condition. One conclusion is that both conditions are genetically heterogeneous and polygenic. For Crohn's disease, implicated genes include *NOD2* and *CARD15*. For ulcerative colitis, genes *IBD1*, *IBD2* and *IBD3* have been identified. It is even postulated that the presence of more than one of these genetic mutations may in fact result in Crohn's disease.

Another similarity between the two diseases is the association of both conditions with a range of non-gastrointestinal autoimmune disorders involving eyes,

joints, skin and liver. The most common association for both ulcerative colitis and Crohn's disease is **ankylosing spondylitis**, which in most cases is associated with the lymphocyte surface antigen HLA-B27. Pericholangitis, in contrast, occurs commonly in ulcerative colitis but is rare in Crohn's disease. This occasionally progresses to **sclerosing cholangitis**.

Infection is believed to play a part in initiating some cases of both ulcerative colitis and Crohn's disease as many cases follow an acute attack of gastroenteritis. Recent experimental work suggests that patients with Crohn's disease may have a highly specific congenital immunodeficiency disorder in which the macrophages secrete unusually low levels of interleukin 8, a cytokine that normally attracts neutrophils early in acute inflammation.

Importantly, tobacco smoking is more common in patients with Crohn's disease, and smoking increases disease recurrence. Ulcerative colitis by contrast is more prevalent in non-smokers.

ULCERATIVE COLITIS

Ulcerative colitis is an inflammatory disorder of the mucosa and submucosa of the **large bowel** only. It is characterised by recurrent acute exacerbations and intervening periods of quiescence or chronic low-grade activity. The severity of symptoms corresponds to the level of disease activity. Extracolonic features affect a small proportion of patients and include anaemia, inflammation of joints (**arthropathy**) and inflammation of the eyes, skin and biliary tract. The disease always involves the rectum but often extends proximally in continuity to involve a variable length of colon. In nearly 20% of cases (but only those with pancolitis, i.e. colitis involving the whole large bowel), the distal end of the ileum becomes secondarily affected; this is described as **backwash ileitis**.

PATHOPHYSIOLOGY OF ULCERATIVE COLITIS

Initially, the colonic mucosa becomes acutely inflamed. Neutrophils accumulate in the lamina propria and within the tubular colonic glands to form small, highly characteristic **crypt abscesses**. Sloughing of the overlying mucosa produces small superficial ulcers. If the inflammatory process persists, the ulcers coalesce into extensive areas of irregular ulceration. Residual islands of intact but oedematous mucosa project into the bowel lumen; these inflammatory lesions are called **pseudopolyps** (see Fig. 28.1). The inflammation is usually confined to the mucosa and submucosa, only extending into the muscular wall and peritoneal surface in **fulminating colitis**.

Acute inflammatory episodes range from several days' to several months' duration. After subsiding, they can recur months or even years later. During quiescent

periods, the acute inflammation resolves and the mucosa regenerates. The lamina propria, however, remains swollen by a chronic inflammatory infiltrate of lymphocytes and plasma cells. The colonic glands show a marked reduction in the number of mucin-secreting goblet cells, histologically termed '**goblet cell depletion**'.

After the disease has been present for some time, **dysplastic changes** can appear in the epithelium. Dysplasia (Latin for 'bad form') involves recognisable changes in epithelial cells indicating early transformation to neoplasia. After prolonged or repeated episodes of inflammation, the epithelium becomes even more dysplastic and may progress to **adenocarcinoma**. The risk of malignancy

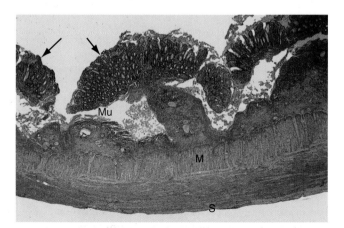

Fig. 28.1 Ulcerative colitis—histopathology
Erosion and undermining of the mucosa **Mu** by the inflammatory process has produced typical pseudopolyps (arrowed). Inflammation spares the muscle wall **M** and serosa **S**. Mucosal glands show reactive and regenerative changes.

Fig. 28.2 Radiological appearances (lateral decubitus) of ulcerative colitis

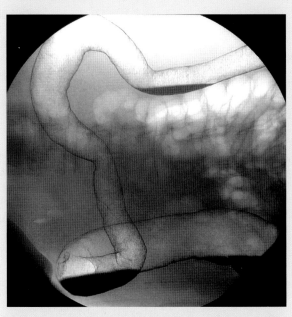

'End-stage' or 'burnt-out' ulcerative colitis in a 49-year-old office worker. He had suffered episodic, but not incapacitating, diarrhoea for 34 years, but presented on this occasion because of urgency and incontinence. Sigmoidoscopy showed only moderate rectal ulceration. This barium enema shows a typical smooth, shortened 'lead pipe' colon, with complete loss of haustration. Note that the film is orientated in the lateral decubitus position. He failed to respond to medical treatment and underwent proctocolectomy and ileostomy.

Box 28.1	Systemic manifestations of ulcerative colitis

Weight loss

- Frequent during exacerbations

Anaemia

- Typically chronic and non-specific (normochromic, normocytic)

Arthropathy

- Sacroiliitis/ankylosing spondylitis or rheumatoid-like arthritis, especially of large joints (approximately 20% of cases)

Uveitis and iritis

- Painful red eye or eyes (approximately 10%)

Skin lesions

- Erythema nodosum, i.e. tender red nodules on the shins (uncommon), pyoderma gangrenosum, i.e. purulent skin ulcers (rare)

Sclerosing cholangitis

- Progressive fibrosis of intrahepatic biliary system leading to cirrhosis, progressive liver failure, jaundice and eventually death (rare)

is greatest for those with early onset and extensive disease, and is approximately 5% after 10 years of colitis. The diagnosis of cancer may be delayed if symptoms are mistaken for a relapse of colitis and are not investigated. Cancers in these patients are often particularly aggressive and occur on average 20 years earlier than in the general population.

In longstanding colitis, the mucosa and submucosa undergo fibrosis, resulting in smoothing out of the haustrations and a shortened colon which has a characteristic radiological appearance, the so-called **lead pipe colon** (Fig. 28.2).

CLINICAL FEATURES OF ULCERATIVE COLITIS

Acute inflammatory attacks are marked by loose blood-stained stools streaked with mucus. This mucus results from inflammation of the recto-sigmoid colonic mucosa. As the extent of inflammation increases, the diarrhoea may become severe. The patient may pass 20 or more loose stools a day, each time preceded by cramping abdominal pain. In many patients, the urge to defaecate

is so precipitate that incontinence occurs unless a lavatory is immediately available. Fear of incontinence keeps many patients at home and may profoundly limit social life and employment. This, rather than the frequency of defaecation, is the worst handicap in ulcerative colitis.

Any attack of ulcerative colitis may progress to the severe form of **fulminant colitis**; the patient may become prostrated by dehydration, severe electrolyte disturbance and blood loss. Occasionally, the colon dilates considerably and eventually patchy necrosis occurs. The patient is systemically ill with high fever, marked tachycardia and dehydration. This process, known as **toxic megacolon**, culminates in perforation and fatal peritonitis unless emergency colectomy is performed.

Ulcerative colitis should probably be regarded as a systemic disorder. It is sometimes accompanied by one or more extra-gastrointestinal manifestations, summarised in Box 28.1. During active phases of the disease, inflammatory markers (erythrocyte sedimentation rate (ESR) and C-reactive protein (CRP)) are elevated and moderate anaemia and hypoalbuminaemia is common. The anaemia is normochromic and normocytic, described as 'anaemia of chronic disease'. A similar non-specific anaemia is found in other chronic inflammatory disorders like rheumatoid disease. Associated arthropathy, eye and skin disorders usually flare up in parallel with the colitis (although rarely they may precede the intestinal symptoms). Treatment of the colitis thus usually improves these complaints. However, the liver-related conditions—sclerosing cholangitis, chronic active hepatitis and bile duct carcinoma—are often independent of colitic activity and are therefore difficult to treat.

CLINICAL EXAMINATION AND INVESTIGATION OF SUSPECTED ULCERATIVE COLITIS

The typical patient referred for investigation of suspected ulcerative colitis is a young adult who gives a history of several weeks of frequent loose stools, later streaked with blood and mucus. The attack often starts with an attack of gastroenteritis or traveller's diarrhoea which fails to settle. Careful questioning often elicits a story of similar previous attacks. There is sometimes a history of associated symptoms like arthropathy or uveitis.

General examination often reveals anaemia but abdominal examination is usually unremarkable. Rectal examination, followed by proctoscopy and sigmoidoscopy, is mandatory to palpate, inspect and, if necessary, biopsy the rectal mucosa. Other diseases of the rectum and anus such as carcinoma and benign solitary ulcer must be excluded. Since ulcerative colitis always involves the rectum and extends proximally for a variable distance, diseased bowel is always accessible to sigmoidoscopic diagnosis. The affected mucosa ranges in appearance from mildly hyperaemic and easily traumatised, to more severe involvement with extensive patchy ulceration. Biopsies should be taken from representative areas. Typically, blood-streaked loose faeces leak down into the lumen during examination.

At least three separate fresh stool samples should be analysed to exclude bacterial or parasitic causes or cytomegalovirus, as these conditions may closely simulate ulcerative colitis but require entirely different treatment.

Proctitis

In ulcerative colitis, the mucosal abnormality usually extends beyond the reach of the rigid sigmoidoscope. However, some patients have inflammation confined to the lower rectum. The mucosa often has a granular appearance and the condition is described as **proctitis** or **granular proctitis**. Its cause is unknown and its course is self-limiting. It tends to recur at times of stress, often at protracted intervals. Proctitis usually responds to short courses of local 5-aminosalicylic acid suppositories (see later), but can occasionally progress into a distal or even a total colitis.

Contrast radiology

If the clinical picture and histological findings are consistent with inflammatory bowel disease, the extent and degree of colonic involvement can be assessed by barium enema examination. Radiological appearances are illus-

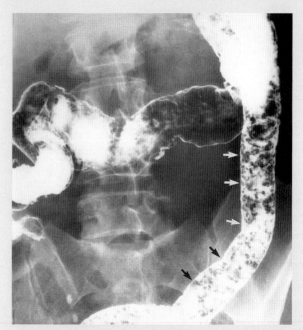

Fig. 28.3 Radiological appearances of ulcerative colitis

Severe and longstanding ulcerative colitis in a man of 50. The whole colon is affected (pancolitis) with loss of the normal haustral pattern. There is extensive pseudopolyp formation, particularly in the descending and sigmoid colon, manifest by multiple small filling defects (arrowed). Prolonged severe ulceration stimulates mitotic activity and is probably responsible for dysplastic changes and eventual malignant change in longstanding severe ulcerative colitis.

trated in Figures 28.2 and 28.3. Contrast radiology is not usually performed in acute disease.

Endoscopy

In an acute situation, an unprepared flexible sigmoidoscopy is usually performed. In non-acute situations, colonoscopy enables direct inspection of the entire colonic mucosa and the taking of multiple biopsies (see Fig. 28.4). It is a useful adjunct (or alternative) to radiological examination and permits excision or biopsy of polyps or other suspicious lesions (e.g. inflammatory pseudopolyps) to exclude malignancy. Furthermore, in patients with longstanding total colitis, colonoscopy with dye spray (e.g. with 0.1% indigo carmine enabling detection of smaller adenomas and flat adenomas) and multiple biopsies is used for annual surveillance for dysplastic change. This group in particular has an increased risk of developing carcinoma which is preventable if adenomas are treated early.

Fulminant ulcerative colitis

Fulminant attacks of ulcerative colitis sometimes occur, with extremely frequent watery, blood-stained stools and

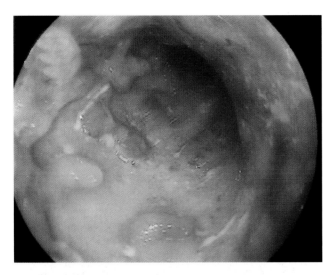

Fig. 28.4 Colonoscopic view of ulcerative colitis
This colon is quiescent with no evidence of current ulceration but inflammatory polyps are seen as memorials to past severe inflammation and ulceration.

severe systemic illness. An attack may progress to toxic dilatation and eventual perforation of the colon. Urgent colectomy may be judged necessary to treat fulminant colitis resistant to medical therapy, or to treat toxic megacolon. Fulminant bloody diarrhoea with prostration may also occur in infective colitis, e.g. *Salmonella* colitis, cholera or amoebiasis, and these diagnoses should be excluded by microbiological examination of the stool.

Whatever the cause, patients with acute colitis require urgent hospital admission and resuscitation including fluid, electrolyte and blood replacement. Sigmoidoscopy and biopsy are performed to establish the diagnosis. Stool is sent for microscopy and culture. Plain abdominal radiography is performed to monitor for dilatation, which might indicate toxic megacolon (defined as a colonic diameter greater than 6 cm in the presence of pyrexia or tachycardia). In the absence of megacolon, plain radiography may demonstrate other features of acute ulcerative colitis as shown in Figure 28.5. A flexible sigmoidoscopy without bowel preparation can be performed to confirm the diagnosis.

Fig. 28.5 Acute ulcerative colitis and toxic megacolon

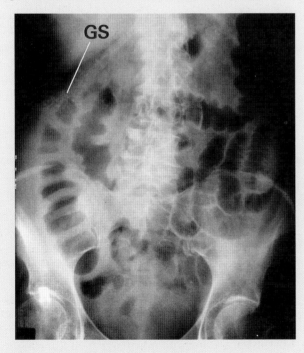

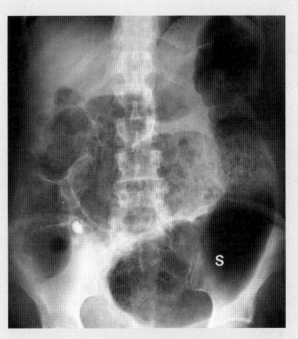

(a) This 44-year-old woman presented with fulminant ulcerative colitis. She was prostrated by frequent diarrhoea and consequent electrolyte abnormalities. This plain supine radiograph shows acute right-sided colitis. The caecum, ascending colon and proximal transverse colon are affected. In this area, there is absence of the normal 'convex outward' pattern and there are thick folds crossing the bowel lumen. This appearance is caused by oedema of the bowel wall; note the incidental finding of gallstones **GS**.

(b) This patient presented in a similar way but became toxic while in hospital undergoing intensive medical treatment. There was an increasing tachycardia, fever and abdominal tenderness. Serial plain abdominal radiographs showed an increasing diameter of the left colon. This film shows the sigmoid colon **S** dilated to 10 cm and in imminent danger of perforation. This is known as toxic dilatation of the colon; it occurs most commonly in ulcerative colitis and usually affects the transverse colon.

MANAGEMENT OF ULCERATIVE COLITIS

The management of ulcerative colitis varies from patient to patient and from episode to episode. The choice of treatment depends on the severity of individual attacks, the amount of colon involved, the extent of chronic symptoms and the risk of long-term complications. The treatment options for ulcerative colitis are summarised in Box 28.2.

Aminosalicylate preparations

Mild attacks of proctitis or proctosigmoiditis are treated locally with 5 aminosalicylic acid (5-ASA) suppositories or enemas, which are more effective in acute proctitis than steroids. Mild attacks of pan-colitis are treated initially with oral 5-ASA preparations. Oral 5-ASA preparations are also employed as maintenance therapy in ulcerative colitis to prevent relapse. Although aspirin and other non-steroidal anti-inflammatories are chemically related to 5-ASA compounds, these drugs should be avoided as they may worsen inflammatory bowel disease. The 5-ASA compounds are discussed further later in this chapter as they are also used in the management of Crohn's disease.

Corticosteroids

Steroid suppositories or enemas (foam or liquid) can also be used for local treatment of rectal inflammation. Short courses of high-dose oral corticosteroids are used for more severe exacerbations (e.g. prednisolone 40 mg daily for 2 weeks then reducing the daily dose by 5 mg weekly). Intravenous administration is advisable in seriously ill patients. There is no evidence that 'bowel rest' (i.e. nil by mouth) and total parenteral nutrition (TPN) are of any value in ulcerative colitis. Immunosuppressive drugs, including **ciclosporin** and **azathioprine**, are often tried in patients who fail to respond to corticosteroids. Azathioprine is also used as a steroid-sparing agent in patients whose disease settles on steroids but flares again as the steroids are reduced.

Other supportive measures

In the acute case, anti-diarrhoeal agents such as codeine phosphate or loperamide should be avoided as they can precipitate toxic dilatation.

Patients with moderately severe chronic disease frequently become anaemic and lose weight, in part because of persistent loss of protein in the stool. These problems may be helped by medical treatment, a diet high in calories and protein, and oral iron supplements.

Surgery for ulcerative colitis

Surgery is required in only about 20% of patients with ulcerative colitis. Colectomy may be needed in the following:

- Urgent treatment of fulminant cases which fail to respond to intensive medical treatment. 'Failure to respond' has no precise definition but, in general, there should be symptomatic improvement after a week of intensive management, and no deterioration within that time
- Acute cases which progress to toxic megacolon, perforation or haemorrhage
- Patients with chronic disabling symptoms of intractable diarrhoea with urgency, recurring anaemia and failure to maintain adequate weight and nutrition
- Children with failure to thrive and retardation of growth (both are exacerbated by corticosteroid therapy)
- Patients with longstanding colitis who develop dysplasia or malignancy

As a general principle, surgery for ulcerative colitis requires removal of the entire large bowel and is curative. There are three main surgical options:

- **Subtotal colectomy with ileostomy** is the safest operation in the emergency situation when the patient is sick and on high-dose corticosteroids. Most of the diseased colon is removed, but the patient is left with an inflamed rectal stump. Months later, when the patient is well, this may be revised to one of the other two surgical options. Alternatively the rectum may be retained and treated with local

---

> **Box 28.2 Main treatment measures for ulcerative colitis**
>
> **Local corticosteroid or 5-ASA preparations** (suppositories, foam or liquid enema)
> - Employed in cases of left-sided active disease
>
> **Systemic corticosteroids**
> - Suppress moderate or severe exacerbations (oral or intravenous administration according to severity of disease)
>
> **Oral (or sometimes rectal) aminosalicylate preparations,** e.g. sulfasalazine, mesalazine (Asacol or Pentasa) or olsalazine
> - Long-term maintenance therapy to minimise relapse
>
> **Surgical removal of the colon**
> - Emergency operation: incipient or actual perforation, serious haemorrhage, failure of fulminant colitis to improve on medical treatment
> - Elective operation: failure of medical treatment, risk of malignancy

therapy plus endoscopic surveillance, although the cancer risk remains

- **Proctocolectomy with permanent ileostomy** is generally only recommended for elderly patients in whom sphincter-preserving procedures are inadvisable
- **Restorative proctocolectomy (ileo-anal pouch, Parks' pouch)** is a sphincter-preserving operation which avoids a permanent ileostomy (see Fig. 27.12).

The entire colon and rectal mucosa is excised and a **pouch** reservoir is fashioned from a loop of terminal ileum. The pouch is brought down into the pelvis and anastomosed to the upper anal canal. A temporary ileostomy is usually left in place for a few months to allow healing of the anastomoses. Many patients have excellent continence and can evacuate their bowels in the normal way

CROHN'S DISEASE

Crohn's disease is a chronic relapsing inflammatory disorder of **any part** of the gastrointestinal tract which predominantly affects younger people. About 60% of patients are under 25 years at the time of initial diagnosis, and on average, symptoms will have been present intermittently for 5 years. A useful website is http://www.crohns.org.uk/

The disease often affects one or more discrete segments of the bowel with intervening parts of the bowel completely spared, unlike the continuous nature of ulcerative colitis. In Crohn's disease, the discontinuous affected areas are known as '**skip lesions**' (see Fig. 28.12, p. 427).

The small bowel alone is affected in 50% of patients, the large bowel alone in 20% and both together in 30%. The terminal ileum is affected most commonly; in up to half of all cases, the disease is confined to the terminal ileum. In the original description of this disease it was named 'terminal ileitis'. Later, when it became clear that other segments of the bowel could also be affected, the name was changed to **regional enteritis**, a term still used in the USA. Crohn's disease also commonly affects the perianal region, whether or not large bowel is involved. Occasionally, the disease involves the stomach, duodenum, oesophagus or mouth.

In contrast to ulcerative colitis, the inflammation involves the entire thickness of the bowel wall (**transmu-**

ral inflammation). Because of this, affected bowel may partially obstruct, fistulate or perforate, whereas this rarely occurs in ulcerative colitis. See Table 28.1 for comparisons between Crohn's disease and ulcerative colitis.

With each exacerbation, previously affected or new areas may become involved. The disease tends to run a protracted and unpredictable course.

PATHOPHYSIOLOGY AND CLINICAL CONSEQUENCES OF CROHN'S DISEASE

The essential pathological feature of Crohn's disease is chronic inflammation of one or more discrete segments of bowel with the inflammation extending diffusely through the entire thickness of the bowel wall. The wall becomes markedly thickened by inflammatory oedema, especially in the submucosa. The epithelium remains largely intact but is criss-crossed by deep **fissured ulcers**. These large serpiginous ulcers and the intervening areas of dome-shaped mucosa and submucosa give a typical 'cobblestone' surface appearance.

Granulomas containing multinucleate giant cells (see Fig. 28.6) are usually scattered throughout the inflamed bowel wall as well as in local lymph nodes. (Although non-caseating granulomas are typical of Crohn's disease,

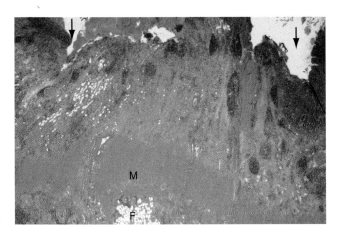

(a)

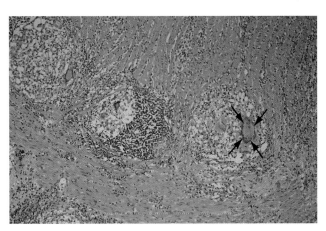

(b)

(a) Inflammation has produced fissure ulcers (arrowed) which extend into the muscle wall **M**. Lymphoid aggregates are also present and the inflammatory process extends into serosal fat **F**.

(b) High-power view showing well-formed granulomas with typical giant cells (arrowed), enabling a confident diagnosis of Crohn's disease to be made.

Fig. 28.6 Crohn's disease affecting the colon—histopathology

they are not always found, and ruptured crypt abscesses in ulcerative colitis may also cause these.) Longstanding inflammation leads to progressive **fibrosis** of the thickened bowel wall, which encroaches on the lumen, producing **elongated strictures**.

Effects of mucosal inflammation

Mucosal inflammation causes diarrhoea which, if the colon is involved, may be streaked with mucus and blood. Luminal narrowing in the small bowel results in partial obstruction that causes grumbling, colicky abdominal pain. There may also be acute episodes of more severe pain and vomiting which precipitate hospital admission. Pain is a prominent feature in Crohn's disease in contrast to ulcerative colitis, since inflamed large bowel does not obstruct in this way.

If the small bowel is inflamed, diarrhoea occurs and digestive and absorptive functions may be adversely affected. Extensive disease results in general malabsorption causing protein-calorie malnutrition, iron and folate deficiency and anaemia. In children, Crohn's disease may cause marked growth retardation. Ileal inflammation disrupts **bile salt reabsorption**. Excess bile salts in the faeces cause colonic irritation (and more diarrhoea) while diminished recirculation of bile salts may result in gallstone formation. Involvement of the terminal ileum may also reduce vitamin B_{12} absorption but serious deficiency usually occurs only after surgical resection.

Effects of transmural inflammation

Crohn's disease causes additional problems if serosal inflammation extends to adjacent structures. If inflamed bowel impinges on the parietal peritoneum, pain becomes localised and more severe, and signs of local peritonitis develop. Indeed, Crohn's disease of the terminal ileum may mimic acute appendicitis. At appendicectomy, the terminal ileum is seen to be inflamed and the bowel wall abnormally thick to palpation. In this case, the terminal ileum should not be excised; a firm diagnosis of Crohn's disease requires histological and microbacterial exclusion of *Yersinia* ileitis (see Ch. 26) as well as tuberculosis. Both may simulate Crohn's, but are completely reversible with medical treatment.

Fulminant colonic Crohn's disease occasionally causes toxic dilatation which is clinically identical to ulcerative colitis but this presentation is rare.

Serosal inflammation may cause a segment of diseased bowel to adhere to nearby abdominal structures. Several complications may occur if these become matted together by the inflammatory process:

- **Adhesions**. These tough, fibrotic post-inflammatory adhesions are rarely symptomatic but constitute a formidable obstacle if operation is needed later

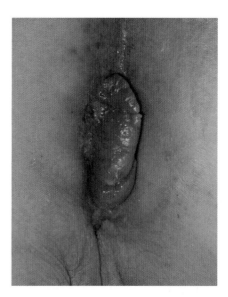

Fig. 28.7 Crohn's 'piles'
This appearance is typical of Crohn's 'piles'. They are pale and oedematous in contrast to ordinary haemorrhoids.

- **Perforation**. Free perforation is rare but a contained perforation may occur which causes localised pericolic or pelvic abscess formation
- **Fistulae**. These may develop between diseased bowel and other hollow viscera causing unusual clinical phenomena. For example, a gastro-colic fistula may result in faecal vomiting; an ileo-rectal fistula may aggravate diarrhoea. Entero-vesical fistulae cause severe urinary tract infections and pneumaturia (passage of 'soda-water' urine), and fistulae between bowel and uterus or vagina lead to vaginal passage of faeces. Entero-cutaneous fistulae between bowel and skin occasionally develop as a complication of bowel resection for Crohn's disease, or spontaneously

Perianal inflammation

Perianal inflammation occurs in 15% of patients with Crohn's disease. Symptoms include recurrent perianal abscesses, characteristic blueish, boggy 'piles' (see Fig. 28.7) and anterolateral anal fissures. The last two are quite distinct from ordinary haemorrhoids and posterior anal fissures. Multiple fistulae commonly develop between rectum and perianal skin and can extend into the labia or scrotum. Fistulae are sometimes so numerous as to cause a 'pepper-pot' or 'watering-can' perineum (see Fig. 28.8). Paradoxically, this is more often associated with small bowel disease than colorectal disease.

Systemic features

Like ulcerative colitis, Crohn's disease is a systemic disorder and has a similar range of non-gastrointestinal manifestations (see Box 28.1, p. 419). In contrast with ulcerative colitis, it is common for patients to feel generally ill

Fig. 28.8 Multiple anal fistulae in Crohn's disease

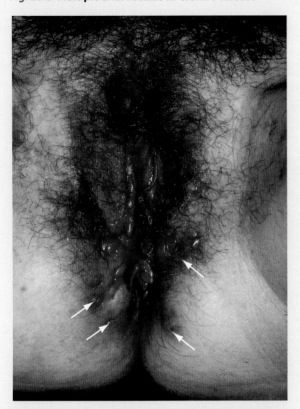

This 30-year-old woman had several 'skip lesions' of Crohn's disease in her small bowel and was troubled by recurrent perianal sepsis. This photograph shows a typical 'pepper-pot perineum', with several fistulous openings (arrowed) seen around the circumference of the anus. Anal skin tags are also visible.

during an acute attack. Specific systemic features affecting skin, joints or the eye are relatively uncommon and not necessarily related to intestinal disease activity.

SYMPTOMS AND SIGNS IN CROHN'S DISEASE

Symptoms of Crohn's disease can be similar to those of ulcerative colitis, particularly when the large bowel is involved (see Table 28.1, p. 417). Diarrhoea is usually less distressing and less likely to contain blood. Other characteristic symptoms of Crohn's disease include cramp-like abdominal pain, weight loss and general malaise. As an aide memoire, think of **pain, weight loss** and **diarrhoea** as symptomatic of Crohn's.

Physical examination may reveal generalised wasting and anaemia and sometimes other features like arthropathy. On abdominal examination, there may be areas of tenderness, an inflammatory mass in the right iliac fossa where omentum wraps around inflamed terminal ileum or the scars of previous surgery. The perianal skin should be examined for fissures, fistulae, Crohn's 'piles' or stenotic scarring from previous disease. Diseased rectal mucosa, with its

typical firm surface nodularity, may be felt on digital examination. Sigmoidoscopic examination is usually normal but there may be mucosal oedema if the rectum is involved. In more severe cases, the typical 'cobblestone' appearance with fissured ulceration may be seen. Biopsies may be positive even when the mucosa is apparently normal.

APPROACH TO INVESTIGATION OF SUSPECTED CROHN'S DISEASE

Investigation of suspected Crohn's disease is similar to that for ulcerative colitis in respect of the large bowel, but follows a different pattern when there is suspected small bowel disease.

Colonoscopy with intubation of the terminal ileum enables a histological diagnosis to be obtained in colonic disease, and also allows biopsies of terminal ileum to be taken, which are often diagnostic. Direct small bowel visualisation by enteroscopy remains difficult to achieve but developments in **capsule enteroscopy** (see Ch. 5) hold promise in this respect.

Barium 'follow-through' is the traditional method of examining the small bowel but better images are sometimes obtained by controlled instillation of barium into the duodenum through a nasogastric tube. Typical radiological appearances of Crohn's disease include narrowing of the lumen due to mural oedema and fibrosis, nodularity and cobblestoning of the mucosal surface, deep fissured ulceration extending into the muscular wall, spiky 'rose thorn' ulcers and possibly evidence of fistula formation. Radiological changes in small and large bowel are shown in Figures 28.9 to 28.11. Note that large bowel abnormalities on barium enema may be difficult or impossible to distinguish from ulcerative colitis.

Isotope scanning using radioactive indium-labelled white blood cells can be useful as an initial assessment of the extent and inflammatory activity of disease and indicates which parts of the bowel to examine further.

As in ulcerative colitis, full blood count, inflammatory markers (ESR and CRP) and liver function tests also give an indication of the disease activity; stool microscopy and culture is always undertaken to exclude an infective cause for diarrhoea.

MANAGEMENT OF CROHN'S DISEASE

The aim of medical therapy in active Crohn's disease is to bring about and maintain remission. The treatments available may be broadly divided into three classes of medication:

Anti-inflammatory agents

● **5-ASA compounds**, as used in ulcerative colitis. These compounds act locally, making it a challenge to deliver the oral medication to inflamed small bowel without gastric inactivation. **Sulfasalazine** (a combination of 5-ASA and a carrier, sulfapyridine) is useful in ulcerative colitis and large bowel Crohn's disease

Fig. 28.9 Radiological appearances in Crohn's disease

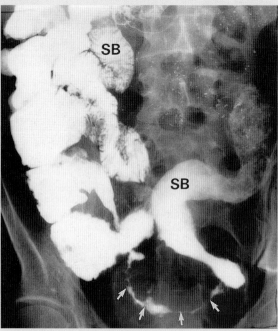

This man of 51 had recurrent attacks of colicky abdominal pain, with diarrhoea and loss of weight. This barium follow-through examination shows one of the characteristic radiological appearances of Crohn's disease. The terminal ileum is extremely narrowed by inflammation of the whole wall thickness (arrowed); this is known as the 'string sign of Kantor' and causes the symptoms and signs of partial obstruction. This film also shows dilatation of small bowel **SB** proximal to the stricture.

Fig. 28.10 Radiological appearances in Crohn's disease

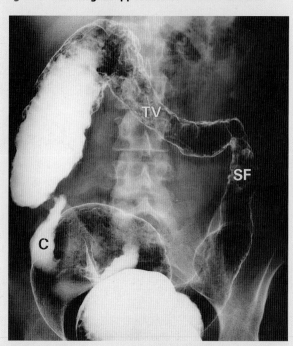

This man of 54 presented with 8 months of diarrhoea and feeling generally unwell. The barium enema shows Crohn's disease of the caecum **C**, transverse colon **TV** and splenic flexure **SF**. The descending colon and sigmoid are normal. Here, the features of Crohn's disease are discontinuous skip lesions with normal bowel between, a ragged luminal outline due to ulceration, and loss of haustration.

since the active ingredient is released by colonic bacteria. However, up to 15% of patients suffer side effects related to the sulfapyridine moiety. Mesalazine is useful for more proximal Crohn's disease as the active compound is released earlier. In other proprietary versions, the active ingredient is coated to enable its release in the terminal ileum and colon. Rectal Crohn's disease can be treated with 5-ASA suppositories or enemas, as used in ulcerative colitis. 5-ASA compounds can be used as maintenance therapy in Crohn's disease but large doses are required

● **Corticosteroids** can act both as systemic agents (e.g. prednisolone) or locally. Budesonide is a new oral steroid which is mostly released in the terminal ileum then rapidly inactivated by the liver after absorption, minimising systemic effects. Corticosteroids act rapidly to control flare-ups, but are little used for long-term maintenance

Immunomodulators

● **Azathioprine and 6-mercaptopurine** are immunosuppressants, sometimes used in more severe

Crohn's disease. They can spare the need for damaging steroids, or they can help maintain remission in patients who relapse on 5-ASA compounds. About 10% of those treated are at risk of bone marrow suppression but those at risk can be predicted by pre-treatment testing

● **Methotrexate** acts both as an anti-inflammatory agent and an immunomodulator but has potentially serious side effects upon liver and bone marrow

● **Infliximab** is a chimeric monoclonal antibody to TNF-α, a mediator of inflammation. It is given by intravenous infusion for acute disease and is usually effective within 2 weeks. The drug can be given at 8-weekly intervals to maintain remission. Risks include developing antibodies to the drug. It should not be used where there is active infection or an abscess

Other supportive treatments

● Antidiarrhoeal drugs (e.g. loperamide) and antispasmodics are used in the chronic situation

● Dietary modification: liquid/low-fibre diets for those with obstructive symptoms, and supplementary calories, iron and vitamins

Fig. 28.11 Radiological appearances in Crohn's disease

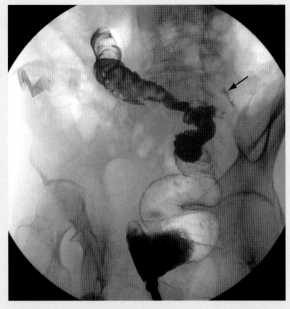 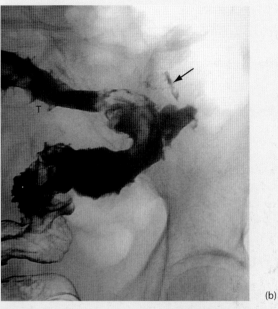

(a) (b)

(a) Double contrast barium enema in a 28-year-old woman who complained of 8 months' history of recurrent abdominal pains and diarrhoea. She had not lost weight. This film shows a 'ragged' segment in the sigmoid colon with narrowing and 'rose thorn' ulcers **T**, better seen in the close-up view in **(b)**. In both views, contrast is visible outside the colon (arrowed). In fact, this is in small bowel because of a fistula between colon and small bowel.

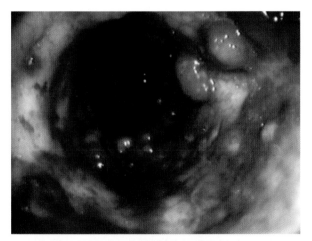 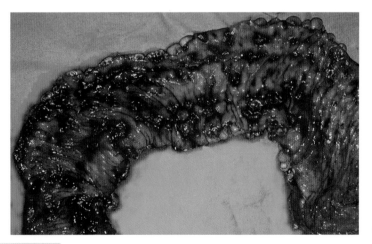

(a) (b)

(c)

Fig. 28.12 Appearances of Crohn's colitis
(a) This is a typical colonoscopic view of florid Crohn's colitis. Note the nodular appearance producing a 'cobblestone' surface with linear ulcers between the nodules, seen more clearly in **(b)**. **(b)** Specimen of Crohn's colon from another patient with similar symptoms. Here 'aphthous type' ulcers are clearly visible. **(c)** Case study—this subtotal colectomy specimen was removed from a man of 54 with a long history of weight loss, diarrhoea and abdominal pain (see barium enema, Fig. 28.10). There are three 'skip lesions' typical of Crohn's disease, in the ascending colon, the transverse colon and the hepatic flexure showing thickening of the wall, cobblestone mucosal surface and narrowing of the lumen.

427

THE ROLE OF SURGERY IN CROHN'S DISEASE

Surgery should not be considered curative in Crohn's disease, unlike ulcerative colitis. This is because operating on one section of bowel does not affect later recurrence elsewhere. Up to 70% of patients with Crohn's disease will eventually need surgery, of whom half will need further surgery within 5 years.

The main indications for surgery can be summarised as follows:

- Acute complications, e.g. abscess, perforation
- Persistent local ileal disease
- Intolerable long-term obstructive and other symptoms, e.g. abdominal pain, perianal disease, general ill-health
- Entero-cutaneous fistulae and symptomatic internal fistulae

The choice of operation depends on the site and extent of disease. The former belief that all disease must be resected has been abandoned. Given the diffuse nature of the disease and likelihood of further operations, as much bowel as possible should be preserved. Surgery for multiple small bowel strictures now involves **stricturoplasty** of each lesion, a technique of enlarging the lumen of diseased bowel without losing potential absorptive length. If the disease is limited, resection of the diseased segment with a small margin of normal tissue may be performed, followed by wide side-to-side anastomosis. **Abscesses** are usually treated by simple drainage, with resection of the affected bowel at the same time or later.

Fistulae between abdominal viscera are treated by removal of the diseased bowel. In contrast, entero-cutaneous fistulae, usually a complication of recent surgery, are a more formidable problem since they are often associated with complicating factors like intra-abdominal infection, gross fluid and electrolyte abnormalities and a hypercatabolic state. Patients with entero-cutaneous fistulae require intensive preparatory medical care and strategic surgical intervention before definitive treatment is possible.

For severe **large bowel disease**, the entire colon is generally removed (pan-proctocolectomy with ileostomy). This is because there are usually several colonic 'skip lesions' and recurrence is likely. Pouch procedures are not generally recommended because of the risk of recurrent disease in the small bowel pouch or reservoir.

Recurrent disease often necessitates further surgery. Careful medical treatment to reduce disease recurrence and hence increase intervals between reoperations is imperative: stopping smoking, 5-ASA preparations, and even azathioprine may be used, particularly if the patient has been left with a short bowel.

OTHER CHRONIC INFLAMMATIONS OF THE COLON

AMOEBIC COLITIS

Entamoeba histolytica is a protozoon parasite responsible for amoebic colitis. It is an endemic bowel commensal in many developing countries but is also found in a few people in developed countries. Most of those infected have no symptoms but they are all carriers. Less than 5% of those infected suffer amoebic colitis. In these, the organism invades the large bowel mucosa, causing chronic relapsing symptoms similar to ulcerative colitis or Crohn's disease. Encysted parasites are shed by carriers in the faeces and infection is readily transmitted to new individuals via contaminated hands or uncooked food.

The incidence of amoebiasis is likely to increase in the West as tourism expands into endemic areas. If sufferers are mistakenly treated with systemic steroids for inflammatory bowel disease, the result may be fatal.

PATHOLOGY OF AMOEBIC COLITIS

Initial penetration of bowel mucosa by the parasite causes small surface erosions. Lateral spread from the depths of the crypts produces **flask-shaped mucosal ulcers**. These are multiple and discrete and are characteristic of amoebic colitis. Amoebae can often be observed near the edge of ulcers on standard histological preparations but can best be demonstrated when stained magenta by the periodic acid–Schiff method. The mucosa between the ulcers is remarkably normal. Large granulomatous colonic lesions also occur. These are known as **amoebomas**.

Occasionally, rampant invasion causes widespread mucosal sloughing and muscle wall involvement. This progresses to local perforation and a pericolic abscess or toxic megacolon leading to massive perforation and generalised peritonitis.

In any case of amoebic colitis, amoebae passing to the liver in the portal veins may occasionally produce **hepatic abscesses**, most frequently in the right lobe. These are usually solitary and are filled with reddish-brown necrotic material, said to resemble anchovy sauce.

CLINICAL FEATURES OF AMOEBIC COLITIS

The disease usually affects the proximal colon, causing colicky abdominal pain, erratic bowel habit with episodes of blood-stained loose stools, and right iliac fossa tenderness. If the distal colon is involved, the patient suffers chronic watery diarrhoea with blood and mucus. When the entire colon is involved there is generalised abdominal tenderness as well as systemic features, e.g. pyrexia and progressive weight loss. A large **amoeboma** may be palpable and must be differentiated from carcinoma or diverticular disease.

If the patient develops an amoebic liver abscess, systemic features become more marked, with general ill-health and a swinging pyrexia with sweating attacks. There is pain in the liver area and an enlarged tender liver on palpation. The abscess may rupture spontaneously into the peritoneal cavity (causing peritonitis) or through the diaphragm into the chest. Secondary lung abscesses may then rupture into the bronchi and the patient coughs up 'anchovy sauce' sputum.

DIAGNOSIS OF AMOEBIASIS

In developed countries, amoebic colitis should always be considered in the differential diagnosis of ulcerative colitis or Crohn's colitis. Amoebic colitis is best diagnosed by microscopic examination of fresh stool specimens; this may reveal trophozoites containing ingested red cells. Sigmoidoscopy often shows small discrete ulcers with normal mucosa between, however rectal disease is less common than involvement of the right side of the colon. Scrapings from the ulcer base placed in warm saline may reveal trophozoites, as may mucosal biopsies, but trophozoites may be undetectable in more than half of the cases.

Liver abscesses cause serological tests for amoebiasis to become positive. The lesions are readily demonstrated by hepatic ultrasound and the diagnosis is confirmed by needle aspiration.

TREATMENT OF AMOEBIASIS

Metronidazole is the drug treatment of choice for amoebic dysentery and is given orally, 800 mg 3 times daily for 5 days, followed by diloxanide 500 mg 3 times daily for 10 days to eradicate cysts. Liver abscesses are treated with metronidazole 400 mg 3 times daily for 5–10 days followed again by diloxanide. Emergency surgery is occasionally necessary in fulminating amoebic colitis or less urgently for large liver abscesses.

MICROSCOPIC COLITIS

This recently described condition is so called because the histology is abnormal but the macroscopic appearance may be normal. It causes chronic watery diarrhoea and is thought to be the cause in up to 5% of patients complaining of this symptom. Its aetiology is still unknown, but a link with non-steroidal anti-inflammatory drugs has been noted. Specific histological findings (collagenous and lymphocytic types) are seen in biopsy specimens, although the colon may look macroscopically normal at colonoscopy. The collagenous type seems to affect predominantly women and patients of either sex between 60 and 80 years of age. Treatment is not very effective: budesonide and bismuth are tried for patients unable to control symptoms with antidiarrhoeal agents.

29 Disorders of large bowel motility, structure and perfusion

INTRODUCTION

Irritable bowel syndrome, chronic constipation and **diverticular disease** all arise from disordered peristaltic function and are at least partly attributable to the highly refined Western diet. These disorders could almost be regarded as endemic in developed societies.

Irritable bowel syndrome causes distressing abdominal discomfort in younger patients, whilst chronic constipation can affect people of all age groups in whom a variety of factors cause slowing of gut transit time. Diverticular disease, in which ageing of the bowel wall predisposes to localised outpouchings, may also be caused by long-term dietary factors. The disorders make substantial demands on the time of family practitioners, physicians and surgeons, yet they are largely preventable. A hundred years ago, they were largely unknown in the West (apart from an obsession with constipation), as they still are in rural communities in developing countries.

In addition to symptoms needing treatment, the main surgical importance of these conditions is that they must be distinguished from inflammatory bowel diseases in the young and large bowel cancer in the older population. They have several symptoms in common:

- Intermittent attacks of abdominal pain, which can be severe
- Erratic bowel habit
- Abdominal bloating and passage of excessive flatus

Sigmoid volvulus is an acute condition resulting from chronic dilatation of the sigmoid colon plus an acute event of twisting of the sigmoid loop on a narrow mesentery, resulting in obstruction and massive dilatation (see Fig. 29.1, p. 434).

Angiodysplasia of the large bowel and **ischaemic colitis** are vascular conditions of the ageing gut, both of which usually present with rectal bleeding and pain.

Again, colorectal cancer has to be excluded as the cause of the bleeding.

MODERN DIET AND DISEASE

EPIDEMIOLOGICAL OBSERVATIONS

Little scientific attention was paid to diet-related disease until the 1970s, although Gaylord Hauser had written on the subject of fibre in the diet in the 1930s. In the 1970s, the ideas of Surgeon Captain T. L. Cleeve, a Royal Navy physician, and later the remarkable epidemiological observations of Denis Burkitt, a long-time missionary surgeon in Africa, began to be published. Now the subject of diet is not only respectable in surgical circles but has made contributions to the understanding, prevention and management of many common diseases. Diseases such as irritable bowel syndrome, diverticular disease and appendicitis, which are common in Western society, are largely unknown in most of the developing world and this difference is almost certainly related to diet. Thus it follows that an accurate dietary history is important in evaluating patients with these conditions, and dietary change is often a fundamental part of their management.

Over millions of years as 'hunter-gatherers', humans subsisted on a staple diet of a wide variety of vegetables and fruits, grains, legumes and nuts, supplemented by occasional meat or fish. The modern human gastrointestinal and metabolic systems are thus perfectly adapted to that diet. During the brief period (in evolutionary terms) of the last 100 years, the average Western diet has changed dramatically, due to affluence, fashion, convenience, food processing and advertising. Since the 1980s there have been similar trends in the more prosperous parts of developing countries, particularly in the cities. The modern diet contains many more calories than the hunter-

---

Box 29.1   **Mechanisms by which refined diet may cause disease**

Slowed gastrointestinal transit time

- Increases duration of contact between stool and bowel mucosa; this increases duration of contact of carcinogens, predisposing to colorectal cancer

Increased intra-abdominal pressure due to straining at stool

- Obstructs venous return making haemorrhoids and varicose veins more likely
- Predisposes to hiatus hernia, inguinal hernia and rectal prolapse

Reduced bulk and more solid consistency of faeces

- Make peristalsis less effective and constipation more likely
- Increase intraluminal pressure, perhaps predisposing to diverticular disease
- Hard stool increases friction, causing anal fissure and perhaps haemorrhoids
- Small stool bulk increases concentration of carcinogens
- May contribute to pathogenesis of appendicitis by obstructing appendiceal orifice

Decreased loss of bile salts in the faeces

- Increased bile salt pool predisposes to gallstone formation
- Increased bile salts in lumen may result in formation of carcinogens

Changes in bacterial flora of the bowel

- May result in formation of carcinogens
- May be implicated in appendicitis

Increased refined carbohydrate intake

- Predisposes to diabetes
- Contributes to excess calorie intake causing obesity

Increased dietary fat intake, particularly saturated animal fats

- Predisposes to atherosclerosis
- Predisposes to gallstone formation
- Contributes to excess calorie intake and obesity

Increased absorption of dietary fat because of reduced binding by fibre

- Increases fat absorption and blood lipid levels

Obesity

- Weakens abdominal wall muscles predisposing to hiatus hernia, abdominal wall hernias and vaginal prolapse
- Predisposes to thromboembolism
- Contributes to musculoskeletal and joint disorders

---

gatherer diet. These are largely in the form of refined carbohydrates and fats, especially saturated animal fats and 'trans' fats found in artificially hydrogenated vegetable oils. Perhaps equally important, the modern diet contains far less unabsorbable fibre residue.

MECHANISMS OF DISEASE CAUSED BY MODERN DIET

Whilst the increase in calories and nutrients has brought benefits, it has also brought problems. The modern diet adversely affects both bowel function and metabolism, particularly of lipids, and this has led to an array of disorders. Box 29.1 outlines the important ways in which modern diet can induce disease and dysfunction. With regard to diseases of the bowel, the most important diet-related factors are likely to be faecal volume and consistency, together with gastrointestinal transit time. The average Western adult passes between 80 and 120 g of firm stool each day with a transit time of about 3 days, although transit time can be as long as 2 weeks in the elderly. In contrast, rural dwellers in the developing world, with a diet similar to that of the hunter-gatherer, pass between 300 and 800 g of much softer stool each day, with an average transit time of less than a day and a half.

Box 29.2   **Foods with a high fibre content**

- Whole-grain and bran-enriched breakfast cereals, e.g. muesli, All-Bran, Weetabix (not cornflakes, puffed rice, etc.)
- Wholemeal bread (not white or 'brown')
- Other wholewheat products, e.g. wholewheat pasta, wholemeal pastry, digestive biscuits
- Other whole grain, e.g. brown rice, cracked wheat
- Pulses of any kind, e.g. haricot beans (including canned baked beans), kidney beans, chick peas, other dried beans and lentils
- Potatoes (skins should be left on)
- Unpeeled fruit and vegetables (actually low in fibre compared with grains and pulses)

INCREASING DIETARY FIBRE CONTENT

An essential part of managing many bowel conditions (other than irritable bowel syndrome) and preventing others is a substantial increase in daily dietary fibre intake. Box 29.2 lists the readily available foods with a high fibre content which can be eaten regularly with little effort or extra expense. Increasing the fibre content of the normal diet almost inevitably leads to reduced consumption of refined carbohydrates and saturated animal fats and lower total energy intake. Patients should be advised to introduce dietary fibre gradually because a sudden increase is likely to cause abdominal discomfort and distension and increased production of flatus. Bulking agents (**ispaghula husk** preparations) can be taken in the early stages to achieve a rapid result whilst avoiding these unpleasant side effects.

IRRITABLE BOWEL SYNDROME

Irritable bowel syndrome (IBS) has only been accepted as a pathological entity in recent years, although Osler coined the term *mucous colitis* in 1892 to describe mucorrhoea (excess mucus in the stool) and abdominal colic often found in patients with psychological problems. Another commonly used name is '**spastic colon**'. The condition is widespread, particularly in young and middle-aged women.

CLINICAL FEATURES OF IRRITABLE BOWEL SYNDROME

Irritable bowel syndrome is a functional gastrointestinal disorder characterised by abdominal pain and altered bowel habit in the absence of identifiable organic pathology. IBS can only be diagnosed clinically (after excluding organic causes) as there are no specific diagnostic tests. A group of experts formalised a diagnostic set of symptoms known as the **Rome II Criteria**. To fulfil a diagnosis of IBS, a patient must have the following symptoms continuously or recurrently for at least 3 months in any one year: abdominal pain relieved by defecation, and a change in stool frequency and consistency. Symptoms supporting the diagnosis include altered stool form, mucorrhoea and abdominal bloating.

The patient typically complains of episodic 'cramping' abdominal pain occurring at any time of day and lasting from 15 minutes to several hours. The pain is unrelated to meals or other obvious provoking factors. It occurs anywhere in the abdomen but tends to arise peripherally, i.e. in either iliac fossa or the epigastrium, and usually recurs in the same general area in any one patient.

Symptoms occur daily for weeks at a time and then resolve for weeks or months, only to return later. The patient may recognise that symptoms are worse at times of stress and are absent during weekends and holidays. The pain may provoke an urge to open the bowels and evacuation may bring some relief from the pain. An erratic bowel habit is a characteristic feature of irritable bowel syndrome. Passage of loose stools alternates with constipation, with small hard stools described as looking like rabbit pellets: but patients are divided into those for whom either diarrhoea or constipation is the predominant problem. Sufferers often complain of abdominal distension and excess flatus.

PATHOPHYSIOLOGY AND AETIOLOGY OF IRRITABLE BOWEL SYNDROME

The pathophysiology of irritable bowel syndrome is poorly understood. Studies of colonic motility show abnormal rises in intraluminal pressure and disordered peristalsis resulting in segmenting, non-propulsive contractions. The small volume of faeces (because of little residual fibre) becomes excessively dehydrated and fragmented. However, some patients with irritable bowel syndrome appear to be hypersensitive to gut distension and their symptoms may be made worse by a high-fibre diet. These patients in particular may benefit from a low-fibre diet with the addition of methylcellulose fibre substitutes that do not ferment, e.g. Celevac. Thus the patient avoids constipation without the usual fermentation and excess gas production associated with a high-fibre diet. There is growing support for the view that at least some IBS is due to food intolerance, particularly wheat protein, and it is worth excluding this in a trial of treatment.

MANAGEMENT OF IRRITABLE BOWEL SYNDROME

The diagnosis is made on the basis of a typical history after excluding organic disorders and often after a trial of treatment. In the younger patient, where carcinoma is unlikely, abdominal and rectal examination (probably including sigmoidoscopy) is all that is required. In IBS, these will be normal except perhaps for mild tenderness to palpation in the area of pain. Other factors that help to exclude inflammatory bowel disease are a normal erythrocyte sedimentation rate (ESR) and C-reactive protein (CRP), and an absence of weight loss, ill-health and tiredness, troublesome diarrhoea or rectal bleeding. In cases of diagnostic difficulty, small bowel radiology and other investigations can exclude Crohn's disease.

Persistent upper gastrointestinal pain should be investigated with gallstones or peptic ulcer disease in mind. In a patient over the age of 50, a diagnosis of irritable bowel syndrome is less likely, and carcinoma and diverticular disease must be excluded by sigmoidoscopy and/or colonoscopy or barium enema before IBS can be confirmed.

Treatment involves reassurance, adjusting the diet to test for wheat intolerance, treating the predominant symptom of constipation or diarrhoea, and antispasmodic drugs such as mebeverine and peppermint oil. Mebeverine plus codeine phosphate (as an analgesic) given immediately an attack comes on produces rapid relief of symptoms and confirms the diagnosis. There is probably little benefit in giving continuous treatment. For selected patients, relaxation therapy or antidepressants such as amitriptyline may be useful.

CONSTIPATION

CLINICAL FEATURES OF CONSTIPATION

Whether or not they consider it a problem, many patients suffer from chronic constipation. Constipation is difficult to define but the essence is a subjective inability to evacuate the bowels with sufficient frequency, ease, completeness or satisfaction. Perception of what is normal varies greatly; some patients insist that daily evacuation is essential whilst others tolerate a bowel movement only once a week.

Constipation is often considered in two groups. The first is **slow transit constipation** where there appears to be a general failure of colonic propulsion. The second, much smaller group includes patients with an **evacuation disorder**. Patients in this group often complain of incomplete rectal evacuation and a sensation of obstructed defaecation: some anatomical disorders responsible (like rectal intussusception) can only be demonstrated on a dynamic X-ray study known as an **evacuation proctogram**. These patients also require specialised anorectal physiological assessment.

From a medical viewpoint, evacuation less than twice a week is abnormal. In the uncomplaining elderly, defaecation may occur much less frequently, causing vague discomfort and anorexia, and predisposing to urinary retention, incontinence and urinary tract infection. Severe constipation alone may lead to **faecal impaction** and **complete bowel obstruction** necessitating admission to hospital. Faecal fluid may intermittently escape past the impacted faecal mass and cause soiling, overflow incontinence or apparent ('**spurious**') diarrhoea.

Abdominal pain may be the presenting symptom of constipation. The pain may be sufficiently severe to precipitate emergency hospital admission with, for example, suspected appendicitis (usually children) or suspected intestinal obstruction (usually the elderly). As many as 25% of patients in these age groups admitted with abdominal pain are eventually diagnosed as suffering from constipation. There is no fever, tachycardia or vomiting, and signs of peritoneal inflammation are absent. There may, however, be mild abdominal tenderness. The faecally loaded left side of the colon often forms a palpable column which indents on palpation and has a putty-like consistency. Rectal examination usually reveals a palpable mass of faeces, although in the elderly the faeces may be impacted higher up. Thus, an empty rectum does not exclude constipation.

PATHOPHYSIOLOGY OF CHRONIC CONSTIPATION

For surgeons, chronic constipation is mainly a problem of children and the elderly. Patients present both as emergencies and in the outpatient clinic. In most cases, the cause is a combination of low-fibre diet, poor fluid intake, obesity, inactivity and persistent failure to respond promptly to the urge to defaecate. Long-term use of **purgative drugs** such as senna derivatives may have an adverse effect on peristalsis. Some drugs, particularly **codeine** and **opiates**, slow large bowel motility, whilst yet other drugs such as **aluminium hydroxide mixtures** and **iron preparations** solidify the stool. Constipation is a characteristic feature of **hypothyroidism** and is also seen in hypo- and **hypercalcaemia**.

MANAGEMENT OF CONSTIPATION

Diagnosis of constipation in children can usually be made on the history and clinical examination; successful treatment confirms the diagnosis. If chronic severe constipation persists in infants despite treatment, the diagnosis of **ultra-short segment Hirschsprung's disease** (see Ch. 50) should be considered. A dietary and drug history should be obtained, and blood tests performed to exclude metabolic causes of constipation. It is vital to differentiate between constipation and early large bowel obstruction in the elderly. In this group of patients, carcinoma or the complications of diverticular disease should be excluded by sigmoidoscopy and barium enema, colonoscopy or CT pneumocolon.

In severe constipation, treatment involves a series of measures used progressively:

- Discontinue constipating medication
- Rectal measures: lubricant glycerine suppositories, small phosphate enemas, stool-softening arachis oil enemas, manual disimpaction (may require general anaesthesia)
- Oral agents (Box 29.3): senna, bisacodyl or osmotic laxatives containing macrogol (polyethylene glycol 3350). A more radical method is to use oral sodium picosulfate (as used in surgical bowel preparation), along with adequate oral or intravenous fluids to avoid dehydration. Note that if powerful oral

---

> **Box 29.3   Oral laxative agents**
>
> - Stimulant/irritant laxatives, e.g. danthron, bisacodyl, senna derivatives
> - Faecal softeners and lubricants, e.g. dioctyl, liquid paraffin
> - Osmotic laxatives, e.g. lactulose, mixtures of magnesium hydroxide or magnesium sulphate
> - Proprietary preparations, e.g. Milpar (liquid paraffin and magnesium hydroxide emulsion)
> - Strong laxatives for single-dose use for bowel preparation or very stubborn constipation, e.g. sodium picosulfate (stimulant), mannitol solution (osmotic)
>
> *Note:* bulking agents do not have a laxative effect in the short term

Fig. 29.1 Sigmoid volvulus
(a) Schematic diagram showing a grossly distended fluid-filled sigmoid colon twisted about its narrow neck, producing a 'closed-loop' obstruction; the loop is beginning to undergo necrosis. **(b)** and **(c) case study**: this 35-year-old man with Down's syndrome presented with a massively swollen abdomen and total constipation. **(b)** Plain abdominal radiograph showing the abdomen filled with the dilated sigmoid loop, confirming the clinical diagnosis of sigmoid volvulus. Note the abdomen was so distended that two films were required to cover the area. The volvulus could not be relieved by gentle passage of a flatus tube. At operation **(c)**, the hugely distended sigmoid emerged from the laparotomy wound. The loop had twisted three times around its narrow base and the colon was of doubtful viability. This sigmoid colon was resected without untwisting the volvulus.

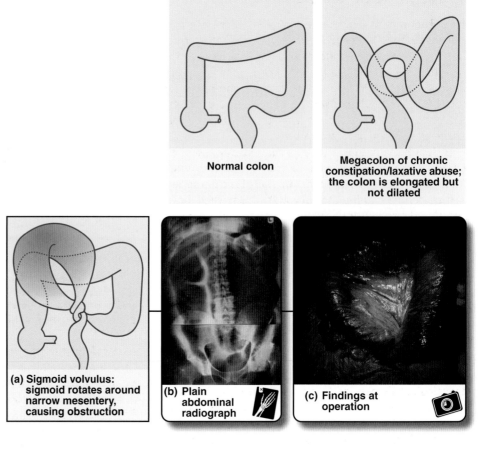

Normal colon

Megacolon of chronic constipation/laxative abuse; the colon is elongated but not dilated

(a) Sigmoid volvulus: sigmoid rotates around narrow mesentery, causing obstruction

(b) Plain abdominal radiograph

(c) Findings at operation

laxatives are given to an obstructed patient, life-threatening perforation of the bowel can occur
● Oral 'maintenance' medications: sodium docusate as a stool softener, lactulose, Fybogel

In milder long-term constipation, dietary measures should be used. Many patients take a high-fibre diet but do not drink enough, failing to recognise that both are necessary to produce the benefits of fibre. Many women fail to gain from a high-fibre diet; clearly, increasing their fibre even more does not improve matters. If the condition is not severe, then eating more figs, apricots and prunes may solve the problem. Otherwise, a low dose of a stimulant laxative taken intermittently may be needed.

SIGMOID VOLVULUS (Fig. 29.1)

PATHOPHYSIOLOGY OF SIGMOID VOLVULUS

Patients with longstanding chronic constipation tend to develop a capacious, elongated and relatively atonic colon, especially in the sigmoid region. This is sometimes described as **acquired** or **idiopathic megacolon**.

Occasionally, a huge sigmoid loop, heavy with faeces and distended with gas, becomes twisted on its mesenteric pedicle (which may be abnormally narrow) to produce a closed-loop obstruction (see Fig. 29.1a–c). If this sigmoid volvulus is not corrected, venous infarction ensues, followed by perforation and catastrophic faecal peritonitis. This full picture is uncommon, but there is often a history of transient episodes of abdominal pain diagnosed as constipation. Some episodes may in fact be sigmoid volvulus that resolves spontaneously as constipation is treated. Note that volvulus of the caecum, small bowel or stomach is unrelated to constipation.

CLINICAL FEATURES OF SIGMOID VOLVULUS

In Western countries, sigmoid volvulus is rarely seen except in the elderly, those with severe learning difficulties, and long-stay patients in mental institutions; these are all groups that readily become faecally loaded. In contrast, it is very common in parts of the world where diet is extremely high in fibre, e.g. parts of Chile.

The patient with sigmoid volvulus is mildly unwell with abdominal distension and a variable degree of abdominal pain. There is absolute constipation (of both faeces and flatus) that has persisted for at least 24 hours. On digital examination, the rectum is empty but capacious. The abdomen is visibly distended and tympanitic to percussion but rarely tender. This is true even if the colon has reached the stage of venous infarction. Once perforation occurs, the full picture of faecal peritonitis will be evident.

MANAGEMENT OF SIGMOID VOLVULUS

Plain abdominal X-ray usually shows a single grossly dilated sigmoid loop, often reaching the xiphisternum (see Fig. 29.1). An erect film may reveal a characteristic 'inverted U' or 'coffee-bean sign' of bowel gas in the upper abdomen, with fluid levels at the same height in the two bowel limbs in the lower abdomen; an abdominal lateral decubitus X-ray may reveal two parallel fluid levels running the length of the abdomen.

If sigmoid volvulus is diagnosed, a sigmoidoscope is gently passed as far as possible into the rectum and a flatus tube inserted through it. The end of the **flatus tube** is then gently manipulated through the twisted bowel into the obstructed loop. If this is successful, there is a gush of liquid faeces and flatus, relieving the obstruction. The flatus tube can be left in situ for 24 hours to maintain decompression, discourage retwisting and allow recovery of the vascular supply of the bowel wall. Despite this, volvulus is likely to recur.

If plain X-ray and sigmoidoscopy do not confirm volvulus but large bowel obstruction is still suspected, an 'instant' **Gastrografin enema examination** is peformed, without bowel preparation. This differentiates volvulus from other causes of obstruction such as carcinoma and diverticular disease, and from pseudo-obstruction. In volvulus, pressure from the enema may cause the bowel to untwist, releasing a torrent of faeces and flatus.

If a volvulus cannot be released, operation is performed urgently. In most cases, the bowel is still viable but sigmoid colectomy is often required to prevent recurrence. A safe alternative procedure is to bring the two divided ends of bowel out on to the abdominal wall to form a **double-barrelled colostomy**, rather than risk a primary anastomosis in this dilated and unprepared colon. For recurrent volvulus, **sigmoid colectomy** or suturing the bowel to the abdominal wall to prevent twisting may be performed electively.

DIVERTICULAR DISEASE

Diverticular disease causes substantial morbidity in the older population, particularly in the West, and is a very common cause for hospital admission and operation. In developed countries, localised outpouchings or diverticula are present in the bowel wall in at least one-third of people over the age of 60. There is strong evidence that this can be caused or aggravated by a chronic lack of dietary fibre but there may also be a genetic element. Females are affected more often than males. (Note that the singular noun is *diverticulum* and the plural *diverticula*, not *diverticulae*; the adjectival form is *diverticular*.)

PATHOPHYSIOLOGY OF DIVERTICULAR DISEASE

In diverticular disease, the colonic muscle wall is thicker than normal because of an excess of elastic tissue be-

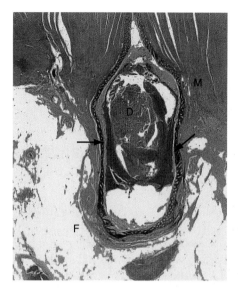

Fig. 29.2 Diverticular disease—histopathology
Low-power view of muscle wall **M** showing a diverticulum lined by mucosa (arrowed) and extending into fat **F**. Faecal material is present within the diverticulum **(D)**.

tween the muscle fibres rather than muscle hypertrophy. This most noticeable pathological abnormality may be related in some way to the pathogenesis. The likely mechanism for the formation of diverticula is functional **hypersegmentation**. In this, two adjoining segments of colon contract at the same time, sending peristaltic waves towards each other. This causes very high luminal pressure in short segments of the colon which forces pockets of mucosa to herniate through weak points in the bowel wall. These potential defects occur where the mucosal blood vessels normally penetrate the wall from outside, between the longitudinal muscle bands (the **taeniae coli**). The sigmoid colon is the section most commonly affected by diverticular disease and the condition extends for a variable distance proximally. Right-sided diverticular disease is more common in Japanese, Chinese and Polynesian races and is particularly common in Hawaii. In the West, isolated diverticula sometimes occur in the caecum and may become inflamed or perforate, but these are probably congenital rather than acquired.

The simple presence of uncomplicated diverticula is unimportant; this asymptomatic condition is known as '**diverticulosis**'. An individual diverticulum may, however, become inflamed as a result of obstruction of its narrow outlet. This results in the formation of a **diverticular abscess**. The abscess effectively lies outside the bowel wall and leads to other complications described below. The microscopic anatomy is demonstrated in Figure 29.2.

COMPLICATIONS OF DIVERTICULAR DISEASE

Diverticular disease may lead to a range of complications:

- Spreading pericolic inflammation
- Pericolic abscess

- Intraperitoneal perforation
- Fistula formation into other abdominal or pelvic viscera
- Bowel-to-bowel adhesions
- Fibrous strictures of bowel
- Acute haemorrhage (which tends to occur in the absence of inflammation)

CLINICAL PRESENTATIONS OF DIVERTICULAR DISEASE AND THEIR MANAGEMENT

The pathological consequences of diverticular inflammation are collectively described as **diverticulitis** and are summarised in Figure 29.4. Most patients with diverticula are asymptomatic, and diverticula are a common incidental finding when the colon is investigated by barium enema or colonoscopy. The typical appearances are shown in Figures 29.3 and 29.4.

Chronic grumbling diverticular pain (see Fig. 29.4b)

This is probably the most common manifestation of diverticular disease and is usually managed in family practices. Peridiverticular inflammation is chronic, low-grade and recurrent. Local irritation provokes bowel wall spasm, causing chronic pain and erratic bowel habit. There is chronic constipation with small pellet-like faeces and episodic diarrhoea. There is little abnormal to find on clinical examination, except perhaps mild left iliac

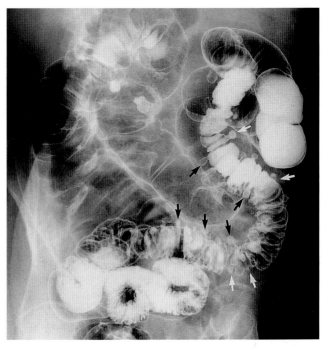

Fig. 29.3 Diverticular disease
Barium enema showing the typical appearance of multiple diverticula (arrowed) in the sigmoid and descending colon in a 77-year-old woman. A few diverticula are also present in the transverse colon.

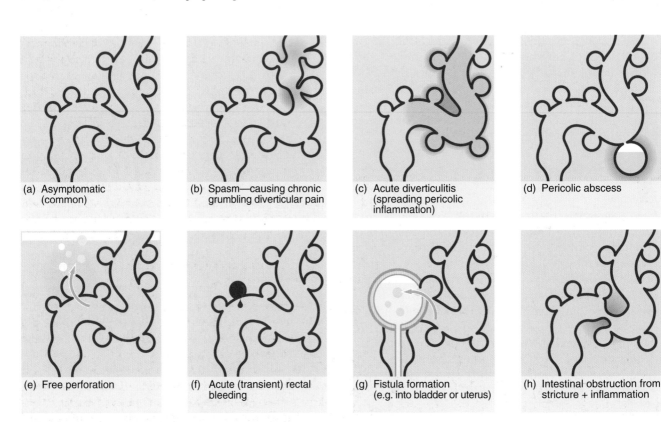

(a) Asymptomatic (common)

(b) Spasm—causing chronic grumbling diverticular pain

(c) Acute diverticulitis (spreading pericolic inflammation)

(d) Pericolic abscess

(e) Free perforation

(f) Acute (transient) rectal bleeding

(g) Fistula formation (e.g. into bladder or uterus)

(h) Intestinal obstruction from stricture + inflammation

    Fig. 29.4 Clinical presentations of diverticular disease

fossa tenderness and faecal loading. Endoscopy or radiological imaging is often performed to confirm the diagnosis and exclude malignancy.

In most patients, symptoms can be relieved by taking a high-fibre diet and bulking agents, although some patients find their symptoms are better on a low-fibre intake.

Acute diverticulitis (i.e. spreading pericolic inflammation, see Fig. 29.4c)

This represents local extension of the inflammation described above. The local inflammation involves the pericolic tissues and parietal peritoneum. Typically, the patient complains of continuous left iliac fossa pain and is systemically ill with a pyrexia and tachycardia, often requiring admission to hospital. Abdominal findings range from mild left iliac fossa tenderness to obvious local peritonitis.

Antibiotic treatment is directed against the usual faecal organisms. In severe cases, a combination of intravenous antibiotics such as ciprofloxacin and metronidazole is used, and the bowel 'rested' by stopping oral intake and giving intravenous fluids. Less severe cases can be managed at home with oral antibiotics.

Pericolic abscess (see Fig. 29.4d)

Pericolic abscess represents a further extension of the pathological process just described. The clinical presentation is similar at first but fails to resolve with antibiotics. The patient suffers persistent pain and tenderness, a swinging pyrexia and incomplete obstruction due to spasm of the bowel wall muscle. Sometimes a pericolic abscess presents as 'pyrexia of unknown origin' or even systemic sepsis (septicaemia). The pericolic abscess may drain spontaneously into the bowel, producing an attack of purulent diarrhoea; the condition then resolves.

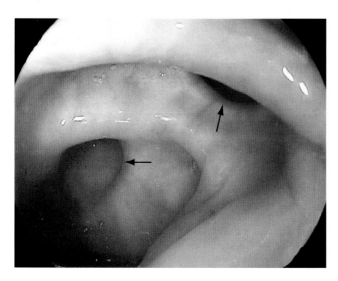

Fig. 29.5 Colonoscopic view of diverticula (arrowed)

Diagnosis of a pericolic abscess can often be made by ultrasonography or CT scan. A contrast enema may show leakage of contrast into the abscess cavity (see Fig. 29.6).

Antibiotic therapy, as for acute diverticulitis, is the first line of treatment. Ideally, this allows the abscess to be contained, and then to drain spontaneously into the bowel. The abscess may also be drained percutaneously under radiological guidance. If this treatment fails, operation is required. This is a major procedure that usually involves diverting the faecal stream via a colostomy, and exploration and drainage of the abscess. In addition, the affected segment of bowel must be removed to prevent recurrence. Note that perforated carcinoma can present in a similar way and histological confirmation of the diagnosis is mandatory. The surgical options are to leave a rectal stump for later reanastomosis (Hartmann's operation, see Ch. 27), or to primarily reanastomose the bowel ends. The latter option is not attempted in the presence of faecal peritonitis or in a frail patient, as the chances of success are remote.

Diverticular perforation (Fig. 29.4e)

A small, asymptomatic diverticular abscess may rupture spontaneously, i.e. perforate, resulting in the escape of gas or bowel contents into the peritoneal cavity. The patient presents with an acute abdomen, the severity of clinical signs depending on the size of the perforation and degree of peritoneal contamination. The perforation may be anything from a pinhole size, allowing only bowel gas and a little fluid to escape, to a hole up to 1 cm in diameter causing generalised faecal peritonitis and potentially fatal sepsis. With small perforations, the symptoms and signs may be little more than those of acute diverticulitis; diagnosis of perforation is confirmed by the presence of free gas under the diaphragm on an erect chest X-ray.

Treatment usually involves immediate parenteral antibiotics to prevent infection, followed by laparotomy to perform peritoneal toilet, diversion of the faecal stream and resection of the diseased bowel, as previously described, although success has been reported with **conservative treatment** for minimal perforations, employing percutaneous placement of a drain and bowel rest.

Fistula formation into other abdominal or pelvic structures (Fig. 29.4g)

Fistula formation occurs when an inflamed diverticulum lies in close proximity to another hollow viscus. An inflammatory adhesion develops between them and the diverticulum then ruptures into the other viscus. Alternatively, an abscess bursts its wall, leaving a persistent channel between the two organs. A fistula between the large bowel and a loop of small bowel (see Fig. 29.7) causes diarrhoea. A vesico-colic fistula causes **pneumaturia** and severe urinary tract infection. A fistula into the

Fig. 29.6 Pericolic abscess due to perforated diverticular disease

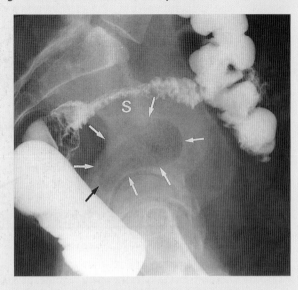
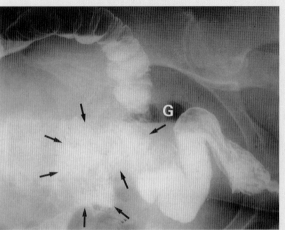

(a)   (b)

Barium enema films from a 49-year-old woman who presented with abdominal pain and tenderness, a mass in the left iliac fossa and a swinging pyrexia. She was treated with antibiotics but the pyrexia failed to settle. **(a)** Right lateral view of the recto-sigmoid region showing marked narrowing of the distal sigmoid **S** due to spasm and inflammatory oedema. The radiolucent area antero-inferiorly (outline arrowed) represents a bubble of gas in a large pelvic abscess. **(b)** Lateral decubitus film (left side upwards) of the same patient taken later during the same examination. This shows barium which has leaked into the abscess cavity (outline arrowed). Note also a fluid level with a gas bubble **G** above it, within the abscess. At laparotomy, a large pericolic and pelvic abscess was found to be walled off. This was drained surgically, the sigmoid colon excised and the end of the descending colon brought out as a terminal colostomy in the left iliac fossa. The rectal stump was oversewn; 3 months later, the bowel was reconnected.

vagina after a previous hysterectomy causes a purulent vaginal discharge. Diverticular disease is the most common cause of these varieties of fistula but they may also be caused by Crohn's disease and sometimes colorectal cancers.

Surprisingly, fistulae rarely show up on barium enema examination. CT scanning may reveal a loss of normal tissue planes between bowel and viscus, and the presence of abnormal gas in the bladder. Diagnosis can also be made on the history, at operation or, in the case of bladder fistula, at cystoscopic examination. Surgical treatment involves excision and histological examination of the affected segment of bowel and repair of the viscus.

Intestinal obstruction (Fig. 29.4h)

Diverticular disease occasionally presents with complete large bowel obstruction due to a combination of acute inflammatory thickening, muscle hypertrophy and spasm. **Incomplete obstruction** is much more common and presents as severe constipation. Chronic diverticular inflammation sometimes causes isolated fibrous strictures, particularly in the sigmoid colon, which cause intermittent bouts of constipation when the stool is dry. When detected radiologically or endoscopically, these strictures must be distinguished from malignancy or Crohn's disease by tissue biopsy.

When acute diverticular inflammation involves the pericolic tissues, small bowel may become involved in the process. Thus, small bowel adynamic disorder may be the presenting feature, with obstruction-like symptoms.

Acute rectal haemorrhage (Fig. 29.4f)

Diverticular disease may present with an episode of acute rectal bleeding, which, unlike the other complications of diverticula, is usually spontaneous and not the result of inflammation. Blood loss is variable but the bleeding almost always stops spontaneously. The patient typically complains of having passed a mass of fairly fresh blood instead of the expected stool and is admitted to hospital urgently. The main differential diagnosis is **ischaemic colitis** but other causes of rectal bleeding such as carcinoma and haemorrhoids must be considered.

Management is rarely surgical but an angiogram and embolisation is sometimes performed by a specialist radiologist if the bleeding is severe. After any necessary resuscitation, the patient is kept under observation for several days, after which it is safe to perform further investigations.

Fig. 29.7 Diverticular fistula into the distal ileum

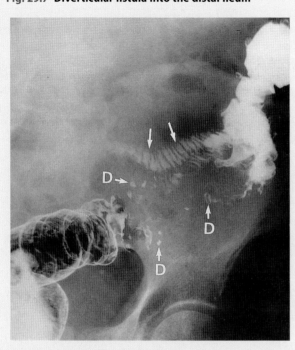

Barium enema of a 61-year-old man with a recently erratic bowel habit, who presented with pain and tenderness in the left iliac fossa. The X-ray shows the sigmoid colon, although part of it is poorly filled with barium which is only seen in the diverticula **D**. There is a loop of small bowel which contains contrast (arrowed), indicating the presence of a colo-ileal fistula caused by peridiverticulitis.

Fig. 29.8 Diverticular stricture in the sigmoid colon

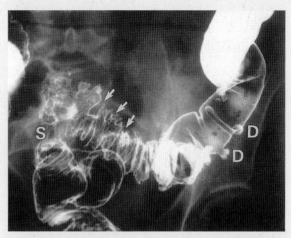

This 64-year-old man suffered several attacks of diverticulitis which settled with antibiotics. This frontal view of a barium enema shows diverticula **D** in the upper sigmoid colon and circular muscle hypertrophy in the distal sigmoid colon (arrowed) typical of diverticular disease. There is a stricture **S** near the recto-sigmoid junction. This stricture does not show the typical 'shouldering' of a carcinoma, although carcinoma could not be excluded on barium enema. Colonoscopy confirmed that it was benign. This patient later had a severe attack of diverticulitis which required surgery and a Hartmann's operation was performed.

Fig. 29.9 Caecal angiodysplasia

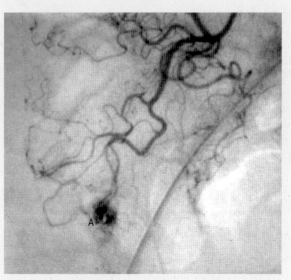

This 66-year-old man had been admitted to hospital on 12 occasions for rectal bleeding or anaemia and received a total of 77 units of blood by transfusion. This selective arteriogram was performed on the most recent admission and shows an abnormal mass of blood vessels **A** in the caecum typical of angiodysplasia. This part of the bowel was resected and the patient had not re-bled 3 years later.

COLONIC ANGIODYSPLASIAS

Colonic angiodysplasias have been recognised as a common cause of acute or chronic rectal bleeding and iron deficiency anaemia since the mid-1970s. The lesions are tiny hamartomatous vascular lesions in the colonic wall, usually in the ascending colon, and produce bleeding out of proportion to their size (see Fig. 29.9). They may also occur in the stomach and small bowel. The origin of colonic angiodysplasias is unknown but since they occur later in life, they are more likely to be acquired and degenerative than congenital.

If bleeding is acute and is occurring rapidly, selective mesenteric arteriography may demonstrate the source of bleeding. In chronic or recurrent haemorrhage, large bowel lesions can be visualised by colonoscopy. This underlines the importance of thorough colonoscopy in patients with unexplained gastrointestinal blood loss. The lesions can often be treated by electrical coagulation via the colonoscope. If this is unsuccessful, the affected segment is resected. Similar lesions occur more rarely in the small bowel and bleed in the same way.

Fig. 29.10 Ischaemic colitis

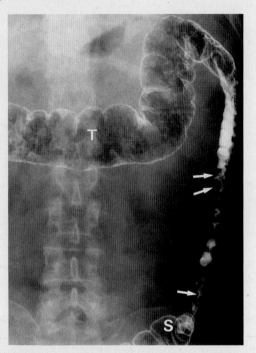

This 72-year-old man presented with a bout of severe abdominal pain 48 hours before this barium enema was performed. Soon after the pain, there was a single episode of fresh rectal bleeding. This film shows typical (though extensive) changes of acute ischaemic colitis, which characteristically involved the proximal descending colon. The transverse colon **T** and sigmoid colon **S** are normal. Note the extremely narrowed lumen of the ischaemic segment and the characteristic thumb-printing (arrowed) caused by mucosal oedema

ISCHAEMIC COLITIS

Ischaemic colitis is another condition of the elderly which usually presents with rectal bleeding. The history is characteristic; there is a bout of cramp-like abdominal pain lasting a few hours, followed by an attack of rectal bleeding. Usually the bleeding is dark red, often without faeces, and occurs one to three times over about 12 hours. The episode then ceases spontaneously. The differential diagnosis includes acute bleeding from diverticular disease, and inflammatory bowel disease. The cause is transient ischaemia of a segment of large bowel, followed by sloughing of the mucosa. The splenic flexure is the most vulnerable. Further attacks occasionally occur but most patients have no further trouble. Investigation by barium enema in the acute stage may reveal colonic oedema in the affected segment (see Fig. 29.10). A rare late complication is fibrotic stricturing of the area originally affected by ischaemia.

Anal and perianal disorders

30

INTRODUCTION

Anal and perianal disorders make up about 20% of general surgical outpatient referrals. These conditions can be distressing and embarrassing, and patients often tolerate symptoms for a long time before seeking medical advice. The common anal symptoms are summarised in Box 30.1 and their interpretation is discussed in Chapter 18.

The range of disorders of the anus and perianal area is illustrated in Figure 30.1. Haemorrhoids and other common benign anal conditions must be distinguished by the clinician from carcinoma of the rectum and the rare carcinoma of the anus. Most anal and perianal conditions can be treated on an outpatient basis, although abscesses, and haemorrhoids that have become strangulated or thrombosed may present as surgical emergencies.

ANATOMY OF THE ANAL CANAL

THE ANAL CANAL

Outside the anal canal at the anal verge, there is normal skin composed of **stratified squamous epithelium** with skin appendages—sweat glands, hair follicles and sebaceous glands. The anal canal proper is about 4 cm long, extending from the lower to the upper border of the internal sphincter (see Fig. 30.2). There are three zones, each with different lining epithelium:

- The lowest or **distal zone** lies between the squamous–mucocutaneous junction and the level of the anal valves at the **dentate (pectinate) line**. This is lined by **non-keratinising** squamous epithelium without skin appendages or glands; the epithelium contains some melanocytes. This area is exquisitely sensitive, for example, to injection
- The **anal transitional zone (ATZ).** This lies between the zone of squamous epithelium below and the columnar mucosal zone above, and extends a variable distance between 0.3 and 2 cm. It consists of transitional epithelium resembling urothelium, 4–9 cell layers thick. Anal glands are present in the submucosa but there is minimal mucin production. Its importance is the unique type of anal carcinoma that develops from it and its apparent viral aetiology
- The upper part of the anal canal is lined by rectal mucosa. On proctoscopic inspection, it is a darker reddish-blue where it overlies the submucosal venous plexus, giving way to the typical pink of colorectal mucosa more proximally. This area of mucosa is relatively insensitive

The mucosa of the upper part of the anal canal is thrown into 6–10 longitudinal folds, known as the **columns of Morgagni**, each containing a terminal branch of the superior rectal artery and vein. The folds are most prominent in the left lateral, right posterior and right anterior sectors where the vessels form prominent **anal cushions**. These are important in fine control of continence. They may become pathologically enlarged to form **haemorrhoids**, which are complex collections of arterioles, arteries, venules, venous saccules and connective tissue. The anal columns are not readily visible on proctoscopy but the transition between glandular rectal mucosa and anal skin is clearly visible. The lymphatics of the upper part of the anal canal drain to the pelvic and abdominal lymph node chain, whereas the lower part of the anal canal drains to the inguinal lymph nodes. All of the anal canal below the dentate line is exquisitely sensitive, for example,

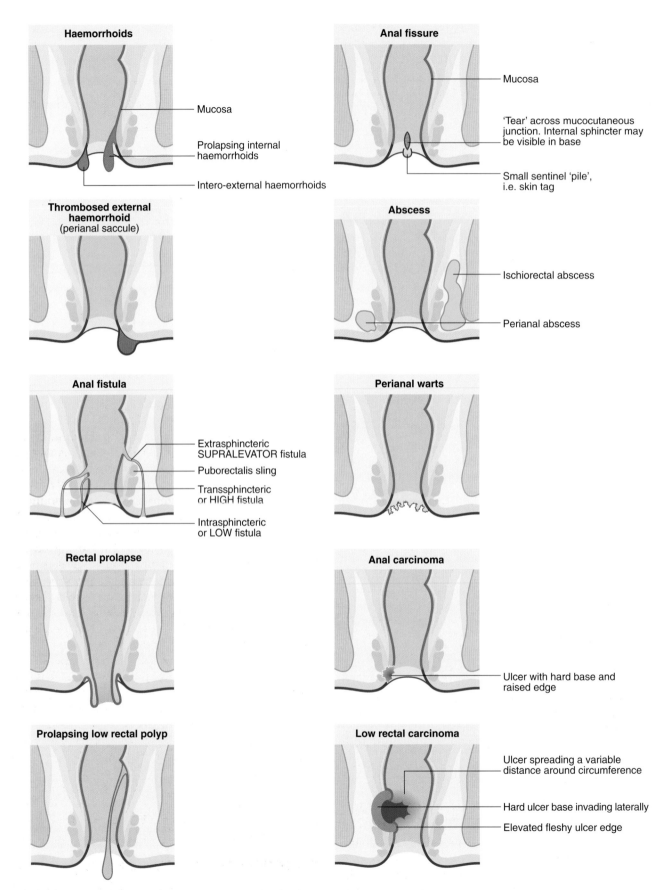

Fig. 30.1 Anal and perianal disorders

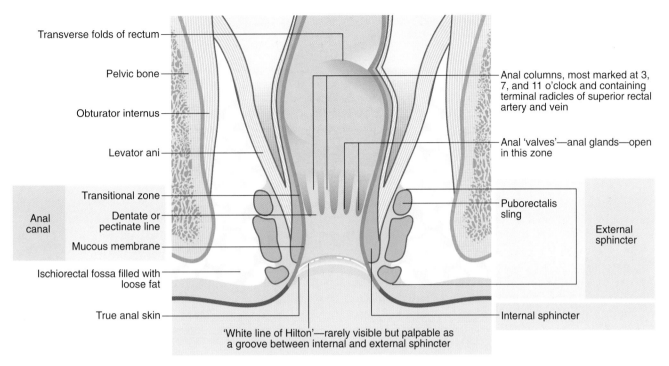

Transverse folds of rectum

Pelvic bone

Obturator internus

Levator ani

Transitional zone

Anal canal

Dentate or pectinate line

Mucous membrane

Ischiorectal fossa filled with loose fat

True anal skin

Anal columns, most marked at 3, 7, and 11 o'clock and containing terminal radicles of superior rectal artery and vein

Anal 'valves'—anal glands—open in this zone

Puborectalis sling

External sphincter

Internal sphincter

'White line of Hilton'—rarely visible but palpable as a groove between internal and external sphincter

Fig. 30.2 Anatomy of the anal canal

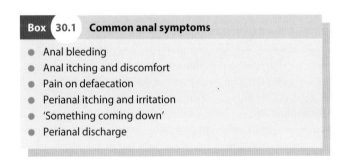

Box 30.1 Common anal symptoms

- Anal bleeding
- Anal itching and discomfort
- Pain on defaecation
- Perianal itching and irritation
- 'Something coming down'
- Perianal discharge

to injection. In contrast, the rectal mucosa is relatively insensitive.

The anal sphincter mechanism has three constituents: the **internal sphincter**, the **external sphincter** and the **puborectalis muscle**. The internal sphincter represents a downward but thickened continuation of the normal rectal wall musculature. The encircling external sphincter and the puborectalis sling (which is part of levator ani) arise from the pelvic floor. Continence is maintained principally by the anal sphincters squeezing the three anal cushions together so that they occlude the lumen. Continence is assisted by the fact that the rectum proximally forms a compliant reservoir to accumulate faeces.

HAEMORRHOIDS

Haemorrhoids (piles) are extremely common, affecting nearly half of the population at some time in their lives. Men tend to suffer more often and for longer periods, whereas women are particularly susceptible in late pregnancy and the puerperium.

PATHOGENESIS OF HAEMORRHOIDS

It is likely that heredity plays a part in predisposing individuals to haemorrhoids. This predisposition is brought to light by pregnancy, constipation or diarrhoea. Lack of fibre in the modern Western diet is probably also a factor. Haemorrhoids are probably initiated by straining to pass small hard stools. Straining raises intra-abdominal pressure and this obstructs venous return, causing the venous plexuses to become engorged. The bulging mucosa is then dragged distally by the hard stool. Furthermore, persistent straining at stool causes the pelvic floor to sag downwards, extruding the anal mucosa and causing a small degree of prolapse. In pregnancy-related haemorrhoids, venous engorgement and mucosal prolapse are probably the main mechanisms. Progesterone mediates venous dilatation, and the fetus obstructs pelvic venous return.

Haemorrhoids may bleed, prolapse or cause slight mucus or faecal leakage, particularly when passing flatus. Bleeding from the arterial component of the anal cushion results in the characteristic bright red rectal bleeding. The venous component causes a problem only if it becomes thrombosed to form a **thrombosed external venous saccule** (sometimes wrongly labelled a perianal haematoma). Haemorrhoids are usually located in the three, seven and eleven o'clock positions when viewed with the patient in the supine lithotomy position. These correspond to the anatomical positions of the anal cushions.

CLASSIFICATION OF HAEMORRHOIDS

Haemorrhoids (piles) are classified into first, second and third degrees according to the extent to which they prolapse

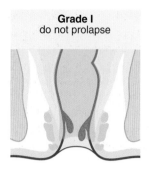
Grade I
do not prolapse

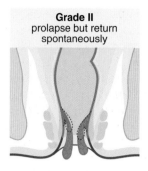
Grade II
prolapse but return
spontaneously

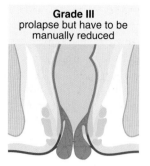
Grade III
prolapse but have to be
manually reduced

Fig. 30.3 **Classification of haemorrhoids**

through the anal canal. **First degree (or grade I) piles** never prolapse; **second degree (grade II) piles** prolapse during defaecation and then return spontaneously into the anal canal; **third degree (grade III) piles** remain outside the anal margin unless replaced digitally (see Fig. 30.3). Most haemorrhoids can be described as 'internal' because they are covered by glandular mucosa. Large neglected haemorrhoids may extend beneath the stratified squamous epithelium so that their lower part becomes covered by skin. These are correctly described as **'intero-external' haemorrhoids**, or more commonly 'external piles'.

SYMPTOMS AND SIGNS OF HAEMORRHOIDS

Haemorrhoids often produce symptoms intermittently. Attacks last from a few days to a few weeks, often with complete freedom from trouble between times. Episodes of constipation are often a precipitating factor.

Any haemorrhoid may **bleed** from stool trauma during defaecation. Large haemorrhoids may **prolapse** and then **thrombose**, causing acute pain if venous return is obstructed by sphincter tone. Longstanding haemorrhoids eventually atrophy, probably by thrombosis and fibrosis, leaving small **skin tags** at the anal margin.

The common chronic or intermittent symptoms of haemorrhoids are:

- Perianal irritation and itching (pruritus ani) caused by mucus leakage. Scratching exacerbates the problem
- Rectal bleeding (fresh blood, on the paper or separate from stool)
- Mucus leakage due to imperfect closure of the anal cushions
- Mild incontinence of flatus also due to imperfect closure of the anal cushions
- Haemorrhoidal prolapse

Most patients reaching the surgeon have already tried various anaesthetic or soothing creams and suppositories, either self-administered or prescribed by the family practitioner. The usual reasons for referral are persistent symptoms or the need to exclude malignancy as a cause of bleeding.

On examination, external piles or skin tags may be visible in the anal area. Digital examination is essential to exclude carcinoma and provides a useful measure of anal tone. Haemorrhoids, however, are not palpable

unless they are large since the contained blood empties with pressure from the examining finger. **Proctoscopy** is needed to demonstrate internal piles, which are seen bulging into the lumen as the proctoscope is withdrawn. **Sigmoidoscopy** is important in patients over 40 years if there is a history of bleeding or any symptoms suspicious of malignancy; occasionally a rectal polyp will be diagnosed in this way. Since piles are so common, they can mask a concomitant underlying diagnosis of cancer.

ACUTE PRESENTATIONS OF HAEMORRHOIDS

Thrombosed or strangulated haemorrhoids present with acute pain and many patients are admitted to hospital as an emergency. These complications are common in the late stages of pregnancy and soon after delivery. The diagnosis of **thrombosed haemorrhoids** is usually obvious on inspection as an oedematous, congested purplish mass is seen at the anal margin. Tight spasm of the anal sphincter makes digital rectal examination extremely painful. **Strangulated haemorrhoids** are even more painful, and the strangulated mass may become necrotic or even ulcerated. Symptomatic relief is provided by several days of bed rest and the application of ice packs and topical anaesthetic gel; this type of conservative treatment may be the most that can safely be offered in late pregnancy. Some surgeons favour urgent haemorrhoidectomy for thrombosed or strangulated piles, accepting the slightly higher risk of complications in exchange for a more rapid return to normal life. Prophylactic antibiotics should be given to cover the operation because of the risk of infection in necrotic tissue. Hospital stay and recovery period are generally shorter with urgent haemorrhoidectomy than with any conservative approach.

CONSERVATIVE MANAGEMENT AND PREVENTION OF HAEMORRHOIDS

The most important means of preventing and treating haemorrhoids is avoiding constipation and ensuring a bulky stool. This is often best achieved by taking a diet high in fibre. The patient should be advised always to heed the call to evacuate. This appears to be associated with a reflex release of lubricating mucus that may be absent later. Many sufferers regularly spend a long time on the lavatory reading; they should be strongly encouraged to avoid straining and to spend minimal time defaecating. A prolonged ritual often leads to further straining at the end of defaecation when a mild haemorrhoidal or mucosal prolapse can be interpreted as incomplete evacuation of faeces. In many patients with symptomatic haemorrhoids, these simple measures are enough to relieve the symptoms. Note that repetitive straining occasionally leads to the formation of a '**solitary ulcer**' on the posterior wall of the proximal anal canal, which may be clinically indistinguishable from a malignant ulcer.

With third degree haemorrhoids, symptoms can often be relieved by the patient replacing the prolapsing haemorrhoids digitally after defaecation.

Many creams, suppositories and other topical preparations are available with or without prescription and are very widely used. Many contain local anaesthetic agents or steroids. They are useful as a temporary measure to help a patient recover from a bout of haemorrhoidal symptoms but do nothing to treat the underlying condition and may even cause local allergic reactions. Overuse causes maceration of the perianal skin and predisposes to secondary infection.

SURGICAL TREATMENTS FOR HAEMORRHOIDS

Injection of sclerosants

First degree haemorrhoids which do not regress with dietary change and avoiding straining, and most second degree haemorrhoids can be treated by sclerosant injections. An irritant solution is injected submucosally around the pedicles of the three major haemorrhoids, in the insensitive upper anal canal. This provokes a fibrotic reaction, effectively obliterating the haemorrhoidal vessels and causing atrophy of the haemorrhoids.

Sclerotherapy can be performed on an outpatient basis and does not require any anaesthetic. The haemorrhoids are first assessed by external inspection, with the patient both at rest and 'straining down'. A proctoscope is then inserted to its full length so that the distal end of the proctoscope lies beyond the external sphincter and projects into the lower rectum (see Fig. 30.4). The instrument is then slowly withdrawn and the haemorrhoids are assessed as they bulge into the lumen. The proctoscope is reinserted as before and 1–3 ml of 5% phenol in oil is injected into each of the three pedicles just beneath the mucosa. Injections must be placed superficially and are painless provided the needle is placed correctly; direct injection into the haemorrhoid would be extremely painful. Sclerotherapy may be repeated on 2–3 occasions at intervals of 4–6 weeks.

Banding

A frequently used alternative to injection for large grade I and for grade II haemorrhoids is the application of rubber bands (**Barron's bands**) to obliterate the haemorrhoidal vessels (see Fig. 30.5). A cone of mucosa just above the haemorrhoidal neck is drawn into the banding

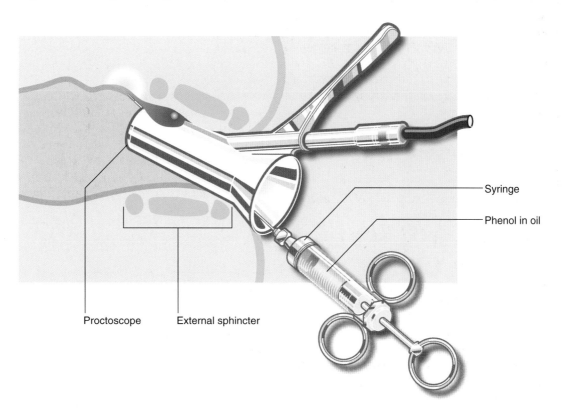

Syringe

Phenol in oil

Proctoscope   External sphincter

Fig. 30.4 Technique of injecting haemorrhoids

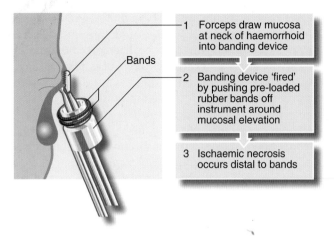

1. Forceps draw mucosa at neck of haemorrhoid into banding device

2. Banding device 'fired' by pushing pre-loaded rubber bands off instrument around mucosal elevation

3. Ischaemic necrosis occurs distal to bands

Bands

Fig. 30.5 Rubber banding technique for haemorrhoids
Note that the haemorrhoid itself is not banded but the band is applied to the blood vessels at its base.

instrument and tight bands released around the base of the cone, constricting the haemorrhoidal vessels. (Note: the bands are **not** placed around the stalk of prolapsing haemorrhoids; this would be unbearably painful because of the somatic innervation of anal skin.) The result of banding is that the haemorrhoid gradually shrinks. The bands separate with time and are passed.

Haemorrhoidectomy

Haemorrhoidal excision is indicated for third degree haemorrhoids, and for lesser degrees when other treatments have failed. The operation most commonly performed is the one described by **Milligan and Morgan** in which the haemorrhoidal masses are excised together with overlying mucosa and some skin (Fig. 30.6). This leaves skin and mucosal defects which heal by secondary intention and

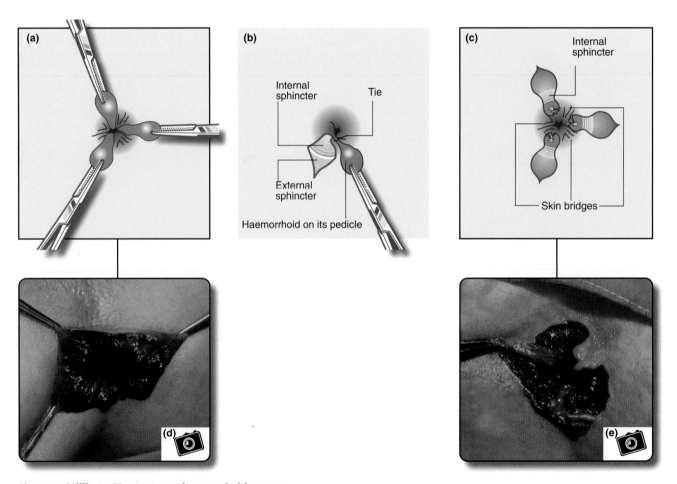

Fig. 30.6 Milligan–Morgan open haemorrhoidectomy
(a) and **(d)** Identification of the main haemorrhoids; the external part of each is clamped with a haemostat and retracted outwards.
(b) Scissors are used to incise the skin around the external haemorrhoid, any excess skin being excised at the same time. The haemorrhoid is then raised on its pedicle by dissection from the external sphincter and the internal sphincter. The pedicle is transfixed and ligated at its base with an absorbable suture. The skin is not closed. **(c)** and **(e)** The process is repeated for the other primary haemorrhoids, ensuring that **skin bridges** are preserved between the areas of resection or else anal stenosis will occur as healing proceeds ('If it looks like a dahlia, it's a failure'). The completed haemorrhoidectomy has a 'cloverleaf' appearance ('if it looks like a clover, it's all over'). After haemostasis is ensured, wounds are dressed with a non-adherent dressing (e.g. Mepitel) and a surgical pad applied, held in place by elasticated net underpants.

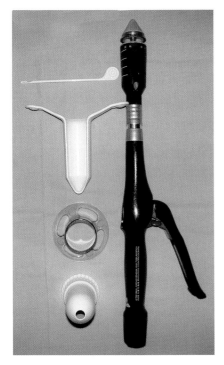

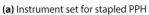

(a) Instrument set for stapled PPH

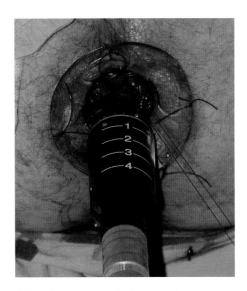

(b) Staple gun about to be inserted after securing haemorrhoids with sutures

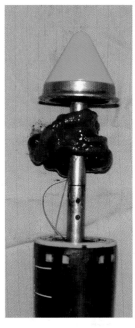

(c) Excised haemorrhoids after firing circular staple gun

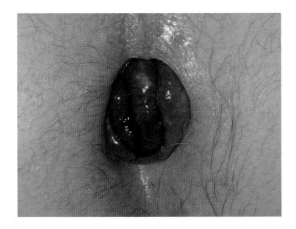

(d) Preoperative picture of prolapsed haemorrhoids (3rd degree)

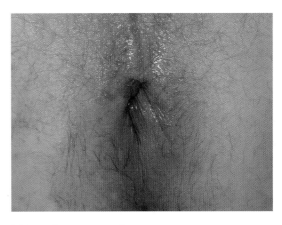

(e) Immediate postoperative appearance

Fig. 30.7 Procedure for prolapse and haemorrhoids (PPH)
This is a minimally invasive surgical treatment for haemorrhoids. It may also be called stapled haemorrhoidectomy or stapled anopexy.

wound contraction. A skin bridge **must** be preserved between each wound to prevent the serious late complication of anal stenosis. **Stapled haemorrhoidectomy** (Fig. 30.7) has gained popularity for large grade II and for grade III haemorrhoids, particularly when mucosal prolapse is a feature. It aims to restore the anatomy of the anal cushions by excising an entire ring of low rectal mucosa, including the engorged neck of the piles. This is a less painful procedure than the open operation and gives equivalent results. The fine staple line remains palpable digitally.

Before either operation, stool softeners such as bulking agents and gentle laxatives should be given to avoid constipation afterwards. The painful early postoperative period can be greatly eased by caudal analgesia given at operation.

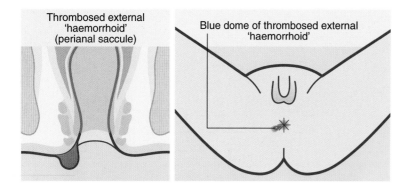

Thrombosed external 'haemorrhoid' (perianal saccule)

Blue dome of thrombosed external 'haemorrhoid'

Fig. 30.8 Thrombosed external haemorrhoid

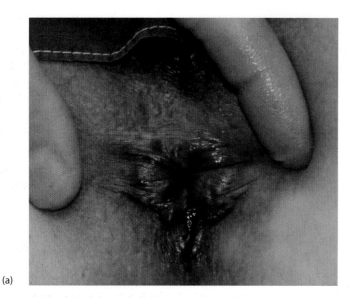

(a)

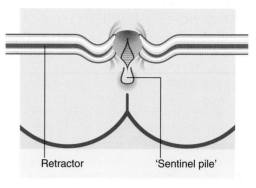

Retractor   'Sentinel pile'

(b)

Fig. 30.9 Anal fissure
(a) Chronic anal fissure with a 'sentinel pile'. Simple fissures are typically posteriorly located, as in this patient. **(b)** Explanatory diagram.

THROMBOSED EXTERNAL HAEMORRHOIDS

A thrombosed external haemorrhoid or **thrombosed external venous saccule** is an acutely painful anal condition (Fig. 30.8). The onset is sudden and, if untreated, there is persistent pain lasting 1–2 weeks, worse on defaecation. On examination, a blue-black hemispherical bulge is seen in the skin near the anal margin. A thrombosed external haemorrhoid is sometimes called a perianal haematoma but this is inaccurate for it is not a haematoma. The condition often occurs in patients with haemorrhoids but is usually seen in isolation.

Most thrombosed external haemorrhoids subside over a few days and patients need only oral analgesia. If pain is severe or prolonged, the thrombosis may be incised and drained under local anaesthesia; some surgeons favour this as a first line therapy.

ANAL FISSURE

An anal fissure is a longitudinal tear in the mucosa and skin of the anal canal, sometimes caused by passing a large, constipated stool. The tear is nearly always in the midline of the posterior anal margin. The fissure causes acute pain during defaecation and sphincter spasm, both of which persist for an hour or longer. The result is fear of defaecation and this aggravates the constipation. There is often a small amount of fresh bleeding at defaecation. This history alone is diagnostic of an anal fissure. On inspection, the fissure is concealed by the anal spasm but a small skin tag (sentinel pile) may be seen at the superficial end of the fissure (see Fig. 30.9). Rectal examination is extremely painful and rarely possible unless the fissure has become chronic.

Patients sometimes manage to tolerate the pain of an acute fissure by using local anaesthetic creams and then present much later with a chronic anal fissure that has been prevented from healing by anal sphincter spasm and repeated tearing open of the healing fissure during passage of stools.

MANAGEMENT OF ANAL FISSURE

Anal fissure can be managed conservatively or operatively. Modern conservative treatment involves the use of topical glyceryl trinitrate (GTN) ointment 0.2–0.4%,

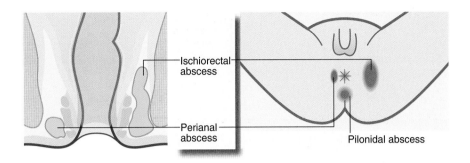

Fig. 30.10 Abscesses in the anorectal region

applied 3 times a day for a month. This causes relaxation of the sphincter spasm and increases blood supply to the fissure, thus allowing healing. Patients need to be warned that it may cause headaches. This treatment can cure most anal fissures. For the rest, diltiazem ointment, a calcium channel blocker, may be successful where GTN has failed. Injection of botulinum toxin into the sphincter complex is another way to cause a temporary 'chemical sphincterotomy'.

Surgery in the form of **lateral submucous (internal) sphincterotomy** brings more immediate relief, but there is a 10–15% incidence of incontinence of flatus following this procedure. Surgeons tend to be reluctant to offer sphincterotomy to women because their sphincters are shorter and less robust, and because occult sphincter injury from childbirth may already have occurred. However, if conservative treatments fail and the patient is suitably informed of the risks, an internal anal sphincterotomy may be performed. This operation involves dividing about a 1 cm length of the lower rim of the internal sphincter via a small lateral incision. For chronic refractory fissures, anal advancement flap operations are sometimes performed; this avoids the damage to the sphincter muscle caused by sphincterotomy. **Lord's anal stretch** used to be performed for fissure, and sometimes for haemorrhoids. It involved manual dilatation of the anal sphincter to 4 fingers' diameter under general anaesthesia. The procedure was found to cause an unacceptable rate of incontinence and has long been abandoned. Anal stretch dilates the external sphincter excessively and produces global damage to the internal sphincter which is exceptionally difficult to correct later.

ANORECTAL ABSCESSES

PATHOPHYSIOLOGY AND CLINICAL FEATURES

Abscesses in the anorectal area are common surgical emergencies. They present with constant and often severe perineal pain and local tenderness.

Anorectal abscesses begin as acute purulent infections of **anal glands**. These lie in the **intersphincteric space** between the internal and external sphincters and drain into tiny pits, the anal crypts, near the dentate line. The ducts are very narrow and duct obstruction may be the factor that initiates the infection. Rarely, an abscess remains confined between the sphincters and an **intersphincteric abscess** results. The only symptom of this may be chronic anal pain, and there is little to find on clinical examination to explain it. The only clue may be localised tenderness on rectal examination.

From the intersphincteric plane, infection tends to spread in one or more of three directions (see Fig. 30.10):

- **Downwards** between the sphincters towards the anal verge, forming a **perianal abscess**. This is the most common presentation and accounts for 80% of anorectal abscesses. The patient presents with a painful, tender, red swelling close to the anal verge
- **Outwards** through the external sphincter into the loose fibro-fatty tissue of the ischiorectal fossa, forming an **ischiorectal abscess**. There is little barrier to spread of infection in this space and a neglected or inadequately treated abscess may become enormous. Ischiorectal abscesses make up about 15% of anorectal abscesses. The patient presents with systemic signs of infection and perineal pain. There is tenderness over the ischiorectal fossa lateral to the anus but there may be no visible redness or swelling; rectal palpation reveals a tender mass lateral to the rectum
- **Upwards** between the sphincters to form a **supralevator abscess**, involving the pararectal tissues above the pelvic floor. These make up less than 5% of anorectal abscesses and present with systemic signs of infection, rectal pain and difficulty in micturition. On rectal examination, a tender mass is often palpable near the tip of the finger

TREATMENT OF ANORECTAL ABSCESSES

If perianal infection is seen very early, oral antibiotic treatment may abort it. The use of antibiotics in this way by general practitioners, coupled with early referral, has reduced the number and severity of cases reaching the surgeon. However, once an abscess is diagnosed, **surgical drainage** is needed; antibiotics are only indicated when there is spreading infection. Drainage is performed under regional or general anaesthesia after the extent of the abscess has been established by careful examination under anaesthesia. An **intersphincteric abscess** is drained via an internal sphincterotomy; **perianal** and **ischiorectal abscesses** are drained via the perianal skin, ensuring all loculations are broken down. A swab of the pus is taken for microbiological diagnosis to differentiate infection by skin pathogens (e.g. *Staphylococcus*) which occur spontaneously, from infections of bowel origin (e.g. *E. coli*) which suggest an underlying fistula. Large ischiorectal abscesses require packing or placement of a drain to keep the neck of the cavity open whilst granulation tissue gradually fills the space from its depths. Further examinations under anaesthesia after a few days are often planned to ensure complete drainage and to inspect for fistulae. Supralevator abscesses are usually more complicated and require complex staged surgical procedures.

Incising a perianal abscess results in complete resolution in about 50% of cases; the other half develop an **anal fistula** (see below). The fistula is usually undetectable at the time of drainage but is recognised by a persistent discharge through the area of the skin incision continuing for several weeks afterwards (see Fig. 18.6).

Differential diagnosis of abscesses in the perianal area includes:

- **Crohn's disease**—may cause multiple abscesses and complex fistulae (see Ch. 28) and must be excluded
- **Hidradenitis suppurativa**—originates in perianal apocrine glands in the skin; it is easily distinguished from deeper perianal abscesses by careful inspection and palpation. There may be multiple infected glands in the natal cleft, groins and sometimes axillae
- **Pilonidal abscess**—occurs in the skin of the natal cleft (see Fig. 30.10) but may mimic a true perianal abscess if near the anal margin; careful examination shows no communication with the anal canal and often the presence of embedded hairs. Treatment is by incision and drainage but further procedures may be required to treat the associated pilonidal sinus (see p. 451)
- **Tuberculous abscess and fistula**—very rare

ANAL FISTULA

Anal fistulae usually develop as a complication of perianal, ischiorectal or supralevator abscesses. A fistula is an abnormal connection between two epithelial surfaces and consists of a chronically infected tract which may become epithelialised. It extends from an **internal opening** at the level of the dentate line, and passes through the site of the previous abscess to an external opening on the perianal skin near the old drainage scar. The communication between abscess cavity and bowel has become established by spontaneous discharge of the enlarging abscess into the bowel either before surgical drainage or after incom-

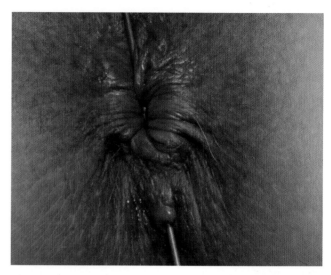

Fig. 30.11 Anal fistula
A probe has been passed from the skin surface through a low anal fistula to emerge in the anal canal at the level of the dentate line. Treatment consisted simply of cutting down onto the probe, thus laying open the fistula along its length. The wound was left to heal by secondary intention.

plete surgical drainage. To minimise the risk of fistula, any abscess in the anal region should be drained early and thoroughly to prevent it progressing.

The patient with a fistula typically complains of intermittent discharge of mucus or pus in the perianal region, which is often faecally stained. On examination, a small papilla of granulation tissue is seen on the skin within 2–3 cm of the anal margin (see Fig. 18.6). Pus may be expressed from it by compressing the underlying tract digitally between papilla and anus. This clinical picture is diagnostic of an anal fistula; often, however, this apparently trivial skin lesion is dismissed as a pustule or an incompletely healed perianal abscess.

Most anal fistulae are simple and relatively superficial, with the internal opening located in a crypt at the level of the dentate line (well below puborectalis), most often in the posterior midline. These are known as **low anal fistulae** (Fig. 30.11). For successful treatment, it is essential to locate the internal opening so the entire tract can be dealt with.

Goodsall's rule helps to predict the course of a low fistula:

- If the external opening is **in front** of an imaginary transverse line across the anus, the fistula is likely to have a short **direct** tract to the anal canal
- If the external opening is **behind** the transverse line, the tract is likely to have a **curved** course towards an internal opening in the posterior midline

Assessment and treatment of fistulae requires general or regional anaesthesia. Examination under anaesthetic

(EUA) is performed first. A malleable probe is gently manipulated through the fistula to try to demonstrate the internal orifice. If this is not found, hydrogen peroxide can be gently injected into the external opening. Provided the fistula is superficial and involves less than half of the sphincter bulk, treatment is by laying open the entire tract by cutting down on to the probe with a scalpel, transecting the anal margin and opening the whole length of the fistula. This is known as **fistulotomy** and involves dividing some of the internal and external sphincter. The wound heals gradually by secondary intention. There should be no loss of faecal continence, but flatus may be less well controlled. Attempts have been made to deal with some fistulae by using tissue glues or fibrin packs but results so far are unimpressive.

If the fistula involves more than half the length of the anal sphincter complex, surgical treatment is difficult and highly specialised because of the need to retain the functional integrity of the sphincters and preserve continence. Where complex fistulae are suspected, the anatomy can be very well defined by **magnetic resonance imaging (MRI)** so that careful staged surgery and appropriate conservative measures can be planned.

In many of the more severe cases, primary surgical cure is not attempted and infection is controlled long-term by placing a soft **seton** or thread through the tract and out through the anus, where it is tied to form a ring. This maintains free drainage of pus and reduces the risk of abscess formation, whilst the seton goes largely unnoticed by the patient. After a long period of quiescence, the seton may be removed with the hope that the tract will close. In the worst cases, where there is extensive destructive involvement of the anal sphincters in the infective process, the only surgical cure is perineal excision of the anal canal and lower rectum, with a permanent colostomy. In exceptional cases, patients may choose this option to improve their quality of life.

Anal fistulae sometimes occur as a manifestation of **Crohn's disease**. Such fistulae tend to be multiple and in the most extreme cases form a 'pepper-pot' perineum (see Fig. 28.8, p. 425).

PILONIDAL SINUS AND ABSCESS

These conditions arise from the skin of the natal cleft rather than the anus. As the name implies, pilonidal sinuses, cysts and abscesses contain **'a nest of hairs'**. They are common in young adults, particularly hirsute men, and are found at the upper end of the natal cleft. Here, between the buttocks, there is often a congenital dimple or pit. Fragments of hair falling from the back or the head accumulate in this nidus. The hairs slowly work their way into the dermis, with the cuticular scales on the hairs acting like the barbs of an arrow. The process is encouraged by the massaging effect of sitting for long periods, for example when driving. Pilonidal sinus is thus common in truck and tractor drivers. They

also occur between the fingers of hairdressers from implantation of their clients' hair (see below).

Pilonidal sinuses tend to run a long indolent course with chronic or intermittent purulent discharge to the skin surface via one or more sinuses. Periodic acute exacerbations may progress to abscesses.

PILONIDAL ABSCESS

The mass of hairs and other skin debris in a pilonidal sinus excites a foreign-body inflammatory reaction, often merely resulting in a mildly or intermittently discharging sinus. If, however, the cavity becomes secondarily infected, an abscess develops and causes acute pain and swelling. Pilonidal abscesses are often multilocular. They sometimes drain spontaneously but rarely heal completely. Many require surgical drainage because of pain.

TREATMENT OF PILONIDAL SINUS
(Figs 30.12 and 30.13)

Definitive treatment aims to eliminate the nidus of hairs and associated cystic cavities, chronic abscesses and sinuses. At operation, obvious plugs of hair are first removed and then the sinus network is explored with probes, often aided by injecting blue dye into the sinuses. The standard operation is to excise an elliptical wedge of tissue, incorporating the mass of sinuses, cysts and overlying skin. The incision may have to extend as deeply as the sacral fascia. The resulting large defect bounded by healthy tissue is then packed and allowed to granulate from the base upwards. Healing takes several weeks but the patient can return home after a few days.

A less extensive surgical method known as **de-roofing** may be preferred. This is shown in Figure 30.13. Another alternative treatment is **phenolisation**. In this, the sinus network is thoroughly curetted under general anaesthesia and then filled with liquefied phenol for a minute or two. Phenol encourages fibrosis and may eliminate the cavity. These treatments are only suitable when fibrosis and scarring are minimal. For complex primary and recurrent cases, various flap operations have been devised. The Limberg rhomboid transposition flap (Fig. 30.13c) has been shown to give good results. The procedure moves healthy skin into the natal cleft, flattening it at the same time.

Despite surgery, pilonidal lesions commonly recur but this may be reduced by careful attention to hygiene. Daily baths and regular shaving of the area are recommended.

OCCUPATIONAL PILONIDAL SINUSES

Pilonidal sinuses occasionally develop in the web spaces between the fingers in hairdressers, caused by implanted hairs from customers. A similar condition occurs in farmers, with hairs implanted from farm animals.

Fig. 30.12 Pilonidal sinus and abscess

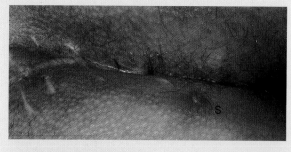

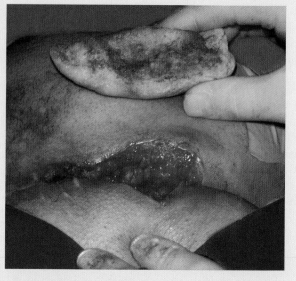

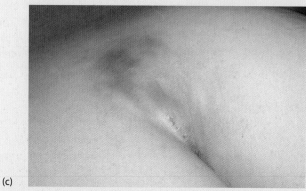

(a) Recurrent pilonidal sinuses. The scar from a previous operation for this condition is visible. There are several tufts of hair emerging from sinuses in the midline and a typical sinus opening **S** to one side. **(b)** At operation, there was an extensive network of sinuses lined with granulation tissue and containing loose hairs. The entire network was excised and the wound 'saucerised' to prevent the cavity healing over. No attempt was made to close the defect as this is usually unsatisfactory because of breakdown or infection. A silicone foam **(F)** dressing was made by mixing the two components and pouring it into the wound. **(c)** Pilonidal abscess in a different patient of 24. This is a common presentation and usually requires formal surgical drainage and curettage of the sinuses.

RECTAL PROLAPSE

Rectal prolapse is mainly seen in young children and the elderly. In children, it is usually a relatively minor and self-correcting problem. In the elderly, it is usually a chronic problem with no easy surgical solution (see Fig. 30.14). In pathophysiological terms, a rectal prolapse is a herniation of the rectum through the pelvic floor. In effect, the mucosa and muscle wall intussuscept through the anal canal. In the early stages, the prolapse occurs only with defaecation and retracts spontaneously. At a later stage, the rectum may prolapse when the patient merely stands up. The patient is thus reluctant to leave home and often becomes socially isolated.

In childhood, rectal prolapse usually occurs around the age of 2 years. It tends to occur during toilet training and causes parental anxiety. Parents should be reassured that the prolapse will return spontaneously after defaecation; gentle manipulation using water-soluble lubricant jelly may be required. These children should be given a high-fibre diet and taught not to strain during defaecation. More sophisticated treatment is rarely required.

In the elderly, rectal prolapse is either remarkably well tolerated or else concealed. The patient becomes accustomed to reducing the prolapse manually after defaecation and rarely complains about it. A high-fibre diet makes little difference to the problem since the anatomical defect will never recover spontaneously. If the prolapse occurs on standing or if incontinence develops, the patient is likely to require surgical treatment. Incontinence is not directly due to the prolapse but to dilatation of the internal anal sphincter by the prolapse.

MANAGEMENT OF RECTAL PROLAPSE

Rectal prolapse can be treated by abdominal or perineal procedures, or a combination of both. The **abdominal** operations include two main types of operation:

- **Suture fixation rectopexy**, where the rectum is mobilised and the mesorectum sutured to the sacral promontory and the presacral fascia
- **Resection rectopexy**, where the rectum is mobilised and sutured in the same way, but a sigmoid colectomy is also performed to try to prevent the constipation that often accompanies suture fixation alone

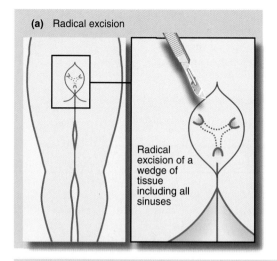
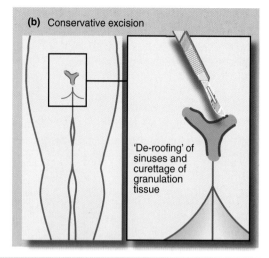
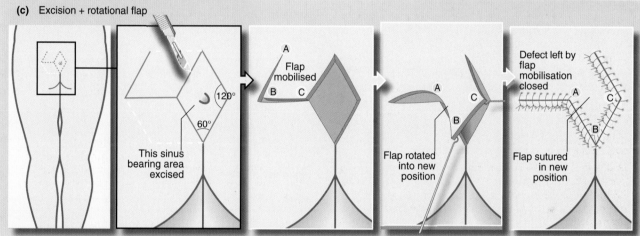

Fig. 30.13 Surgical treatment for pilonidal sinus

The most popular **perineal** procedure is **Delorme's operation,** which involves a perineal excision of the redundant rectum.

FAECAL INCONTINENCE (Table 30.1)

The process of maintaining continence is complex, involving higher behavioural control, sensory and motor pathways and the anal sphincter mechanisms. In addition, the rectal reservoir must function effectively. The continence mechanism has evolved to cope principally with semi-solid faeces and may fail if the stool is otherwise. Declining mobility may be a factor: mild incontinence that would be otherwise be manageable may become a problem where debility and immobility impair the patient's ability to move to the toilet when required.

Incontinence is socially debilitating. It is surprisingly common but to some degree concealed. It particularly affects some younger women and many elderly people. Incontinence presents in varying degrees: first to flatus, then to fluid and finally to solids as control is progres-sively lost. Social embarrassment forces patients to alter their lifestyles so that they never stray far from a lavatory, using constipating agents like loperamide or simply staying at home all day. Assessment of the severity of incontinence should include information about these coping strategies, which patients or carers may be too embarrassed to volunteer. Standard rating scales can be used to assess incontinence and compare treatments, e.g. the Cleveland Clinic faecal incontinence scale.

Young faecally incontinent patients are mostly female and usually suffer from **anorectal incontinence**. In the elderly, the aetiology is usually multifactorial.

Anorectal incontinence

The main functional abnormality in anorectal incontinence is weakness of the external anal sphincter and the pelvic floor muscles. This is sometimes due to direct injury from trauma or surgery but most cases were previously labelled idiopathic. It is now recognised that the most important cause of sphincter dysfunction in women is obstetric injury. Repeated childbirth, episiotomies or difficult forceps deliveries increase the risk. The mechanism is probably via traumatic **pudendal neuropathy** leading to atrophy of sphincteric and pelvic floor muscles. It is now known that even chronic straining at stool may cause pudendal neuropathy. In old age, degenerative changes in the spinal cord appear to be the principal cause of muscle atrophy.

If sphincters have been physically damaged, surgical sphincter repair may be undertaken but results are not always predictable or long-lasting. Continuous sacral

nerve stimulation, where an implanted 'pacemaker' promotes increased sphincter tone, can be attempted. As a last resort, a colostomy may allow the patient a better quality of life.

ANAL WARTS (CONDYLOMATA ACUMINATA)

Warts in the perianal region (see Fig. 30.15) have the same pathology and viral aetiology (human papillomavirus, HPV) as warts elsewhere and are generally transmitted by sexual activity. Just as cervical cancer is linked to specific strains of HPV infection, anal warts are an indicator of an increased risk of carcinoma of the anal canal by virtue of their common aetiology. Immune suppression, for example in patients with organ transplants or with HIV infection, can accelerate the development of severe and rapidly developing anal warts and progression to malignant change.

In small numbers, anal warts can be treated by topical applications of **podophyllin**. When large numbers are present, surgical excision under general anaesthetic is the only practical option. This involves meticulous excision of each individual wart by electrocautery. The normal skin between the warts is carefully preserved to avoid delayed healing or the disastrous complication of anal stenosis. Carefully mapped biopsies can also be undertaken to monitor for dysplastic change.

SQUAMOUS CELL CARCINOMA OF THE ANUS

EPIDEMIOLOGY

The annual incidence of anal cancer in women and the general population is about 1 : 100 000; however, in

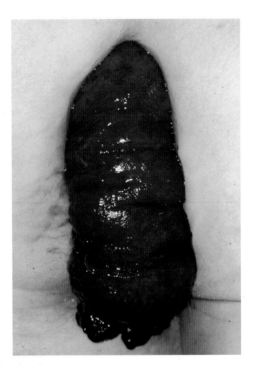

Fig. 30.14 Rectal prolapse
This complete rectal prolapse was in an 80-year-old woman. It emerged spontaneously whenever she stood, causing considerable discomfort and inconvenience, to say the least!

Table 30.1 Causes of faecal incontinence

Underlying problem	Disorders
Anorectal incontinence—pudendal neuropathy (previously known as 'idiopathic faecal incontinence'), anal sphincter and pelvic floor damage	Obstetric damage, operative damage, radiation damage, rectal prolapse, high anal fistula
Colorectal disease	Inflammatory bowel disease; polyps and tumours in rectum and anal canal
Faecal quality	Diarrhoea from any cause including infective; faecal impaction with overflow diarrhoea and incontinence
Rectal reservoir and sensation	Inflammatory bowel disease
Brain and higher cerebral functioning	Neurological disorders—dementias, psychological disturbances, impaired consciousness
Sensorimotor pathways	Spinal injury; neurological disorders
Mobility and access to toilet	Enforced bed rest or impaired mobility

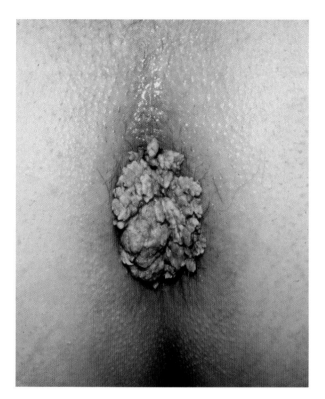

Fig. 30.15 Anal warts (condylomata acuminata)

men who have sex with men and who are HIV negative, the incidence markedly increases to 35 : 100 000. In HIV-positive men who have sex with men, the incidence is an estimated 60–70 : 100 000. This sharp increase in these groups of mainly non-keratinising cancers arising in the transitional zone is largely due to heightened rates of infection with HPV and the effects of immunosuppression fostering its progress. An effective vaccine has now been developed for HPV and, if administered in the early teens, should prevent infection and its consequences.

CLINICAL FEATURES

The symptoms of anal carcinoma are similar to those of haemorrhoids and other familiar benign anal conditions, namely fresh rectal bleeding, anal pain, discomfort and discharge. Later, incontinence can result from involvement of the anal sphincter. The patient may ignore the symptoms for a period and the doctor may initially overlook the diagnosis. On digital rectal examination, a localised firm or hard ulcer or a growth with an irregular surface and edge may be palpable and there may be surrounding woody induration. The lesion is usually visible on proctoscopy and the diagnosis confirmed by biopsy. Palpation of the groins may reveal hard, matted involved inguinal nodes. Anal canal carcinoma also metastasises to superior rectal (intra-abdominal) lymph nodes, reflecting the mixed drainage of the anal canal.

Until the 1980s, the standard treatment was surgical **abdomino-perineal resection** of rectum and anus with a permanent end colostomy in the left iliac fossa. Now, **chemoradiotherapy** is the primary treatment of choice as improved cure rates for non-surgical therapy have emerged. This also has the benefit of sparing the anal sphincter.

OTHER RARE ANAL NEOPLASMS

The anal canal is the third most common site for **malignant melanomas** after the skin and the eye. These cause non-specific anal symptoms of discomfort and bleeding and diagnosis may thus be delayed. These melanomas are usually non-pigmented and biopsy evidence is needed to make a firm diagnosis. Treatment outcomes, however, are poor. **Adenocarcinoma** of the rectum may extend distally into the anal region, and rarely **basal cell carcinomas** may occur here.

LOW RECTAL POLYPS AND CANCER

Rectal **adenomas** may sometimes develop a long pedicle and be dragged down into the anal canal. They may be mistaken for haemorrhoids if it appears at the anal verge. This emphasises the importance of proper investigation of patients with persistent haemorrhoid-like symptoms by palpation, proctoscopy and sigmoidoscopy. Treatment of low polyps is by excision with a diathermy snare, and histological examination to check for malignancy and completeness of excision.

Adenocarcinomas arising low in the rectum sometimes present with anal bleeding and discharge. Again, these symptoms should be properly investigated rather than dismissed as haemorrhoids.

PROCTALGIA FUGAX

Proctalgia fugax is a neuropathic type of pain which often manifests as brief episodes of severe lancinating pain in the perineum with sphincter spasms at unpredictable times but often at night. It usually occurs independently of conditions such as anal fissure, complicated piles and anal or rectal neoplasms; the patient may be convinced that cancer is the cause and may suspect that the doctor thinks it is 'all in the mind'. The cause is unknown but is believed not to be psychological. Whilst it is difficult to cure, reassurance and recommending ice packs or warm baths may help. If this fails, therapy with amitriptyline or gabapentin may be successful in controlling symptoms.

PRURITUS ANI

Anal itching can be distressing. It is generally caused by mucus leakage and may occur without significant haemorrhoids; even a minute quantity of leaking mucus or faecal material causes profound irritation. Patients generally try to self-medicate with a variety of creams. However, these tend to increase skin maceration and worsen the problem. Pruritus can be helped greatly if the perineum is washed and dried after defaecation using plain water. Washing the perianal area with soap can aggravate the symptoms, so it is best avoided. All topical creams should be stopped. Sometimes pruritus ani is worsened by a high-fibre diet, and a lower-residue, drier stool may lessen the problem.

Thoracic surgery

31

INTRODUCTION

Although most respiratory disease is managed by non-surgical methods, non-cardiac thoracic surgery includes the diagnosis and management of a range of benign and malignant thoracic wall and intrathoracic conditions including chest trauma, oesophageal reflux and tumours (also managed by some upper gastrointestinal surgeons), and various mediastinal disorders. This chapter deals with surgical respiratory problems and mediastinal disorders. The principles of oesophageal surgery are covered in Chapter 22 and chest trauma in Chapter 17.

INVESTIGATIVE TECHNIQUES

IMAGING

Computerised tomography (CT) of the chest now offers high-resolution images of the entire lung fields in cross-section and provides quantitative information about tissue density in all parts of the chest. Most pathological lesions can thus be diagnosed with a fair degree of confidence. In particular, the progress of apparently benign intrapulmonary masses can be followed accurately with serial CT scans, thus avoiding unnecessary surgical resection.

For staging bronchogenic carcinoma, CT scanning is invaluable. Positron emission tomography (PET) is also being evaluated for its potential to provide improved diagnostic accuracy for intrathoracic malignancy.

LUNG FUNCTION TESTS

Formal lung function tests are mandatory before chest surgery and serve two main purposes:

- Measurement of **air flow** into and out of the alveoli, i.e. FEV_1, FVC, peak air flow, total lung capacity, alveolar ventilation
- Measurement of **gas diffusion** across the alveolar–capillary interface, i.e. tests that usually involve measuring the rates of diffusion of carbon monoxide

Lung function tests provide a detailed portrait of the physiological effects of the particular chest disease and can be used to demonstrate changes over time or as a result of treatment. When surgery is contemplated, lung function tests are employed to assess the ventilatory capacity to withstand chest wall incision or lung resection.

BRONCHOSCOPY

Bronchoscopy gives direct access for biopsy of lesions within the airways and, with **transbronchial biopsy**, provides access to lesions in the lung parenchyma. In many centres, diagnostic bronchoscopy is performed mainly by chest physicians using flexible instruments, with the more difficult and potentially complicated cases passing to thoracic surgeons. Flexible bronchoscopy is performed under similar conditions to gastroscopy, using topical local anaesthesia and sometimes intravenous sedation.

Rigid bronchoscopy

Direct visual access to the large airways first became possible with the rigid bronchoscope. Its limitations included the need for general anaesthesia, the technical difficulty in achieving a thorough, reliable and satisfactory examination, and limited access to the airways beyond lobar level. Rigid bronchoscopy remains a useful tool for certain therapeutic manoeuvres, e.g. removing inhaled foreign bodies and aspirating inspissated mucus causing postoperative lung or lobar collapse; the latter, however, is now best achieved with a flexible bronchoscope.

Despite the popularity of rigid bronchoscopy in some centres, its use is certain to decline for most applications in the face of competition from flexible bronchoscopy.

Flexible bronchoscopy

There has been steady progress in the development of flexible bronchoscopes employing fibre optics and micro-chip cameras. Endoscopes have become narrower (yet with larger biopsy channels), more manoeuvrable and capable of producing better-quality colour images. The instruments can be introduced using local anaesthetic sprays or via an endotracheal tube already in situ. Access to airways can easily be achieved to the level of individual lung segments, and adequate-sized biopsies can be obtained of masses lying within the airway or in the adjoining lung parenchyma, the latter by transbronchial needle biopsy under X-ray guidance.

PLEURAL ASPIRATION AND PERCUTANEOUS BIOPSY

In the case of pleural effusion, pleural aspiration may be performed for cytological examination using a standard wide-bore needle and syringe. Blind pleural biopsy can be performed at the same time using an **Abrams needle**. Many deeper intrathoracic masses are amenable to percutaneous biopsy under X-ray or CT guidance.

MEDIASTINOSCOPY

The mediastinoscope is used to biopsy paratracheal and sometimes subcarinal lymph nodes. The instrument is a rigid tube incorporating fibreoptic light guides; it is inserted via a skin incision above the suprasternal notch and passed caudally along the plane of the pretracheal fascia (see Fig. 31.1a and b). The route passes close to the superior vena cava on the right, the innominate artery, the arch of the aorta and the left atrium anteriorly, the descending aorta on the left and the recurrent laryngeal nerves posterolaterally on each side. All these structures are at risk of damage and, although rare, this must be explained to the patient (and the information recorded) as part of obtaining consent. Mediastinoscopy gives access to the entire middle and posterior mediastinum except for the subaortic fossa (the area below the arch of the aorta which often contains lymph nodes). Access to this area is obtained by anterior mediastinotomy.

THORACOSCOPY

This is the thoracic equivalent of laparoscopy or 'keyhole' surgery and is sometimes known as **video-assisted tho-racoscopic surgery** or **VATS**. Rigid instruments for viewing and operating are inserted through small incisions in the chest wall and the image is displayed on a monitor so that the whole team can view the procedure.

VATS is an established minimally invasive technique for both diagnosis and therapy. It is the technique of choice for most pleural surgery such as pleural biopsy, pleurectomy, stapling of bullae and evacuation of early empyema thoracis. It can also be carried out to sample mediastinal lymph nodes and to perform cervical (thoraco-dorsal) sympathectomy. Other applications such as lobar resection and thoracic hiatus hernia repair need further appraisal.

ANTERIOR MEDIASTINOTOMY

Anterior mediastinotomy (see Fig. 31.1c), a form of mini-thoracotomy, may be used to obtain tissue from lesions in the anterior mediastinum, e.g. thymic tumours. The approach may be made via the left or right of the sternum, either intercostally or by resection of a costal cartilage.

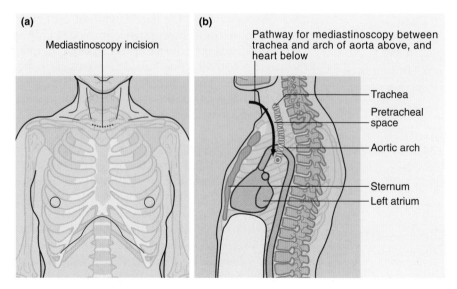
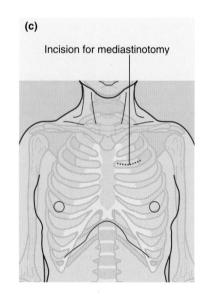

(a) Mediastinoscopy incision

(b) Pathway for mediastinoscopy between trachea and arch of aorta above, and heart below

- Trachea
- Pretracheal space
- Aortic arch
- Sternum
- Left atrium

(c) Incision for mediastinotomy

Fig. 31.1 Mediastinoscopy and mediastinotomy
(a) and **(b)** Mediastinoscopy for investigation of the posterior mediastinum. **(c)** Mediastinotomy.

Left anterior mediastinotomy affords good access for diagnostic biopsy of masses in the subaortic fossa.

THORACOTOMY

Thoracotomy, described on page 460, gives full access for biopsy of paratracheal, subcarinal and hilar lymph node groups, the great vessels, oesophagus, lung and pericardium and is used when less invasive procedures are inadequate or have failed. Immediate examination of frozen sections of specimens taken during surgery is often helpful in determining the extent of surgery required and the completeness of resection achieved.

THERAPEUTIC PROCEDURES

TRACHEOSTOMY

PRINCIPLES OF TRACHEOSTOMY

A tracheostomy (see Figs 31.2, 31.3) is an artificial opening into the trachea and is performed to provide a secure airway when the pharyngeal airway or larynx needs to be bypassed. With time, an epithelialised fistula develops between the skin and trachea which allows tracheostomy tubes to be changed and the airways cleaned without difficulty.

Indications for tracheostomy include:

- Permanent functional obstruction of the upper airway, e.g. carcinoma of larynx
- Temporary or potential upper airway obstruction, e.g. facial fractures, major head and neck operations

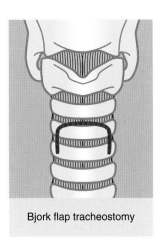
Bjork flap tracheostomy

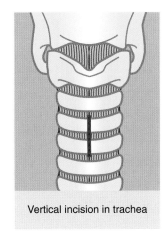
Vertical incision in trachea

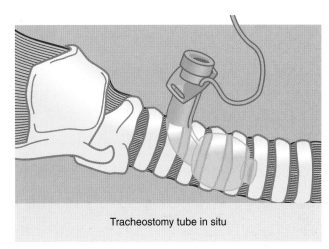
Tracheostomy tube in situ

Fig. 31.2 Tracheostomy placement

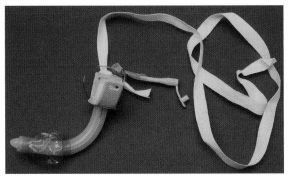

(a)

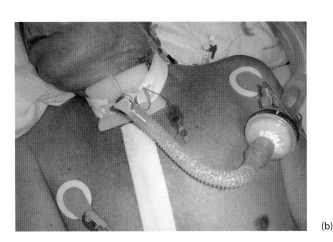

(b)

(a) Disposable tracheostomy tube. Note the distal balloon which is inflated via the small tube to provide a snug fit inside the trachea.

(b) Patient being ventilated via an elective tracheostomy after cardiac surgery.

Fig. 31.3 Tracheostomy

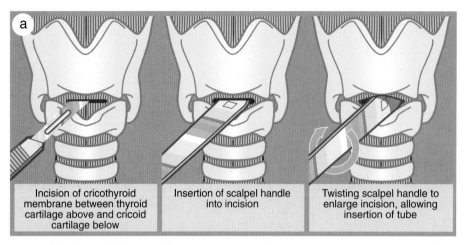

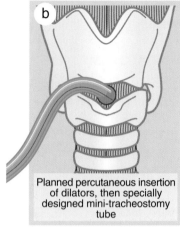

Incision of cricothyroid membrane between thyroid cartilage above and cricoid cartilage below	Insertion of scalpel handle into incision	Twisting scalpel handle to enlarge incision, allowing insertion of tube	Planned percutaneous insertion of dilators, then specially designed mini-tracheostomy tube

Fig. 31.4 Cricothyroidotomy
(a) In a dire emergency, this life-saving procedure can be rapidly employed to gain time. **(b)** Modern mini-cricothyroidotomy can be performed percutaneously by making a small incision through the cricothyroid membrane and progressively dilating it with graduated dilators before insertion of a specially constructed small-diameter tube, e.g. Minitrach or Quicktrach. These are used in accident victims and often in intensive care units.

• Patients requiring long-term ventilatory support. In these, prolonged endotracheal intubation is likely to cause permanent laryngeal damage and prevent swallowing and speech. Tracheostomy also provides continuous access to the lower airways for bronchial aspiration and toilet

Tracheostomy should be a planned procedure performed in the operating room under general anaesthesia. It is not an emergency procedure for patients with upper airway obstruction. For these patients endotracheal intubation or cricothyroidotomy (see Fig. 31.4) should be used.

COMPLICATIONS OF TRACHEOSTOMY

• **Haemorrhage** caused by erosion of the innominate (brachiocephalic) artery or vein
• **Tracheo-oesophageal fistula**, particularly where a nasogastric tube is in place
• **Displacement of the tracheostomy tube** may occur before a 'fistula' is established, making it difficult to reintubate the trachea
• **Tracheal stenosis**, usually the result of prolonged use of a high-pressure cuff

THORACOTOMY

POSTEROLATERAL THORACOTOMY

Posterolateral thoracotomy is the standard approach for lung and oesophageal resections as well as for surgery of the descending aorta. The incision is sited below the inferior angle of the scapula, latissimus dorsi is divided and the chest is entered through the bed of the (unresected)

fifth or sixth rib. If necessary, the incision can be extended into the abdomen (thoraco-abdominal incision) so that the operative field extends above and below the diaphragm, e.g. for oesophago-gastrectomy or thoraco-abdominal aortic aneurysm.

LATERAL THORACOTOMY

Lateral thoracotomy involves an incision extending between anterior and posterior axillary lines. It is used for limited access, most often for surgical treatment of pneumothorax.

ANTERIOR THORACOTOMY

This is used for diagnostic biopsy. It is less likely to cause post-thoracotomy neuralgia than other thoracotomy approaches.

THORACOSCOPY

As mentioned earlier, this is the thoracic equivalent of laparoscopy or 'keyhole' surgery and is sometimes known as **video-assisted thoracotomy**. Rigid instruments for viewing and operating are inserted through small incisions in the chest wall and the image is displayed on a monitor.

As with laparoscopic surgery, these techniques are evolving and being evaluated and the indications and contraindications are gradually emerging. For some applications, such as thoraco-dorsal sympathectomy and pleural biopsy, thoracoscopy is the treatment of choice, whilst for others, e.g. lobar resection, hiatus hernia repair, further appraisal is needed.

Disadvantages of thoracoscopic techniques include:

- Thoracoscopic operations often take much longer than equivalent open procedures (e.g. pleurodesis, pleurectomy, stapling of apical bullae)
- The completeness of thoracoscopic excision of malignant lesions is difficult to evaluate
- Post-thoracotomy neuralgia may complicate thoracoscopy incisions

MEDIAN STERNOTOMY

Median sternotomy or 'sternal split' gives wide access to the heart and the entire anterior mediastinum including the great vessels. It is the standard incision for coronary artery bypass surgery as well as for excision of thymic lesions and large retrosternal parathyroid tumours and, occasionally, resection of a goitre with massive retrosternal extension.

SPECIFIC THORACIC DISORDERS

PROBLEMS AFFECTING THE PLEURAL SPACE

Between the chest wall and the lung is a potential space, the pleural cavity, lined by mesothelium. The pleura lining the chest wall is known as **parietal pleura** and that covering the lung as **visceral pleura**. The pleural space normally contains a minute amount of serous fluid which lubricates the movement of the opposed shiny pleural surfaces and causes them to adhere by surface tension. This, and the negative pressure that would result if the surfaces were separated, keep the lungs expanded. Disease or injury may result in accumulation within the pleural cavity of air (**pneumothorax**), fluid (**pleural effusion**), pus (**empyema**) or blood (**haemothorax**), causing potentially serious (or even fatal) disturbances of respiratory and, in some cases, cardiovascular function. Pus in the pleural cavity, as in any other location, must be drained before infection can be controlled.

The basic principles of pleural drainage are illustrated by the management of pneumothorax. The management of pleural effusion, empyema and haemothorax involves variations of the technique to accommodate the particular pathologies of such fluid collections.

PNEUMOTHORAX

Spontaneous pneumothorax usually results from rupture of a bulla on the pleural surface of the lung. This is a congenital air-filled cavity which communicates with the bronchial tree. Rupture causes air to escape into the pleural space and the lung to collapse. **Traumatic pneumothorax** usually results from blunt chest injury, often as a result of rib fractures penetrating the visceral pleura. Sharp penetrating chest injury, e.g. stab wounds, may also be responsible. Different types of pneumothorax are illustrated in Figure 31.5.

A pneumothorax requires **treatment** under the following circumstances:

- When the lung volume is compromised by more than about 25% as calculated on a PA chest X-ray
- If the pneumothorax is increasing in size
- When a small pneumothorax is having a disproportionate effect on lung function because of pre-existing lung disease
- Where there is a tension pneumothorax

Sometimes, if the site of air leakage acts as a one-way valve, a **tension pneumothorax** is created. The valve effect allows air to escape into the pleural space but not to return to the airway, causing collapse of the lung on the affected side. Rising intrapleural tension pressure pushes the mediastinum towards the opposite side, compressing and compromising the contralateral lung and obstructing systemic venous return. The physiological upset is extreme and poses an immediate threat to life so the condition must be treated urgently.

Treatment of pneumothorax

Aspiration
An uncomplicated pneumothorax in an otherwise fit patient can often be treated by aspiration. A 20 ml syringe

Fig. 31.5 Classification of pneumothorax
(a) In closed pneumothorax the pleural defect closes spontaneously, leaving a fixed amount of air in the pleural space. **(b)** In open pneumothorax there is free passage of air via an open defect in the visceral pleura. **(c)** In tension pneumothorax the pleural defect acts as a flap valve allowing progressive entry of air into the pleural space, collapsing the lung and pushing the mediastinum to the opposite side.

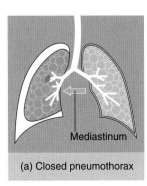
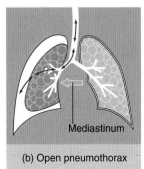
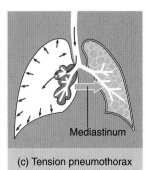

(a) Closed pneumothorax   (b) Open pneumothorax   (c) Tension pneumothorax

1 Local anaesthesia

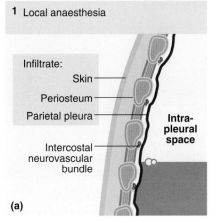

Infiltrate:

Skin

Periosteum

Parietal pleura

Intra-pleural space

Intercostal neurovascular bundle

(a)

2 Make 2 cm transverse incision just above upper border of chosen rib

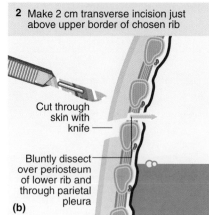

Cut through skin with knife

Bluntly dissect over periosteum of lower rib and through parietal pleura

(b)

3 Position large chest drains (28–30 F diameter)

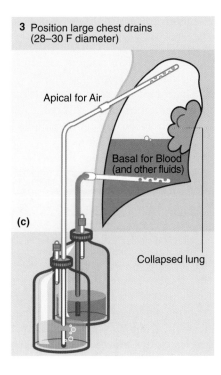

Apical for Air

Basal for Blood (and other fluids)

Collapsed lung

(c)

Fig. 31.6 Technique of intercostal tube drainage of chest (tube thoracostomy)
- Inject local anaesthetics to block sensitive structures and intercostal nerve and give time for this to take effect
- Make 2 cm incision near upper border of rib and parallel to it
- Bluntly dissect intercostal muscles down to parietal pleura with artery forceps. Stay near upper border of rib to avoid intercostal vessels
- Palpate lung with gloved index finger to free adhesions and ensure free entry for the drain
- Remove trocar from large-bore chest drain tube (at least 28 F gauge); 16 F can be used for pneumothorax alone. Grasp distal end with artery forceps and guide drain into chest in an apical or a basal direction according to purpose. *Never* insert a chest drain with the trocar in position as this is highly dangerous
- Attach drain to an underwater seal and suture drain to chest wall. Snug the skin around the drain with a purse string suture. Apply airtight dressing around the tube and tape tube to chest wall. Sit patient up to 45°
- Take a chest X-ray to confirm position of tube

is connected to a three-way tap and a needle. The needle is inserted into the pneumothorax via an intercostal approach and 20 ml of air aspirated. The tap is turned to exclude the needle and the air evacuated from the syringe. This is repeated until no more air can be withdrawn. Progress is monitored by chest X-ray. The process can be repeated, but formal tube drainage may become necessary if the pneumothorax continues to recur.

In the case of **tension pneumothorax**, rapid emergency relief can be obtained by plunging a large needle into the pleural space via an intercostal space. However, a formal apical chest drain must be inserted soon afterwards.

Intercostal tube drainage

The technique of intercostal chest drainage is described in Box 39.1 and Figure 31.6; see also Figure 31.7. For treatment of a pneumothorax, a single apical drain is used which may be of small size, e.g. 16F gauge.

Intercostal tube drains must be connected to an apparatus which prevents lung collapse due to air flowing into the chest as a result of negative intrapleural pressure. The usual arrangement is to connect the chest drain via a flexible tube to a water bottle, attaching it to a rigid tube

secured below the water level; this forms an underwater seal, allowing air or fluid to leave the chest cavity but not return. The bottle is placed below the level of the patient so that gravity creates a small vacuum. As the patient breathes, excess air and fluid in the pleural space are gradually expelled into the bottle, and air bubbles out of the exhaust tube. If there is an air leak from the lung via a breach in the visceral pleura, this is manifest by continued bubbling in the bottle and failure of the lung to expand. Continuous suction should then be applied to the outlet of the underwater seal for a few days; this usually enables the lung to expand and adhere to the chest wall, thereby remaining inflated and blocking the site of the air leak.

Patients with intercostal drains must be transported with care to prevent reflux of fluid into the chest. At one time it was recommended that chest tubes should be clamped when patients were to be moved but this advice is now rarely given because if drainage tubes are clamped, the drain fails and lung collapse can occur. When a patient is transported, one attendant should be in charge of the drainage bottle to ensure that it does not tip over and that it always remains below the level of the patient.

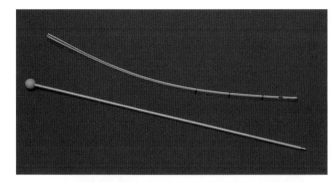

(a)

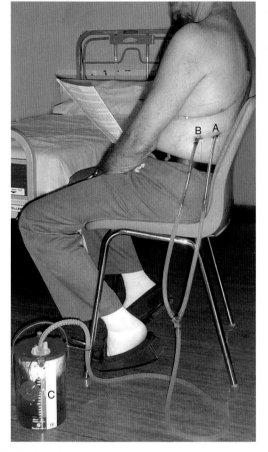

(b)

Fig. 31.7 Chest drain
(a) 30 F gauge tube (10 mm) with stylet removed (and thrown away!). Note the radiopaque line and the side holes near the tip. **(b)** Case study—post thoracotomy and lobar resection of lung for cancer. This patient has two chest drains in situ, an **A**pical drain for **A**ir and a **B**asal drain for **B**lood. Both are connected to an underwater seal, **C**, to prevent inflow of air that would cause a pneumothorax.

Intercostal drains are removed when their purpose is complete. In all cases the lung must be fully expanded. For pneumothorax, cessation of bubbling in the bottle for 24 hours is an indication for removal; for fluid drainage, the duration varies according to the underlying problem.

Treatment of persistent or recurrent pneumothorax

More extensive surgical intervention may be required for persistent or recurrent pneumothorax. Approaches

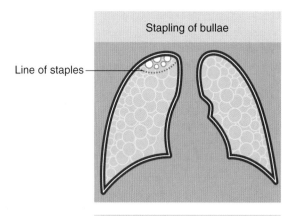

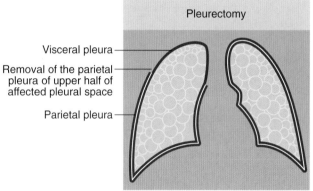

Fig. 31.8 Surgical approaches for treatment of persistent pneumothorax

include stapling of bullae to prevent air leakage, and pleural abrasion or pleurectomy. The latter causes the visceral pleura to adhere permanently to the bare chest wall (see Fig. 31.8).

EXCESS PLEURAL FLUID

There is normally only a very small amount of fluid lying between visceral and parietal pleura. This may substantially increase in response to lung disorders secondarily affecting the pleura (e.g. infection, inflammation, primary lung cancers, metastatic cancer of breast) or as a result of primary pleural disorders such as mesothelioma. The fluid may be a watery transudate (e.g. in heart failure) or an exudate of variable viscosity (e.g. due to pleural infection).

Indications for draining a pleural effusion include:

- **Diagnostic**
  —empyema
  —suspected malignancy
  —traumatic haemothorax
- **Therapeutic**
  —removing the compressive effects of a large pleural fluid collection on the lung
  —draining pus from an empyema
  —arresting haemorrhage from damaged intercostal vessels causing haemothorax

Uncomplicated pleural effusions are usually drained via a large-bore (30 F gauge) tube inserted towards the base of the pleural cavity in the most practical dependent position. If the fluid collections are loculated, more than one drain may be required.

Malignant effusions

Malignant effusions (e.g. from breast cancer) usually recur after simple drainage and need to be treated in other ways. Methods include:

- Stimulating **adhesion formation** between visceral and parietal pleura (**pleurodesis**). This can be achieved by aspirating the fluid, injecting an irritant such as tetracycline and maintaining tube drainage until permanent adhesions have developed. An alternative is to perform **pleural abrasion**. Via a small thoracotomy, the parietal pleura is widely abraded using a surgical swab. Again, chest drainage allows adhesions to form between the two layers of pleura with permanent prevention of effusion. This and the following technique both obliterate the pleural space
- **Parietal pleurectomy**. This open thoracotomy operation involves the stripping of the parietal pleura which results in diffuse adhesion of the lung surface to the chest wall (see Fig. 31.8b)
- **Pleuro-peritoneal shunting** using a tubular device connecting the two cavities. This is implanted beneath the skin and incorporates a one-way valve. The excess pleural fluid is manually 'pumped' from the pleural space into the peritoneal space by the patient several times a day where it is then reabsorbed via the abdominal peritoneum. This may be the treatment of choice in patients with a short life expectancy

EMPYEMA

When pleural fluid becomes infected, pus accumulates in a loculus within the pleural cavity; this is known as an **empyema**. In the early stages, an empyema can be treated by dependent intercostal tube drainage with irrigation if necessary; early loculi may respond to lytic treatment with urokinase. In chronic cases, a thick fibrous wall or **cortex** gradually forms around the pus-filled space. Treatment options then include prolonged closed tube drainage, or open tube drainage involving removal of a segment of rib, and surgical 'decortication' of the entire abscess wall (see Figs. 31.9, 31.10). This releases the entrapped lung and tethered chest wall and diaphragm, thus allowing the lung to re-expand.

HAEMOTHORAX

Following chest trauma, blood may accumulate in the pleural space. This is usually drained via two large drains, one apically and one basally located. A similar strategy is employed after open chest surgery. However, recently clotted blood will not drain successfully and a clotted haemothorax may require evacuation through a thoracoscope. Thoracotomy may sometimes be required. Later, clot liquefies and may be removed by drainage. Removing blood allows the lung to expand against the chest wall and helps to arrest continuing haemorrhage from intercostal vessels. Persistent or increasing drainage of blood indicates continuing intrathoracic bleeding which often necessitates surgical intervention. Continued bleeding is usually from the systemic circulation (e.g. intercostal or great vessels) rather than from lung parenchyma.

LUNG ABSCESS

Lung abscesses have become much less common with effective antibiotic treatment of pulmonary infections. Onset of symptoms may be insidious with clinical features including a swinging pyrexia, foul-smelling sputum and the finding of a cavitating shadow on chest X-ray. Primary lung abscess may follow bacterial lung infection,

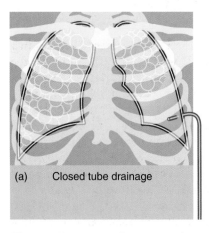

(a)   Closed tube drainage

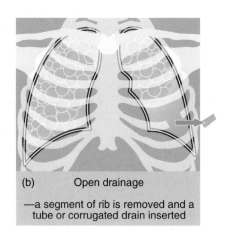

(b)   Open drainage

—a segment of rib is removed and a tube or corrugated drain inserted

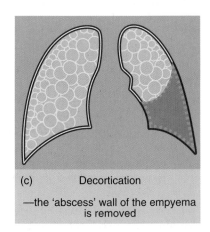

(c)   Decortication

—the 'abscess' wall of the empyema is removed

 Fig. 31.9 Treatment of empyema thoracis

Fig. 31.10 Empyema thoracis

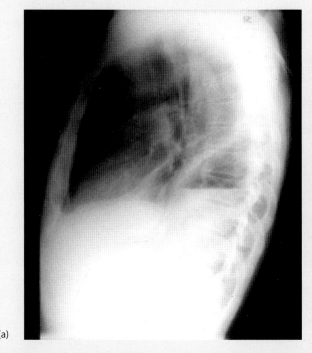

(a)

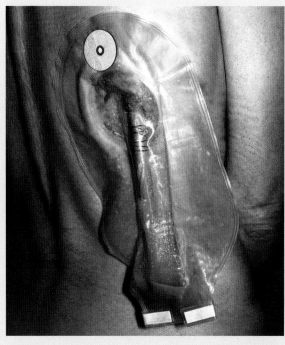

(b)

This 51-year-old man underwent a thoraco-abdominal oesophagogastrectomy for proximal gastric cancer. He suffered a small intrathoracic anastomotic leak and developed an intrapleural empyema, shown by the fluid level in **(a)**. **(b)** Drainage of empyema. A section of rib overlying the cavity was resected and a large red rubber tube was inserted to give dependent drainage into a bag. The drain was gradually shortened as the cavity closed. This patient was alive and well 15 years later.

most commonly with *Staphylococcus aureus*, beta-haemolytic streptococci, *Pseudomonas* or *Klebsiella*.

Secondary lung abscess may follow aspiration of gastric contents or occur in lung segments distal to a bronchial obstruction caused by a centrally placed neoplasm (usually squamous cell carcinoma) or inhaled foreign body.

Lung abscesses are usually treated with antibiotics alone but occasionally a cavity requires drainage. Drains are usually placed percutaneously under ultrasound or CT guidance.

CANCER OF THE LUNG

Lung cancers arise as primary bronchogenic tumours or as metastatic deposits from cancers elsewhere in the body. Of the primary tumours, only 20% will not have metastasised by the time of presentation. Lymph nodes in the hilar area are usually involved first, followed by other mediastinal nodes. Bone and brain are common sites of distant metastatic spread and may be responsible for initial presentation.

Primary lung cancers are classified into **small cell tumours** (10–15%) and **non-small cell tumours** (85–90%). Small cell tumours (often called 'oat-cell carcino-

mas' from their histological appearance) are thought to originate from pulmonary APUD cells. Non-small cell tumours are derived from bronchopulmonary tissues and include squamous cell carcinoma (almost always related to smoking), adenocarcinoma and large cell or undifferentiated carcinomas, and broncho-alveolar cell tumours. Many lung cancers grow rapidly and assessment should not be delayed if surgery is contemplated.

STAGING OF LUNG CANCER AND ITS IMPLICATIONS

TNM staging of lung cancer is fundamental to planning appropriate treatment. The staging system follows the general TNM pattern and is shown in Figure 31.11.

In staging bronchogenic carcinoma, CT scanning is invaluable. Intravenous injections of contrast improve its reliability by enabling blood vessels to be discriminated reliably from lymph nodes. The likelihood of enlarged lymph nodes being malignant increases with size, from 7% for nodes less than 1 cm in diameter to 40% for nodes 1–2 cm in diameter and 66% for nodes larger than 2 cm.

The role of surgery in the management of lung cancer varies according to the type of tumour, the known

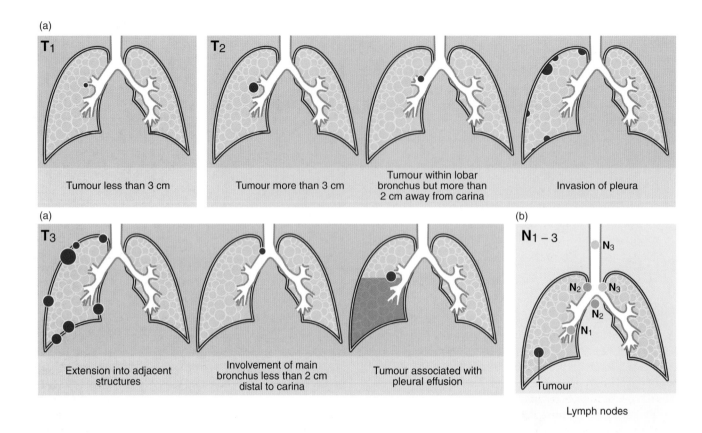

Fig. 31.11 Tumour staging using the TNM classification
(a) Tumour size and extent. **(b)** Lymph node involvement.

responsiveness of the tumour type to other therapies (i.e. radiotherapy and chemotherapy), the general state of respiratory function and the age and fitness of the patient for major surgery. As a general principle, surgery is reserved for patients who are potentially curable. Surgery usually involves removing one or more affected lung lobes (**lobectomy**) or the whole lung (**pneumonectomy**), sometimes with resection of involved chest wall.

For carcinoma in nodal stage N_0 (no nodal involvement) or N_1 (metastasis to ipsilateral hilar or peribronchial nodes only) with no known distant metastases (M_0), excising the primary tumour and local nodes by lobectomy or pneumonectomy (with or without chest wall resection) gives a 5-year survival of about 50%. N_2 disease is diagnosed when there are metastases to ipsilateral mediastinal or subcarinal lymph nodes or both. When diagnosed preoperatively (e.g. by mediastinoscopy and biopsy), complete resection is possible in less than 10% of patients and 5-year survival following resection is only 2%.

N_3 disease is defined by metastases in contralateral mediastinal lymph nodes, scalene or supraclavicular lymph nodes. If N_2 or N_3 disease (or M_1 disease with distant metastases) is confirmed during initial staging, the results of surgery are so poor that it is rarely offered and other methods of palliation need to be considered. If

preoperative staging of mediastinal lymph nodes is negative but N_2 disease is discovered at thoracotomy (occult N_2 disease), 50% of patients can undergo a histologically complete resection and this subgroup would expect a 5-year survival of 30%.

For disease too advanced for useful surgery, radiotherapy can increase life expectancy and provide effective palliation for troublesome complications such as lobar collapse, haemoptysis, superior vena caval obstruction or symptomatic metastases in brain or bone. Radiotherapy has also proved useful for managing symptomatic tumour recurrence after surgery. The role of adjuvant chemotherapy in treating lung cancer is currently under scrutiny.

SURGICAL TREATMENT OF LUNG CANCER

Surgical treatment of operable lung cancer involves wide resection of the primary cancer with sampling of loco-regional (mediastinal) lymph nodes to establish accurate TNM staging. Accurate pathological staging of the surgical specimen influences the decision to employ adjuvant chemotherapy or radiotherapy.

The standard surgical approach is via a postero-lateral thoracotomy. For lobectomy, one or more lobes are excised. Each lung has three 'surgical' lobes; the right has upper, middle and lower lobes, the left has upper, lingular and lower lobes. In pneumonectomy, the entire lung is removed.

The empty thoracic space left by resection is soon taken up by hyperinflation of the remaining lung tissue, mediastinal shift and elevation of the hemidiaphragm.

Apart from treatment of malignant disease, indications for lung resection include:

- **Trauma**—major sharp injury to a lobe or lung, or cases of blunt trauma where a bronchus has been ruptured
- **Infection**—consequences of infection including bleeding due to bronchiectasis or secondary fungal infection of a persistent, antibiotically 'sterilised' abscess cavity
- **Benign tumours**—if curative excision via bronchotomy is impracticable
- **Lung transplantation**—transplantation of a single lung is sometimes performed for non-malignant disease when there is minimal respiratory reserve and one lung is significantly more affected than the other. Bilateral lung transplantation is performed in patients with lung diseases involving infection, e.g. cystic fibrosis or bronchiectasis. Heart–lung transplantation is offered when both lungs and heart are irreparably damaged, e.g. Eisenmenger's syndrome (see Ch. 14)

DISORDERS OF THE MEDIASTINUM

Disorders of the mediastinum of surgical importance are summarised in Figure 31.12.

ANTERIOR MEDIASTINUM

Retrosternal thyroid

Rarely, the thyroid gland is ectopically located in the anterior mediastinum where it may become enlarged by any of the processes discussed in Chapter 49. Alternatively, an inferior extension of a normally located thyroid gland may spread retrosternally into the anterior mediastinum as a result of similar pathological changes. The adverse effects of retrosternal thyroid enlargement are usually related to progressive displacement of the trachea. Sudden enlargement of retrosternal thyroid tissue caused by haemorrhage can threaten the airway. Most retrosternal thyroids can be removed through a standard thyroidectomy collar incision and only rarely is a median sternotomy required.

Thymus

The thymus causes few pathological problems with the exception of the rare thymic tumour (**thymoma**) which may be benign or malignant. Distinguishing between the two is difficult on histological grounds and diagnosis has to be based on morphological characteristics, such as the presence of a capsule. For malignant thymomas, surgical excision is the only treatment and achieves a 5-year survival rate of about 65%.

Myasthenia gravis is an unusual clinical condition associated with certain thymic tumours or thymic hyperplasia. After thymectomy, the paroxysmal fatigue of myasthenia is usually improved and the need for anticholinesterase therapy reduced. However, the symptoms are rarely completely eliminated.

Parathyroid

Benign and malignant parathyroid tumours usually occur in the neck but may occasionally occur anywhere between the retrothyroid area and the arch of the aorta. If retrosternal lesions are suspected, exploration of the anterior mediastinum accompanied by thymectomy permits the abnormal parathyroid tissue to be removed. Note that thymectomy alone can be performed via a collar incision.

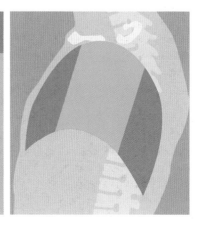

Anterior mediastinum (between sternum and pericardium)	Middle mediastinum (pericardium and its contents and lymph nodes)	Posterior mediastinum (posterior to pericardium)
• Retrosternal thyroid • Parathyroid hypertrophy or tumour • Thymoma • Lymph node enlargement • Aneurysm of ascending aorta • Hernia through foramen of Morgagni • Germ cell tumour (seminoma/teratoma)	• Lymph node enlargement • Mediastinal cysts	• Neurogenic tumours • Aneurysm of descending aorta • Hiatus hernia • Congenital hernia through foramen of Bochdalek

Fig. 31.12 Disorders of the mediastinum

MIDDLE MEDIASTINUM

This contains the pericardium and hila of both lungs. Disorders requiring surgical intervention include:

- **Lymph node enlargement**—bronchogenic malignancy or lymphoma are the most common causes. Tumour type may be defined by biopsy, and the extent by CT scanning
- **Aneurysms**—those of the ascending aorta or the arch of the aorta are usually degenerative but may also appear as a late complication of aortic trauma or dissection. Syphilitic aneurysm is now rare
- **Developmental cysts**—these include pericardial, bronchogenic, enterogenous and cysts of uncertain origin. Mediastinal cysts occasionally become infected and even more rarely undergo malignant change
- **Germ cell tumours**—primary or secondary teratoma or seminoma occasionally occur. These tumours are diagnosed by histology or raised serum markers and can usually be treated successfully with chemotherapy

POSTERIOR MEDIASTINUM

The posterior mediastinum lies behind the pericardium. Surgery may be required for the following conditions:

- **Aneurysms of the descending aorta**
- **Benign tumours of neurological origin**—these may be bilobed and extend into the spinal canal
- **Diaphragmatic hernia**—hiatus hernia is common but is not always associated with gastric reflux. Most sliding hernias can now be treated with acid-reducing drugs, weight loss and other simple advice (see Ch. 22). The more unusual para-oesophageal or rolling hiatus hernia may lead to gastric infarction and many believe its presence is an indication for surgery. Congenital herniation into the posterior mediastinum (hernia of Bochdalek) is very rare. Discussion continues as to whether hiatus hernias requiring surgery should be approached from above or below the diaphragm

Hernias and other groin problems

32

INTRODUCTION

This chapter describes the clinical presentation and diagnosis of lumps and swellings in the groin along with the specific conditions causing these problems. Other hernias of the anterior abdominal wall (ventral hernias) are considered near the end of the chapter, whilst problems and disorders of the male genitalia, the penis, testis and scrotum, are covered in the following chapter.

Groin lumps and swellings account for about 10% of general surgical outpatient referrals. In both sexes, the most common lumps in the groin are **hernias**, mainly inguinal but also femoral. Both are caused by abdominal contents protruding through a defect in the abdominal wall. In the male, the normal testicular descent is from the abdomen to the scrotum via the inguinal canal, and this area remains potentially vulnerable throughout life; inguinal hernias are therefore much more common in males. If large, an **inguinal hernia** may present as a scrotal lump rather than a groin lump, but it is obvious on examination that it arises in the groin. In the female, the uterine round ligament pursues a course similar to the spermatic cord in the male; this explains the occurrence of inguinal hernias in females. The femoral canal, below the inguinal ligament, is another potential weakness in the abdominal wall and may give rise to a **femoral hernia**, particularly in women.

Enlarged lymph nodes due to infection or malignancy also cause groin lumps or swellings. Less common are vascular abnormalities such as a **saphena varix** or a **femoral artery aneurysm**. Very rarely nowadays, a **psoas abscess** may track down beneath the inguinal ligament to present in the groin. This used to be a common complication of tuberculous disease of the spine but is now more often a result of infection tracking down from a perforation in the left colon.

The anatomy of the groin provides a good starting point for understanding surgical problems in this area and is explained in Figure 32.1.

When a patient presents with **pain** in the groin as the main symptom, a frequent cause is a newly developed inguinal hernia. If symptoms are more acute and severe, there may be a strangulated inguinal or femoral hernia. Perhaps more commonly, the cause is believed to be a **groin strain** brought on by excessive or unaccustomed exercise. This condition is poorly understood but most cases recover gradually without treatment.

LUMPS IN THE GROIN

CLINICAL EXAMINATION

Lumps in the groin may be painful and tender, so care is needed in examination. In any case, the groin and scrotum must both be examined to discover the anatomical origin of the swelling. Lumps in the groin are examined in the same way as lumps elsewhere but there are some special points to note as follows:

- Examine the patient both standing and lying
- Examine for the presence of a cough impulse and test the reducibility of the lump
- Demonstrate the relationship of the origin of the lump to the inguinal ligament and the pubic tubercle

Position for examination

The patient must be examined both standing and lying. When standing, intra-abdominal pressure increases, making a hernia more visible. If the patient is asked to cough while the lump is palpated, intra-abdominal pressure is transmitted through the abdominal wall and an expansile **cough impulse** is felt in a hernia. Smaller

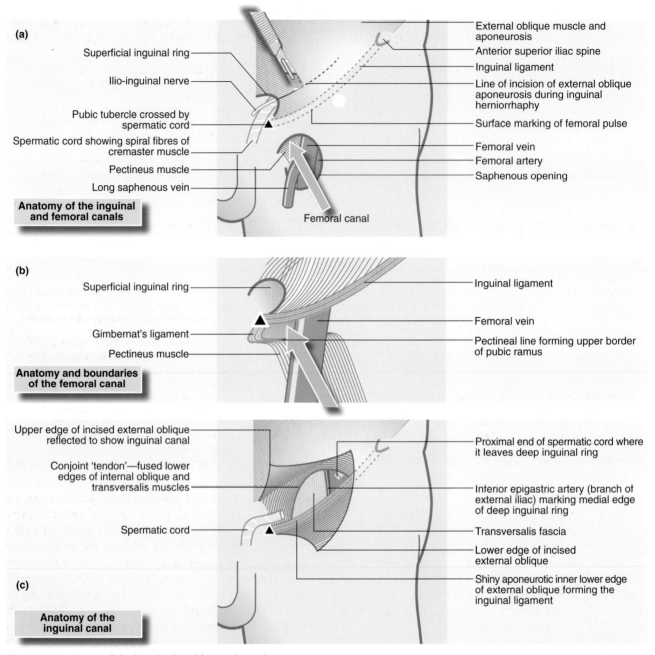

(a)

Superficial inguinal ring

Ilio-inguinal nerve

Pubic tubercle crossed by spermatic cord

Spermatic cord showing spiral fibres of cremaster muscle

Pectineus muscle

Long saphenous vein

Anatomy of the inguinal and femoral canals

External oblique muscle and aponeurosis

Anterior superior iliac spine

Inguinal ligament

Line of incision of external oblique aponeurosis during inguinal herniorrhaphy

Surface marking of femoral pulse

Femoral vein

Femoral artery

Saphenous opening

Femoral canal

(b)

Superficial inguinal ring

Gimbernat's ligament

Pectineus muscle

Anatomy and boundaries of the femoral canal

Inguinal ligament

Femoral vein

Pectineal line forming upper border of pubic ramus

Upper edge of incised external oblique reflected to show inguinal canal

Conjoint 'tendon'—fused lower edges of internal oblique and transversalis muscles

Spermatic cord

Proximal end of spermatic cord where it leaves deep inguinal ring

Inferior epigastric artery (branch of external iliac) marking medial edge of deep inguinal ring

Transversalis fascia

Lower edge of incised external oblique

Shiny aponeurotic inner lower edge of external oblique forming the inguinal ligament

(c)

Anatomy of the inguinal canal

Fig. 32.1 Structure of the inguinal and femoral canals
(a) The entire groin area. The surface marking of the femoral pulse is shown, midway between the pubic symphysis and the anterior superior iliac spine; the deep ring lies 2.5 cm above it. **(b) Structure of the femoral canal**—the abdominal opening seen from below. **(c) Structure of the inguinal canal.** The inguinal canal displayed by incising the anterior wall (external oblique aponeurosis) as in the first stage of open repair; the spermatic cord has been removed for clarity.

inguinal hernias may reduce spontaneously on lying down, and a scrotal varicocoele (see Ch. 33) will empty when the patient is supine.

Consistency and reducibility

Hernias are usually soft and 'squishy' but the most reliable diagnostic sign is whether the lump reduces spontaneously when the patient lies flat or can be reduced with gentle manipulation by the patient or clinician. Most inguinal hernias are at least partly reducible, although long-standing hernias gradually become irreducible because of adhesions within the sac. These are said to be **incarcerated**, i.e. chronically irreducible. If bowel is present within a large hernia sac (and the hernia is not strangulated), auscultation will usually reveal bowel sounds. In contrast, femoral hernias are nearly always **irreducible** and have no cough impulse since the femoral canal is so narrow (see Table 32.1).

Table 32.1 Summary of groin lumps and swellings and their clinical features

Disorder	Anatomical/developmental basis	Clinical features
a. Inguinal hernia Direct	Simple bulging of abdominal contents resulting from inadequate support by weak or ruptured posterior wall of inguinal canal (transversalis fascia)	Discomfort; lump usually disappears on lying down; risk of incarceration if large but low risk of strangulation
Indirect	Passage of abdominal contents, often including bowel, through inguinal canal towards scrotum or labium majus	Potential for incarceration and strangulation; much more common in men
b. Femoral hernia	Abdominal contents, often including bowel, migrate into femoral canal	Rarely has a cough impulse; rarely reducible; high rate of strangulation; more common in women
c. Inguinal lymphadenopathy	Inguinal nodes drain lower limb, abdominal wall below umbilicus, anal canal, scrotal skin, penis (but not testes, which drain to para-aortic and para-iliac nodes)	Enlarged nodes indicate infection, lymphoma or metastases from primary lesion in drainage area
d. Saphena varix	Dilatation of long saphenous vein superficial to deep fascia before it enters the femoral vein	Can be mistaken for femoral hernia but empties on pressure and disappears on lying down, unlike femoral hernia; varicose veins present in the leg
e. Femoral artery aneurysm	Dilatation of common femoral artery just below inguinal ligament	Found in patients over 65 years, mostly male; classic clinical sign is expansile pulsation; could be mistaken for femoral hernia
f. Psoas abscess (this is not discussed in detail in this book)	Classically, a tuberculous abscess of lumbar vertebra tracking down inside sheath of psoas muscle; occasionally a pyogenic abscess originating within the abdomen presents via the same route	TB presents as swelling or 'cold abscess' below inguinal ligament; rare nowadays but may be confused with lymph nodes; pyogenic abscess typically 'hot'; rarely may be due to abscess from renal stones

A **strangulated** inguinal hernia can be readily diagnosed by finding an irreducible hernia in the correct anatomical position; the lump is tender and often red. Conversely, strangulated femoral hernias are usually very small and unimpressive, often no more than the size of a grape, yet have serious consequences. Strangulated hernias, particularly femoral hernias, sometimes present with abdominal pain or signs of obstruction but without localised pain. This emphasises the importance of examining the hernial orifices in every patient with an acute abdomen.

Enlarged inguinal lymph nodes vary in consistency, number and size depending on the pathological cause; they are not of course reducible. A **saphena varix** is very soft and completely disappears on palpation or if the patient lies down, refilling when pressure is released or if the patient stands. The limb on that side nearly always has substantial varicose veins. A saphena varix also exhibits a cough impulse. **Femoral artery aneurysms**, however, are firm and pulsatile. These vascular conditions must be diagnosed correctly as injudicious operation could be catastrophic!

Relationship to the inguinal ligament

The site of the lump in relation to the inguinal ligament needs to be identified. The ligament is not visible but stretches between two palpable bony prominences, the **anterior superior iliac spine** laterally and the **pubic tubercle** medially (see Fig. 32.1a). The pubic tubercle is higher than might be imagined from the skin contour, lying 2–3 cm above the groin crease. The iliac spine is easy to locate but the pubic tubercle can be difficult, especially in obese patients. It is best found by palpating along the upper border of the pubic symphysis, outwards from the midline (care is needed in the male as the spermatic cord can be tender where it crosses the pubic tubercle). This is a kinder method than invaginating the scrotum with the index finger from below (see Fig. 32.2).

As shown in Figure 32.3, inguinal hernias always originate **above** the inguinal ligament, whereas femoral hernias, saphena varices and femoral artery aneurysms always arise **below** it. Enlarged inguinal **lymph nodes** are usually situated below the inguinal ligament. The rare **psoas abscess** has its origins out of reach, well above the inguinal ligament and posteriorly, but it tracks down within the psoas sheath to present below the inguinal ligament.

Direct and indirect inguinal hernias (Fig. 32.4)

Distinguishing between direct and indirect inguinal hernias may be clinically difficult and is of little practical

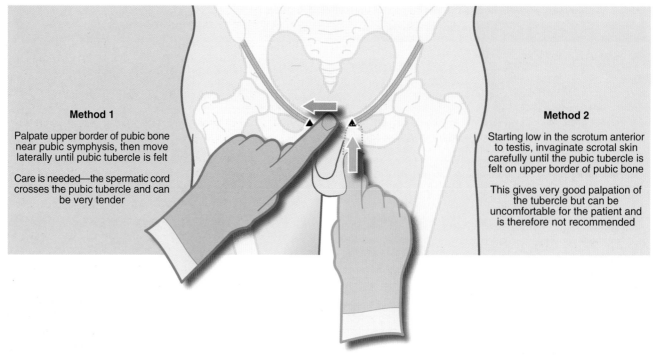

Method 1

Palpate upper border of pubic bone near pubic symphysis, then move laterally until pubic tubercle is felt

Care is needed—the spermatic cord crosses the pubic tubercle and can be very tender

Method 2

Starting low in the scrotum anterior to testis, invaginate scrotal skin carefully until the pubic tubercle is felt on upper border of pubic bone

This gives very good palpation of the tubercle but can be uncomfortable for the patient and is therefore not recommended

Fig. 32.2 Digital palpation of the pubic tubercle
Note that method 2 is not recommended.

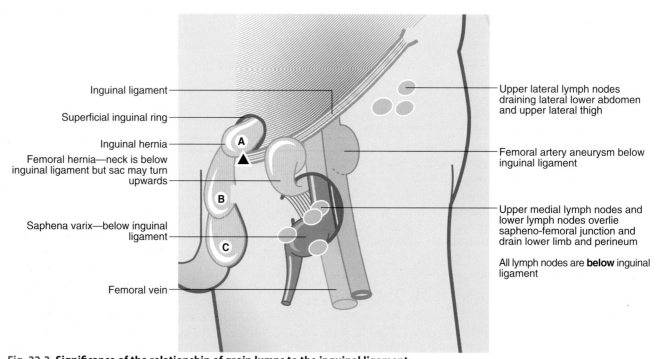

Inguinal ligament

Superficial inguinal ring

Inguinal hernia

Femoral hernia—neck is below inguinal ligament but sac may turn upwards

Saphena varix—below inguinal ligament

Femoral vein

Upper lateral lymph nodes draining lateral lower abdomen and upper lateral thigh

Femoral artery aneurysm below inguinal ligament

Upper medial lymph nodes and lower lymph nodes overlie sapheno-femoral junction and drain lower limb and perineum

All lymph nodes are **below** inguinal ligament

Fig. 32.3 Significance of the relationship of groin lumps to the inguinal ligament
A, **B** and **C** are stages in the enlargement of an indirect inguinal hernia. Note that the neck is above the inguinal ligament. A direct inguinal hernia enlarges forwards in position **A**, but occasionally extends into the scrotum.

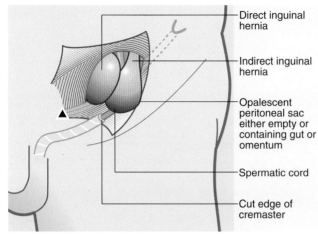

Direct inguinal hernia

Indirect inguinal hernia

Opalescent peritoneal sac either empty or containing gut or omentum

Spermatic cord

Cut edge of cremaster

Fig. 32.4 Direct and indirect inguinal hernias
A direct inguinal hernia bulges medially to the inferior epigastric artery and is not usually attached to the spermatic cord. An indirect inguinal hernia leaves the deep inguinal ring lateral to the artery and lies *within* the cremaster muscle covering the cord.

importance. Despite this, it is a useful exercise in eliciting clinical signs and frequently comes up in student examinations! The patient's age is perhaps the most useful indicator of the likely type of inguinal hernia, with indirect hernias most frequent under the age of 50 and direct hernias more common after that age.

By definition, an **indirect inguinal hernia** is one in which the hernial sac lies within the spermatic cord, leaving the abdomen via the deep (internal) inguinal ring to pass along the inguinal canal, exiting through the superficial (external) ring. Thus, if the hernia can be completely reduced, finger pressure over the deep ring (midway between the pubic symphysis and the pubic tubercle, which is 2.5 cm above the femoral pulse, see Fig. 32.1a) will prevent it reappearing on coughing. In contrast, a **direct inguinal hernia** leaves the abdomen through a weakness or split in the **transversalis fascia**, the posterior wall of the inguinal canal, emerging directly through the superficial ring. This lies medial to the deep ring and so cannot be controlled by digital pressure over it. In practice, this test is often unreliable.

Inguinal and femoral hernias

Differentiating an inguinal from a femoral hernia may sometimes be problematic but is important as it will determine the surgical approach used and the operation performed. The key is the position of the hernia in relation to the inguinal ligament. An inguinal hernia, emerging from the superficial ring, has its origin above the inguinal ligament, often descending over the pubic tubercle. A femoral hernia originates below the inguinal ligament. Rarely it becomes large, and tends to be deflected upwards and may seem to arise above the inguinal ligament. This explains the importance of careful examination to determine the origin of the neck of any groin hernia.

INGUINAL HERNIA

Inguinal hernia is one of the most common conditions seen in general surgical clinics. In a typical district general hospital, inguinal hernias account for about 7% of surgical outpatient consultations and about 12% of operating theatre time.

As shown in Figure 32.5, inguinal hernias in males are by far the most common type of groin hernia. Inguinal hernias occur eight times more often in males because of the abdominal wall deficiency caused by testicular descent. Femoral hernias are rare in males, comprising only 2.5% of groin hernias. Even in females, inguinal hernias are the most frequent (twice as common as femorals). Femoral hernias are twice as common in females as in males.

Inguinal hernias occur at any age. In childhood they always have a developmental origin and are particularly common in premature infants. In males, hernias appear most often before the age of 5 and after middle age. A smaller peak occurs in the late teens and early twenties. Hernias in these young men probably result from a congenital predisposition, exacerbated by work or sport. Most inguinal hernias should be repaired early to reduce the long-term risk of strangulation and the need for emergency operation. The exception is small, easily reducible direct hernias in elderly men or those with substantial comorbidity.

ANATOMICAL CONSIDERATIONS

The surgical anatomy of the inguinal canal is shown in Figure 32.1c. The external oblique aponeurosis (or fascia) forms the anterior wall of the inguinal canal. In the diagram, it has been split obliquely from the external ring along the line of its fibres for about 5 cm laterally and the cut edges reflected upwards and downwards to expose the inguinal canal. This is how it would appear after the first stage of an inguinal hernia repair operation.

The internal oblique and transversus abdominis muscles are deficient above the medial half of the inguinal ligament, with the D-shaped defect normally filled with the **transversalis fascia**. Transversalis is particularly strong here and forms the posterior wall of the inguinal canal, providing the only restraint to herniation of the abdominal contents in this area. Arching over this, the inferior borders of the two muscles fuse to form the conjoint musculature and tendon which extends from the lateral half of the inguinal ligament to the pubic crest.

The spermatic cord passes through the deep ring, a defect in the transversalis fascia at the most lateral part of the muscular defect. The **inferior epigastric artery** passes upwards from the external iliac immediately medial to it. Thus, the **deep (internal) ring** is bounded by the inguinal ligament below, conjoint musculature above and laterally, and the inferior epigastric artery

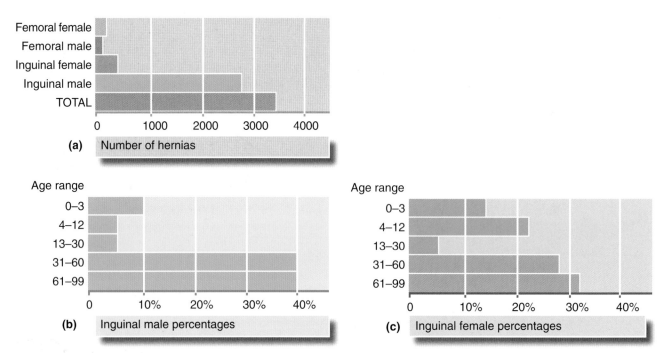

Fig. 32.5 Relative annual incidence of inguinal and femoral hernias in East Anglia (UK)
(a) Number of hernias by type and sex. The percentage of each type is shown in brackets. **(b)** Incidence of inguinal hernias in males by age. **(c)** Incidence of inguinal hernias in females by age.

medially. At operation, a direct or indirect inguinal hernia is defined by its position in relation to the inferior epigastric artery.

MECHANISMS OF INGUINAL HERNIA FORMATION

As described previously, inguinal herniation may be direct or indirect. In either case, the herniated abdominal contents are contained within a sac of peritoneum. In an **indirect hernia**, the peritoneal sac may represent a patent or reopened processus vaginalis. It may extend as far as the tunica vaginalis and surround the testis. It is easy to accept that indirect hernias have a congenital origin in children or in young muscular men, but this is less convincing in older men where muscular and connective tissue ageing must play a part.

Direct hernias tend to bulge forwards and rarely enter the scrotum. They are usually found in older patients with deficient muscles and weak transversalis fascia. The neck of a direct sac tends to be broad, in contrast to the narrow neck of an indirect hernia, confined as it is by the borders of the deep ring. Consequently, indirect inguinal hernias are more liable to strangulate. Occasionally, a direct hernia occurs suddenly after physical effort. In this case, the transversalis fascia has split, causing the sudden appearance of what is known in lay terms as a 'rupture'.

It should be noted that an indirect and a direct hernia can occur together on the same side—a **pantaloon hernia**. A hernial mass may consist merely of peritoneum and

associated extraperitoneal fat, but the sac usually contains omentum or small bowel. Less commonly, the sac contains large bowel or appendix, or rarely bladder. Occasionally, the contents of the sac are diseased, e.g. large bowel carcinoma, an inflamed appendix (acute appendicitis) or peritoneal tumour metastases. This disease may be the reason for the emergency presentation and the operation at which the condition is discovered.

Sometimes a retroperitoneal viscus 'slides' down the posterior abdominal wall and herniates directly (occasionally indirectly) into the inguinal canal, dragging its overlying peritoneum with it. Thus, the visceral contents of a **sliding hernia** lie behind and outside the peritoneal sac (see Fig. 32.6). Diagnosis can only reliably be made at operation.

Rarely, herniation occurs through a fascial defect in the linea semilunaris at the lateral border of rectus abdominis. The hernial sac comes to lie interstitially, i.e. between the layers of internal and external oblique or transversus abdominis. This is known as a **Spigelian hernia**. It has some of the clinical characteristics of an inguinal hernia but the bulge lies higher than the position of an inguinal hernia and may be difficult to palpate because it is covered by one or more layers of the abdominal wall (see Fig. 32.7).

NATURAL HISTORY OF INGUINAL HERNIA

Inguinal hernias usually develop slowly, although exacerbated by any condition which persistently raises intra-

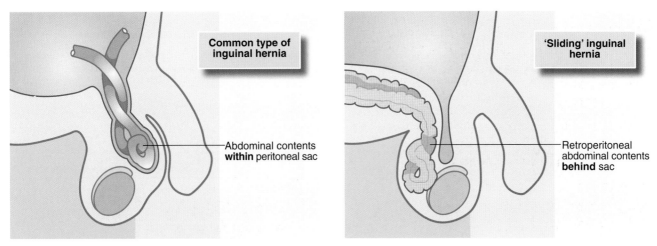

Fig. 32.6 Common and sliding inguinal hernias

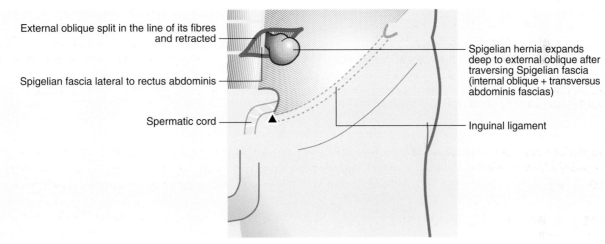

Fig. 32.7 Spigelian hernia

abdominal pressure, e.g. obesity, constipation, straining at micturition or chronic coughing; continued heavy lifting probably has a similar effect. In adults, a single episode of increased intra-abdominal pressure, such as an extreme bout of heavy lifting, may 'rupture' the abdominal wall, resulting in the sudden appearance of a direct hernia. In infants, a period of severe coughing or crying may precipitate an acute indirect hernia which may become irreducible.

In adults, the peritoneal sac and its contents are usually completely reducible into the abdominal cavity. Reduction usually occurs spontaneously when the patient lies down, but larger hernias may need manipulating by the patient. In general, the longer a hernia remains and the larger it becomes, the more difficult it is to reduce and the greater the likelihood of fibrous adhesions forming within the sac. A chronically irreducible hernia which is not strangulated is described as **incarcerated**. However, the term is often used inaccurately when a clinician is uncertain whether an acutely irreducible hernia is strangulated. In patients presenting as emergencies, is safer to assume such a hernia is strangulated until proved otherwise.

Hernial strangulation

Inguinal hernias may become irreducible or strangulated at any time; those with a narrow neck that are difficult to reduce or which intermittently cause pain are at special risk. Strangulation occurs if the hernial contents become constricted by the neck of the sac or by twisting. Obstruction of venous return then leads to swelling and later to arterial obstruction. If strangulation is not relieved by manual or operative reduction, **infarction** follows. A strangulated inguinal hernia first becomes irreducible and then tender and later red. Symptoms and signs of bowel obstruction develop over the next few hours, followed by peritonitis if the bowel perforates (Fig. 32.8).

MANAGEMENT OF INGUINAL HERNIAS

Inguinal hernias in adults should ideally be repaired by **herniorrhaphy**, although there is evidence that small,

Fig. 32.8 Strangulated inguinal hernia—case study

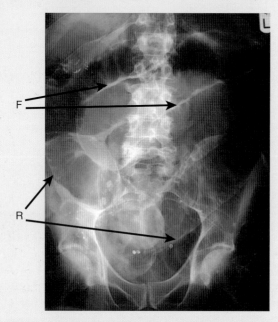

This 40-year-old man presented with symptoms and signs of distal small bowel obstruction evidently due to a strangulated inguinal hernia. At first, the abdomen, though distended and tympanitic, was not tender. However, during resuscitation, the abdomen became tender. This X-ray shows a clear outline of the outside of parts of the small bowel **R**, representing Rigler's sign. A false Rigler's sign is seen in other parts **F**; this is where two loops of thickened small bowel lie in contact.

Fig. 32.9 Inguino-scrotal hernia—case study

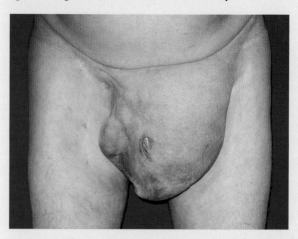

This man of 76 lived alone and only presented to a doctor when he had increasing difficulty controlling the direction of his micturition. His penis had disappeared altogether as the hernia had enlarged. The right testis is visible in the scrotum but the left side of the scrotum is filled with a large hernia. At operation, the abdominal wall defect was surprisingly small and was easily repaired by a standard method.

reducible direct hernias in older men can safely be left alone. Performing elective repair reasonably soon after diagnosis reduces the risk of strangulation and minimises stretching of the abdominal wall musculature.

Hernia operations are usually performed under general anaesthesia, although epidural or spinal anaesthesia may be used in patients with poor cardiovascular or respiratory function. Many surgeons favour repair under local anaesthesia for most cases; certainly if age or infirmity makes anaesthesia hazardous, this is a safe option. With time, an enlarging hernia may become **irreducible**. Urgent operation is not essential provided there are no symptoms attributable to the hernia. Some patients give a history of episodes in which the hernia becomes temporarily irreducible. These episodes may be accompanied by local pain and tenderness or even symptoms of bowel obstruction (vomiting, colicky abdominal pain, distension and absolute constipation). These warning episodes should be taken as an indication for early operation. More severe and prolonged symptoms of this nature usually precipitate emergency admission to hospital, in which case strangulation must be assumed to be the diagnosis (the expression strangulation prompts rapid action!) and

operation performed urgently, preferably within 4 hours to maximise the chance of saving ischaemic bowel.

Very large 'wheelbarrow' hernias are invariably of long standing and are found mainly in elderly men (see Fig. 32.9). They only present when size becomes a handicap, if bowel strangulates within the hernia or if the anatomical distortion interferes with micturition. Bowel adhesions may make operation difficult and postoperative wound infections are common. Despite this, surgery for strangulation cannot be avoided. If the hernia is not strangulated, a bag truss (see later) to support the hernia may be an appropriate treatment.

Inguinal herniorrhaphy and herniotomy

Until recently, the standard open techniques of herniorrhaphy were mostly based on Bassini's 19th century extraperitoneal approach. Many variations have been described but all remove the peritoneal sac or reduce it into the abdomen and then employ non-absorbable sutures or mesh to repair the abdominal wall. Success with these methods of herniorrhaphy is undoubtedly operator-dependent and, in competent hands, most standard techniques give satisfactory results and reasonably low recurrence rates. The lowest reported recurrence rates of this type of repair, around 2.5% at 10 years, were from the Shouldice hernia clinic in Canada using the **Shouldice** variation of a Bassini repair, but the technique is difficult to learn and recovery is both painful and prolonged.

In recent years, the **Lichtenstein** technique has overshadowed the various Bassini and other techniques and

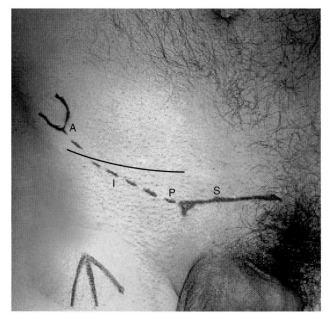

(a)

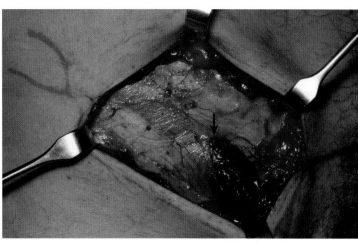

(b)

(a) Skin markings demonstrating the upper border of the pubic arch **S**, the anterior superior iliac spine **A**, the pubic tubercle **P** and the inguinal ligament **I**. Note the side of the planned operation has been marked with an arrow on the thigh to ensure the correct side is operated upon. The line of incision is shown as a solid line.

(b) The dissection down to the external oblique aponeurosis. The external (superficial) ring is arrowed.

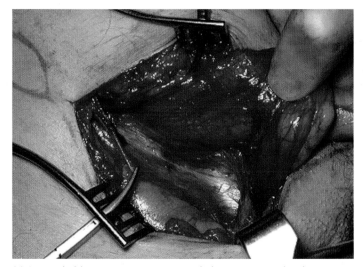

(c)

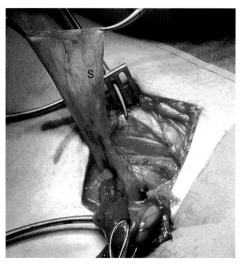

(d)

(c) External oblique aponeurosis opened, demonstrating the shiny inguinal ligament, which is its inturned lower edge.

(d) The indirect hernia sac **S** dissected out from the spermatic cord and held upwards before ligation and excision. The inferior epigastric artery and vein lie at the medial border of the deep inguinal ring.

Fig. 32.10 Technique of mesh hernia repair (continued on next page)

has widely become the preferred standard operation. This operation is similar to the Bassini up to the point of repair. It then employs a **no tension** technique, using a patch of non-absorbable open-weave **mesh** to repair and reinforce the defect rather than suturing muscle and fascial layers together under tension. Figure 32.10 shows the principles of the Lichtenstein mesh type of inguinal hernia repair.

The mesh technique has several distinct advantages:

- The technique is easily learned and trainee surgeons can reliably produce good results
- Postoperative pain is substantially less, allowing increased mobility and early return to normal activities such as work and driving
- Recurrence rates appear to be exceptionally low

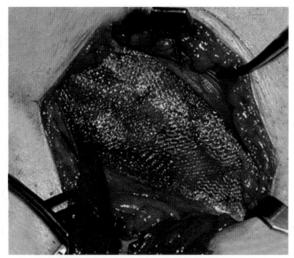

(e)

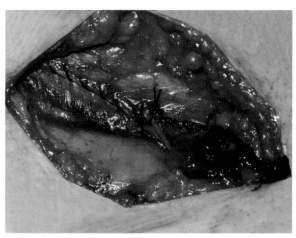

(f)

(f) External oblique closed to recreate the inguinal canal before skin closure.

(e) Polypropylene mesh is cut to shape before insertion and sutured in place along the inguinal ligament and, in this case, tacked to the surface of the internal oblique with 'starry sky' sutures.

Fig. 32.10 Technique of mesh hernia repair—cont'd

Having a foreign body implanted might be expected to increase the risk of infection but in practice it is exceptionally rare.

In infants, the patent processus vaginalis is merely ligated and excised (**herniotomy**); formal repair of the abdominal wall defect is usually unnecessary. If the defect is enormous, a single stitch should be used on the medial side to narrow the deep ring.

Complications

Early complications of herniorrhaphy include scrotal haematoma or wound infection. Most surgeons employ prophylactic antibiotics for mesh repairs but there is little solid evidence of benefit. Late complications include recurrence (see below), chronic **groin pain** due to inadvertent trapping of the ilio-inguinal or another nerve in the repair, and **testicular atrophy** caused by inadvertent damage to the testicular artery, usually with diathermy, or overtightening of the deep ring. Testicular atrophy is a particular problem with recurrent hernias. In patients with obstructed and strangulated hernias, the first step towards minimising complications is to ensure that the patient is fully resuscitated; more patients die of fluid and electrolyte problems than of delaying an operation by a few hours.

Recurrence

Inguinal hernias recur in 2–25% of cases over a lifetime. The rate is greatly increased when inadequate attention has been given to operative principles. Operations for recurrent hernia are often more difficult and have a higher potential for complications (including further recurrence) than a primary repair. Recurrence is an important problem that has been addressed by improved techniques that have substantially reduced recurrence rates.

The causes of inguinal hernia recurrence include:

- Inappropriate technique—Bassini type repairs have as much as a 25% recurrence rate in the long term
- Operator inexperience—Shouldice and laparoscopic repairs have a long learning curve
- Technical failure—failure to recognise and remove an indirect sac at operation; insufficient coverage of the defect; suture or mesh failure
- Missed diagnosis of a concomitant femoral hernia
- Inherently poor musculature, chronic cough, urinary obstruction, constipation or resumption of heavy work too soon after repair may be a factor in some recurrences. It is important to screen for underlying problems and address them before hernia surgery

Laparoscopic inguinal hernia repair

Laparoscopic repair of inguinal hernias by a transperitoneal or retroperitoneal route is becoming popular. It offers less postoperative pain and a slightly quicker return to normal activities but has a slightly higher risk of major complications compared to open techniques for primary hernia repair. The method is recommended for repair of recurrent hernias, having the advantage of allowing the mesh to be placed in virgin territory, and also for bilateral repair, when both sides can be repaired through the same

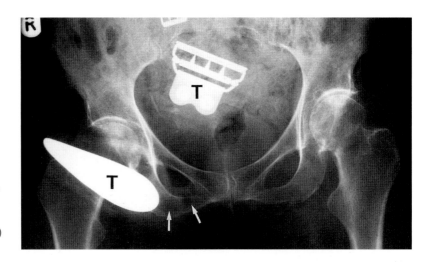

Fig. 32.11 Truss with unreduced inguinal hernia
X-ray of the pelvis in an 82-year-old woman following a fall causing a fractured neck of the left femur. She happened to be wearing a truss **T** for a longstanding, large right inguinal hernia. This was not kept reduced by the truss as indicated by the presence of bowel gas (arrowed) in the inguinal area.

three small incisions. There is a long learning curve for laparoscopic repair and the recurrence rate may be slightly higher than the Lichtenstein technique. Laparoscopic repair is described in Chapter 11.

Postoperative care and return to normal activities

Most inguinal hernias are now repaired on a day case basis although some patients stay in hospital overnight to allow early recovery under controlled conditions.

During the first postoperative week, patients should avoid activities likely to strain the repair, such as heavy lifting or driving a car. Over the next 2 or 3 weeks, they should gradually return to normal activity, including usual sexual activity. Time to return to work depends on the physical nature of the job and whether activities cause pain, but usually varies from 2 to 4 weeks.

Trusses (see Fig. 32.11)

A **truss** may be used to control certain types of hernia when surgery is inappropriate or unacceptable to the patient. Pressure trusses made of padded webbing have superseded various spring contraptions, but can be safely used only if the hernia is easily reducible and can be kept reduced and free of symptoms. For very large hernias which cannot be reduced, a 'bag truss' can be used to support the hernia. Most trusses are ill-fitting and ineffective and are better avoided if possible.

FEMORAL HERNIA

A femoral hernia is formed by a protrusion of peritoneum into the potential space of the femoral canal. The sac may contain abdominal viscera (usually small bowel) or omentum. Forty percent of femoral hernias present with strangulation. The incidence is higher in women (Figs 32.5 and 32.12) and increases with age. It is likely

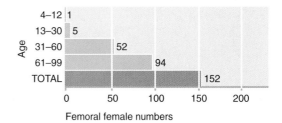

Fig. 32.12 Annual incidence of femoral hernias in females by age in East Anglia

that the portal of the femoral canal is larger in women, possibly as a result of a smaller muscle bulk of iliopsoas and pectineus. Increased intra-abdominal pressure and other factors related to pregnancy may also be important in females since the incidence of femoral hernia is higher in parous than nulliparous women. In both sexes, femoral hernia is assumed to be acquired; no evidence of a congenital sac has ever been found. Thus, femoral hernias, unlike inguinal hernias, are rare in children.

CLINICAL FEATURES OF FEMORAL HERNIA

The anatomy of the femoral canal is shown in Figure 32.1b, page 470. A femoral hernia is usually small, appearing as a lump immediately below the inguinal ligament and just lateral to its medial attachment to the pubic tubercle. Since the femoral canal is narrow, a cough impulse can rarely be detected, and the hernia is usually irreducible. Thus, small femoral hernias may be difficult to distinguish from other lumps arising in the femoral canal such as a lipoma or enlarged Cloquet's lymph node. However, a hernia is deeply fixed whereas the others tend to be more mobile. Note that 40% of femoral hernias present as emergencies with strangulation.

Fig. 32.13 Richter's hernia—case study

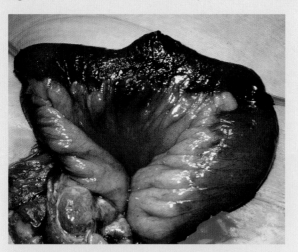

This 71-year-old woman presented with symptoms and signs of incomplete small bowel obstruction; these included vomiting, abdominal distension and colicky abdominal pain, but she continued to pass flatus. She had a 2 cm femoral hernia which was not tender. At operation, only a part of the wall of the ileum was trapped in the hernia. The photograph shows bruising around the area trapped in the hernia. Luckily, the bowel was viable and did not need resection. The hernia was repaired before closure.

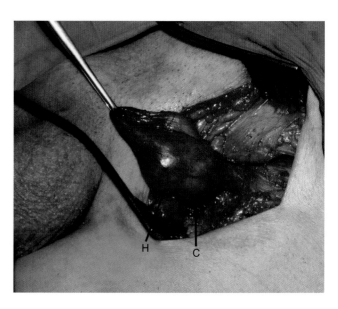

(a)

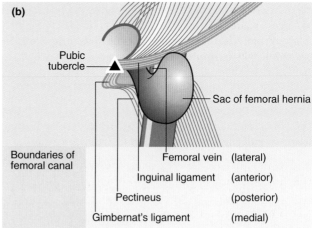

Pubic tubercle

Sac of femoral hernia

Boundaries of femoral canal

Femoral vein (lateral)

Inguinal ligament (anterior)

Pectineus (posterior)

Gimbernat's ligament (medial)

Fig. 32.14 Femoral hernia
(a) An average-sized femoral hernia **H** at operation. The patient's genitalia are to the left of the photograph. The line of the inguinal ligament is marked with an interrupted line and the opening of the femoral canal is seen at **C**. **(b)** The four margins of the femoral canal.

Strangulated femoral hernia

In contrast to strangulated inguinal hernia, there are often no obvious localising symptoms and signs in strangulated femoral hernia, and the classic presenting features are those of distal small bowel obstruction. The diagnosis of strangulated femoral hernia is easily missed unless the femoral region is carefully examined for a lump.

In nearly 30% of strangulated femoral hernias, only a portion of the bowel circumference is trapped in the hernial sac. Although the bowel lumen remains patent and the patient continues to pass flatus, peristalsis is sufficiently disrupted for other signs of obstruction to occur, notably vomiting. This is known as **Richter's hernia** (see Fig. 32.13). Resuscitation and urgent operation are required as for completely strangulated hernias.

MANAGEMENT OF FEMORAL HERNIA

The abdominal orifice of the femoral canal is small and indistensible. Consequently, abdominal contents finding their way into the canal strangulate much more readily than they do in inguinal hernias. Thus, all femoral hernias, even if asymptomatic, should be repaired without delay. Use of a truss is pointless as these hernias are not reducible.

Elective repair is performed by first isolating, emptying and excising the peritoneal sac (see Fig. 32.14). The femoral canal is then closed with a non-absorbable plug or sutures placed between pectineus fascia and inguinal ligament. The canal can be exposed by several different methods. The most common are the **femoral** or low approach, the **Lotheissen** or high approach, via the posterior wall of the inguinal canal, and the **McEvedy** or pararectus extraperitoneal approach. The last is virtually a laparotomy and is rarely employed. Occasionally a femoral hernia containing bowel cannot be safely reduced via a local approach, or bowel of doubtful viability escapes back into the abdominal cavity. In either case, a laparotomy incision is required in addition.

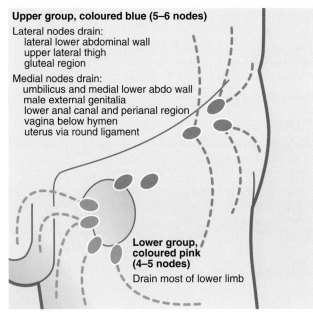

Upper group, coloured blue (5–6 nodes)

Lateral nodes drain:
  lateral lower abdominal wall
  upper lateral thigh
  gluteal region

Medial nodes drain:
  umbilicus and medial lower abdo wall
  male external genitalia
  lower anal canal and perianal region
  vagina below hymen
  uterus via round ligament

Lower group, coloured pink (4–5 nodes)
Drain most of lower limb

Fig. 32.15 Superficial inguinal lymph nodes of the groin
The lower group lie around the termination of the long saphenous vein. Both upper and lower groups drain to the external iliac nodes.

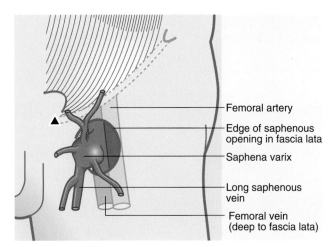

Femoral artery
Edge of saphenous opening in fascia lata
Saphena varix
Long saphenous vein
Femoral vein (deep to fascia lata)

Fig. 32.16 Saphena varix

ENLARGED INGUINAL LYMPH NODES

The lymph nodes of the inguinal region are clustered into the three anatomical groups shown in Figure 32.15. These drain the lower abdominal wall and lower back, perineum (including vulva and vagina), anal canal, penis and scrotal skin and the whole lower limb. The testes are derived from the retroperitoneal area and hence drain to the upper para-aortic nodes within the abdomen rather than inguinal nodes.

Inguinal lymph nodes may become secondarily enlarged as a result of local disease in their field of drainage. Examples include infections of the foot, skin diseases, sexually transmitted infection or tumours. Inguinal lymph node enlargement may also be part of a generalised lymphadenopathy in lymphoma or a systemic infection such as glandular fever or AIDS. Inguinal nodes may also become involved in tuberculosis. Multiple small firm ('shotty') nodes are commonly found, especially in men, and are accepted as normal if less than 1 cm in diameter. These nodes probably result from minor infections of the lower limb, and are easily palpable in males because males tend to have less subcutaneous fat.

CLINICAL FEATURES OF ENLARGED INGUINAL LYMPH NODES

Enlarged inguinal lymph nodes present with pain or with a lump in the groin but are often discovered incidentally. When they are small, it can be difficult to determine clinically whether nodes are abnormal. Enlarged lymph nodes are recognised by their anatomical position and by excluding hernias or vascular abnormalities. Enlarged nodes are usually mobile but become fixed to the surrounding tissues when infiltrated by tumour. If doubt exists as to whether the nodes are enlarged, ultrasound scanning will usually give a definitive answer and can be used to guide percutaneous needle biopsy. In general, nodes smaller than 1 cm are unlikely to be malignant.

If enlarged and fixed inguinal lymph nodes are confirmed, the history may need to be reviewed for clues as to the origin. A history of systemic manifestations of lymphoma, TB or acquired immunodeficiency syndrome (AIDS) should be sought. These include malaise, periodic fevers and weight loss. There may be a history of a 'mole' or 'wart' having been removed, even many years before. If this was a malignant melanoma or squamous carcinoma, it could now have metastasised. Other symptoms of tumours that metastasise to inguinal lymph nodes should be sought; for example, anal pain or bleeding might indicate an anal carcinoma, and an unretractable foreskin may hide a penile carcinoma.

The examination should include palpating lymph nodes in the neck and axillae, and palpating the liver and spleen. The skin of the whole drainage field should be examined closely, paying particular attention to the back, perineum and feet, including between the toes and beneath the toenails. The examination may reveal infection, squamous cell carcinoma or malignant melanoma. Rectal examination is mandatory to exclude anal carcinoma. A blood test for human immunodeficiency virus (HIV) may be indicated.

If enlarged lymph nodes cannot be explained by simple local factors or a systemic illness, nodes should be sampled for histological examination. If metastatic malignancy is suspected, fine needle aspiration or needle core biopsy is appropriate, but if lymphoma is likely, a node should be

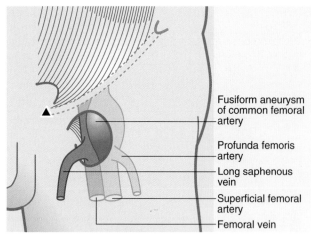

Fusiform aneurysm of common femoral artery

Profunda femoris artery

Long saphenous vein

Superficial femoral artery

Femoral vein

Fig. 32.17 Femoral artery aneurysm

surgically removed or be subject to an open biopsy to obtain substantial tissue for histological typing. Sometimes, histology shows only non-specific reactive changes. The patient usually recovers fully and a diagnosis is never made.

SAPHENA VARIX

A saphena varix is a dilatation of the long saphenous vein in the groin, just proximal to its junction with the femoral vein (see Fig. 32.16). The varix is caused by valvular incompetence at this point; there are usually substantial varicose veins elsewhere in the long saphenous system.

The varix can reach the size of a golf ball or even larger. On examination, the swelling is soft and diffuse. The diagnostic feature is that it empties with minimal pressure and refills on release ('the sign of emptying'). A cough impulse is invariably present. If these physical signs are not sought and the patient is only examined standing, the varix can be mistaken for a solid mass.

Treatment is high saphenous ligation, as for saphenofemoral reflux associated with varicose veins (see Ch. 43).

FEMORAL ARTERY ANEURYSM

Femoral aneurysms are uncommon as a cause of lumps in the groin. They may occur as part of a generalised aneurysmal disease involving the abdominal aorta, iliac and lower limb arterial system but can also occur in isolation. Diagnosis is made on clinical examination; the lump lies below the midpoint of the inguinal ligament (see Fig. 32.17) and has a characteristic expansile pulsation. Distinguishing an aneurysm from a femoral hernia is clearly vitally important. The management of aneurysms is discussed in Chapter 42.

GROIN PAIN

ACUTE PAIN

Conditions causing acute groin pain are strangulated inguinal or femoral hernias; conditions causing scrotal pain are listed in Box 33.1 (p. 488). 'Groin strain' is a difficult entity to understand and often seems to affect professional sports people. It starts acutely but often becomes chronic; the diagnosis is one of exclusion. A newly-appeared inguinal hernia may cause groin pain, often on sitting, yet be too small to detect clinically. Unfortunately, there is no dependable test for an early hernia other than laparoscopy, although ultrasound in experienced hands is fairly reliable.

CHRONIC PAIN

Chronic pain in the groin that occurs without any clues in the history and without swelling is difficult to diagnose and treat. Groin pain may be caused by **inflamed inguinal lymph nodes** secondary to infection in their field of drainage. **Strained muscle attachments** to the bony pelvis sometimes cause groin pain; this particularly affects the hip adductor attachments near the pubic tubercle and usually follows extreme physical activity. Groin pain may also be **referred** from a diseased hip joint. An early **inguinal hernia** sometimes causes groin pain before the hernia becomes clinically detectable.

VENTRAL HERNIAS

Ventral hernias include epigastric, umbilical and paraumbilical hernias. Ventral incisional hernias occurring through previous surgical or traumatic wounds are considered in Chapter 12.

EPIGASTRIC HERNIAS (see Fig. 32.18)

These are herniations through defects in the linea alba, anywhere between xiphoid process and umbilicus. They are four times more common in males and are often tiny, with a defect less than 0.5 cm. Most are symptomless but the presence of a lump and sometimes episodic sharp pain on exertion are the presenting complaints. Treatment is by direct suture repair if the hernia is small. Larger hernias may require a tension-free mesh repair.

UMBILICAL AND PARAUMBILICAL HERNIAS

Umbilical hernias in infants and children are discussed in Chapter 51. **Paraumbilical hernias** are acquired rather than congenital. They occur in all age groups but are five times more common in females. The abdominal wall defect is in the linea alba, generally above the umbilical cicatrix. The swelling often lies above the umbilicus, with

Fig. 32.18 Epigastric hernia
This man of 28 had an unusually large epigastric hernia that caused pain on exercise. It was situated in the midline, midway between the xiphisternum and the umbilicus.

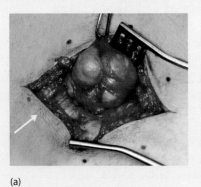 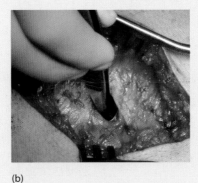 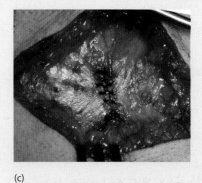

(a)

(b)

(c)

(a) 'Mushroom-like' epigastric hernia mass protruding through the linea alba (fibres indicated by arrow).

(b) Relatively small defect in linea alba after mobilising and reducing the hernia.

(c) After edge-to-edge repair of defect using continuous non-absorbable nylon suture.

the umbilicus itself covering the lower part of it. These hernias become progressively bigger and have a tendency to strangulation. Surgical repair is the treatment of choice.

Umbilical hernias in adults are the third most common abdominal hernia after inguinal and femoral hernias. They occur more commonly in females, and obesity and poor muscle tone are predisposing factors. The hernias range from asymptomatic small protrusions, through larger, occasionally painful lumps, to very large, irreducible and intermittently painful swellings. Strangulation is constantly a risk and most cases are best offered surgical repair; this is by direct suture or the use of prosthetic mesh for large defects.

33 Disorders of the male genitalia

DISORDERS OF THE SCROTAL CONTENTS

INTRODUCTION

Abnormalities of the scrotal contents include disorders of any of the normal scrotal contents (i.e. the testis and its coverings) and the spermatic cord as well as inguino-scrotal hernias (see Ch. 32). Distinguishing between them is usually a matter of simple clinical examination. The diagnosis that must not be missed is the testicular tumour. Other problems include inflammation, hydro-coeles and cysts, maldescent or torsion of the testis and testicular trauma, as well as varicocoele. Male sterilisation is also covered in this chapter. Disorders of the female genitalia are usually seen by gynaecologists and are not covered here.

CLINICAL EXAMINATION OF SCROTAL LUMPS AND SWELLINGS

A lump or swelling in the scrotum may be:

- A solid or cystic mass arising from one of the components of the scrotal contents or spermatic cord. These anatomical structures include testis, epididymis, epididymal appendage, vas deferens and pampiniform venous plexus
- A collection of fluid in the tunica or processus vaginalis (**hydrocoele**)
- An inguinal hernia extending along the embryological path of testicular descent

The important disorders of the scrotum and its contents are summarised in Table 33.1, together with their ana-tomical and clinical significance.

The origin of a scrotal lump

The first clinical objective is to determine whether the swelling arises in the groin, in the spermatic cord itself or in the scrotum. This is achieved by palpating the sper-matic cord at the neck of the scrotum. In the case of a hernia, the spermatic cord is much greater in diameter than normal and the hernia can be shown to communi-cate with the abdominal cavity by the presence of an impulse on coughing or by reducing the hernia. Sper-matic cord swellings (varicocoele or cyst) are usually easy to recognise. If the lump is purely scrotal, the spermatic cord is normal in diameter.

Testicular and epididymal lumps

When the abnormality is scrotal, an attempt should be made to palpate the testis and epididymis separately, and to find their relationship to the lump. If the testis is enlarged or there is a lump within it, this must be regarded as a primary tumour until proven otherwise. Testicular swellings due to lymphoma, leukaemia or granulomatous infections (e.g. tuberculosis or syphilitic gumma) tend to be softer but this is an unreliable sign. Any testicular pathology may cause a little fluid to accumulate in the

Table 33.1 Summary of disorders of the scrotum and its contents and their clinical features

Disorder	Anatomical/developmental basis	Clinical features
1. TESTICULAR DISORDERS		
a. Incompletely descended testis (see also Ch. 51)	Failure of complete descent from retroperitoneal site into scrotum; testis may be arrested at any point of descent or in an ectopic site	Mainly a problem of infancy and childhood and requiring orchidopexy; possible cause of lump in groin; predisposition to malignancy; fertility may be impaired
b. Torsion of testis	Rotation of testis in scrotum; twisting of the spermatic cord results in venous obstruction which may culminate in infarction; recurrent incomplete torsion may occur	Complete torsion causes severe acute scrotal pain (and sometimes abdominal pain); partial torsion may cause episodic pain
c. Inflammation of epididymis or testis	'Epididymo-orchitis' is a term often used incorrectly for acute epididymitis. Usually caused by common urinary tract pathogens or sexually transmitted organisms Acute orchitis is often viral (mumps) Chronic orchitis may be caused by tuberculosis or syphilitic gumma	Acute epididymitis is painful; must be distinguished from testicular torsion; usually associated with UTI Testicular pain and swelling Usually presents as painless testicular enlargement
d. Malignant testicular tumours	Derived from germ cells of testis; metastasise via lymphatics to para-iliac and para-aortic nodes or via bloodstream, commonly to lung	Present as painless swelling of testis usually with small secondary hydrocoele
2. DISORDERS OF OTHER SCROTAL CONTENTS		
a. Hydrocoele	Abnormal collection of fluid in space around testis; in children may still be in communication with peritoneal cavity (communicating hydrocoele)	Presents as a painless scrotal swelling which transilluminates; testis may be difficult to palpate within it until fluid is drained
b. Haematocoele	Collection of blood around testis; usually early result of trauma or surgery	Presents like a hydrocoele after trauma but does not transilluminate
c. Varicocoele	Dilatation of pampiniform venous plexus of spermatic cord	Presents as a scrotal swelling separate from testis and epididymis; feels like a 'bag of worms'; disappears on lying down, thus patient must be examined standing
d. Epididymal cyst and spermatocoele	Cysts derived from epididymal tissue	Epididymal cyst presents as a scrotal swelling which transilluminates; separate from the testis, often multiloculated Spermatocoele is unilocular, sometimes bilateral, in cord or epididymis and may be transilluminable
e. Torsion of hydatid of Morgagni	Torsion of epididymal appendage	Occurs in children; may present late as a small hydrocoele; in the acute phase, presents as scrotal pain and oedema and may simulate testicular torsion

tunica vaginalis resulting in a small **secondary hydrocoele**. This rarely interferes with testicular palpation.

Lumps in the epididymis (cysts, chronic epididymitis or, rarely, tuberculous granulomata) are discrete from but attached to an otherwise normal testis. Tiny focal lumps in the epididymis are rarely clinically important. Infective lesions cause diffuse and usually painful thickening of the epididymis, whereas epididymal cysts are almost always located at the upper pole. Epididymal cysts are filled with clear fluid and therefore transilluminate. **Transillumination** (Fig. 33.3) is demonstrated by shining a strong beam of light from a torch or fibreoptic cable through the scrotum in a partly darkened room. If the lesion is fluid-filled, it will glow (except in the case of blood). About 10% of cysts in the epididymis, and most of those in the cord, are filled with an opalescent fluid containing spermatozoa. These **spermatocoeles** also sometimes transilluminate brilliantly.

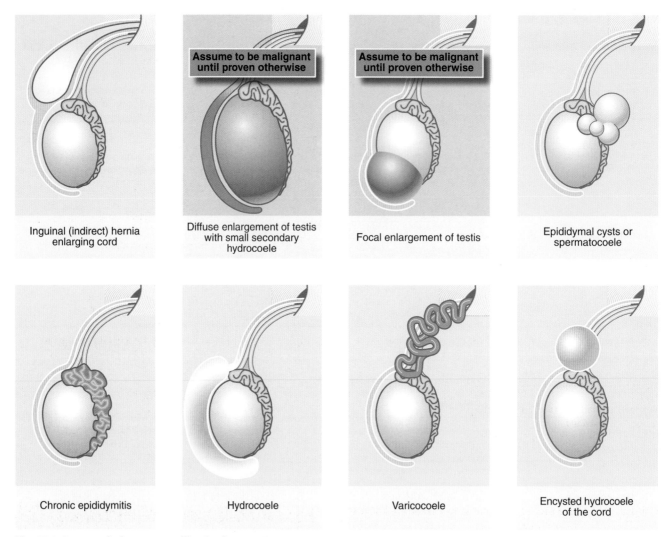

Inguinal (indirect) hernia enlarging cord

Assume to be malignant until proven otherwise

Diffuse enlargement of testis with small secondary hydrocoele

Assume to be malignant until proven otherwise

Focal enlargement of testis

Epididymal cysts or spermatocoele

Chronic epididymitis

Hydrocoele

Varicocoele

Encysted hydrocoele of the cord

Fig. 33.1 Causes of a lump or swelling in the scrotum

Other scrotal lumps and swellings

Slow accumulation of fluid within the tunica vaginalis produces a **primary hydrocoele** surrounding the testis. These are common in the elderly and are often ignored by the patient until they become very large (300 ml or more) because they do not cause pain. The testis is not palpable separately from the swelling but occasionally the hydrocoele is lax enough to allow the testis to be palpated through it; more often the hydrocoele is too tense for this. Diagnosis is confirmed if the swelling transilluminates.

In young boys, the tunica vaginalis may sometimes remain in continuity with the peritoneal cavity via a **patent processus vaginalis**. This is so narrow that herniation does not occur but it allows peritoneal fluid to accumulate by gravity during the day. This causes a scrotal swelling which may disappear overnight, and is known as a **communicating hydrocoele**.

Abnormalities of the spermatic cord are usually varicocoeles or cysts. **Varicocoeles** are common, often asymptomatic, and represent dilatation of the venous network

making up the pampiniform plexus. They feel like a 'bag of worms' on palpation and disappear in the supine position. **Cysts of the cord** are usually small, spherical and transilluminable. They represent either an **encysted hydrocoele** arising from a remnant of the processus vaginalis or a **spermatocoele**.

SCROTAL PAIN

ACUTE PAIN

If there is acute scrotal pain, **testicular torsion** must always be excluded clinically since the torted testis can be saved if operation is performed promptly; an exploratory operation is mandatory if torsion of the testis cannot be confidently excluded. Torsion occurs mainly in adolescents but occasionally in young adults. The main differential diagnosis at all ages is acute bacterial epididymitis. Torsion of an epididymal appendage (hydatid of Morgagni) produces symptoms similar to testicular torsion in

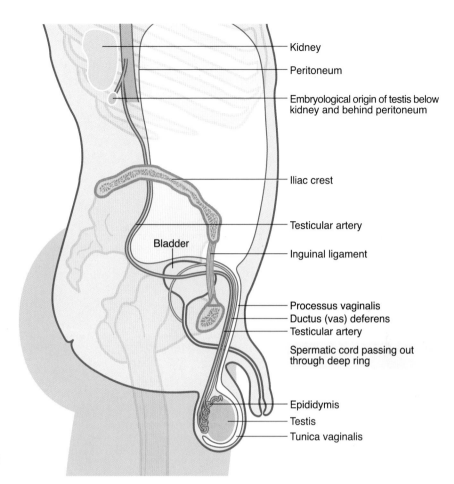

Kidney

Peritoneum

Embryological origin of testis below kidney and behind peritoneum

Iliac crest

Testicular artery

Bladder

Inguinal ligament

Processus vaginalis
Ductus (vas) deferens
Testicular artery

Spermatic cord passing out through deep ring

Epididymis
Testis
Tunica vaginalis

Fig. 33.2 Embryological descent of the testis
The testicular artery marks the line of descent of testis towards the scrotum. In the embryo, the arterial supply is direct from the aorta and this persists even when the testis has reached the scrotum.

children but these are less severe; surgical exploration is usually still required to exclude it. A traumatic haematocoele is also associated with acute pain but the trauma or surgery that preceded it will point to the likely diagnosis.

CHRONIC PAIN

Chronic scrotal pain is most often due to **inflammation**. It can often be traced back to a vasectomy, although the precise cause is often obscure and the treatment often ineffective. Patients present weeks or months after the operation, complaining of localised tenderness at the operation site or a general ache in one side of the scrotum. If there is a small tender lump due to a stitch granuloma, this is usually cured by excision.

Pain is also a feature of chronic bacterial epididymitis, which usually follows an acute episode.

Recurrent, incomplete **testicular torsion** may cause transient episodes of severe pain in the inguino-scrotal region or poorly defined lower abdominal pain. In these cases, the anatomical relationship of the testis to the tunica vaginalis is often abnormal so the testes lie **horizontally** rather than vertically when the patient is standing. These 'bell-clapper' testes are susceptible to torsion.

INFLAMMATION OF THE EPIDIDYMIS AND TESTIS

EPIDIDYMITIS

The most common inflammatory disorder of the scrotal contents is bacterial epididymitis. This is usually secondary to a urethral infection that has been conducted proximally via the vas deferens. The primary infection is either a urinary tract infection with coliforms (in the 50–65 age group) or a sexually transmitted infection with *Chlamydia* or *Neisseria gonorrhoeae* (common in the 15–30 age group). Epididymitis is often incorrectly referred to as orchitis or epididymo-orchitis. The testis is rarely infected, although the surrounding inflammation may cause testicular tenderness. The differential diagnosis includes sperm leakage following vasectomy causing a **sperm granuloma**, and **vasitis nodosa**. Vasitis nodosa is an uncommon nodular lesion of the vas deferens, usually following vasectomy or sometimes prostatectomy or herniorrhaphy.

Epididymitis is painful and usually begins acutely. It may present as a surgical emergency and be clinically indistinguishable from testicular torsion. On examination of a patient with acute epididymitis, the affected side of the scrotum and its contents are swollen, oedematous

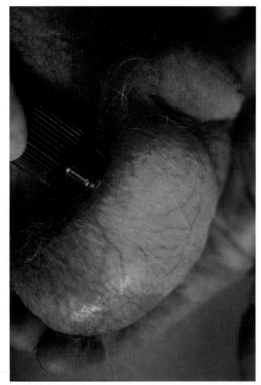

Fig. 33.3 Transillumination of a scrotal cyst
This 30-year-old man complained of a swelling in the right scrotum. On clinical examination there is a 3 cm soft rounded swelling at the upper pole of the epididymis. A confident diagnosis of epididymal cyst can thus be made.

Box 33.1 Common causes of acute pain in the scrotum

Torsion of the testis
- Sudden onset of unilateral scrotal pain with or without poorly localised abdominal pain
- In early cases, the testis is high in the scrotum and exquisitely tender, and the cord is thickened; later these signs are often obscured by oedema
- The opposite testis may lie horizontally (bell-clapper testis)

Torsion of the epididymal appendage (hydatid of Morgagni)
- Nearly always in children
- Sudden onset of unilateral scrotal pain; the testis hangs normally. There is a tenderness only at its upper pole and minimal overlying oedema

Acute epididymitis
- Moderate or severe scrotal pain and tenderness with marked redness and oedema
- Often preceded by symptoms of urinary tract infection; urine usually contains white cells, nitrites and organisms

Haematocoele following trauma or scrotal surgery (e.g. vasectomy)
- History may be diagnostic although torsion is sometimes precipitated by trauma

---

and tender, and the scrotal skin is red and warm. It may be difficult to palpate the testis and epididymis separately once the infection has become established. Epididymitis must never be diagnosed in a boy under 15 in the absence of urinary symptoms or a proven urinary infection or urethritis. Such an 'acute scrotum' must be explored to exclude torsion (see p. 486).

Treatment of acute epididymitis is initially with bed rest for pain relief and at least 1 month of an appropriate broad-spectrum antibiotic. The infecting organism is often not identified but attempts should be made to pin it down using urine cultures, blood cultures or culture of urethral discharge after prostatic massage. Ofloxacin is often favoured on a 'best-guess' basis as it covers both *Chlamydia* and Gram-negative organisms. This antibiotic is continued if culture confirms sensitivity of the organisms.

Persistent or chronic epididymitis may cause the patient to suffer chronic scrotal tenderness. Chronic epididymitis may also result from inadequate antibiotic treatment of an acute episode.

Tuberculous epididymitis

Tuberculosis may involve the epididymis via bloodstream spread from a pulmonary focus. A tuberculous urinary tract infection can spread to the epididymis, with epididymal swelling as the presenting complaint. Typically, the whole length of the epididymis is thickened, non-tender and 'cold'. In contrast to bacterial epididymitis, the epididymis can be readily distinguished from the testis on palpation. If untreated, the testis may also become involved.

Diagnosis requires the analysis of serial early morning urine specimens (EMUs) for mycobacteria or, more reliably, histological examination of percutaneous needle biopsies. If tuberculosis is confirmed, a search must be made for pulmonary and urinary tract disease (see Ch. 38).

ORCHITIS

Primary bacterial orchitis is rare and may result from pyogenic infection in the genital tract or elsewhere in the body. **Tertiary gummatous syphilis** may involve the testis, producing diffuse non-tender enlargement. This is now extremely rare and there is usually a history of primary and secondary lesions. Sometimes a gumma is found unexpectedly during investigation of a suspected testicular tumour.

Viral orchitis is most often caused by **mumps**. In post-pubertal males, bilateral mumps orchitis produces

Fig. 33.4 Testicular hydrocoele

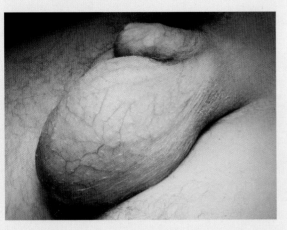

This man of 67 had a painless swelling of the left side of the scrotum for several years that was slowly enlarging. On examination, the swelling was confined to the scrotum and did not involve widening of the cord at the neck of the scrotum which might indicate a hernia. The testis was not palpable separately from the swelling, and the swelling transilluminated, confirming the diagnosis.

infertility in 50% of cases; elevated follicle-stimulating hormone (FSH) blood levels following orchitis usually indicate the patient is infertile. Mumps orchitis manifests 4–6 days after the onset of parotitis with extreme testicular tenderness and an inflammatory hydrocoele. Treatment is directed at symptomatic relief. Other viruses affecting the testis include Coxsackie, human immunodeficiency virus (HIV), Epstein–Barr, varicella and, in earlier times, smallpox.

HYDROCOELE

PRIMARY HYDROCOELE

A hydrocoele is an excessive collection of fluid within the tunica vaginalis, i.e. in the serous space surrounding the testis. Like the peritoneal cavity, the tunica vaginalis normally contains a small amount of serous fluid which is produced and reabsorbed at the same rate (Fig. 33.4).

In infants and children, a hydrocoele is usually an expression of a patent processus vaginalis (PPV). Provided there is no hernia present, hydrocoeles below the age of 1 year usually resolve spontaneously. For older children, ligation of the PPV is required.

Primary hydrocoeles may develop in adulthood, particularly in the elderly, by slow accumulation of serous fluid, presumably caused by impaired reabsorption. These hydrocoeles can reach a huge size, containing several hundred millilitres of fluid. The lesions are otherwise asymptomatic. The swelling is soft and non-tender on examination and the testis cannot usually be pal-

pated. The presence of fluid is demonstrated by transillumination.

Note that a secondary hydrocoele may develop in response to tumour or inflammation of the testis. In most cases, the hydrocoele is small and the testis can easily be palpated to reveal the primary abnormality.

Management

If a testicular tumour is a possibility, a hydrocoele must not be aspirated as malignant cells can be disseminated via the scrotal skin to its lymphatic field. If tumour cannot be excluded clinically, ultrasonography is indicated. Provided there is no suspicion of tumour, the hydrocoele can be **tapped**, i.e. aspirated with a needle and syringe. Clear straw-coloured fluid and a palpably normal testis confirm the diagnosis; otherwise surgical exploration of the testis is needed.

After aspiration of a primary hydrocoele, fluid reaccumulates over the following months and periodic aspiration or operation is needed. For younger patients, operation is usually preferred, whereas the elderly or unfit can have aspirations repeated whenever the hydrocoele becomes uncomfortably large. Sclerotherapy is an alternative; after aspiration, 6% aqueous phenol (10–20 ml) together with 1% lidocaine for analgesia can be injected and this often inhibits reaccumulation. Several treatments may be necessary.

HYDROCOELE OF THE CORD

Rarely, a hydrocoele develops in a remnant of the processus vaginalis somewhere along the course of the spermatic cord. This hydrocoele also transilluminates, and is known as an **encysted hydrocoele of the cord** (see Fig. 33.1). In females, a multicystic **hydrocoele of the canal of Nuck** sometimes presents as a swelling in the groin. It probably results from cystic degeneration of the round ligament.

FOURNIER'S SCROTAL GANGRENE

Occasionally, elderly men develop an acute unilateral infection within the tunica vaginalis which rapidly extends outwards to cause spreading gangrene of the scrotal skin (see Fig. 33.5). It is a form of **necrotising fasciitis** and does not involve the testes. There is often associated systemic sepsis. The underlying causes are varied and include pre-existing primary hydrocoele, genitourinary trauma, either accidental or iatrogenic, perirectal abscess and urethral stricture. Predisposing factors include diabetes mellitus, corticosteroids, chemotherapy and alcohol abuse. The infecting organism is principally an anaerobe but there is often synergistic aerobic infection. Treatment is urgent and includes intravenous antibiotics and surgical excision of all the necrotic tissue, with the wound being left open to heal by secondary intention.

Fig. 33.5 Fournier's scrotal gangrene

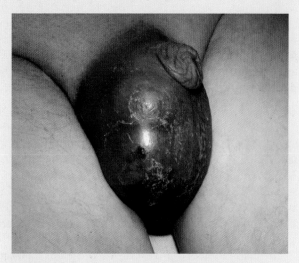

This 81-year-old man presented with scrotal pain and a rapidly rising temperature. The right side of the scrotum was red and oedematous on admission to hospital; within 2 hours, the black necrotic areas seen at the lower pole appeared and rapidly extended. He was treated with intravenous antibiotics and wide surgical excision to remove all necrotic tissue. The patient had a pre-existing hydrocoele. He recovered completely.

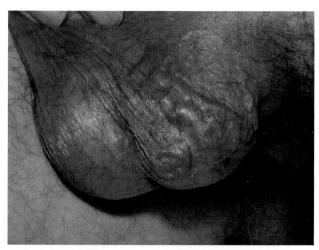

Fig. 33.6 Varicocoele
Note the 'bag of worms' appearance.

EPIDIDYMAL CYST AND SPERMATOCOELE

Multiple cysts may develop in the upper pole of the epididymis and present as a painless scrotal swelling (see Fig. 33.1). One cyst is usually larger than the others. Epididymal cysts affect a slightly younger age group than hydrocoeles. The testis can be palpated separately from the cysts, which lie near the upper pole of the testis. Epididymal cysts transilluminate.

Less common is the **spermatocoele**, a single cyst containing spermatozoa, which may be bilateral. Spermatocoeles usually occur in the head of the epididymis and may present like a third testis. They are clinically similar to epididymal cysts but may or may not transilluminate. Occasionally they occur in the spermatic cord. They probably arise from the **rete testis** (a plexus of spaces upon which the seminiferous tubules converge) and the 10–20 small ductuli efferentes connecting the rete testis to the epididymis; thus surgical excision may cause obstruction to the passage of sperm. If a patient wishes to remain fertile and the cysts are bilateral, excision may be contraindicated.

VARICOCOELE

A varicocoele (see Figs 33.1 and 33.6) represents dilatation and tortuosity of the veins of the pampiniform plexus of the spermatic vein in the spermatic cord. The cause is unknown, but since the condition is much more common on the left (90%), it may result from the different venous drainage on the two sides. On the left, the testicular vein drains into the high-pressure renal vein, whereas the right testicular vein drains directly into the inferior vena cava.

Varicocoele is common, affecting as many as 10% of young adult males. It is usually asymptomatic but is often discovered during general physical examination for infertility. Varicocoele increases scrotal temperature, which may inhibit normal sperm function and eventually cause testicular atrophy. In the supine position, the distended veins collapse and are impalpable. Varicocoele is best diagnosed if the patient is examined while standing, when the varicocoele feels like 'a bag of worms'.

Rarely, a varicocoele may be caused by obstruction of the left renal vein by an invading renal adenocarcinoma. Such varicocoeles do not collapse when the patient lies supine. If the history of varicocoele is short, particularly in the elderly, or if it is on the left side, then ultrasound investigation for renal adenocarcinoma may be appropriate.

In adults, surgical treatment of varicocoele is only indicated for the relief of pain or the treatment of low sperm count (oligospermia). In the child or adolescent, treatment is advised to preserve spermatogenesis. The treatment can be laparoscopic, clipping the veins where they lie posterior to the sigmoid colon, or open surgical ligation can be performed at or above the groin level. Embolisation of testicular veins can be performed percutaneously via the femoral vein; this may become the treatment of choice in the future.

TESTICULAR TUMOURS

Testicular tumours are relatively uncommon, making up about 1.5% of male cancers, but they are the most common cancer in men in their third and fourth decades. They are important because curative treatment is now available for most of them. The lymphatic drainage of the testis, and hence the route of lymphatic metastases, is to the intra-abdominal nodes and is determined by the embryology of testicular descent (see Fig. 33.2). Note that this is different from that of the scrotal skin, which drains towards the inguinal nodes.

About 1 new case of testicular malignancy occurs in 20 000 males per annum, and half already have metastases by the time of presentation. Undescended testes are at least 30 times more likely to become malignant, although the individual risk is still low. These tumours are usually seminomas.

More than 90% of primary testicular tumours are derived from **germ cells**, the rest being classified by the World Health Organization as **sex cord/gonadal stromal tumours** which includes Leydig, Sertoli and granulosa cell tumours. Germ cell tumours are categorised as **seminomas**, derived from spermatocytes, or **teratomas**, derived from multipotent germ cells. Strictly speaking, teratomas fall within the category of **non-seminomatous germ cell tumours** (NSGCTs), but teratomas make up the vast majority of this group, with the rest being a small number of undifferentiated embryonal cell carcinomas, choriocarcinomas or tumours of mixed cell type. Germ cell tumours of the testis are in general fast-growing, aggressive tumours that metastasise initially to intra-abdominal lymph nodes and subsequently via the bloodstream to the lungs.

Non-germ cell **Leydig cell tumours**, derived from the gonadal stroma, often present with excess hormone secretion rather than a testicular lump. This causes precocious puberty in a child and testicular feminisation in an adult.

The testes may also be secondarily involved in more widespread malignancy such as lymphoma, chronic lymphocytic leukaemia or, in children, acute lymphoblastic leukaemia. These rarely present as lumps in the testis but the surgeon may be asked to perform a testicular biopsy as part of the monitoring process.

PATHOLOGY OF TESTICULAR TUMOURS

Seminomas

Seminomas—derived from spermatocytes—make up more than half of malignant testicular tumours (Fig. 33.7). They occur mainly between the ages of 20 and 45 years with a peak incidence at 35 years. The cut surface of seminomas is typically pale, creamy-white and **homogeneous**. Histologically, the tumour cells are uniform and tightly packed. A distinct but rare form of seminoma, the **spermatocytic seminoma**, occurs between the ages of 50 and 70 years and almost never metastasises.

Teratomas

Teratomas are slightly less common than seminomas and their peak incidence is a decade earlier. Since they are derived from multipotent cells, teratomas may contain tissue from all three germ cell layers: ectoderm, mesoderm and endoderm. Teratomas exhibit a wide range of differentiation. Differentiated and intermediate tumours contain a collection of tissues resembling mature adult tissues: in particular, squamous epithelium (ectodermal), cartilage and smooth muscle (mesodermal), and respiratory epithelium (endodermal). Consequently, the cut surface of teratomas often appears **variegated**, with cystic areas and patches of necrosis and haemorrhage; this is easily distinguished from seminoma with the naked eye.

Undifferentiated germ cell tumours are regarded as variants of teratoma and are generally known as **non-seminomatous germ cell tumours**. In some of these tumours, described as **embryonal carcinomas** in the USA, no organoid elements are evident. Another variant contains tissues with malignant syncytiotrophoblastic and cytotrophoblastic features. These are known as **trophoblastic teratomas** or **choriocarcinoma**. Some germ cell tumours contain mixed cell types with areas of poorly differentiated teratoma and areas of seminoma, but one or other tumour type usually predominates. These mixed tumours behave as teratomas and should be treated as such.

Box 33.2 shows the current classification of primary malignant testicular tumours used in the UK. Other classifications are used in other countries. All classifications are frequently updated as new information emerges.

Fig. 33.7 Seminoma

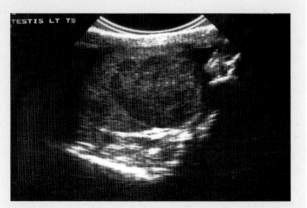

This ultrasound scan was performed on a 23-year-old man with a short history of an enlarged testis. There was no clinical sign of a hydrocoele. The scan shows a solid mass involving the whole testis with no evidence of fluid. The scan is fairly homogeneous, suggesting seminoma. Teratomas tend to be more variegated but a definitive diagnosis requires surgical exploration.

Box 33.2   Classification of malignant testicular tumours*

- Seminoma
- Differentiated teratoma (TD)
- Malignant teratoma intermediate (MTI)
- Malignant teratoma undifferentiated (MTU)—also known as embryonal tumour
- Subvariant: Malignant teratoma trophoblastic (MTT) also known as choriocarcinoma
- Yolk sac tumour

* Testicular Tumour Panel and Registry of the Pathological Society of Great Britain and Ireland. Unlike the WHO classification, this groups all non-seminomatous tumours under the heading of teratoma

---

CLINICAL FEATURES OF TESTICULAR TUMOURS

A malignant testicular tumour usually presents as a painless, progressively enlarging testicular lump. If the capsule becomes involved, a **secondary hydrocoele** may develop but this is usually small and does not hinder palpation of the lump.

Both seminoma and teratoma spread via lymphatics to para-aortic nodes at the level of L1/2. Spread is then proximally along the lymphatic chain and thoracic duct to the supraclavicular nodes and systemic circulation. Lung secondaries are particularly common in teratomas. Poorly differentiated testicular tumours metastasise early and may present as enlarged abdominal or cervical lymph nodes or with symptoms of lung metastases. The primary testicular lesion may be very small or even impalpable.

A solid testicular lump **must** be assumed to be a tumour until proven otherwise. The history is rarely helpful but may include an episode of trauma which merely drew attention to the lump. On examination, the testis is either diffusely enlarged or contains a discrete lump which is firm and non-tender. A small hydrocoele may be present. Systemic examination may reveal evidence of metastases. Malignant cervical nodes will be palpable but enlarged para-aortic nodes can rarely be palpated unless they are huge. Inguinal nodes are not involved unless the tumour has spread to the scrotal skin. This is rare except when biopsy or orchidectomy has been performed through a scrotal incision, which is bad surgical practice if malignancy is suspected.

INVESTIGATION AND TREATMENT OF TESTICULAR TUMOURS

The outlook for treated testicular tumours, even with metastases, is often good. Cure rates have improved dramatically over the past 30 years with the use of CT scanning and tumour markers for staging and monitoring the disease and with the evolution of scientifically based treatment protocols. Investigation and treatment usually take place in parallel. The aims are to confirm the diagnosis, to detect any metastases and stage the disease, and to treat according to the stage.

The first investigation is **ultrasonography** of the scrotal contents. If this confirms a solid testicular mass, direct surgical exploration will be required, as described on below. Preliminary staging investigations are usually performed beforehand, including **chest X-ray** or CT chest to look for hilar node involvement and lung secondaries (see Fig. 33.8), and blood levels of **tumour markers** (see below). Tumour markers are useful for tracking residual or recurrent tumour metastases because blood levels correlate closely with tumour bulk. A preoperative measurement is important as it may become negative later; serial postoperative measurements help monitor disease progress and the impact of therapy.

Tumour markers

Human chorionic gonadotrophin (beta-hCG) is secreted by syncytiotrophoblastic cells and levels may rise in any tumour type, particularly poorly differentiated germ cell tumours. **Alpha-fetoprotein** (AFP) is produced by yolk sac elements. About 75% of patients with metastatic teratoma have elevated AFP levels but this marker is not expressed in seminoma. **Lactic dehydrogenase** (LDH) is elevated in more than half of all patients with metastatic seminoma. Tumour markers are repeated at intervals during follow-up and are invaluable for predicting the appearance of new metastases.

Surgical exploration

Orchidectomy is the only appropriate treatment for the primary tumour and is usually performed as part of the diagnostic process. The surgical approach involves an exploratory operation performed via an inguinal incision to avoid involving the scrotal skin. The spermatic cord is temporarily clamped to preclude venous spread of tumour cells and the testis is brought out for visual examination and palpation. If the testis is obviously malignant, orchidectomy is then performed, dividing the cord at the internal inguinal ring. If there is any diagnostic doubt, a testicular biopsy is taken and examined immediately by frozen section. The other testis is usually unaffected and can be preserved. Further treatment is planned according to tumour type and stage.

Imaging for staging

If malignancy is confirmed, computed tomography is performed to establish the sites and degree of involvement of abdominal, thoracic and pelvic lymph nodes. CT may demonstrate pulmonary metastases that are not shown on chest X-ray. A standard method of staging testicular tumours is shown in Figure 33.9 and Box 33.3.

Fig. 33.8 Metastatic testicular tumours

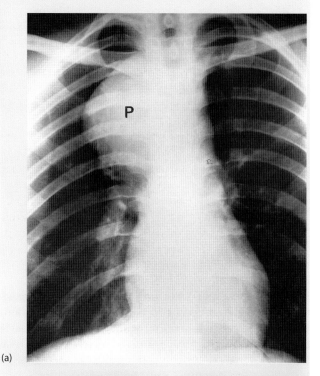

(a)

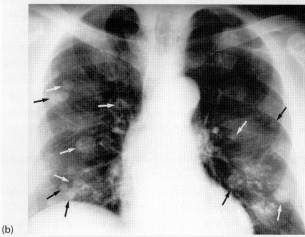

(b)

(a) This 24-year-old man presented with a small testicular lump. An orchidectomy was performed and the cut surface of the tumour was cystic and haemorrhagic. Histology confirmed the expected diagnosis of testicular teratoma. This chest X-ray shows a large mediastinal mass which represents a grossly enlarged paratracheal lymph node **P**. Para-aortic node involvement occurs in teratoma but not seminoma. This patient's disease was defined as stage III because the disease had not become extralymphatic.

(b) Multiple bilateral pulmonary metastases (arrowed) in a 27-year-old man with a testicular swelling. The cut surface of the orchidectomy specimen was homogeneous and histology confirmed seminoma. Pulmonary metastases occur in both teratoma and seminoma, and in either case indicate stage IV disease.

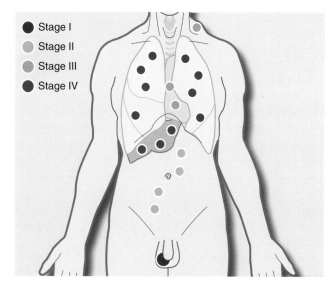

Stage I
Stage II
Stage III
Stage IV

Fig. 33.9 Stages of spread of testicular tumours

Box 33.3 Stages of spread of testicular tumours

Stage I
- Tumour confined to testis

Stage II
- Retroperitoneal lymph node involvement
  —IIa nodes < 2 cm
  —IIb nodes 2–5 cm
  —IIc nodes > 5 cm

Stage III
- Metastasis above the diaphragm confined to lymph nodes

Stage IV
- Extralymphatic metastases (usually lungs and liver)

Management of seminoma

For stage I seminoma, i.e. disease confined to the testis, some oncologists recommend no further treatment after orchidectomy. Seminoma is, however, very radiosensitive and many advise para-aortic radiotherapy as there is a 30% relapse rate with orchidectomy alone. For stages IIa and b (i.e. abdominal lymphadenopathy up to 5 cm diameter), radical radiotherapy to the ipsilateral para-aortic and iliac nodes gives a cure rate of about 95%. Oligospermia of the contralateral testis may occur even if the latter is lead-shielded but this is usually transient. There is also a vogue for single-dose chemotherapy with **carboplatin** for all stages, avoiding radiotherapy altogether. For more advanced disease, chemotherapy is nearly always indicated.

Management of teratomas and other non-seminomatous germ cell tumours

Up to 25% of patients with stage I disease would relapse within a year of orchidectomy without further treatment. 493

Radiotherapy has no curative role in these types of tumour. Further treatment for stage I disease therefore has three options:

- Immediate chemotherapy
- Retroperitoneal lymph node dissection
- Surveillance and treatment if metastases occur

In the USA, lymph node dissection is often employed and provides a good cure rate but risks ejaculatory failure from autonomic nerve damage. In the UK, meticulous surveillance is the preferred option. Chemotherapy for relapse is virtually always successful and thus the 75% of patients that do not relapse are spared additional treatment.

Chemotherapy is indicated for all patients with known metastatic disease, including those in whom the only evidence of metastatic disease is elevated tumour markers. Results of chemotherapy for metastatic disease were transformed in the 1970s by the use of **cisplatin**. The Einhorn regimen, originating from Indiana, combined this with **vinblastine** and **bleomycin** and gave even better cure rates of 70%. Later, **etoposide** replaced vinblastine (bleomycin, etoposide, cisplatin—'**BEP**') increasing overall cure rates to 85%. Three-quarters of patients with teratomas and other non-seminomatous germ cell tumours have **low-volume disease**, and in these cure can be expected in 95%.

Long-term surveillance

After chemotherapy, surgical debulking ('salvage') of residual lymph node masses is occasionally indicated. In the long term, tumour markers and sequential CT scans are used to monitor the success of treatment. Recurrent disease can often be successfully treated by radiotherapy, chemotherapy or surgery.

Fertility

Many patients with testicular tumours are already subfertile at presentation, and chemotherapy is likely to adversely affect fertility. Patients need to be counselled carefully about fertility and, if required, semen can be collected and stored before treatment so that artificial insemination or in vitro fertilisation may be performed later. However, the success rate is poor.

Treatment of testicular tumours is summarised in Box 33.4.

THE MISSING OR ECTOPIC TESTIS

Scrotal examination may reveal the absence of one testis or both testes. This is relatively common in children and is usually due to **incompletely descended testes**. In adults, previous **orchidectomy** should of course be excluded. This is often performed bilaterally for treating

---

| Box | 33.4 | Treatment of testicular tumours |

1. Removal of the affected testis—usually performed as part of the diagnostic process
2. No further treatment given if stage I disease (i.e. no metastases) but meticulous surveillance with tumour markers and CT scans required
3. Radiotherapy—local irradiation alone for moderate abdominal lymph node metastases in seminoma (stages IIa and IIb)
4. Chemotherapy with BEP (bleomycin, etoposide and cisplatin)—for all cases of metastatic teratoma, and metastatic seminoma beyond stage IIb
5. Debulking surgery for lymph nodes treated by chemotherapy—sometimes necessary

---

metastatic prostatic cancer or unilaterally for torsion associated with a necrotic testis or during surgery for recurrent inguinal hernia.

Occasionally, an adult testis may become displaced upwards towards the inguinal canal following trauma or surgery (e.g. hernia repair); this is known as a **trapped testis**. The testis is normal in size but is fixed in position by adhesions. If trauma was the cause and there were other major injuries, the scrotal injury may have been overlooked.

Trauma, including operative trauma during operations for hernia or incompletely descended testis, may damage the blood supply and cause **testicular atrophy**. The resulting testis is abnormally small and soft. When both testes are small, the cause is usually hypoplasia, androgen insufficiency or hormonal therapy for prostatic carcinoma.

MALDESCENT OF THE TESTIS

The testis may fail to descend normally from the posterior abdominal wall into the scrotum, where it should lie at birth in a full-term infant. This problem is common in infants but is sometimes discovered incidentally in adults. In developed countries, the condition is usually identified at screening during early childhood and surgically corrected (by orchidopexy) at a young age (see Ch. 51); to best preserve spermatogenesis, the testis should be surgically placed in the scrotum by the age of 2 years.

An impalpable testis is very rarely truly absent but most often lies somewhere along the normal path of testicular descent (see Fig. 33.2), usually at the external ring, sometimes in the inguinal canal itself and occasionally within the abdomen. Alternatively, it may be found in an **ectopic** position, commonly in the superficial inguinal pouch just above the external inguinal ring. **Incompletely descended testes** (often called undescended testes) are often small and atrophic and, as most are histologically dystrophic, are moderately predisposed to malignant change; indeed an inguinal mass may sometimes be a testicular tumour occurring in an incompletely descended testis. The testis needs to be successfully relocated in the scrotum before the age of 10 to avoid any increased risk of malignancy.

Occasionally, an absent testis is not recognised until adulthood, in which case it may present in one of three ways:

- A 'missing' testis—confirmed if a blind-ending vas is found at groin exploration. Laparoscopy appears to be the best investigation to search further if no vas is found
- A groin lump—the testis or a testicular tumour
- Groin pain due to acute or recurrent torsion

TORSION OF THE TESTIS OR EPIDIDYMAL APPENDAGE

TESTICULAR TORSION (see Fig. 33.10)

In infants, the newly descended testis and its investing tunica vaginalis are mobile within the scrotum. These testes may undergo **extravaginal torsion** which presents as a hard, swollen testis. Later in childhood, the testis becomes suspended in the scrotum in a near vertical position, anchored by the spermatic cord and by attachments to the posterior wall of the scrotum. This attachment prevents rotation of the testis. Minor anatomical variations can produce a narrow-based pedicle with a horizontal ('bell-clapper') testicular lie, which allows the testis to become twisted about its axis within the tunica vaginalis (**intravaginal torsion**). When this occurs, the veins in the pampiniform plexus become compressed, causing venous congestion. After a few hours, venous infarction will occur unless the torsion is corrected. Trauma during sport may sometimes initiate the process of torsion, and there have been reports of successful manual untwisting of the testis on the sports field. In general, however, torsion of the testis is a surgical emergency requiring prompt diagnosis and urgent surgical treatment if the testis is to be saved.

Testicular torsion presents with a sudden onset of severe testicular pain often accompanied by poorly localised central abdominal pain and sometimes vomiting. The abdominal pain occurs because the testis retains its embryological nerve supply within the abdomen. In the early stages of torsion, the affected testis is tender, slightly swollen and drawn up into the neck of the scrotum where the cord may be palpably thickened. With these features, the diagnosis is seldom in doubt. At a later stage, the overlying scrotal skin tends to become red and oedematous, making accurate palpation difficult. At this point, torsion may be difficult to distinguish clinically from acute epididymitis and the scrotum must be explored surgically.

TORSION OF THE EPIDIDYMAL APPENDAGE (HYDATID OF MORGAGNI)

A small embryological remnant at the upper pole of the testis is known as the hydatid of Morgagni (see Fig. 33.11). This may undergo torsion and produce symptoms similar to those of testicular torsion, out of proportion to the size of the infarcted tissue. Infarction of the hydatid is of no consequence except that it must be distinguished from testicular torsion.

MANAGEMENT OF SUSPECTED TESTICULAR TORSION

Differentiating between acute epididymitis and torsion can be difficult; if a firm diagnosis cannot be reached, surgical exploration is mandatory. Investigations are of little value: both radionuclide studies and Doppler ultrasound examination may be employed to show testicular blood flow but results can be misleading. If torsion is seen at an early stage, it is sometimes possible to untwist the testis without operation. The testis is gently rotated outwards, if necessary using local anaesthetic infiltration in the cord. Successful reduction relieves the emergency, but the testis should be surgically secured as soon as practicable to prevent recurrence.

CASE STUDY

Fig. 33.10 Torsion of the testis

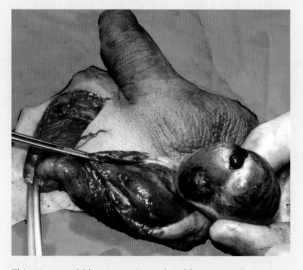

This 15-year-old boy experienced sudden severe lower abdominal pain extending to the scrotum during a football match. A provisional diagnosis of torsion was made and the scrotum explored within 2 hours of the onset of pain. At operation, the testis was twisted $2^1/_2$ times around on its cord (arrowed) and was near infarction. On untwisting, however, it soon regained normal colour. Both testes were fixed to prevent future torsion.

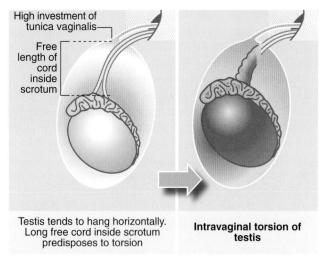

High investment of tunica vaginalis

Free length of cord inside scrotum

Testis tends to hang horizontally. Long free cord inside scrotum predisposes to torsion

Intravaginal torsion of testis

Pedunculated hydatid of Morgagni predisposes to torsion of hydatid

Torsion of hydatid of Morgagni

Fig. 33.11 **Torsion of the testis and hydatid of Morgagni**

In most cases, urgent operation is imperative as delay leads to testicular necrosis after about 8 hours. A scrotal incision is made and the testis is examined and untwisted. If the testis is black and fails to recover its colour, it is necrotic and should be removed to prevent it inducing a sympathetic contralateral orchiopathy. If some colour is restored, biopsy can be performed to check for viability; otherwise the testis is best left, although it may later atrophy. The untwisted testis is then sutured to the tunica vaginalis or placed into a dartos pouch to prevent recurrence. Both testes should be secured since predisposition to torsion is usually bilateral.

TRAUMA TO THE TESTIS

The testes may be injured during contact sports or fights. The dense fibrous capsule which invests the testis (tunica albuginea) may remain intact or it may split but the testis is extremely painful in either case. If the tunica remains intact, a **testicular haematoma** results; if it splits, the testicular parenchyma bursts and bleeds into the tunica vaginalis cavity, resulting in a **haematocoele**.

If pain is severe and persistent, the scrotum can be explored surgically. Pain from a testicular haematoma can be relieved by incising the tunica albuginea. Evacuating a haematocoele, however, may be impossible because blood tends to infiltrate the tissues. If the haematocoele can be evacuated, a rupture of the tunica albuginea is best repaired.

MALE STERILISATION

Male sterilisation by vasectomy is a simple, effective method of birth control. It can be performed under local anaesthesia at little cost and requires no special equipment. The essential prerequisite is that the couple involved should have completed their family, since reversal is technically difficult and unreliable. A technique of vasectomy is illustrated in Figure 33.12.

Most procedures involve removing a section of the vas (ductus) deferens and ligating or cauterising the cut ends. For medico-legal reasons, the nature of the excised portion is often confirmed histologically. Spermatozoa remain in the proximal duct system for several months after vasectomy. Thus, the operation cannot be considered a success until at least two successive sperm counts are negative. These need to be performed about 1 month apart, after 20–25 ejaculations. Despite correct operative technique and negative sperm counts, there is still a late failure rate of about 1 case in every 500. Failure suspected of resulting from spontaneous reconnection of the vas should be proved by a positive sperm count. This is because of the problem of determining paternity in the case of unexpected pregnancy!

Early complications of vasectomy include postoperative scrotal haematoma (usually operator error) and wound infection. Later, failure of sterilisation may become apparent or a **sperm granuloma** may present as a tender scrotal swelling near the cut end of the vas for which further excision is usually required. Chronic debilitating pain can occur in the testis and the patient must be warned of this possibility at the time of consent. The patient must also be warned of the possibility of spontaneous reversal.

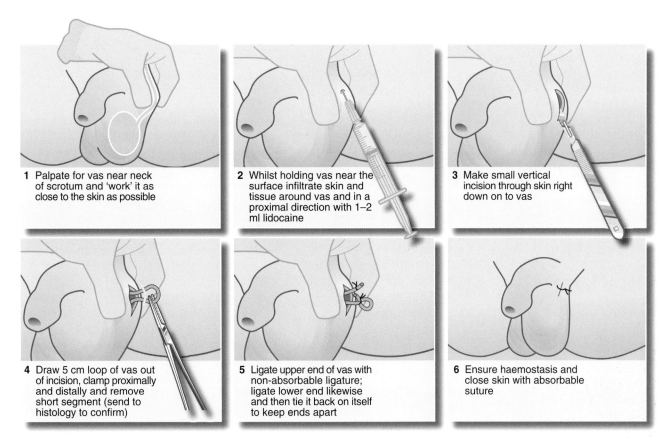

1 Palpate for vas near neck of scrotum and 'work' it as close to the skin as possible

2 Whilst holding vas near the surface infiltrate skin and tissue around vas and in a proximal direction with 1–2 ml lidocaine

3 Make small vertical incision through skin right down on to vas

4 Draw 5 cm loop of vas out of incision, clamp proximally and distally and remove short segment (send to histology to confirm)

5 Ligate upper end of vas with non-absorbable ligature; ligate lower end likewise and then tie it back on itself to keep ends apart

6 Ensure haemostasis and close skin with absorbable suture

Fig. 33.12 Technique of vasectomy
Note that each side is dealt with separately.

DISORDERS OF THE PENIS

Problems with the foreskin (prepuce) are common and form the majority of surgical disorders of the penis. Other disorders are uncommon in adults but the most serious is carcinoma. In children, penile disorders are either developmental or minor inflammatory conditions; these are discussed in Chapter 51. Disorders of the foreskin include **balano-posthitis** (inflammation of the glans and foreskin), **phimosis** (stricture of the preputial meatus), **paraphimosis** (acute constriction of the glans by a tight retracted foreskin) and **balanitis xerotica obliterans** (idiopathic sclerosis of the foreskin).

Carcinoma of the penis is uncommon but obviously important. **Peyronie's disease** (idiopathic fibrosis of the corpora cavernosa) is now a frequent presentation in urological outpatient clinics (see below). Exclusion of cancer is usually the first prerequisite.

FORESKIN PROBLEMS IN ADULTS

PHIMOSIS

The most common complaint is that the foreskin will not fully retract, causing pain on intercourse. Such phimosis is usually caused by fibrosis of the foreskin and may be due to chronic or recurrent low-grade *Candida* infection. Phimosis is aggravated by attempts at retraction which cause minor tears of the inner epithelial lining, inducing further inflammation and fibrosis. The condition may be accompanied by stenosis of the urethral meatus, also due to recurrent inflammation and fibrosis. Treatment usually involves circumcision but a preputioplasty or reshaping operation is sometimes successful.

BALANO-POSTHITIS (BALANITIS)

The term balano-posthitis refers to overt inflammation of the glans penis and foreskin (Greek: *balanos* gland, *posthe* foreskin); it is the correct term but the short form 'balanitis' has passed into common usage. The condition occurs most commonly in children. Inflammation alone is most often caused by *Candida* or faecal bacteria, but this problem rarely reaches the surgeon.

Balanitis xerotica obliterans is a fibrotic condition of the foreskin of unknown aetiology and is probably analogous to lichen sclerosus of the vulva in females. It produces a thickened, stenosed, often depigmented foreskin which is often adherent to the glans. Circumcision is usually curative. As many as 25% of children with phi-

497

mosis have this condition. The process can involve the urethral meatus and this may cause stenosis, sometimes requiring meatotomy or meatoplasty at the same time. More rarely it results in a urethral stricture likely to require urethroplasty.

PARAPHIMOSIS

If a phimotic foreskin is forcibly retracted, the tight meatal band may lodge in the coronal sulcus making reduction impossible. This is known as paraphimosis. Progressive oedema of the glans penis and foreskin then exacerbates the difficulty of reduction. It may occur at any age, but is particularly common in elderly men in whom the foreskin is not correctly pulled forwards after retraction for catheterisation or washing the glans (nurses and junior doctors are the main culprits). Paraphimosis also occurs in children and adolescents experimenting with foreskin retraction or cleaning beneath it. In most cases, the foreskin can be reduced by firm manual compression of the glans and foreskin. Local anaesthetic jelly is applied first for lubrication and pain relief. Sometimes, it may be necessary to incise the tight ring under local or general anaesthesia to effect reduction. **Preputioplasty**, in which the band is incised longitudinally and the skin sutured transversely, can often be performed at the same time to solve the problem in the long term. If not, circumcision or preputioplasty is usually performed at a later date when the oedema and inflammation have resolved.

CIRCUMCISION

Circumcision is or has been a widespread practice in some communities for religious or other cultural reasons. From a strictly scientific or medical standpoint, however, it is difficult to support as a health measure, although there is some evidence that circumcision reduces the risk of urinary tract infections, as well as sexually transmitted infections including HIV. It also reduces the frequency of the rare carcinoma of the penis. Routine circumcision for recurrent balanitis, phimosis and even paraphimosis in children has largely gone out of favour as most cases respond to local treatments or to preputioplasty. Misguided circumcision in babies may predispose to ammoniacal nappy rash and meatal stenosis.

Circumcision should be reserved for unresolved phimosis, recurrent balanitis and sclerosis from balanitis xerotica obliterans. The surgical technique is shown in Figure 33.13. During the operation, the urethral meatus should be checked for stenosis. If present, a meatotomy may be required. An occasional early postoperative complication is haemorrhage which usually requires surgical re-exploration. Postoperative bleeding can best be prevented by meticulous haemostasis at operation.

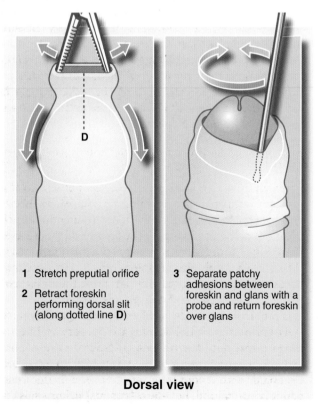

1 Stretch preputial orifice

2 Retract foreskin performing dorsal slit (along dotted line **D**)

3 Separate patchy adhesions between foreskin and glans with a probe and return foreskin over glans

Dorsal view

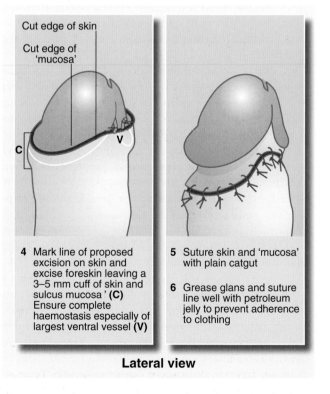

4 Mark line of proposed excision on skin and excise foreskin leaving a 3–5 mm cuff of skin and sulcus mucosa ' **(C)** Ensure complete haemostasis especially of largest ventral vessel **(V)**

5 Suture skin and 'mucosa' with plain catgut

6 Grease glans and suture line well with petroleum jelly to prevent adherence to clothing

Lateral view

Fig. 33.13 Technique of circumcision

Fig. 33.14 Carcinoma of the penis

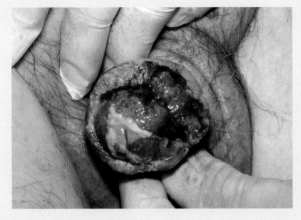 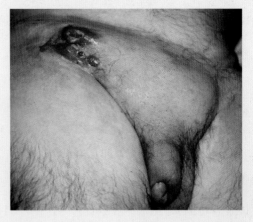

(a) (b)

(a) An obvious carcinoma of the penis, revealed when the foreskin is retracted. **(b)** Unfortunately, this patient already had extensive spread to the inguinal lymph nodes.

PEYRONIE'S DISEASE

This disease of unknown aetiology occurs in young to middle-aged adults. Some cases are thought to result from penile trauma during sexual activity and some cases are associated with Dupuytren's contracture of the palmar fascia. Slowly progressive asymmetrical fibrotic plaques develop in the fascia surrounding the corpora cavernosa of the penis. The corpus spongiosum including the glans is spared. The plaques may become calcified and visible on X-ray. The condition causes the penis to bend towards the affected side on erection, making intercourse difficult and painful. There may be spontaneous partial resolution with time.

Severe cases require surgery. **Nesbit's operation** involves creating pleats in the corpus on the contralateral side. Another approach involves excision of the plaques, which are replaced by a patch of tunica vaginalis. Either procedure may restore symmetrical erection, although with Nesbit's procedure the condition and subsequent surgery result in a shorter penis. Penile prosthetic implants may be required if erection is inadequate for satisfactory sexual intercourse. 'Medical treatments', i.e. steroid injections or radiation, are of no benefit.

CARCINOMA OF THE PENIS

Carcinoma of the penis is rare in developed countries and almost unknown in circumcised males. Poor hygiene and accumulation of smegma are suspected aetiological factors but there is growing evidence of a viral aetiology linked to that of carcinoma of the uterine cervix in females (human papilloma virus).

Histologically, the tumours are squamous cell carcinomas, usually well differentiated, which arise from the inner surface of the foreskin or the glans penis in the region of the coronal sulcus. The tumour invades locally and tends to penetrate the distal urethra (Fig. 33.14a). Metastatic spread is to inguinal lymph nodes (see Fig. 33.14b). **Erythroplasia of Queyrat** is the term given to severe dysplasia and carcinoma in situ of the glans that may represent a precursor of invasive carcinoma.

Most cases of carcinoma of the penis are found in the elderly. The disease is usually well advanced before an irregular lump, bleeding or discharge is noticed. In uncircumcised males, the lesion may be hidden by the foreskin. Figure 33.15 illustrates staging of the disease.

Surgical excision usually requires at least partial amputation of the penis, and block dissection of the inguinal lymph nodes if they are involved. Radiotherapy can be used in stage I disease if the urethra is not involved and for palliation in stage IV disease.

PRIAPISM

Priapism is an abnormally prolonged penile erection lasting 4 hours or more. It is usually painful and occurs without sexual stimulation, nor does it resolve after ejaculation. The abnormality affects only the **corpora cavernosa** and is caused by a disturbance of the mechanisms that control penile detumescence. The corpus spongiosum surrounding the urethra and forming the glans penis is not affected and the glans remains flaccid.

There are two main types of priapism. **High-flow (arterial) priapism** occurs when an artery ruptures into the lacunar spaces of the corpora cavernosa. This is often associated with trauma and is relatively uncommon. Compared with venous priapism, there is less tumescence and it is less painful. **Low-flow (venous) priapism** is due to prolonged corporeal venous stasis caused by occlusion

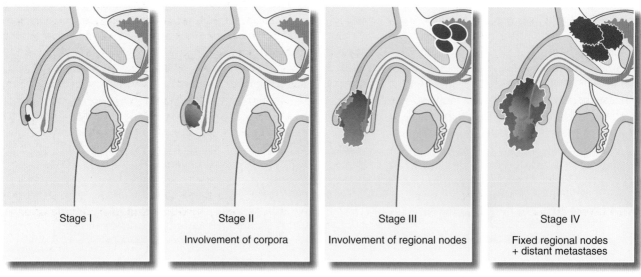

Stage I	Stage II	Stage III	Stage IV
	Involvement of corpora	Involvement of regional nodes	Fixed regional nodes + distant metastases

Fig. 33.15 Stages in the spread of carcinoma of the penis

Box 33.5   Causes of priapism

- Drugs used for intracavernosal injection for erectile dysfunction
  - papaverine
  - phentolamine
  - alprostadil (synthetic prostaglandin E_1)
- Psychotropic medications
  - chlorpromazine, trazodone and thioridazine
  - citalopram (a selective serotonin reuptake inhibitor)
- Hormones
  - tamoxifen
  - testosterone
- Antihypertensives
  - hydralazine
  - prazosin
  - calcium channel blockers
- Anticoagulants
  - warfarin and heparin
- Recreational drugs
  - cocaine
  - marijuana
  - ecstasy
  - ethanol abuse
- Miscellaneous drugs
  - hydroxyzine (an antihistamine)
  - metoclopramide
  - omeprazole
- Pro-thrombotic or hypercoagulable diseases
  - leukaemia and multiple myeloma
  - sickle cell disease and thalassaemia
  - total parenteral nutrition
  - Fabry disease
  - dialysis
  - vasculitis
  - fat embolism
  - asplenia
- Neoplastic disease causing direct invasion or venous outflow obstruction
  - prostate cancer
  - bladder cancer
  - haematological (leukaemia)
  - renal carcinoma
  - melanoma
- Neurogenic problems
  - spinal cord injury
  - spinal anaesthesia
  - spinal cord stenosis (i.e. trauma to the medulla)
  - autonomic neuropathy and cauda equina compression
- Other rare causes
  - malaria
  - amyloidosis
  - recent infection with *Mycoplasma pneumoniae*
  - gout
  - carbon monoxide poisoning
  - black widow spider bites

of the venous outlet mechanism (veno-occlusive priapism). This eventually results in penile ischaemia. It is very painful and, unless treated, results in long-term fibrosis and impotence (loss of the ability to achieve an erection). In veno-occlusive priapism, tissue changes that will lead to fibrosis are already evident within 24 hours, whereas there is no such change in arterial priapism.

The most common cause of priapism is a side effect of injected intracavernosal drugs used to treat erectile dysfunction. Other veno-occlusive causes include thromboembolic or hypercoagulable states such as sickle cell disease, polycythaemia or thalassaemia. Rarely, priapism can be the presenting feature of leukaemia in children. Other causes are listed in Box 33.5.

Treatment of veno-occlusive priapism must be prompt in order to avoid long-term erectile problems. Ice packs and external compression are a useful temporising measure but will not give long-term relief. Oral terbutaline, a beta-2-adrenergic receptor agonist, produces detumescence in about a third of patients. A first dose of 5 mg is followed by a second similar dose 15 minutes later. If this is not successful, the next step is usually intracavernous injection of an alpha-adrenergic agonist. This should be the first line treatment when the effects of papaverine need to be reversed. Aspiration of blood from the cavernosa is the next step. If these measures are unsuccessful, operative management by means of a surgical shunt may be necessary but results are sometimes disappointing.

34 Symptoms, signs and investigation of urinary tract disorders

INTRODUCTION

Urinary tract disorders are common and comprise a significant part of the workload of family practitioners, general physicians, paediatricians and surgeons. In recent decades, the specialty of urology has become well established but despite this, many general surgeons still deal with urological problems, especially in smaller hospitals, where they make up about 25% of the general surgical workload.

Disorders of the prostate account for at least half the workload in urological surgery. The main conditions are benign prostatic hyperplasia, which affects about 10% of ageing males in Western countries, and prostatic carcinoma, which is now the second most common cancer in men. The remaining surgical disorders of the kidney and urinary tract can be divided into five broad groups: tumours, stone disease (**urolithiasis**), infections, congenital abnormalities and, finally, local and systemic disorders which secondarily involve the urinary tract.

This chapter deals with the symptoms, signs, approach to investigation and diagnosis of urinary tract disease. The various disease entities are then discussed in the following five chapters.

SYMPTOMS OF URINARY TRACT DISEASE

Urinary symptoms may be caused by disease intrinsic to the urinary tract or else by disease of other structures.

URINARY SYMPTOMS CAUSED BY INTRINSIC DISEASE OF THE URINARY TRACT

Outflow of urine from the kidney may sometimes become impeded by obstruction of the urinary tract, and this may secondarily interfere with renal function. If there is chronic obstruction to bladder outflow or bilateral upper tract obstruction, the patient may develop renal failure, often without any localising symptoms.

Benign prostatic hypertrophy is the most common prostatic disorder, and usually presents with symptoms of bladder outflow obstruction (i.e. disorders of micturition or urinary retention or both) and sometimes with haematuria. Prostatic obstruction predisposes to bladder infections or stones, and the patient may present with symptoms of these.

Carcinoma of the prostate is undoubtedly becoming more common. It may present with bladder outflow obstruction similar to benign prostatic disease hypertrophy or it may be discovered at an asymptomatic stage at a medical check-up, either by digital rectal examination (DRE) or a blood test (prostate specific antigen, PSA). Many cases are first diagnosed because of symptoms of metastases, such as bone pain.

Chronic prostatitis may be bacterial or abacterial and usually presents with a chronic perineal ache and often aching testes (properly called **prostatodynia**). In the acute form, bacterial prostatitis may present as a systemic illness (or even Gram-negative septicaemia) with urinary symptoms and an exquisitely tender prostate. Occasionally, a prostatic abscess develops.

The important urinary tract tumours, stone diseases and infections are briefly outlined in Table 34.1. Any of these disorders may present with haematuria. Some of the conditions cause urinary obstruction and abdominal

Table 34.1 Pathophysiology and clinical features of urinary tract tumours, stones and infections

Disease	Pathophysiology	Clinical features
TUMOURS		
Renal cell carcinoma (also known as renal adenocarcinoma and formerly as 'hypernephroma')—fairly common	Occurs in adults. Derived from renal tubular cells	Presents either incidentally (e.g. on CT scan) or with symptoms of haematuria, a mass or constitutional signs such as pyrexia or polycythaemia or is asymptomatic
Nephroblastoma (Wilms' tumour; see Ch. 51—rare	Developmental origin; usually diagnosed before age 5	Presents as an abnormal mass with or without pain and haematuria
Transitional cell carcinoma (TCC)—common	May arise in transitional epithelium anywhere in urinary tract from pelvicalyceal system to urethra, but most commonly in bladder	Usually presents with haematuria. Predisposes to urinary tract infections. May cause ureteric obstruction
Squamous cell carcinoma (very uncommon)	Arises in metaplastic squamous epithelium. Secondary to chronic stone or schistosomal irritation, especially in bladder. Also arises *de novo* in squamous epithelium of distal urethra (very rare)	As for transitional cell carcinoma
Adenocarcinoma of bladder (very rare)	Arises from columnar epithelium of urachal remnant	As for transitional cell carcinoma
STONE DISEASE		
In general	Stones in situ may cause irritation of urinary tract epithelium	Present as pain or haematuria or recurrent infection
Stones may develop in pelvicalyceal system or bladder. Pelvicalyceal stones can pass into the ureter—very common	Chronic—renal stones may cause chronic pelviureteric or ureteric obstruction either directly or by causing fibrotic strictures. Acute—renal stones may cause ureteric obstruction as they pass down the tract	Present with chronic pain (due to back pressure) or recurrent infection. Present as acute colicky pain often with renal tenderness (renal or ureteric colic). Infection may supervene, destroying the kidney if untreated
INFECTIONS		
'Common' infections due to bowel organisms	Infection develops either via bloodstream (haematogenous) or else lower urinary tract stasis predisposes to infection	Typically present with dysuria and frequency with or without haematuria. Any urinary tract abnormality or stasis predisposes to infection. Ascending infection may cause pyelonephritis, i.e. infection of kidney and renal pelvis
Tuberculosis (uncommon)	Kidney involvement via bloodstream from pulmonary or other primary disease. May spread via urine to ureters and bladder	May present as haematuria, persistent sterile pyuria, or as an incidental finding in pulmonary tuberculosis
Urinary schistosomiasis (also known as bilharzia)—very common in in some developing countries; probably the world's most common cause of haematuria	Induces chronic inflammation and fibrosis in bladder wall leading to gross bladder distortion, stones and squamous cell carcinoma	Presents with haematuria and various symptoms of infection and bladder fibrosis
Urethritis	Usually caused by sexually transmitted infections, e.g. gonococcus or *Chlamydia*	Presents with urethral discharge and dysuria

pain. The severity and character of the pain are determined by the site and degree of obstruction and, perhaps most importantly, the rapidity of onset. Disorders which cause urinary stasis also predispose to urinary tract infection.

Many different congenital abnormalities may involve the kidneys, ureters, bladder, urethra and genitalia, either alone or in combination. Most of the serious abnormalities are recognised at birth or in early childhood. The exceptions are **polycystic disease** and **medullary sponge kidney**, which usually present in adulthood. Less serious congenital abnormalities such as duplex systems may predispose to urinary tract infections because of abnormal flow dynamics. These abnormalities may be discovered at any age during the investigation of recurrent urinary tract infections. Congenital disorders which present mainly in adulthood are discussed in Chapter 39 and those presenting mainly in childhood in Chapter 51.

URINARY SYMPTOMS CAUSED BY NON-URINARY DISEASE

The urinary tract sometimes becomes secondarily involved in local inflammatory conditions such as Crohn's disease or diverticular disease. Fistulae may form, resulting in the passage of flatus or faeces in the urine or both (pneumaturia and faecuria). Retroperitoneal fibrosis, diverticulitis, tumours of the prostate, cervix or colon, and sometimes aortic or iliac aneurysms may secondarily involve the ureters and cause upper urinary tract obstruction.

THE COMMON SYMPTOMS OF URINARY TRACT DISEASE

These fall into eight categories:

- Abdominal pain
- Passage of blood in the urine (**haematuria**)
- Pain associated with micturition (**dysuria**)
- Disorders of micturition such as frequency or hesitancy
- Retention of urine (acute or chronic)
- Urinary incontinence
- Passage of bowel gas in the urine (**pneumaturia**)
- Passage of blood in the semen (**haemospermia**)

The pattern of symptoms usually suggests the diagnosis and guides appropriate investigations. The following section explains how the various symptoms relate to the underlying causes.

ABDOMINAL PAIN

Most urinary tract diseases cause symptoms that are obviously referable to the urinary tract. Urinary tract disorders may, however, cause abdominal pain without urinary symptoms; the diagnosis is then not so obvious and other characteristic clinical features must be sought.

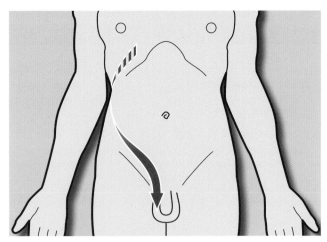

Fig. 34.1 Renal pain and its referral

PAIN ARISING FROM THE KIDNEYS AND UPPER TRACT

Both renal inflammation and stretching of the renal capsule cause pain in the renal angle, the posterior space between the lowest rib and the iliac crest. This area may also become tender to palpation or percussion.

Renal stones, tumours or polycystic disease may cause dull and persistent loin pain even without obstruction.

In acute infections such as pyelonephritis (affecting renal pelvis and kidney) or bladder infection, the pain is severe and is usually associated with systemic features and urinary tract symptoms.

Acute upper ureteric obstruction and distension of the pelvicalyceal system produce excruciating loin pain. The pain is colicky (resulting from powerful ureteric peristalsis) and often radiates to the hypochondrium (right or left upper quadrant of the abdomen) or groin (see Fig. 34.1). When obstruction is low in the ureter, the pain may radiate to the genitalia. This pain is known as **renal** or **ureteric colic**.

PAIN ARISING FROM THE BLADDER

Pain originating in the bladder (e.g. in cystitis) is felt in the suprapubic area. Pain may be referred to the penis or vulva if the bladder trigone is involved. In adults, clear-cut urinary symptoms such as dysuria and frequency are usually also present, but children may have no localising symptoms or complain only of pain, making the diagnosis less obvious. Dysuria is usually the predominant symptom of urethral disorders, but pain arising in the male urethra (e.g. in sexually transmitted infections) is usually referred to the tip of the penis. Finally, the pain of prostatic inflammation (prostatitis) is usually felt deep in the perineum. The prostate is tender on rectal examination in the acute but not the chronic form.

PAIN SIMULATING URINARY TRACT DISEASE

Pain from other abdominal pathology may sometimes mimic pain arising from the urinary tract. Acute appendicitis may present with suprapubic pain, and biliary tract pain may be referred to the right thoraco-lumbar region, while posterior duodenal ulcers and pancreatic disease may cause pain in the central lumbar region. An expanding or leaking abdominal aortic aneurysm may sometimes mimic the pain of urinary tract disease, particularly if a ureter is compressed. Diseases of the thoraco-lumbar spine, such as metastatic cancer, tuberculosis, spondylosis and disc lesions, may also simulate upper urinary tract disorders. Suspected renal colic with a local rash is usually due to shingles (herpes zoster); the rash may not appear for several days after the onset of pain; perineal zoster may cause retention of urine. In women, pain arising from the ovaries or genital tract (e.g. pelvic inflammatory disease) may be confused with bladder pain.

HAEMATURIA

Patients may notice blood or even clots in the urine (**frank haematuria**) and this needs to be distinguished from urethral bleeding. More often, blood is discovered on 'dipstick' testing or microscopy of a midstream urine specimen (**microscopic haematuria**). Haematuria is often episodic rather than persistent, whatever the cause. 'Dipstick' testing for haematuria is extremely sensitive and yields many false positive results. Thus a positive dipstick result should be confirmed by urine microscopy, and if confirmed, freshly voided urine should be examined for malignant cells by exfoliative cytology.

CAUSES OF HAEMATURIA (see Fig. 34.2 for renal causes)

Tumours are a common cause of frank and microscopic haematuria and must be suspected, even if another possible cause is found. Haematuria from tumours is typically painless. However, carcinoma in situ, a dysplastic condition with a high probability of progression to frank carcinoma, usually presents with irritative voiding, dysuria and haematuria. Irritation from infection or stones may also cause bleeding, but this is usually accompanied by pain or dysuria. If the urethra is obstructed by prostatic enlargement, straining at micturition may cause bleeding from dilated veins at the bladder neck.

Trauma to a normal kidney may cause frank haematuria if considerable force has been applied, but microscopic haematuria is common after minor trauma in contact sports and rarely indicates a significant injury. Enlarged kidneys are more susceptible to trauma, whatever the primary pathology. In hydronephrosis or polycystic kidneys, minor blunt trauma may cause gross haematuria.

Sometimes urine becomes red with haemoglobin rather than blood. In young people this may be induced by vigorous exercise such as jogging (**exercise haemoglobinuria and haematuria**). These patients are believed to have defective red cell membranes which makes them more vulnerable to trauma. Exercise haemoglobinuria is self-limiting and requires no treatment.

Haematuria also occurs in renal parenchymal inflammations such as glomerulonephritis or arteritis. Renal haematuria may also be caused by microemboli settling in the kidneys, as in atrial fibrillation or infective endocarditis. Any urinary tract disorder with a potential for haematuria is more likely to be revealed when a patient is on anticoagulant therapy or develops a bleeding diathesis.

DIAGNOSTIC FEATURES OF HAEMATURIA

Gross bleeding results in the passage of clots. The stage of micturition at which blood appears is sometimes diagnostically useful. Blood from the kidneys, ureters or bladder wall will completely mix with the urine, and be present throughout the urinary stream. Urethral bleeding may leak out independently of micturition, or be seen only at the beginning or end of the urinary stream. Blood arising from the bladder neck or posterior urethra may sometimes present as terminal haematuria.

Haematuria on dipstick testing should be confirmed by urine microscopy for red blood cells, which can also check for infection by culture and sensitivity. Microscopic haematuria may represent a significant lesion anywhere in the urinary tract and must be taken seriously; however, a significant cause is found in only 5–25% of patients.

DYSURIA

Dysuria describes pain or discomfort on micturition, often accompanied by difficulty in voiding. The pain is often described as 'burning' or 'scalding'. Any irritation of the urethra may cause dysuria. The most common cause is urinary tract infection, but urethral instrumentation, or the presence of a catheter, also commonly causes dysuria.

DISORDERS OF MICTURITION

The normal bladder has a capacity of 350–500 ml. When this is reached, the detrusor muscle undergoes reflex contraction, initiating the desire to void. Micturition is normally initiated by conscious sphincter relaxation; a voluntary detrusor contraction then empties the bladder completely.

FREQUENT MICTURITION

Urinary frequency is defined as the frequent passage of small quantities of urine, but with a normal daily urine volume. If severe, frequency may sometimes result in incontinence.

There are five main causes of frequent micturition:

- **Bladder irritation**—infection is the most common cause and is usually accompanied by dysuria. The

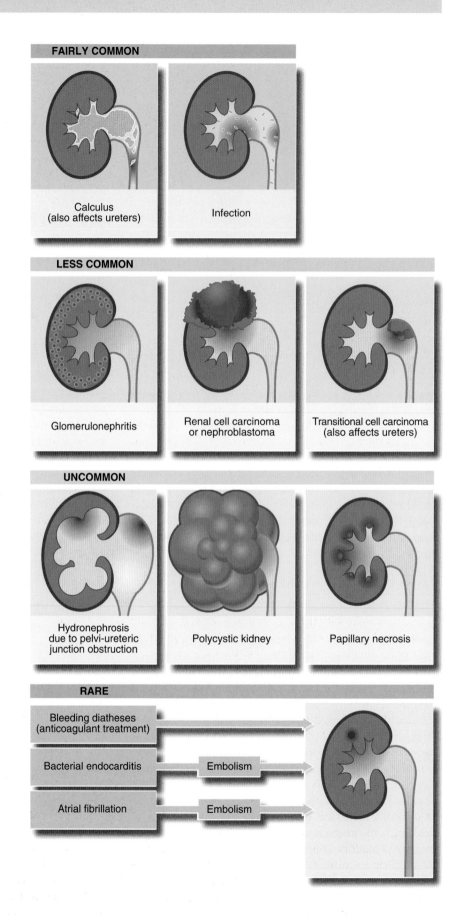

Fig. 34.2 Renal causes of haematuria

patient feels an almost constant need to pass urine regardless of the amount of urine in the bladder. It should be remembered that carcinoma in situ of the bladder may give rise to similar symptoms

- **Incomplete emptying of the bladder**—this is most commonly caused by bladder outlet obstruction as in prostatic hypertrophy, but it may also be caused by neurological disorders such as multiple sclerosis or spinal trauma. Voiding is incomplete so the bladder soon reaches full capacity again. The increased volume of residual urine in the bladder after micturition predisposes to infection
- **Overactive bladder (detrusor instability)**—in this condition, the voiding reflex is activated before the bladder is properly filled. Small volumes of urine are thus passed more frequently. This may be associated with bladder outflow obstruction
- **Small or indistensible bladder**—this is a rare cause of frequency and may be due to surgical resection, inflammatory fibrosis such as tuberculosis, schistosomiasis, idiopathic interstitial fibrosis or scarring following radiotherapy
- **Psychosomatic frequency**—this characteristically occurs during the daytime and not at night

Frequency must be distinguished from **polyuria**, in which the amount of urine produced is excessive and normal voiding volumes are passed at more frequent intervals. Polyuria is usually accompanied by **polydipsia** (excessive drinking). Excess urine production is not a surgical problem; it most commonly results from untreated diabetes mellitus, less commonly from renal failure and occasionally from diabetes insipidus.

NOCTURIA

Nocturia describes the need to pass urine at night. The patient may wake with the urge to void hourly, if not more frequently. Nocturia usually accompanies frequency or polyuria. Patients with cardiac failure may experience nocturia as peripheral oedema is returned to the general circulation in the supine position and renal perfusion is thereby increased. Elderly patients in particular, elaborate more urine at night due to enhanced renal blood flow when recumbent. Thus they may pass more urine at night than in the daytime. Some class II calcium channel antagonists are associated with nocturnal polyuria.

URGENCY

Urgency is the sudden desire to void, which, if ignored, may result in incontinence. Urgency results from irritation of the bladder neck as in cystitis, or from the abnormal entry of urine into the proximal urethra as in prostatic enlargement. If the bladder is overfilled as a result of outlet obstruction, spasms of abnormally high detrusor pressure can cause urgency or even incontinence. Other urinary symptoms are usually present.

HESITANCY

Difficulty in initiating micturition, known as hesitancy, usually occurs in males. In extreme cases, the patient may have to stand for several minutes before urinary flow begins. The usual cause is prostatic obstruction, which prevents entry of sufficient urine into the proximal urethra to initiate sphincter relaxation. Hesitancy may occur in young males because the bladder neck will not relax. The symptom is common, and often intermittent and situational, e.g. in a urinal when other men are nearby; the problem is psychosomatic rather than organic.

POOR URINARY STREAM

The urinary stream is often reduced when there is urethral narrowing. The most common cause is prostatic enlargement or bladder neck hypertrophy, which may limit the urine flow to a dribble despite straining. A poor stream may also be caused by a urethral stricture, in which case other urinary symptoms may be minimal or absent.

POST-MICTURITION DRIBBLING

With this symptom, urine flow does not cease completely at the end of micturition. Dribbling may simply involve the leakage of a few drops of urine or it can be so severe as to amount to incontinence. Post-micturition dribbling may result from abnormal sphincter function, but is usually due to incomplete emptying of the urethra by a weakened bulbospongiosus muscle. This symptom is not indicative of prostatic obstruction. When occurring in isolation in women, it may denote weakness of the pelvic floor muscles. Urine trapped below a healthy sphincter and above a urethral stricture dribbles out after bladder emptying but more commonly presents with terminal dribbling.

LOWER URINARY TRACT SYMPTOMS (LUTS)

This term encompasses the symptoms of hesitancy, poor stream, terminal dribbling and incomplete bladder emptying with frequency, nocturia, urgency and urge incontinence. Although these occur in prostatic obstruction, similar symptoms also occur in bladder neck obstruction, urethral stricture, bladder calculi and lower urinary tract infection. The severity of symptoms can be estimated using the International Prostate Symptom Score (see Box 35.1, p. 518).

RETENTION OF URINE

Urinary retention means the inability to void when the bladder is full. It occurs when the sphincter is unable to relax or when there is proximal urethral obstruction. Both factors may occur together.

ACUTE RETENTION

In its simplest form, acute urinary retention can occur in normal individuals, usually males, particularly postoperatively. At this time, fluid overload, drugs, pain, the supine posture, anxiety or embarrassment are responsible. Similar factors may precipitate an episode of acute retention in individuals with asymptomatic prostatic enlargement. Occasionally acute retention is caused by an obstructing blood clot (**clot retention**) or stone.

In the female, acute retention can occur after abdominal surgery, perhaps as a side effect of anaesthetic or analgesic drugs. It may also occur in pregnancy if the enlarging uterus becomes wedged in the pelvis at about 14 weeks' gestation. An ovarian cyst or uterine fibroid of similar dimensions may also cause obstruction of this type. Other possible causes include neurological disorders such as sacral nerve injury or herpes zoster and multiple sclerosis.

CHRONIC RETENTION

Chronic retention may occur with abnormalities of structure or function of the bladder muscle or sphincter mechanism. Less commonly, it is caused by persistent urethral obstruction. In chronic retention, voiding of urine is often incomplete. The problem progresses until the residual volume approaches maximum bladder capacity. Voiding then usually occurs by 'overflow' and the bladder tends to become abnormally distended. When obstruction is prolonged and severe, the bladder muscle hypertrophies, bladder diverticula may develop, and back pressure on the kidneys may cause uraemia and renal failure. At any stage, complete cessation of flow, i.e. **acute-on-chronic retention**, may be precipitated by overfilling (often alcohol-induced), urinary tract infection or severe constipation. The most common cause of chronic retention is bladder outflow obstruction caused by a thickened bladder neck or prostatic enlargement. It may also be caused by lower spinal neurological problems, e.g. central protrusion of lumbar intervertebral discs damaging the S2, 3, 4 innervation of the detrusor.

URINARY INCONTINENCE

Involuntary passage of urine is a distressing and socially debilitating symptom. It may occur in a variety of disorders with a structural or functional abnormality of the bladder or sphincter mechanism. The normal bladder has a capacity of approximately 350–500 ml. During filling, the detrusor muscle relaxes so that the intravesical pressure does not rise until bladder capacity is approached. Once the bladder is filled, voiding occurs by detrusor contraction and sphincter relaxation. Both are mediated via a spinal reflex at the level of S2, 3, 4. Superimposed on this system is an inhibitory mechanism under cortical (conscious) control, which delays voiding if it is socially

---

Box 34.1	Causes of incontinence

Loss of cortical control
- Cortical disease
- Spinal cord disease, i.e. supra-sacral neurogenic bladder

Abnormalities of the sacral reflex mechanism
- Sacral neurogenic bladder
- Overactive bladder
- Infection producing bladder hyperactivity
- Hypotonic bladder

Detrusor or sphincter abnormalities
- Stress incontinence
- Post-prostatectomy
- Tumour invasion
- Urethral trauma
- Contracted bladder
- Rare congenital abnormalities

---

inappropriate. Conscious control, including nocturnal control, develops during early childhood. Nocturnal incontinence is known as **enuresis**.

The pathophysiology of incontinence can be divided into three categories based on disorders of structure and function which are described below and summed up in Box 34.1. Some disease processes may produce incontinence by more than one mechanism.

LOSS OF CORTICAL CONTROL

Loss of inhibitory control over reflex voiding may occur in disease of the cortex, such as the dementias, or in disease of the spinal cord above the sacral reflex level, such as multiple sclerosis. Traumatic paraplegia is a common cause of complete loss of cortical control. The resulting incontinence may be described as **supra-sacral neurogenic bladder**. The bladder fills to normal capacity and then empties spontaneously, more or less completely, leaving little residual urine.

DISORDERS OF SACRAL REFLEX CONTROL OF DETRUSOR AND SPHINCTER FUNCTION

If the sacral reflex arc is damaged on its afferent or efferent sides, reflex contraction of the detrusor and relaxation of the sphincter are lost. This may occur in low spinal trauma or systemic or nearby disease such as myelomeningocoele, diabetic neuropathy or invasive pelvic tumours. The bladder consequently becomes grossly distended and urine passively overflows causing constant **dribbling incontinence**. This can be alleviated considerably by regular manual emptying of the bladder, achieved by applying abdominal pressure, or more effectively by intermittent self-catheterisation (ISC). This form of incontinence may be described as a **sacral neurogenic bladder**. The large residual volume of urine strongly predisposes to infection, which must be prevented if possible.

In some patients, typically middle-aged women, the reflex control of detrusor activity becomes hypersensitive so that the voiding reflex is initiated when the bladder volume is well below full capacity. The cause is unknown. This hypersensitivity results in small volumes of urine being passed frequently, and often so precipitously as to produce **urge incontinence**. The condition is known as **irritable bladder syndrome** or **detrusor instability**, a minor but distressing form of incontinence.

Bladder infection produces excessive sensory irritation and activation of the voiding reflex. In young children and the elderly, this may be responsible for incontinence without the usual symptoms of infection.

Persistent bladder outflow obstruction—prostatic enlargement—causes progressive stretching of the bladder and in some way damages the voiding reflex. The result is a hugely distended, flaccid, **hypotonic bladder**. Dribbling overflow incontinence may persist even when the obstruction has been removed.

STRUCTURAL ABNORMALITIES OF THE BLADDER OR SPHINCTER

Many disorders may directly interfere with normal detrusor or sphincter function. In some cases, an additional contributory factor is damage to the afferent or efferent components of the neurogenic reflex mechanism.

The most common condition in this category is **stress incontinence**, in which the sphincter is weak. Any sudden increase of pressure on the bladder (while coughing, sneezing or laughing, for example) causes small quantities of urine to leak out. Stress incontinence is usually seen in parous women and results from pelvic floor damage during childbirth. There is often a degree of uterine prolapse and cystocoele.

Prostatectomy (transurethral or open) may damage the sphincter, as may locally invasive tumours or pelvic fractures which involve the proximal urethra. Tuberculosis, radiotherapy and **interstitial cystitis** in its severest form may cause severe bladder contraction and frequency to the point of incontinence.

Incontinence is a feature of several rare congenital abnormalities such as epispadias or an ectopic ureter opening below the sphincter mechanism. These should be excluded in a child who fails to develop continence.

PNEUMATURIA

Pneumaturia is the passage of gas mixed with urine. It is caused by perforation of gut into the urinary tract or, rarely, vice versa, resulting in fistula formation. The commonest causes are diverticular disease and Crohn's disease, although it sometimes occurs in carcinoma of the colon or bladder (see Fig. 34.3). Gross urinary tract infection is inevitable. The patient typically complains of symptoms of urinary infection (dysuria and frequency) and may also describe bubbles or even faeces in the urine.

HAEMOSPERMIA

Haemospermia describes the presence of blood in semen. It is usually innocent but can be caused by prostatitis or a stone in an ejaculatory duct. In the older male patient it is a rare presenting symptom of prostatic carcinoma.

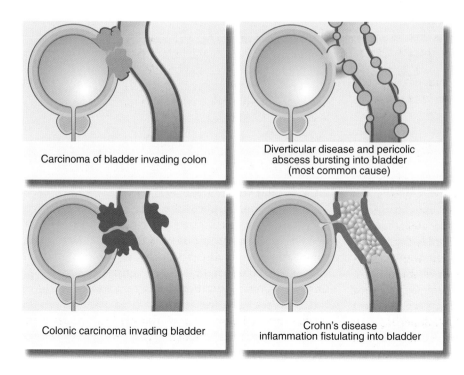

Carcinoma of bladder invading colon

Diverticular disease and pericolic abscess bursting into bladder (most common cause)

Colonic carcinoma invading bladder

Crohn's disease inflammation fistulating into bladder

Fig. 34.3 Causes of vesicocolic fistula and pneumaturia

APPROACH TO THE DIAGNOSIS OF URINARY SYMPTOMS

SPECIAL POINTS IN THE HISTORY

A detailed history of the urinary tract symptoms should be taken, together with a general history to elucidate any systemic causes or contributing factors, e.g. diabetes or multiple sclerosis. A full history of medication, both past and present, should be recorded.

In patients with haematuria, the occupational history may be important. Exposure to aniline dyes and other industrial chemicals that were once widely used in the rubber and cable industries greatly increased the risk of transitional cell carcinoma of the urinary tract. Tobacco smoking has been calculated to cause 50% of bladder cancers.

Haematuria can also be caused by infestation with *Schistosoma*, which is endemic in parts of the Middle East and Africa and is transmitted by water snails. A history of residence or travel in affected regions should therefore be sought. Similarly, tuberculosis is common in developing countries and can easily be overlooked in immigrants.

PHYSICAL EXAMINATION

GENERAL EXAMINATION

A full general examination should pay special attention to a sallow complexion and signs of weight loss which may indicate uraemia, particularly if accompanied by a uriniferous smell and scratch marks indicating itching. Blood pressure must be measured in every case as hypertension may be a feature of pyelonephritis, renal artery stenosis, polycystic kidneys or glomerulonephritis.

ABDOMINAL EXAMINATION

Abdominal inspection may reveal asymmetry due to a huge renal mass; this may be a nephroblastoma in a child or polycystic kidneys in an adult. In chronic retention, a large, sometimes lopsided bladder may be visible. The loins should be carefully inspected from behind; a subtle fullness may indicate a renal mass or a perinephric abscess.

A bimanual technique is used when examining the abdomen for kidney enlargement. One hand palpates the subcostal region anteriorly while the other hand is placed in the renal angle posteriorly to push the kidney forward on to the palpating hand. The kidneys are impalpable unless they are enlarged or displaced, except in a very thin patient. A renal mass will usually move with respiration and, because it is retroperitoneal with bowel lying anteriorly, should also have an overlying area of resonance on percussion. The main causes of an enlarged kidney are hydronephrosis, polycystic disease, renal cell carcinoma and, in children, nephroblastoma (Wilms' tumour). Loin tenderness is uncommon in non-acute renal disorders except in chronic perinephric abscess. Tenderness is usually found in acute conditions, such as pyelonephritis or acute obstruction. Renal tenderness can be distinguished from vertebral tenderness by gently tapping the spinous processes. This will cause pain if the tenderness is vertebral.

The lower abdomen is palpated for an enlarged bladder. A distended bladder is felt as a soft mass arising from the pelvis, sometimes asymmetrically. It is dull to percussion, and pressure on it may induce an urge to void; bladder distension is easily confirmed on ultrasound examination. A suprapubic mass in the male usually indicates urinary retention, but occasionally it is a colonic carcinoma or a huge bladder tumour or stone. In the female, ovarian masses, pregnancy or uterine fibroids are more common causes of a suprapubic mass than urinary retention.

Auscultation along the 12th rib posteriorly may reveal the bruit of renal artery stenosis.

RECTAL EXAMINATION

Rectal examination should be performed in both sexes. In females, a vaginal examination may also be indicated. In the male, the prostate is palpated per rectum for size, shape and consistency (see Fig. 34.4). The normal prostate is about 3 cm in diameter and weighs 10–15 g. When moderately enlarged, it is approximately the size of a golf ball and weighs about 30–40 g; when greatly enlarged, it may weigh as much as 800 g. When it is this large, its upper edge may be out of reach of the examining finger. Note that most prostatectomy operations leave a capsular remnant so that the prostate is still palpable after prostatectomy and may be of a firmer consistency. Note that it is impossible to make an accurate assessment of the volume of the prostate digitally (see Fig. 34.5).

The severity of prostatic obstructive symptoms depends not on the prostatic diameter but on the extent of encroachment upon the urethra. In some cases, an enlarged median lobe lying posteriorly above the bladder outlet may act as a flap valve, intermittently obstructing urine outflow.

On palpation, the normal prostate has a smooth surface and a firm consistency and is divided into two lateral lobes by a midline groove. In prostatic hyperplasia, enlargement is usually symmetrical, and the midline groove is maintained. Consistency remains normal. In contrast, a prostate infiltrated with carcinoma is irregular and asymmetrical. There are often hard nodules, and the median groove may be lost. In advanced cases, the tumour may be felt invading laterally into the pelvis or posteriorly around the rectum. Digital examination can help distin-

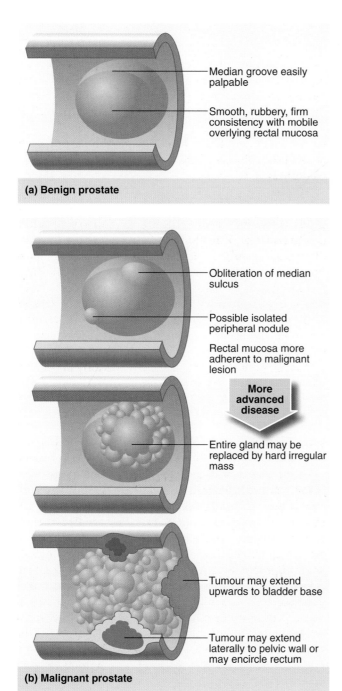

Median groove easily palpable

Smooth, rubbery, firm consistency with mobile overlying rectal mucosa

(a) Benign prostate

Obliteration of median sulcus

Possible isolated peripheral nodule

Rectal mucosa more adherent to malignant lesion

More advanced disease

Entire gland may be replaced by hard irregular mass

Tumour may extend upwards to bladder base

Tumour may extend laterally to pelvic wall or may encircle rectum

(b) Malignant prostate

Fig. 34.4 Palpation characteristics of the prostate
(a) Benign. **(b)** Malignant.

guish benign from malignant prostatic enlargement in gross cases, but if carcinoma is suspected, **transrectal ultrasound scanning (TRUS)** using a rectal probe is performed, together with multiple needle biopsies under ultrasound guidance. Note, however, that there is a 2% risk of systemic sepsis and the procedure needs to be covered with a single dose of a prophylactic antibiotic, e.g. gentamicin.

Prostatic tenderness is uncommon and may indicate prostatitis.

INVESTIGATION OF SUSPECTED URINARY TRACT DISEASE

In common conditions like prostatic hyperplasia or urinary tract infection, the diagnosis is usually evident from the history and examination. Investigation is limited to confirming and refining the diagnosis before treatment is initiated. Symptoms such as haematuria, however, suggest several diagnostic possibilities and other diagnoses must be excluded.

A simple approach to investigation of urinary tract disease is to consider the following questions:

- Are any blood tests likely to be helpful in diagnosis?
- What urine tests are indicated?
- Where is the lesion?

ARE ANY BLOOD TESTS LIKELY TO BE HELPFUL IN DIAGNOSIS?

The blood tests that can be useful in diagnosing urinary tract disease are summarised in Box 34.2.

When prostate cancer is suspected, **prostate specific antigen (PSA)** levels should be estimated and fractionated into **free PSA**, **total PSA** and their **ratio**. The free PSA is more likely to be raised in carcinoma and is a reliable indicator if the level is markedly elevated. In biopsy-proven prostatic cancer, persistently raised PSA levels above 20 are likely to indicate metastatic disease. However, the level may be normal in the presence of a small-volume cancer.

Total PSA rises with age and, in benign hyperplasia, tends to rise in proportion to prostate mass. Acute retention, urinary tract infection, any urethral instrumentation or biopsy of the prostate causes elevation of the PSA for up to 6 weeks; standard digital rectal examination does not affect PSA level.

WHAT URINE TESTS ARE INDICATED?

Any urinary symptoms should prompt collection of a clean **midstream urine (MSU) specimen** for microscopy and bacteriology. Microscopy will show the presence or absence of significant numbers of red blood cells (**microscopic haematuria**), white cells (**pyuria**) and bacteria (**bacteriuria**). However, the cells can lyse if the specimen is kept overnight at room temperature.

Bacteriuria of more than 5×10^5 per cubic millimetre is considered to indicate significant infection. The urine is cultured to identify the organisms, and the organisms are tested for antibiotic sensitivity. Culture-negative urine (**sterile pyuria**) is characteristic of urinary tract tuberculosis, urinary stone, bladder tumour, prostatitis or (most commonly) a partly treated urinary tract infection. In sterile pyuria, three early morning urine specimens should be examined for acid-fast bacilli and cultured. **Bacteriuria without significant pyuria** usually indicates

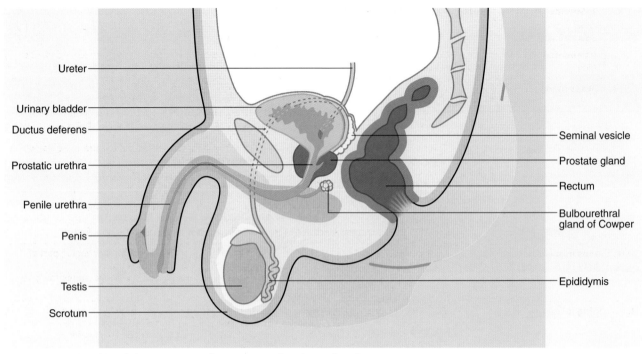

Fig. 34.5 Relationship of the prostate to the rectum and peritoneal cavity

---

Box 34.2 Blood tests useful in diagnosing urinary tract disease

Full blood count

- Hypochromic microcytic anaemia: chronic iron deficiency anaemia due to haematuria (rare)
- Normochromic normocytic anaemia: chronic renal failure (lack of erythropoietin), chronic inflammatory disorders, e.g. tuberculosis
- Polycythaemia: renal adenocarcinoma
- Leucocytosis: infection

Erythrocyte sedimentation rate (ESR) and C-reactive protein (CRP)

- Raised in chronic and acute infections, renal adenocarcinoma and retroperitoneal fibrosis

Urea, electrolytes and creatinine

- Impaired renal function in bilateral obstructive uropathy or chronic renal failure associated with hypertension, diabetes, etc.

Prostate specific antigen

- Raised in metastatic carcinoma of prostate. A normal level does not exclude prostatic carcinoma. Moderate elevations occur in benign disease, especially with acute retention of urine, urinary tract infection and following urethral instrumentation or prostatic biopsy

Alkaline phosphatase (bone isoenzyme)

- Raised in multiple bony metastases from any type of tumour

Calcium, phosphate, uric acid and parathyroid hormone levels

- Useful investigations in stone disease

---

contamination of the urine specimen. **Casts** found on microscopy suggest a nephritic (renal inflammatory) process. The presence of epithelial cells indicates perineal contamination of the specimen, a common problem in females and infants.

Urine cytology is a useful screening test for urothelial tumours in people at high risk, particularly those who have been exposed to industrial carcinogens. The test has a high positivity in carcinoma in situ and poorly differ-entiated tumours. Cytology needs to be performed on freshly voided urine. Some centres with an efficient local service use cytology for long-term follow-up of patients with treated bladder cancer.

WHERE IS THE LESION?

Investigations for localising urinary tract pathology are summarised in Table 34.2.

Table 34.2 Summary of investigations for localising urinary tract pathology

Investigation	Indications	Findings
Plain erect abdominal X-ray ('KUB' film)	Follow-up of radiopaque stones (Incidental finding)	Renal calcification; stones in kidney, ureter and bladder Abnormal renal size, shape and position
Ultrasound scanning	Renal masses Suspected upper tract obstruction Symptoms of bladder outflow obstruction	Differentiates solid from cystic renal lesions Shows dilatation of renal pelvis or ureters Estimates bladder volume after micturition; bladder wall thickness; complications of upper tract obstruction
	Transrectal ultrasound (TRUS) for assessing prostatic symptoms or enlargement	Useful for assessing the size of the gland and guiding biopsy needles
	Chronic renal disease and chronic urinary obstruction	Thickness of renal cortex
	General investigation of urinary symptoms	Morphology of upper tracts and bladder
	Investigation of urethral strictures	Definition of stricture and periurethral fibrosis
Intravenous urography (with or without tomography)	Haematuria	If tumour present, may show non-functioning part of cortex and/or distorted anatomy
	Suspected urinary tract stone	Back pressure effects of obstruction on upper tract; position of stone
CT scanning (plus intravenous contrast)	Renal mass suspicious of tumour	Abnormal mass and blood supply typical of renal tumour
	Palpable loin mass; differentiation of a pelvic mass from a prostatic or bladder tumour	Size, nature of lesions and extent of invasion
	Loin pain	Definition of cause particularly in calculous disease
Special contrast examinations of upper tract, e.g. retrograde or percutaneous (antegrade) ureterography	Obstruction of upper urinary tract not shown by other means	Site and perhaps nature of obstruction
Micturating cystography	Recurrent urinary tract infections or 'failure to thrive' in children	Severity of vesicoureteric reflux
Radionuclide renal scans	Definition of renal bloodflow, function or morphology. Diagnosis or follow-up of upper tract obstruction	Renal morphology, excretory function (total and differential), presence and sites of obstruction
	Vesicoureteric reflex	Indirect evidence of vesicoureteric reflux
Radionuclide bone scans	Bone pain in prostatic carcinoma	Bony metastases
Cystourethroscopy (with or without biopsy or bladder resection)	Haematuria Investigation of bladder neck obstruction and treatment, e.g. transurethral resection of bladder neck or prostate	Urothelial tumours of urethra or bladder Visual inspection of bladder neck and prostate
	Treatment of bladder stones	Litholapaxy (stone crushing)
Ureteroscopy	Ureteric problems, particularly stones	Direct visualisation of ureter and guidance for instrumentation to destroy or retrieve stones
Urine flow rate	Measurement of urinary flow in bladder outlet obstruction. Poor flow indicates obstruction or poorly functioning detrusor	Assessment before and after prostatectomy or bladder neck incision
Cystometrography (usually video)	Investigation of incontinence Sometimes used in assessment of bladder outflow obstruction and results of treatment	Nature of incontinence To confirm bladder outflow obstruction in equivocal outflow obstruction To demonstrate overactive bladder (detrusor instability) in irritative voiding
Renal arteriography	Occasional use in renal tumours	Demonstrating abnormal tumour blood supply (rarely used nowadays) Therapeutic embolisation for bleeding or pain in inoperable tumours

Suspected upper tract lesions

Ultrasound

Renal ultrasound is a valuable non-invasive technique for investigating a suspected renal mass. Ultrasound is particularly useful in differentiating solid from cystic lesions, and for demonstrating dilatation of the renal pelvis. If bladder pathology is suspected, the bladder can easily be examined at the same time. The bladder is particularly well seen if it is distended with urine; patients should be advised to take copious fluids before the investigation is performed. Ultrasound can demonstrate stones in the kidney or bladder even if they are radiolucent (urate), but can rarely demonstrate a stone in the ureter.

Intravenous urography

Intravenous urography (IVU) is the traditional radiographic technique for demonstrating the urinary tract, although it provides poor assessment of function. Comparative renal function is best investigated by radionuclide scanning.

IVU involves intravenous injection of a contrast medium which is rapidly filtered by the glomeruli and excreted. This radiopaque solution opacifies the urinary system, demonstrating the renal parenchyma, the renal pelvis and the ureteric anatomy. The cortical concentration of contrast (**nephrogram**) gives an indication of the size, shape, thickness and bilateral symmetry of the renal cortex.

Cysts and tumours of the kidneys are usually revealed by the distortion of normal anatomy they cause, although they are often indistinguishable from each other by this investigation. Tumours opacify with contrast to a variable extent and sometimes show a characteristic 'vascular blush'.

If the collecting system (renal pelvis, calyces and ureter) is dilated, this is usually easily seen, and the level of an obstruction can often be demonstrated. When obstruction is almost complete, films may have to be taken at long intervals since back pressure delays cortical excretion.

Congenital abnormalities of the pelvicalyceal system, such as duplex systems, are often found incidentally. Transitional cell tumours may show as filling defects in collecting systems or bladder. If an abnormality is seen in the kidney or renal pelvis, **renal tomography** can be performed during the same examination to reveal more structural detail (see Ch. 5). If renal excretion is poor as in chronic renal failure, IVU examination yields poor images. In addition, the contrast material may lead to further impairment of renal function. Similarly, in diabetic nephropathy intravenous contrast may precipitate acute renal failure. In such cases, retrograde pyelography is the investigation of choice, if available.

In the initial assessment of urological symptoms, the imaging investigation of choice is ultrasound, although

IVU is a better option in stone disease or when greater detail of the ureters is required.

CT scanning

In urology, CT scanning is usually performed after injection of intravenous contrast. This helps distinguish renal malignancy from hamartomas or other benign diseases. It can also distinguish the rare **angiomyolipoma** of the kidney. Modern spiral and multislice CT machines give more rapid image capture and better definition. In renal cell carcinoma, CT can demonstrate direct spread of tumour thrombus along the renal vein and into the inferior vena cava so that surgery can be better planned. Enlarged lymph nodes may be diagnosed and biopsied percutaneously and the liver examined for metastases. CT may demonstrate that the malignancy is so advanced as to be inoperable, saving the patient a fruitless operation. In bladder or prostatic cancer, CT can aid staging by demonstrating whether the disease is **organ-confined**. Increasingly, spiral or multislice non-contrast CT is indicated for the investigation of stone disease, particularly ureteric colic.

Special contrast investigations

Ascending ureterography, in which contrast is injected directly up the ureters via a cystoscope, is especially useful for defining ureteric tumours. Its use has considerably declined, however, as radiological experience and technologies have advanced.

Radionuclide scanning

Radionuclide scanning techniques can be used to assess differential renal function. They are particularly useful in monitoring renal function after relief of obstruction. They can demonstrate renal scars and are a non-invasive method of demonstrating vesicoureteric reflux in children.

Suspected lower tract lesions

Radiography and ultrasound

Ultrasound examination has largely replaced IVU as the standard investigation for lower tract disease. Modern high-resolution ultrasound equipment can demonstrate tumours, cysts and other abnormalities of bladder and prostate shape and volume, but can seldom define lesions smaller than 5 mm. Ultrasonography can also define the size, shape and position of stones in the kidney. In addition, it can be employed to estimate the volume of residual urine where there is any degree of bladder outlet obstruction. **Transrectal ultrasound** can help assess the size of the prostate as well as allowing directed biopsies of abnormal areas. In addition, it can help achieve representative biopsies of all areas of the prostate, in which a minimum of eight representative samples is required.

Cystourethroscopy

Cystourethroscopy (cystoscopy), using rigid or flexible instruments, is an important diagnostic and therapeutic tool for disease of the urethra, prostate and bladder. Flexible cystoscopy can usually be performed under local anaesthesia on an outpatient basis.

A similar but longer rigid instrument, the **ureteroscope**, can now be used for retrieving stones from the ureter, and a flexible ureteroscope allows passage to the kidney and treatment of calyceal stones by laser lithotripsy.

When a bladder tumour or urethral pathology is suspected, **cystoscopy** is the investigation of choice. Flexible cystoscopy allows the same 'instant' availability as outpatient flexible sigmoidoscopy. It allows direct visual examination, but if biopsy and immediate treatment are known to be required, rigid cystoscopy is usually performed under general or regional anaesthesia; this also permits deep bimanual palpation (eua).

Other investigations

If clinical examination suggests local spread of a bladder or prostatic tumour, **CT** or **MRI scanning** may be used to assess the extent of invasion. In carcinoma of the prostate, **radionuclide scanning** is the most accurate non-invasive method for diagnosing bony metastases.

In perineal injuries and pelvic fractures, **urethrography** is the best investigation for assessing suspected urethral rupture and may be combined with **suprapubic contrast cystography**. It is also used for urethral stricture examination. For suspected urethral obstruction, **contrast urethrography** or urethral ultrasound can be used to localise the site of obstruction or stricture. If a colovesical fistula is suspected, **barium enema** may demonstrate the colonic lesion responsible (but rarely the fistula itself).

Urine flow rate provides a quick assessment of the degree of outflow obstruction and can be used after treatment to assess change. It is easily measured and can be plotted simultaneously on a graph as voiding progresses. The patient simply passes urine into a funnel leading to the machine, although it should be noted that urine volumes voided below 100 ml can be misleading. When incontinence and bladder instability are being investigated, **cystometrography** is usually performed as a video-cystogram and this is combined with urodynamic measurements to assess the relationship between bladder pressure and volume. It is particularly useful in the case of high-pressure bladders with outlet obstruction and in diagnosing urge and stress incontinence in women.

35 Disorders of the prostate

INTRODUCTION

Benign hyperplasia and carcinoma are the most common prostatic disorders and they have an increasing importance in an ageing population. Inflammation and infection of the prostate (**prostatitis**) is a less common condition that occurs in a younger age group and is clinically rather poorly defined.

ANATOMY

The normal prostate gland is about 3 cm long and 3 cm in diameter and weighs about 10–15 g. The gland is situated immediately below the bladder neck so that the first 3 cm of the urethra lies within the gland (see Fig. 35.5, p. 524). Thus, the walls of the proximal urethra are composed of glandular tissue and this part is known as the **prostatic urethra**. The urethra then passes through the muscle of the pelvic floor that also constitutes the distal sphincteric mechanism. Prostatic hyperplasia or carcinoma may cause local urethral obstruction, and carcinoma may invade and disrupt the sphincter mechanism.

The posterior aspect of the gland is palpable rectally (see Fig. 35.4, pp. 521, 522) and a **median groove** can usually be identified. This groove is described as dividing the gland into two lateral lobes. The median groove tends to be obliterated in advanced prostatic carcinoma but is usually exaggerated in benign hypertrophy.

When the prostatic urethra is examined cystoscopically, an important landmark is the **veru montanum** (urethral crest), an elongated mound on the posterior wall. The size and prominence of the veru may vary considerably. At its midpoint is a small depression that may be visible, into which the two **ejaculatory ducts** open. The posterior part of the gland lying above the ejaculatory ducts is known as the **median lobe**. If this becomes hypertrophied it may form a pedunculated mass in the floor of the bladder (often described as the surgical 'middle lobe'); this may act as a flap valve and obstruct the bladder outlet.

As seen in Figure 35.1, the bulk of the normal prostate consists of up to 50 peripheral **glandular lobules**. These converge into about 20 separate ducts that open into the prostatic urethra lateral to the veru montanum. In addition to this glandular tissue proper, there is a zone of small para-urethral glands immediately adjacent to the urethra, the **transition zone**.

From middle age onwards, the transition zone tends to enlarge to cause **benign prostatic hyperplasia**. At the same time, the peripheral glandular tissue becomes compressed to form a fibrous outer 'surgical capsule'. In contrast, carcinoma of the prostate arises most often in the peripheral glandular tissue, tending to spread outwards into adjacent structures more often than obstructing the centrally located urethra. Even after prostatectomy, carcinoma may arise in the glands of the remnant of the peripheral zone.

The normal prostate gland is surrounded by a filmy **true capsule** of little surgical significance; outside this is a rich venous plexus which, in turn, is invested by a dense fascial sheath. During open or endoscopic prostatectomy, it is important not to disturb this venous plexus as it is a common source of haemorrhage during and after the operation. There are direct venous connections between the prostatic plexus and the vertebral extradural venous plexus which provide an easy route for blood-borne dissemination of prostatic cancer. Posteriorly, the prostatic fascial sheath is fused with the dense **fascia of Denonvilliers**. This provides something of a barrier against direct spread of cancer from the prostate to the rectum and vice versa.

BENIGN PROSTATIC HYPERPLASIA

Benign prostatic hyperplasia (BPH) affects half of all men aged 50, and the proportion increases with advancing age

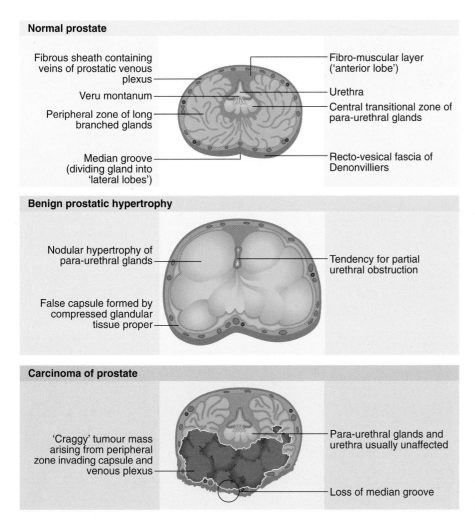

Normal prostate

Fibrous sheath containing veins of prostatic venous plexus

Veru montanum

Peripheral zone of long branched glands

Median groove (dividing gland into 'lateral lobes')

Fibro-muscular layer ('anterior lobe')

Urethra

Central transitional zone of para-urethral glands

Recto-vesical fascia of Denonvilliers

Benign prostatic hypertrophy

Nodular hypertrophy of para-urethral glands

False capsule formed by compressed glandular tissue proper

Tendency for partial urethral obstruction

Carcinoma of prostate

'Craggy' tumour mass arising from peripheral zone invading capsule and venous plexus

Para-urethral glands and urethra usually unaffected

Loss of median groove

Fig. 35.1 Horizontal sections through normal, hypertrophic and malignant prostate glands

such that BPH is universal at 70 years. Approximately half of those with BPH have either no symptoms or mild symptoms acceptable to the patient and his family. In about 50% of men over 60, however, hyperplasia produces sufficient symptoms for treatment to be considered.

PATHOPHYSIOLOGY OF BENIGN PROSTATIC HYPERPLASIA

In pathological terms, the para-urethral transition zone glands undergo **nodular hyperplasia**. This causes progressive symmetrical enlargement of the gland up to several times its normal size. Patients occasionally present with a gland of 150 g but most are less than 50 g. The largest glands (of up to 800 g) may be fibrosarcomatous. The prostatic glandular tissue proper is compressed peripherally to form a false or surgical capsule. Occasionally, the process is predominantly fibrotic, resulting in a small dense gland. Similar symptoms and signs of bladder outflow obstruction may be caused by the apparently independent disorder of **bladder neck hypertrophy and fibrosis**. Bladder outflow obstruction can be caused

entirely by enlargement of the prostatic gland, by bladder neck obstruction or by a combination of the two.

The size of the prostate cannot be estimated reliably by digital examination and is best assessed by ultrasound. However, there is little relationship between prostatic volume and symptoms, and the presence of a large prostate without symptoms is no indication for treatment. Urine flow rate is determined by the calibre and length of the prostatic urethra and by detrusor contractility, not by prostatic bulk. Prostatic urethroscopy provides further anatomical detail but no functional information.

CLINICAL FEATURES OF BENIGN PROSTATIC HYPERPLASIA

The symptoms of bladder outlet obstruction are summarised in Box 35.1. Symptoms usually develop gradually until eventually they interfere with daytime activity and sleep. **Acute retention** of urine may occur suddenly at any time and is commonly precipitated by bladder overfilling after excessive fluid intake. It is also a hazard of many general surgical or orthopaedic operations on older men

---

| Box | 35.1 | **Symptoms of bladder outlet obstruction** |

Symptoms formally assessed using the International Prostate Symptom Score (I-PSS). Each symptom is graded from 1 to 5 (up to 6 for nocturia) for the previous month. Total indicates severity of symptoms: 0–7 = mild; 8–19 = moderate; 20–35 severe

- Incomplete bladder emptying after urination
- Frequency—need for urination again after less than 2 hours
- Intermittent flow—stopping and starting during urination
- Urgency—difficult to postpone urination
- Weak stream—often made worse by a full bladder or by straining
- Straining to begin urination
- Nocturia—number of times needing to urinate per night

Other symptoms (not scored)

- Hesitancy, worse with a full bladder or at night
- Post-micturition dribbling
- Double micturition ('pis-à-deux')

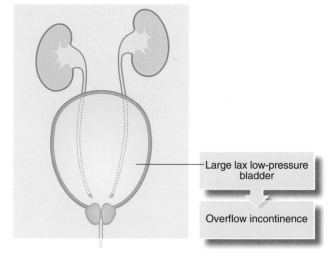

Fig. 35.2 Atonic bladder due to outlet obstruction

and also of pelvic or perineal operations after adolescence. In some patients, the severity of prostatic symptoms fluctuates from month to month (and even perhaps with the season!), making it difficult to decide whether an operation is necessary.

COMPLICATIONS OF BLADDER OUTLET OBSTRUCTION

Prostatic obstruction can progressively interfere with the patient's ability to empty his bladder but only 20–30% of patients have progressive symptoms and 50% remain unchanged over a 5-year period. In the progressive cases, the volume of **residual urine** gradually increases over weeks and months (i.e. chronic retention) and the intravesical pressure rises. The threshold for the voiding reflex is therefore reached more quickly and calls to void become more frequent. The stagnant residual urine is prone to infection, which exacerbates the symptoms. In chronic retention, the bladder becomes vastly distended and atonic, leading to **overflow incontinence** (see Fig. 35.2). In other cases, the detrusor muscle undergoes hypertrophy in an attempt to overcome the outflow obstruction. The normally smooth bladder lining then becomes trabeculated. Eventually, muscle fibre bundles are replaced by non-contractile fibrous tissue; this may explain why some patients fail to improve after the prostatic obstruction is relieved. With a further rise in pressure, the depressions between the muscle bands deepen (sacculation) and eventually form **bladder diverticula**. Urinary stasis in the diverticula predisposes to stone formation (see Fig. 35.3).

A small proportion of patients with bladder outlet obstruction experience little in the way of local symptoms. In these, rising intravesical pressure can be transmitted back into the ureters and kidneys causing hydronephrosis and **progressive renal parenchymal damage**. Patients often present with systemic illness or symptoms such as anorexia, apparently of non-renal origin. The renal failure may be accompanied by anaemia, dehydration, acidosis and infection. Bladder outflow obstruction in these patients is easily overlooked unless the bladder is examined for distension.

MANAGEMENT OF BENIGN PROSTATIC HYPERPLASIA

The principles of management of bladder outlet obstruction believed to be due to benign prostatic hyperplasia are outlined in Box 35.2.

Diagnosis

A detailed history is first taken to assess the nature of the symptoms and how much they interfere with the patient's life. The International Prostate Symptom Score sheet helps in assessing the overall impact of symptoms (Box 35.1). This, together with the patient's general condition, are the principal factors determining the need for treatment. The abdomen is examined for bladder size and the prostate palpated rectally. These clinical examinations, however, will reveal only gross abnormalities.

The next step is to investigate the effects of outlet obstruction on the bladder by measuring the **urinary flow rate** and estimating the **volume of residual urine** using ultrasound examination. This is reliable, quick, non-invasive, safe and cheap. When urinary symptoms are severe but residual volume is insignificant, the alternative diagnosis of an **irritable bladder** should be investigated. Cystometrography is more complex and involves

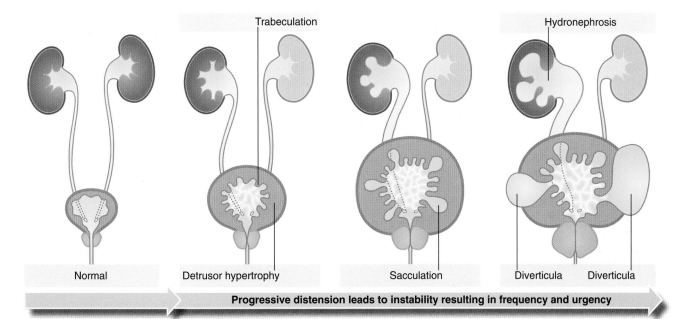

Fig. 35.3 Back-pressure effects of bladder neck obstruction

Box 35.2 **Management of chronic bladder outflow obstruction**

- Assess the symptoms and the likely need for treatment from the history, particularly how much the symptoms bother the patient
- Estimate the severity of bladder outlet obstruction by ultrasound and by measuring urine flow rate or cystometrography
- Investigate any disturbance of upper tract function and structure with renal function tests and ultrasound
- Exclude urinary tract infection by urine microscopy and culture
- Exclude prostatic carcinoma clinically, biochemically (prostate specific antigen) and by transrectal diagnostic ultrasound; if necessary, perform guided needle biopsy of abnormal areas
- Treat renal failure and other systemic problems
- Consider whether catheter drainage of the bladder is desirable

- Cystoscope the patient to rule out other pathology and to define the anatomical problem
- Discuss with the patient what can be offered and at what risk, i.e. drug treatment, transurethral resection of prostate (TURP), laser vaporisation or enucleation or, as a last resort, long-term catheterisation
- Implement appropriate non-surgical treatments

If operation becomes necessary, diagnose the cause and extent of obstruction by cystoscopy, then either:
- Resect benign prostatic hyperplasia, divide bladder neck hypertrophy transurethrally, or obtain biopsy material by TURP if carcinoma seems likely and prior confirmation has been negative
or
- Consider any other operative measures such as open prostatectomy or excision of diverticula where appropriate

---

measuring the filling and emptying pressures of the bladder but it may be invaluable if doubt remains about the nature of the problem.

Renal function is assessed by estimating serum urea, creatinine and electrolytes. If these are abnormal, further metabolic investigations may be necessary and renal tract ultrasound is mandatory.

A **midstream specimen of urine** should be examined by microscopy and culture as urinary infection alone may be responsible for the presenting symptoms or may have precipitated an episode of urinary retention. In addition,

if surgery is intended, it is important that infection is eradicated because of the risk of perioperative sepsis and secondary haemorrhage.

If the prostate feels nodular on palpation, carcinoma should be suspected, particularly if the serum **prostate specific antigen** (PSA) is elevated. Transrectal ultrasound scanning of the prostate (TRUS) and needle biopsy of suspicious areas should be performed even if prostatectomy is planned because a preoperative diagnosis of carcinoma is likely to alter the plan of management. Marked elevation of serum PSA level is diagnostic of prostatic cancer but a mildly elevated PSA may be due to benign disease or infection. A normal result does not, however, exclude cancer.

Relief of chronic retention and obstructive effects on the kidney

In chronic retention associated with a large volume of residual urine (750 ml or more), abnormal renal function or upper tract dilatation on renal tract ultrasound, the patient is usually catheterised for a period to drain the bladder. This allows detrusor tone to recover over the course of a few days. Drainage also allows any reversible component of renal failure to correct itself; it may take 3 weeks of catheter drainage to improve biochemical renal function tests, after which spontaneous improvement is unlikely. Initially, fluid and electrolyte balance is monitored and restored if necessary by infusing intravenous fluid. In patients with chronic outflow obstruction and obstructive renal failure, catheterisation may produce a **massive diuresis** and this should be anticipated and treated appropriately. Such patients may need blood transfusion, intravenous antibiotics and other preparatory measures before surgery can be contemplated.

Cystoscopy

Despite the above investigations, the anatomical nature of the bladder outlet obstruction can only be accurately assessed by direct cystoscopic examination. At the same time, the bladder can be examined for other problems such as trabeculation, diverticula, tumours and stones. In patients with complications from bladder outlet obstruction or severe symptoms not responding to medical treatment, transurethral resection (TUR) or laser enucleation of the obstruction is performed under the same anaesthetic (see *TURP*, below). In elderly or unfit patients, placement of a **urethral stent** may be considered. However, these devices are prone to problems of displacement, haemorrhage, local irritation and blockage. Only very occasionally are patients too unfit for some form of intervention. It is now rarely necessary to leave a patient with a long-term catheter; in this event a suprapubic catheter is far preferable to a urethral catheter because of the ease of changing it and much greater patient comfort.

Drug treatments

Finasteride or **dutasteride** blocks the enzyme 5-alpha reductase from converting testosterone to dihydro-testosterone and thus reduces the size of hyperplastic prostate glands. A 6-month trial of treatment is required; if successful, symptoms may improve to the extent that surgery can be delayed or avoided. Some herbal remedies such as **saw palmetto** contain naturally occurring 5-alpha reductase substances. The place of finasteride and similar drugs in managing prostatic hyperplasia is still being defined but they can reduce the rates of surgical intervention and acute retention.

Alpha-adrenergic A_1 receptors are present in the bladder neck and prostate. If bladder neck hypertrophy or a prostate less than 50 g is responsible for the symptoms, selective alpha-adrenergic blocking drugs may enable the prostatic urethra to open more readily, relieving symptoms. Newer drugs, e.g. tamsulosin or alfuzosin, have fewer side effects than earlier drugs such as prazosin. Combination therapy with alpha-adrenergic blocking drugs and 5-alpha reductase inhibitors may be more beneficial in some patients.

Transurethral resection of prostate (TURP) and other transurethral treatments

Transurethral prostatectomy has lower postoperative mortality and morbidity than open retropubic prostatectomy and requires a shorter hospital stay. Whilst TURP remains the standard for prostatic surgery, various other physical treatments have given varying degrees of success. Cryo-prostatectomy (freezing the gland), cold punch prostatectomy, microwave thermotherapy and transurethral needle ablation (TUNA) are obsolete procedures. **Holmium laser enucleation of prostate (HOLeP)** yields at least equivalent results to TURP with the added benefit of reduced blood loss. In addition, larger glands can be enucleated than can reasonably be resected, thus avoiding the need for open retropubic prostatectomy. **Laser ablation techniques** (using KTP-green light and holmium lasers) can be valuable in special circumstances such as a patient on warfarin and have shown promising results approaching those of TURP.

The aim of transurethral prostatectomy is to remove the bulk of the prostate but leave the compressed but normal peripheral tissue. This protects the subcapsular venous plexus which might otherwise bleed catastrophically. In TURP a series of 'chips' or strips of tissue are excised with the resectoscope using a cutting diathermy wire loop; the chips drift into the bladder out of the way. A transparent isotonic irrigation solution is used during the process and this washes away blood and debris to allow continuous visibility. Some irrigation fluid is inevitably absorbed, so sterile **glycine solution** is most often used instead of water as it does not cause haemolysis. If large volumes are absorbed, this causes dilutional hyponatraemia and hyperammonaemia along with drastic plasma electrolyte changes, producing the **TUR syndrome**. Various isotonic sugar solutions can now be safely used as alternatives. The enlarged gland is progressively sliced away as shown in Figure 35.4, taking great care to preserve the sphincter mechanism immediately distal to the veru montanum. The prostatic chips are always examined histologically and may reveal unsuspected carcinoma.

When obstruction is caused by bladder neck hypertrophy, the prostate is not usually resected but the bladder

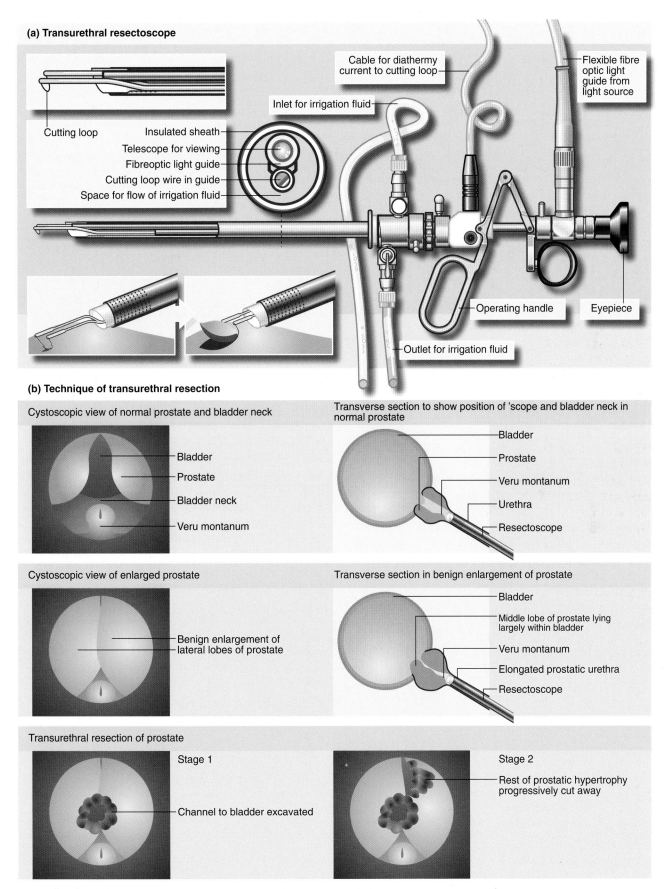

Fig. 35.4 Transurethral prostatectomy
(a) Transurethral resectoscope. 'Divots' or chips are cut by squeezing the handle towards the eyepiece while turning the diathermy current on. This 'cheese-wires' the cutting loop through tissue. (b) Technique of transurethral resection.

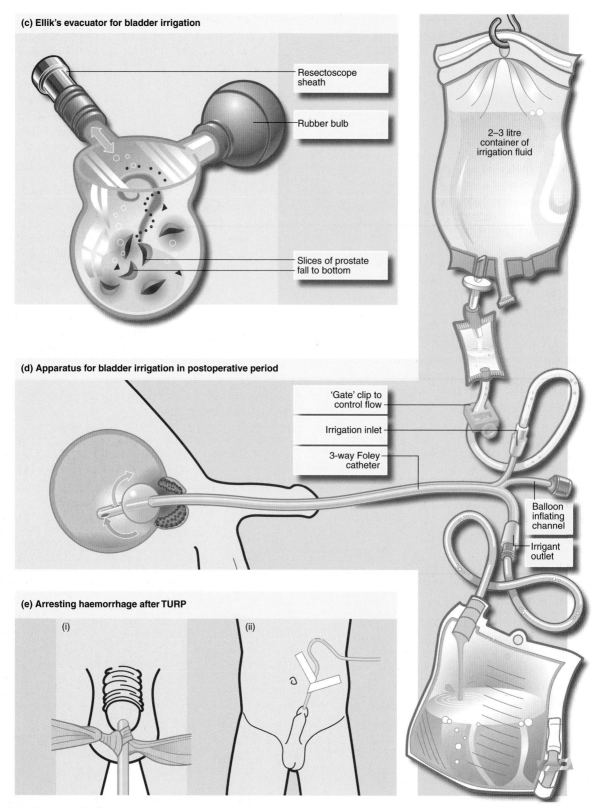

Fig. 35.4 Transurethral prostatectomy

(c) Ellik's evacuator for bladder irrigation. The instrument is completely filled with irrigation fluid and then attached to the resectoscope sheath which is left in the bladder after withdrawal of the main instrument. Squeezing the bulb flushes fluid alternately in and out of the bladder, bringing the cut prostatic slices with it which then settle to the bottom of the glass container. **(d)** Apparatus for bladder irrigation in the postoperative period. The rate of fluid flow is adjusted to be fast enough to prevent clotting within the bladder. In practice the effluent should be pink rather than red. **(e)** Arresting haemorrhage after TURP. Excessive bleeding after transurethral resection can often be controlled by inserting a special large balloon catheter and exerting traction on the catheter for 20 minutes (but not more). Tension is maintained by (i) tying a swab around the catheter, or (ii) attaching the catheter to the anterior abdominal wall with adhesive tape.

neck muscle is divided by making a longitudinal incision (bladder neck incision, BNI) using a diathermy point via the resectoscope. This operation is also effective where the obstruction is caused by a small prostate (< 30 g).

Retropubic prostatectomy

Open prostatectomy is used when the gland is so large that transurethral resection is not practicable or on the odd occasion where there are accompanying bladder diverticula or huge stones.

Complications of TURP and open prostatectomy

Prostatectomy usually disrupts the mechanism at the bladder neck which normally prevents semen entering the bladder during ejaculation. Thus, patients usually fail to ejaculate through the penis after prostatectomy (**retrograde ejaculation**), although the sensation of orgasm is unaffected. This affects 75% of patients and it is essential that the patient is informed and accepts this possible side effect beforehand. Maintaining fertility is not usually important in this older age group, but should the need arise, urine can be filtered to recover sperm for artificial insemination. **Erectile impotence** follows TURP in 5–10%, a similar rate to other major operations in the pelvis or perineal area; patients must be informed of this before consent to operation is obtained. **Urethral strictures** develop in 1–10% of cases, reflecting the relatively large instruments used and the employment of potentially harmful urethral catheters.

Minor **haematuria** can be expected during the first few weeks after prostatectomy. Secondary haemorrhage (due to infection or unsuspected cancer) can be more profuse and may cause **clot retention**, i.e. retention of urine caused by obstructing blood clot. Recovery of complete urinary continence is sometimes delayed following prostatectomy but there is only occasional permanent damage to the sphincter mechanism.

Long-term catheterisation or stenting

Operation greatly improves the quality of life in most patients. Even in patients over 80, perioperative morbidity and mortality are acceptably low. Nevertheless, a small proportion of severely debilitated, immobile or demented patients are better managed by long-term suprapubic or urethral catheterisation, changed regularly by the family practitioner or in the hospital department (see catheter management, below). An alternative is in-situ urethral stenting, although this currently has a high rate of failure and other complications.

ACUTE URINARY RETENTION AND ITS MANAGEMENT

Acute urinary retention may occur in patients with long-standing symptoms of bladder outlet obstruction; indeed in the majority of men with chronic retention, acute retention is the first presentation. It is often precipitated by overfilling of the bladder, faecal loading or urinary tract infection but infarction of the gland substance may play a role in some cases. Acute retention is a common cause of emergency surgical admission. It is also a frequent early complication after any major operation, especially in males, and may occur at any age even without bladder neck hypertrophy or prostatic enlargement. Management of postoperative acute retention is described in Chapter 12.

DIAGNOSIS OF ACUTE RETENTION

In a patient with no urine output, acute retention must be distinguished from anuria. However, the diagnosis is usually not difficult—the patient in retention is acutely distressed with abdominal or perineal pain and a readily palpable bladder. A brief history of previous similar episodes, previous urological surgery or accidental injury should be sought in case special treatment is required. If the problem is uncomplicated, a more complete history can be delayed until after the pain is relieved by catheterisation.

CATHETERISATION

Acute retention is usually treated by urethral or suprapubic catheterisation. Suprapubic catheterisation is no more demanding of the trained junior doctor or patient than urethral catheterisation (Figs 35.5, 35.6). In either case, strict aseptic precautions must be taken to avoid introducing infection. Urethral catheterisation may prove difficult in patients with a history of previous difficult catheterisation, prostatectomy or urethral stricture or the finding of a non-retractile foreskin. For a patient with pelvic trauma and a suspected urethral fracture, suprapubic catheterisation is mandatory. Inserting a suprapubic catheter is quick and safe provided the bladder is palpably distended but should be avoided if there is a history of bladder tumour. If the problem appears complex, an experienced opinion should be sought early on before risking urethral damage by unwise attempts at urethral catheterisation. A surgeon with urological training may elect to carry out cystourethroscopy and appropriate surgical treatment as a single scheduled procedure if catheterisation is not urgent.

EVALUATING THE UNDERLYING CAUSE AND ANY PRECIPITATING FACTORS

A catheter is usually left in situ for a day or two after relieving the acute retention until the patient has been fully assessed. At this point, the decision is whether to attempt a **trial without catheter** or **TWOC** (i.e. test whether the patient can void urine satisfactorily when the catheter is removed, or clamped off in the case of a suprapubic catheter) or whether to proceed directly with surgi-

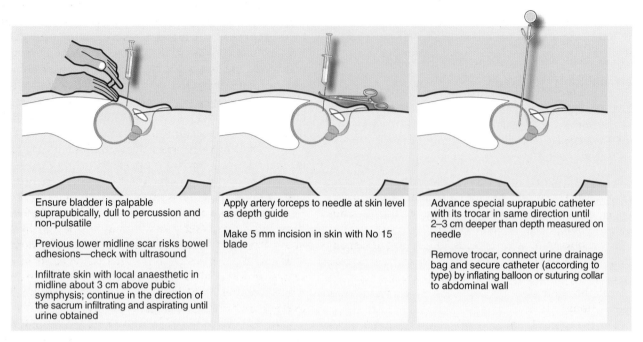

Ensure bladder is palpable suprapubically, dull to percussion and non-pulsatile

Previous lower midline scar risks bowel adhesions—check with ultrasound

Infiltrate skin with local anaesthetic in midline about 3 cm above pubic symphysis; continue in the direction of the sacrum infiltrating and aspirating until urine obtained

Apply artery forceps to needle at skin level as depth guide

Make 5 mm incision in skin with No 15 blade

Advance special suprapubic catheter with its trocar in same direction until 2–3 cm deeper than depth measured on needle

Remove trocar, connect urine drainage bag and secure catheter (according to type) by inflating balloon or suturing collar to abdominal wall

Fig. 35.5 Suprapubic catheterisation

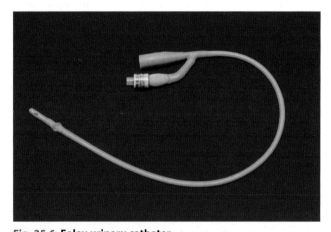

Fig. 35.6 Foley urinary catheter
The most commonly used self-retaining catheter. The main tube is made of latex, silicone-coated latex, silicone rubber or plastic. After passing the catheter into the bladder, the distal balloon is inflated with water or saline according to its capacity, usually between 5 ml and 20 ml, and a drainage bag attached to the distal end of the catheter.

cal or other treatment. Any urinary tract infection must be vigorously treated before a trial without catheter or an operation.

Common indications for cystourethroscopy and early prostatectomy or bladder neck resection are:

- A huge volume of retained urine released by catheterisation—indicates chronic retention
- Raised levels of plasma urea and creatinine which improve after catheterisation—indicates chronic obstructive uropathy
- Previous episodes of acute retention
- Bladder outflow obstruction caused by carcinoma of prostate
- Failure of 'trial without catheter'
- Presence of vesical (bladder) calculi
- Acute retention in combination with a history of prostatism sufficient in itself to warrant surgery

'TRIAL WITHOUT CATHETER'

If appropriate, the catheter should be removed either around midnight or very early in the morning so that if the trial is unsuccessful, a catheter can be replaced before the patient's and the surgeon's bedtime. Success is judged if the patient can pass reasonable volumes of urine with each voiding, i.e. more than about 100 ml. Even if passing good volumes, the patient must be examined at intervals to ensure that the bladder is not distending with retained urine which would indicate chronic retention with overflow. Unsuccessful trial without catheter is an indication for cystourethroscopy and probable surgical treatment on the next available operating list. Approximately 50% will pass urine successfully, although many (up to 50%) will have a further period of retention within 1 year. Men with low flow rates, large residual volumes and palpably large prostates are more likely to develop further retention.

INDWELLING CATHETERS AND THEIR MANAGEMENT

The majority of patients with permanent catheters are elderly men with bladder outflow obstruction in whom surgery is either contraindicated or has failed. Indications for permanent catheterisation include:

- Patient unfit for prostatectomy
- Incontinent, elderly patient who is severely debilitated, demented or immobile
- Incontinence due to external sphincter damage caused by previous prostatectomy or invading carcinoma
- 'Sacral neurogenic bladder', e.g. in multiple sclerosis

Improvements in urological care, anaesthesia and perioperative care have meant that many more patients can tolerate prostatectomy safely and are no longer condemned to long-term catheterisation.

For the rare patient who needs long-term catheterisation, either the **urethral** or the **suprapubic** route may be used. An indwelling suprapubic catheter (inserted directly through the abdominal wall) is likely to have fewer complications.

For either type, the major problems are **recurrent catheter blockage** and **infection**. Catheters readily become blocked by epithelial debris or by gradual accretion of calculus. Modern silicone or silicone-coated 'long-term' catheters are better in this respect but must still be changed regularly (every 10–12 weeks) to avoid this. In most cases, they can be changed at home by the general practitioner or community nurse using full sterile precautions and antibiotic cover to prevent systemic sepsis. Once infection becomes established in the presence of a catheter, it is difficult to eradicate. However, low-grade infection is almost constantly present in elderly patients and causes little discomfort. Antibiotics should be prescribed only if local symptoms become troublesome, if systemic signs of infection develop or when the catheter is changed.

CATHETERS IN PARAPLEGIC PATIENTS

In paraplegic patients, ureteric reflux predisposes to recurrent upper urinary tract infections. Established infections lead to progressive renal failure and death at an early age. For these patients, special care must be taken to avoid introducing infection, and urine specimens should be regularly microscoped and cultured and any infections treated promptly. **Intermittent catheterisation** rather than an indwelling catheter may be a better form of management, provided it is performed correctly; in many cases, patients successfully perform intermittent self-catheterisation.

CARCINOMA OF THE PROSTATE

PATHOPHYSIOLOGY OF PROSTATIC CARCINOMA

Carcinoma of the prostate is common after the age of 65 years and is becoming increasingly common in the two decades before that age. The rising incidence is partly but not entirely explained by an enormous increase in early cases discovered on screening, particularly in the USA. The rise may also be related to high meat and fat consumption. East Asians living on a predominantly vegetarian diet have the lowest incidence of prostate cancer. There is some evidence that prostate cancer is more common in men who have fewer ejaculations over their lifetime.

Carcinoma usually arises in the **peripheral** prostatic glands rather than in the para-urethral tissue and thus is often slow to intrude on the urethra and become symptomatic. For the same reason, malignant change occurs in the **pseudocapsule** of compressed peripheral glandular tissue remaining after prostatectomy for benign hyperplasia. Prostatic cancers are nearly all **adenocarcinomas** with variable degrees of differentiation reflected in the aggressiveness of local and metastatic spread. The exception is carcinoma of the prostatic ducts. This is urothelial in origin and behaves like bladder cancer.

Most adenocarcinomas are well differentiated and contained within the capsule, slowly invading adjacent prostatic tissue and sometimes involving the bladder neck or sphincter mechanism. In many cases, the prostate is already enlarged by benign hyperplasia. Prostatic cancer metastasises to pelvic lymph nodes and via the bloodstream to bone (for which it has a particular affinity) and other organs. Tumour cells enter the subcapsular venous plexus which drains directly into the spinal venous system. This may explain the frequent occurrence of bone metastasis in the pelvis and spinal column. The average survival time after diagnosis of metastases is about 2 years.

Until recently, a higher proportion of patients in the UK, in contrast to the USA, have presented with either locally advanced or metastatic disease and are therefore incurable. However, in recent years with greater public awareness and PSA testing, men are now being seen with earlier organ-confined and potentially curable disease.

Most prostatic cancers secrete a glycoprotein, **prostate specific antigen** (PSA), which is detectable in the blood even when the tumour remains confined within the gland. More advanced tumours appear to produce greater amounts and hence higher blood levels of PSA. Other prostatic conditions (e.g. hyperplasia, prostatitis) may cause elevation of PSA but levels over 10–15 nanograms/ml are likely to be caused by cancer, provided urinary infection can be eliminated as a cause.

Most tumours depend on the presence of male sex hormones for their growth and are rendered quiescent, at least for a time, by surgical or chemical castration. Localised tumours may be so slow-growing as to be effectively dormant but an unknown proportion of these will later metastasise. The main prognostic indicators are the presenting PSA level, the PSA velocity (i.e. the rate at which it rises) and the histological grading. These factors have complicated the debate about the value of screening for prostatic cancer and the appropriateness of radical 'curative' surgery for localised asymptomatic disease. Prostate cancer screening has not yet been recommended in the UK and Australia and there is little evidence that it is worthwhile.

Many patients have asymptomatic, localised or dormant disease diagnosed incidentally at TURP for presumed benign disease. At autopsy, one-third of men over 50 and 90% of men over 90 dying of other causes have microscopic cancer in the prostate and it can be assumed that this is true for the population at large. The natural history of such occult cancers is unknown and it seems that many do not progress to become clinically relevant. Some elderly patients with occult metastatic disease suffer

troublesome non-specific symptoms, e.g. malaise and fatigue, which may be dismissed at first if prostatic cancer is not considered in the differential diagnosis. Even after characteristic local symptoms appear, the disease often pursues a prolonged course and many patients over 70 years die *with* their prostate cancer rather than from it. On the other hand, 50% of patients aged less than 70 years with moderately or poorly differentiated cancers will eventually die from the disease and a greater proportion will develop significant morbidity. Patients who suffer other life-threatening co-morbid conditions should be offered an 'active monitoring' policy unless their metastases are symptomatic. A carcinoma of low histological grade that comprises less than 5% of prostatic volume can safely be left untreated but followed up with PSA monitoring. An untreated intracapsular lesion (T_1, T_2) takes about 7 years to progress to extracapsular spread.

Symptoms and signs of prostatic cancer depend on the degree of local and systemic spread. Clinical staging is most commonly based on the TNM system (see Fig. 35.7). See also Table 35.1 for the incidence of positive pelvic lymph nodes. The palpation characteristics of the malignant prostate are illustrated in Figure 35.4 (pp. 521, 522).

SYMPTOMS AND SIGNS OF PROSTATIC CANCER

Patients with stage T_1 or T_2 tumours may be asymptomatic. They may be discovered incidentally or on a routine health check, or present with lower urinary tract symp-

Table 35.1 Incidence of positive pelvic lymph nodes according to T category

T category	%
T_1 (focal)	2
T_2 (diffuse)	20
T_3	25
T_4	50
T_5	85

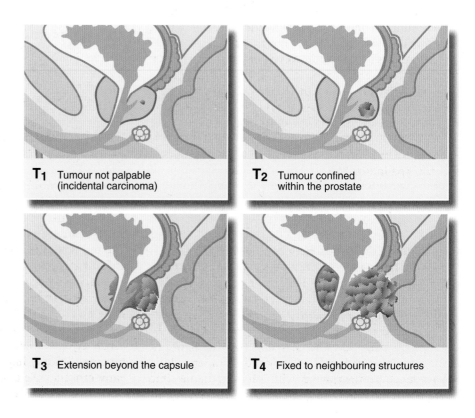

T_1 Tumour not palpable (incidental carcinoma)

T_2 Tumour confined within the prostate

T_3 Extension beyond the capsule

T_4 Fixed to neighbouring structures

Fig. 35.7 TNM staging system for prostatic cancer

toms identical to those of benign hyperplasia. Provided the PSA is below 20, systemic spread is unlikely. Those with T_3 and T_4 tumours may present in the same way but many develop other local symptoms from advancement of the primary, e.g. encirclement of the rectum or occlusion of ureters, and present with renal failure. Patients with nodal disease (N^+) may have symptoms from local compression (swollen legs) and impaired lymphatic drainage (penile and genital oedema). Unfortunately, T_3 and T_4 lesions have often already metastasised by the time of presentation (M^+) and present with symptoms of these metastases such as bone pain, pathological fractures or spinal cord compression. Some patients present with pathological fractures of the spine or neck of femur. Thus older men presenting to a doctor with **backache** should always have a rectal examination and PSA assay. In more advanced cases, non-specific symptoms of malaise, fatigue, weight loss and anaemia may develop and escape recognition for many months. Respiratory problems from pulmonary carcinomatous lymphangitis are an uncommon presentation.

Rectal examination will usually reveal the primary diagnosis. On palpation of a T_1 tumour, the prostate appears normal or smoothly enlarged by benign hyperplasia; stage T_2 presents typically with a nodular, asymmetrical surface, and stage T_3 with a large, hard, irregular gland with evidence of extension beyond the capsule or into the seminal vesicles. A tumour fixed to bone or adjacent pelvic organs is stage T_4. Once cancer spreads outside the prostatic capsule, characteristic symptoms and signs develop and the prognosis becomes substantially worse. Local spread may involve the rectum (causing changes in bowel habit) or the bladder neck and ureters (causing incontinence, impotence or rarely obstructive renal failure). At this late stage, the tumour is obvious on rectal palpation. In very advanced cases where cancer has invaded laterally to involve the pelvic walls or encircle the rectum, the pelvis may appear 'frozen' solid with tumour. Some patients develop major deep venous thrombosis affecting the lower limb.

Modes of presentation of carcinoma of the prostate are summarised in Box 35.3.

APPROACH TO INVESTIGATION OF SUSPECTED PROSTATIC CARCINOMA

Obstruction of the bladder outlet by the prostate is usually caused by benign disease but may be caused by carcinoma. Unless the prostate feels malignant or there are obvious bony metastases, it may be impossible to distinguish between them clinically. **Transrectal ultrasonography** is used to image the prostate irrespective of the findings on palpation and to guide transrectal needle biopsy if necessary. Serum PSA should be measured but results must be interpreted with caution, taking into account that modestly rising levels with advancing age are

---

Box 35.3 Modes of presentation of carcinoma of the prostate

- Asymptomatic—screening by rectal examination and PSA
- Asymptomatic—incidental finding of nodular prostate on digital rectal examination
- Symptoms of bladder outflow obstruction—tumour suspected by finding nodular prostate on rectal examination or a suspiciously raised serum PSA or found on histology after TURP
- Symptoms of spread to surrounding pelvic tissues, e.g. change in bowel habit, loss of continence, recent impotence, ureteric obstruction
- Symptoms of bony metastases, e.g. bone pain, malaise, anaemia, pathological fractures

---

accepted as normal. Unfortunately, a normal PSA result cannot exclude carcinoma confined to the gland; PSA is normal in 25% of such cases. Substantially elevated PSA usually indicates aggressive localised disease or metastatic disease. False positive results sometimes occur in benign prostatic hyperplasia or inflammation (prostatitis). If carcinoma can be effectively excluded, any obstruction may be treated in the usual way by TURP and the specimens examined histologically. At prostatectomy, carcinoma is suspected if the gland lacks the usual clear plane of cleavage.

If a patient has skeletal pain, X-rays and radionuclide bone scans are indicated. On X-ray, prostatic bony metastases are typically **sclerotic** or osteoblastic (i.e. dense, appearing white on X-rays) rather than **lytic** (as in most other bony secondaries), giving the characteristic patchy 'cotton-wool' appearance shown in Figure 35.8. Some lesions, however, are radiolucent. An isotope bone scan can reveal metastases even when a plain X-ray is normal.

MANAGEMENT OF PROSTATIC CARCINOMA

Screening

Prevention would be ideal but this is impossible whilst the cause remains unknown. Screening is continuing to be evaluated for detecting early, potentially curable disease. Ideally, clinicians would **avoid treating** cancers unlikely to advance, would **ablate** cancers confined to the gland (stages T_1 or T_2; N_0, M_0) but which would be expected to advance, and would provide long-term **palliation** for locally advanced tumours (stage T_3; N_0, M_0) and metastatic disease (stages T_{1-4}; N^+ and/or M^+). Uncertainty will remain, however, until it becomes possible to accurately predict which local cancers will advance to become clinically important, as well as recognise which early cancers have already metastasised and progressed beyond cure. In the USA the growing trend towards

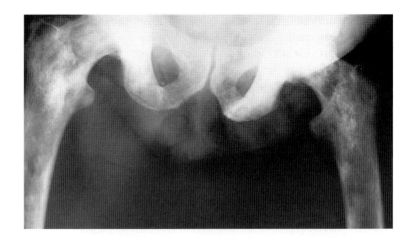

Fig. 35.8 Osteosclerotic bony metastases from prostatic carcinoma

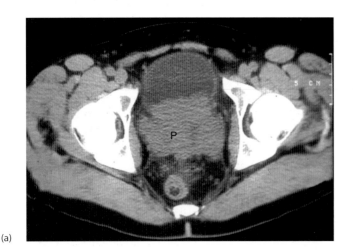

(a)

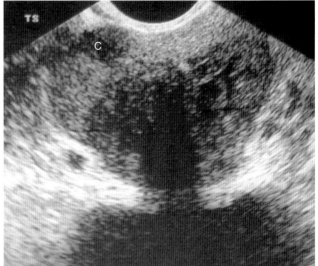

(b)

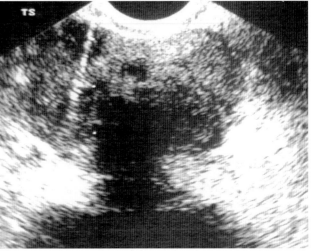

(c)

Fig. 35.9 Carcinoma of the prostate
(a) CT scan showing a large carcinoma of the prostate **P** invading extensively into the bladder anteriorly and posteriorly towards the rectum. This was a late and aggressive form of the disease and the patient lived less than 1 year. **(b)** and **(c)** Ultrasound guided biopsy. **(b)** Transrectal ultrasound scan of prostate showing a small cancer **C** within the peripheral zone and an acoustic shadow beyond it. The larger central zone is enlarged by benign hypertrophy. **(c)** After transrectal biopsy. The white line represents bubbles of air left after successful needle biopsy of the tumour.

aggressive treatment of all operable cancers (by total pros-tatectomy) is leading to a perception of falling mortality despite increased prevalence. If confirmed in the longer term, this suggests that surgical intervention may be gen-uinely curative.

Early-stage disease (stages T_1 or T_2; N_0, M_0)

Total prostatectomy or radical radiotherapy is potentially curative for organ-confined disease, i.e. disease confined to the prostate or 'true' stage T_1 and T_2, and there is enthusiasm for radical local treatment at specialist centres. If external beam radiation therapy is chosen, it is delivered so as to provide a high local tumour dose without adversely affecting the rectum. A fall in PSA level to 1.0 or less within 12 months of treatment is an indication of success. Unless this occurs relapse can be expected. There is a revival in the use of radioactive seed implants (**brachytherapy**) as an alternative to external beam therapy; the seeds can be placed accurately under ultrasound control and provide the necessary high but localised dosage.

The standard management for patients with low-grade, impalpable, organ-confined prostate cancer remains **active monitoring** until there is evidence of increased disease activity (rising PSA, detectable nodule on palpation). This gives outcomes equivalent to radical treatment for all and spares many patients the side effects of radical treatment. There is now evidence of improved survival with radical treatment in patients with moderate to high-grade organ-confined disease compared to active monitoring.

Radical prostatectomy entails risks such as incontinence or impotence, although reduced complications are claimed for advanced surgical techniques, including robotic-assisted radical prostatectomy. Patient selection for radical treatment is important in terms of the cancer characteristics (staging, PSA level and tumour volume) as well as patient characteristics (comorbidity, age, sexual function and patient preference). Patients must be fully counselled in the range of treatment options and their complications.

Locally advanced disease (stages T_3 or T_4, N_0, M_0)

For patients presenting with bladder outlet symptoms, standard transurethral resection may relieve urinary symptoms; TURP may, however, risk permanent incontinence if the tumour has invaded the sphincter mechanism or the nerves controlling it. Further treatment then depends on local practice and patient preference. Locally advanced primary disease (stage T_3) is usually treated by **neoadjuvant** radiotherapy (before the principal therapy) or adjuvant radiotherapy, with or without hormone therapy.

Metastatic disease (stage N^+ and/or M^+)

Many patients still present with metastatic disease. In these, the aim of treatment is to control symptoms and to retard the progression of disease. For patients presenting with bladder outlet symptoms, standard transurethral resection or 'channel TUR' usually restores urinary flow.

Most prostatic cancers are androgen-dependent, at least initially, and hormonal manipulation is the mainstay of treatment of advanced disease. Local radiotherapy is frequently effective for treating painful metastases. Pathological fractures in the sclerotic metastases of prostatic cancer are much less common than in lytic metastases of other cancers. This is fortunate since the dense bone is more difficult to cut and drill than normal bone if internal fixation is needed.

Hormonal therapy

There are now three main treatment options:

- **Removal of both testes by subcapsular orchidectomy**. This is a quick and simple scrotal operation and removes about 95% of the testosterone synthesised (the rest is from the adrenals), producing an immediate fall in plasma testosterone. The testicular capsules are left in situ and these fill with blood clot and preserve the scrotal contour. There are few side effects other than hot flushes and sexual dysfunction, and no serious long-term sequelae.

  Diethylstilbestrol is a synthetic oestrogen and in the early days was the standard treatment for symptomatic prostate cancer. Diethylstilbestrol suppresses luteinising hormone releasing hormone (LHRH) secretion from the hypothalamus and may also be cytotoxic to prostatic cancer cells in its own right. Although effective, it was found to have a high rate of serious thromboembolic side effects and has now largely been abandoned in favour of other methods of achieving similar ends. However, it remains an alternative to orchidectomy, either as primary treatment or as a salvage treatment after other methods have failed. The dose must not exceed 3 mg a day and precautions must be taken to reduce the increased risk of thrombosis.

- **Monthly injections of depot LHRH agonists (LHRHa)**. LHRH or **gonadorelin** analogues such as goserelin are at least as effective as orchidectomy but are expensive and have to be given parenterally, at least initially. The drugs need to be administered at intervals ranging from 4 weeks to 12 weeks. Therapy causes initial **stimulation** of luteinising hormone (LH) release from the pituitary, which in turn causes increased testicular testosterone secretion for up to 2 weeks. This is followed by **inhibition** of LH release by competitively blocking the receptors, resulting in an 'anorchic' state. As with orchidectomy, hot flushes and sexual dysfunction are the major side effects. Many patients experience a 'flare' of symptoms in the first 2 weeks, aggravating bone pain or spinal cord compression. For this reason, the first dose is usually covered by anti-androgen therapy (e.g. cyproterone acetate or flutamide). There is probably no advantage in continuing combined gonadorelin and anti-androgen therapy because the anti-androgen contributes to the hormone resistance of the tumour by blocking androgen receptors. In addition, anti-androgens are hepatotoxic.

- **Anti-androgen drugs such as cyproterone acetate or flutamide**. These block the binding of

Fig. 35.10 Local effects of advanced prostatic carcinoma

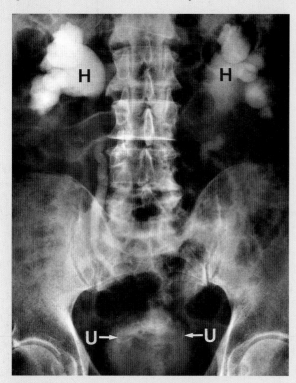

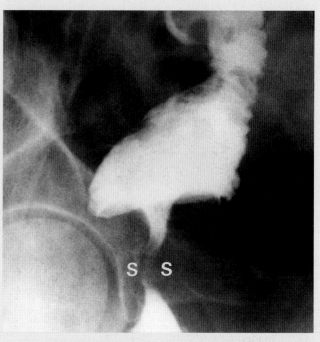

(a) Intravenous urogram from an elderly man with advanced prostatic carcinoma. He presented with renal failure due to retroperitoneal spread of tumour which had caused bilateral distal ureteric obstruction. Note the gross bilateral hydronephrosis **H**; the distal ureters can be seen to narrow at **U**; this is better shown on the original film.

(b) Barium enema from a 76-year-old man with known prostatic carcinoma who developed a change in bowel habit. The tumour has compressed and invaded the rectal wall circumferentially causing a marked stricture **S**.

dihydrotestosterone to its receptor at cellular level and, in contrast to LHRH antagonists, block both testicular and adrenal testosterone. Flutamide may preserve the potential for sexual arousal for longer, though with occasional side effects of diarrhoea and gynaecomastia; this may be the preferred treatment for younger patients with advanced disease. Cyproterone acetate can lead to depression and thromboembolic complications but is effective in suppressing hot flushes.

Almost inevitably, prostatic cancer eventually escapes its androgen dependency and becomes **refractory** to hormonal treatment. The mechanism is unknown but occurs at a mean of 2 years after commencing treatment in M^+ and 5 years in $N^+ M^0$ disease. When this occurs, secondary treatment with diethylstilbestrol may be of value. Bone metastases can sometimes be palliated by intravenous radioactive strontium. Non-hormone chemotherapy has little to offer, and often only symptomatic and general palliative measures can be offered. The principles and techniques of palliative care are described in Chapter 13.

The management of prostatic carcinoma is summarised in Box 35.4.

PROSTATITIS

Bacterial prostatitis is an uncommon inflammatory disorder of the prostate usually caused by coliforms, *Chlamydia* or *Neisseria*. Mycoplasma may also have a role. It occurs in acute and chronic forms. Urinary tract infection or instrumentation may be a predisposing factor. Prostatitis can present acutely or in a chronic form.

ACUTE PROSTATITIS

Acute prostatitis is characterised by perineal pain and fever. Prostatic swelling may also cause bladder outflow obstruction and urinary frequency. The prostate is exquisitely tender on rectal examination and prostatic massage is inadvisable as it may precipitate bacteraemia.

Initial treatment is with intravenous antibiotics such as gentamicin until the patient is apyrexial and then a quinolone antibiotic orally for 6 weeks. Infective prostatitis may be the first presentation of diabetes mellitus.

Box 35.4 **Management of prostatic carcinoma—summary**

Histological diagnosis

- By ultrasound-guided transrectal biopsy (TRUS) or after TURP for symptoms of bladder outlet obstruction

Staging

- If radical treatment is contemplated—rectal examination, PSA, transrectal ultrasound, CT or MRI scanning for local spread and lymph node involvement

Treatment by stage

- At any stage, transurethral resection ('channel TUR') for persistent bladder outlet obstruction

- Stages T_1 and T_2—a choice of active monitoring or radical local treatment, i.e. prostatectomy or radiotherapy
- Stage T_3—radiotherapy, often with neoadjuvant or adjuvant hormonal therapy
- Stage T_4
    —anti-androgen therapies (e.g. bilateral orchidectomy) plus radiotherapy for painful bony metastases or spinal cord compression
    or
    —drug treatment with gonadorelins
    or
    —drug treatment with anti-androgen drugs, e.g. cyproterone acetate, flutamide, bicalutamide

CHRONIC PROSTATITIS

Chronic prostatitis presents with chronic, low-grade perineal and suprapubic pain. Symptoms and signs are often vague and ill defined and the diagnosis is sometimes made on inadequate grounds. Around 5% of cases are due to chronic bacterial infection, most commonly by coliforms, whereas in 95% no infective cause can be defined.

Other theories of causation have been proposed, such as autoimmunity and intraprostatic urinary reflux.

Treatment is with appropriate antibiotics according to culture and sensitivity of prostatic fluid obtained after prostatic massage. Anti-inflammatory drugs may be used in addition to or instead of antibiotics, particularly in the non-infective cases; alpha-adrenergic blockers may also be employed.

36 Tumours of the kidney and urinary tract

INTRODUCTION

Two types of cancer arise from the renal parenchyma: renal cell carcinomas and nephroblastomas. **Renal cell carcinomas** (also known as renal adenocarcinomas and sometimes by the old names of hypernephroma and Grawitz tumour) are confined to adults. **Nephroblastomas** (Wilms' tumours) are developmental in origin and present in infancy or early childhood. These are described in Chapter 51. Occasional benign renal tumours also occur, e.g. oncocytoma, adenoma and angiomyolipoma (see Box 36.1).

Tumours of the transitional cell epithelium lining the urinary tract (urothelium) are very common. They may arise anywhere in the tract, including the pelvicalyceal system of the kidney, the ureters, the bladder and occasionally the urethra. Pelvicalyceal tumours are generally uncommon but occur frequently in some parts of the world, e.g. Balkan nephropathy. These **transitional cell carcinomas** occur exclusively in adults and are most common in the bladder. **Squamous cell carcinomas** sometimes occur in the urinary tract and probably arise from metaplastic squamous epithelium caused by chronic irritation from stones or schistosomiasis. Squamous cell carcinomas also occasionally arise in the squamous epithelium at the urethral meatus. Very rarely, an **adenocarcinoma** may develop in the bladder from glandular epithelial remnants of the embryological **urachus** or a **sarcoma** may develop from connective tissue elements.

RENAL CELL CARCINOMA

PATHOLOGY OF RENAL CELL CARCINOMA

Renal cell carcinoma accounts for about 3% of adult malignancies and is twice as common in males as in females. It rarely develops before puberty but may occur at any age thereafter, with the peak incidence between 50 and 70 years. Renal cell carcinoma, like prostate, breast and colon cancer, mainly occurs sporadically but there are rare familial forms, e.g. von Hippel–Lindau disease. The only proven environmental risk factor is tobacco use.

Renal cell carcinoma originates in the renal tubules. The tumour cells are characteristically large and polygonal, with clear cytoplasm representing accumulation of glycogen and lipid. For this reason, these tumours are sometimes known pathologically as **clear cell carcinomas**. In other variants, the cells are granular and stain more intensely.

Renal cell carcinomas vary in their grade of malignancy. Small isolated tumours are often found at autopsy. Many pathologists regard tumours of less than 2 cm as virtually benign as they rarely display local invasion or distant metastases. Bilateral tumours are present in about 5% of cases. Large tumours invade surrounding tissues and may metastasise to para-aortic lymph nodes. Advanced renal cell carcinoma characteristically extends into the lumen of the renal vein and into the inferior vena cava ('tumour thrombus'—see Fig. 36.1). Distant spread is typically to lung, liver and bone. Lung metastases are often typical discrete 'cannonball secondaries'. Isolated metastases occasionally develop in the brain, bone and elsewhere.

STAGING OF RENAL CELL CARCINOMA

Stage I tumours are confined by the renal capsule; stage II tumours have penetrated the renal capsule but remain confined by Gerota's perinephric fascia; stage III tumours have renal vein involvement or nodal spread; stage IV have distant metastases.

CLINICAL FEATURES OF RENAL CELL CARCINOMA

The classic presentation of renal cell carcinoma is with the triad of **haematuria**, **a mass** and **flank pain**; although all three features occur in only about 15% of cases (see Figs 36.2, 36.3), one is present in 40% of patients. Com-

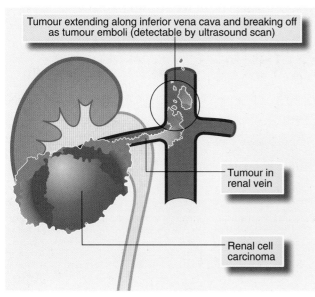

Fig. 36.1 **Venous spread of renal cell carcinoma**

Tumour extending along inferior vena cava and breaking off as tumour emboli (detectable by ultrasound scan)

Tumour in renal vein

Renal cell carcinoma

| Box | 36.1 | **Histological classification of adult renal tumours of the Union Internationale Contre le Cancer (UICC)** |

A. Malignant

1. Conventional clear cell carcinoma
2. Papillary or tubulo-papillary renal carcinoma
3. Chromophobe renal carcinoma
4. Collecting duct carcinoma

B. Benign

1. Oncocytoma
2. Papillary or tubular adenoma
3. Angiomyolipoma (may be neoplastic or hamartomatous)

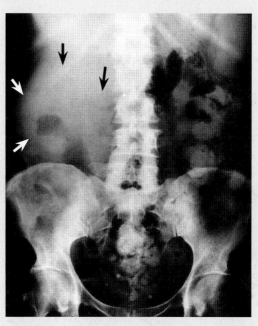

Fig. 36.2 **Renal cell carcinoma: plain radiography**

This 50-year-old man presented with painless haematuria. The plain abdominal film shows a large soft-tissue mass in the right loin which obscures the psoas shadow (arrowed). Later investigation showed this to be a renal cell carcinoma.

| Box | 36.2 | **Presenting features of renal cell carcinoma** |

Common presentations

- Frank haematuria
- Microscopic haematuria often discovered incidentally
- Loin pain
- Renal mass
- Incidental finding on imaging

Uncommon presentations

- Iron deficiency anaemia
- Polycythaemia
- Hypertension
- Hypercalcaemia due to parathormone-like protein production
- Pyrexia of unknown origin
- Elevated erythrocyte sedimentation rate
- Secondary lesions (e.g. 'cannonball' lesions on chest X-ray, pathological fractures)

monly, diagnosis is made **incidentally** by discovering a tumour on ultrasonography or CT scanning. Renal cell carcinomas often reach a large size before discovery owing to their retroperitoneal position; unfortunately, tumours larger than 8 cm have an 80% chance of having already metastasised.

Renal cell carcinoma can also present in a variety of unusual ways. Some tumours secrete excess **erythropoietin** which causes polycythaemia; **hypertension** may result from excess renin production. Similarly, ectopic production of a parathormone-like protein may cause **hypercalcaemia**. Renal cell carcinoma may cause pyrexia and should be considered in patients with a pyrexia of unknown origin. The erythrocyte sedimentation rate (ESR) is elevated in most cases. As with many other malignancies, metastases may be the presenting feature: for example, 'cannonball' secondaries discovered on a chest X-ray.

Common and uncommon presenting features of renal cell carcinoma are summarised in Box 36.2.

APPROACH TO INVESTIGATION OF SUSPECTED RENAL CELL CARCINOMA

When a renal cell carcinoma is suspected, ultrasonography is the first investigation and has superseded intravenous urography. Ultrasound investigation reliably distinguishes simple benign cysts from solid masses

Fig. 36.3 Renal cell carcinoma: IVU

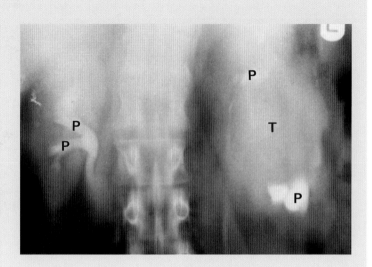

Tomogram taken during intravenous urography of a 58-year-old woman presenting with haematuria. The shape of the pelvicalyceal system **P** on the right is normal, but on the left it is grossly distorted by a tumour **T** in the middle of the kidney which proved to be a renal cell carcinoma.

Fig. 36.4 Renal cell carcinoma: CT scan

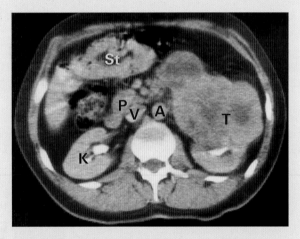

A 62-year-old man presented with left loin pain and a palpable loin mass. This CT scan shows a huge left renal tumour **T**; note the variable density of the tumour caused by areas of necrosis and haemorrhage. Note also the normal right kidney **K**, aorta **A**, pancreas **P**, inferior vena cava **V** and distal stomach **St**.

that are most likely to be tumours and is an accurate method of demonstrating tumour thrombus in the inferior vena cava. CT scanning is used to stage the disease by assessing invasion of perinephric tissues and by demonstrating regional lymph node or liver metastases (see Fig. 36.4).

Arteriography is still occasionally employed in the case of solitary unilateral or bilateral tumours to assess the prospects for segmental resection. Renal tumours have a characteristic circulatory pattern distinct from normal kidney (see Fig. 36.5a). Arteriography is also employed if therapeutic embolisation is being considered to reduce the vascularity of a tumour a few days before surgery.

A full blood count is performed to look for anaemia or polycythaemia and a chest X-ray taken to look for pulmonary metastases (see Fig. 36.5 b, c). No other preoperative investigations are usually required.

MANAGEMENT OF RENAL CELL CARCINOMA

In most patients, the kidney involved by tumour is excised (**nephrectomy**). Most surgeons prefer an anterior transperitoneal approach. This allows clinical staging of the disease, permits control of the inferior vena cava and provides access to the renal artery and vein during extensive resections. A posterolateral thoraco-abdominal approach may be employed to allow early access to the inferior vena cava and renal arteries if the tumour is large. Wherever possible, the resection should be radical, with kidney, perinephric fat and lymph nodes taken *en bloc*. There is probably no role for radiotherapy, chemotherapy or hormonal therapy, although immunotherapy with interleukins or interferon may help, despite their toxicity. Increasingly, radical nephrectomies are performed laparoscopically, allowing shortened hospital stay and earlier return to normal activity.

Renal cell carcinoma is unusual in that surgical removal of isolated pulmonary or cerebral metastases occasionally results in cure. These isolated metastases may present many years after the primary surgery. For palliation of multiple metastases, chemotherapy or immunotherapy is sometimes used but treatment is generally ineffective.

Fig. 36.5 Renal cell carcinoma—case study: arteriography and radiography

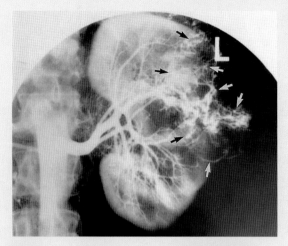

(a)

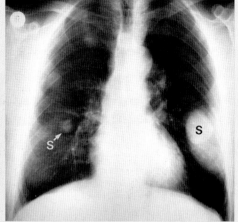

(b)

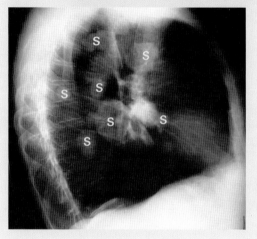

(c)

This 68-year-old woman presented with haematuria. A renal mass was demonstrated on intravenous urography. Before CT scanning was developed, renal arteriography was often used in the diagnosis of renal cell carcinoma and to display its arterial supply as an aid to surgery. **(a)** This left renal arteriogram outlines the normal renal vessels but also shows a large crescentic mass of abnormal vessels (outline arrowed in white) typical of renal cell carcinoma. Only the residual part of the tumour vasculature is demonstrated, the rest having been destroyed by necrosis within the tumour. Unfortunately, this patient had already developed pulmonary metastases, as shown in the chest X-rays (b) and (c). **(b)** PA and **(c)** lateral chest X-rays showing multiple 'cannonball' secondary lesions **S** of various sizes. These are typical of renal cell carcinoma.

TRANSITIONAL CELL CARCINOMA

EPIDEMIOLOGY AND AETIOLOGY OF TRANSITIONAL CELL CARCINOMA

Tumours of urothelium are common. Histologically, they are nearly all transitional cell carcinomas (TCC); other than rarities, the rest are squamous cell carcinomas (7%) and adenocarcinomas (1%). Most arise primarily in the bladder but they also occur in the pelvicalyceal system and ureters and rarely in the urethra. Pan-urothelial transitional cell carcinoma occasionally develops in the renal pelvis, ureter, bladder and urethra but not necessarily simultaneously. Urothelial tumours are uncommon below the age of 50 and the incidence increases with age. Men are affected three times more often than women. TCC is at least four times more common than renal cell carcinoma; TCC of the renal pelvis is generally less common than parenchymal renal tumours. TCC occurs with a similar frequency to gastric cancer in men and about one-quarter the frequency of lung cancer.

Cigarette smoking is associated with a fourfold increase in incidence of urothelial tumours; this is probably mediated by urinary excretion of inhaled carcinogens. Urothelial cancers have been strongly associated with exposure to industrial carcinogens, once widely used in the rubber, cable, dye and printing industries. The likely carcinogens, benzidine, nigrosine and beta naphthylamine, are now banned in most countries but tumours can develop as long as 25 years after exposure and so a detailed occupational history should be taken in suspected cases. Hairdressers with prolonged exposure to various aniline dyes may also be at risk. Prolonged exposure to carcinogens causes a 20–60 times increase in risk of developing urothelial cancer. These carcinogens are excreted in the urine and the more prolonged presence of urine in the bladder compared with the rest of the tract probably explains why urothelial tumours most often arise in the bladder.

PATHOLOGY OF TRANSITIONAL CELL CARCINOMA

Well-differentiated TCCs histologically resemble normal transitional epithelium. Less well-differentiated tumours become increasingly unlike their tissue of origin so that the most anaplastic tumours can only be classified as urothelial because they are known to have arisen in the urinary tract. The degree of differentiation tends to be reflected in the tumour morphology as visualised at cystoscopy. Well-differentiated tumours form papillary frond-like lesions, whereas more aggressive tumours form plaque-like lesions which invade underlying muscle and surrounding tissues.

Most aetiological factors act on the whole urothelium, predisposing it to malignant transformation. Consequently, urothelial tumours are often **multifocal** and there may already be multiple tumours at the time of presentation. An affected individual is at high risk of developing further tumours despite complete eradication of an earlier tumour. When the primary tumour is in the pelvicalyceal system or ureter, there is a high risk of tumours developing later in the urothelium distal to the primary. About 50% of patients with upper tract urothelial tumours will ultimately develop bladder urothelial tumours. This was thought to result from 'seeding' of tumour cells shed from the proximal lesion but is more likely due in some way to the effect of carcinogens and the multicentric nature of the disease.

A sinister form of transitional cell carcinoma is **in situ carcinoma**. This presents with frequency and dysuria, aptly named 'malignant cystitis'. In the male these symptoms are often misdiagnosed as bacterial prostatitis. These lesions desquamate easily and have a high pick-up rate on urine cytology. Untreated, they infiltrate rapidly.

CLINICAL FEATURES OF TRANSITIONAL CELL CARCINOMA

TCC usually presents with painless haematuria (see Fig. 36.6). An upper tract lesion may cause **ureteric colic** (clot colic) and long stringy clots may be seen in the urine. If bleeding is gross, clots may cause ureteric obstruction. Rapid bleeding from a bladder tumour may cause **clot retention**, i.e. acute retention of urine due to clot obstruction. Bladder tumours arising near a ureteric orifice commonly obstruct one ureter, causing **hydronephrosis**. Rarely, bilateral obstruction causes uraemia. Bladder tumours also predispose to infection, and unexplained recurrent urinary tract infections need investigating to exclude TCC as a cause. Tumour invasion near the bladder neck may cause incontinence but this is usually preceded by haematuria or infection.

INVESTIGATION OF SUSPECTED TRANSITIONAL CELL CARCINOMA

Confirmed haematuria in the absence of infection must be investigated. A renal cell carcinoma which causes haematuria can usually be demonstrated by ultrasound. Intravenous urography outlines the upper tracts, and a filling defect in the collecting system or ureter is suspicious of a urothelial tumour (see Fig. 36.7).

Ultrasound and IVU is followed by cystoscopy, which is the only reliable method for examining the lining of the bladder and urethra. If there is an upper tract tumour, cystoscopy may reveal blood emerging from one of the ureteric orifices. When bladder tumours are found, diagnosis and initial therapy go hand in hand. Where possible, lesions are completely excised down to muscle using a **transurethral resectoscope** (transurethral resection of

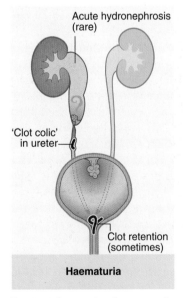
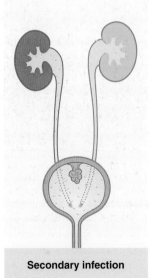
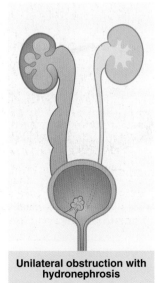
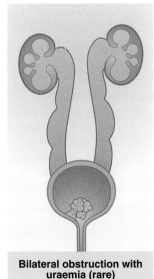

| Haematuria | Secondary infection | Unilateral obstruction with hydronephrosis | Bilateral obstruction with uraemia (rare) |

Fig. 36.6 Presenting features of urothelial tumours

Fig. 36.7 Urothelial tumours at different sites

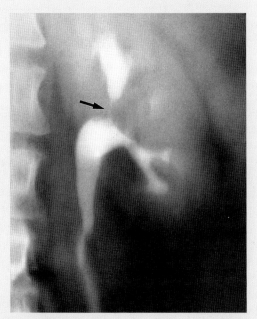

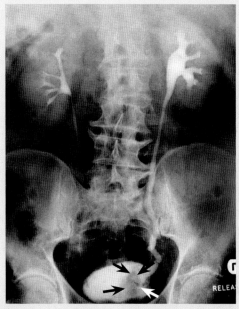

(a) Case study 1: This woman of 64 presented with persistent microscopic haematuria; a left renal tomogram during intravenous urography showed a stricture in the upper pelvicalyceal infundibulum (arrowed) caused by a urothelial tumour.

(b) Case study 2: This 67-year-old man complained of loin pain and haematuria. On the left side of this intravenous urogram there is hydronephrosis and ureteric obstruction caused by a bladder tumour visible at the vesicoureteric orifice (arrowed).

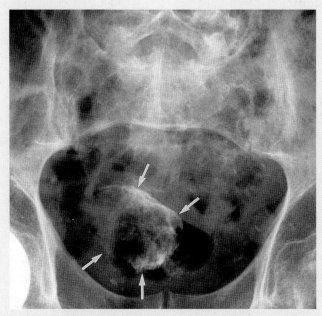

(c) Case study 3: This 84-year-old man presented with recurrent urinary tract infections. This plain X-ray of the pelvis shows a huge calcified lesion in the bladder (arrowed), typical of calcification on the surface of a long-standing bladder tumour. In a woman, this appearance would more likely be due to a calcified uterine fibroid.

bladder tumour, TURBT). The resected tissue is then sent for histological examination. This defines the degree of **differentiation** and the depth of tumour **invasion** into the bladder wall. Benign tumours do occur in the bladder, for example 'inverted papillomas' or polyps with intestinal metaplasia, but they are excessively rare. The term papilloma implies that a lesion is benign and it should not be used for what is almost invariably a well-differentiated papillary transitional cell carcinoma.

STAGING OF TRANSITIONAL CELL TUMOURS OF THE BLADDER

Staging of bladder tumours is achieved mainly by cystoscopic examination and palpation under anaesthesia, combined with histological examination of resected specimens. For small and superficial lesions, histology will show the extent of bladder wall invasion and whether the tumour has been completely removed. Lesions near a ureteric orifice that appear to be superficial should be treated as having invaded underlying muscle. For larger or deeper lesions, palpation of the bladder under general anaesthesia (EUA) bimanually between a finger in the rectum and a hand on the anterior abdominal wall should be performed before and after resection of the tumour. This gives an idea of the extent of bladder wall penetration and spread into the pelvis. However, clinical 'bimanual examination' can be misleading, especially in the obese, and CT scanning is a more reliable indication of spread into the bladder wall or beyond. Note however that CT scanning can be misleading if performed soon after a TURBT.

The Union Internationale Contre le Cancer's TNM clinical system widely used in staging bladder tumours is illustrated in Figure 36.8 (the 'T' applies to the clinical stage of the tumour). In addition, some pathologists grade bladder tumours according to P and G pathological criteria. **The 'P' system** (small p for the biopsy specimen and capital P for the whole specimen) classifies the extent of invasion on gross anatomical and histological grounds. **The 'G' system** grades the lesion according to the degree of histological differentiation (G1 = well differentiated, G2 = moderately differentiated and G3 = poorly differentiated or undifferentiated). Thus, as an example, a pathologist may report a biopsy as pT_2, G3. The pathological staging system is more precise than the clinical system alone.

MANAGEMENT OF TRANSITIONAL CELL CARCINOMA

Bladder tumours

Transitional cell tumours of the bladder display a range of morphological types ranging from small, discrete, often multiple, frond-like lesions through to extensive papilliferous or flat tumours. The first type is usually at a very early invasive stage and such lesions were formerly known as papillomas before their malignant potential was fully realised. Solitary T_a or T_1 tumours without evidence of widespread carcinoma in situ have a 50% chance of not recurring after treatment. Four-quadrant biopsy of the rest of the bladder can help in formulating a treatment plan and estimating prognosis. If papillary tumours coexist with carcinoma in situ (CIS), however, the long-term prognosis is ominous. These patients are usually treated by immunotherapy with a course of intravesical BCG to stimulate local immunity. However if CIS persists, then total cystectomy is the treatment of choice.

The initial management of bladder tumours is usually aimed at complete removal of tumour tissue by cystoscopic **transurethral resection**, even with large lesions. Further management then depends on the stage of tumour spread determined by examination under anaesthesia, CT scanning and histological staging.

As shown in Figure 36.9, bladder tumours classified as T_a or T_1 and sometimes T_2 can usually be completely resected. Single-dose **intravesical chemotherapy** with mitomycin C or epirubicin has been shown to reduce the recurrence rate after the initial TURBT in T_a or T_1 disease. T_1 lesions are notoriously recurrent and if they recur repeatedly, weekly courses of intravesical chemotherapy or BCG is the treatment of choice. For T_3 lesions, the preferred treatment in a fit patient is **total cystectomy**. The tumour can sometimes be downstaged before surgery by neoadjuvant systemic chemotherapy of the CMV or M:VAC types. Radiotherapy should be reserved for the unfit or older patient, or for relapse after initial cystectomy or initial systemic chemotherapy. There is no proven role for radiotherapy in superficial lesions.

When total cystectomy is necessary, some method of **urinary diversion** is required. The classic operation involves the isolation of a segment of ileum; both ureters are then anastomosed into one end of the ileal segment, creating an **ileal conduit**, whilst the other end is opened onto the abdominal wall as a urostomy. An earlier operation in which both ureters were diverted into the sigmoid colon has long been abandoned because of electrolyte disruption and a high risk of carcinoma at the ureterocolic anastomoses. Nowadays, most urinary diversions are into a **continent pouch** (a neo-bladder) constructed from a segment of ileum or large bowel and anastomosed to the urethra.

T_4 tumours are usually incurable; even total cystectomy rarely eliminates the entire lesion. Radiotherapy offers palliation and is valuable for controlling pain and haematuria.

Transitional cell tumours of the upper tract

TCCs of the pelvicalyceal system and ureter are uncommon. Treatment usually requires excision of the whole upper tract on the affected side including kidney, ureter and a cuff of bladder wall surrounding the distal ureter.

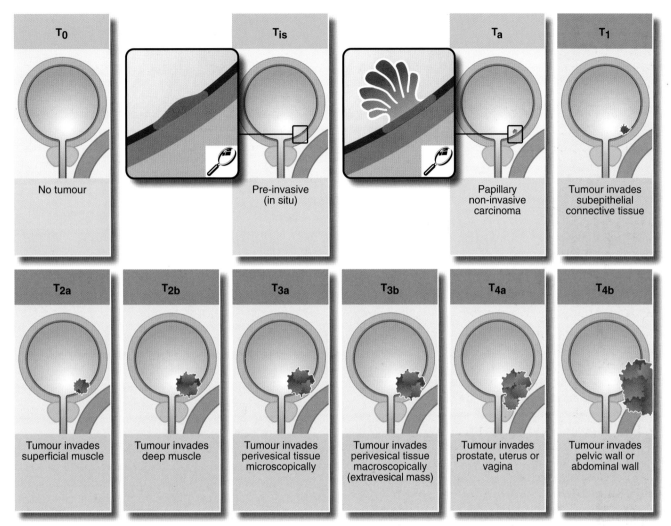

Fig. 36.8 UICC system for staging bladder tumours
Note that ureteric involvement usually classifies a tumour as T_{3a} or T_{3b}.

However, some small, isolated renal pelvic tumours can be dealt with endoscopically via a nephroscope passed percutaneously into the pelvicalyceal system or by laser ablation via a fibreoptic flexible ureteroscope.

Urethral tumours

Bladder tumours occasionally involve the urethra by direct spread. Very rarely a primary lesion occurs in the urethra; a pre-existing urethral stricture may be a predisposing factor. Management is by urethroscopic coagulation. Mitomycin C incorporated into urethral lidocaine gel can also be used. The surrounding penile vasculature allows early spread of the tumour via the bloodstream and thus the ultimate prognosis is poor.

Unusual tumours of the urinary tract

The uncommon **squamous cell carcinoma** of the urinary tract is diagnosed and treated along similar lines to TCC. As previously mentioned, many develop as a com-plication of schistosomiasis. Distal urethral lesions are managed in the same way as penile carcinoma (see Chapter 33).

Adenocarcinoma is rare but can occur anywhere in the bladder, most often in a urachal remnant at the vault. Tumours of this type can often be removed by segmental resection of the bladder.

Follow-up and control of recurrent disease

Patients who have had potentially curative treatment for urothelial tumours (i.e. bladder stages T_1 to T_3 and all upper tract lesions) must be followed up for life. The goal is to detect recurrence of the original tumour and to diagnose new primary lesions at an early stage, bearing in mind the fact that the environmental factors that induced the initial lesion predispose the remaining urothelium to malignant change. It is not always easy to distinguish between small recurrences and new primaries; all of them tend to be labelled 'recurrences'.

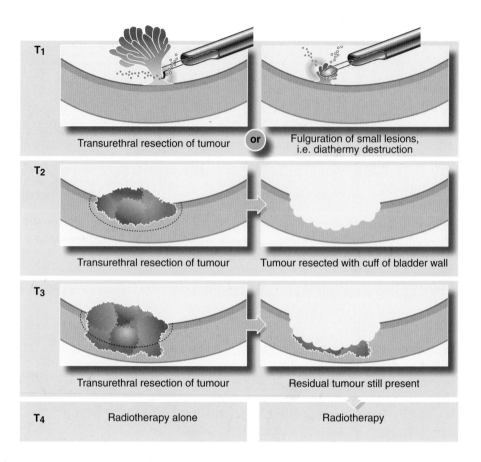

Fig. 36.9 Cystoscopic management of bladder tumours—summary

Follow-up involves regular 'check' cystoscopies. Initially, these are performed at 3-month intervals and the interval is gradually extended to once a year if no further tumour is discovered. Flexible cystoscopy under local anaesthesia is employed for surveillance if there is a low risk of recurrence. This is quicker and more convenient than the former practice of repeated rigid cystoscopy under general anaesthesia but is not yet a suitable method of treating recurrences. After several years free of tumour, cystoscopy may be replaced by annual **urine cytology**. However, this is unreliable for patients known to have well-differentiated papillary lesions. In these, dipstick testing for blood may be more useful. There is currently a vogue for using nuclear protein tumour markers which can pick up 50% of tumour recurrences; however, the reliability of the method needs to be improved before it can replace existing methods. Urine cytology may also be used for screening normal individuals with a high occupational risk.

Recurrent lesions are managed in the same way as the initial lesion, i.e. according to the stage of bladder wall invasion. The exception is when the initial treatment involved radiotherapy. For these patients, cure of recurrent cancer is improbable and palliative surgery ranging from TURBT to total cystectomy may be necessary to treat intractable problems such as severe haemorrhage.

Stone disease of the urinary tract

37

INTRODUCTION

Stone disease is second only to prostatic disease in the overall urological workload. Stones may occur in all parts of the urinary tract, including the pelvicalyceal system of the kidney, the ureter, the bladder and even sometimes the urethra. Stones most commonly provoke symptoms due to obstruction or by predisposing to urinary tract infections.

The pattern of stone disease has changed markedly over the last 150 years. Bladder stones were once extremely common, particularly in children, and were one of the few conditions successfully treated by surgery before the advent of anaesthesia and antisepsis. 'Cutting for stone', or **lithotomy** (*lithos* = stone), was often performed by itinerant surgeons. They used a perineal approach to the bladder, placing the patient in the manner still described as the **lithotomy position**. A **bladder sound** (i.e. a curved bougie) was placed via the urethra into the bladder to locate the stone. Meanwhile, fascinated onlookers held down the wretched patient for the surgeon's theatrical ministrations. The operation was often completed in seconds!

Nowadays, upper tract calculi are much more common than bladder calculi and the incidence is rising. The stones range from the uncommon **staghorn calculus** (Fig. 37.2—7% of stones) which fills the pelvicalyceal system, to small stones developing in the pelvicalyceal system that may migrate and obstruct the ureter. Acute ureteric obstruction causes severe pain and presents as the surgical emergency known as **ureteric colic**. Most stone disease is, however, asymptomatic or else presents non-urgently to the outpatient clinic.

In developed countries stone disease in childhood is now rare. As shown in Figure 37.1, stone disease has a peak incidence in early adulthood and declines slowly thereafter. Males are affected two and a half times more often than females. Right and left upper tracts are equally affected. There is also a high incidence of recurrent stones.

PATHOPHYSIOLOGY OF STONE DISEASE

CHEMICAL COMPOSITION

Urinary calculi consist of crystalline compounds with a small proportion of matrix material similar to ground substance. It is likely that most stones form around a nidus of organic material, e.g. necrotic renal papilla or infective debris. One constituent often predominates but sometimes there is a mixture. In other cases, the central nucleus of the stone and the surrounding bulk of the stone are each composed of different materials. Thus, it is often difficult to reconcile the chemical classifications used in different analytical studies. Table 37.1 provides a simple chemical classification showing the relative frequency of the different types of stone as well as their important clinical characteristics and aetiology. Calcium is present in at least 90% of stones, either as oxalate or phosphate compounds or both.

MECHANISMS OF STONE FORMATION

Calcium-containing stones

In patients with stones containing calcium (the majority of cases) no specific underlying abnormality is discovered. Some excrete excessive calcium (**idiopathic hypercalciuria**) without being hypercalcaemic; in these, there may be increased intestinal absorption of calcium leading to increased urinary excretion. Experimental evidence suggests that some patients in this group are deficient in a urinary factor that prevents stone formation. Such a factor has not yet been defined.

Idiopathic stone disease is probably caused not by a single factor but by the interaction of several factors. The

541

following examples illustrate some of these. Bladder stones composed of **urate** were once common in boys in England and are still common in some parts of Africa, Turkey and India. They are believed to be due to the combined effects of deficiency of protein, vitamin A and trace elements, gastroenteritis and dehydration. All of these factors conspire to produce a small volume of concentrated acid urine which encourages uric acid to precipitate. Another factor is **prolonged immobilisation**, e.g. after multiple fractures or paraplegia, which causes generalised skeletal decalcification and increased calcium

excretion. If there is also poor fluid throughput and incomplete bladder emptying, stone formation is likely. Inadequate fluid intake probably plays a part in the aetiology of many urinary tract stones.

Stones caused by excessive urinary excretion of a stone constituent

A minority of patients are found to have an underlying disorder responsible for excessive urinary excretion of the main constituent of the stone. Examples include **hyperparathyroidism** (calcium), **hyperoxaluria** (oxalate), **gout** (uric acid), **cysteinuria** (cysteine stones) and **xanthinuria** (xanthine stones).

Other predisposing factors

A specific predisposing factor can be detected in a further minority of cases:

- **Chronic infection**. Infection, particularly with urea-splitting bacteria (e.g. *Proteus*), predisposes to magnesium–ammonium–phosphate stones
- **Urinary stasis**. There may be obvious or occult **urinary stasis** of the upper tract (e.g. **hydronephrosis** or rarely, **horseshoe kidney**) or the lower tract (e.g. **prostatic hypertrophy** or **neurogenic bladder**). Stasis becomes a particularly important predisposing factor when associated with recurrent or chronic infection

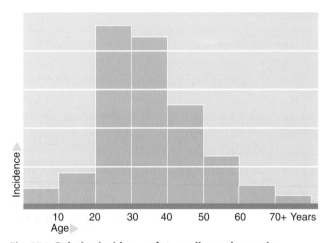

Fig. 37.1 Relative incidence of stone disease by age in developed countries

Table 37.1 Chemical composition, clinical features and aetiology of urinary tract stones

Chemical composition	%	Clinical features	Aetiology
Calcium oxalate	40	Three types of stone are described: —small smooth 'hemp-seed' stones —small irregular 'mulberry' stones —small spiculated 'jack' stones	Most cases are idiopathic; predisposing factors include urinary stasis, infection and foreign bodies. Some are due to metabolic disorders: —hyperparathyroidism —hyperoxaluria (rare inherited disorder)
Mixed calcium oxalate and phosphate stones	15	As above	Some are due to disorders associated with hypercalcaemia, e.g. sarcoidosis, multiple metastases, multiple myeloma, milk-alkali syndrome, overtreatment with vitamin D
Calcium and phosphate	15	As above	Some of these patients excrete abnormally large amounts of calcium (idiopathic hypercalciuria but without hypercalcaemia)
Magnesium ammonium phosphate	15	Typically large 'staghorn' calculi of pelvicalyceal system and some bladder stones	Chronic infection with organisms capable of producing urease, typically *Proteus*. Urease splits urea, forming ammonia if the urine is alkaline
Uric acid	8	Stones tend to absorb yellow and brown pigments. Pure stones are radiolucent	Occur in primary gout and hyperuricaemia following chemotherapy for leukaemias or myeloproliferative disorders. Childhood urate bladder stones occur in some developing countries when urine pH is low
Cysteine or xanthine	2	Excess urinary excretion of cysteine or xanthine. Pure stones are radiolucent	Autosomal recessive inherited disorders

- Idiopathic (most common)
- Stasis of urine, e.g. congenital abnormalities, chronic obstruction
- Chronic urinary infection (urea-splitting organisms, e.g. *Proteus*, cause alkaline urine and the development of magnesium–ammonium–phosphate stones, typically the 'staghorn' calculi of the renal pelvis—see Fig. 37.2)
- Excess urinary excretion of stone-forming substances, e.g. idiopathic hypercalciuria (calcium stones), hyperparathyroidism (calcium stones), hyperoxaluria (oxalate stones), gout (uric acid stones), cysteinuria (cysteine stones), xanthinuria (xanthine stones)
- Foreign bodies, e.g. fragments of catheter tubing, self-inserted artefacts, parasites (schistosome ova)
- Fragments of diseased tissue, e.g. renal papillary necrosis
- Multifactorial, e.g. prolonged immobility, children in the developing world

- Incidental finding on X-ray
- Loin pain
- Ureteric colic
- Painful passage of small stones via urethra
- Cystitis
- Pyelonephritis
- Haematuria
- Impaired renal function

Urinary tract stones produce their injurious effects in three main ways:

- By obstructing urinary flow
- By predisposing to infection
- By causing local tissue irritation and damage

OBSTRUCTION OF URINARY FLOW

Pelvicalyceal obstruction

Obstruction of one or more renal calyces causes local urinary obstruction (**hydrocalyx**) and typically leads to chronic or recurrent loin pain. Similar pain may also be caused by chronic, incomplete obstruction of the pelvi-ureteric junction (PUJ) or ureter. The result is **hydrone-phrosis**, i.e. dilatation of the renal pelvis, both intrarenal and extrarenal. More severe obstruction may lead to progressive renal parenchymal damage and impaired renal function; if both kidneys are affected, the patient may develop renal failure.

Passage of stones into the ureter

If small renal stones pass into the ureter, there are several possible outcomes:

- Stones may pass to the bladder and exit via the urethra causing minor symptoms. The patient may intermittently pass 'gravel' or 'sand' (see Fig. 37.3) and experience dysuria and sometimes haematuria
- Stones may pass into the bladder and act as a nidus there for development of a larger bladder stone. Bladder stones occasionally cause bladder outlet obstruction and urinary retention
- A stone may impact in the ureter causing chronic partial obstruction and eventually hydroureter. This typically presents as loin pain but, surprisingly, may be asymptomatic
- A stone may impact in the ureter, causing sudden complete obstruction. The patient experiences extremely severe, unilateral colicky pain (**ureteric colic**) often with loin pain and tenderness due to renal distension

- **Foreign bodies**. Diseased tissue such as necrotic renal papillae (occurring in diabetes or analgesic nephropathy) may calcify. If a papilla sloughs into the renal pelvis, it can act as a nidus for calculus formation. Similarly, **foreign bodies** in the bladder act as foci for calcification. These may be inserted by the patient (e.g. ballpoint pen caps or hair clips) or be left behind after instrumentation or surgery (e.g. sutures, catheter fragments). **Schistosome ova** are responsible for bladder stones in some developing countries
- **Dietary causes**. These probably include overconsumption of dairy products. In areas with a high calcium content in the water, there is a slight increase in stone formation

Predisposing factors in stone formation are summarised in Box 37.1.

The clinical problem of discrete urinary stones should not be confused with calcification of the renal paren-chyma, which can be a feature of tuberculosis and medul-lary sponge kidney. These and similar diseases can usually be diagnosed on their characteristic X-ray appearance.

CLINICAL FEATURES OF STONE DISEASE

The nature of the adverse effects depends on the size, morphology and site of the stone(s). Many stones cause no symptoms but represent a potentially serious problem. Other stones produce marked pathological effects which present with acute or chronic symptoms or are discovered incidentally on investigation of unrelated symptoms. The presentation of stones in the urinary tract is summarised in Box 37.2.

Fig. 37.2 Plain abdominal X-rays showing staghorn calculi

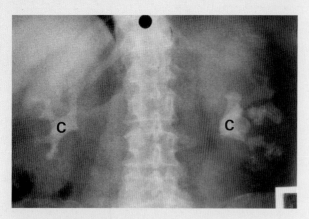

(a) Asymptomatic bilateral 'staghorn' calculi **C**, found incidentally in a 61-year-old woman.

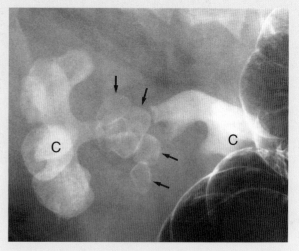

(b) Huge 'staghorn' calculus **C** in upper middle parts of the right kidney; an incidental finding in a 69-year-old woman during barium enema examination; note also the multiple radiopaque faceted gallstones (arrowed), also asymptomatic!

Fig. 37.3 Recurrent urinary tract stones
This man aged 40 had a 2-year history of passing small stones and 'gravel' in the urine.

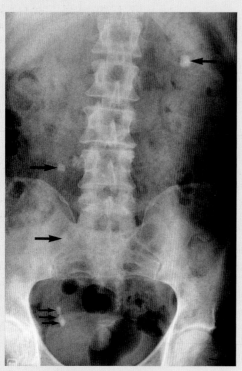

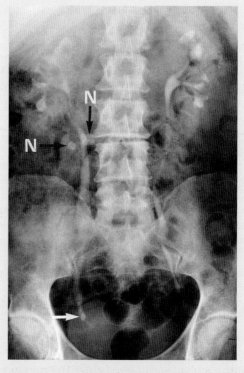

(a) Plain abdominal X-ray showing what appear to be several stones (arrowed) in the right ureter and in the upper pole of the left kidney.

(b) Intravenous urogram (IVU) of the same patient showing partial obstruction at the lower end of the right ureter (arrowed); note that two of the radiopaque objects on the right side lie outside the area of contrast and thus probably represent calcified mesenteric lymph nodes **N** rather than ureteric stones; metabolic studies showed that this patient has idiopathic hypercalciuria.

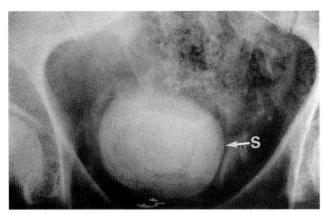

Fig. 37.4 Bladder stone
Plain X-ray showing massive bladder stone **S** in an 85-year-old man with benign prostatic hypertrophy and recurrent urinary tract infections; such stones are rare nowadays.

PREDISPOSITION TO INFECTION

Urinary tract stones predispose to infection by causing urinary stasis, by preventing proper 'flushing' of the tract and by providing niches in which bacteria multiply. Pelvicalyceal or ureteric stones may cause **acute pyelonephritis** and occasionally **perinephric abscess**. Bladder stones predispose to cystitis and ascending infections (see Fig. 37.4).

LOCAL IRRITATION AND TISSUE DAMAGE

Stones may present because of their irritant effects on local tissues. Simple inflammation may cause bleeding and thus present as **haematuria**. Chronic inflammation may lead to fibrosis; if this occurs at a narrow part of the tract, typically the PUJ or ureter, a **stricture** may form. Prolonged irritation of the bladder mucosa by stone may cause **squamous metaplasia** and eventually **squamous carcinoma**.

INVESTIGATION AND MANAGEMENT OF SUSPECTED URINARY TRACT STONES

APPROACH TO INVESTIGATION

When investigating a patient with urinary tract stones, the objectives are:

- To confirm a stone is present
- To locate the stone or stones
- To evaluate any deleterious effects of the stone(s) on renal function and urinary tract morphology
- To identify any structural disorders of the urinary tract acting as local predisposing factors
- To identify any metabolic predisposing factors

- Obstruction of urinary flow
- Infection
- Persistent, recurrent or severe pain
- Stones likely to cause future obstruction or infection
- Small 'metabolic' stones likely to grow rapidly in size
- In patients where colic could be disastrous, e.g. airline or military pilots
- Patients with a solitary kidney

METHODS OF INVESTIGATION

In general, the above objectives will be met by performing the following investigations. For convenience, they are conducted concurrently:

- Urine dipstick testing, microscopy, culture and sensitivities
- Tests of renal function, i.e. plasma urea, electrolytes and creatinine estimation
- Plain abdominal X-ray ('KUB'). Around 90% of stones are radiopaque because they contain calcium. Urate stones are radiolucent
- In acute cases, 'emergency' intravenous urogram (IVU). This consists of a pre-injection plain film of the abdomen and pelvis (KUB) and a further film 20 minutes after injection of radiopaque contrast and after micturition, with the patient prone (face down). Note: this is not the same as a full IVU with prior preparation. Figure 37.5 shows an IVU with the effects of stone obstruction. Urate stones show as filling defects on excretory films and look deceptively similar to a tumour. Many units now use CT scanning instead of IVU
- Renal ultrasonography. This demonstrates hydronephrosis as well as the stones themselves
- Special contrast techniques. These are occasionally required when other techniques do not give the required information, e.g. percutaneous (antegrade) pyelography or ascending (retrograde) ureterography
- Biochemical analysis of any recovered stones
- Tests for metabolic disorders (for recurrent stones), i.e. serum calcium, phosphate, oxalate, uric acid and alkaline phosphatase; 24-hour urinary excretion of calcium, uric acid and cysteine

INDICATIONS FOR STONE REMOVAL (Box 37.3)

The finding of a urinary tract stone is not an automatic indication for its removal or destruction. The exception is in airline or military pilots in whom ureteric colic could prove disastrous. The usual indications for stone removal are summarised in Box 37.3. Small stones in the pelvicalyceal system often remain unchanged and asymptomatic

Fig. 37.5 Emergency IVU in ureteric colic
This 37-year-old man presented with left ureteric colic.

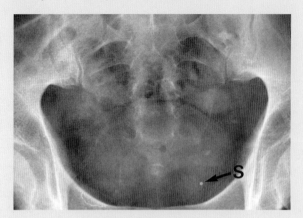

(a) Part of the 'control' film showing a small radiopacity **S**, probably a stone, in the area of the left vesicoureteric junction.

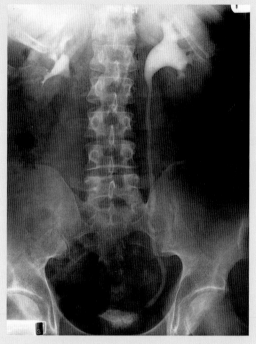

(b) IVU taken 20 minutes after injection of contrast showing dilated left pelvicalyceal system and contrast-filled ureter down to the area of the stone. This confirms an obstruction at the vesicoureteric junction.

for many years and can safely be monitored by annual radiography. Stones of 5 mm or less in diameter often pass right through the tract, although in doing so they may produce severe but short-lived symptoms of ureteric colic, haematuria or dysuria.

METHODS OF STONE REMOVAL

Stones can be removed by endoscopic methods, open surgery or a variety of percutaneous and other less invasive techniques. The choice of technique depends on the size, nature and site of the stone, the availability of expertise and special equipment, and whether there is a need to correct congenital or acquired structural abnormalities.

Cystoscopic techniques

Cystoscopic methods (Fig. 37.6) are suitable for most bladder stones and for impacted stones in the lower third of the ureter. Bladder stones can be broken into small fragments (**litholapaxy**) using a **lithotrite**, a modification of a cystoscope incorporating stone-crushing jaws. The fragments are then washed out by irrigation. Stones can also be fragmented by directly applied pulsed ultrasound, laser or other energy sources via a cystoscope.

A **ureteroscope** can be used to examine the lower part of the ureter and assist with stone removal. The ureteric orifice is first dilated cystoscopically and then the slender rigid ureteroscope is passed (see Fig. 37.7a). It can be used to help capture elusive stones with a Dormia basket (declining in popularity) or used to apply energy via ultrasonic, electrohydraulic, lithoclast probes or laser fibre directly to the surface of a stone in order to destroy it. **Flexible ureteroscopes** allow access into the renal pelvis and calyces so that stone fragmentation can be achieved using holmium laser probes.

Open surgical removal of renal or ureteric stones is rarely performed nowadays as renal stones can usually be removed by percutaneous methods or else fragmented by extracorporeal lithotripsy (see below). Ureteric stones can often be extracted or fragmented by ureteroscopy or be treated by lithotripsy, with or without prior stent placement. A **ureteric stent** is usually introduced after repeated instrumentation of the ureter to assist drainage or to prevent any stone displaced upwards from reimpacting in the ureter. If an impacted stone is causing complete ureteric obstruction and leading to marked proximal dilatation, or if there is infection, a **percutaneous nephrostomy** should be inserted without delay (see Fig. 37.8, p. 549) to preserve renal function.

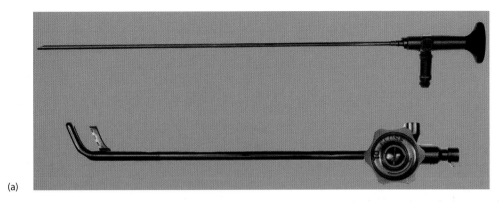

(a)

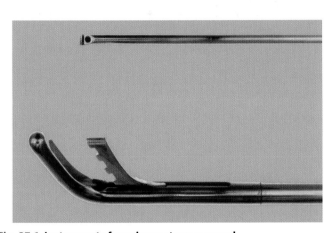

(b)

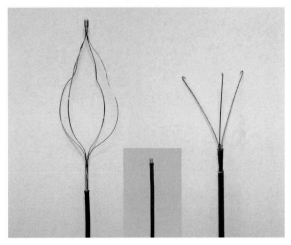

(c)

Fig. 37.6 Instruments for urinary stone removal
(a) Lithotrite. The telescope (above) fits through the centre of the lithotrite, allowing a direct view as the stones are crushed between the jaws. Note: the jaws are closed before passing the instrument into the bladder via the urethra. **(b)** Close up of tip of lithotrite and telescope. **(c)** Dormia basket and grasping forceps. The Dormia basket (centre and left) is advanced beyond the stone in the ureter and then opened by advancing the centre wire from the proximal end. When open (left), the whole instrument is gradually withdrawn until the stone lodges within the wire basket. The centre wire is then withdrawn further until the stone is firmly held within the basket and the whole instrument withdrawn complete with stone. The trident grasper (right) operates in a similar way, grasping the stone as the wire is retracted.

Open surgical methods

Before today's minimal access methods of removing or destroying urinary tract stones, open surgery was often required. For the pelvicalyceal system **pyelolithotomy** was performed; for the ureter, **ureterolithotomy**; and for some bladder stones, **cystolithotomy**. 'Invasive' surgery is employed nowadays when the appropriate techniques are not available, are not indicated or have failed. Open stone removal is also indicated at the same operation if an elective correction of an anatomical abnormality which predisposes to stone formation is being performed. Examples are bladder diverticula, pelviureteric junction obstruction or ureteric stricture.

Percutaneous techniques of stone removal

Direct percutaneous access to the renal pelvis can be obtained under local anaesthesia using radiological or ultrasound guidance. This allows a track to be created from the skin of the loin into the pelvicalyceal system

(**nephrostomy**), through which progressively larger instruments can be passed. Small stones can be retrieved using a Dormia basket or a steerable grasping tool. Larger stones can be broken into fragments with electrohydraulic or other probes, after which the fragments can be lifted out with special instruments (see Fig. 31.7b). The nephrostomy track closes spontaneously after a short period.

Non-invasive stone removal technique (Fig. 37.7)

Extracorporeal shock wave lithotripsy (ESWL) is a non-invasive method of destroying stones using externally applied shock waves which pass into the patient to shatter the stone. The ultrasound beam is usually transmitted via water pads and focused on the stone by ultrasound or X-ray. The stone fragments are passed out in the urine and may cause ureteric colic or ureteric obstruction. For this reason, a ureteric stent is often placed before lithotripsy of a large stone (> 1.5 cm) to prevent obstruction with stone fragments. The ureter dilates around the stent and stone debris is passed more easily after stent removal.

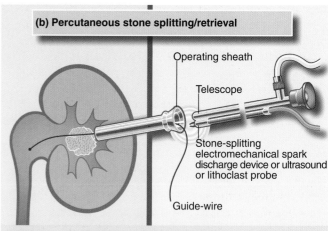

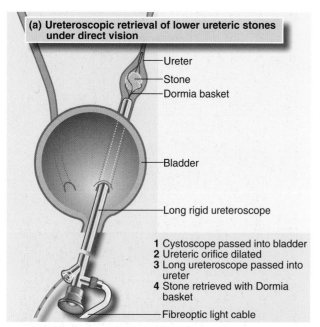

(a) Ureteroscopic retrieval of lower ureteric stones under direct vision

- Ureter
- Stone
- Dormia basket
- Bladder
- Long rigid ureteroscope
- Fibreoptic light cable

1 Cystoscope passed into bladder
2 Ureteric orifice dilated
3 Long ureteroscope passed into ureter
4 Stone retrieved with Dormia basket

(a)

(b) Percutaneous stone splitting/retrieval

- Operating sheath
- Telescope
- Stone-splitting electromechanical spark discharge device or ultrasound or lithoclast probe
- Guide-wire

1 Needle passed through skin into renal pelvis
2 Guide-wire passed through needle into ureter
3 Hollow dilators passed sequentially over guide-wire until large bore operating sheath can be placed
4 Stone progressively broken into fragments by mechanical shock, spark discharge or other energy-emitting probe applied to surface of stone
5 Stone fragments removed with forceps under direct vision

(b)

(c) Extracorporeal Shock Wave Lithotripter (ESWL) Photograph by kind permission of Siemeus UK

(c)

Fig. 37.7 Current methods of urinary tract stone removal

MANAGEMENT OF ACUTE URETERIC COLIC

Ureteric colic occurs when a stone causes sudden obstruction of a ureter. It presents typically with a sudden onset of severe unilateral pain radiating from one loin to the groin or tip of the penis. The pain is due to waves of ureteric peristalsis, and episodes may last from several minutes to half an hour. At the peak of the pain, the patient writhes in agony. Indeed, the pain of ureteric colic can be so severe and incapacitating that military pilots known to have stones are grounded until the stones are removed. Most patients are seen urgently by their family practitioner or brought straight to the accident and emergency department. Non-steroidal anti-inflammatory drugs given as suppositories or injection have largely replaced intramuscular opiate analgesia to settle the pain. NSAIDs are more effective, longer-lasting and without risk of addiction or legal compromise. The usual drug of choice is diclofenac. Morphine should be avoided as it tends to provoke or prolong ureteric spasm and pain. The patient may have become pain-free by the time of first examination by the surgical staff, but the pain history is usually diagnostic. Occasionally, ureteric colic is not as severe but is more persistent, in which case it may mimic other acute abdominal conditions.

INVESTIGATION OF URETERIC COLIC

Ureteric colic almost always causes **microscopic haematuria**, and the first investigation is 'dipstick' testing of the urine for blood; if positive it should be confirmed on microscopic examination. A positive result reinforces the diagnosis. An IVU or CT scan should then be performed urgently to confirm or refute the diagnosis (see Fig. 37.5, p. 546).

The characteristic radiological features on IVU of acute ureteric obstruction are:

- **Delay** of all phases of passage of contrast through the kidney and collecting system on the affected side; the more severe the obstruction, the longer the delay. If there appears to be no excretion, further films are taken every few hours for about 24 hours; usually contrast will eventually pass into the system, demonstrating the site of obstruction
- **Dilatation** of the collecting system above the point of obstruction

TREATMENT OF URETERIC COLIC

Most patients with ureteric colic initially require strong analgesics. These are usually non-steroidal anti-inflammatory drugs given by suppository or injection. Many patients settle on a single dose but two or three doses may be required. In most cases, the stone gradually passes down the ureter and into the bladder. Each stage of movement may be accompanied by an attack of colic. If a stone is retrieved, it should be chemically analysed. If there is **complete obstruction** of the ureter, or infection above an obstructing stone, urgent intervention is usually required to prevent renal damage. Immediate treatment may involve placing a percutaneous nephrostomy tube to drain the renal pelvis (see Fig. 37.8) or placing a stent beside the stone to allow urinary drainage or else removal of the stone endoscopically. After nephrostomy or stent placement, the stone sometimes passes spontaneously but more often further treatment is required later. In cases with persistent pain that do not need immediate intervention, plain abdominal X-rays will usually record changes in the position of the stone. If the stone is very large, it may have to be surgically removed. If the stone appears to be small enough to pass spontaneously, yet fails to progress, the patient can safely be allowed home if the criteria for urgent intervention mentioned above are not

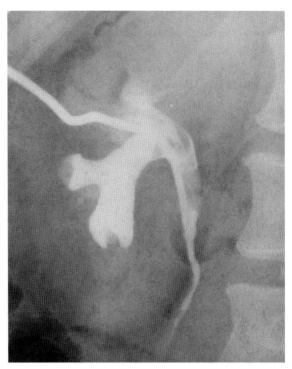

Fig. 37.8 Percutaneously placed nephrostomy drainage tube
A ureteric stone caused complete ureteric obstruction and the patient suffered continuing pain and developed a fever. Urgent drainage was required to prevent renal damage from a combination of obstruction and infection.

fulfilled. The patient can be reviewed after a week or two with a plain abdominal X-ray and a decision taken then about any need for intervention.

LONG-TERM MANAGEMENT OF UROLOGICAL STONE DISEASE

MANAGEMENT OF METABOLIC ABNORMALITIES

Hyperparathyroidism is the only stone-forming metabolic abnormality that can be corrected by surgical treatment (parathyroidectomy). It is diagnosed by an elevated plasma calcium, lowered plasma phosphate and an elevated plasma parathormone level. Most patients are also hypercalciuric.

Dietary hypercalciuria should be treated by reducing the intake of milk, cheese, butter, bread and pastry. Local tap water and bottled water imbibed by the patient should have its calcium level checked. **Idiopathic hypercalciuria** can be treated with thiazides. Urate stones dissolve in alkaline urine and treatment may involve alkalinising the urine with potassium citrate. **Primary oxaluria** is very rare; secondary oxaluria only occurs with huge intakes of tea, coffee, chocolate, strawberries or rhubarb.

The drug **allopurinol** may be given for hyperuricaemia (gout) and is routinely given during chemotherapy for leukaemia. Allopurinol inhibits xanthine oxidase, an enzyme involved in synthesis of uric acid. Allopurinol can be used in hyperuricaemia (see below) and may also prevent nidus formation in urine around which calcium crystals deposit during stone formation.

LONG-TERM FOLLOW-UP OF PATIENTS WITH URINARY TRACT STONES

For many patients, a symptomatic urinary tract stone manifests as an isolated episode with no apparent predis-posing cause. Long-term follow-up for these patients is not usually required. Patients with stones that do not need removing or with recurrent stones require long-term follow-up with regular plain abdominal X-rays. Stones that enlarge during follow-up, that cause symptoms or obstruct need removing. Any patient with stone disease should be advised to increase fluid intake; dietary advice based on stone composition may also help. Drinking excessive fluids during a bout of ureteric colic however is misguided and is likely to cause an increase in pain.

Urinary tract infections

38

INTRODUCTION

Urinary tract infections are a common problem in surgery. They may be responsible for urinary tract symptoms that present to the clinician for diagnosis or for abdominal pain that is not obviously urological. More often, urinary tract infection is a secondary problem. It may occur after operation, particularly if a urinary catheter has been employed, or it may complicate surgical disorders of the urinary tract such as tumours or stones. Most infections are caused by common bacteria of faecal origin.

Urinary tract infections may also be caused by more unusual organisms, in particular *Mycobacterium tuberculosis*. In its early stages, urinary tract infection with the tubercle bacillus may produce the same symptoms and signs as ordinary bacterial infection. Tuberculosis can be easily overlooked unless specifically sought.

On a world-wide basis, other organisms are more important causes of urinary tract infection, most notably the trematode *Schistosoma*. One variety of this causes severe bladder disease in some developing countries.

Infections of the urethra are usually transmitted by sexual intercourse. Gonococci and *Chlamydia* are the organisms most commonly involved. A late result of gonorrhoea in males or its inappropriate treatment may be a fibrous **urethral stricture**.

Other urethral strictures

The most common cause of urethral stricture is **trauma**. This may follow prolonged catheterisation, instrumentation of the urethra or pelvic fractures with urethral involvement. Although most are not infective in origin, urethral strictures are covered in this chapter.

COMMON BACTERIAL INFECTIONS OF THE LOWER URINARY TRACT

PATHOPHYSIOLOGY OF LOWER URINARY TRACT INFECTIONS

The common infections of the urinary tract, i.e. those caused by faecal organisms, involve either the **bladder** or the **upper tract** (kidney, pelvicalyceal system and ureter) or both together.

The bladder is the area infected most often, with females being particularly susceptible. Probably half of all females are affected at one time or another. Infection rate rises with pregnancy and with increasing age. In females, the infecting organisms probably enter via the short urethra, which is only 3 cm long. Organisms easily spread from the perineal skin, particularly during sexual intercourse.

Normally, the bladder is flushed clean by the frequent passage of newly produced urine, preventing the multiplication of bacteria in the urinary tract. Stasis of urine for any reason—such as incomplete bladder emptying, dehydration or immobility—interferes with this mechanism and predisposes to infection. Urethral instrumentation greatly predisposes to infection in either sex.

CLINICAL FEATURES OF LOWER URINARY TRACT INFECTIONS

Typical symptoms of bladder infection are **dysuria**, **frequency**, **urgency** and a sensation of **incomplete bladder emptying**. The term 'cystitis' is often used by patients to

---

Box 38.1   Presentations of bladder infection

- Dysuria with frequency and urgency of micturition (very common)
- Lower abdominal pain (common—usually children or young adults)
- Unexpected development of incontinence (common in the elderly)
- Development of enuresis (bed-wetting) in a previously 'dry' child
- Non-specific ill-health in previously well infants or the elderly (including pyrexia of unknown origin and systemic sepsis)

---

mean symptoms included in this list; however, infection is not always the cause and the term is probably best avoided to prevent confusion. Even when infection is present, symptoms may be trivial or absent and this may make diagnosis difficult. Abdominal pain may be the only symptom; consequently, most patients with abdominal pain should have their urine tested as a matter of course.

In the elderly or the very young, there are often no localising symptoms, and the patient is just non-specifically unwell. Recurrent fever in a child can result from urinary infection. In any ill patient in these age groups, the urine must be sent for examination before antibiotics are given. A sudden onset of **enuresis** or **urinary incontinence** in children or the elderly should also suggest bladder infection.

The different presentations of bladder infection are summarised in Box 38.1.

BACTERIOLOGICAL DIAGNOSIS OF LOWER URINARY TRACT INFECTIONS

Urinary tract infection is confirmed by examining a 'midstream' specimen of urine (MSU). If the specimen cannot be examined quickly, it should be refrigerated or it will become of no diagnostic value in a few hours. The specimen is examined microscopically for white blood cells ('pus cells') and bacteria. The specimen is also cultured to identify the causative organism and determine antibiotic sensitivity. Bacterial contamination of urine specimens is common; a 'significant' infection is therefore defined as one in which pus cells are abundant and there are more than 100 000 (10^5) organisms per millilitre of urine. Enteric organisms are almost always responsible, the usual culprits being *Escherichia coli*, *Proteus* spp., *Enterococcus faecalis* and *Pseudomonas* (the last particularly in debilitated and catheterised patients). *Staphylococcus saprophyticus* is an important cause of uncomplicated bladder infection in young sexually active females.

Significant numbers of pus cells in the urine without bacterial growth most commonly result from patients taking antibiotics. If this is not the case, a stone, tumour, prostatitis or tuberculosis must be suspected and investigated. Infection often causes frank or occult haematuria; this only warrants further investigation if it persists after the infection is treated.

Some female patients experience typical symptoms of urinary infection but despite multiple laboratory examinations, no evidence of bacterial infection of urine is found. Non-specific urethral inflammation from the trauma of intercourse may be responsible; this is probably the cause of 'honeymoon cystitis'.

MANAGEMENT OF BLADDER INFECTIONS

Antibiotic therapy is the principal treatment for bladder infection, initially chosen on a 'best-guess' basis if treatment is urgent. An MSU specimen should be collected for microscopy, culture and sensitivities (M, C & S) before therapy is commenced. If the initial antibiotic choice is inappropriate or unsuccessful, then the results of urine culture may suggest a more suitable alternative. The MSU should be repeated several days after completion of the course of antibiotics if there is doubt whether the infection has been eliminated or in complicated cases.

Patients who have had urinary tract infections should be encouraged to increase their fluid intake. Indeed, this is often effective in dealing with early or mild symptoms and will probably allow mild infections to resolve without drugs.

In **pregnancy**, the ureters and renal pelvis dilate under the effect of circulating progestogens and become more susceptible to infection. Where bladder infection is suspected, the urine should be tested and evidence of significant bacterial growth treated with appropriate antibiotics, whether or not the patient is symptomatic. This is because of the risk of infection ascending to the upper tracts. The antibiotic used must be safe for use in pregnancy and non-teratogenic, e.g. a cephalosporin. Trimethoprim is also safe but may deplete folate. Standard texts such as the *British National Formulary* give specific information on prescribing in pregnancy and should be consulted.

RECURRENT BLADDER INFECTIONS

Patients likely to suffer recurrent infections tend to fall into three groups:

- The elderly, debilitated and infirm
- Young and middle-aged women
- Patients with urinary tract abnormalities predisposing to infection

Those in the first two groups can usually be managed without surgery.

The elderly, debilitated and infirm

These patients often have a multiplicity of simple predisposing factors such as constipation, incontinence, an indwelling catheter, poor fluid intake and diminished resistance. Correction of these problems and good nursing care (e.g. regular changes of indwelling catheter) may break the pattern. Antibiotic-resistant bacteria are often a problem in this group of patients because of previous courses of antibiotics.

Young and middle-aged women

Many of these patients can be helped by simple hygiene measures. These include 'wiping from front to back' after micturition or defaecation, frequent and complete emptying of the bladder, increasing urine flow by raising fluid intake, and emptying the bladder soon after intercourse.

Patients with urinary tract abnormalities predisposing to infection

Abnormalities should be suspected in children or young men with a single episode of urinary infection, particularly if they fail to respond to simple measures, and anyone with recurrent urinary infections. These patients require investigation (e.g. ultrasonography, intravenous urography) and are often found to have a structural abnormality or pathological condition which encourages bacterial proliferation. Bladder stone or prostatic hypertrophy is commonly responsible. These predisposing conditions can often be corrected surgically. In the rest, however, no predisposing factor can be found.

As with isolated episodes of infection, recurrent infections are treated with antibiotics, but bacteriological investigation assumes a greater importance. Some patients may need long-term, low-dose antibiotics to prevent recurrence.

The 'urethral syndrome'

This syndrome is only found in women and is characterised by episodic or persistent dysuria, frequency or urgency. Urinary symptoms occur without demonstrable infection or local anatomical abnormality such as uterine prolapse. The cause is not known and the condition may be indistinguishable from recurrent urethral trauma due to sexual intercourse. Urethral dilatation under general anaesthesia may be successful in relieving symptoms, although the mechanism is obscure. If it fails, urethroscopy should be performed to look for a urethral diverticulum. Dysuria may also be a symptom associated with **atrophic vaginitis** in perimenopausal and postmenopausal women; this may be relieved by topical application of oestrogens to the introitus and vagina.

Some patients, particularly women and girls, experience persistent or recurrent low-grade symptoms, notably frequency and urgency. No cause is found, although some cases can be attributed to habit or to psychogenic or psychosexual factors.

Box	38.2	**Presenting features of acute pyelonephritis**

- Unilateral loin pain and tenderness
- Poorly localised abdominal pain and discomfort
- Dysuria plus cloudy, strong-smelling urine
- Haematuria
- Pyrexia and tachycardia
- Systemic sepsis (especially young children and the elderly)

UPPER URINARY TRACT INFECTIONS

PATHOPHYSIOLOGY OF UPPER URINARY TRACT INFECTIONS

Infections of the pelvicalyceal system and renal parenchyma (**acute pyelonephritis**) arise by upward extension of a lower tract infection or via the bloodstream (haematogenous).

Ascending infections occur most commonly when there is an abnormality causing ureteric reflux or stasis. Such conditions include ureteric obstruction, abnormal peristalsis (as in megaureter) and congenital incompetence of the cysto-ureteric antireflux mechanism. During pregnancy, ureters dilate under hormonal influences and this may increase the incidence of upper urinary tract infections.

Infection is often haematogenous when there is urinary stasis in the upper tract. Common causes are stones in the renal pelvis or obstruction of the pelviureteric junction (PUJ). In such cases, lower tract infection is a secondary phenomenon.

The factors initiating a renal infection are often unknown but pre-existing renal damage is a strong predisposing factor.

Pathological examination of an acutely infected kidney shows extensive neutrophilic infiltration of the renal parenchyma, often with small abscesses. Usually only one kidney is involved and the causative organisms are enteral, as in other urinary tract infections.

CLINICAL FEATURES OF UPPER URINARY TRACT INFECTIONS

The classic clinical features of acute pyelonephritis are unilateral loin pain and tenderness (see Box 38.2). The patient is generally unwell with systemic features of infection, i.e. pyrexia and tachycardia. The urine is usually cloudy, and microscopy and culture confirm the presence of pus cells and bacteria. There may also be typical symptoms of bladder infection. Often, the symptoms and signs are less specific and the patient presents with unilateral

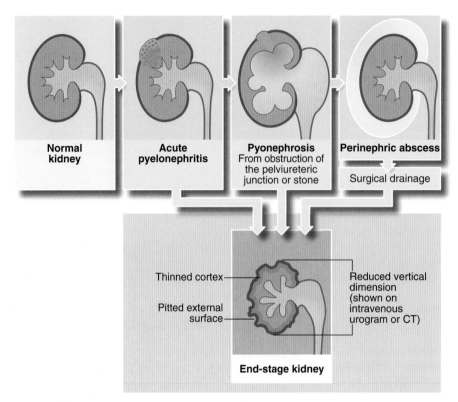

Fig. 38.1 Consequences of untreated renal infection

abdominal pain or discomfort. This may be mistaken for early acute appendicitis unless the urine is examined. Pyelonephritis may present without localising signs, especially in infants and the elderly, but patients are more unwell than in bladder infection and may even develop signs of systemic sepsis.

MANAGEMENT OF UPPER URINARY TRACT INFECTIONS

Diagnosis is made on the basis of clinical symptoms, signs and urine examination. Blood is also taken for culture when there are systemic signs of infection.

Treatment is with antibiotics, initially on a 'best-guess' basis, based on local microbiological advice. Dosage and route of administration depend on the severity of the illness; severe cases are treated with intravenous antibiotics.

Once the acute illness has been successfully treated, further investigation, usually ultrasonography and intravenous urography, may be indicated in the search for predisposing factors. In children, investigation should include a contrast micturating cystogram or equivalent radionuclide scintigram to identify ureteric reflux (see Chapter 51).

COMPLICATIONS OF ACUTE PYELONEPHRITIS
(see Figs 38.1 and 38.2)

Pyonephrosis

Severe infections may be complicated by obstruction of the pelviureteric outlet, resulting in accumulation of pus in the renal pelvis. If untreated, this will destroy the renal parenchyma. Treatment involves surgical or percutaneous drainage followed by correction of the obstruction.

Perinephric abscess

If infection develops in the presence of a large 'staghorn' calculus, the accumulating pus may discharge through the renal capsule into the surrounding fat, resulting in a perinephric abscess (Fig. 38.2). This presents as a slowly expanding mass in the loin, often with only low-grade local and systemic symptoms. Urine investigation will reveal pyuria, whilst ultrasound and radiology will show a non-functioning renal mass containing fluid-filled areas. A large renal calculus may also be seen. A perinephric abscess sometimes develops as a result of **haematogenous infection** of a traumatic perinephric haematoma. The treatment of perinephric abscess is drainage, often followed later by nephrectomy of the end-stage kidney. The diagnosis should be considered in elderly patients with sepsis from an unknown source. If a perinephric inflammatory mass partially resolves, it can result in **xanthomatous pyelonephritis**, a solid mass often suspected of malignancy and hence removed surgically.

URINARY TRACT INFECTION IN THE CATHETERISED PATIENT

Even with the best of care, almost all catheterised patients eventually develop bacteriuria. Antibiotic treatment should be employed only if there are systemic signs of

Fig. 38.2 Perinephric abscess

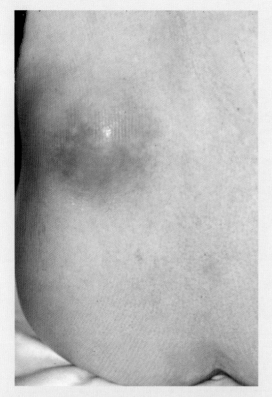

This woman of 55 presented with a 3-week history of left loin pain and 48 hours of rigors. The photograph shows a large abscess surrounding the left kidney, 'pointing' in the posterior loin. A plain abdominal film showed a staghorn calculus in the kidney and isotope studies showed no function in that kidney. The abscess was drained percutaneously and she was treated with antibiotics. The kidney was later removed.

infection, otherwise there is a risk of generating bacteria that are ever more resistant to antibiotics.

GENITOURINARY TUBERCULOSIS

PATHOPHYSIOLOGY OF GENITOURINARY TUBERCULOSIS

About 4% of patients with tuberculosis have involvement of the genitourinary system. In developed countries, incidence is highest in debilitated elderly patients, often with a history of treated tuberculosis and in patients with HIV infection. The other vulnerable group comprises immigrants from developing countries where tuberculosis is endemic.

Mycobacteria reach the kidney or epididymis via the bloodstream, causing typical centrally caseating granulomatous lesions which may later calcify (see Fig. 38.3). From the kidney, direct spread may occur to the ureter

(causing a fibrous stricture) or to the bladder. Tuberculosis of the bladder usually begins around a ureteric opening and spreads more widely to cause patchy ulceration of the bladder wall and later fibrotic contraction. Young adults are most commonly affected and, as mentioned, there is a seriously increased incidence among patients with acquired immune deficiency syndrome (AIDS). These and other patients 'living rough' are poorly compliant with treatment and provide a reservoir of infection for others.

CLINICAL FEATURES AND INVESTIGATION OF GENITOURINARY TUBERCULOSIS

Urinary tract tuberculosis is often asymptomatic and is diagnosed during investigation of 'sterile pyuria'. If symptoms are present, the usual ones are painless urinary frequency, nocturia and sometimes haematuria. There may also be systemic features such as weight loss and night sweats, and respiratory symptoms if the lungs are affected.

When urinary tuberculosis is suspected, at least three early morning urine (EMU) specimens must be sent to the laboratory to be stained and cultured for tubercle bacilli (also known as acid-fast bacilli, AFB). The entire volume of the first urine passed in the morning is collected and centrifuged to concentrate the small number of organisms. Culture usually takes 6–8 weeks but unfortunately a negative result does not exclude urinary tuberculosis. Any acid-fast bacilli cultured need to be identified to exclude non-tuberculous varieties. If there is a red patch around a ureteric orifice at cystoscopy, this can be biopsied and examined histologically for caseating granulomas and stained for tuberculosis organisms, thus accelerating the diagnostic process. Blood is tested for anaemia, lymphocytosis and elevation of the erythrocyte sedimentation rate (ESR), and for biochemical indicators of renal function. A chest X-ray is taken to search for pulmonary disease. Renal calcification may be seen on plain abdominal X-ray (such as the control film of an intravenous urogram), while urography may show renal abnormalities or ureteric strictures.

MANAGEMENT OF GENITOURINARY TUBERCULOSIS

Chemotherapy is the mainstay of treatment, as for pulmonary tuberculosis, with the choice of agents made according to the local prevalence of particular strains of the organism and the results of culture and sensitivities. Surgery may be required later to treat ureteric strictures or a contracted bladder, or to excise damaged kidney tissue (partial or total nephrectomy). For ureteric tuberculosis, corticosteroids are usually given along with antituberculous chemotherapy to reduce the risk of stricture formation. Plasma urea and creatinine should be moni-

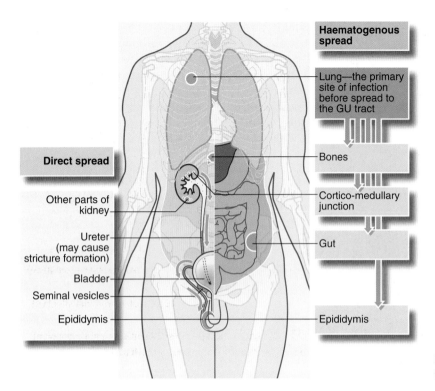

Fig. 38.3 Spread of tuberculosis to the genitourinary tract

tored during the usual 6 months of therapy and signs of upper tract dilatation sought with periodic ultrasound examinations.

SCHISTOSOMIASIS

Schistosomiasis (bilharzia) is the most important parasitic disease of the urinary tract. It causes chronic inflammatory lesions in the bladder which lead to severe fibrotic damage. Schistosomiasis also predisposes to stone formation and squamous carcinoma of the bladder.

Three *Schistosoma* species, *S. haematobium*, *S. mansoni* and *S. japonicum*, have a wide tropical distribution and are important human pathogens. The most destructive bladder disease, however, is caused by *S. haematobium*. This species is endemic to tropical and North Africa (particularly the Nile valley), and is also found in some Middle Eastern and southern European countries. More effective treatment with **praziquantel** has dramatically reduced the reservoir of infection and consequently the incidence of cases in Egypt, but treatment is relatively expensive and has made little impact in Sudan. Increasing world-wide travel makes it likely that the disease will be seen more frequently in travellers from Western countries.

The schistosome has a sophisticated life cycle which depends on poor sanitation. Humans (the main definitive host) are infected by working or bathing in contaminated water. The free-swimming adult forms (**cercaria**) penetrate the skin, usually of the feet, and pass through the venous circulation and lungs to the systemic arterial cir-

culation, which disseminates them throughout the body. In the hepatic portal veins, male and female worms mate. The females, crammed with fertilised ova, then find their way via the mesenteric veins to the venous plexuses of the pelvic viscera, notably the bladder, where the ova are released. Aided by lytic enzymes, the ova then pass through the bladder wall into the urine and thence to the external environment.

On reaching water, the ova release mature ciliated forms (**miracidia**) which enter the intermediate host, a species of freshwater snail. The miracidia mature in the snail's liver before they are released as a new generation of adult cercarial worms. At this point, they are ready to enter human hosts, thus completing the life cycle.

CLINICAL PRESENTATIONS OF SCHISTOSOMIASIS

Initial skin penetration may cause mild local inflammation. Soon afterwards, the phase of haematogenous spread may cause general malaise, low-grade pyrexia and eosinophilia. About 2 months later, ova invading the bladder mucosa cause local inflammation, and manifest as frequency and haematuria at the end of micturition. The early symptoms may be trivial and may pass unnoticed in low-grade infestations.

The main bladder damage caused by schistosomiasis is due to an intense chronic inflammatory reaction to dead ova which have not passed out in the urine and become sequestered in the mucosa. Small granulomatous 'pseudotubercles' develop around each ovum and these

- Skin rash at site of cercarial penetration
- Low-grade systemic illness with eosinophilia
- Urinary frequency and terminal haematuria
- Chronic inflammation of the bladder
- Bladder fibrosis and contracture
- Bladder stones
- Squamous cell carcinoma (two-thirds of carcinomas) or transitional cell carcinoma (one-third) of the bladder

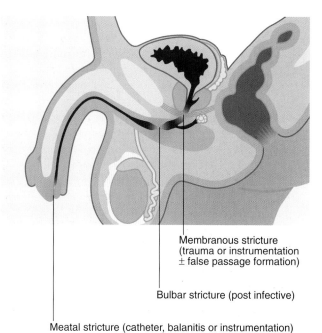

Membranous stricture
(trauma or instrumentation
± false passage formation)

Bulbar stricture (post infective)

Meatal stricture (catheter, balanitis or instrumentation)

Fig. 38.4 Common sites of urethral strictures

later become fibrotic and calcified. Heavy or recurrent infestations result in a variety of destructive lesions including **ulcers**, **papillomata**, **cysts**, **giant granulomata** and **severe bladder contracture**. All predispose to secondary bacterial infection and formation of bladder stones. Squamous metaplasia is common and strongly predisposes to **carcinoma**: two-thirds of these are squamous and one-third transitional cell.

The clinical features of urinary schistosomiasis are summarised in Box 38.3.

MANAGEMENT OF SCHISTOSOMIASIS

Bladder or ureteric calcification is almost diagnostic of schistosomiasis. Diagnosis is confirmed either by microscopic examination of urine for ova (these are best found in the last few millilitres of a mid-morning specimen of urine) or more reliably by cystoscopic biopsy of bladder lesions. Serological tests may also be of value in travellers from the developed world without previous exposure.

Treatment is much simplified nowadays using the drug **praziquantel**. This is given in two doses of 20 mg/kg body weight on 1 day, 6 hours apart. **Metrifonate** is an alternative treatment if praziquantel is unavailable. Surgery is occasionally necessary later to correct or palliate residual deformities of the lower urinary tract.

About 5% of the world's population is affected by various forms of schistosomiasis and prevention must be the cornerstone of disease control. Improved sanitation and clean water supplies are essential. Ironically, the rapid expansion of water conservation and irrigation schemes has tended to spread the disease to previously unaffected populations. Effective treatment of affected individuals can substantially reduce the pool of infection and the number of new cases.

URETHRAL INFECTIONS AND STRICTURES

URETHRAL INFECTIONS

The only clinically significant infections of the urethra are sexually transmitted diseases. The most common are **gonorrhoea** and '**non-specific urethritis**', the latter usually

caused by chlamydial infection. The acute condition usually presents with a urethral discharge and dysuria. The surgical importance of urethritis, particularly gonococcal urethritis, is that it may lead, months or years later, to a fibrous stricture in the posterior urethra. Fortunately, these strictures are becoming less common as effective primary antibiotic therapy is more readily available. However, in recent years multi-antibiotic resistant strains have begun to emerge, particularly in the Far East.

Serological tests for gonorrhoea and *Chlamydia* are relatively unreliable and have largely been abandoned. The standard tests for diagnosis now involve molecular amplification (PCR, LCR) which can be done on urethral swabs and first-catch urine samples.

URETHRAL STRICTURE

Urethral strictures are now most commonly caused by inflammation resulting from **iatrogenic trauma**. Transurethral resection for prostatic surgery is the most common cause. Catheterisation with latex catheters in patients with poor tissue perfusion is another common cause, particularly urinary catheterisation during cardio-pulmonary bypass for cardiac surgery. These iatrogenic strictures involve the distal urethra or the meatus but strictures may also be a complication of traumatic instrumentation, in which case the membranous urethra is most vulnerable (see Fig. 38.4). A small proportion of strictures result from urethral tearing or rupture following displaced pelvic fractures. These usually require open surgical reconstruction.

The characteristic symptom of urethral stricture is a progressive diminution in urinary stream. If there is any associated chronic urinary retention, this may be accompanied by symptoms of bladder outlet obstruction, i.e. frequency and urgency. Diagnosis is made by direct inspection using a cystourethroscope.

Strictures may be short, elongated or multiple. An effective treatment involves **stretching** the scar tissue by repeated self-dilatation. This technique, performed once a week for 2 years, keeps the urethra open long enough for fibroblasts to remodel around it. An alternative with tight strictures is to **cut the stricture** longitudinally with a urethrotome under direct urethroscopic vision, and follow this by repeated dilatation. Recurrence after treatment is not only frequent, but almost to be expected, so skilled urological follow-up is desirable. More complicated strictures may require **open surgical treatment**: for example, excision of a short stricture and end-to-end anastomosis of the urethra. For some, **inlays** of oral mucosa or post-auricular skin may prove successful.

Urethral strictures may cause lifelong disability, and most can be avoided by extreme care of the urethra during catheterisation and urethral instrumentation. 'Routine' catheterisation appears to be an irresistible temptation to all but urologists. As a general rule, the urethra should not be catheterised or interfered with unless absolutely essential. Sick patients should be catheterised only with a silicone-coated urethral catheter or else a suprapubic catheter employed to minimise local trauma. Any catheter or other urological instrument should be placed gently with minimal force or else under direct vision. If urethral catheterisation proves difficult, an alternative means should be found or the procedure abandoned rather than risk urethral damage by forceful instrumentation.

Congenital disorders and diseases secondarily involving the urinary tract

39

CONGENITAL URINARY TRACT DISORDERS

INTRODUCTION

Serious congenital disorders of the kidneys and urinary tract nearly all present at birth or in early childhood; these are described in Chapter 52. The exception is **polycystic kidney** which may present in juveniles but presents more commonly in adulthood. There are also a number of lesser abnormalities of the upper tract which interfere with normal flow dynamics and predispose to infection, e.g. duplex systems or medullary sponge kidney. These are usually discovered during investigation of recurrent infections or incidentally. Finally, asymptomatic abnormalities such as unilateral renal agenesis, renal cysts or horseshoe kidney may be discovered incidentally during investigations (e.g. for hypertension) or during surgery. With advancing age, a large proportion of the population develops benign renal cysts of varying size; these are usually of no clinical consequence.

A systematic summary of congenital disorders that present after childhood is given in Table 39.1.

POLYCYSTIC KIDNEYS

Adult polycystic kidney disease (PCKD) is an autosomal dominant disorder characterised by multiple bilateral cysts of the renal parenchyma (see Fig. 39.1). The cysts slowly expand, compressing the renal parenchyma, and may lead to disruption of local control of blood pressure and eventually to deteriorating renal function. Polycystic kidneys have three main variants:

- A rare infantile form also affecting the liver; affected children often die when young

- A serious adult form which manifests in middle age with hypertension or progressive renal failure. It is the commonest cause of inherited renal failure. Kidneys can appear normal on ultrasound scanning up to about age 20
- A less serious adult form usually found incidentally in later life with almost normal renal function. Patients are usually hypertensive

Thus, adult polycystic kidney may present with **hypertension** or progressive **chronic renal failure**. The enlarged cystic kidneys may cause loin pain or may be discovered incidentally on abdominal examination. These kidneys are particularly vulnerable to even minor trauma and **haematuria** is a common presentation.

Some of those affected with polycystic disease also have multiple cysts in the liver and sometimes in the pancreas. They present with massive abdominal swelling due to gross liver enlargement. There is no specific treatment for polycystic kidney disease and despite good conservative management about 50% of patients will eventually require dialysis or renal transplantation. Surgical 'deroofing' of cysts, as may be appropriate in the management of solitary renal cysts (see below), is not appropriate here and often makes matters worse.

MEDULLARY SPONGE KIDNEY

This is caused by cyst-like dilatation (**ectasia**) of the collecting ducts of the renal medulla and may affect one or both kidneys. The cysts tend to become calcified, giving a characteristic radiographic appearance of streaky linear calcification of the renal papillae (see Fig. 39.2). On excre-

559

Table 39.1 Congenital abnormalities of the urinary system presenting after childhood

Nature of abnormality	Presentation
KIDNEY	
Medullary sponge kidney Cystic dilatation of collecting ducts of one or more medullary pyramids (the sub-units of the medulla) in one or both kidneys	May be found incidentally or during investigations for urinary infection. Cysts tend to become calcified and have characteristic X-ray appearance
Adult polycystic kidney Autosomal dominant disorder with multiple cysts throughout the parenchyma	Usually presents after age 30 with chronic renal failure, hypertension, haematuria or recurrent urinary tract infections
Solitary cysts Usually develop at one pole	Often an incidental finding. May present with loin swelling or pain
Horseshoe kidney Fusion of lower poles of kidneys preventing normal developmental ascent	Often found incidentally but may cause hydronephrosis due to pelviureteric obstruction
Ectopic kidneys and abnormalities of rotation Due to failure of developmental ascent	Found incidentally or during investigation of complications such as pelviureteric obstruction
PELVICALYCEAL SYSTEM AND URETERS	
Ureterocoele Cystic dilatation of intravesical part of ureter due to stenosis of ureteric orifice	Incidental finding or may cause infection or symptoms of obstruction
Duplex systems Partial or complete duplication of a ureter	Often an incidental finding or cause of recurrent infection
BLADDER AND URETHRA	
Urachal abnormalities Cyst, sinus, abscess, secondary malignancy	Cysts and sinuses may present in adulthood as a result of persistence of urachal remnants. Adenocarcinoma sometimes develops in the urachal remnant

tion pyelography (IVU), the tubular ectasia can be demonstrated as a 'flare' in the renal papilla. Marked degrees of medullary sponge kidney predispose to recurrent infection and stone formation because of intrarenal stasis of urine but patients rarely present before adulthood. Minor degrees of change are often seen on IVU without causing symptoms.

DUPLEX SYSTEMS

The urinary collecting system may be duplicated to a greater or lesser extent. Duplication is usually complete proximally but may be incomplete distally. Lesser degrees of duplication are usually asymptomatic and may be discovered by chance on IVU. Complete duplex ureter is relatively common and may result in renal damage from infection, reflux or obstruction (see Fig. 39.3). The ureter draining the **upper pole** (upper moiety) of the kidney is often inserted ectopically into the urethra (or vagina in a girl), resulting in continuous incontinence. Otherwise it joins the bladder ectopically **below** the orifice of the lower pole ureter. The orifice is often tightly stenosed, resulting in obstruction. This causes back pressure on the kidney, and dilatation of the distal ureter known as a **ureterocoele**. The upper moiety may not show up on an IVU because of damage to that part of the kidney.

The ureter draining the **lower moiety** may have a defective distal antireflux mechanism, predisposing to infection and renal parenchymal damage. The typical IVU picture is of calyces that look like a 'drooping daffodil'.

SOLITARY RENAL CYSTS

Isolated cysts of the renal parenchyma (see Fig. 39.4) are a common developmental abnormality and though rarely

achieve with ultrasonography. Malignancy in association with a solitary cyst is very rare; if it does occur, it may show up as calcification in the cyst wall. Occasionally simple cysts cause pain or swelling. For these, aspiration alone is of no value as the cysts rapidly refill. If intervention is required, cysts should be deroofed laparoscopically (in contrast to treatment of polycystic disease). **Hydatid disease** of the kidney should always be excluded before undertaking any surgical procedure on a 'renal cyst' to treat loin pain or ureteric obstruction, as inadvertent puncturing of cysts can lead to intraperitoneal spread.

HORSESHOE KIDNEY

This abnormality is caused by embryological fusion of the two developing kidneys at their lower poles. Normal renal ascent in fetal life is prevented by the inferior mesenteric artery arising from the abdominal aorta, so that the isthmus of the kidney comes to lie across the aorta at the level of the third or fourth lumbar vertebra. The condition is usually a chance finding on IVU investigation (where the diagnostic feature is medially directed calyces—see Fig. 39.5) or else at abdominal aortic surgery, when it may cause serious operative difficulties. Horseshoe kidney is sometimes associated with pelviureteric junction obstruction, the symptoms of which may lead to the diagnosis. Occasionally, a horseshoe kidney first causes problems during pregnancy.

RENAL ECTOPIA AND OTHER RENAL ABNORMALITIES

A variety of other renal abnormalities may be found unexpectedly on investigation or at surgery. These include ectopic kidneys (see Fig. 39.6), rotational abnormalities, unilateral agenesis, aplasia or hyperplasia. These abnormalities may confuse the diagnosis and sometimes result in surgical mishap, e.g. excision of a pelvic kidney mistaken for an ovarian tumour. Note that transplanted kidneys are usually deliberately sited in the iliac fossa!

URACHAL ABNORMALITIES (see Fig. 39.7)

During fetal development, the urogenital sinus communicates with the allantois via the urachus. Occasionally, this tract persists as a **fistula** between bladder and umbilicus. Sometimes the fistula does not open until adulthood. Similarly, a remnant may form a blind urachal **sinus** that opens at the umbilicus or result in a urachal **cyst** in the midline of the lower abdomen. These structural abnormalities may then become infected. Very rarely, an **adenocarcinoma** develops in a urachal remnant in the bladder vault or in other urachal remnants.

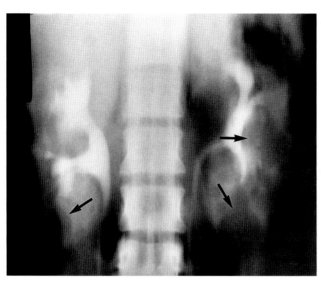

Fig. 39.1 Polycystic kidneys
IVU tomogram from a 52-year-old woman with hypertension and microscopic haematuria; both kidneys exhibit multiple lucent areas in the nephrogram representing cysts (arrowed) and the pelvicalyceal systems are slightly compressed.

Fig. 39.2 Medullary sponge kidney

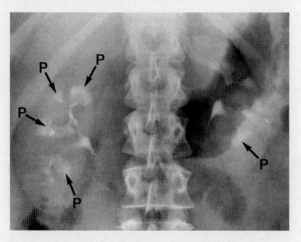

Bilateral medullary sponge kidney on an IVU from a 55-year-old woman with recurrent urinary tract infections; the renal papillae **P** have a typical 'flared' appearance and retain contrast because of the dilated collecting ducts. No radiopacity was visible on the control film although it can be seen in a considerable proportion of cases because of calcification in the ectatic ducts of the papillae.

symptomatic, can be found in a large proportion of the population in later life. They are usually recognised incidentally during renal ultrasound or IVU investigation. Their importance lies in distinguishing them from solid tumours and hydatid cysts, which is usually easy to

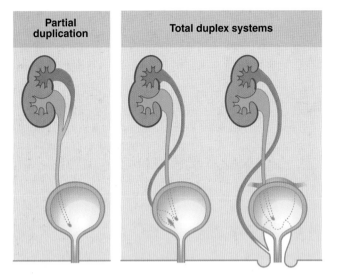

(a) Partial and total duplication. In a total duplex system (right), the ureter from the upper renal moiety may open into the urethra or vagina (i.e. wholly ectopic). Such an ectopic ureter causes continuous incontinence and presents early in life. Otherwise, it opens inferiorly in the bladder (centre). The orifice is often stenosed and a **ureterocoele** results (dilated lower end of ureter). Vesicoureteric reflux often occurs via the **upper** ureteric orifice back into the **lower** renal moiety.

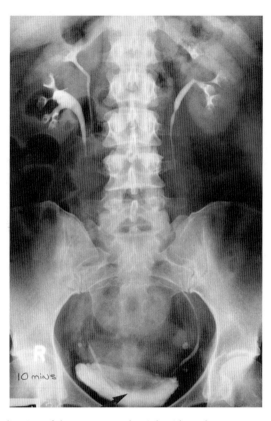

(b) Duplication of the ureters on the right side; only one ureter can be seen passing as far as the bladder. The vesicoureteric junction is associated with a small, elongated ureterocoele (arrowed).

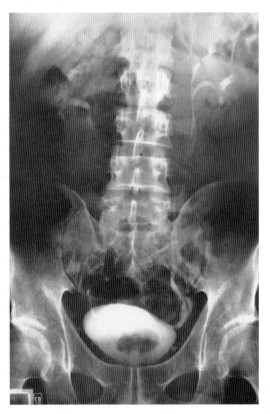

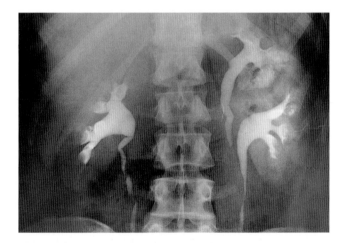

(d) Partial duplication on the left side, the upper moiety of which exhibits the medullary sponge abnormality; this 25-year-old man presented with multiple ureteric stones, and the other abnormalities were incidental findings.

(c) Complete left duplex system with both ureters visible all the way down to the bladder.

Fig. 39.3 Duplex systems

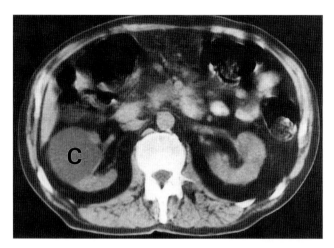

(a) CT scan showing right renal cyst **C**. This was a chance finding in a woman of 45 under investigation for pancreatic pain. No treatment was necessary.

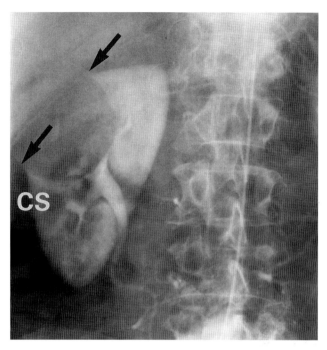

(b) Another solitary renal cyst found by chance, this time on an aortogram. In this film, contrast has been injected into the aorta ('flush aortogram') rather than selectively; the typical animal-like 'claw sign' **CS** of a simple cyst (arrowed) is demonstrated.

Fig. 39.4 Solitary renal cyst

DISEASES SECONDARILY INVOLVING THE URINARY TRACT

INTRODUCTION

A variety of abdominal disorders such as tumours, inflammatory bowel disease, aneurysms and retroperitoneal fibrosis may secondarily involve the urinary tract, as may iatrogenic (surgical) damage. These conditions affect the urinary tract by obstructing one or both ureters or occasionally by causing a fistula between bowel and urinary tract. Obstruction of one ureter alone may not be symptomatic although it may cause loin pain or predispose to infection; bilateral involvement usually presents with acute or chronic renal failure.

Of tumours outside the urinary tract, advanced **carcinoma of the uterine cervix** most commonly produces bilateral ureteric obstruction because of the close anatomical relationship of the ureters to the cervix. This cancer may also ulcerate anteriorly into the bladder causing a **vesico-vaginal fistula**. This anatomical closeness makes the ureters vulnerable to trauma even at straightforward hysterectomy. Abdominal and particularly laparoscopic-assisted hysterectomy can be associated with damage to the ureter, causing stenosis and hydronephrosis or a uretero-vaginal fistula. An iatrogenic vesicovaginal fistula can also occur as a result of surgery. Carcinoma of the ascending or rectosigmoid colon may obstruct the right or left ureter respectively although this

is surprisingly rare. Most ureteric damage in relation to large bowel cancer results from colectomy operations.

Inflammatory disease which involves the bowel serosa may extend to involve nearby structures such as the ureters and bladder and this may lead to fistula formation. This is important in **Crohn's disease and diverticular disease**. A fistula between bowel and urinary tract presents as severe urinary infection, often with pneumaturia or faecuria.

An expanding abdominal mass may compress one or both ureters and cause symptoms from partial obstruction; sometimes **aorto-iliac aneurysms** are responsible. An 'inflammatory' aneurysm near a ureter is likely to cause obstruction. This variant occurs in about 5% of aortic aneurysms. The cause is unknown but the effect is to produce retroperitoneal fibrosis across the anterior surface of the aneurysm. A much more common cause of ureteric dilatation is **pregnancy**, in which bilateral megaureter results from the effects of progestogens. The main clinical significance of bilateral megaureter of pregnancy is that it predisposes to upper tract infection. Thus, significant bacteriuria in pregnancy, symptomatic or not, should be treated with antibiotics. Retention of urine can be caused by a pelvic mass such as a pregnancy of around 14 weeks or an ovarian lesion of similar size.

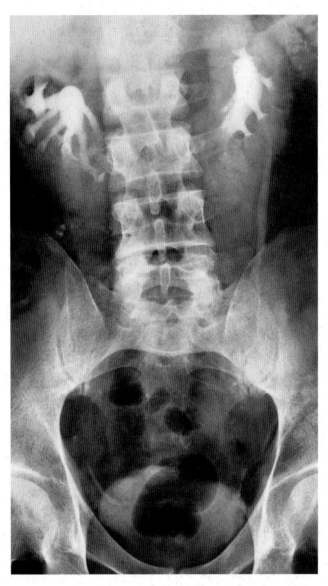

(a)

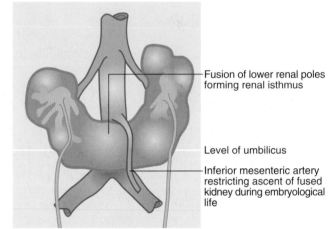

Fusion of lower renal poles forming renal isthmus

Level of umbilicus

Inferior mesenteric artery restricting ascent of fused kidney during embryological life

(b)

Fig. 39.5 Horseshoe kidney

Horseshoe kidney shown on IVU from a 51-year-old woman with recurrent urinary tract stones; the pelvicalyceal systems are oriented obliquely and converge inferiorly because the isthmus is stretched over the vertebral column. Each pelvis and ureter is more medially placed than normal and the whole renal mass lies much lower than would normal kidneys. The isthmus of a horseshoe kidney can rarely be demonstrated by IVU or ultrasound but can easily be imagined in this image.

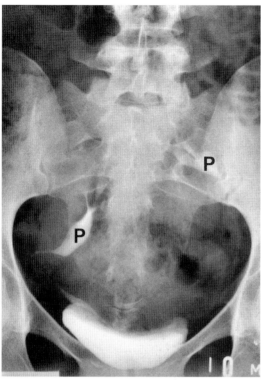

(a) A 48-year-old woman with recurrent urinary tract infections; IVU shows abnormal pelvicalyceal systems **P** of bilateral pelvic kidneys.

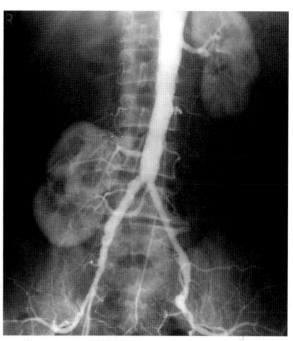

(b) Right pelvic kidney discovered incidentally during arteriography for severe claudication. Its blood supply can be seen to arise from the distal aorta and iliac artery. The patient needed an aorto-femoral bypass but when faced with the technical difficulties, agreed to conservative management of her claudication.

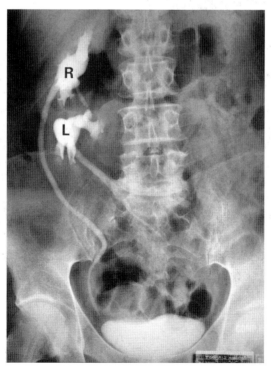

(c) Another middle-aged woman with recurrent urinary tract infections; the left kidney **L** is ectopically located on the opposite side and is fused to the right kidney **R** ('crossed renal ectopia').

Fig. 39.6 Ectopic kidneys

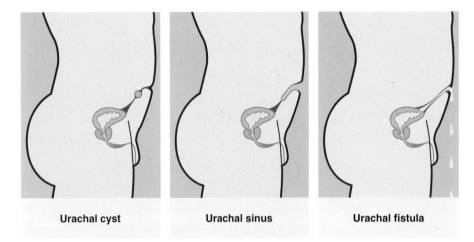

Urachal cyst   Urachal sinus   Urachal fistula

Fig. 39.7 Urachal abnormalities

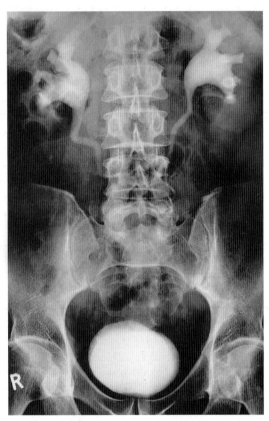

Fig. 39.8 Retroperitoneal fibrosis
This man of 62 presented with back pain. The IVU shows bilateral hydronephrosis due to ureteric compression; note how the ureters are tapered and characteristically drawn medially by the fibrotic process.

RETROPERITONEAL FIBROSIS (RPF)

This relatively rare and obscure condition is characterised by progressive, intense fibrosis of the connective tissue lying posterior to the peritoneal cavity. About 50% of cases turn out to be caused by retroperitoneal spread of malignant disease. In the rest, the cause is unknown in many (i.e. idiopathic), but some rarely used drugs such as **methysergide** can induce the condition or it may be associated with an inflammatory aortic aneurysm. Retroperitoneal fibrosis sometimes causes hypertension via its effect on the kidneys.

Retroperitoneal fibrosis compresses both ureters, causing bilateral hydronephrosis and eventually renal failure. Sometimes it is associated with inferior vena caval obstruction. Diagnosis is usually made on IVU, which shows bilateral hydronephrosis (see Fig. 39.8). The fibrotic process also draws the ureters closer together in the midline. The ESR is characteristically elevated.

Treatment usually involves a preliminary trial of high-dose steroids and insertion of **double-J stents** to maintain upper tract function whilst awaiting improvement. Surprisingly, ureters compressed by retroperitoneal fibrosis can usually be catheterised with ease. If medical treatment fails, the next step is usually dissection from the retroperitoneal tissue of the ureters (**ureterolysis**), which are then resited within the peritoneal cavity in an attempt to prevent recurrent obstruction. A biopsy of the retroperitoneal tissue should be taken to exclude malignancy and to confirm the diagnosis. If obstruction recurs, corticosteroid therapy may suppress the condition. Aortic grafting is indicated if a substantial aneurysm is present.

Pathophysiology, clinical features and diagnosis of vascular disease affecting the limbs

40

INTRODUCTION

The term 'peripheral vascular disease' (**PVD**) is often employed to mean obstructive ('obliterative') disease of major lower limb arteries causing ischaemia. However, a range of vascular disorders can cause symptoms in upper and lower limbs, and a broader definition should include any disease of arteries, veins or lymphatics outside the heart. Vascular-related problems are so much more common in the lower limb that this chapter concentrates on the lower limb; upper limb symptoms are outlined in Table 40.5.

Patients with symptomatic vascular limb disorders may present to any medical specialty and some require urgent action, e.g. those with acute ischaemia of a limb or a painful abdominal aneurysm. Thus all clinicians need to understand the principles of diagnosis and the scope and timing of treatment. This chapter covers the **pathophysiology** of vascular insufficiency of limbs, the details of **taking a history and examining patients** with suspected vascular disease, particularly of the limbs, and the process of reaching a broad, 'first stage' diagnosis.

VASCULAR INSUFFICIENCY OF THE LIMB (Table 40.1)

Arterial insufficiency and venous insufficiency are useful terms to describe symptomatic dysfunction of a limb's vasculature. The terms do not indicate one specific pathophysiology and either type may be acute or chronic. As examples, **acute arterial insufficiency** means an inadequate supply of arterial blood to the limb over a period of hours or days, whereas **chronic venous insufficiency** means inadequate venous drainage from the limb for several weeks or more. Vascular disorders of the limbs are caused mainly by atherosclerosis, arterial thromboembolism, aneurysms, complications of diabetes mellitus, and thrombotic and varicose disorders of the venous system. In some cases, limbs can be affected by remote disease. For example, thrombus originating in the heart or other proximal site can detach and be swept distally until it lodges and obstructs the vessel, a process known as **embolism**. In many patients, especially the elderly, several causes may interact. Conversely, the same disease process can manifest differently in different patients (see Table 40.2 for the various manifestations of popliteal aneurysm).

SYMPTOMS AND SIGNS IN THE LIMB

An accurate initial diagnosis of vascular-related symptoms depends almost entirely on skilled and methodical clinical evaluation rather than on special investigations. Preliminary assessment of the suspected vascular patient takes into account obvious major risk factors (Table 40.3). Detailed history taking is covered in Table 40.4 and examination in Figure 40.1. During the clinical assessment, the student or doctor tries to decide if the problem is arterial, venous or lymphatic, or has some other cause. The symptoms and signs are best interpreted in the light of the likely underlying patho-

physiology and investigations are chosen according to the nature of the problem and the perceived urgency of treatment.

The principal symptoms and signs of lower limb vascular disease are pain, changes in skin texture, colour and temperature, tissue loss including ulceration, and swelling. The diagnostic importance of each of these is outlined in the following sections. The upper limb is affected by a largely different range of disorders that produce a diverse set of signs and symptoms with only a small degree of overlap (see Table 40.5).

Table 40.1 Pathophysiology of arterial and venous insufficiency: the clinical consequences of vascular diseases affecting the lower limb*

Basic disease	Pathophysiological process	Clinical manifestations
Atherosclerosis and embolism causing ischaemia		
Atherosclerotic narrowing of large distributing arteries	Arterial supply inadequate to supply muscles during exercise Arterial supply inadequate even at rest, with relative ischaemia of all tissues. Risk of pressure ulceration. Healing severely impaired Limb is critically ischaemic; risk of limb necrosis in 6–8 hours unless urgently revascularised Thrombotic occlusion of atherosclerotic artery; clinical features as acute critical ischaemia	**Intermittent claudication**—muscle pain on walking, quickly relieved by rest **Chronic severe ischaemia**—rest pain in foot, worse at night. Onset sudden, or chronic over a few days or weeks. Skin pale/red/purple **Acute critical ischaemia**—more extreme manifestation of severe ischaemia, often with patchy gangrene or ischaemic ulcers **Acute-on-chronic ischaemia**—sudden onset of acute ischaemia in patient with chronic ischaemia
Embolism arising from atherosclerotic lesions in carotid arteries	Atherosclerotic debris or platelet thrombi migrate distally and occlude cerebral arteries	**Transient ischaemic attacks** (TIAs) and strokes from carotid disease
Embolism from heart	Masses of thrombus detach and impact at arterial bifurcations, occluding flow	**Acute severe ischaemia** of upper or lower limb, brain or intestine. Often pre-existing atrial fibrillation or recent myocardial infarction
Diabetes mellitus		
The 'diabetic foot' (neuro-ischaemic foot)	Accelerated atherosclerosis and neuropathy in an unpredictable mixture. Loss of sensation predisposes to injury and ulceration Lesions often complicated by pyogenic infection	Foot lesions (often painless)—deep ulceration in pressure areas, necrotic toes. Assume atherosclerotic ischaemia unless foot pulses palpable. Infection spreads rapidly, causing limb-threatening necrosis and systemic sepsis. Needs early and vigorous treatment Resistance to infection impaired in diabetics
Venous disorders		
Thromboembolism Acute deep venous thrombosis (DVT) May be complicated by **pulmonary embolism**	Spontaneous thrombosis in deep veins of calf or thigh; may propagate to ilio-femoral veins. Obstructs venous return causing swelling and warmth. Venous gangrene in extreme cases	**Pain and swelling of calf and ankle**, often with calf tenderness. Thigh swollen if ilio-femoral veins thrombosed. Associated with risk factors, particularly immobility. Leg usually blueish or normal colour
Chronic venous insufficiency Post-thrombotic limb and venous eczema	Late complication of DVT. Spontaneous recanalisation of occluded veins damages valves causing incompetence (reflux) and local venous hypertension. Similar features in gross superficial venous insufficiency in varicose veins	**Chronic brawny oedema** of leg often with narrow ankle due to lipo-dermatosclerosis ('champagne bottle leg'). Skin atrophic, scaly and pigmented and gaiter area above ankle vulnerable to chronic ulceration after minor trauma

* Aneurysms are covered in Chapter 42 and varicose veins and thrombophlebitis in Chapter 43.

Table 40.2 Symptoms and signs of popliteal aneurysm: different clinical consequences of a similar underlying disorder

Clinical presentation	Pathophysiology
Asymptomatic—pulsatile swelling in popliteal fossa discovered by patient, by chance or during examination of patient with vascular problem	Often part of multi-aneurysmal disease. Examine for other aneurysms—other popliteal fossa, abdomen, femoral arteries
Acute ischaemia	Thrombosis of aneurysm or distal embolisation of clot from within aneurysm
Chronic ischaemia	Gradual occlusion of aneurysm or arterial runoff by thrombus or atherosclerosis
Apparent deep venous thrombosis (DVT)—swelling, cyanosis of leg	Large aneurysmal swelling occludes popliteal veins. May lead to DVT
Rupture of aneurysm	Sudden pain and swelling behind knee; swelling and pain in leg; evidence of distal ischaemia

Table 40.3 Preliminary assessment of the vascular patient for obvious risk factors

Factors to assess first	Significance
Major risk factors for arterial disease—'GASD'	
Gender	Men affected by atherosclerosis and aneurysms 10 years earlier than women
Age	Peripheral atherosclerosis rare below 55 years—most common age 60–70. DVT unlikely below 20
Smoking cigarettes	Risk of atherosclerosis proportional to 'pack-years' smoked; PVD unlikely in people who have never smoked
Diabetes (especially type 2)	Premature and accelerated atherosclerosis, predominantly more distally in limb. 25% of PVD patients are diabetic compared with 2–3% of general population Peripheral neuropathies (sensory, motor and autonomic) Reduced resistance to infection
Other risk factors	
Hypertension	Predisposes to atherosclerosis, stroke and aneurysm expansion
Hypercholesterolaemia and hypertriglyceridaemia	Risk factors for atherosclerosis. Some inherited types have major adverse effects
Obesity and sedentary lifestyle	Difficult to quantify but likely to be significant factors

PAIN

Most limb pain is due to trauma or musculoskeletal disorders such as arthritis rather than vascular disease. In a patient with lower limb pain, where peripheral ischaemia is the working diagnosis a full cardiovascular workup is necessary (see Table 40.4 and Fig. 40.1).

- **Lower limb**—where symptoms are caused by vascular disease, patients may have itching and aching associated with varicose veins, have exercise-related pain, or experience more severe and constant pain caused by chronic obliterative arterial disease. Where the history is short, acute ischaemia may be the cause
- **Upper limb**—pain from vascular causes is uncommon. Aching and swelling may be caused by subclavian vein thrombosis. Claudication due to chronic arterial obstruction is rare and acute ischaemia is usually due to arterial embolism. Thoracic outlet syndrome is also rare. The brachial plexus may be compressed as it passes between the clavicle and first rib (or extra cervical rib) causing nerve root symptoms. Even less commonly, the condition may cause arterial or venous obstruction at the thoracic outlet

INTERMITTENT CLAUDICATION

Chronic lower limb arterial insufficiency presents most commonly as muscular pain on walking. The history is very characteristic: pain begins at a reproducible distance, is worse walking uphill and increases if walking continues, forcing the patient to stop. Symptoms usually pre-

Table 40.4 History taking in suspected limb arterial or venous disease

History of presenting complaint—limb symptoms	Important features of the history
Symptoms and signs Pain Changes in skin texture Changes in skin colour (including gangrene) Changes in skin temperature Ulceration and tissue loss Swelling Loss of sensation	**Detailed history of each symptom:** **Where?** Upper/lower limb; one or both; which part of the limb; precipitating/relieving factors; extent of changes **When?** When did it start; sudden or gradual onset; progress—getting worse or better; worse during day or night **Initiating factors?** Preceding activity or event, e.g. trauma/excess exercise **Exacerbating factors?** e.g. exercise/posture **Relieving factors?** e.g. Hanging leg out of bed/elevation/analgesics **Nature of symptoms?** Severity; periodicity, i.e. continuous or intermittent **Pain?** Site/severity/timing/precipitants/onset/radiation **Impact of symptoms?** What is the patient prevented from doing (working/walking/sleeping/sitting comfortably) **Disability?** e.g. impaired grip; heavy arm **Recent trauma to limb?** e.g. fracture and treatment, dislocation, soft tissue trauma
Past medical history	**Important features of the history**
General cardiovascular history **Peripheral vascular disease** Arterial Venous Related history	Venous or arterial thromboses; bleeding tendency Intermittent claudication; previous limb surgery—bypass operations; angioplasty; arterial thrombosis Varicose veins/previous surgery; thrombophlebitis; DVT or pulmonary embolism; arm swelling; trauma + immobilisation, e.g. lower limb fracture/treatment/ligament injury (predisposing to silent DVT) In claudication—back problems and surgery (possible cauda equina claudication) Cervical rib; hypothyroidism Pre-existing lymphatic disorder of limb (e.g. primary lymphoedema)
Cardiac disease Manifestations Interventions	Ischaemic heart disease; (angina, MI) Heart failure (chronic lower bilateral limb oedema) Hypertension; valvular disease; arrhythmias Medication/thrombolysis Coronary angiography/angioplasty /pacemaker Cardiac surgery, e.g. CABG; valve surgery
Cerebrovascular disease Manifestation Interventions **Renal failure** **Rheumatological disease**	Ischaemic/haemorrhagic stroke; transient ischaemic attacks (TIAs) Medication; carotid artery surgery/angioplasty Acute or chronic renal failure ± dialysis Collagen/vascular disease: Raynaud's; rheumatoid disease Scleroderma; other connective tissue disorders; vasculitis
Miscellaneous contributing factors Lower limb paresis or deformity Haematological disorders	Predisposes to pressure ulcers: stroke or congenital spinal problems, e.g. spina bifida Thrombophilias, e.g. thrombocythaemia, factor V Leiden mutation, antithrombin III, protein C or S deficiency; polycythaemia vera
Drug history Is patient taking:	Antihypertensives (ACE inhibitors, beta-blockers, calcium channel blockers, diuretics); anti-platelet drugs (aspirin, clopidogrel, etc.) Anticoagulants (e.g. warfarin); a statin
Social history Smoking Exercise Employment	Smoker/ex-smoker/passive smoker; how many pack-years Physically fit; regular exercise Do symptoms impact on work; how does occupation impact on symptoms
Family history Hereditary cardiovascular disease?	Cardiac, PVD, aneurysm, arterial or venous thrombosis

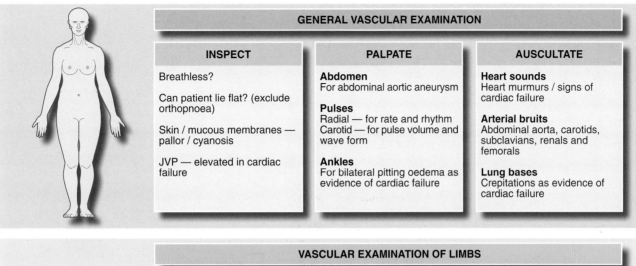

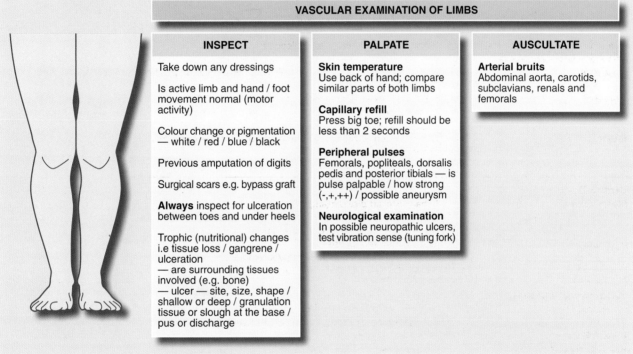

Fig. 40.1 Examination of the vascular patient

dominate in one limb and the patient commonly begins to **limp**, accounting for the name 'intermittent claudication' (Latin: *claudicare* to limp). The pain subsides within a minute or two of stopping and recurs at the same walking distance. The pain is almost always in the calf, wherever the level of arterial obstruction, but may extend into the thigh or even buttock in aorto-iliac obstruction. If associated with male impotence, this is known as **Leriche syndrome**.

After a thorough history has been taken, there is only one condition that might reasonably be mistaken for 'true' claudication; this is **cauda equina claudication** or **pseudo claudication**, caused by compression of the cauda equina in the spinal canal by central disc protrusion or spinal canal stenosis. In this condition, lower limb pain

is also brought on by exercise but there are important differences, see Table 40.6.

ISCHAEMIC REST PAIN

With more severe arterial obstruction, ischaemic pain occurs when the patient is in bed or even when sitting. Termed **rest pain** for obvious reasons, this is usually felt in the skin of the foot and is very severe and burning in character. It occurs mostly at night because of several factors working together: loss of gravity assistance to arterial supply, reduction in cardiac output at rest, and reactive dilatation of skin vessels to warmth. The pain is characteristically relieved to a degree by hanging the leg over the side of the bed or even walking around and is

Table 40.5 Summary of signs and symptoms of vascular disease of the upper limb

Sign or symptom	Underlying disorder	Other clinical features
Swelling of arm and/or forearm		
	Axillary vein thrombosis Predisposing causes: Unaccustomed use of arm overhead, e.g. decorating Excess weight lifting Cervical rib or congenital bands obstructing vein Too narrow a space between first rib and clavicle	Blueness and heaviness of arm; later, prominent collateral veins over delto-pectoral area. Symptoms usually abate spontaneously but early thrombolysis worth considering
Colour change		
Acute whiteness or blueness	Embolism (causes as lower limb) Trauma to brachial artery, e.g. supracondylar fracture	Acute ischaemia—hand cold, painful, loss of sensation and motor function
White finger(s)	Raynaud's disease (common): fingers go white then turn blue then red, often in response to cold. Due to vasospasm—pathogenesis unknown Secondary Raynaud's phenomenon (rare); underlying disorders include: Limited cutaneous scleroderma (CREST) Mixed connective tissue disease Sjögren's syndrome Systemic lupus erythematosus Vibration white finger due to power tool use	Recurrent symptoms especially in cold weather. May lead to atrophy of finger tips but rarely major tissue loss As Raynaud's disease
Red painful fingers	Reflex sympathetic dystrophy post trauma following fracture, especially forearm	Pain, redness, disability in arm
Pain		
Vascular	Substantial subclavian arterial narrowing. Rarely symptomatic because of excellent upper limb collaterals. Acute ischaemia—most commonly embolism of cardiac thrombus; sometimes acute-on-chronic thrombosis (see acute ischaemia above)	Muscle pain on exercise— arm 'claudication'. Low systolic pressure Acute pain of vascular origin plus other features of ischaemia—pulselessness, pallor, paralysis, loss of sensation
Neuro-vascular	Thoracic outlet syndrome— 95% neurological symptoms, 5% arterial—lower trunk symptoms affecting C8/T1 most common. Rare and difficult to diagnose	Chronic pain—usually musculo-skeletal but may be due to thoracic outlet syndrome

not completely relieved by analgesics, even large doses of morphine. Patients often present after tolerating this severe pain for several weeks but eventually it becomes intolerable. There are often ischaemic skin changes or tissue loss such as gangrene and ulceration (see below). The term **critical ischaemia** implies that loss of part of the limb is inevitable unless it is revascularised. Beware of the trap in **diabetic patients** with neuropathy—**severe ischaemia may be painless**. Associated disruption of small vessel autonomic control may mean a severely ischaemic foot is warm and red rather than cold and white or blue. In the absence of palpable pulses, only arteriography will reveal the truth.

In **acute critical ischaemia** of sudden onset, the pain is similar to rest pain. However, if blood flow to the periphery is very low, pain may be absent in the distal most severely affected area, which becomes numb or has diminished sensation (paraesthesia) due to nerve ischaemia. However, severe pain is present proximally where the tissue is less ischaemic. By this time, the patient has muscle pain on moving the foot or paralysis due to muscle ischaemia. It is vital to recognise acute arterial insufficiency as it rapidly progresses to irreversible necrosis without timely treatment.

DEEP VENOUS THROMBOSIS

In deep venous thrombosis, swelling and heaviness are the usual presenting symptoms. Any pain is always less severe than in severe ischaemia. At its greatest, it amounts to acute onset calf aching, made somewhat worse by walking. Physical examination alone usually distinguishes between the two conditions. In deep vein thrombosis, the limb is warm not cold, pulses are detectable (by

Table 40.6 **Comparison between cauda equina claudication and arterial claudication**

Arterial insufficiency	Cauda equina syndrome
History	
'Fixed' claudication distance	'Variable' claudication distance
Pain exacerbated by walking uphill	Pain often absent when walking uphill; often better when cycling
No history of low back problems	History of low back problems
Pain disappears after 1–2 minutes rest	Pain takes 15–30 minutes to subside
Examination	
Absent peripheral pulses and low ankle pressure in affected limb	Pulses usually present and ankle pressure normal
No evidence of a lower motor neurone (LMN) lesion	Evidence of an LMN lesion such as diminished or absent lower limb tendon reflexes
Duplex ultrasound scan or arteriography shows arterial obstruction	CT or MRI scanning of the spinal canal is diagnostic, demonstrating a narrow spinal canal or disc protrusions impacting on the cauda equina

palpation or Doppler flow detector) and there is no colour change (except in very severe cases). Swelling is often a feature of deep venous thrombosis but is not found in acute arterial ischaemia.

SKIN CHANGES

Changes in **skin texture**, **colour**, **pigmentation** or **temperature** (and their distribution) help to distinguish between limb vascular disorders. In chronic conditions, the epidermis and dermis may become thin and atrophic because of deficient oxygenation and nutrition; these are termed **trophic changes**.

In arterial insufficiency, whatever the level of obstruction, the trophic effects are most evident at the extreme periphery, i.e. the foot and toes or the hand. In contrast, the changes caused by chronic venous insufficiency are most severe around the medial side of the ankle above the malleolus (the 'gaiter area'), almost never on the foot. Furthermore, in venous disease, the cutaneous fat around the ankle may become thinned by atrophy and indurated (hardened) by fibrosis. These changes as a whole are termed **venous eczema** or **lipo-dermatosclerosis** or, less accurately, **fat necrosis**. The leg above the ankle is usually oedematous and in extreme cases, when combined with constriction at the ankle, gives rise to a **champagne bottle leg** (see Fig. 43.1c).

CHANGES IN SKIN COLOUR AND TEMPERATURE

Colour change alone may suggest the underlying disease process, particularly if temperature change is also considered (see Table 40.7). Many people, particularly the elderly, suffer from cold feet in cold weather; if both feet are pale or blueish when cold but are painless with normal pulses, this falls within the normal range of arteriolar constriction for temperature conservation. If pathological, the cause may be due to a **vasospastic disorder** such as Raynaud's disease although this more commonly affects the hands.

The acutely cold white foot

The main pathological reason for a foot becoming acutely cold and white is a sudden complete arterial occlusion by thrombosis or embolism. This event is usually spontaneous but precipitating events such as trauma or frostbite will be evident from the history. Ischaemia is usually unilateral unless the abdominal aorta or both iliac arteries become obstructed. There are ischaemic tissue changes in the foot reaching a variable distance up the leg.

The cardinal clinical features of acute critical ischaemia are:

- **Pain**—severe but variable in intensity; affects distal part of limb
- **Pallor** of the extremity. The ischaemic area is initially white or it may be blueish but blanches on pressure with slow capillary refill. Later, if necrosis occurs, it becomes blue and non-blanching (**fixed pigmentation**)
- **Pulselessness** of the extremity. Foot pulses are absent and popliteal and femoral pulses may be lost, according to the level of arterial occlusion
- **Perishing coldness**—most extreme at foot (or hand)
- **Paraesthesia** (reduced sensation) or **anaesthesia** of the periphery. This only occurs if ischaemia is severe

Table 40.7 Interpretation of colour and temperature change in limbs

Colour of limb	Signs	Interpretation
White (see also Buerger's test, Fig. 40.4)	If cold with pulses	Physiological or vasospastic disorder
		Chronic ischaemia
	If cold without pulses	Acute ischaemia
	Asymptomatic	Constricted venules
Blue or cyanotic	Painful, absent pulses	Acute or chronic ischaemia
	Swollen	DVT
Red	Intact skin, warm	Cellulitis or the diabetic ischaemic trap (see above)
	Superficial gaiter area ulceration, little pain	Chronic venous insufficiency
	Ulceration in foot or ankle plus severe pain; cold with absent pulses	Severe ischaemia
Brown	In gaiter area ± ulcer	Chronic venous insufficiency
Black	Toes or distal foot	Necrosis or gangrene
Temperature	**Other signs**	**Interpretation**
Cold	White (compare other limb)	See 'white' above
Warm or hot	Swollen	DVT
	Indurated, oedematous skin	Cellulitis
	Ulcerated distally in diabetic + absent foot pulses	The diabetic ischaemic trap—do an arteriogram
	Always hot—patient puts feet in fridge to cool them	Erythromelalgia; unknown aetiology

Fig. 40.2 Frost-bite

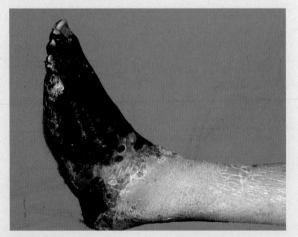

Ischaemic necrosis of the forefoot in an elderly tramp who slept overnight outside in a very low temperature in winter. Note that less tissue is usually lost than initially appears likely. Nevertheless, below knee amputation was later performed in this case.

- **Paralysis** of calf muscles. The patient is unable to flex or extend the toes or ankle. This only occurs if ischaemia is extreme. Pain may disappear at this stage

(As an aide memoire, the features of acute limb ischaemia are known as the six P's: Pain, Pallor, Pulselessness, Perishing coldness, Paraesthesia, Paralysis. Not all of these are present all of the time; anaesthesia and paralysis are dire prognostic features.)

Colour change in venous thrombosis

Noticeable colour change is unusual in deep venous thrombosis but massive pelvic vein thrombosis may cause changes sometimes mistaken for arterial occlusion. Such extensive thromboses are now unusual and occur mainly in high-risk patients. Massive thrombosis was once more common, especially during late pregnancy or the early puerperium. The condition was known as **white leg of pregnancy** or **phlegmasia alba dolens**. The whole of the lower limb is painful, pale and massively swollen. In contrast to the findings in arterial occlusion, the limb is warm and pulses are detectable despite the oedema. A rare but more serious variant is **blue leg** or **phlegmasia caerulea dolens**, which represents incipient venous infarction.

The chronically cold foot (Fig. 40.2)

Blue toes

In chronic arterial insufficiency with severe claudication or rest pain, the onset of a dusky skin colour in the toes or foot suggests developing tissue necrosis (**pre-gangrene**). If finger pressure is applied to the ischaemic skin, the rate of colour return gives some indication of skin perfusion. However, many elderly people with blueish

Fig. 40.3 Necrosis from severe ischaemia

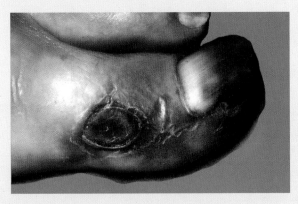

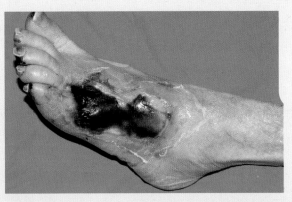

(a)

(b)

(a) Sudden thrombosis of an atherosclerotic superficial femoral artery ('acute-on-chronic' occlusion) led to acute ischaemia, manifesting as rest pain and necrosis of big toe.

(b) Embolism of thrombus from left atrium into femoral artery led to severe ischaemia and necrosis of skin within 6 hours. Embolectomy was performed as early as possible. The photograph shows the resulting acute ischaemic ulcer of dorsum of foot.

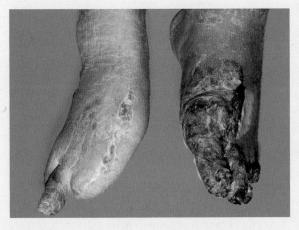

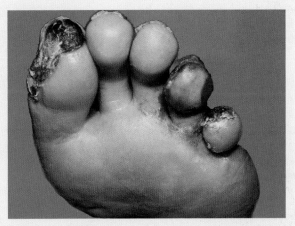

(c)

(d)

(c) Left foot shows signs of severe chronic ischaemia with dry gangrene. Right foot has healed following successful femoro-popliteal bypass grafting and local amputation.

(d) Typical patchy distal necrosis following spontaneous embolism of thrombus from within an abdominal aortic aneurysm.

cool feet with few symptoms have a slow refill time; these patients rarely have arterial disease and this can easily be excluded by Doppler ankle pressure measurement.

Black toes

Necrosis in chronic ischaemia may be patchy and localised if there is a developed collateral circulation (Fig. 40.3). Such necrosis is usually confined to toes or a limited part of the forefoot. The necrotic area slowly becomes hard, black and mummified (**dry gangrene**) and may eventually separate spontaneously from the viable tissue. However, there is always a risk that the necrotic area can become infected. The tissue then becomes boggy and ulcerated and the infection and gangrene spread proximally, particularly in diabetics. This **wet gangrene** requires urgent treatment, often with a combination of revascularisation and amputation.

Redness

Redness of the skin indicates that oxygenated blood is present in the capillaries. This implies there is no venous congestion or obstruction. With ischaemia, there is reactive dilatation of the microvasculature to hypoxia, a physiological attempt to extract the maximum oxygen from whatever blood is reaching the area. Thus severely ischaemic skin may feel cool but, paradoxically, be red.

Buerger's test for severe ischaemia (Fig. 40.4) involves high elevation of the leg for a minute or two. If the peripheral arterial pressure is inadequate to overcome the effects of gravity, the entire foot becomes white. When the leg is hung down, it gradually becomes blueish-red as blood flow returns. This test is easily misinterpreted—even in normal people, the foot will blanch somewhat with elevation.

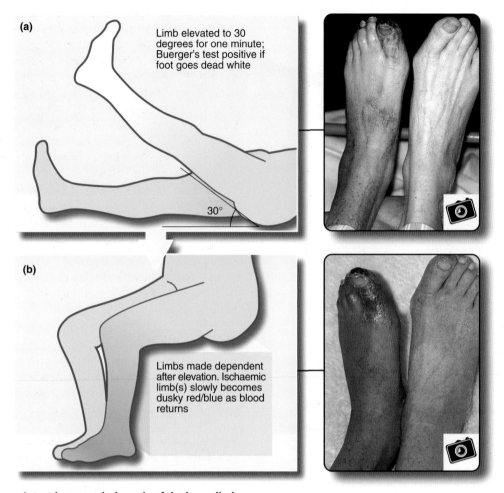

(a) Limb elevated to 30 degrees for one minute; Buerger's test positive if foot goes dead white

30°

(b) Limbs made dependent after elevation. Ischaemic limb(s) slowly becomes dusky red/blue as blood returns

Fig. 40.4 Buerger's test in severe ischaemia of the lower limb
Buerger's test is only truly positive when limbs are severely ischaemic. This 78-year-old man had severe ischaemia of both legs with the left being critically ischaemic. **(a)** In the first stage, one or both feet are elevated. Both feet go pale but the right is dead white. The left big toe is seen to be necrotic distally. **(b)** In the second stage, with dependency, both feet go blueish red, most marked on the left.

The warm foot

Inflammatory dilatation of the microcirculation also causes skin redness, but the skin is warm and slightly swollen because of enhanced blood flow. An example is low-grade bacterial **cellulitis** which may be seen in diabetes or chronic venous insufficiency or may arise unexpectedly. Note that if infection develops in a severely ischaemic limb, the usual signs of inflammation may not develop and the extent of infection may be underestimated. If the blood supply is later restored, signs of inflammation appear.

Abnormal pigmentation

Brown pigmentation around the gaiter area is often caused by superficial or deep **chronic venous insufficiency** due to gross reflux in varicose veins or a **post-thrombotic limb**. In the latter, valves in the deep veins have been disrupted by inflammation, organisation and recanalisation following deep venous thrombosis.

The valves thus become incompetent and allow **deep venous reflux**. This prevents the leg muscles acting as an effective venous return pump and leads to chronic venous insufficiency. In gross superficial or deep venous reflux, standing erect causes venous stagnation, increased venous pressure in the leg (**venous hypertension**) and chronic leg swelling. Red cells extravasate into the tissues and form haemosiderin deposits which cause brown skin pigmentation. This, accompanied by dry, scaly, atrophic skin, is described as **varicose** or **venous eczema** (see Fig. 40.5).

ULCERATION

LOWER LIMB ULCERS (Box 40.1)

Chronic ulceration of the lower limb is a common problem, particularly in the elderly. These ulcers are usually managed by general practitioners and community nurses with only the more difficult cases being referred

Fig. 40.5 Skin changes of chronic venous insufficiency

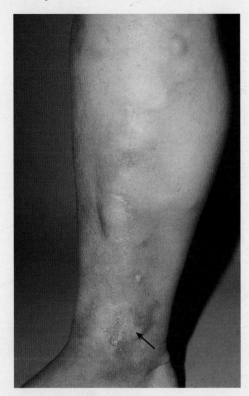

This 53-year-old woman suffered a deep vein thrombosis during her second pregnancy many years earlier. The leg is pigmented around the ankle and this tissue is woody on palpation (lipo-dermatosclerosis). The scar of a healed varicose ulcer is seen above the medial malleolus (arrowed).

Box 40.1 Causes of chronic leg ulcers

- Chronic venous insufficiency
  —Previous deep venous thrombosis (post-thrombotic limb)
  —Varicose veins (superficial venous insufficiency)
  —Combined deep and superficial insufficiency
  —Congenital reflux—defective deep vein valves
- Chronic arterial insufficiency
- Diabetic neuropathy (often called neuro-ischaemia) or other sensory neuropathies
- Pressure sores
- Vasculitis, e.g. in rheumatoid disease and other collagen diseases
- Tropical ulcers involving bacterial or fungal infections, tuberculous ulcers. Ulcers common on feet of surfers— likely combination of trauma and infection
- Malignant tumours

---

to a dermatologist or vascular surgeon. Many are venous in origin, either a complication of varicose veins or a late complication of deep venous thrombosis. The majority of the rest are caused by arterial insufficiency or diabetic neuro-ischaemia and a few by vasculitis or ulcerating tumours. In developed countries, infection rarely plays a primary role but various tropical ulcers and tuberculosis are important causes in developing countries. In intractable cases, persistent ulceration may be due to a combination of factors, e.g. local trauma, diabetic neuropathy and obliterative atherosclerosis.

Effective treatment of leg ulceration depends on clinical evaluation of the patient's general condition first, then the following factors, discussed in detail below:

- History of the origin and evolution of the ulcer
- The site of the ulcer
- The characteristics of the ulcer
- The nature of the surrounding tissues
- Relevant regional findings

History of the ulcer

Details of the initial skin lesion and the circumstances in which it occurred may provide diagnostic clues. **Minor trauma** such as an injury or an insect bite may be the initiating incident but failure to heal can usually be attributed to abnormal skin nutrition. The common causes include chronic venous insufficiency, arterial ischaemia and diabetic neuropathy. The ulcer often begins insidiously with minor breakdown in a patch of atrophic skin. In venous insufficiency, the leg is often oedematous and the skin may 'weep' plasma.

The duration of the ulcer, its healing, and subsequent recurrence or change in extent or distribution give further clues to the diagnosis. **Ischaemic ulcers** present early because pain soon becomes intolerable (except in diabetics with coexisting neuropathy and ischaemia) and the ulcer refuses to heal (Table 40.8). In contrast, post-thrombotic and varicose ulcers are not usually severely painful and commonly fluctuate between healing and breakdown. Very rarely, squamous carcinoma develops in a long-standing ulcer and is recognised by proliferative change at the ulcer margin. These are sometimes known as **Marjolin's ulcers** and were first described following burns which failed to heal (Fig. 40.6). Primary skin malignancies on the leg may ulcerate, but these usually begin as a cutaneous lump.

If a patient with a leg ulcer has claudication or rest pain, this suggests an ischaemic cause (Fig. 40.7). Neuropathic or mixed diabetic ulcers tend to be painless because of sensory neuropathy (which may be the main predisposing cause). A history or strong suspicion of previous deep venous thrombosis makes venous insufficiency the likely cause.

Site of the ulcer

The site of the ulcer on the lower limb may point to its cause. Post-thrombotic and varicose ulcers arise typically

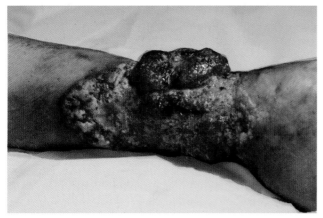

Fig. 40.6 Squamous carcinoma developing in a chronic venous ulcer
This very rare transformation, sometimes known as Marjolin's ulcer, followed 34 years of continuous venous ulceration. The leg was amputated below knee and the patient cured.

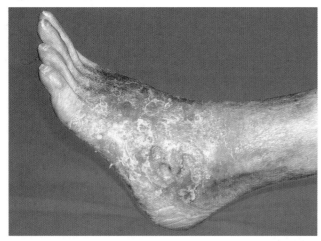

Fig. 40.7 Chronic ischaemic ulcers
This elderly man had intolerable pain in his foot, worse at night for 7 weeks. Note the foot is red and there are multiple ulcers over the lateral malleolus.

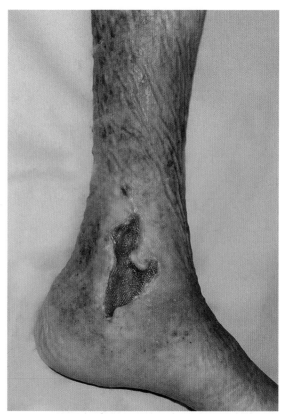

Fig. 40.8 Venous (varicose) ulcer
This longstanding ulcer is typical of venous ulceration by its site, the medial gaiter area of the ankle, its relative painlessness and the presence of venous eczema surrounding it. The visible corrugations in the skin above the ulcer are caused by four-layer compression bandaging.

just above the medial malleolus (the 'gaiter' area) and may extend circumferentially around the leg (Fig. 40.8). They rarely occur in other sites. Diabetic (neuropathic) ulcers always occur on the foot either as perforating ulcers on the sole beneath the metatarsal heads or at other bony prominences; these include the toes, the ball of the great toe and the malleoli (see Fig. 41.10, p. 594).

Ulcers due to arterial insufficiency may occur anywhere below the mid-calf, including the usual sites of venous or diabetic ulcers. **Pressure ulcers** occur mainly in debilitated, elderly or unconscious patients, especially at the back of the heel (see Fig. 12.10). Even a few minutes in one position on a hard casualty trolley or operating theatre table may initiate skin necrosis in an already ischaemic limb. Pressure ulcers usually begin as a well-circumscribed patch of skin discoloration, which becomes

necrotic and later ulcerates. The heels of vulnerable patients should be nursed carefully and regularly inspected to avoid this complication. Treatment of pressure ulcers is difficult and prolonged and it is best to prevent them.

Characteristics of the ulcer

Most ulcers are shallow, involving only the skin and subcutaneous fat. Diabetic ulcers, however, tend to penetrate deeply into the foot, where there is underlying necrotic and infected tissue. The base of any ulcer usually contains slough and fibrin but granulation tissue may be visible beneath. The slough should not be removed unless arterial insufficiency can be excluded, as this could aggravate ischaemia. If there is proliferating tissue in the ulcer, this should be biopsied.

The edge of most chronic lower limb ulcers slopes towards the base with no specific diagnostic features, although epithelial proliferation growing inwards from around the edge suggests healing. Diabetic foot ulcers have a characteristic 'punched-out' edge with abrupt transition from normal skin to the necrotic crater. On the sole, diabetic ulcers have a hyperkeratinised edge in response to excess local pressure during walking caused by distor-

Table 40.8 Main characteristics of ischaemic versus venous ulcers

	Ischaemic ulcer	Venous ulcer
Pain	Yes, unless neuropathic	Minimal; not intolerable
Duration	Less than 6 weeks	Often months or years
Past history	Cardiac ischaemia/coronary artery bypass graft common	DVT; severe varicose veins
Limb signs Swelling	Not swollen unless patient has been sleeping in a chair to relieve pain	Usually non-pitting plus pitting oedema unless effective bandaging in place
Temperature	Usually cold	Usually normal or warm
Pulses	Absent; low Doppler pressure	Present; normal Doppler pressure

Table 40.9 Causes of swelling of the lower limbs

Unilateral swelling	Bilateral swelling
a. Local causes	
	'Sluggish venous return', e.g. immobility, pregnancy, prolonged sitting in a chair, inefficient calf muscle pump (e.g. paralysis due to polio or hemiplegia) Lymphatic obstruction by filariasis (in tropical Africa and Asia)
Chronic venous insufficiency Destruction of valves in deep venous system following venous thrombosis (post-thrombotic limb)—superficial venous reflux	May be bilateral
Congenital lymphatic aplasia or hypoplasia, e.g. Milroy's disease	May be bilateral
Acute obstruction of venous return, e.g. deep venous thrombosis Chronic cellulitis (usually streptococcal)	
b. Regional causes	
	Left ventricular failure Venous obstruction by pelvic mass, e.g. advanced pregnancy, ovarian cyst, pelvic malignancy Lymphatic obstruction by malignant involvement of inguinal or more proximal nodes, or after block dissection or radiotherapy Inferior venal caval obstruction
c. Systemic causes	
	Congestive or right-sided cardiac failure Hypoalbuminaemia, e.g. malnutrition, nephrotic syndrome Fluid overload

Fig. 40.9 Swollen limbs due to venous obstruction

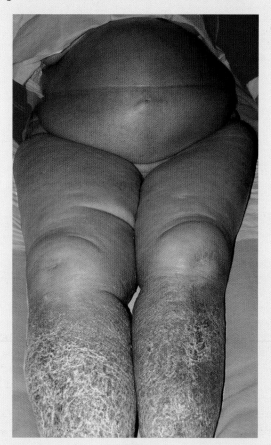

Lower limb swelling due to pelvic compression caused by a massive ovarian tumour. After excision of the tumour, the limbs gradually returned to near normal over a period of 6 months.

tion of the foot. Malignant ulcers may have a raised margin.

Nature of the surrounding tissues

The characteristics of the surrounding tissues indicate the background upon which the ulcer has formed. These characteristics include colour, e.g. chronic venous pigmentation, texture, e.g. induration, and perfusion (shown by temperature, blanching response, venous filling and Buerger's test), as well as swelling.

Regional features

Regional examination should search for diagnostic clues, e.g. peripheral pulses, inguinal lymphadenopathy (infection or malignancy), varicose veins and deep or superficial venous thrombosis.

LIMB SWELLING

Swelling of the lower limb may be unilateral or bilateral. The causes are summarised in Table 40.9. If bilateral, this suggests a 'central' cause such as heart failure. Systemic causes, and conditions listed under 'sluggish venous return' cause bilateral swelling. Unilateral swelling is more likely to present to a surgeon. The other causes tend to produce swelling of only one limb. Most causes of unilateral swelling are chronic and painless, except for acute deep venous thrombosis and cellulitis.

Managing lower limb arterial insufficiency, the diabetic foot and major amputations

41

INTRODUCTION

The surgical management of arterial disease only began in the 1950s, employing special techniques uncommon in general surgery such as angiography, thrombo-endarterectomy and arterial bypass surgery. The specialty of **peripheral vascular surgery** has evolved since then, with increasing cooperation in patient management between surgeons and interventional radiologists, ultrasonographers and vascular physicians. There has been a growing realisation that peripheral atherosclerosis is a marker for coronary and cerebrovascular atherosclerosis and the best medical management takes in the systemic nature of the condition as well as dealing with the local problem.

Chronic arterial insufficiency of the lower limb presents at any point along a scale of severity ranging from mild intermittent claudication brought on by vigorous exercise to gangrene of a large part of a limb. Between these two extremes are increasing severities of claudication, rest pain and ischaemic skin changes (including ulceration), or any combination of these.

Symptoms of claudication often develop suddenly, presumably signalling the acute event; they may evolve over days or weeks or even arise so gradually as to be hardly noticed. Once present, symptoms and signs of claudication are likely to remain stable (in about one-third of cases) or get better (in about half the cases). However, if ischaemia is extreme, and particularly if infection is present, progression is likely. In the advanced stages, the **critically ischaemic limb** is one which will undoubtedly be lost unless the blood supply is restored.

CHRONIC LOWER LIMB ISCHAEMIA

INTERMITTENT CLAUDICATION

SYMPTOMS OF INTERMITTENT CLAUDICATION

Intermittent claudication is the characteristic symptom complex of chronic lower limb ischaemia and the typical pain pattern is nearly always present. The patient experiences cramping pain in the lower limb muscles on walking. The calf is almost always involved first and is usually the only part involved. If there is more proximal arterial disease, the pain may ascend to the thigh or even the buttock if walking continues. In nearly all cases, resting allows the pain to resolve within a minute or two, after which the patient can walk a similar distance before the pain recurs. An individual's **claudication distance** may range from 30 to several hundred metres. Once established, the distance remains remarkably constant under similar conditions, e.g. on flat ground and at the same speed. Pain is worse on walking uphill and may be absent downhill or when walking slowly.

The first symptoms appear unexpectedly and are often attributed to musculoskeletal causes. The patient usually seeks medical advice only when symptoms have persisted for several weeks or more. Two-thirds of patients are male and most are aged 50–70 years; females are on average 10 years older. There is often a history of **myocardial ischaemia** in the form of angina or myocardial infarction or a history of coronary artery surgery or angioplasty. Nearly all are **cigarette smokers** or ex-smokers or live in a house with smokers. Non-smokers affected invariably have other risk factors. Most are hypertensive. Diabetes is a powerful risk factor: 25% of patients with claudication or severe ischaemia have the condition compared with 2–5% of the general population. In a few cases, claudication may be exacerbated by polycythaemia or by beta-adrenergic blocking drugs prescribed to control hypertension.

PHYSICAL SIGNS OF INTERMITTENT CLAUDICATION

Peripheral pulses are usually absent on the affected side but local examination is otherwise unremarkable. The dorsalis pedis, posterior tibial and popliteal pulses are almost invariably absent, and the femoral pulse is weak or absent in about 30% of patients. Trophic (nutritional) skin changes are unusual except in patients towards the 'severe ischaemia' end of the scale. In these, there may be evidence of nail thickening and peripheral skin atrophy and Buerger's test may be positive; hair loss is probably of no significance. General systematic examination should seek other signs of atherosclerosis; these may have an important bearing on management and prognosis.

NATURAL HISTORY OF INTERMITTENT CLAUDICATION

About one-third of patients experience spontaneous remission of all or most of their symptoms over a year or two without any treatment. It is well established that stopping cigarette smoking greatly improves the chance of remission. Another third remain stable in the long term with tolerable symptoms. The remaining third are either severely disabled by walking restriction or else progress to more severe ischaemic symptoms like rest pain. Indeed, only about 10% of the total would progress to necrosis and amputation if untreated.

Epidemiological studies show that patients with intermittent claudication have only half the life expectancy of unaffected people of the same age. Most die of ischaemic heart disease or stroke. Indeed, intermittent claudication is now regarded as a powerful marker for coronary atherosclerosis and patients carry the same level of risk of sudden death as those who have suffered a previous myocardial infarction. A diagnosis of claudication carries a 5-year mortality of around 25%, nearly all from cardiovascular causes.

SEVERE ISCHAEMIA

Severe lower limb ischaemia most commonly presents without a history of claudication but it may sometimes develop after a period of deteriorating claudication. In general, these patients are older and less physically active than typical claudicants.

The first manifestations of severe ischaemia develop in the foot and include:

- Intolerable rest pain initially at night, later becoming continuous
- Trophic skin changes—atrophic shiny red skin of the leg; ischaemic ulcers between the toes, in pressure areas of the foot or on the leg
- Patchy necrosis of the toes or skin of the foot
- Positive Buerger's test
- Failure of trivial injuries to heal
- Extreme vulnerability of ischaemic feet to pressure sores

If untreated, a very small proportion improve and lose their pain, but the majority smoulder on with intolerable pain or progress to extensive necrosis. Once the deeper tissues of the foot become necrotic, local defences are overwhelmed and infection spreads widely in the vulnerable ischaemic tissue, especially in diabetics. This results in wet gangrene and, ultimately, death from sepsis and multi-organ dysfunction. This sequence of events is rarely permitted to run its full course since rest pain is so severe and signs of systemic inflammatory responses become so obvious that vascular reconstruction or amputation becomes essential.

Critical ischaemia

Critical ischaemia occurs when arterial insufficiency is so severe that it threatens the viability of the foot or leg. This has been defined formally by a European consensus document as follows: persistently recurring rest pain requiring regular analgesia for more than 2 weeks, or ulceration or gangrene affecting the foot, plus an ankle systolic pressure of less than 50 mmHg (in diabetics, absent ankle pulses on palpation replace pressure measurement as calcification may render pressures artificially elevated).

In acute ischaemia, limb viability may be critically compromised from the outset, but in chronic arterial insufficiency, critical ischaemia usually develops gradually over days or weeks. The usual underlying cause is blood flow restriction caused by progressive obliterative atherosclerosis exacerbated by secondary thrombosis.

MANAGING LOWER LIMB ISCHAEMIA

INVESTIGATION OF CHRONIC LOWER LIMB ARTERIAL INSUFFICIENCY

The extent to which investigation is pursued in a patient with symptoms of lower limb ischaemia depends on whether the clinical picture suggests interventional treatment is likely to be necessary. As a minimum, most patients with claudication should have resting ankle systolic pressures measured in the clinic to confirm the diagnosis and a full blood count to exclude polycythaemia or thrombocythaemia. Resting ankle systolic blood pressure can be measured using a **Doppler ultrasound blood flow detector**. Normal pressure is slightly above brachial systolic whilst patients with claudication usually range from 50 to 120 mmHg. Results are sometimes expressed as a ratio, the **ankle/brachial pressure index** (ABPI), with normal values from 0.8 to 1.2. Also in the clinic, it is simple to walk the patient along a corridor to measure claudication distance, although this may not be practical in a busy clinic. Note, however, that Doppler pressure measurements can be misleading. Considerable experience is needed in taking and interpreting the measurements, and radical treatment should not be based solely on a random ankle pressure measurement. In practice, the patient's severity of symptoms is usually the driving force behind decisions about intervention.

The vascular laboratory

Severe claudicants are often investigated in a vascular laboratory, if available, as this can provide useful objective information about blood flow under exercise conditions. Vascular laboratory assessment provides a useful baseline against which to measure improvement or deterioration (see below). Tests vary in type and complexity but the basic test is usually to measure the ankle systolic pressure before and after the patient has exercised on a treadmill (see Fig. 41.1). A fall in ankle pressure after exercise gives an indication of the severity of arterial disease and the recovery rate provides an indication of collateral compensation. This type of test is particularly useful where doubt exists about the diagnosis of claudication.

Another test that may be performed in the vascular laboratory or the radiology department is **duplex Doppler scanning** for arterial stenoses and occlusions.

Arteriography (see Ch. 5)

Arteriography should be reserved for patients thought to require intervention in the form of angioplasty or reconstructive surgery. It provides a map of the arterial system (see Fig. 41.2), showing sites and severity of vessel stenoses and occlusions, including the quality of inflow (arteries feeding the area of concern) and the runoff (distal arteries beyond the main obstruction supplying the lower part of the limb) (see Fig. 41.3). Arteriography is sometimes used wrongly by non-specialists as a way of assessing chronic arterial insufficiency. Arteriography does not measure the rate of blood flow to the tissues or the dynamic circulatory responses to exercise; it helps only with the mechanics of revascularisation. Traditional arteriography is performed via direct vessel puncture but this carries some risk. Many centres are now using either CT or MR-based imaging systems for diagnosis.

APPROACH TO MANAGEMENT OF CHRONIC LOWER LIMB ARTERIAL INSUFFICIENCY

The treatment options for chronic lower limb ischaemia range from conservative or 'expectant' treatment for most, to extensive reconstructive operations for the few with severe ischaemia. Treatments are summarised in Box 41.1.

Conservative management

For patients with intermittent claudication, management starts with **lifestyle measures** such as stopping smoking,

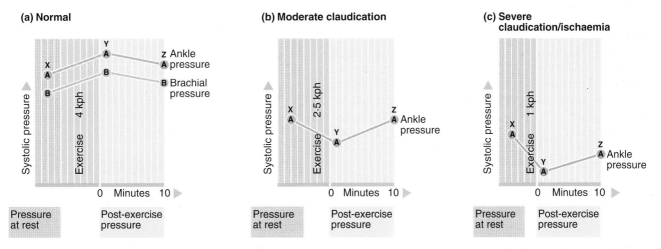

Fig. 41.1 Ankle pressure responses to exercise in intermittent claudication
X = systolic pressure at rest (A = ankle pressure; B = brachial pressure), Y represents pressure immediately after treadmill exercise (duration indicated by the breadth of the shaded zones) and Z = the pressure 10 min later. **(a)** Normal ankle pressure response to exercise. **(b)** Response in moderate claudication, i.e. reduced resting ankle pressure, reduced exercise tolerance, ankle pressure fall and recovery within 10 min. **(c)** Response in severe claudication or more severe ischaemia.

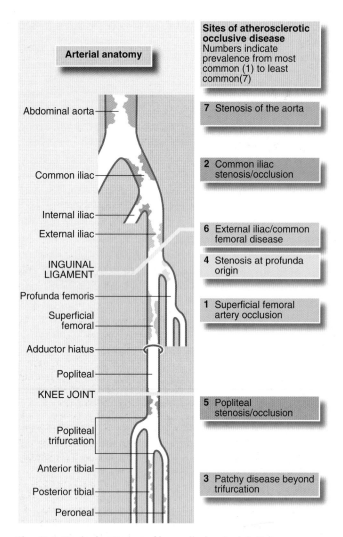

Sites of atherosclerotic occlusive disease
Numbers indicate prevalence from most common (1) to least common(7)

Arterial anatomy

Abdominal aorta

7 Stenosis of the aorta

Common iliac

2 Common iliac stenosis/occlusion

Internal iliac

External iliac

6 External iliac/common femoral disease

INGUINAL LIGAMENT

4 Stenosis at profunda origin

Profunda femoris

Superficial femoral

1 Superficial femoral artery occlusion

Adductor hiatus

Popliteal

KNEE JOINT

5 Popliteal stenosis/occlusion

Popliteal trifurcation

Anterior tibial

Posterior tibial

3 Patchy disease beyond trifurcation

Peroneal

Fig. 41.2 Typical patterns of lower limb arterial disease

Box 41.1 Treatment options for chronic lower limb ischaemia

Mild to moderate claudication

- No active treatment except advice to stop smoking, exercise regularly, take statin and aspirin, lose weight
- Balloon angioplasty

Disabling claudication

- Balloon angioplasty
- Reconstructive arterial surgery

Critical ischaemia

- Intravenous drug therapies such as prostacyclin
- Lumbar sympathectomy (surgical or by phenol injection)
- Balloon angioplasty
- Reconstructive arterial surgery
- Amputation (below, through or above knee)
- Terminal pain relief

---

attention to diet (reduced fat, more fruit and vegetables, weight reduction) and systematic exercise. Cigarette smoking is both a primary risk factor in the aetiology of atherosclerosis and a secondary risk factor in causing deterioration, or occlusion or stenosis of angioplasty or graft after reconstruction. Symptoms of claudication are more likely to resolve without treatment if the patient ceases smoking by the process of collateral development. However, the overall success rate of persuading patients to give up smoking is low; others in the household should also be encouraged to give up smoking to help motivate the patient.

Medical management is also important, with attention to blood pressure control and regular prescription of an anti-platelet agent (usually aspirin) and a statin (even if cholesterol levels are normal). These measures aim to reduce mortality by treating systemic atherosclerosis including cardiac and cerebrovascular disease, as well as encourage the gradual development of collateral vessels. Treatment with the phosphodiesterase inhibitor, **cilostazol**, has been shown to provide a small but measurable increase in walking distance in several clinical trials. It does however have a significant side effect profile which is likely to limit its usefulness.

For claudication, the degree of handicap is assessed clinically by careful history-taking and perhaps by walking with the patient. There is a marked trend towards purely conservative treatment these days, given that many patients recover function satisfactorily and this recovery is more durable than intervention. The choice of treatment depends on the degree of handicap, the patient's willingness to give up smoking, the potential for treating the pattern of atherosclerosis and finally the patient's overall preference. Further investigation is then planned accordingly. Severe and critical ischaemia are usually clear indications for revascularisation (or amputation) since the symptoms cannot be tolerated in the long term.

Mild to moderate claudication

Most patients with mild or moderate claudication do not require revascularisation and are optimally managed with best medical management and lifestyle advice. The symptoms often improve spontaneously over 6–18 months, especially if the patient stops smoking, exercises regularly and loses excess weight. Simple advice to walk more slowly and use a walking stick will often greatly extend the claudication distance. The use of a structured and supervised programme of exercise has been clearly shown to produce a sustained increase in the patient's walking distance. Care of the feet and appropriate footwear should be strongly emphasised.

Investigation of this group of patients is unnecessary apart from baseline ankle pressure measurements and a full blood count to exclude polycythaemia and thrombocythaemia. In polycythaemia vera, soft thrombi can

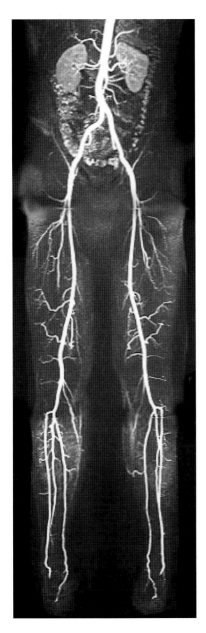

(a)

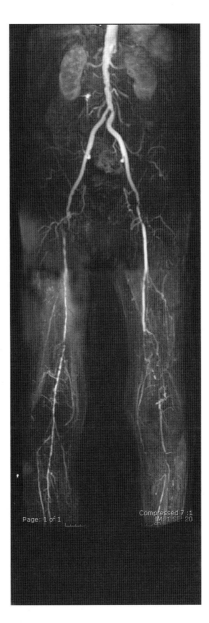

(b)

Fig. 41.3 Arteriograms comparing the normal with typical patterns of arterial obstruction affecting the lower limbs
(a) This magnetic resonance angiogram is entirely normal, showing smooth, regular arterial walls, all branches intact and three normal infrainguinal arteries below knee on each side. **(b)** This composite subtraction arteriogram was performed because the patient suffered bilateral severe claudication. The aorta is irregular and narrowed by atherosclerosis from above the renal arteries to the bifurcation. The common, internal and proximal external iliacs are smooth and normal but the right external iliac is occluded and the left stenosed. Both profunda femoris arteries are occluded. The superficial femoral arteries are both diseased and occluded distally. On the left side, collaterals are visible around the knee area. The infrageniculate vessels are diseased on both sides with stenoses and occlusions. Reconstruction would have been extensive, difficult and risky and hence conservative management alone was undertaken, in the absence of rest pain or tissue loss.

develop in the lower limb and cause arterial insufficiency. Systemic manifestations of atherosclerosis such as hypertension, angina or arrhythmias should be investigated and treated as appropriate.

Disabling claudication

The main indication for imaging is symptoms severe enough to warrant radiological or surgical intervention. Disabling claudication is usually an indication for treatment unless the patient is too unfit even for angiography. This may include marked exercise restriction in younger patients or markedly worsening symptoms, especially if associated with proximal arterial obstruction (as shown by absent femoral pulses) as this is often relatively easily

treated by angioplasty. Treatment is usually by angioplasty or sometimes reconstructive surgery.

TECHNIQUES OF REVASCULARISATION FOR CHRONIC ARTERIAL INSUFFICIENCY

Angioplasty

Angioplasty involves percutaneously introducing a guide-wire into a remote artery and advancing it until it lies across the stenosis. A balloon catheter is then passed over the guide-wire and manoeuvred into position (see Fig. 41.4). The balloon is finally inflated to a high pressure (5–15 atmospheres), crushing the atheroma into the arterial wall and relieving the obstruction. Success is

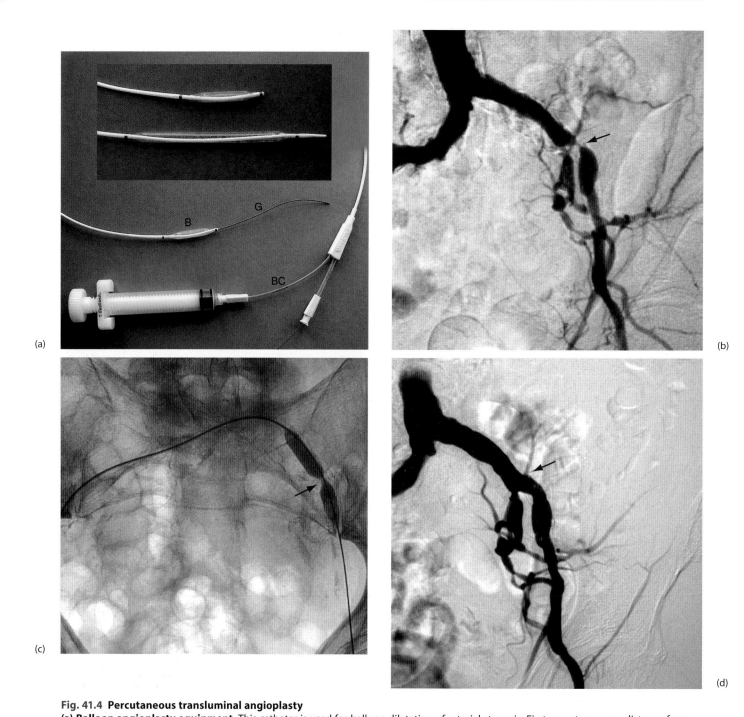

Fig. 41.4 Percutaneous transluminal angioplasty
(a) Balloon angioplasty equipment. This catheter is used for balloon dilatation of arterial stenosis. First, an artery some distance from the stenosis (usually the femoral) is punctured with a needle. A flexible guide-wire **G** is passed through the needle, along the artery and manipulated across the stenosis. The catheter is then threaded over the guide-wire until the distal balloon **B** (which can be inflated only to a predetermined diameter) lies within the stenosis. The balloon is then inflated to high pressure using a special syringe attached to the balloon channel **BC**. Note the radio-opaque markers at each end of the balloon to allow it to be sited radiographically.
(b) Arteriogram showing a tight stenosis at the distal end of the left common iliac artery (arrowed). **(c)** Catheter access proved impossible via the left femoral artery, so a guide-wire was passed from the right femoral, over the bifurcation and across the stenosis. An angioplasty balloon catheter was then guided across the stenosis. As it was inflated the 'waist' caused by the arterial stenosis became clearly visible (arrowed). With further inflation to 4 atmospheres pressure, the waist disappeared. **(d)** Appearance of the arteries post angioplasty. This procedure was completed in under an hour on a day-case basis under local anaesthesia and proved durable over several years.

very operator dependent and the treatment is most effective for isolated short stenoses. With increasing experience, longer stenoses and occlusions in smaller vessels can be tackled, avoiding the need for major surgery. Unfortunately, the method is less useful for distal calf arteries although results in this area continue to improve. A similar technique is widely used for treating coronary artery stenoses as an alternative to coronary artery bypass surgery (see Ch. 44). Angioplasty of the lower limb arteries will often provide symptom improvement for a few years but disease progression limits long-term efficacy.

Arterial reconstructive surgery

Arterial reconstructive surgery began in the 1950s with the open removal of atheromatous plaques and associated thrombus from the aorta and iliac arteries. This technique, known as **thrombo-endarterectomy**, is technically difficult and time-consuming. It has largely been replaced by bypass grafting, although endarterectomy remains the standard operation for carotid artery stenosis (see below) and for isolated common femoral artery occlusions.

Arterial bypass grafting was first developed during the Korean War to treat arterial trauma using homografts from human cadavers. The initial results were excellent but the grafts eventually suffered from aneurysmal dilatation and rupture. This led to the introduction of synthetic graft materials for large arteries, and these are now available in a wide variety of shapes, sizes and types of cloth. Knitted polyester (Dacron) is the most popular and is the standard graft material for treating aorto-iliac obstruction. Many of these grafts are now sealed with gelatin or other proteins to minimise porosity. For smaller arteries, autogenous **long saphenous vein** from the leg provides the best bypass conduit, provided it is of suitable diameter and is not damaged by thrombosis. Vein has the additional benefit that it is inherently resistant to infection, a useful attribute when treating patients with infected lower limb wounds and ulcers.

The recognition that conservative treatment may be as good as intervention for claudication, and the availability and success of angioplasty has meant that the volume of bypass grafting for arterial occlusive disease has fallen dramatically. Reconstructive arterial surgery is now largely reserved for severely ischaemic limbs, either chronic or acute, if angioplasty is unsuitable or has proved unsuccessful.

The most common bypass procedures are synthetic 'trouser' grafting for aorto-iliac (supra-inguinal) disease and femoro-popliteal bypass grafting, preferably using saphenous vein, for infra-inguinal disease (see Figs 41.5 and 41.6). However, a range of other bypass procedures and endarterectomy techniques sometimes have to be employed to cope with non-standard disease.

Aorto-iliac disease

The most common operation for aorto-iliac obstruction is the insertion of a trouser graft or 'Y' graft (see Fig. 41.5) between the aorta and the common femoral arteries just below the inguinal ligament. Each 'trouser leg' is sewn to a femoral artery, and the diseased vessels are left in situ posteriorly. For patients whose physiological reserve is poor, this can be a demanding operation. In this situation, an **extra-anatomic synthetic graft** may be less challenging. Examples include a **cross-over graft** to supply blood from one femoral artery to another or an **axillo-bifemoral graft**, supplying blood to both femorals from one axillary artery via a subcutaneous route.

Femoro-popliteal disease

The superficial femoral artery is a common site of obstruction that can often be relieved by a bypass graft linking the common femoral artery to the popliteal artery; this is known as autogenous **femoro-popliteal bypass grafting** (see Fig. 41.6). The usual technique is to dissect out the long saphenous vein from groin to knee and ligate its tributaries, then reverse the graft proximal to distal so the valves do not obstruct flow. An anastomosis is then performed at each end. Arm veins can be used if there is no suitable leg vein. Synthetic materials (e.g. PTFE or Dacron) are a less satisfactory alternative; these have a lower long-term patency rate, particularly when they cross the knee joint. A vein graft is therefore nearly always the first choice.

An alternative method leaves the long saphenous vein in situ and destroys the valves with a **valvulotome** (see

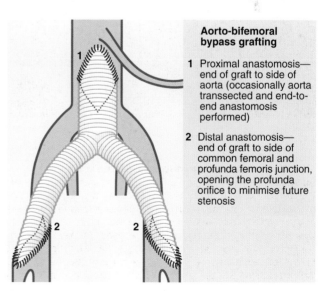

Aorto-bifemoral bypass grafting

1 Proximal anastomosis—end of graft to side of aorta (occasionally aorta transsected and end-to-end anastomosis performed)

2 Distal anastomosis—end of graft to side of common femoral and profunda femoris junction, opening the profunda orifice to minimise future stenosis

Fig. 41.5 Aorto-bifemoral bypass for aorto-iliac disease using a trouser or 'Y' graft
A Dacron bifurcation graft or prosthesis is used to bypass the aorto-iliac segment when it is occluded or stenosed, or to replace it when aorta and iliacs are aneurysmal. In the latter case, the distal anastomoses are to the iliac arteries *not* the femorals so as to maintain pelvic perfusion.

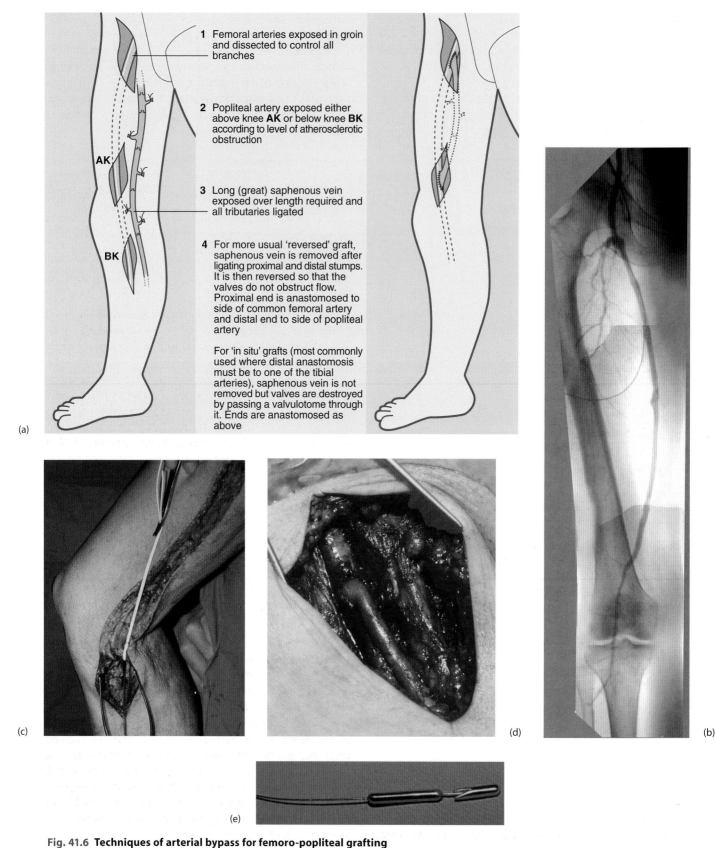

1 Femoral arteries exposed in groin and dissected to control all branches

2 Popliteal artery exposed either above knee **AK** or below knee **BK** according to level of atherosclerotic obstruction

3 Long (great) saphenous vein exposed over length required and all tributaries ligated

4 For more usual 'reversed' graft, saphenous vein is removed after ligating proximal and distal stumps. It is then reversed so that the valves do not obstruct flow. Proximal end is anastomosed to side of common femoral artery and distal end to side of popliteal artery

For 'in situ' grafts (most commonly used where distal anastomosis must be to one of the tibial arteries), saphenous vein is not removed but valves are destroyed by passing a valvulotome through it. Ends are anastomosed as above

Fig. 41.6 Techniques of arterial bypass for femoro-popliteal grafting
(a) Technique of femoro-popliteal grafting. (b) Composite arteriogram showing patent femoro-popliteal bypass after operation. (c) Long saphenous vein exposed in the thigh where it will be left in situ after destroying the valves with a valvulotome. The below knee popliteal artery is held in the white sling. (d) The vein graft anastomosed end-to-side to the common femoral artery in the groin. (e) Head of Hall's valvulotome used to destroy valves for in situ grafting.

| Box **41.2** | **Complications of arterial surgery** |

- Complications of generalised arteriopathy: acute myocardial ischaemia, cerebrovascular accidents, renal failure, intestinal ischaemia—early or late
- Haemorrhage: arterial or venous—early
- Thrombosis of reconstructed vessels or graft leading to profound distal ischaemia (usually a technical fault)—early
- Embolism into limb vessels or renal vessels (particularly aneurysm surgery)—early
- Graft infection—early or late
- False aneurysm formation—late
- Progressive atherosclerotic lower limb ischaemia—late

Fig. 41.6e). For distal bypasses, this has the advantage that the vein tapers from proximal to distal. By this method, bypasses down to the tibial or even dorsalis pedis artery or smaller foot arteries can be performed for distal disease. These are known as **infrapopliteal** or femorodistal grafts and are used only for severe ischaemia because of the higher risk of graft occlusion.

The complications of arterial surgery

These are summarised in Box 41.2.

Intravenous and intra-arterial drug therapies

There is little in the way of drug therapy that has any substantial effect in relieving claudication or severe isch-aemia, nor have any yet been discovered that can reliably reverse atherosclerosis, although **rosuvastatin** has recently shown some potential in this regard.

Several research programmes are looking into stimulating new vessel formation in unreconstructable limbs using locally applied intra-arterial growth factors but these are still some distance from everyday clinical practice.

Sympathectomy

Blood flow in the skin (but not muscle) is controlled by the sympathetic nervous system. Thus, even if the overall arterial supply is inadequate, early rest pain in the skin may sometimes be relieved by sympathetic blockade. It is not beneficial in claudication as muscle blood flow is not improved.

Sympathectomy can be performed by surgical excision of part of the lumbar sympathetic chain or, much more commonly and less invasively, by translumbar injection of 6% aqueous phenol. This is known as **chemical sympathectomy** and is performed under local anaesthesia with radiographic control.

Unfortunately, only about 15% of patients with severe ischaemia obtain sufficient relief of symptoms to avoid a reconstructive operation or amputation and there appears to be no reliable way of selecting in advance those who will benefit; sympathectomy is, however, certain to fail in the presence of tissue loss (gangrene). Sympathectomy is most likely to succeed in early rest pain but may also help heal ulcers where moderate ischaemia co-exists with another factor such as chronic venous insufficiency.

ACUTE LOWER LIMB ISCHAEMIA

PATHOPHYSIOLOGY OF ACUTE LOWER LIMB ISCHAEMIA

The lower limb (or upper limb) may become acutely isch-aemic as a result of **embolism** or **thrombosis**. If a large embolus impacts in a major distributing artery, the distal blood supply is abruptly cut off. If the distal arteries are not atherosclerotic, no alternative collateral network will have developed and the ischaemia is therefore all the more severe.

Embolism

Most large emboli originate in the heart, as a result of **atrial fibrillation** or **mitral stenosis** or both (left atrial thrombus), or of **myocardial infarction** (mural thrombus). Emboli usually impact at branching points where the arterial lumen abruptly narrows. Common sites are the aortic bifurcation (**saddle embolus**), the common femoral bifurcation and the popliteal trifurcation. Aortic or popliteal aneurysms can also be the source of distal embolism when thrombus accumulated within the sac travels distally (see Figs 41.8 and 41.9).

Thrombosis

Acute ischaemia may develop if an essential distributing artery, already narrowed by atherosclerosis, becomes completely obstructed by secondary thrombosis of its lumen (**acute-on-chronic occlusion**). Another cause is thrombosis of a **popliteal aneurysm**. Occasionally, **widespread thrombosis** occurs in normal arteries causing acute ischaemia. This used to be well recognised as a complication of the high-oestrogen contraceptive pill when it was in common use, but similar widespread thrombosis is sometimes seen as a complication of **blood disorders** including polycythaemia vera, thrombocythaemia or leukaemias.

Acute thrombotic occlusion causes the most catastrophic results when it occurs in particular sites, namely the popliteal artery (which has few useful collaterals), the external iliac/common femoral arterial trunk (the axial

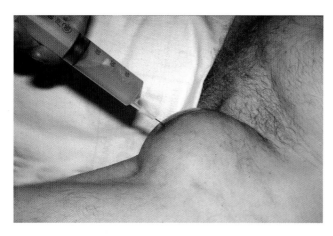

Fig. 41.7 Lymphocoele in groin following graft to femoral artery
Any operation in the region of the inguinal lymph nodes can interfere with lymphatic drainage and cause an accumulation of lymph known as a lymphocoele. In this case, the lymphocoele was aspirated periodically and finally stopped refilling about 2 months after the original operation. In fact, aspiration probably does not hasten the natural process of resolution.

Fig. 41.8 Embolic occlusion of popliteal arteries

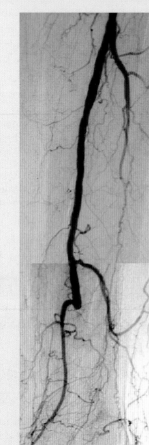

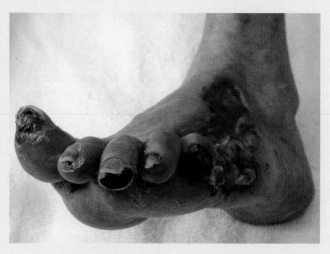

(b)

(a) Angiogram showing the thigh and upper leg arteries in a woman of 70 who presented with rest pain for 48 hours and necrosis of the dorsum of her foot and black toe tips for 24 hours. The left popliteal is occluded with a sharp cut-off typical of embolism. The patient was in atrial fibrillation and the likely source of the embolus was the left atrium. She underwent a successful embolectomy, but because of the delay, a below-knee fasciotomy was performed to prevent compartment syndrome. (b) The foot ulcer 3 weeks after revascularisation. The ulcer gradually healed completely.

(a)

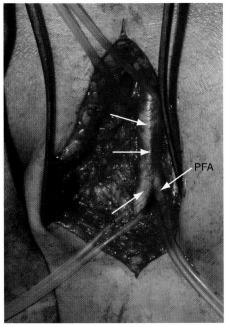

(a)

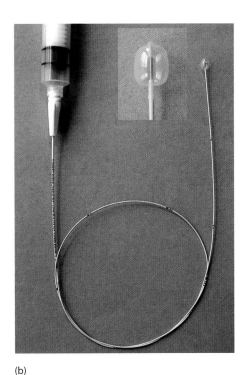

(b)

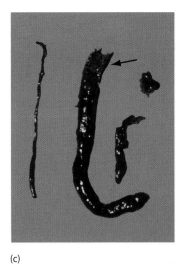

(c)

Fig. 41.9 Femoral artery embolectomy
(a) Surgical exposure of the femoral artery bifurcation, usually performed under local infiltration anaesthesia. The common femoral artery **CFA**, the profunda femoris **PFA** and the superficial femoral artery **SFA** are dissected cleanly and silicone slings placed around each artery. A transverse arteriotomy is made just proximal to the bifurcation (position arrowed). **(b)** A Fogarty balloon catheter is passed distally, the balloon is gently inflated and the catheter withdrawn to extract embolic and thrombotic material. This is performed in stages until the catheter can be passed to ankle level and back-bleeding occurs. **(c)** Embolic material removed at operation from the superficial femoral artery and beyond using a Fogarty catheter. Note the paler embolic material (arrowed) and the darker thrombus propagated beyond it.

blood supply of the lower limb) or the profunda femoris (if the superficial femoral artery is already occluded).

CLINICAL FEATURES OF ACUTE LOWER LIMB ISCHAEMIA

The clinical features of acute severe lower limb ischaemia are listed in Box 41.3. The condition usually presents as a sudden onset of pain, coldness and pallor, extending from the foot for a variable distance up the leg. If the blood supply is completely cut off, nerve ischaemia causes **loss of sensation** and then muscle **paralysis** after an hour or two (the **six Ps**—see Ch. 40, p. 573). It is crucial that acute severe arterial occlusion is recognised quickly as the viability of the limb is in immediate danger and urgent steps need to be taken to revascularise it. Unfortunately, the urgency is not always appreciated by the patient, nursing staff or inexperienced doctors. Even if successful revascularisation occurs, ischaemic changes may already be irreversible and there is a serious risk of muscle necrosis and permanent nerve injury due to **reperfusion injury** and **compartment syndrome** (see Ch. 17).

Later, necrosis becomes obvious as the affected area becomes mottled, dusky blue and discoloured. After about 24 hours, the skin becomes blistered; tissue death is now irreversible and limb loss inevitable. These changes always involve the foot but may extend proximally (though rarely above the knee). The upper limit of the necrotic area is usually well demarcated from the proximal viable tissue.

PRINCIPLES OF MANAGING THE ACUTELY ISCHAEMIC LIMB

It is important to plan the management of a patient with acute lower limb ischaemia at the outset. The window of opportunity before necrosis occurs is likely to be short and any delay or procrastination is likely to increase the morbidity or mortality. Treatment is best carried out by cooperation between vascular surgical and radiological experts so that the full range of appropriate and timely treatment can be offered. As a first step, the patient should be anticoagulated with a bolus dose of 5000 U of **intravenous heparin** plus 150 mg oral aspirin to prevent propagation of thrombus proximal and distal to the occlusion. If the diagnosis is later confirmed as embolism, oral anticoagulation is usually continued after surgery.

Box 41.3   Clinical features of acute severe lower limb ischaemia

Risk factors predisposing to embolism or thrombosis

- Recent chest pain or other evidence of myocardial infarction
- History of rheumatic heart disease
- History or finding of atrial fibrillation
- Previous arterial embolism
- History of intermittent claudication or other symptoms of peripheral arterial disease (thrombosis)
- Polycythaemia vera (prone to intravascular thrombosis)
- Popliteal aneurysm in contralateral limb (possible thrombosis or embolism in affected limb)
- Aortic aneurysm (possible source of embolism)

Symptoms suggesting acute lower limb ischaemia

- Sudden onset of continuous pain, usually in one periphery. Note: may be painless in diabetic neuropathy
- Sudden and persistent coldness, usually in one periphery

- Sudden numbness or paraesthesia, usually in one periphery

Signs of acute lower limb ischaemia

- Pallor or blueness of the periphery; in late cases, the fixed pigmentation of necrosis or skin blistering
- Unexpected coldness of the peripheral part of one or (less commonly) both legs
- Absent lower limb pulses (particularly if known to have been present before)
- Poor peripheral capillary return after pressure blanching
- Strongly positive Buerger's test (pallor on elevation, slow return of redness on dependency)
- Progressive paralysis and foot drop (late sign)
- Ankle pulses undetectable by Doppler or very low ankle systolic pressure

---

THROMBOSIS OR EMBOLISM?

Distinguishing clinically between thrombosis and embolism is unreliable, although the history may provide some clues. Evidence of mitral stenosis, an arrhythmia or recent myocardial infarction suggests embolism, whereas a history of claudication or a pro-thrombotic blood disorder points to thrombosis. Examining the affected limb cannot distinguish embolism from thrombosis but the other limb provides clinical evidence of the condition of the peripheral arteries. If the other limb is well perfused with good peripheral pulses and a normal ankle systolic pressure, then embolus is more likely. If a **saddle embolus** has lodged at the aortic bifurcation then both limbs may be ischaemic, although one side is usually affected more than the other. The popliteal fossa must always be palpated to exclude a **thrombosed popliteal aneurysm**. A full blood count should be performed to exclude predisposing blood disorders and blood grouped and screened for antibodies if surgery is contemplated.

If clinical signs are strongly in favour of embolism, immediate surgical embolectomy may be undertaken, performing on-table **arteriography** if necessary. In most cases, however, the first intervention is not surgery but arteriography. This nearly always demonstrates whether embolism or thrombosis is the diagnosis or if there is an occluded popliteal aneurysm; it will also show which distal vessels are patent. Unfortunately, expediency is often the excuse for omitting arteriography, but this may place the patient at greater risk and removes the possibility of minimal access treatment with thrombolysis and/or clot aspiration.

If acute-on-chronic thrombosis is the problem, immediate radiologically-guided clot aspiration followed by angioplasty may be undertaken if technically possible. Alternatively, if the limb is judged likely to remain viable for 12 hours, **thrombolysis** may be undertaken, followed by angioplasty of any revealed underlying stenoses. However, thrombolysis is falling out of favour, chiefly because of its limited clinical efficacy and also the fairly high risk of causing haemorrhagic stroke. If the patient is unsuitable for angioplasty or thrombolysis, urgent reconstructive surgery should be performed if feasible. Most patients needing arterial reconstruction for acute ischaemia require a **femoro-popliteal** or **femoro-tibial bypass** (see Fig. 41.6, p. 588).

EMBOLECTOMY

Embolectomy is often performed under local anaesthesia but the patient and theatre should be prepared for general anaesthesia in case it becomes necessary; full monitoring should be undertaken from the outset. The patient is usually already anticoagulated with intravenous heparin and an anti-platelet agent. A groin incision provides access to the arterial system; the femoral artery bifurcation is exposed, all the vessels are temporarily clamped and an incision (**arteriotomy**) is made in the common femoral artery (Fig. 41.9). This may reveal the obstructing clot. A **Fogarty balloon catheter** is then passed gently into each main vessel in turn, both proximally and distally. When the catheter has been passed into the artery for 10 cm or so, the balloon is inflated gently and the catheter drawn back to sweep out any obstructing clot. This process is repeated at 10 cm intervals until the distal limit is reached. The operation is successful if clot is retrieved and blood flows back ('**back-bleeding**') from each vessel as it is unclamped. If the embolectomy catheter will not pass easily, this usually indicates acute-on-chronic thrombosis. Immediate arteriography and surgical treatment are required as delay carries a high rate of limb loss and death.

THE DIABETIC FOOT

Managing diabetic foot problems often involves the surgeon as part of a multi-disciplinary diabetic team (vascular surgeon, diabetologist, podiatrist, orthopaedic surgeon, orthotist).

PATHOPHYSIOLOGY OF THE DIABETIC FOOT

Diabetic patients are particularly prone to serious ulceration and infection of the feet. The underlying disorder is either neuropathy, obliterative atherosclerosis or both together. Type 2 diabetic patients appear to be at greater risk than type 1, but remember **there is no such thing as mild diabetes**. All diabetic patients need to be screened for potential complications of diabetes.

Several factors may contribute to diabetic foot problems:

- **Neuropathy.** Microangiopathy is believed to cause peripheral neuropathies which affect motor, sensory and autonomic nerves. Affected **motor nerves** supply the small muscles of the foot; the consequent unmodified traction of the calf muscles distorts the morphology and weight-bearing characteristics of the foot. **Sensory neuropathy** lessens pain sensation and hence awareness of potential injury from ill-fitting footwear and foreign bodies in shoes. Damaged **autonomic nerves** disrupt vascular control and cause loss of sweating. Ulceration and infection in neuropathic feet are often painless and for this reason tend to be neglected by the patient
- **Arteriovenous communications.** These open beneath the skin, perhaps diverting nutrient flow away from it. Damaged tissue thus heals poorly and is vulnerable to infection, even if the injury or pressure damage is only minor. This may also explain why an ischaemic diabetic foot can be warm and pink
- **Arterioles.** In a few cases, these become narrowed and restrict capillary perfusion
- **Impaired intermediary tissue metabolism** and a glucose-rich tissue environment. Both of these favour bacterial growth and spreading infection
- **Obliterative atherosclerosis.** Diabetics have a markedly increased predisposition and are at greater risk of arterial insufficiency. In fact 1–5% of the general population have diabetes, but 25% of patients with lower limb ischaemia have diabetes. Atherosclerotic disease in diabetic patients follows the usual pattern (although often more distal) but tends to develop at a younger age

IDENTIFYING THE CAUSES OF DIABETIC FOOT PROBLEMS

Most diabetic foot problems can be identified as being either primarily neuropathic or primarily atherosclerotic but some patients have elements of both. This makes diagnosis and management more difficult. The term 'neuro-ischaemic' foot is sometimes used to cover both types of problem but is not clinically precise. Typically, the **neuropathic foot** is painless, red and warm with strong pulses, whereas the **atherosclerotic foot** without neuropathy is pale, painful, cold and pulseless. However, when both conditions occur together, **the diabetic trap** is that the limb can be seriously ischaemic yet painless, warm and pink. If the foot is neuropathic and pulseless, only **arteriography** or arterial duplex scanning will demonstrate the arterial insufficiency.

Patients most at risk of neuropathic foot complications are elderly, poorly controlled, maturity-onset (type 2) diabetics and younger patients with longstanding type 1 diabetes. Similarly, patients with diabetic renal or retinal complications appear to have an increased risk of foot problems. Recognising the **'at-risk' foot**, i.e. the neuropathic foot, before trouble strikes is fundamental, as virtually all neuropathic foot complications can be prevented with proper patient education and regular inspection and chiropody (podiatry) (Box 41.4).

Management of atherosclerotic ischaemia is similar in diabetic and non-diabetic patients. For mixed disease, the arterial insufficiency must nearly always be treated first if there is to be any hope of healing.

Box 41.4   The problem of the diabetic foot

- 'Diabetic gangrene is not heaven-sent but earth-born' (Joslin 1934)
- There is no such thing as 'mild' diabetes; all diabetics are potentially at risk
- Four out of five patients with diabetic foot problems have type 2 diabetes
- Foot problems are responsible for 47% of days spent in hospital by diabetics
- Diabetic foot problems are responsible for 12% of all hospital admissions in (internal) medicine
- In diabetics with new foot ulcers, 90% have peripheral neuropathy (compared with 20% in a diabetic control group), whereas only 14% have peripheral arterial disease compared with 10% in controls (Miami 1983–4)
- Patients with diabetic foot problems are incapacitated for an average of 16 weeks
- Diabetic foot problems are largely preventable
- Care and prevention of diabetic foot problems require specialist surveillance and management by a dedicated team; foot ulceration in diabetics represents a failure of medical management

CLINICAL PRESENTATIONS OF DIABETIC FOOT COMPLICATIONS

Foot complications of diabetic neuropathy present in four main ways (see Fig. 41.10):

- **Painless, deeply penetrating ulcers.** These usually develop in pressure areas caused by distortion of foot morphology, often beneath the first or fifth metatarsal head. The infecting organism is usually *Staphylococcus aureus*. The infection and necrosis tend to spread through the plantar spaces and along the tendon sheaths. Infection and local venous thrombosis appear to be the predominant factors in causing tissue destruction
- **Chronic ulceration of pressure points** and sites of minor injury. Skin perfusion is otherwise adequate
- **Extensive spreading skin necrosis** originating in an ulcer and associated with superficial or deep

infection. This develops very rapidly and spreads proximally, threatening both limb and life
- **Painless necrosis of individual toes.** These first turn blue, then later become black and mummified, and may eventually be shed spontaneously. This usually occurs in mixed neuropathy and atherosclerosis and the management hinges on whether local amputations will heal or whether arterial reconstruction is needed

MANAGEMENT OF NEUROPATHIC FOOT COMPLICATIONS

CONTROL OF INFECTION

After excluding ischaemia and as a general rule, control of infection is the first priority in the management of the diabetic foot. Minor foot lesions in the diabetic should always be taken seriously and treated early with **oral**

Fig. 41.10 Foot complications of diabetes

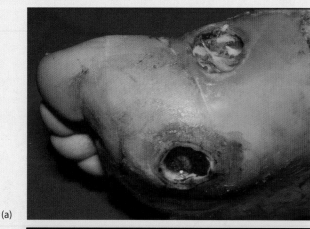

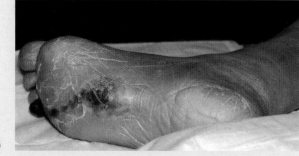

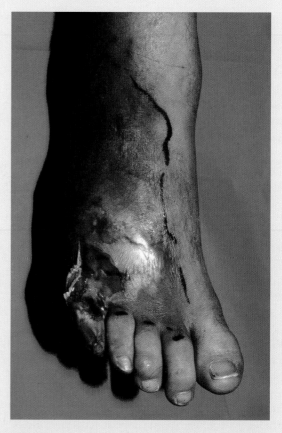

(a)

(b)

(c)

(a) Chronic penetrating ulcers in a 60-year-old man with maturity-onset diabetes. He had no evidence of major vessel disease but had signs of neuropathy. The deep ulcer beneath the head of the first metatarsal is characteristically surrounded with a thick keratin margin, and the ulcer on the medial side of the foot has an exposed tendon in its base. **(b)** This patient has a combination of neuropathy and arterial insufficiency. This foot was painless despite spreading necrosis and a collection of pus in the sole of the foot. He underwent femoro-popliteal bypass and local excision of dead tissue and healing was eventually complete. **(c)** This man of 34 presented with a neglected infection in his foot. He had severe neuropathy but no arterial disease. The entire dorsum of his foot was necrotic and he had to undergo a primary below-knee amputation. This complication would have been entirely avoidable had he sought and received treatment earlier.

antibiotics (including cover for anaerobic organisms) and frequent local cleansing and dressing.

If there is any sign of spreading infection or systemic involvement (i.e. pyrexia, tachycardia or loss of diabetic control), the patient should be admitted to hospital for more intensive treatment. This includes parenteral antibiotics, elevation, excision of any necrotic tissue and attention to blood glucose control.

REMOVAL OF NECROTIC TISSUE

Surgery may involve anything from simple **desloughing** of an ulcer to major amputation (see Fig. 41.11). If per-

formed correctly, these surgical procedures result in complete and rapid healing. If good foot care is available, it is rare that amputation of more than single toes is required. Before debridement, careful consideration needs to be given to assessing the arterial inflow and to improving it if necessary to maximise the chances of wound healing.

PREVENTION OF THE DIABETIC FOOT

All clinicians dealing with diabetics should place the highest priority on prevention. All diabetic patients should be screened for peripheral neuropathy and, for

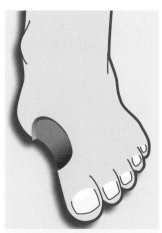
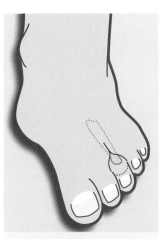
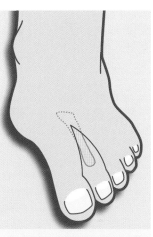
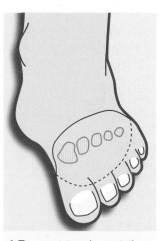

1 Excision of all necrotic tissue from ulcer, which is left to granulate

2 Digit amputation using racquet-shaped incision; toe is removed with both phalangeal bones and cartilage is nibbled from metatarsal (shaded)

3 Filleting of digit and metatarsal if infection has spread more deeply. A cake-slice is taken out of the foot and the wound left unsutured to heal by granulation (see (b))

4 Transmetatarsal amputation

(a)

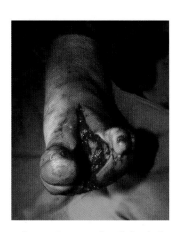

(b)

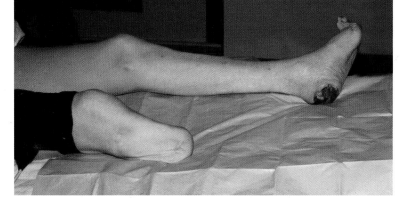

(c)

Fig. 41.11 Operations on the diabetic foot

(a) Types of local amputation. **(b)** This patient had a neuropathic ulcer and necrotic toes but no arterial disease. The second and third metatarsals have been excised, together with all the necrotic tissue, in a 'cake slice' procedure. The wound was left open to heal by secondary intention, eventually giving a remarkably good functional result. **(c)** This elderly man suffered from a combination of neuropathy and obliterative atherosclerosis. He was blind as a result of diabetic complications. The right leg was eventually amputated below knee because of spreading infection, but the left was saved by angioplasty of stenoses in the iliac and superficial femoral arteries, together with local surgery to remove necrotic tissue. Note the typical 'clawed foot' and distorted sole of motor neuropathy. Note also that the great toe has already been amputated. The heel has not yet been debrided.

those at risk, detailed advice on self-care given and high-quality chiropody provided. Careful attention should be given to footwear to correct abnormal pressure patterns. Special insoles or even special shoes may

need to be made by an orthotist or surgical fitter. Careful follow-up and regular monitoring by a diabetic specialist nurse or clinic can successfully anticipate trouble.

LOWER LIMB AMPUTATION

Where practicable, strenuous efforts should be made to preserve limbs by reconstructive surgery or interventional radiological techniques. This is because the functional results of successful revascularisation are far better than even the best major amputation. Mobility with artificial limbs is disappointing, especially in the elderly or infirm. However, amputation cannot be avoided in patients where revascularisation is technically impossible (particularly in diffuse distal arterial disease), or if there is substantial tissue necrosis and a functionally useless foot, or deep spreading infection is present.

LEVEL OF AMPUTATION

Two principles guide the level of amputation (see Fig. 41.12):

- The amputation must be made through healthy tissue. If not, there is a high risk of wound breakdown and chronic ulceration, requiring further amputation at a higher level. When amputation is for (uncorrected) peripheral ischaemia, it is almost always necessary to amputate at mid-tibial level or above to ensure healing

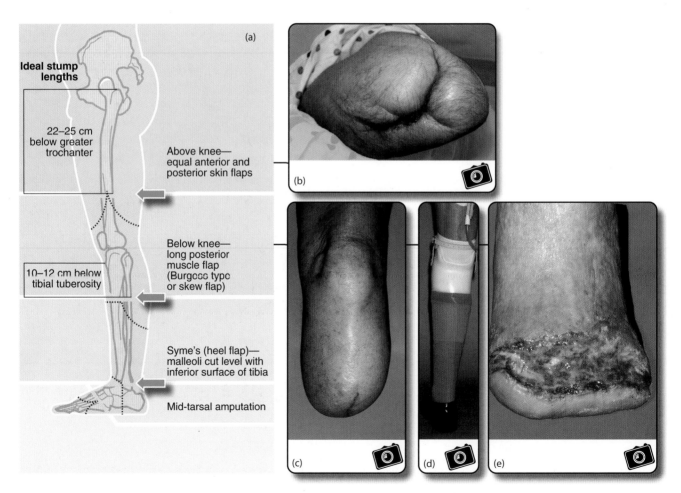

Ideal stump lengths

22–25 cm below greater trochanter

Above knee— equal anterior and posterior skin flaps

10–12 cm below tibial tuberosity

Below knee— long posterior muscle flap (Burgess type or skew flap)

Syme's (heel flap)— malleoli cut level with inferior surface of tibia

Mid-tarsal amputation

Fig. 41.12 Lower limb amputations
(a) Sites of election for lower limb amputations. **(b)** Above-knee stump in a diabetic patient. Unfortunately the original above-knee wound broke down and necrotic muscle had to be excised. The wound was left open and had nearly healed by secondary intention two months later. **(c)** A well-healed below-knee stump at 6 weeks. The operation used a long posterior muscle flap and equal length 'skew' skin flaps. **(d)** The same patient fitted with a modular below-knee prosthesis retained by a close-fitting socket and a small strap above the knee. Note the urinary catheter. **(e)** Breakdown of below-knee stump because of inadequate arterial blood supply.

● The choice of amputation level must take into account the fitting of a prosthetic limb. For this purpose, the mid-tibia (**below-knee**) and lower femoral levels (**above-knee**) are preferred. If the knee joint can be saved, the functional success of a prosthesis is much better. With improved prostheses, through-knee amputation is possible but healing rates are poor; most surgeons and prosthetists prefer above-knee to through-knee amputation; the above-knee site of election has a better healing rate and easier prosthetics than through-knee

The traditional 'guillotine' amputation of the battlefield simply sliced off the limb, leaving the wound to heal by secondary intention. This reduced the risk of fatal gas gangrene or tetanus but the outcome for fitting a prosthetic limb was poor.

There have been considerable developments in amputation techniques in recent decades, particularly in the use of **myoplastic flaps**. For below-knee amputations, a long posterior flap of muscle and skin is wrapped forward over the amputated bone and sutured in place. This results in more reliable healing and a suitably shaped and cushioned stump. A more recent variation, the Robinson '**skew flap'** technique, uses a long posterior muscle flap but equal skin flaps. The healing rate is no better but the stump is better shaped for early prosthetic fitting. With these techniques and in experienced hands, 70% or more of below-knee amputations for ischaemia will eventually heal even without revascularisation, thus preserving the knee joint. Modern below-knee prostheses are **modular** in construction and weight is borne mainly on the patellar tendon.

For above-knee amputations, myoplastic flaps are used in which the bony amputation level is proximal to the musculo-cutaneous amputation level. This allows the muscles to be sutured over the exposed bone end. The short anterior and posterior skin flaps are then closed over the muscle.

42 Aneurysms and other peripheral arterial disorders

ANEURYSMS (see Table 42.1)

PATHOLOGY

An aneurysm is defined as a localised area of pathologically excessive arterial dilatation. For the abdominal aorta, an antero-posterior (AP) diameter of 3 cm is generally accepted as defining an aneurysm. In some patients with aneurysmal disease, all the major arteries are increased in diameter (arteriomegaly) and one or more becomes truly aneurysmal. Aneurysms of the abdominal aorta and the iliac, femoral and popliteal arteries have often been labelled as complications of atherosclerosis but it is more likely that the primary disorder is **degeneration of the elastin and collagen** of the arterial wall. Atherosclerosis within aneurysms may be a less important secondary factor or it may simply be that the two pathologies share several risk factors. Aneurysms are relatively uncommon; they are found mainly in males over 70 years of age, and even less commonly in women in whom they present an average of 10 years later. At least a quarter of these patients have more than one aneurysm.

Degenerative aneurysms are usually **fusiform** in shape, slowly expanding in diameter. As the aneurysm becomes larger, the vessel wall thins, expansion accelerates and the risk of rupture increases. The majority of abdominal aortic aneurysms involve only the infrarenal aorta; some extend distally to involve one or both common iliac arteries; sometimes there are separate aneurysms of internal iliac arteries (see Fig. 42.1). A few extend proximally to become **thoraco-abdominal aneurysms**.

CLINICAL PRESENTATION OF ANEURYSMS (see Table 42.1)

Aorto-iliac aneurysms are often found **incidentally**. The patient may notice a pulsatile abdominal mass or a pulsatile mass may be discovered on abdominal examination. An aneurysm may also be noticed incidentally on radiological investigation for some other disorder—as calcification on a plain abdominal X-ray, as an obvious aneurysm on CT or, most commonly, on ultrasound scanning for obstructive urinary symptoms (see Fig. 42.2).

Despite this, nearly half of the cases that reach surgeons present because of symptoms of **leakage or rupture** into the retroperitoneal tissues. This mode of presentation carries a very high mortality. Several studies have shown that the total community and hospital mortality after rupture is more than 85% whereas elective treatment can have a mortality rate of around 5%. There is a growing recognition that **ultrasound screening** for aneurysms in older men is effective in allowing timely treatment before they rupture; national screening has now been accepted by the UK National Screening Committee

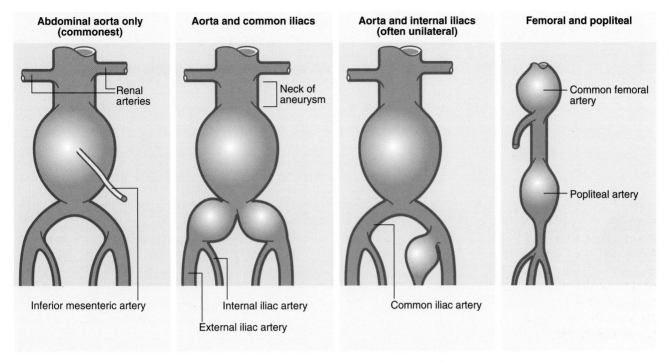

Abdominal aorta only (commonest)

Renal arteries

Inferior mesenteric artery

Aorta and common iliacs

Neck of aneurysm

Internal iliac artery

External iliac artery

Aorta and internal iliacs (often unilateral)

Common iliac artery

Femoral and popliteal

Common femoral artery

Popliteal artery

Fig. 42.1 Patterns of aneurysm formation
About 25% have more than one aneurysm either in continuity (common iliac, internal iliac, thoraco-abdominal) or not (femoral 10%; popliteal 20%; thoracic 5%). Abdominal aortic aneurysms rarely extend above the renal arteries. External iliacs are never aneurysmal.

Table 42.1 Clinical presentation and pathophysiology of aortic, iliac, femoral and popliteal aneurysms

Clinical presentation	Pathophysiology
Asymptomatic—discovered incidentally as pulsatile mass in abdomen, groin or popliteal fossa, on abdominal X-ray, CT or ultrasound scan	Progressive aneurysmal dilatation. May be self-limiting if hypertension and smoking controlled
Symptomatic—abdominal or back pain with tender aneurysm. Needs urgent surgery	Rapidly expanding aneurysms cause pressure on adjacent structures
Sudden death—acute, usually fatal, cardiovascular collapse. Often misdiagnosed as myocardial infarction	Sudden rupture of aneurysm only detected at autopsy or in the dissection room
Leaking/ruptured aneurysm—ill-defined back or abdominal pain often simulating ureteric colic or other abdominal emergency. Diagnostic if accompanied by transient collapse. Sometimes a history of recent similar episodes. Pulsatile abdominal mass palpable in 50%	Dilatation and thinning of the wall of an aneurysm leading to leakage of blood into retroperitoneal tissues—usually leads to catastrophic rupture within hours
Symptoms and signs of **acute severe leg ischaemia**; often pulsatile popliteal aneurysm on contralateral side	Sudden thrombotic occlusion of aneurysmal popliteal artery
Complete arterial occlusion—sudden distal ischaemia affecting lower limb due to embolism of thrombus from within aneurysm	Thrombotic occlusion of popliteal artery
Screening—discovered on population screening or opportunistic screening for aneurysm	

for implementation (2006). **Pain** is the most common symptom of a leaking aneurysm. The patient often gives a history of transient or more persistent **cardiovascular collapse** (fainting, hypotension) which should alert the clinician to the probable diagnosis. The clinical picture ranges from an 'acute abdomen' to abdominal or back pain of up to a week's duration and the diagnosis is usually confirmed by finding a pulsatile abdominal mass. Intraperitoneal rupture and often extraperitoneal rupture are rapidly fatal and are frequently an unrecognised cause

Fig. 42.2 Abdominal aortic aneurysm

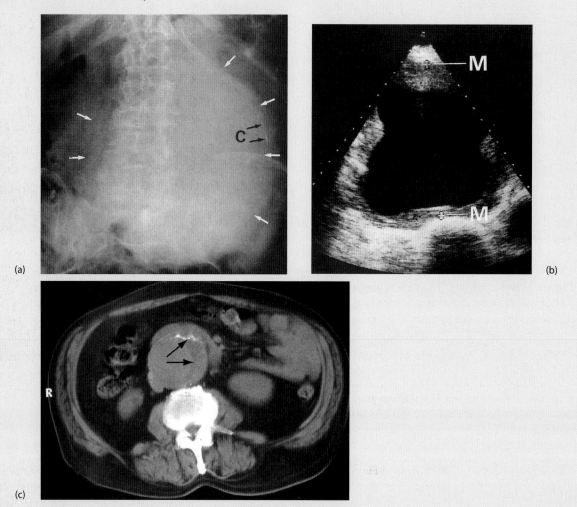

(a)

(b)

(c)

(a, b) This very obese 64-year-old man complained of continuous aching back pain for 2 weeks. **(a)** Plain abdominal X-ray showing huge abdominal aneurysm (outlined by arrows). Note calcification **C** along its left-hand aspect. **(b)** Abdominal ultrasound scan of the same patient. This shows the aneurysm is 11.5 cm in maximum antero-posterior diameter, as measured between the markers **M, M**. **(c)** CT scan of a different patient with a 6 cm AAA. The thrombus lining the wall can clearly be seen (arrowed). Calcification is visible in the anterior wall where the third part of the duodenum is closely applied to it. Rarely, a primary aorto-duodenal fistula develops at this point.

of **sudden death** in the elderly, with the cause of death often wrongly attributed to myocardial infarction.

Femoral and popliteal aneurysms are relatively uncommon and usually present as a pulsatile mass. The larger they become, the more likely complications are to ensue. Femoral aneurysms occasionally rupture causing pain and massive swelling in the groin. Popliteal aneurysms are liable to undergo thrombosis or cause embolism, causing an **acutely ischaemic leg** (see Table 40.2). In any patient presenting with an acutely ischaemic leg, it is vital to exclude this diagnosis as successful treatment often requires thrombolysis in addition to surgery. Popliteal aneurysms can also rupture and cause a variety of presentations listed in Table 40.2.

PRINCIPLES OF MANAGEMENT OF ANEURYSMS

INDICATIONS FOR OPERATION (see Box 42.1)

For **asymptomatic** aneurysms, the risk of rupture increases almost exponentially as the aneurysm dilates. Most vascular surgeons would consider operating on abdominal aortic aneurysms of 5–5.5 cm or more in diameter or those that expand more than 0.5 cm a year; 6 cm is generally considered to be critical since 40% of such aneurysms can be expected to rupture over the following 2 years.

If there are **symptoms** such as back pain or abdominal pain, or signs of tenderness that can be attributed to the

Box 42.1 **Indications for operating on abdominal aortic aneurysms**

Leaking or ruptured aneurysms—if patient's state and general fitness permit

Symptomatic aneurysms—aneurysms causing pain (particularly if tender), ureteric obstruction or embolism

Expanding aneurysms—aneurysms that enlarge at a rate of more than 0.5 cm in 1 year

Size—most arterial surgeons now recommend operation on aneurysms of 5.5 cm diameter or greater, or any saccular aneurysm

Fig. 42.3 Thoracic aneurysm

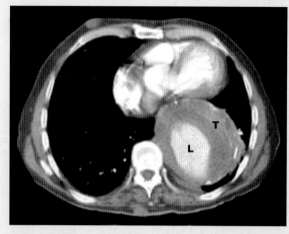

This man of 75 has had lifelong neurofibromatosis with multiple superficial lumps, particularly on the scalp. This bears no relevance to his aneurysms. Eight years before this scan, he had an emergency grafting of his ruptured abdominal aortic aneurysm. This thoracic aneurysm was discovered on a regular follow-up chest X-ray. This transverse CT scan shows a huge aneurysm of the descending thoracic aorta. The lumen L is filled with blood but the sac is lined with laminated thrombus T. This aneurysm was successfully treated with a stent graft.

aneurysm, imminent rupture must be assumed and urgent operation performed.

A **leaking or ruptured** abdominal aortic aneurysm (AAA) is a surgical emergency. Less than half the patients reach hospital alive, and only about half of these survive. The majority of patients die of shock before reaching the operating theatre or else of myocardial infarction or acute renal failure after operation. The true mortality of rupture is thus more than 85%. On the other hand, the mortality after elective operation or endovascular repair (EVAR, see p. 602) for aneurysm can be less than 5%. Thus, the decision to operate electively on a known aneurysm depends on the estimated risk of rupture. Indications for operation are summarised in Box 42.1.

INVESTIGATION OF ANEURYSM (see Fig. 42.2)

Non-ruptured AAA

For asymptomatic aneurysms considered too small to warrant operation, ultrasonography is used for periodic **monitoring**, with referral to a surgeon once the size reaches an index diameter (usually 5 or 5.5 cm) or is seen to expand more than 0.5 cm in a year.

Where elective operation is planned, CT scanning is often used to show the relationship of the aneurysm to the renal arteries; the 5% of cases where the aneurysm extends above the renal arteries require a **thoraco-abdominal** operative approach and the operation carries a greater risk. CT can also show if iliac arteries are aneurysmal and if the aneurysm is **inflammatory** (i.e. has a thick layer of inflammatory tissue on its anterior surface that makes surgery technically difficult). Representative CT slices are usually taken through the chest to ensure the thoracic aorta is not aneurysmal (Fig. 42.3); if there is a **thoracic aneurysm**, the management plan will have to accommodate it, according to size and position. If an aneurysm patient requiring surgery also has evidence of lower limb **ischaemia**, some form of arteriography is usually necessary in case a combined reconstruction is required.

Leaking or ruptured AAA

Any patient with a suspected leaking or ruptured AAA should be treated as a true surgical emergency but not necessarily by immediate transfer to the nearest operating theatre. There is good evidence that the survival rate increases when ruptured AAAs are treated by a specialist team of surgeons and anaesthetists, and this may mean transfer to a different centre. Over-aggressive blood pressure resuscitation of the hypotensive patient may convert a stable contained leak into a free rupture, and many clinicians support the use of **permissive hypotension** to facilitate transfer (see Ch. 15), i.e. not treating relative hypotension whilst the patient remains conscious and free from cardiac symptoms. The principle of permissive hypotension has increased the time available for transfer and/or further investigation.

Provided the patient with a leaking AAA is not demonstrating signs of cardiovascular instability, a CT scan can be valuable in helping to plan treatment. CT can demonstrate the relationship of the aneurysm to the renal and visceral arteries and show any secondary iliac aneurysms; sometimes other abdominal pathology is shown that influences the decision to operate, e.g. liver metastases. In units equipped to undertake emergency endovascular repair (EVAR, see below), CT can show whether this is practicable in a particular individual.

Table 42.2 Comparison of conventional and endovascular therapy for aortic aneurysm

	Conventional surgery	Endovascular therapy
Mortality related to procedure	Approximately 5%	1.7%
Length of hospital stay	7–10 days	2–4 days
ITU/HDU care needed	Likely	Unlikely
Overall cost	£6500	£8000
Anatomical constraints	Distance between AAA and renal arteries can be less than 15 mm	Needs 15 mm of relatively normal aorta below renals
Past medical history	More difficult with previous surgery or peritonitis	Unaffected by previous abdominal surgery
Follow-up	Discharge at 3 months. Rescan after 5–7 years. Reintervention unlikely	Frequent CT and ultrasound for life. Reintervention rates high but improving

PRINCIPLES OF ANEURYSM SURGERY

The dilated aneurysmal segment is surgically corrected by means of a graft. Most patients currently undergo open surgery, but minimally invasive stent-graft placement (endovascular repair, EVAR) via the femoral artery is becoming an option for a proportion of aorto-iliac aneurysms. The indications and relative merits of each technique are shown in Table 42.2. **Tube grafts** or **bifurcation grafts** of synthetic material (usually Dacron) are used for aorto-iliac and femoral aneurysms, whilst **autogenous saphenous vein** is preferred for popliteal aneurysms.

Open abdominal aortic aneurysm surgery (Fig. 42.4)

For abdominal aneurysms, the standard open approach is a long midline or a transverse abdominal incision. The aorta is usually reached via the peritoneal cavity or sometimes via an extraperitoneal approach. The patient is usually anticoagulated peroperatively with intravenous heparin to prevent distal thrombosis, and the iliac arteries and the infrarenal aorta are clamped (see Fig. 42.5). The aneurysm is incised longitudinally and any clot within it removed. Bleeding lumbar arteries opening into the posterior aortic wall are closed with sutures.

The graft is sutured within the aneurysmal sac at the proximal end, and within the sac or more distally at the distal end. The aneurysm sac is left in situ and later closed around the graft. This technique is known as **inlay grafting**: it allows separation of the graft from the intestine, reducing the risk of an aorto-intestinal fistula arising later from the graft anastomoses. Proximally, the graft is sutured just above the upper limit of the aneurysm to (relatively) normal aortic wall. Placement of the distal end depends on the extent of the aneurysm. It may be located within the aorta near its bifurcation, in which case a straight tube graft is used (most commonly), or more distally to iliac vessels. In this case a bifurcation graft ('trouser graft') is necessary.

Endovascular aneurysm repair (see Fig. 42.6)

Endovascular aneurysm repair (EVAR) is a minimally invasive surgical technique employing combined stent-grafts. In the UK, NICE has approved the technique but has recommended that clinicians ensure patients fully understand the long-term uncertainties and potential complications associated with the procedure, including the risk of endovascular leaks, the possibility of secondary intervention and the need for lifelong follow-up.

Most cases are undertaken under general anaesthesia but many can be done under local anaesthesia. The procedure can be performed in a normal operating theatre using a mobile X-ray image intensifier or in a specialist endovascular suite. The **stent-graft** consists of a self-expanding metal framework with a non-porous cloth covering; it is supplied in a constrained state and measures around 8 mm in diameter. When in situ, the main body of the device resembles a pair of trousers with one leg cut off.

Two short transverse incisions are used to access the common femoral arteries in the groin. The main device is passed into one femoral artery and guided proximally using radiological guidance to its position below the renal arteries. An angiogram is performed to check that the device can release below the renals. The constraining mechanism is then removed and the stent opens up and expands against the vessel wall. An approach is then made via the contralateral femoral artery; a guide-wire is passed proximally to enter the main graft body through the short 'cut-off' leg. The second limb of the stent-graft is then completed by passing a covered stent over the guide-wire and securing it into the main body of the graft and the iliac artery. After completion, the device looks

Fig. 42.4 Abdominal aortic aneurysm

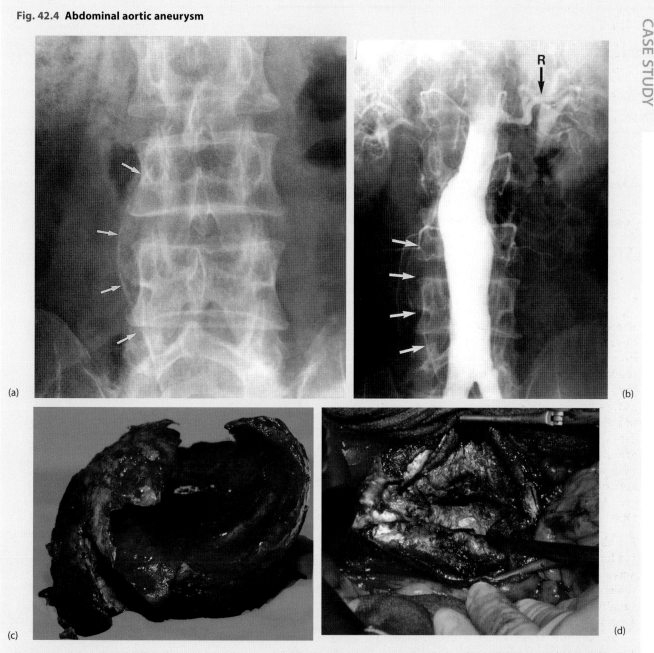

(a)

(b)

(c)

(d)

(a–c) A 70-year-old asymptomatic man in whom a pulsatile abdominal mass was an incidental finding. (a) Plain antero-posterior abdominal X-ray showing a mildly radiopaque mass in the midline with a line of calcification down its right-hand margin (arrowed). (b) Arteriogram from the same patient showing fusiform dilatation of the aorta beginning 2.5 cm below the origins of the renal arteries **R**. Note the calcification (arrowed) in the outer wall corresponding to that in (a); the space between this and the lumen of the aneurysm consists of old lamellated thrombus. (c) This cast of thrombus was removed from within the aortic aneurysm at operation; note the false lumen and concentric lamellae of thrombus progressively laid down as the aneurysm expanded over many months. (d) This shows the aneurysm sac opened at operation on a different patient who had complained of chronic back pain. The posterior wall of the aorta is completely deficient in part and the anterior longitudinal ligament is visible in its base.

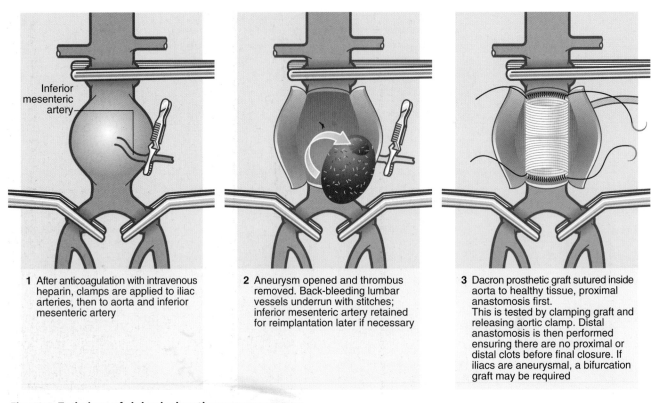

1 After anticoagulation with intravenous heparin, clamps are applied to iliac arteries, then to aorta and inferior mesenteric artery

2 Aneurysm opened and thrombus removed. Back-bleeding lumbar vessels underrun with stitches; inferior mesenteric artery retained for reimplantation later if necessary

3 Dacron prosthetic graft sutured inside aorta to healthy tissue, proximal anastomosis first.
This is tested by clamping graft and releasing aortic clamp. Distal anastomosis is then performed ensuring there are no proximal or distal clots before final closure. If iliacs are aneurysmal, a bifurcation graft may be required

Fig. 42.5 Technique of abdominal aortic aneurysm surgery

like a complete pair of trousers and extends from the renal arteries to the common iliacs.

Other applications of EVAR
Open surgical repair of **thoracic aneurysms** carries a mortality of 10–20% and a high morbidity but many can be repaired by EVAR using just two small groin incisions.

Even **ruptured aneurysms** (abdominal or thoracic) can sometimes be repaired using this technique, often using local anaesthesia. **Traumatic aortic transsections** have also been successfully treated with endovascular therapy. Advances continue to be made in EVAR technology so that more complex cases can be managed via the endovascular route.

UPER LIMB PROBLEMS (see Table 40.5, p. 572)

UPPER LIMB ISCHAEMIA

Ischaemia of the upper limb is rare. This is both because atherosclerosis is uncommon in the arteries supplying the upper limb and also because there is a rich collateral blood supply via the scapular anastomoses that can bypass occlusive disease of the subclavian artery. Upper limb ischaemia usually occurs when the subclavian artery is compressed at the thoracic outlet or when emboli obstruct the brachial or more distal arteries. Occasionally, vasospastic disorders such as severe Raynaud's disease cause digital ischaemia. Embolic disease has similar causes, presentation and treatment as embolism affecting the lower limbs (see Ch. 41).

THORACIC OUTLET COMPRESSION

The subclavian artery and vein and the brachial plexus pass through the space between the first rib and the clavicle. If this space becomes unduly narrow, neurological or arterial symptoms may appear; either of these can be part of the **thoracic outlet syndrome**. Neurological symptoms are much more frequent than arterial symptoms but either variety of thoracic outlet syndrome is rare. Congenital causes include upward pressure exerted by a **cervical rib** that lies above the first rib, or by fibrous bands (Fig. 42.7). The gap may be encroached upon by acquired causes including a healed clavicular fracture, excess muscle development or other unknown means.

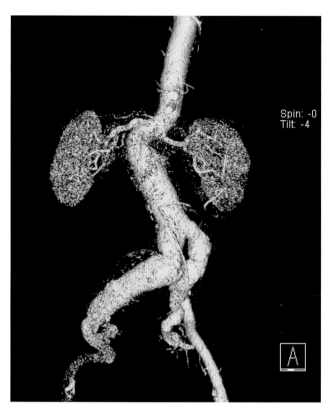

(a) Pre-procedure CT scan showing lumen of aorto-iliac aneurysm, suprarenal aorta and kidneys. On this view, the much larger diameter of the aneurysmal aortic wall is not visible.

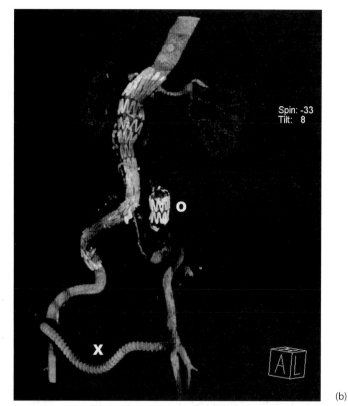

(b) Post-procedure CT scan showing the stent-graft in position extending from the right common iliac to just above the renal arteries. In this case, there were technical problems placing a bifurcation graft and so the left common iliac origin was deliberately blocked with an occluding stent **O** and the left lower limb was revascularised with a crossover femoro-femoral graft **X**.

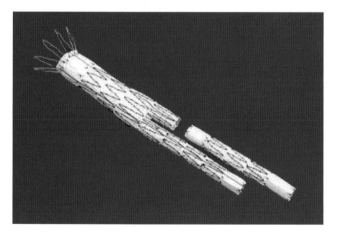

(c) Typical two-piece stent graft. Note the body and one limb are in one piece and the other limb is fitted afterwards. Note also the retaining wires at the proximal end.

Fig. 42.6 Endovascular aneurysm repair

Neurological symptoms of thoracic outlet syndrome usually cause deficits in the T1 nerve root distribution (wasting and weakness of small muscles of hand; paraesthesia of inner forearm and hand). Symptoms of arterial compression include upper limb 'claudication' in people who habitually work with their arms above their heads, as the artery becomes further compressed in this posture.

In longstanding cases of subclavian artery compression, the artery beyond the stenosis often becomes dilated into an aneurysm (**post-stenotic dilatation**) which may collect thrombus. This may later embolise into the brachial artery causing acute ischaemia.

Occasionally the diagnosis of arterial compression is made by finding a lower blood pressure in the affected

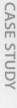
Fig. 42.7 Cervical rib causing subclavian artery compression

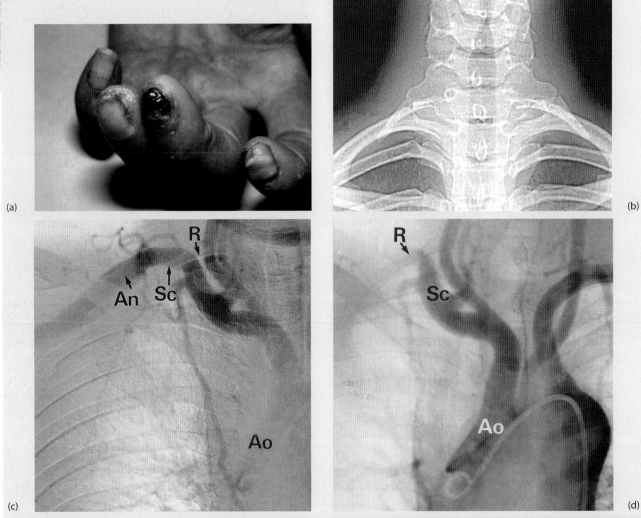

(a) This 65-year-old butcher complained of a sudden onset of extreme pallor, coldness, weakness and paraesthesia in his right hand and forearm when handling meat in the cold room. **(b)** Plain X-ray of thoracic outlet showing bilateral cervical ribs. **(c, d)** Arch arteriography. **(c)** With the shoulder adducted, there is normal blood flow through the subclavian artery **Sc**. Note the presence of a cervical rib **R** and dilatation of the subclavian artery just distal to it. This was a post-stenotic aneurysm **An** containing thrombus, which gave rise to distal embolism. The aorta is labelled **Ao**. **(d)** With the shoulder abducted and externally rotated ('the army saluting position'), subclavian blood flow is completely obstructed by the cervical rib; note the 'pigtail' arteriogram catheter in the aorta **Ao**.

arm which varies with arm posture; obstruction can be confirmed by arteriography. Most cases, however, are not so straightforward. Overall, the diagnosis of thoracic outlet syndromes is difficult and is best performed in specialist centres with appropriate input from neurologists, surgeons, radiologists and physiotherapists.

Operative intervention is becoming less common as conservative management improves. If indicated, treatment is by excision of a cervical rib if present or else excision of the first rib, together with division of any obstructing bands. A post-stenotic subclavian aneurysm should be resected and replaced with a graft.

SUBCLAVIAN STEAL SYNDROME

This unusual syndrome is caused by obstruction of the subclavian artery proximal to the origin of the vertebral artery. In consequence the subclavian is fed by retrograde flow from the vertebral artery via the carotids and circle of Willis. This situation remains tenable and asymptomatic until there is excessive demand by the upper limb. At that point, blood becomes diverted ('stolen') from the cerebral circulation causing transient cerebral ischaemia. Figure 42.8 illustrates a classic example. Treatment is to bypass the obstruction with a graft.

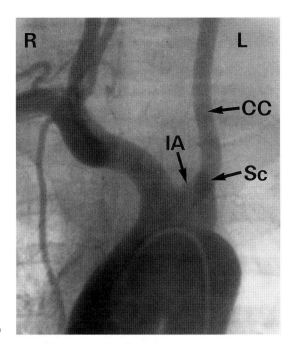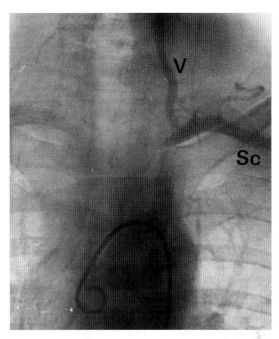

(a)

(b)

Fig. 42.8 Subclavian steal syndrome

Subtraction angiograms from a 55-year-old house-painter who complained of dizziness when painting walls and ceilings. **(a)** Aortic arch (with 'pigtail' arteriogram catheter visible) showing normal right innominate artery with its subclavian and common carotid branches. On the left, the arterial anatomy is anomalous, with the common carotid **CC** arising from a left innominate artery **IA** rather than direct from the aorta. The left subclavian artery **Sc** appears to be occluded beyond a short stump. **(b)** X-ray exposure taken 4 seconds later; the aortic arch and its branches are now clear of contrast, but contrast has appeared in the left vertebral artery **V**, flowing downwards from the circle of Willis. This has flowed onwards to fill the left subclavian artery **Sc** retrogradely. Thus there is complete obstruction of a segment of the left subclavian artery proximal to the origin of the vertebral artery, and the vertebral artery now supplies the left upper limb at the expense of the cerebral circulation. The results in episodes of transient cerebral ischaemia at times of high vascular demand from the left upper limb.

EXTRACRANIAL CEREBRAL ARTERIAL INSUFFICIENCY

Strokes are common world-wide and about 1 million strokes occur each year in the UK. Extracranial atherosclerosis is common and is probably responsible for about a quarter of all strokes. The **common carotid bifurcation** is the area most affected by atherosclerosis, although obstructive disease often affects the distal internal carotid in the **carotid siphon**. The vertebral arteries are the next most commonly affected extracranial arteries. Less frequently, the orifices of the **great vessels** become obstructed where they branch from the aortic arch.

Atherosclerotic carotid stenosis is an important cause of stroke, and strokes are often heralded by a transient ischaemic attack (TIA) or a minor stroke. This recovers spontaneously without serious disability but the risk of recurrent stroke in recently symptomatic patients like this with severe carotid stenosis is as high as 28% over the course of the next two years.

CAROTID ARTERY INSUFFICIENCY

PATHOPHYSIOLOGY OF CAROTID ARTERY DISEASE

Carotid artery disease often results in **stenosis**, with cerebral blood flow becoming impaired when luminal narrowing exceeds about 70% (Fig. 42.9). Cerebral autoregulation of blood flow is able to compensate up to this degree of stenosis. Rough atherosclerotic plaques without gross narrowing may also be the source of **platelet emboli**. Small emboli may cause **transient ischaemic attacks** (including transient blindness, known as **amaurosis fugax**), with symptoms lasting for less than 24 hours. In contrast, large emboli or embolism into critical areas cause major strokes. **Asymptomatic** stenoses may be discovered on investigation of **carotid bruits** or as part of general investigation before major arterial surgery elsewhere in the body.

Fig. 42.9 Carotid artery disease

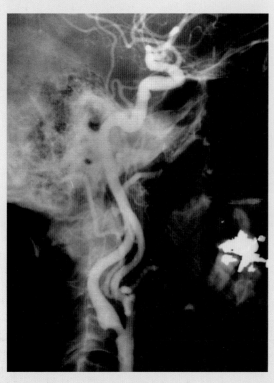
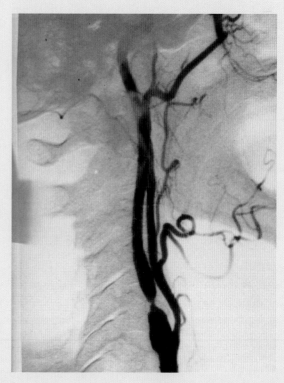

(a)

(b)

(a) This 71-year-old man suffered two transient episodes of left hemiparesis in one week ('TIAs'). Carotid angiography shows a localised 50% stenosis of the internal carotid artery just distal to the common carotid bifurcation; this degree of stenosis alone would not explain the symptoms. Note the typical post-stenotic dilatation immediately beyond the stenosis. The rest of the cerebral arterial system appears normal. At operation, an ulcerated atheromatous plaque was found, which was undoubtedly the source of emboli that caused the transient ischaemic attacks. Endarterectomy was performed and the patient has been entirely well since. Studies in the USA and Europe have shown surgery is definitely better than medical management in patients with a 70% or greater stenosis. **(b)** Subtraction film from a carotid angiogram in a different patient. This shows a 90% stenosis in the internal carotid artery which is haemodynamically significant, causing cerebral ischaemia.

INVESTIGATION OF SUSPECTED CAROTID ARTERY DISEASE

A minority of patients suffering transient ischaemic attacks or stroke are found to have a **bruit** on auscultation of the carotid arteries. However, this finding does not indicate the degree of narrowing; a significant stenosis may be silent, as of course is complete occlusion.

Patients with strokes, transient ischaemic attacks and asymptomatic carotid bruits should initially be investigated urgently for carotid stenosis by non-invasive means, ideally in a dedicated clinic. The preferred method is **duplex Doppler scanning**, an ultrasound technique which allows simultaneous imaging of the carotid arteries and measurement of blood flow velocity. The measured rise in velocity allows the degree of stenosis to be estimated. If there is a high-grade stenosis in symptomatic disease (i.e. over 70%), surgical intervention is the treatment of choice. With skilled duplex examination, many surgeons feel that conventional **carotid angiography** that was once the standard investigation is no longer necessary

or desirable, particularly as this invasive technique carries a definite risk of stroke. Some centres now use magnetic resonance angiography as a less invasive form of imaging but it can overestimate the degree of stenosis.

TREATMENT OF CAROTID ARTERY DISEASE

Medical versus surgical or radiological intervention

The choice of treatment for symptomatic carotid artery stenosis consists of **medical** anti-platelet therapy (with aspirin 75–150 mg or clopidogrel 75 mg daily), surgical **endarterectomy** (i.e. removing the obstructing disease and thrombus) or, latterly, minimally invasive **stenting**. Carotid endarterectomy enjoyed an enormous uncontrolled vogue in the 1970s and 1980s for treating transient ischaemic attacks, completed stroke and asymptomatic carotid stenosis, particularly in the USA, but the role of surgery became much clearer after publication of major randomised studies from Europe and the USA in 1998. These scientific comparative studies showed that surgery reduced the stroke rate more than medical therapy only in patients with carotid stenosis of greater than 70%. In such high-grade stenoses, surgery reduced the annual stroke rate from about 6% in the medically treated group to about 1.5%. However, the trials also showed a substantial risk of stroke or death resulting from surgery of between 6 and 8%. Recent work suggests that patients with 50% or greater stenosis may benefit from surgery. Certainly, for patients suffering repeated symptoms but with lower levels of stenosis, cogent arguments can be made for intervention.

Unfortunately, surgery does not reduce the long-term mortality from carotid artery disease even in high-grade stenosis. The mortality rate of about 5% per annum over 5 years is comparable in medically and surgically treated patients, taking the operative mortality of 2–3% into account.

Acute symptoms

There is an increasing body of evidence that any symptoms referable to potential carotid disease, even a minor TIA, should be investigated as an emergency. This is because carotid endarterectomy is effective at preventing threatened future strokes if performed within 2 weeks of the herald symptoms. This benefit halves if patients are left untreated for 6 weeks or longer.

Asymptomatic carotid stenosis

The role of surgery in the treatment of patients with **asymptomatic** carotid disease remains controversial. Recent trials indicate that even in the hands of surgeons with low complication rates, 15 asymptomatic carotid stenoses need to be treated to prevent a single stroke. The comparable figure for symptomatic disease is about 6 operations.

Technique of endarterectomy

Currently, about 2000 carotid endarterectomies are performed annually in the UK. At present, seven males are treated for stenosis for every three females. The usual operation is **endarterectomy**. The operation may be under general or local anaesthesia. The carotid bifurcation is incised lon-gitudinally after clamping the carotid arteries and anticoagulating the patient. A temporary **shunt** is commonly used to maintain cerebral perfusion; this involves inserting one end of a tube into the common carotid below the stenosis and the other into the internal carotid above the stenosis, bypassing the operation site. The stenotic plaque is then dissected out and the carotid closed by direct suture (if the artery is large) or patched using vein or synthetic material sutured into the wall to maintain the diameter. Carotid surgery carries an appreciable risk of mortality or cerebral complications such as stroke (around 3–5%) which needs to be taken into account when auditing individual departmental results and when comparing groups of patients treated medically and surgically.

Carotid angioplasty and stenting

Angioplasty with or without stenting is well established for treating peripheral and coronary artery disease but is relatively novel for carotid stenosis. Potential advantages include the lack of a neck incision, lower rates of haematoma formation and cranial nerve damage, and shorter hospital stays, but **disadvantages** include the risk of embolism during the procedure and possibly a higher rate of late restenosis. In a randomised trial comparing **angioplasty** and surgery, the 30-day outcome was the same, with a death or stroke rate of 10%. Three-year follow-up suggested both treatments were equally effective for preventing stroke. A new trial, the International Carotid Stenting Study (ICSS), is currently under way to examine **angioplasty plus stenting**.

The technique of carotid stenting involves passing a guide-wire from the femoral artery to the area of stenosis in the carotid artery. A filter or basket at the end of the guide-wire is opened like an umbrella to catch debris to prevent it embolising to the brain and causing a stroke. A balloon-tipped catheter is then fed over the guide-wire to the target area and inflated to a high pressure to compress the plaque into the wall of the artery. The balloon is withdrawn and a self-expanding stent is guided to the area and released. The filter and balloon catheter are finally removed.

ARTERIAL INSUFFICIENCY IN OTHER ORGANS

MESENTERIC ISCHAEMIA

Blood supply to portions of the bowel may be compromised in four main ways:

- **Strangulation**. This is a mechanical problem presenting as bowel obstruction and is described in detail in Chapter 19. It may be the result of a **hernia** (see Ch. 32), **volvulus** of small or large bowel or **fibrous bands** resulting from previous surgery (see Ch. 12)

- **Acute thrombotic or embolic obstruction** (Fig. 42.10). This is analogous to acute thrombosis or embolism of the lower limb as described in Chapter 41. The cause is usually superior mesenteric artery occlusion and the condition presents as an 'acute abdomen' (see Ch. 19)
- **Transient ischaemia**. This presents as inflammation of the bowel characterised by abdominal pain and rectal bleeding. The condition is known as **ischaemic colitis** and is discussed at the end of Chapter 29
- **Chronic mesenteric artery insufficiency**. This rare condition presents with gross weight loss and

Fig. 42.10 Acute mesenteric ischaemia

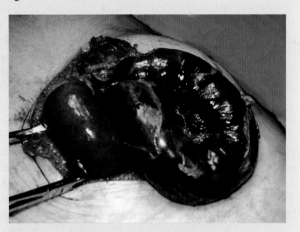

This woman of 77 presented with moderate abdominal pain and circulatory collapse requiring vigorous resuscitation. She was in atrial fibrillation and was acidotic. Mesenteric embolism was suspected and was confirmed at operation. Unfortunately, as often happens, the entire mid-gut territory, between 20 cm along the jejunum to the mid-transverse colon was necrotic and no beneficial procedure was possible.

abdominal pain following eating; it is analogous to intermittent claudication due to arterial insufficiency in the lower limb and is described in the next section

Chronic mesenteric ischaemia

The rare condition of chronic mesenteric ischaemia or 'gut claudication' occurs when the visceral blood supply is restricted to a point where it remains adequate at rest but becomes inadequate during active digestion. This occurs when there is gross atherosclerotic narrowing of all three main mesenteric vessels (coeliac, superior mesenteric and inferior mesenteric arteries). These patients present with severe epigastric pain on eating which causes

'fear of food'. There is always **gross weight loss** and sometimes an epigastric bruit can be heard on auscultation.

Diagnosis is by arteriography with lateral views allowing the origins of the three main vessels to be seen. Treatment is by surgical reconstruction of the origins of one or more mesenteric arteries.

RENAL ISCHAEMIA

RENAL ARTERY STENOSIS

Pathophysiology of renal artery stenosis

This relatively uncommon condition arises in two main ways. In children and young adults, the cause is **fibromuscular hyperplasia**. In older patients, **atherosclerosis** is the usual cause. Renal artery stenosis may present with hypertension (ischaemia of one or both kidneys causes poor perfusion, thus activating the renin–angiotensin system) or functional renal impairment. It is sometimes discovered incidentally on urography as a non-functioning or poorly functioning kidney.

Fibromuscular hyperplasia responds well to balloon dilatation, which often results in the blood pressure returning to normal. Atherosclerosis may be treatable by balloon angioplasty or reconstructive surgery but the effect on hypertension is unpredictable; renal function, however, may improve, particularly in patients with a short history of hypertension or if the renal artery stenosis is bilateral.

It is important that renal artery stenosis is recognised in patients needing aortic reconstructive surgery, whether for occlusive or aneurysmal disease. This is because hypotension during the operation may initiate thrombotic occlusion of narrowed renal arteries and cause postoperative renal failure. Renal artery stenosis may need to be treated before operation by balloon dilatation, or by reconstruction at the same time as the aortic operation.

COMPLICATIONS OF ARTERIAL SURGERY

The specific complications of arterial surgery are summarised in Box 41.2 (p. 589) and discussed in detail below. Local complications include **haemorrhage**, **embolism**, **thrombosis**, **graft infection** and **false aneurysm** formation.

SYSTEMIC COMPLICATIONS OF ARTERIAL SURGERY

Patients undergoing arterial surgery are subject to all the usual complications of major surgery. In addition, they invariably have **generalised atherosclerotic arteriopathy** to a greater or lesser degree, rendering them vulnerable to serious or fatal cardiovascular complications during

the perioperative period. Patients with obliterative disease are more likely to have serious cardiac disease than those with aneurysms. For aortic and other major arterial operations, prolonged general anaesthesia, **aortic clamping** and heavy operative blood loss place extra stress on a compromised cardiovascular system.

Common systemic perioperative complications of arterial surgery include myocardial infarction, cardiac failure, acute arrhythmias, strokes, renal failure and intestinal ischaemia. To minimise the risk of these complications, preparation for elective arterial surgery must include thorough preoperative cardiovascular assessment and sometimes treatment of cardiac abnormalities. Any preexisting medical condition such as cardiac failure or

Fig. 42.11 Late formation of new aneurysm after aneurysm surgery

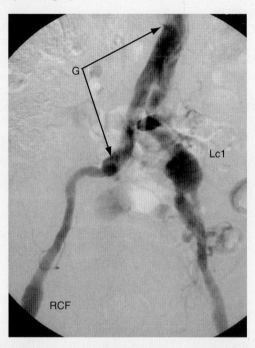

This arteriogram was performed for claudication 10 years after a trouser or 'Y' graft for abdominal aortic aneurysm. The trouser graft **G** is opacified and a new aneurysm has appeared in the left common iliac artery **LCI** beyond the graft. A small aneurysm is also seen in the right common femoral **RCF**. Neither was large enough to require surgery but periodic follow-up was continued using ultrasound. Obliterative disease responsible for the claudication was found in the superficial femoral arteries distal to this film.

hypertension should be stabilised under expert advice. Patients also require intensive monitoring both during and after operation. Peroperatively, this usually includes central venous and peripheral arterial catheterisation for accurate pressure measurements. For patients with severe myocardial disease, trans-oesophageal ultrasound helps estimate cardiac output and guide fluid replacement. These and other high-risk patients should be closely monitored during the early postoperative period in an intensive care or high-dependency unit so that complications can be recognised and treated early.

LOCAL COMPLICATIONS OF ARTERIAL SURGERY (Fig. 42.12)

HAEMORRHAGE

During surgical access to the affected arteries, nearby veins are vulnerable to tearing even when great care is taken in dissection. For example, iliac veins cross deep to the iliac arteries and are often adherent to them. Venous tears are more alarming than arterial ones because veins are very thin-walled and friable and difficult to repair. They are often inaccessible and thus lacerations can be difficult to identify and control; such tears usually result in massive blood loss.

Completing a satisfactory arterial anastomosis is demanding under the best of conditions, but it is made even more difficult if there are friable diseased vessels and calcified atherosclerotic plaques, as is so often the case. In the high-pressure arterial system, any defect is quickly revealed and blood sprays everywhere once clamps are released. Fortunately the arterial system can be remarkably forgiving and small leaks are quickly plugged by platelets if swabs are held in place for a few minutes. If blood loss is massive (10–25 units), platelets and coagulation factors are consumed and haemostasis is progressively impaired (**consumption coagulopathy**). Standard blood transfusions are of little help except as volume replacement, since stored blood lacks functioning platelets and clotting factors. In this deteriorating situation (and preferably in anticipation of it), infusing **platelet concentrates** and **fresh-frozen plasma** provides the main answer. In situations where bleeding is difficult to control by sutures or packing, one of several different **organic-based glues** can be helpful in sealing bleeding areas. Patients are usually heparinised peroperatively before the arteries are clamped to prevent distal thrombosis. This does not usually cause a problem with haemostasis later, but if necessary the effect can be reversed by injecting **protamine**.

There is a growing trend for the regular use of **cell-saving devices** intraoperatively to cope with anticipated heavy blood loss. These enable the patient's spilled blood to be collected, washed, concentrated and reinfused, minimising the use of stored blood. Unfortunately, clotting factors are lost in the process.

Early postoperative haemorrhage is uncommon, provided adequate haemostasis is achieved before completing the operation and closing the wound. When bleeding does occur, it usually results from a pinhole leak at the anastomosis or a slipped ligature. Haemorrhage is manifest by generalised signs of **hypovolaemia**, by progressive abdominal distension or, in the lower limb, by swelling beneath the wound. Postoperative haemorrhage occasionally stops spontaneously following transfusion of blood and clotting factors, but if blood loss continues, further operation must not be delayed.

EMBOLISM

In aneurysm surgery, embolism is usually caused by dislodging fresh or organised thrombus from within the aneurysmal sac. It is largely preventable by clamping the outflow vessels before the aneurysm is manipulated. Large emboli that lodge in femoral vessels can be retrieved

CASE STUDY

Fig. 42.12 Complication of arterial surgery

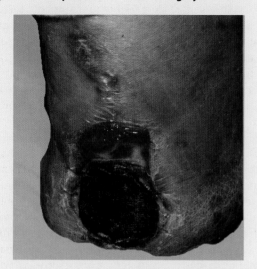

This patient was admitted to hospital with a ruptured aneurysm. He suffered arterial thrombosis of the lower limb during operation, and a thrombectomy to relieve it left him with an ischaemic foot. Poor attention to heel pressure relief during the early postoperative period led to this heel necrosis, which took several months to heal.

with a Fogarty balloon catheter, but the more common case of fragmented distal embolism may cause infarction of digits or even the whole foot ('**trash foot**'). Infarction caused by this distal embolism is irreversible and usually necessitates some form of amputation later. If the embolisation occurs during **carotid** artery dissection under general anaesthesia, the event is not usually apparent until the patient wakes up and is found to have suffered a stroke. Under local anaesthesia, embolic events may be immediately detectable.

THROMBOSIS

Thrombosis of the reconstructed vessels is a major potential problem in arterial surgery. It rapidly leads to profound distal ischaemia and results in loss of the limb unless urgently corrected.

Sluggish flow leads to thrombosis and may arise for a variety of technical reasons as follows:

- Unrecognised arterial stenosis or occlusion proximal or distal to the reconstruction causing poor inflow or runoff
- Faulty anastomotic technique causing stenosis or partial luminal obstruction
- Dissection of the layers of the distal vessel wall resulting in a loose flap of tunica intima and media which acts as a 'flap valve' occluding the lumen
- Twisting or kinking of a graft
- In situ thrombosis during arterial clamping

Thrombosis usually occurs in the first few hours after operation and becomes manifest by deterioration in the colour, temperature and pulses of the affected limb from the satisfactory state initially achieved at operation. Urgent reoperation is usually required. The judicious use of preoperative anti-platelet agents and/or inhibitors of the coagulation system can help prevent this complication. It is good practice to spend spend time at the end of the operation ensuring satisfactory flow in the reconstruction and good peripheral perfusion, as well as securing haemostasis. This can avoid the need for reoperation to deal with a thrombosed graft or to arrest haemorrhage in the middle of the night.

GRAFT INFECTION

Infection of a synthetic graft is uncommon but can be a devastating complication. It may occur in the early postoperative period or at any time months or years later. The infecting organisms are usually from the patient's own intestine. Infection is minimised by avoiding opening bowel, meticulous asepsis and haemostasis, and perioperative antibiotic cover. Antibiotics are normally given intravenously at anaesthetic induction and over the first 24 hours postoperatively. A cephalosporin (e.g. cefotaxime or cefuroxime), or a combination of gentamicin and flucloxacillin is usually suitable; where MRSA is prevalent, specific agents such as vancomycin are routinely employed as well. In addition, protein-coated Dacron grafts can be soaked in an anti-staphylococcal antibiotic before placement, e.g. rifampicin.

Graft infection should be suspected if there is recurrent pyrexia and malaise or a persistently discharging wound sinus; occasionally, the wound breaks down, exposing the infected graft. Major graft infection, particularly when involving an anastomosis, has a bleak prognosis even when treated, the eventual outcome often being death from sepsis or anastomotic breakdown with catastrophic bleeding. Standard treatment is to restore the distal circulation with an **extra-anatomic graft** (e.g. axillo-bifemoral) which bypasses the infected area, and remove the infected graft. In early graft infection without anastomotic breakdown, prolonged graft irrigation with antibiotics can be successful on its own.

FALSE ANEURYSM FORMATION

A false aneurysm is the result of a slow anastomotic leak or a leak from an arterial puncture (e.g. for coronary artery stenting) that is confined by surrounding tissues. A slowly expanding blood-filled cavity results, which eventually ruptures or undergoes thrombosis. A false aneurysm usually presents as a palpable pulsatile mass. Occasionally a false aneurysm at an upper anastomosis of a graft with the abdominal aorta leaks into the overlying duodenum. This produces an **aorto-duodenal fistula** and presents with major haematemesis. Aorto-duodenal fistula may also result from graft infection. False aneurysms were formerly much more common because of the gradual breakdown of the silk suture materials used at the time, but suture durability has greatly improved since the introduction of polyester and polypropylene sutures.

LONG-TERM FOLLOW-UP AFTER ARTERIAL SURGERY

All patients with obliterative atherosclerotic disease are liable to progression of the disease and new ischaemic events. In fact, the risk of sudden cardiovascular death in patients with claudication is the same as that of a patient who has suffered a non-fatal myocardial infarction! All patients should be on 'best medical treatment' for atherosclerosis if possible, i.e. a statin, aspirin or clopidogrel, blood pressure control and, if diabetic, tight control of blood sugar.

Most patients are followed up long-term after surgery or angioplasty to monitor deterioration, to detect new disease and to enable timely intervention if needed. Femoro-popliteal vein grafts can be examined at intervals using duplex Doppler scanning. Such **graft surveillance** can detect early graft stenoses, enabling them to be treated and the graft preserved, although the efficacy of this is not proven. Aneurysm patients after open operation, on the other hand, can be discharged from regular follow-up 3 months after operation if there are no complications; however, they should be rescanned by ultrasound at 5-yearly intervals for new abdominal aneurysms (Fig. 42.11). Stent-graft follow-up needs to be more rigorous as the devices are not as securely fixed in position as conventional grafts that are sewn in place. EVAR patients generally undergo CT scanning every 6 months to look for leaks around the graft (**endoleaks**), but as devices have become more reliable there is a move towards 6-monthly ultrasound scans and yearly CT scans.

43 Venous disorders of the lower limb

VENOUS THROMBOSIS AND THE POST-THROMBOTIC LIMB

ANATOMY OF THE LOWER LIMB VENOUS SYSTEM

Blood is drained from the lower limb via two separate systems. The **deep venous system** drains the deep tissues of the foot and muscles of the lower leg and thigh. These deep veins lie within the mass of lower limb muscles and include the large **soleal venous sinuses**. Muscle contraction during walking and other exercise provides an essential mechanism for pumping blood back towards the heart against gravity (**the muscle pump**). Reverse flow is prevented by numerous valves in the system.

The skin and tissues superficial to the deep fascia drain mainly into the **superficial venous system** which comprises two main vessels, the **long (great) saphenous vein** and the **short (small) saphenous vein**. The long saphenous vein receives tributaries from the antero-medial aspect of the limb (and lower anterior abdominal wall), and penetrates the fascia lata in the groin to drain into the (deep) femoral vein. The short saphenous vein drains the posterior part of the leg and passes through the deep fascia of the calf to flow into the popliteal vein, also part of the deep venous system. There is a network of other interconnecting superficial veins that will drain venous blood from the limb if long or short saphenous veins are surgically removed or ablated. The superficial system has no muscular pump to aid venous return but valves normally prevent retrograde flow, particularly at the sapheno-femoral and sapheno-popliteal junctions. A number of **perforating veins** drain blood from the superficial system into the deep system; valves on these normally ensure the one-way flow. Most of the perforators are on the medial part of the leg above the ankle but there is a fairly constant '**Hunterian perforator**' in the medial mid-thigh.

PRESENTATION AND CONSEQUENCES OF VENOUS THROMBOSIS (Table 43.1)

Thromboembolic disease and its consequences are common and include acute deep vein thrombosis (DVT), pulmonary embolism and superficial thrombophlebitis ('phlebitis'). Deep venous thrombosis in the lower limb most commonly occurs as a complication of a major operation, lower limb fractures, myocardial infarction or other severe illness. In the past, DVTs were common after childbirth but early mobilisation has considerably reduced the incidence. About one-third of DVTs present with no apparent cause and these are usually managed by physicians. Many of these patients have a detectable **prothrombotic state**. The risk factors, clinical presentations and management of acute DVT and pulmonary embolism are discussed in Chapter 12.

Deep venous thrombosis in the lower limb is an acute local problem with the added risk of a potentially fatal pulmonary embolism. However, it may also cause major **long-term complications** in the lower limb. The severity of post-thrombotic problems generally reflects the extent of the original DVT. The affected extremity is known as a **post-thrombotic limb** or, less accurately, a **post-phlebitic limb**.

A high proportion of patients undergoing major operations or who suffer lower limb fractures can be shown by

Table 43.1 A summary of lower limb venous disorders

Basic disease	Pathophysiological process	Clinical manifestations
Varicose veins— incompetent valves in veins connecting deep and superficial venous systems; often begins with sapheno-femoral valve incompetence	Failure of muscle pump means blood is forced from deep venous system to superficial system through incompetent valves causing slowly progressive tortuous dilatation of superficial veins. Venous hypertension may cause chronic skin changes and sometimes ulceration. Women more often affected than men; varicosities often first appear during pregnancy	Slowly progressive development of prominent purple, dilated, tortuous superficial veins. Patient often complains of aching, especially after long period of standing. Patients may be upset by cosmetic appearance or, if there is a family history, fear of progression or ulceration. Pain relieved by elevation. Dilated vessels are vulnerable to trauma and may bleed profusely
Superficial venous thrombosis (i.e. thrombophlebitis) usually occurs in tortuous dilated varicose veins; more common in pregnancy. Occasionally affects normal veins in **thrombophlebitis migrans** occurring in patients with visceral malignancy	Spontaneous thrombosis in superficial veins; excites an inflammatory response in the vessel wall and surrounding tissues	Rapid onset of acute, highly localised pain and tenderness, associated with varicose veins. Overlying skin red and oedematous; underlying veins hard and nodular. Infection is not a feature so antibiotic treatment is illogical
Deep venous thrombosis— predisposed to by previous DVT, pregnancy, oestrogen therapy, major surgery, trauma, obesity, abdominal or pelvic malignancy, immobility and increasing age. May be complicated by pulmonary embolism	Thrombosis in deep venous system of calf; may propagate proximally into ilio-femoral veins. Can obstruct venous return in both short and long term. Spontaneous recanalisation may cause deep vein valvular incompetence, i.e. chronic venous insufficiency, and local venous hypertension. This obstructs capillary flow and inhibits metabolic exchange; leakage of red cells causes subcutaneous deposition of haemosiderin. Combined effects cause atrophy of skin and subcutaneous fat, fibrosis, poor healing and predisposition to ulceration	Classic acute presentation is pain and swelling of calf and ankle with calf tenderness. Dorsiflexion may cause pain (Homans' sign). Leg usually warm and normal in colour but pulses may be impalpable due to oedema. If ilio-femoral veins involved, thigh also swollen. Late complication is post-thrombotic limb with chronic brawny oedema and narrow ankle due to lipodermatosclerosis. Skin atrophic, scaly and pigmented (varicose/venous eczema). Skin above medial malleolus most vulnerable to chronic ulceration after minor trauma

sensitive radionuclide techniques to develop asymptomatic thrombi in calf veins despite no clinical evidence of thrombosis. Such 'silent' thromboses may explain the later occurrence of typical post-thrombotic changes in patients who give no history of an acute thrombotic episode.

PATHOPHYSIOLOGY OF POST-THROMBOTIC PROBLEMS

Provided fatal pulmonary embolism has not occurred, deep venous thromboses gradually undergo **organisation** and the **veins recanalise**. In the process, valves in the deep veins can be damaged and become incompetent, thus allowing reflux, leading to **chronic deep venous insufficiency**. The syndrome usually takes years to develop although it can develop in a matter of months. If the interval is prolonged, it becomes easy to ignore this important reason for trying to prevent deep venous thrombosis in hospital patients!

Recanalisation may not occur at all or else is incomplete in patients in whom the proximal veins have been completely occluded by thrombus. This results in venous outflow obstruction, the consequences of which are more marked and appear sooner than if occlusion had been incomplete.

In the normal adult limb, venous pressure at the ankle while standing is about 125 cm of water. This pressure falls markedly during walking as a result of the calf pump. In contrast, in the post-thrombotic limb, where deep venous valves allow reflux or, worse still, veins remain occluded, ankle venous pressure remains high during calf muscle activity. This leads to incompetence of valves in the perforating veins. Blood is forced into the superficial system causing local venous hypertension, disrupting the normal vascular dynamics of the skin and subcutaneous tissues. This may result in impaired skin vitality and healing ability. Characteristic local signs of a gross post-thrombotic limb are listed in Box 43.1 (see Fig. 43.1).

The following factors probably contribute to the clinical features:

- Venous stagnation restricts arterial replenishment of capillary blood

- Arteriovenous shunts beneath the affected skin divert blood away from the dermal capillaries
- Venous hypertension causes dilatation of the local venules and the capillary network, allowing plasma proteins to leak into the interstitial spaces. Fibrin

polymerises forming **pericapillary cuffs** which may interfere with metabolic exchange between blood and tissues

Post-thrombotic syndrome should also be suspected when a patient presents with lesser degrees of skin change of this type. The majority, however, will prove to have only superficial venous insufficiency.

Box 43.1 Signs of a gross post-thrombotic limb

- Chronic lower leg **swelling** with brawny oedema
- **Varicose veins** with incompetent perforating veins
- Inflammation and haemosiderin **pigmentation** in the area above the medial malleolus (the 'gaiter' area) and other parts of the lower half of the leg. This is known as **varicose or venous eczema** and may be complicated by low-grade cellulitis
- Active or healed venous **ulceration** above the medial malleolus
- **Lipodermatosclerosis** around the ankle (replacement of soft subcutaneous fat with firm collagenous scar tissue). This causes the 'champagne-bottle leg' with oedema above and a narrow atrophic ankle below

---

INVESTIGATION OF VENOUS INSUFFICIENCY

When a patient presents with ankle ulceration, a chronically swollen limb or typical skin changes of venous insufficiency around the ankle, **chronic venous insufficiency** may be suspected. This is due to superficial venous reflux, deep venous reflux (post-thrombotic or congenital absence of valves) or a combination of both.

The diagnostic pathway depends on responses to the following questions:

1. Is the condition venous in origin? This is suggested by a history of DVT, prolonged bed rest in the past or lower limb fractures, or a finding of varicose veins or

Fig. 43.1 Post-thrombotic limbs and venous eczema

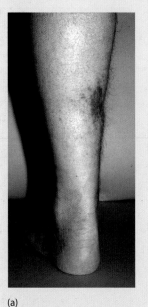

(a)

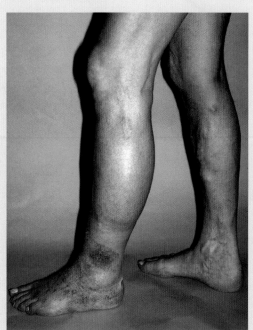

(b)

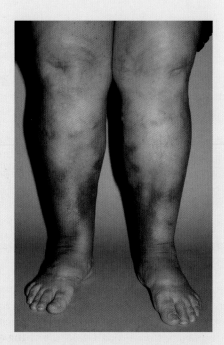

(c)

(a) Healed venous ulcer showing local loss of subcutaneous fat and surrounding pigmentation. **(b)** Man of 66 with no history of DVT showing marked swelling of the left leg with pigmentation in the lateral gaiter area representing venous eczema. The right leg has moderate varicose veins; the blue discoloration around both ankles is an age change due to dilated venules and is of no clinical consequence. On colour duplex ultrasound examination, there was evidence of deep venous thrombotic damage in the left leg. **(c)** Bilateral post-thrombotic limbs in a woman of 57 with gross venous eczema, fat atrophy, signs of healed venous ulceration and varicose veins.

Fig. 43.2 Venous ulceration

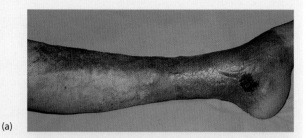

(a)

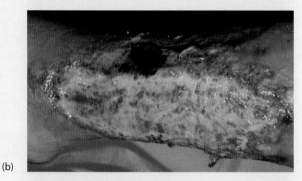

(b)

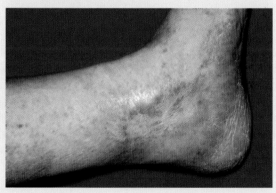

(c)

(a) Post-thrombotic limb with marked venous pigmentation and a chronic ulcer which heals and breaks down periodically. **(b)** Chronic venous ulcer in a post-thrombotic limb. The ulcer is virtually circumferential and represents a serious management problem. **(c)** Chronic ulcer that healed several years before, following a Cockett's operation, an open procedure for subfascial ligation of perforators, the scar of which is visible. This operation and endoscopic variations in the SEPS procedure are rarely performed nowadays.

a 'champagne-bottle' leg (i.e. proximal limb swelling due to oedema and distal narrowing due to fat atrophy and fibrosis). If the condition is not venous, another cause of ulceration and swelling should be sought

2. Is there superficial venous insufficiency (Fig. 43.2), deep venous insufficiency, or a combination of both?

3. How much of a contribution is made by superficial venous insufficiency? (This is likely to respond to surgery, unlike deep venous reflux)

When there are small areas of skin change or ulceration which correlate with the degree of superficial venous incompetence, these can be treated surgically as uncomplicated varicose veins, although ideally the anatomy needs to be imaged. If there are marked skin changes, the anatomy of the deep venous system and the competence of valves in the deep veins need investigation. Skilled assessment with **duplex colour-flow Doppler ultrasound** is now the 'gold standard' investigation.

MANAGEMENT OF POST-THROMBOTIC PROBLEMS

The main post-thrombotic problems requiring active treatment are chronic ulcers and sometimes, acute cellulitis.

Venous ulcers

Ulcers may develop spontaneously but are more commonly initiated by minor trauma which fails to heal, often complicated by secondary infection.

The majority of venous ulcers can be healed by non-operative methods, provided treatment is applied effectively and assiduously. Even if operative treatment is required, conservative measures should be used to prepare the limb. These include reducing swelling by multi-layer bandaging, removing necrotic tissue from the ulcer base and controlling cellulitis. The systolic pressure in the lower leg should be measured relative to the upper limb. If the pressure in the lower limb is less than 80% of that in the upper limb (the ankle-brachial pressure index) the arterial circulation should be fully assessed before compression is applied. Support and compression of the skin and superficial tissues is the mainstay of treatment. This may be provided by elastic bandages or correctly sized graduated compression stockings. In either case, the aim is for pressure to be greatest at the ankle (up to 40 mmHg), reducing progressively up the limb. Great care must be taken to ensure that pressure does not cause ischaemia or abrasions over tendons or bony prominences. The main contraindication to the use of compression is severe chronic ischaemia, where pressure could further reduce arterial input. Most venous ulcers can be rapidly healed while keeping the patient ambulatory by competent multi-layer bandaging (the Charing Cross technique uses four layers), avoiding the need for hospital care unless complications occur or skin grafting is required.

Spreading cellulitis should be treated with systemic antibiotics. Infection confined to the ulcer is treated by excision of dead tissue if necessary and simple dressings such as saline soaks; use of antiseptics may retard granulation tissue and epithelialisation. Simple microbial colonisation rather than invasive infection does not require treatment. Local applications of antibiotics have no place in the management of ulcers.

Surgical treatment may be indicated, particularly if there is superficial venous incompetence. Varicose veins should be ligated or removed unless there is gross deep venous incompetence. There is good evidence that effective treatment of superficial venous reflux will reduce the time to healing for ulcers and it also halves the recurrence rate. More controversial is surgical disruption or ligation of incompetent perforating veins, even if performed by subfascial endoscopic surgery (SEPS). Intractable or large ulcers may require skin grafting once the ulcer base is clean.

Long-term care and prevention

The uncomplicated post-thrombotic limb is debilitating enough to the patient, who is often elderly, without the added complication of chronic venous ulceration.

As soon as the condition is recognised, the patient should be encouraged to use appropriate graduated compression stockings and to take great care to avoid even minor trauma to the limb, especially to the gaiter area above the medial malleolus.

For minor venous insufficiency, well-fitting class I **compression elastic stockings** or tights provide adequate support but care should be taken that they fit well and that there is no proximal constricting band to impair venous return. In more severe venous insufficiency, class II or III compression stockings are valuable and may reverse the tissue damage or at least arrest its progress. In addition, they provide protection from minor trauma. Ideally they should be worn at all times except in bed. The importance of correctly fitted stockings should be emphasised; ideally, they should be supplied by an experienced surgical fitter.

In many patients, effective elastic support will be required for life. Even so, further episodes of cellulitis or ulceration are likely to occur.

AXILLARY VEIN THROMBOSIS

Axillary vein thrombosis is an uncommon condition and is the upper limb equivalent of DVT; it is usually managed by (internal) physicians, but patients sometimes reach the surgeon. The condition usually presents with a sudden onset of swelling, and aching pain in the whole arm. On examination, the hand, forearm and arm are swollen with a bluish tinge. Sensation is preserved. In most patients, no cause is found, but the condition can occur as a manifestation of visceral malignancy (**thrombophlebitis migrans**), or a blood disorder with raised viscosity, such as polycythaemia vera. It is likely that most cases result from external compression of the subclavian vein between the first rib (or a cervical rib) and the clavicle. The space may be congenitally narrow or physical activity such as weight lifting may cause local trauma. The usual treatment is anticoagulation to prevent propagation of thrombus and to encourage spontaneous clot lysis. Predisposing disorders should be sought. A few patients benefit from surgical excision of the first rib.

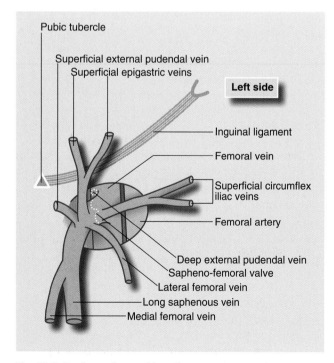

Fig. 43.3 Sapheno-femoral junction—anatomy

Pubic tubercle
Superficial external pudendal vein
Superficial epigastric veins
Left side
Inguinal ligament
Femoral vein
Superficial circumflex iliac veins
Femoral artery
Deep external pudendal vein
Sapheno-femoral valve
Lateral femoral vein
Long saphenous vein
Medial femoral vein

Box 43.2	Initial examination of varicose veins

- **Severity**—Examine the extent and severity of varicose veins with the patient standing. Many patients attend with unsightly 'spider veins' which are not varicose. Others attend for advice because they are worried they will develop ulcers ('like my mother')
- **Skin changes**—Examine the leg for swelling, ulcers and varicose eczema. If present, could indicate a post-thrombotic limb
- **Long or short saphenous**—Examine the distribution of varicose veins. Are there varicosities above knee, indicating probable sapheno-femoral incompetence? Could these be short saphenous system varicosities, i.e. postero-lateral calf veins feeding towards popliteal fossa where short saphenous may be palpable

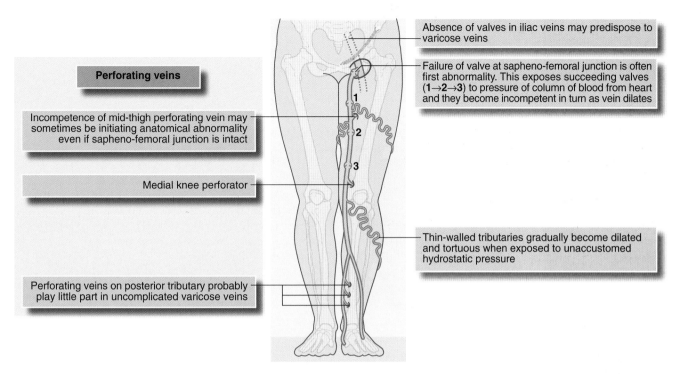

Perforating veins

Absence of valves in iliac veins may predispose to varicose veins

Failure of valve at sapheno-femoral junction is often first abnormality. This exposes succeeding valves (**1→2→3**) to pressure of column of blood from heart and they become incompetent in turn as vein dilates

Incompetence of mid-thigh perforating vein may sometimes be initiating anatomical abnormality even if sapheno-femoral junction is intact

Medial knee perforator

Thin-walled tributaries gradually become dilated and tortuous when exposed to unaccustomed hydrostatic pressure

Perforating veins on posterior tributary probably play little part in uncomplicated varicose veins

Fig. 43.4 Pathophysiology of varicose veins

VARICOSE VEINS

Varicose veins are dilated, tortuous and prominent superficial veins in the lower limb (see Fig. 43.5). Varicose veins are very common, being present in about 20% of people aged 20 and increasing to 80% at 60 years. Nevertheless, only about 12% of those affected have symptoms or develop complications. Varicose veins are one of the most common reasons for referral to a surgeon in developed countries, particularly when improved medical services are able to cope with the volume of more serious disease and where expectations for treatment are higher. The condition appears to be a product of the upright posture.

PATHOPHYSIOLOGY OF VARICOSE VEINS

Abnormal communication between the deep and superficial venous systems appears to be the essential factor in the development of varicose veins. In most patients the process probably begins with failure of the valve at the sapheno-femoral junction. When this happens, an uninterrupted column of blood from the heart progressively dilates the veins down the leg (see Fig. 43.5a). Varicose veins usually develop slowly over 10–20 years, so that in most cases surgical treatment is not urgent. The long saphenous system is involved in about 90% of cases and the short saphenous system in 25% (some have both systems involved).

Women are affected about six times more often than men, with the majority of varicose veins developing during or soon after the second or third pregnancy. An important factor is probably the high level of progesterone which causes changes in the structure of collagen (which may not later recover fully), as well as smooth muscle relaxation. Pressure on the pelvic veins by the enlarging uterus may contribute by restricting venous return.

In some patients, hereditary factors appear to play a part, especially in men, and particularly in those who develop varicose veins in their teens. Predisposing anatomical factors may include congenital lack of valves in the iliac veins or abnormal vein wall elasticity. Deep venous thrombosis plays little part in causing simple varicose veins. Rarely, multiple congenital arteriovenous fistulae (Klippel–Trenaunay and other syndromes) cause gross varicose veins. In these patients, there is gigantism of the lower limb and often venous ulceration (see Ch. 46). A technique of examining varicose veins is shown in Figure 43.6.

SYMPTOMS AND SIGNS OF VARICOSE VEINS

The most common complaints related to varicose veins are:

- Aching legs, usually after standing all day
- Poor cosmetic appearance, especially in summer when the legs are exposed
- Fear of future leg ulcers ('like my mother had')
- Fear of varicosities progressing

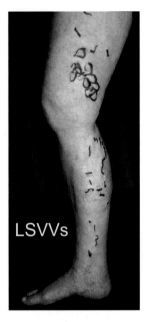

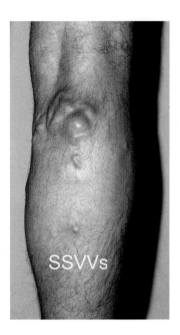

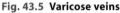

(a)

(b)

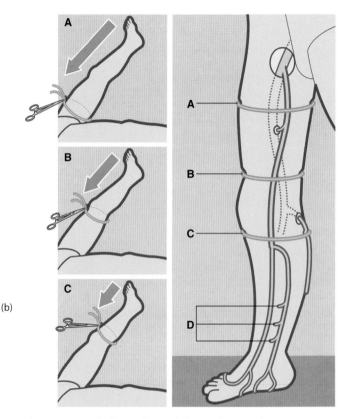

Fig. 43.5 Varicose veins
(a) Typical varicosities in the long saphenous territory (LSVVs) evident both above and below knee and most prominent on the medial side of the limb. The indelible black markings were made immediately prior to surgery by the operating surgeon with the patient standing. **(b)** Typical short saphenous varicosities (SSVVs), which do not extend above the knee. These veins could not be controlled with an above-knee tourniquet and there was gross reflux evident on hand-held Doppler examination, confirmed on colour duplex Doppler scanning.

- Bleeding or worry about varicosities bleeding, particularly if traumatised
- Varicose eczema or ulcers
- Ankle oedema
- Recurrent superficial thrombophlebitis

MANAGEMENT OF VARICOSE VEINS

Many patients who consult a surgeon because of unsightly vascular markings on their legs do not have varicose veins. Instead, these are often 'spider veins' or dilated superficial venules (**reticular veins**). Cosmetic treatment includes covering cosmetics and superficial laser or micro-sclerotherapy using injected sclerosants. Many patients have longstanding varicose veins with no complications, and merely seek reassurance that they will not ulcerate in the future. Surgical treatment is not usually necessary for these patients but advice can be given to elevate the legs when sitting and to wear supporting elastic stockings when standing for long periods.

INDICATIONS FOR SURGICAL TREATMENT OF VARICOSE VEINS

Surgical treatment for varicose veins is to a large extent cosmetic or to prevent future complications, and opera-

Fig. 43.6 A technique of examining varicose veins
Elevate limb and ensure veins are emptied by massaging distal to proximal. Apply tourniquet **tightly** around upper thigh **A** then stand patient up. Does tourniquet prevent veins filling and removing it cause rapid filling from above? If so, main communication is at the sapheno-femoral junction. If veins fill rapidly with tourniquet in place, repeat the test with tourniquet above the knee **B**. If this controls filling, then main communication is mid-thigh perforator. If this tourniquet fails to control filling, repeat below knee **C**. If this controls filling, communication is likely to be short saphenous-popliteal or medial knee perforator incompetence. If no tourniquet controls filling, communication is probably by one or more distal perforating veins, often post-thrombotic in origin **D**. Note that 80% of varicose veins involve the long saphenous system, sometimes with short saphenous incompetence as well.

tion can be planned at leisure. The main medical indications for treating varicose veins are **aching legs** after standing, relieved by elevation or in bed at night (particularly with unilateral ankle oedema), **haemorrhage** from a varicose vein, **superficial thrombophlebitis** and **venous skin changes** due to superficial venous insufficiency. All of these can be treated with support bandages or stockings, but surgery is often preferable.

Injection sclerotherapy (e.g. Fegan's technique) is used for treating small cosmetically unattractive varicose veins below the knee but is unsuitable for major varicosities, particularly in the thigh. The techniques of injection sclerotherapy and surgery for varicose veins are shown in Figure 43.7.

(a) Injection sclerotherapy for minor varicose veins (after Fegan)

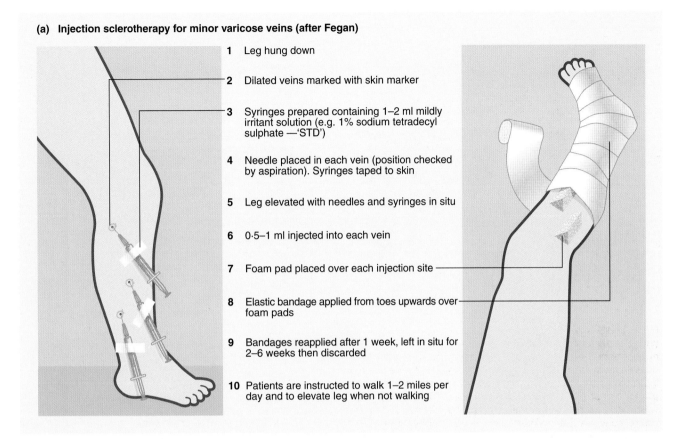

1 Leg hung down

2 Dilated veins marked with skin marker

3 Syringes prepared containing 1–2 ml mildly irritant solution (e.g. 1% sodium tetradecyl sulphate —'STD')

4 Needle placed in each vein (position checked by aspiration). Syringes taped to skin

5 Leg elevated with needles and syringes in situ

6 0·5–1 ml injected into each vein

7 Foam pad placed over each injection site

8 Elastic bandage applied from toes upwards over foam pads

9 Bandages reapplied after 1 week, left in situ for 2–6 weeks then discarded

10 Patients are instructed to walk 1–2 miles per day and to elevate leg when not walking

(b) Operations for varicose veins

(i) HIGH SAPHENOUS LIGATION

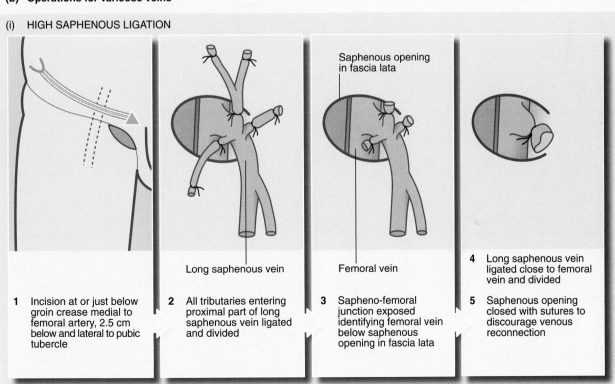

Saphenous opening in fascia lata

Long saphenous vein

Femoral vein

1 Incision at or just below groin crease medial to femoral artery, 2.5 cm below and lateral to pubic tubercle

2 All tributaries entering proximal part of long saphenous vein ligated and divided

3 Sapheno-femoral junction exposed identifying femoral vein below saphenous opening in fascia lata

4 Long saphenous vein ligated close to femoral vein and divided

5 Saphenous opening closed with sutures to discourage venous reconnection

Fig. 43.7a Treatment of varicose veins

(b) Operations for varicose veins

(ii) LONG SAPHENOUS STRIP

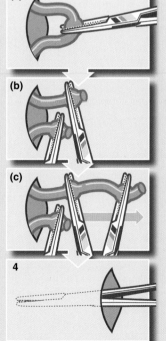

1 The stripper is a long flexible wire with a bullet-shaped knob on the 'business' end. The entry vein (proximal or distal, according to choice) is prepared as shown and the narrow end of the stripper passed down or up the long saphenous vein until it can be brought out to the surface within 15 cm below knee, not to the ankle as was done in the past

2 Stripping is usually downward. The vein is ligated to the wire at the bullet end and the narrow end is pulled smoothly and firmly, tearing off tributaries and any perforators on the way, emerging with the complete vein bunched up on the stripper

3 The wounds are closed and the limb firmly bandaged to minimise subcutaneous bleeding. Patients should be warned to expect postoperative bruising

(iii) AVULSION OF VARICOSITIES

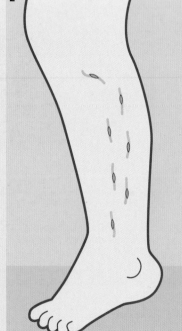

1 Before operation, all varicosities are marked by the surgeon with the patient standing, using an indelible spirit based fibre-tipped pen

2 Very small incisions are made over the marks in a longitudinal direction, or transverse around the knee. As much vein as possible is pulled out ('nick and pick') as follows:

(a) Vein grasped with artery forceps or special vein hook

(b) Second forceps applied and vein divided

(c) One end is drawn out of wound gently and further traction applied by means of another forceps

3 The vein will eventually break and bleeding is controlled by finger pressure. The process is repeated for the other end of vein

4 Forceps can be passed subcutaneously to retrieve nearby varices thus reducing the number of incisions required

5 Each wound is left open or closed neatly with 'steristrips' or a fine suture, and non-adherent gauze applied to each one. The limb is bandaged firmly from the foot to the upper thigh using crepe

Fig. 43.7b continued Surgical treatment of varicose veins

Newer techniques of treating varicose veins

Newer techniques of treating main trunk varicose veins carry the advantage of avoiding a groin incision. These include ablation of the main incompetent superficial vein by **laser** or **radiofrequency ablation**, or by **foam sclerotherapy**. Results appear comparable with surgery in general but long-term evaluation is awaited.

PERIOPERATIVE MANAGEMENT OF THE PATIENT HAVING VARICOSE VEIN SURGERY

Varicose veins must be **marked out** on the legs before operation. This should be done by the surgeon who will actually do the operation. An indelible marker must be used so that marks are not washed off by the patient or by skin preparation in the operating theatre. The patient must stand, often for some minutes, to allow the veins to fill, and marking should be performed in this position. Most surgeons mark all the prominent veins that are visible or palpable. Extra marks are often added for areas needing special surgical attention such as suspected perforating veins. Duplex scanning may be employed to assist marking.

Any patient with a history of venous thrombosis, whether deep or superficial, should be prescribed **low-dose subcutaneous heparin**. Patients with other risk factors for deep venous thrombosis, especially obese patients, should have the same prophylactic treatment. The first dose of heparin should be given 1–2 hours before operation.

Immediately after operation, non-adherent dressings are applied to all the incisions and the whole leg is bandaged firmly with an elastic bandage. The patient should then be mobilised and encouraged to walk about. Twenty-four hours later, all dressings can be removed and the bandage exchanged for a graduated elastic stocking. On return home, patients should keep as active as possible, walking on a treadmill or outside the house for a few hundred metres or cycling a kilometre or two, several times a day for the first 2 weeks. When the patient is sitting, the legs should be elevated, and the patient should get up and walk around about every half-hour. All these measures are designed to discourage venous stagnation and venous thrombosis. Most patients can return to work after 1 week and can drive a car 24 hours after operation. The patient should be warned that the legs will be bruised when the bandages are removed.

44 Cardiac surgery

This chapter is intended to give a flavour of the range and scope of work performed by cardiac surgeons and to provide an introduction to larger reference texts for those seeking greater detail. Heart and lung transplantation is discussed in Chapter 14.

INTRODUCTION AND CARDIOPULMONARY BYPASS

Surgery of the heart has fascinated surgeons for many years. However, up until the 1950s, only a very limited range of cardiac procedures was possible. These included **closed mitral valvotomy** for mitral stenosis and several ingenious methods of closing atrial septal defects in the beating heart. More extensive cardiac surgery became a reality when cardiopulmonary bypass was successfully employed in 1953. For the first time, a patient could be sustained artificially, with the heart and lungs bypassed. Meanwhile surgery could take place in a motionless, blood-free field. Since then, the specialty of cardiac surgery has expanded and developed rapidly.

Hardly any cardiac operations are now performed without bypass and those that are, are mostly palliative procedures for congenital heart disease. The early emphasis in cardiac surgery on uncomplicated operations for congenital heart disease has shifted markedly towards more ambitious techniques for treating acquired heart disease as a result of evolution in cardiopulmonary bypass. More recently, some coronary artery surgery is being performed via small incisions without bypass in the beating heart. This is in keeping with the move towards minimal access in other areas, but further development is needed before it can become generally available.

For most cardiac surgery on bypass, a bloodless field is created by clamping the ascending aorta just proximal to where the aortic cannula returns arterial blood from the bypass machine (see Fig. 44.1). Since there is no coronary arterial blood supply, the myocardium becomes anoxic and would be at risk of infarction; this potential ischaemic damage has to be minimised by reducing the metabolic demands of the heart as follows (see also Table 44.1):

- The electrical and mechanical action of the heart is **arrested** by the high potassium content of a cardioplegic solution (16 mmol/L KCl), see Table 44.1
- The myocardium is **cooled** to between 4 and 12°C

Several actual and potential problems arise when blood is exposed to the extracorporeal circuit of a cardiopulmonary bypass machine:

- The clotting cascade is activated, causing **intravascular coagulation** of blood. This is prevented by anticoagulation with high-dose heparin (300 IU/kg) given systemically before the heart is cannulated. After the patient is weaned off cardiopulmonary bypass, the extracorporeal circuit is removed and the heparin reversed with **protamine sulphate**
- Clotting factors and platelets are consumed within the extracorporeal circuit (mainly within the oxygenator) leading to a bleeding diathesis. Blood products may be needed to reverse this
- The complement cascade and other mediators involved in inflammation are activated to a variable extent

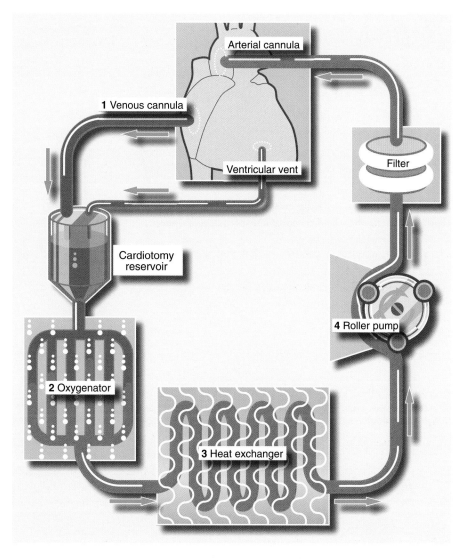

Fig. 44.1 The standard circuit for cardiopulmonary bypass

1. Systemic venous blood is siphoned into a reservoir by gravity from the right atrium (or from the superior and inferior vena cavae) via a venous cannula
2. Venous blood leaves the reservoir and passes through a membrane oxygenator
3. Blood next passes through a heat exchanger to cool or rewarm the blood as necessary
4. The oxygenated and temperature-controlled blood is pumped under pressure through a filter and into the systemic arterial circulation, usually via the ascending aorta by a roller pump

Note: Snares are placed around both superior and inferior vena cavae to occlude them and prevent air from entering the right-sided cardiac chambers and locking the gravity siphon. When the patient is on bypass, any of the four cardiac chambers can be opened for surgical access.

Table 44.1 Constituents of a typical infusate for cold cardioplegia (St Thomas's solution)

Constituent	Quantity
Sodium chloride	110.0 mmol/L
Potassium chloride	16.0 mmol/L
Magnesium chloride	16.0 mmol/L
Calcium chloride	1.2 mmol/L
Sodium bicarbonate	10.0 mmol/L
Procaine	16.0 mmol/L

ASSESSING RISK IN CARDIAC SURGERY

Cardiac surgery can be perceived as being particularly risky but since the range of procedures performed is small, the discipline is relatively easy to audit. In the UK, all cardiac surgical units are now expected to under-take detailed audit. Results are compared between units, allowing appropriate standards to be developed and maintained. Since many patient-related factors can affect the outcome of cardiac surgery in addition to surgical and anaesthetic skill, several scoring systems have been devised to try to predict the mortality and morbidity risk for an individual undergoing a particular operation. The systems generally aim to predict the risk of perioperative death by taking into account the surgical procedure, its urgency and any pre-existing comorbidities. None is completely reliable but the **Parsonnet scoring system** and **Euroscore** (Table 44.2) are perhaps the most widely used and are based on actual outcomes in large numbers of patients. The total score for an individual predicts a likely mortality for a particular operation. For example, a 77-year-old female with a history of claudication undergoing emergency coronary artery surgery has a standard Euroscore of 4 + 1 + 2 + 2 = 9. This equates to an operative mortality risk of 9%.

Table 44.2 Risk stratification for cardiac surgery—the European System for Cardiac Operative Risk Evaluation (Euroscore)

Risk factors		Score
Patient-related factors		
Age	For each 5 years over 60	1
Gender	Female	1
Chronic lung disease	If treated with long-term bronchodilators or steroids	1
Arteriopathic patient	Intermittent claudication, carotid stenosis > 50%, previous or planned reconstruction of limb arteries or carotids	2
Neurological dysfunction	Severely affecting ambulation	2
Renal	Plasma creatinine > 200 µmol/L preoperatively	2
Previous cardiac surgery	Requiring opening of the pericardium	3
Active endocarditis	Currently on antibiotic treatment for endocarditis	3
Critical preoperative state	Ventricular tachycardia/fibrillation/aborted sudden death/cardiac massage	3
	Preoperative ventilation/inotropic support/intra-aortic balloon pump	
	Acute renal failure (anuria or oliguria < 10 ml/hour)	
Cardiac-related factors		
Unstable angina	Angina at rest requiring i.v. nitrates until arrival in anaesthetic room	2
Left ventricular dysfunction	Moderate—Left ventricular ejection fraction (LVEF) 30–50%	1
	Poor—LVEF < 30%	3
Recent myocardial infarction	< 90 days ago	2
Pulmonary hypertension	Systolic PA > 60 mmHg	2
Operation-related factors		
Emergency	Surgery performed before beginning of next working day after urgent referral	2
Operations other than CABG only	Major cardiac procedure other than, or as well as CABG	2
Surgery on thoracic aorta	Ascending, arch or descending aorta	3
Post-infarction septal rupture	Requiring rapair	4

CONGENITAL CARDIAC DISEASE

TYPES OF CONGENITAL HEART DISEASE

Congenital heart disease occurs in about 2 per 1000 live births and falls into two main groups: those with and those without cyanosis.

CYANOTIC HEART DISEASE

Cyanotic heart disease exists when there is mixing of systemic arterial and venous blood through a predominantly **right-to-left cardiac shunt**. The most common examples are:

- **Tetralogy of Fallot**—the four features are ventricular septal defect (VSD), pulmonary artery stenosis, right ventricular hypertrophy and an aorta which overrides the ventricular septum, thus receiving blood from both ventricles
- **Transposition of the great arteries**—the pulmonary artery arises from the left ventricle and the aorta from the right ventricle
- **Tricuspid atresia**—absence of a functional tricuspid valve

- **Truncus arteriosus**—the pulmonary artery and aorta fail to develop separately
- **Total anomalous pulmonary venous drainage**—pulmonary venous blood drains into the right side of the heart
- **Eisenmenger's syndrome**—increased pulmonary blood flow caused by a pre-existing left-to-right shunt (see next section) causes severe pulmonary hypertension later in life, resulting in spontaneous reversal of the shunt so that flow reverses to become right-to-left

ACYANOTIC HEART DISEASE

Acyanotic congenital heart disease may involve:

- A shunt from left to right sides of the heart (e.g. via an atrial or ventricular septal defect) or a ductus arteriosus which persists in its patent antenatal state (PDA)
- Failed or incomplete embryological development of parts of the heart or great vessels without shunting, e.g. coarctation of the aorta

MANAGEMENT OF CONGENITAL HEART DISEASE

Surgical management of congenital heart disease aims to palliate the adverse effects or correct the defects mechanically, or else both in sequence.

Early in the history of cardiac surgery, palliation was often all that could be offered. Later, palliation was sometimes followed by a second-stage corrective operation when the child was larger. Nowadays, corrective procedures are usually offered at the outset, as operations have become more customary, myocardial protection is more predictable and operative risks are lower.

PALLIATING CONGENITAL CARDIAC DISORDERS

When pulmonary blood flow is **reduced** (as in tricuspid atresia, tetralogy of Fallot or pulmonary artery stenosis), palliation aims to increase pulmonary flow by creating a shunt between the systemic arterial circulation and the pulmonary artery (see Fig. 44.2).

When pulmonary blood flow is **too great** (e.g. VSD or truncus arteriosus), the aim is to reduce the pulmonary flow by artificially narrowing the main pulmonary artery by external banding.

CORRECTING CONGENITAL CARDIAC DISORDERS

Surgical correction of congenital heart disease is based on accurately identifying the lesion or lesions, then performing procedures which restore the normal flow and func-

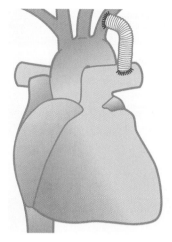

Fig. 44.2 Palliation of tetralogy of Fallot
Modified Blalock–Taussig shunt.

tioning of the heart. Correction may be mechanically straightforward as in the following procedures:

- Closing a persisting ductus arteriosus (PDA)
- Resecting the narrowed segment of descending aorta in coarctation of the aorta
- Closing an atrial or ventricular septal defect

In other cases, correction may be complex, for example in total correction of Fallot's tetralogy or correction of **anomalous pulmonary venous drainage**. Procedures such as these should only be performed in specialist paediatric cardiac surgical units.

ACQUIRED HEART DISEASE

The different types of acquired heart disease are listed in Table 44.3.

CORONARY HEART DISEASE (see Table 44.4 for clinical presentations)

PATHOPHYSIOLOGY

Coronary heart disease (ischaemic heart disease) is nearly always atherosclerotic in origin, with subintimal thickening caused by deposition of cholesterol-containing lipids, together with hyperplasia of media smooth muscle cells which migrate into the subintimal area. Together, these changes reduce the luminal diameter. Since blood flow through a vessel is related to the fourth power of the radius (Poiseuille's Law), only a small change in cross-sectional area in these small arteries is needed to cause a dramatic reduction in coronary artery blood flow. When coronary artery disease is assessed on angiography, a 50% reduction in diameter shown in two different planes is regarded as significant.

Acute coronary ischaemia is usually brought on by thrombosis of already narrowed coronary arteries, in some cases precipitated by haemorrhage into atherosclerotic plaques.

The world-wide distribution of coronary atherosclerosis is patchy. It is predominantly a disease of developed countries, affecting both locally born people and certain immigrants with a genetic predisposition. Men are at greater risk than women, with 45% of men over 65 having some manifestation of the disease. Areas of particularly high incidence include Scotland and Finland. The rates in some countries, notably the USA, have been falling in recent years, largely as a result of reduced cigarette smoking and perhaps changes in other habits such as diet and exercise.

Risk factors for coronary atheroma (and atherosclerosis elsewhere) include unfavourable hereditary cholesterol and lipid profiles, cigarette smoking, diabetes, hypertension, obesity and a sedentary lifestyle (and perhaps a life of severe unrelieved stress).

The presentation of coronary heart disease is outlined in Table 44.4.

Table 44.3 Types of acquired heart disease

Type	Pathophysiology	Clinical presentation
Ischaemic heart disease	Usually caused by coronary atherosclerosis and rarely by spasm, embolism or trauma	1. Reversible ischaemia presenting as angina 2. Painless or silent ischaemia discovered incidentally 3. Myocardial infarction
Valvular heart disease, affecting aortic, mitral, tricuspid or pulmonary valves	1. Congenital valve disorders (e.g. bicuspid aortic valve) predisposing the valve to later malfunction, degeneration or disease 2. Rheumatic valvular heart disease—mitral valve most common; also affects aortic valve (occasionally follows rheumatic fever, causing thickening and tethering of leaflets, shortening of mitral valve chordae and valve calcification) 3. Secondary involvement of valves caused by disruption of nearby structures: —aortic dissection involving the aortic valve —myocardial infarction involving the papillary muscles —myocardial ischaemia leading to scarring and contraction of the papillary muscles —autoimmune disorders, e.g. Libman–Sacks endocarditis —'metabolic' defects, e.g. Marfan's syndrome 4. Infective endocarditis, usually on diseased valves	a. Disordered valve function —valve stenosis restricts blood flow —valvular incompetence causes reflux of blood b. Accumulation of 'vegetations' or thrombus which may embolise into the peripheral arterial tree c. Infection of vegetations or thrombus (bacterial endocarditis) —systemic symptoms (fever, anorexia, weight loss) —deteriorating valve function —infected systemic embolism to brain, kidneys, etc.
Disease affecting the great arteries Aorta	1. Aortic dissection within the media resulting from atherosclerosis or cystic medial necrosis 2. Aneurysm (connective tissue degeneration, syphilis, trauma, infection) 3. Traumatic transsection	a. Acute severe chest pain b. Acute severe hypovolaemic shock with collapse or sudden death
Pulmonary artery	Peripheral deep venous thrombosis detaches and passes through the heart to impact in the pulmonary arteries	a. Acute occlusion by pulmonary embolism—may be silent, symptomatic or 'massive' and fatal b. Recurrent embolism may cause pulmonary hypertension
Pericardial disease	1. Pericardial constriction (scarring or tumour) 2. Pericardial effusion	Signs of constrictive pericarditis: systemic venous congestion with hepatomegaly and ascites; often atrial fibrillation Retrosternal pressure; muffled heart sounds; cardiac tamponade if acute and severe

CONTROL OF PREDISPOSING FACTORS

The first step in treatment is usually an attempt to persuade the patient to modify risk factors known to contribute to disease progression. There are two motives here: firstly, if progression can be arrested, physiological development of collateral blood supply can proceed; this means that intervention may become unnecessary. Secondly, the risk of re-occlusion of any form of revascularisation procedure is increased if risk factors, particularly cigarette smoking, continue to be active. Indeed, it has been shown that, on average, patients who continue to smoke after surgery gain no benefit from coronary artery bypass grafting (CABG). Smokers who fail to improve have thus suffered the risk and discomfort of surgery and at the same time squandered limited hospital resources. Nothing can yet be done about hereditary factors, but smoking, obesity and inactivity can be tackled. The benefits of lowering blood lipid levels are well established. Statins are widely used for this but have other beneficial effects including reducing arterial wall inflammation.

Table 44.4 Presentation of coronary artery disease

Presentation	Secondary effects	Clinical effects
Ischaemic damage discovered incidentally in an asymptomatic patient	Potential risk of further MIs; developing complications of ischaemic heart disease; increased risk when performing an unrelated operation	Found incidentally, e.g. on ECG
A past history of myocardial infarction (MI)	Risk of further MIs; complications of ischaemic heart disease (IHD); risk during unrelated operation	History of typical pain (but note that 25% of MIs are painless)
Angina pectoris	Mortality/morbidity risks of unrelated operations increased	Typical pain brought on by exercise, anxiety or excitement
Complications of myocardial infarction	1. Rupture of part of the heart	Rupture of external wall of left ventricle Septal rupture causing a ventricular septal defect Papillary muscle rupture causing mitral or tricuspid regurgitation
	2. Fibrosis or scarring following myocardial infarction	Generalised fibrosis may cause cardiac failure through loss of contractile myocardium Localised fibrosis of an infarcted ventricular wall may cause a **ventricular aneurysm** Discrete fibrosis near a valve may cause tethering of a mitral leaflet resulting in mitral regurgitation Mural scars may disrupt the conducting system causing ventricular arrhythmias
	3. Mural thrombus may accumulate on a subendocardial infarct as an early response to injury	Thrombus may detach and cause systemic arterial embolism, e.g. to brain, lower limb or superior mesenteric artery; usually an early complication of myocardial infarction (1–6 weeks)

MANAGEMENT OF CORONARY ARTERY DISEASE

Coronary artery disease can be managed conservatively ('medical management') or by interventions employing percutaneous techniques or surgical bypass grafting of coronary arteries. The anatomy of the coronary arteries is shown in Figure 44.3.

Percutaneous angioplasty techniques

A range of percutaneous minimal access techniques have been developed since the early 1980s to expand stenoses or recanalise occluded coronary arteries; these are usually performed by cardiologists. The mainstay of treatment is **percutaneous transluminal coronary (balloon) angioplasty (PTCA)**. Intra-coronary artery stents are being increasingly used in the ballooned segments in certain cases and a reduced restenosis rate has been claimed. These are expensive, particularly drug-eluting stents which are coated with a drug such as sirolimus or paclitaxel to minimise restenosis. Indications for the various stents need to be clearly defined by appropriately randomised trials.

When performed expertly, these techniques cause little disruption to the patient's life and recovery is rapid. However, set against this, there remains a definite early failure rate and a substantial medium-term restenosis rate (> 30% for bare-metal stents and approximately 10–15%

for drug-eluting stents at 6 months). In addition, the patient and a surgical team have to be prepared to carry out an emergency operation at the time of angioplasty if things go wrong. This means tying up resources which are only occasionally required. With improving medium-term results, the main indication for PTCA is for first-time intervention for relieving symptomatic single or double coronary artery stenoses.

Coronary artery bypass grafting (CABG)

Coronary artery bypass grafting is usually indicated in two categories of patient:

- Patients with symptomatic angina not relieved by medical therapy or who are intolerant of it. This is by far the largest group. Most are operated upon electively, but those with crescendo angina may need urgent or emergency surgery
- Patients in categories believed to have a better prognosis after surgery than with medical therapy. Studies in the USA and Europe suggest improved survival after surgery is likely in patients with the following morphological characteristics:
  —Stenosis of the left main stem coronary artery (before it bifurcates into anterior descending and circumflex arteries)

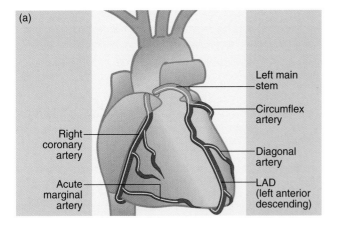

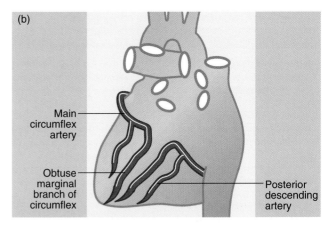

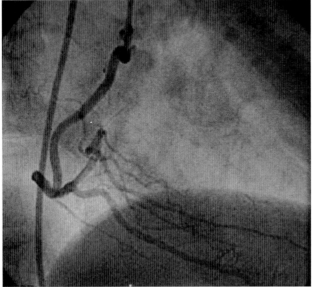

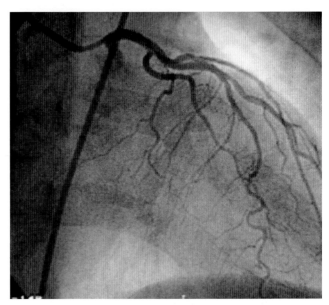

(ci)

(cii)

Fig. 44.3 Anatomy of the coronary arteries
(a) Anterior view of coronary arteries.
(b) Posterior view of coronary arteries.
(c) Selective coronary angiography (AP views as in (a)):
    (i) Normal right coronary artery
    (ii) Normal left coronary artery

—Triple-vessel disease in conjunction with impaired left ventricular contractility (i.e. disease of the right coronary, the left anterior descending and the circumflex arterial systems)
—Two-vessel disease which includes a proximal stenosis in the left anterior descending coronary artery

The results of CABG are encouraging, with between 85% and 90% of patients relieved of angina without the need for medication. A further 5% are substantially improved but require anti-anginal drug therapy.

Surgical technique (Fig. 44.4)
The aim of CABG is to bypass occlusive disease and provide a new source of inflow for the patent distal coronary arteries. Occlusive coronary artery disease is usually situated in the proximal third of the epicardial coronary arteries. This fortunate morphology enables the distal end of bypass grafts to be anastomosed to patent recipient arteries beyond the main disease. Saphenous vein bypass grafts are employed as conduits from the ascending aorta or else a nearby left internal mammary artery is mobilised and attached to the distal coronary artery.

Prosthetic materials give poor results for CABG and are generally not used. Early conduits were almost exclusively reversed autologous long (great) saphenous vein. However, long-term patency is poor, with 50–70% occluding within 10 years of surgery. Long-term patency is better when the left internal mammary artery is grafted onto the left anterior descending coronary artery (see Fig. 44.4). This graft seems to be particularly resistant to occlusion (90%

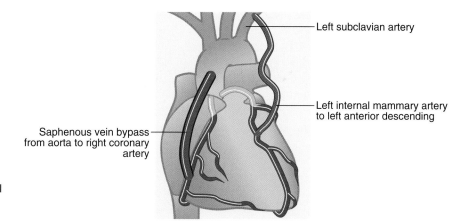

Left subclavian artery

Left internal mammary artery
to left anterior descending

Saphenous vein bypass
from aorta to right coronary
artery

Fig. 44.4 Methods of coronary artery bypass grafting
Note that an explanted autogenous radial artery may be used as a bypass graft instead of saphenous vein.

patency at 10 years) and is the current choice for grafting to this site. Other arteries have also been used for CABG including the radial artery, the right gastro-epiploic artery and the inferior epigastric artery. A combination of left internal mammary grafting to left anterior descending artery and saphenous vein grafts to the other vessels remains the current surgical favourite.

In elective patients, the overall mortality risk of CABG surgery is close to 1%; in addition there is a 2% chance of stroke (especially after a previous stroke). Mortality rates for CABG are higher in patients with pre-existing heart failure as well as those requiring emergency operations. The rate also rises with increasing age.

In order to minimise the potentially damaging problems of cardiopulmonary bypass noted earlier, and also the cognitive deficit that probably follows all such operations, there is a vogue for revascularising the ischaemic heart without bypass. However, operating conditions are more demanding and this may affect the accuracy of anastomoses and increase the occlusion rate of grafts and thereby prejudice the success rate of the procedure in abolishing ischaemia. So far, randomised studies comparing CABG on pump and off pump have failed to demonstrate significant benefit for off pump procedures.

Other types of surgery for ischaemic heart disease

Other forms of surgery in addition to CABG may be required for complications of myocardial infarction. These carry a higher risk than isolated CABG surgery and include:

- Excision of a left ventricular aneurysm—mortality about 5%
- Replacement or repair of a mitral valve leaking as a result of ischaemia—mortality 5–8%
- Surgical identification and ablation of a ventricular arrhythmic focus—mortality 10–15%
- Emergency repair of a post-myocardial infarction ventricular septal rupture—mortality 20–40%

- Post-CABG heart failure necessitating ventricular support (intra-aortic balloon pump) or cardiac transplantation—mortality about 15% at 1 year

VALVULAR HEART DISEASE

Valvular heart disease manifests with symptoms or signs of **stenosis**, with restricted blood flow across the valve, or **regurgitation** where the valve becomes incompetent, allowing blood to escape back through the valve when it should be closed. There has been a trend towards conserving the native valve where possible, but where regurgitant or stenosed valves are unsuitable for conservative treatment, valve replacement is the alternative.

MITRAL VALVE DISEASE

Mitral stenosis following rheumatic fever can be successfully treated by **valvotomy** (separation of fused valve leaflets), provided surgery is performed before calcification has made the leaflets immobile. In the early days of cardiac surgery, Cutler and Levine (1925) introduced semi-closed, blind mitral valvotomy, with mechanical dilatation of the valve orifice performed via the left auricular appendage. With the heart still beating, the auricle was opened, a finger or mechanical device inserted and the valve rapidly dilated. Symptomatic relief was usually reasonable, but the valvotomy was often incomplete or caused splits in the leaflets themselves rather than between them. The procedure often had to be repeated at intervals of a few years. Later, direct **open valvotomy** under cardiopulmonary bypass became popular. More precise and long-lasting results could be achieved by this method. More recently, there has been a return to closed valvotomy, with percutaneous trans-septal balloon dilatation of the stenosed valve. This can achieve reasonable functional results with minimal upset to the patient.

In regurgitant valvular disease, surgical valve repair is possible in most patients but has been most successfully employed for treating myxomatous or degenerate regurgitation of the mitral valve. This conservative technique has a lower perioperative risk than valve replacement and better preserves left ventricular function. Thus, the overall functional result may be better than valve replacement. Repair techniques may also be employed for a diseased tricuspid or aortic valve. Only where valvotomy or repair is inappropriate or has failed are valves replaced.

VALVE PROSTHESES (Fig. 44.5)

There are two types of prosthesis for replacing heart valves, man-made and tissue grafts. Many types of man-made mechanical valves have been tried, ranging from the original 'ball-in-cage' type, through tilting discs to bi-leaflet prostheses (see Fig. 44.5). The mechanical demands on replacement heart valves are extreme. They must cause minimal restriction to blood flow when open, yet prevent reflux when closed; they must be biocompatible, non-thrombogenic, resistant to infection and, most demanding of all, capable of opening and closing 70 times a minute for many years without mechanical failure. Modern mechanical valves are durable but thrombogenic and generally require lifelong anticoagulation. Anticoagulation carries its own risk with a mortality of about 2% over 5 years. Even with effective anticoagulation, there is a small risk of arterial embolism.

Replacement tissue valves may be either **homografts** (human) or **xenografts** (animal origin). Xenografts are almost exclusively harvested from pigs. In general, tissue valves are less thrombogenic (anticoagulation is not nec-essary) but more prone to failure through degeneration as time goes by. In patients over the age of 60 years receiving an aortic bioprosthesis, the freedom from structural valve degeneration at 10 years exceeds 90%. Homograft (human) valves are believed to be resistant to early degeneration and are preferred for young patients to avoid the need for long-term anticoagulation.

Infection of valve prostheses is devastating but fortunately rare. The risk is least for homograft valves. Prosthetic valve endocarditis carries a very high mortality and needs protracted treatment, often requiring the explantation (removal) of the infected prosthesis.

INDICATIONS FOR VALVE SURGERY

The key to successful valvular heart surgery is to carry it out at the most appropriate moment in the natural history of the disease, when risks of surgery are least and potential benefits greatest, i.e. before irreversible ventricular dysfunction has occurred.

In aortic or mitral valve stenosis, surgery is indicated when patients become symptomatic. In aortic or mitral valve regurgitation, surgical intervention is advised when there is evidence of left ventricular dilatation in asymptomatic patients.

PERICARDIAL DISEASE

Pericardial inflammation may result in constriction of the pericardium. World-wide, this occurs most commonly in tuberculosis. Constrictive pericarditis may also occur in certain autoimmune conditions such as rheumatoid

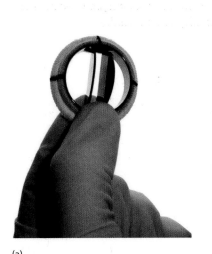
(a)

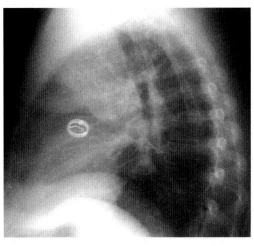
(b)

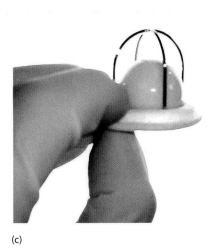
(c)

Fig. 44.5 Mechanical prosthetic valves
The two main types of mechanical valve are shown here. **(a)** A bi-leaflet valve—used in 90% of patients requiring a mechanical prosthesis. **(b)** A lateral chest X-ray showing a tilting disc mitral valve prosthesis in situ. **(c)** A ball and cage type of valve (Starr–Edwards—rarely used these days). These valves variously have metal or plastic balls. Lifelong anticoagulation is mandatory for all patients receiving mechanical valve prosthesis.

arthritis or following pericardial trauma or mediastinal radiotherapy. Pericardial constriction impairs blood filling of the cardiac chambers and typically this causes equalisation of diastolic pressures in all four chambers of the heart. Clinical signs are those of pulmonary and systemic venous congestion, together with a low cardiac output. Surgical treatment involves excision of the entire pericardium.

DISEASE OF THE THORACIC AORTA

Surgical disorders of the thoracic aorta include:

- Aortic dissection
- Thoracic aneurysms
- Aortic trauma

AORTIC DISSECTION

In aortic dissection, blood leaks from the lumen to split the media and flow along a false lumen for variable distances proximally and/or distally. The intimal flap may occlude any of the aortic branches or disrupt the aortic valve. The likely aetiology is degeneration of elastin and collagen in the media. Dissection occurs most commonly in the ascending aorta (65%), but also in the aortic arch (10%), or in the descending thoracic aorta just distal to the ligamentum arteriosum (20%).

Dissection is classified according to the part affected; the most widely used method is the **Stanford system**. Type A indicates that only the ascending aorta is involved while type B describes the situation when any other part of the thoracic aorta is affected. An alternative classification method is that of De Bakey (see Fig. 44.6).

Without surgery, Stanford type A dissection carries an 80% mortality in the first month; with surgical management this falls to less than 20%. The operation involves resecting the ascending aorta and replacing it with a synthetic tube graft. If the dissection reaches the aortic valve, it is likely to be disrupted, causing acute severe regurgitation and perhaps occluding the coronary artery origins. In such cases, the valve will need resuspending or replacing.

Uncomplicated type B dissections have a 20% mortality at 30 days, and the outcome is similar whether surgically or medically managed. Medical management is by control of hypertension. Surgery is required in type B dissections which are complicated by aortic rupture, occlusion of vital branches, progressive dissection or, later, by aneurysm formation. Note that abdominal aortic aneurysms occur years later in about 50% after thoracic aortic dissection.

THORACIC ANEURYSMS

Aneurysmal dilatation of the thoracic aorta may occur in the ascending part (Fig. 44.7), the arch or the descending part. There is a risk of rupture similar to that found in abdominal aortic aneurysms and surgical intervention is usually recommended when the aneurysm reaches a diameter of 6 cm. Replacing the descending aorta, particularly when there is thoraco-abdominal disease, threatens the main blood supply of the spinal cord (the artery of Adamkiewicz at about T10) so that paraplegia complicates 10–30% of these operations. Various methods of monitoring and prevention are being developed. There is a growing trend towards employing endoluminal stent-grafts for appropriate thoracic aneurysms with the promise of lower morbidity and mortality.

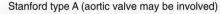
Stanford type A (aortic valve may be involved)   Stanford type B

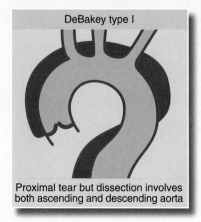

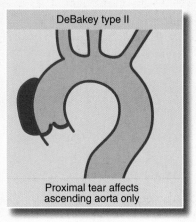

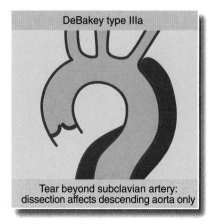

DeBakey type I — Proximal tear but dissection involves both ascending and descending aorta

DeBakey type II — Proximal tear affects ascending aorta only

DeBakey type IIIa — Tear beyond subclavian artery: dissection affects descending aorta only

Fig. 44.6 Thoracic aortic dissection

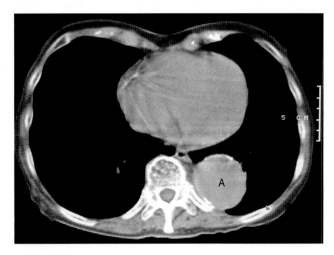

Fig. 44.7 Thoracic aortic aneurysm
CT scan of chest showing a 5 cm aneurysm of the descending thoracic aorta **A**.

TRAUMA TO THE THORACIC AORTA

This may result from blunt or sharp injury. Blunt aortic trauma is usually associated with severe deceleration as occurs in head-on impact in road traffic collisions. The common injury is partial or complete transsection of the aorta at the junction between the arch and the descending aorta close to the ligamentum arteriosum. Complete transsection with free rupture is rapidly fatal; partial transsection with an intact adventitia and a contained haematoma is liable to rupture at any time and must be diagnosed to enable early emergency treatment. There is an increasing trend towards treating these with intraluminal stent grafts placed via the femoral artery. Late aneurysm formation may also occur in those patients who survive an untreated occult aortic transsection.

PULMONARY EMBOLISM

Emergency surgical removal of a massive pulmonary embolism has become increasingly rare with the introduction of effective thrombolytic agents. Nowadays, there are only a few indications for emergency pulmonary embolectomy. These usually relate to situations where thrombolytic therapy might carry unacceptable risks, e.g. after recent surgery or during pregnancy. The operation is carried out under cardiopulmonary bypass.

In some patients with recurrent pulmonary embolism, the pulmonary vasculature becomes progressively obliterated and they eventually develop **chronic thromboembolic pulmonary hypertension**. Life expectancy is significantly shortened when the mean pulmonary artery pressure exceeds 30 mmHg. This condition was previously treated by heart and lung transplantation but pulmonary endarterectomy is now increasingly being offered.

Disorders of the breast

INTRODUCTION TO BREAST DISEASE

Virtually every woman with a breast lump, breast pain or discharge from the nipple fears that she has cancer. The anxiety that results is made up of three components: the unknown course of the disease, the threat of mutilation and the fear of dying. Previously, this often prevented women from seeking early medical advice but in recent years public awareness and media publicity about self-examination and screening (see Ch. 6) and the possible advantages of early treatment have encouraged earlier presentation.

Individual anxiety may be heightened by knowledge of friends' or relatives' experiences of breast cancer or a recent 'celebrity diagnosis', and reassurance of the 'worried well' is an important aspect of managing breast disease.

The possible effects of breast surgery on sexual attractiveness and femininity are often uppermost in a woman's mind, so consideration must be given to this and other psychological aspects of breast disease. Breast care nurses can help provide psychological support at each stage of investigation and treatment.

Rates of referral to breast clinics have increased dramatically over the past decade, reflecting easier access, widespread breast screening and changes in public awareness and attitudes to breast cancer. Despite the fears of those patients being referred, less than 15% turn out to have cancer in the UK. The other 85% includes some with benign breast disease and others that fall within the normal range of breast anatomy and physiology (see Box 45.1).

SYMPTOMS AND SIGNS OF BREAST DISEASE

Patients often present complaining of symptoms and sometimes of signs (see Fig. 45.1). Two-thirds complain of a lump or an area of lumpiness (see Table 45.1). Many do not have a discrete mass, but rather an area of **focal nodularity** which represents a prominent area of glandular tissue, i.e. an **abnormality of normal development and involution (ANDI)**. The distinction may be evident on clinical examination, but further evaluation with ultrasound is often needed.

SPECIAL POINTS IN HISTORY TAKING

A careful and detailed history can provide important clues as to the underlying pathology of a breast problem.

Age has an important bearing on the probability of different breast disorders being present (see Fig. 45.2); in particular the risk of malignancy rises with age. The **duration of symptoms** should be established at the outset; cancers are usually slow-growing and likely to have been present for several years, whilst cysts can appear rapidly, sometimes almost overnight. Benign conditions such as fibroadenosis and fibroadenomas may present with lumps that **fluctuate with the menstrual cycle** or have decreased in size since first noticed by the patient. They are also more likely to be associated with **pain and tenderness** than a malignant lesion.

A **previous history** of breast conditions, particularly malignancy (or breast biopsies showing premalignant

SYMPTOM OR SIGN	CLINICAL SIGNIFICANCE
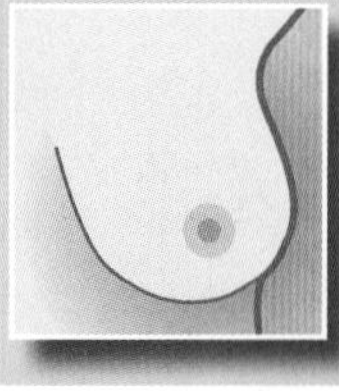 **1. Pain**	
Varying with menstrual cycle	Suggests a physiological cause such as premenstrual syndrome or fibroadenosis. Both are responsive to treatment
Independent of menstrual cycle	Not diagnostic but may occur in carcinoma, fibroadenosis or infection
Refer non-urgently if pain not responding to treatment	
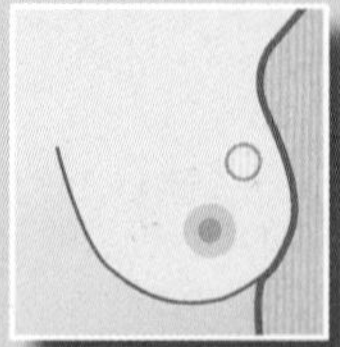 **2. Lump in the breast**	
Hard lump	A discrete mobile lump with a smooth surface is most likely to be a fibroadenoma or a fibroadenotic cyst. An ill-defined margin and any suggestion of tethering to superficial or deep structures strongly suggest carcinoma but are sometimes due to non-infective inflammation or fat necrosis
Refer urgently	
Firm, poorly defined lump or lumpiness	Suggests fibroadenosis, especially if outline is difficult to distinguish from normal breast tissue or if the breast is generally lumpy. Risk of malignancy small but see referral guidelines opposite
Refer urgently if: **Lump enlarging or other features of malignancy** **Over 30 years of age and lump persists after next period** **Family history of breast cancer** **Post menopausal** **Previous breast cancer** **Males over 50, unilateral lump** **Refer non-urgently if:** **Under 30 years of age** **Unexplained persistent symptoms**	
Soft lump	Usually a lipoma or occasionally a lax cyst
3. Skin changes in the breast **Refer urgently**	
Skin dimpling or tethering	Sometimes a subtle sign but highly suggestive of carcinoma
Visible lump	Cyst, carcinoma or phylloides tumour. Cysts can appear with alarming speed
Peau d'orange (appearance of orange peel)	Over a lump, this is virtually pathognomonic of carcinoma. It is due to tumour invasion of dermal lymphatics causing dermal oedema. However, it may occur over an infective lesion
Redness	Usually infection, especially if skin is hot. Sometimes a feature of mammary duct ectasia. Beware inflammatory carcinoma
Ulceration	Neglected carcinoma in the elderly (often slow-growing)
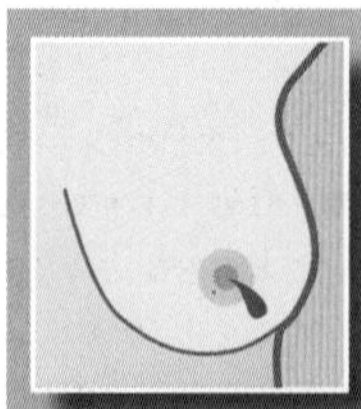 **4. Nipple disorders**	
Recent inversion or change in shape	Suggests a fibrosing underlying lesion such as a carcinoma or mammary duct ectasia but can be malignancy
Refer urgently	
'Eczema' (rash involving nipple or areola, or both)	If unilateral and persistent, this is the classic sign of Paget's disease of the nipple, a presentation of breast cancer
Refer urgently if not responding to treatment	
Nipple discharge	
Milky	Pregnancy or hyperprolactinaemia
Clear	Physiological
Green	Perimenopausal, duct ectasia, fibroadenotic cyst
Refer only if other signs or symptoms	
Blood-stained	Possible carcinoma or intraduct papilloma
Refer urgently	

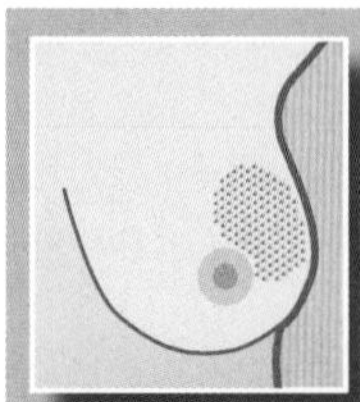

Fig. 45.1 Symptoms and signs of breast disease (see also Figs 45.3–45.5)

UK NICE guidelines for urgent and non-urgent referral to a specialist are indicated on a pink background.

Table 45.1 Frequency of different presenting symptoms of patients in a breast clinic

Symptom	Frequency
Breast lump	35%
Painful lump or lumpiness	33%
Pain alone	15%
Nipple discharge	5%
Nipple retraction	5%
Family history of breast cancer	3%
Breast distortion	2%
Swelling/inflammation	2%

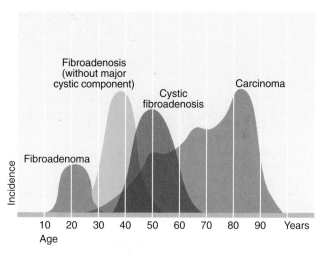

Fig. 45.2 Age incidence of common breast disorders

Box 45.1 Types of breast disease of surgical importance

Malignant neoplasms

- Ductal adenocarcinoma
- Lobular adenocarcinoma
- Sarcoma
- Metastasis from other tissues

Benign tumour-like lesions

- Fibroadenoma
- Intraduct papilloma
- Lipoma

Disordered physiological responses of breast tissue (abnormalities of normal development and involution, ANDI)

- Fibroadenosis (also known as fibrocystic disease, benign mammary dysplasia and chronic mastitis)

Mammary duct ectasia

- Chronic periductal inflammatory reaction due to retained duct secretions

Infections

- Cellulitis and breast abscess
- Subareolar abscesses in mammary duct ectasia

Box 45.2 Risk factors for breast cancer

- Increasing age
- Family history (number of first- and second-degree relatives, their age of onset and bilaterality, known *BRCA1/BRCA2* mutations)
- Previous history of breast cancer or carcinoma in situ
- Early age of menarche (age < 12 years
- Late age of menopause (age > 55 years)
- Late age at first full-term pregnancy (age < 20 years protective)
- Nulliparity
- Previous breast biopsies showing non-malignant abnormalities
- Hormonal therapy—oral contraceptive pill or HRT
- Radiation at a young age (mantle irradiation for lymphomas, atomic bomb survivors)

See also http://info.cancerresearchuk.org/cancerstats/types/breast/riskfactors/#reproductive

Trauma from seatbelt injuries has increased in recent years and patients should be asked whether they have had any episodes of bruising of the breast followed by the appearance of a lump.

Drug history, particularly of the oral contraceptive pill (OCP) or hormone replacement therapy (HRT), should be recorded, including the duration and how recently the drug has been used. These drugs modulate the hormonal environment of breast tissue and tend to increase the risk of breast cancer. Other hormone-related risk factors for cancer include late age at first full-term pregnancy, lower parity (number of pregnancies) and early age of menarche and late age of menopause. Enquiry should be made about a **family history** of breast or ovarian cancer, including number of first- and second-degree relatives, age of

change), cysts or fibrocystic change, can be an important indicator of the likely nature of any current breast problem. It is important to remember that the greatest single risk factor for breast cancer is a previous history of the condition, however long ago (1% risk per year), see Box 45.2. There is also recent evidence that patients with recurrent benign breast disorders are more liable to breast cancer.

637

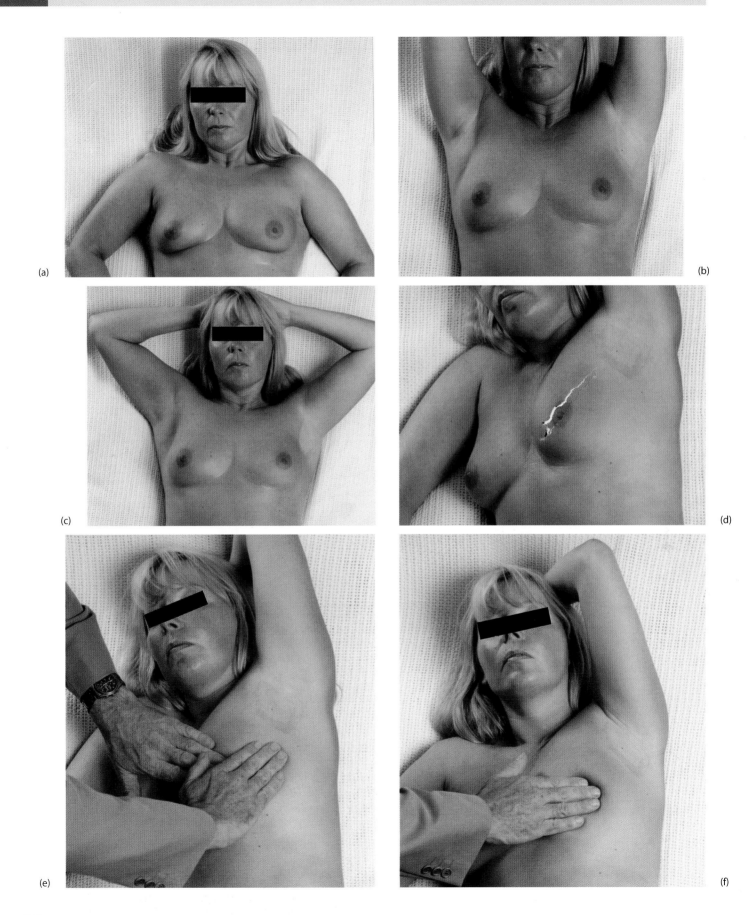

(a)

(b)

(c)

(d)

(e)

(f)

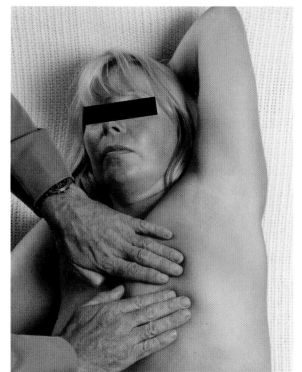

(g)

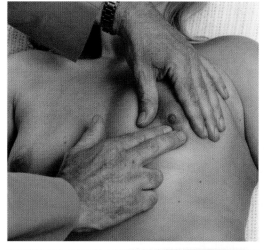

(h)

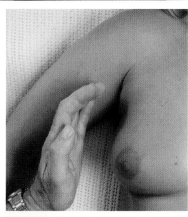

(i)

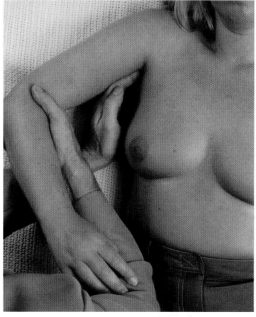

(j)

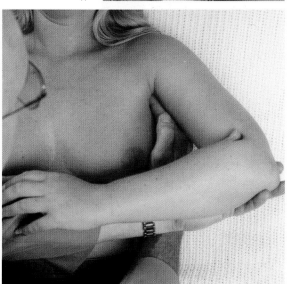

(k)

Fig. 45.3 Technique of breast examination

Inspection: the breasts should be inspected for asymmetry, skin tethering and dimpling and changes in colour. This should be performed with the patient sitting comfortably, pressing hands on hips **(a)**, lifting arms in the air **(b)**, and pressing hands on top of the head **(c)**. *Palpation*: the patient should sit on an examination couch as shown in **(d)**, with the backrest at about 45° and rolled slightly to the contralateral side. The arm on the side to be examined should be elevated and the head rested on the pillow. The effect of these manoeuvres is to spread the breast over a greater area of the chest wall. The flat of the right hand is used to palpate the breast circumferentially by quadrants **(e)**–**(g)**. The central part of the breast and the axillary tail must also be palpated. If there is a history of nipple discharge, the areola is pressed in different areas **(h)** to identify the duct from which it emanates and therefore the segment involved. Finally the **axillary lymph nodes** are palpated as shown in **(i)**, **(j)** and **(k)**. The left axilla is palpated with the right hand **(k)** and the right axilla is palpated with the left hand **(j)**. It is important to relax the axillary muscles by supporting the weight of the patient's arm as shown. The fingers of the examining hand are firmly held in a curve **(i)**, pressed high into the apex of the axilla against the chest wall and drawn downwards. The hand will then 'ride over' any enlarged axillary nodes.

onset and bilaterality. Some families are known to have mutations in the tumour suppressor genes *BRCA1* or *BRCA2* which strongly predispose to breast and other cancers.

EXAMINATION OF THE BREASTS

There are several accepted methods for examining the breasts; one is shown in Figure 45.3. All areas of the breast must be examined, with particular attention to the axillary tail and retroareolar regions. Breast examination involves six distinct manoeuvres:

- Observation with the patient sitting up
- Observation with the patient raising and lowering her arms
- Examination of the nipples
- Systematic palpation of each breast
- Palpation of the axillae and supraclavicular fossae
- General examination for signs of distant metastases

During inspection, the signs to be looked for are listed in Figure 45.1. The technique of palpating the breast may need to be modified according to the shape and size of the patient. Palpation with the flat of one hand is usual, but it may be more appropriate to examine large breasts between two hands. Most of the breast tissue lies in the central and upper outer zones, which are more reliably palpated if the patient is turned somewhat laterally so the breast being examined lies uppermost on the chest wall.

Palpation may be done in one of three accepted routines: **circumferentially**, starting at the nipple then moving in progressively larger circles; **radially** from the nipple outwards like the spokes in a wheel; or by **sectors**, examining each quadrant in turn. The axillary lymph nodes are palpated whilst the other hand supports the weight of the patient's arm (Fig. 45.3 j and k). This helps relax the muscles and aids assessment of the nodal groups **(medial, lateral, anterior, posterior and apical)**. Note, however, that clinical assessment of axillary nodes has a 30% false positive rate and a 30% false negative rate.

A history of **nipple discharge** can often be confirmed by applying pressure over the appropriate part of the breast near the areola. Discharges which are not obviously blood-stained should be tested for blood using urinalysis dipsticks. In addition, a smear preparation should be examined for cytological abnormalities.

Lumps

During the examination the patient should be asked to point out any lump she is worried about. The normal breast has a wide range of textures, from soft through nodular to hard. This means that clinical evaluation alone of what appears to be a lump or lumpiness is unreliable; the texture of the rest of the breast must be taken into account. When a lump is found, its characteristics should be defined (see Box 45.3), in particular whether it is a discrete or dominant mass or whether it is an area of focal nodularity or 'thickening'. If there is a discrete mass, does it appear to be benign or is it suspicious for malignancy? (The characteristic signs of breast cancer are shown in Fig. 45.4.) Note that even for breast specialists, clinical exami-

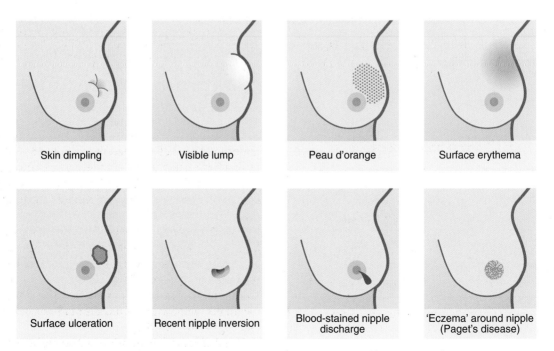

Skin dimpling	Visible lump
Peau d'orange	Surface erythema
Surface ulceration	Recent nipple inversion
Blood-stained nipple discharge	'Eczema' around nipple (Paget's disease)

Fig. 45.4 Characteristic signs of breast cancer

Fig. 45.5 Carcinoma of the breast

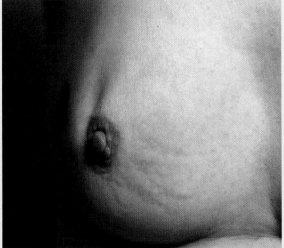

(a)

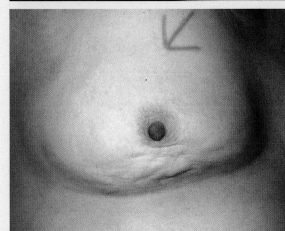

(b)

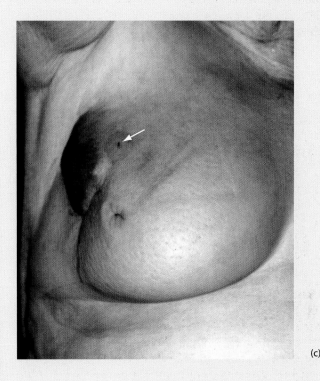

(c)

(a) and **(b)** Characteristic skin dimpling over breast carcinomas. This may be a subtle sign and only be visible in tangential light.
(c) Nipple retraction and widespread 'peau d'orange' resulting from a large central breast carcinoma. Peau d'orange is caused by a combination of cutaneous infiltration by tumour and skin oedema (and occasionally by infection). Locally advanced breast cancer may cause distortion of the breast. The colour change and ulceration are uncommonly seen and only occur in neglected cases. Note also the puncture wound of a core biopsy (arrowed). There was no obvious axillary node enlargement.

Box 45.3	Clinical characteristics of a breast lump

- Solitary or multiple
- Size—in centimetres
- Location—quadrant of breast or clock face
- Contour—smooth and round/ovoid (likely to be benign) or firm/hard (probable malignancy)
- Mobility—mobile (likely to be benign) or fixed (probable malignancy)
- Associated changes—skin/nipple retraction, skin tethering, bloody nipple discharge, erythema
- Axillary lymphadenopathy—enlarged and mobile or enlarged and fixed

nation alone has a sensitivity (i.e. ability to detect abnormalities that are present) of only 65–80%. In one evaluation system, increasing levels of clinical suspicion can be graded E1 to E5; an E3 designation may prompt a core biopsy even if the radiological findings are not suspicious.

Skin tethering (as opposed to direct infiltration) can be a subtle sign and is accentuated by raising the arms above the head to put the suspensory ligaments of the breast under tension. Deep fixation can be assessed by checking the degree of mobility of the lump over the pectoralis major with the muscle both relaxed and tensed (see Figs 45.4 and 45.5).

The differential diagnosis of a discrete breast mass falls into one of five possibilities:

- Cyst
- Fibroadenoma
- Focus of fibrocystic change or fibroadenosis
- Fat necrosis (rare)
- Carcinoma

The probability of a particular diagnosis is to some extent age dependent (see Fig. 45.2). Only 3% of breast cancers occur under the age of 30 years but a discrete lump in a patient over 65 years should be considered to be a cancer until proved otherwise.

Paget's disease of the nipple

Some patients with breast carcinoma present with eczema-like reddening and thickening of the skin of the nipple and areola, together with fissuring and ulceration. This condition is more common in the elderly and is known as Paget's disease of the nipple.

INVESTIGATION OF BREAST DISORDERS

'One-stop' clinics allow rapid and comprehensive preliminary assessment of patients. **Triple assessment** includes clinical examination, breast imaging and biopsy (when indicated) on the same day. This has an overall accuracy of 99.6% when performed by experienced personnel, meaning that the chances of missing a cancer are less than 1%; patients shown not to have cancer can usually be discharged from the clinic. If there is a clinically suspicious lump and needle biopsy is negative or equivocal, diagnostic **excision biopsy** should be performed. The discrete lump is completely excised and the specimen examined histologically.

Imaging

Mammography (breast radiography) is the main method of radiological assessment of the breasts and forms the basis of breast cancer screening programmes (see Ch. 6). In women over the age of 40 years, it has a sensitivity of 88%. In younger women, it is less sensitive because the breast tissue is more dense; it is rarely performed under the age of 35 years. During mammography, the breast is compressed firmly between two transparent plastic plates. This spreads the tissue and makes it easier to detect any mass lesion. Radiological views are taken in two directions, medio-lateral oblique (MLO) and cranio-caudal (CC). Focused magnified views can be taken to better display an abnormal area. Conventional film-screen mammography is being replaced with digital mammography which permits enhancement of the image (Fig. 45.6).

Four features are looked for on a mammogram:

- The presence of a mass lesion
- Microcalcification
- Architectural distortion
- Asymmetry

A typical carcinoma appears as a **spiculated** mass lesion (dense regions with radiating lines) which may have associated malignant-type microcalcification (Fig. 45.7). When fine granular microcalcification is seen within a spiculated lesion this is virtually pathognomonic of a cancer. The tumour is sometimes radiologically detectable as small as 2–3 mm, long before it becomes palpable.

Benign-type microcalcification is coarse and 'chunky' (Fig. 45.8) whilst malignant-type microcalcification is finer and linear or granular (Fig. 45.7b). Fine branching microcalcification is characteristic of **ductal carcinoma in situ (DCIS)**. Architectural distortion and asymmetry are more subtle radiological signs that should be viewed with suspicion.

Ultrasound has long been used to distinguish solid mass lesions from cysts and for this it has a specificity of 100%. Modern B-mode ultrasound machines enable benign breast lesions to be distinguished from malignant lesions with a sensitivity for cancer of 85%. Ultrasound can accurately measure the size of a cancer (correlating well with the pathological measurements, Fig. 45.9) and it is also used to guide percutaneous needle biopsies (including cyst aspiration) (Fig. 45.10).

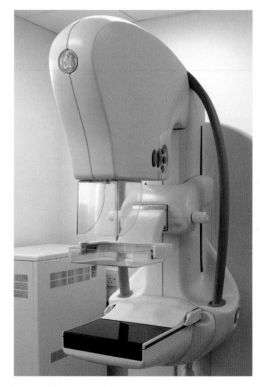

Fig. 45.6 Digital mammography machine

Fig. 45.7 Carcinoma of the breast on mammography

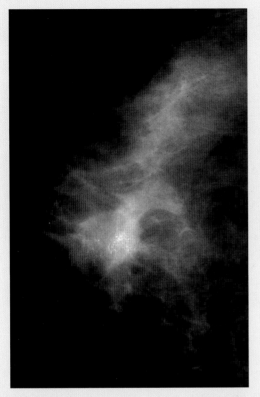

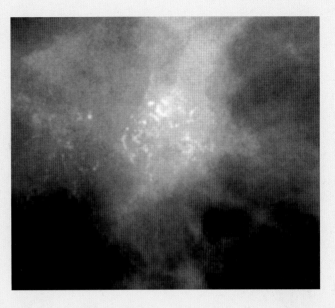

(a)

(b)

This 58-year-old woman presented with a 2-week history of a non-tender lump in the left breast. Clinical examination confirmed a hard irregular mass without skin dimpling, and a palpable left axillary node. **(a)** This image shows a cranio-caudal view of the left breast with a dense opacity lying centrally. It has an irregular border with radiating spicules typical of a carcinoma. **(b)** Enlarged view of the carcinoma showing typical malignant-type microcalcification. This contrasts with the coarser calcification occurring in benign breast conditions (see Fig. 45.8c).

Biopsy

All palpable and non-palpable image-detected mass lesions are biopsied under image guidance, as are any suspicious areas of calcification. Specimens for **fine needle aspiration cytology (FNAC)** are obtained using a 21 gauge needle attached to a syringe to which suction is applied manually while the tip of the needle is passed several times through the lesion. The needle contents are ejected onto a microscope slide and the aspirate can be immediately examined and graded C1–C5 (see Box 45.4). FNAC has a sensitivity of 95% for detecting malignancy but cannot distinguish between in situ and invasive cancers. By contrast, **core biopsy** has a sensitivity of 98%. The tissue architecture is preserved so that invasion can be confidently diagnosed and tumours can be pathologically graded. Many clinicians prefer core biopsy to FNAC because of this improved diagnostic value. After core biopsy, patients need to return later for the results, which has the advantage that any bad news can be broken in a

Box 45.4	Reporting categories for fine needle aspiration cytology

C1—inadequate specimen
C2—benign
C3—suspicious but probably benign
C4—suspicious and probably malignant
C5—malignant

phased manner. If needle biopsy is negative or equivocal, a discrete lump should be completely excised with a wide margin of apparently normal breast tissue and the specimen examined histologically. This procedure, **excision biopsy**, can also form the first step in controlling local disease.

Eczematous lesions suspicious for Paget's disease of the nipple can be 'punch' biopsied under local anaesthesia in the clinic.

Fig. 45.8 Fibroadenoma of the breast

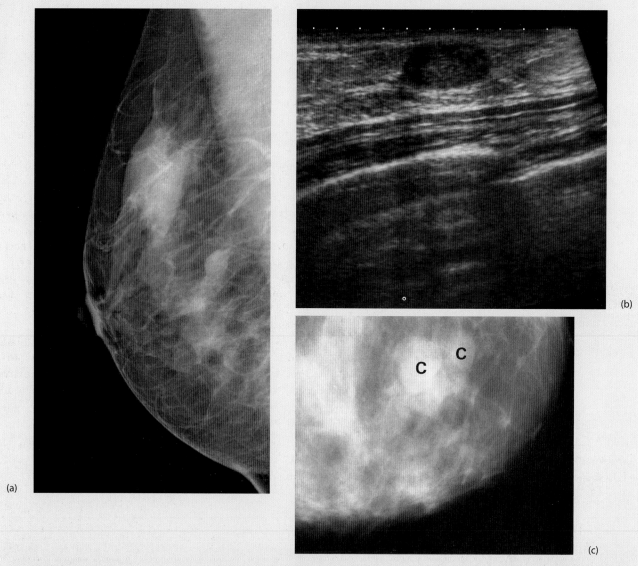

(a)

(b)

(c)

This 35-year-old patient presented with a 3-month history of a lump in the upper aspect of the left breast which was slightly tender at the time of menstruation. Clinical examination revealed a smooth round mobile mass which was firm and very mobile. **(a)** This mammogram shows simple lobulated mass lesion in the upper part of the breast with a well-defined border. These appearances are suggestive of a benign lesion (in this case a fibroadenoma). **(b)** This image shows the ultrasound appearances of the lesion in **(a)**; it is a well-defined solid lesion with regular internal echoes and no posterior enhancement (compare with Fig. 45.10b). The lesion is 'broad' rather than 'tall' and is typical of a fibroadenoma. **(c)** An enlarged mammographic view of a different fibroadenoma in an older woman showing the much coarser calcification associated with benign breast lesions compared with carcinoma.

BREAST CANCER

INTRODUCTION

In Western societies, about 1 in 10 women will develop breast cancer (i.e. a lifetime risk of 10%) and 1 in 18 will die from it. In the UK, 41 000 new cases are diagnosed annually and approximately 14 000 die each year from the disease (about 270 per week). World-wide, there are approximately half a million deaths from breast cancer but, in spite of an increasing global incidence, mortality rates have gradually fallen as a result of earlier diagnosis and improved treatments, including advances in hormonal therapy.

Fig. 45.9 Carcinoma of the breast on ultrasound

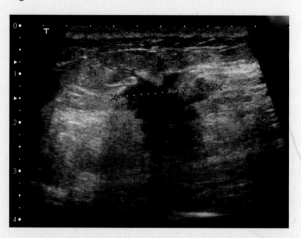

Ultrasound scan of the patient shown in Fig. 45.7 a and b. This shows a hypoechoic mass lesion extending the width of the blue dotted line. It has an irregular border and some internal echoes. The lesion is characteristically 'tall', i.e. deep, and there is acoustic shadowing deep to the lesion. This image should be contrasted with the appearances of a benign fibroadenoma (Fig. 48.8b).

Clinical examination alone is unreliable in diagnosing or excluding breast cancer, partly because the clinical features of benign and malignant breast conditions can be similar. A family practitioner in the UK sees on average only two breast cancer cases a year, but many suspected cases need specialist referral to ensure this diagnosis is not missed.

In the UK, all patients with symptoms suspicious of cancer are referred immediately to specialists and have to be seen within 2 weeks. Ideally, breast referrals should be seen in a 'one-stop' triple assessment diagnostic clinic.

EPIDEMIOLOGY

Breast cancer is not a new disease; it was recognised by the ancient Egyptians and mastectomy was certainly performed in Roman times. Nowadays, breast cancer is predominantly a disease of Western society but differences in incidence are more likely to be due to environmental than racial differences. The disease is relatively uncommon in Japan, but Japanese immigrants to the United States acquire local incidence rates within two generations.

Breast cancer rates are rising fastest in those Asiatic countries where Western lifestyles have been adopted. The rise is most likely to be due to changes in reproductive practice, including deferring childbirth until past 30 years

Fig. 45.10 Breast cyst

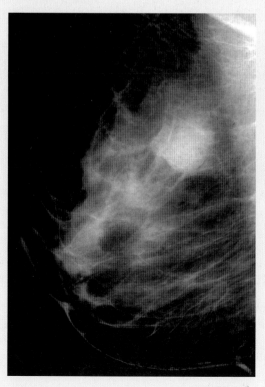

(a)

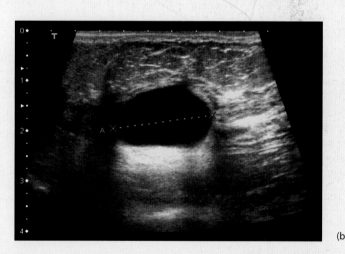

(b)

This 42-year-old woman presented with a tender lump in the superior aspect of the right breast. There was a previous history of breast cysts. Examination revealed a smooth, round and slightly fluctuant mass. **(a)** Mediolateral oblique view mammogram showing a well-defined lesion with circumscribed margins in the upper part of the breast. The appearances are of a benign lesion. **(b)** Complementary ultrasound examination reveals an anechoic mass with sharp, well-defined margins and posterior acoustic enhancement. This is diagnostic of a simple cyst.

of age, smaller families, and prolonged use of the oral contraceptive pill.

There is a progressive rise in the incidence of breast cancer with age from about 25. The rise is steepest between the ages of 40 and 55 with a slight levelling off until about the age of 70. After that there is another fairly steep rise that continues into old age (see Fig. 45.2). Indeed, breast cancer is the commonest cause of death in women aged between 40 and 50 years.

Genetic factors

The aetiology of breast cancer is multifactorial, with genetic factors being relatively more important in pre-menopausal women and environmental factors more so after the menopause. Many patients have a family history of breast cancer, but only 5–10% of all breast cancer is hereditary and in these cases it is transmitted in an autosomal dominant fashion. Mutations in two tumour suppressor genes, *BRCA1* and *BRCA2*, are known to confer a genetic predisposition to breast cancer: a mutation in either of these leads to an 80–90% lifetime risk of developing the disease.

Certain features make it more likely that a patient with the disease has one of these gene mutations. These are the presence of bilateral breast cancers, disease onset under 40 years of age and three or more first-degree relatives affected. If breast and ovarian cancer occur in the same patient, this suggests a *BRCA1* mutation. Some carriers of these mutations elect to have prophylactic bilateral mastectomies, which reduce the cancer risk by more than 90%. Others opt for close surveillance.

Hormonal factors

The growth of most breast cancers is promoted by oestrogens, hence reproductive physiology and behaviour influence breast cancer risk. It has long been known that nulliparous women are at greater risk of breast cancer. Ramazzini commented in 1703 that breast cancer was common in Catholic nuns who as 'Vestalis Virgines' were prone to 'horrendis mammarium canceris'. A first full-term pregnancy under 20 years halves the risk of breast cancer compared with one between 30 and 35 years or nulliparity. A first full-term pregnancy delayed until over the age of 35 years further increases the risk. Prolonged breast-feeding has a small protective effect.

The interval between menarche and menopause is known as the **oestrogen window** and is a measure of cumulative exposure to endogenous oestrogen. The longer this interval, the higher the breast cancer risk. A natural or a 'medical' menopause under 40 years reduces breast cancer risk by two-thirds. Prolonged use of the **oral contraceptive pill** increases the risk of breast cancer by over 20% and by even more among women aged over 45 who continue to use it. Combined **hormonal replacement therapy** (HRT) increases cancer risk by only a small amount whilst oestrogen-only HRT has a negligible effect, even with extended use.

Environmental factors

Exposure to irradiation in the teenage years may initiate some breast cancers which are promoted by other factors years later. Female survivors of the atomic bombs of Hiroshima and Nagasaki have a high risk of developing breast cancer, as do those who have received extended irradiation for Hodgkin's disease. Women exposed to large numbers of chest X-rays for monitoring tuberculosis (which occurred in the days before modern chemotherapy) have a moderately increased risk of breast cancer.

An individual's risk of breast cancer can be reduced by avoiding obesity, minimising use of exogenous hormones and avoiding excessive alcohol. It has been convincingly demonstrated that a woman's risk of breast cancer rises by 6% for each regular daily unit of alcohol consumed. Surprisingly, no link has been shown between smoking and breast cancer.

PATHOLOGY

Tumour types

Almost all cancers of the breast are adenocarcinomas and arise from the terminal duct/lobular unit. Seventy-five per cent of cancers originate from the ductal component and are designated invasive **ductal carcinomas** of 'no special type' (NST) (Fig. 45.11). About 10% of invasive cancers arise from the lobular component and are called **lobular carcinomas**. These have similar behaviour and prognosis to ductal carcinomas but can be difficult to see on a mammogram. Microscopically these tumours are characterised by a linear arrangement of cells, so-called 'Indian filing' (Fig. 45.11b). A few invasive carcinomas have both ductal and lobular features and are termed 'mixed' tumours. Nowadays, most tumours are tested for hormone receptor status. Oestrogen receptor (ER) status determines how tumours respond to adjuvant hormonal treatment.

The remaining 12–15% of breast cancers are known as **'special types'** and generally have a better prognosis. These are all well differentiated and include several distinct histological types:

- Tubular—prominent tubule formation (6%)
- Mucoid—high mucoid production (5%)
- Medullary—prominent lymphocytic infiltrate (3%)
- Papillary—composed of papillary structures (1–2%)

In situ carcinoma

Most breast cancers develop from an in situ or non-invasive precursor known as **ductal carcinoma in situ** or **DCIS**. With the roll-out of breast screening programmes there has been a substantial increase in the number of non-invasive breast cancers detected. **High-grade DCIS is**

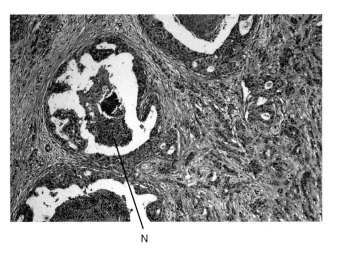

(a)

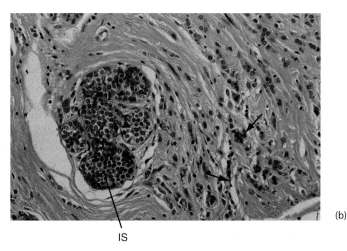

(b)

N   IS

Fig. 45.11 Breast adenocarcinoma—histopathology
(a) Ducts to the left of the picture contain highly atypical epithelium, with central necrosis **N**, a type of in situ ductal carcinoma also known as *comedocarcinoma*. On the right of this micrograph is invasive ductal carcinoma composed of many small glandular structures diffusely invading breast tissue. **(b)** In situ **IS** and invasive lobular carcinoma. Malignant cells tend to be less atypical than in ductal carcinoma and do not form glands, but often invade in 'single-file' (arrowed). Intracellular mucin is also characteristic of this variant of breast carcinoma.

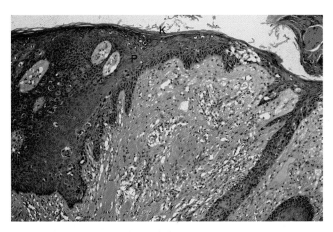

(a)

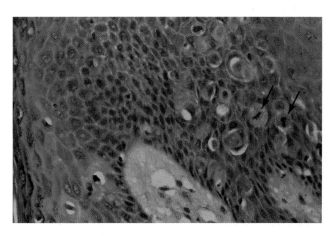

(b)

Fig. 45.12 Paget's disease of the nipple—histopathology
(a) Nipple epidermis containing numerous malignant Paget's cells **P** which have spread from an underlying in situ ductal carcinoma. The epidermis and keratin layer **K** show associated changes. **(b)** High-power view of Paget's cells showing intracellular mucin and mitotic activity (arrowed).

often identified by areas of microcalcification on a mammogram without a mass lesion. These have a 25% chance of progressing to invasion within 5–10 years. **Low-grade DCIS** is found in up to 15% of autopsies, suggesting that at least some non-invasive cancers do not progress to invasion.

Tumour grade

Breast carcinomas are graded histologically for biological aggressiveness; this helps with estimating the prognosis and with treatment planning. Ductal cancers are ranked into grades I, II or III on the Bloom–Richardson scale. Three elements are scored for each tumour: the degree of tubule formation, the amount of nuclear pleomorphism and the number of mitoses. The higher the combined score, the higher the grade and the worse the prognosis. Higher grade tumours tend to infiltrate blood and lymphatic vessels which increases the chance of lymph node and haematogenous metastases. Unfortunately, grade III tumours are relatively more common in younger premenopausal women. Also, the larger the tumour, the worse the grade tends to be.

Paget's disease of the nipple

In Paget's disease, the epidermis becomes infiltrated by neoplastic cells arising from an underlying ductal carcinoma which reach the surface by intra-epithelial spread along the mammary ducts (Figs 45.12 and 45.13).

NATURAL HISTORY OF BREAST CANCER

Individual breast cancers vary greatly in their behaviour, with an unpredictable natural history that limits the impact of early detection by screening. Estimates of tumour doubling times suggest that many cancers have been present for 4–6 years before diagnosis.

There are two main theories about the biological dissemination of cancer as applied to the breast. **Halsted** proposed in the 1880s that cancer spreads sequentially from a focus in the breast to regional lymph nodes and then into the bloodstream to produce haematogenous metastases. In other words, distant spread occurs only after lymph nodes have been invaded and their filtration capacity has been overwhelmed. On this basis, loco-regional control by radical mastectomy and/or radiotherapy would cure most patients. By contrast, **Bernard Fisher's** research between 1957 and 1970 challenged Halsted's concept that mandated radical cancer surgery and presented evidence that breast cancer might be systemic early in its inception, long before the primary cancer is detectable. Furthermore, disseminated cancer cells could represent potential metastases throughout the life of the patient and it is these that ultimately determine the patient's fate. In practice, 30% of node negative breast cancer patients eventually relapse with distant metastases, thus supporting Fisher's theory. It follows therefore that for treatment to be curative it would have to be effective against widely disseminated (systemic) disease.

In fact, both Halsted's and Fisher's theories appear to apply in different situations, and breast cancers may show either of these biological behaviours. Poorly differentiated cancers in younger women are more likely to have distant micrometastases at the time of diagnosis and carry a higher chance of recurrence and death. Conversely, cancers in older patients often have low metastatic potential even when locally advanced. In these patients, screening may detect tumours before systemic spread has occurred and which remain potentially curable.

PRINCIPLES OF MANAGEMENT OF BREAST CANCER

The overall prognosis for breast cancer patients has not changed substantially over the past few decades, but the duration of disease-free survival and to a lesser extent the overall survival rate have improved. Over the past 20 years, 10-year survival rates have increased from 55% to

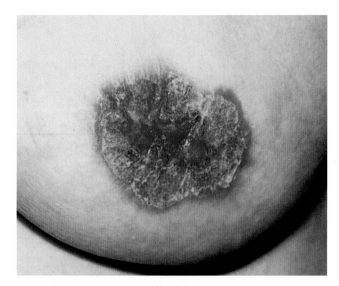

Fig. 45.13 Paget's disease of the nipple

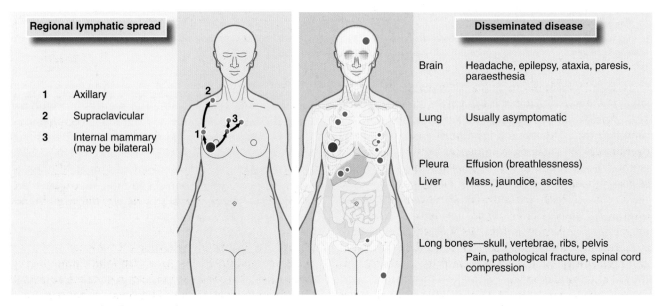

Regional lymphatic spread		Disseminated disease	
1	Axillary	Brain	Headache, epilepsy, ataxia, paresis, paraesthesia
2	Supraclavicular	Lung	Usually asymptomatic
3	Internal mammary (may be bilateral)	Pleura	Effusion (breathlessness)
		Liver	Mass, jaundice, ascites
		Long bones—skull, vertebrae, ribs, pelvis	Pain, pathological fracture, spinal cord compression

Fig. 45.14 Common sites of spread of breast carcinoma

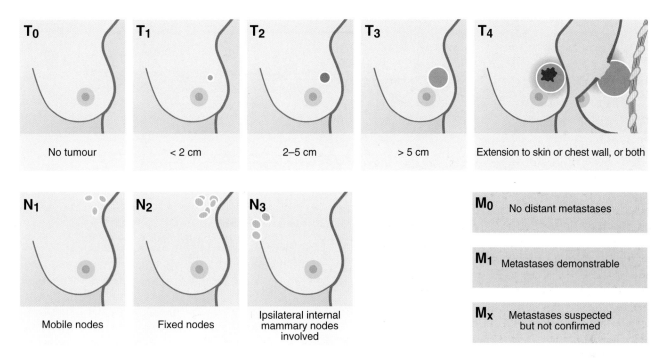

T0	**T1**	**T2**	**T3**	**T4**
No tumour	< 2 cm	2–5 cm	> 5 cm	Extension to skin or chest wall, or both

N1	**N2**	**N3**
Mobile nodes	Fixed nodes	Ipsilateral internal mammary nodes involved

M0 No distant metastases

M1 Metastases demonstrable

Mx Metastases suspected but not confirmed

Fig. 45.15 **Staging system for breast cancer using TNM classification**

74% and 20-year survival from 44% to 64%. Some of this improvement is due to earlier detection causing **lead-time bias**, but most of it is due to improved adjuvant therapy which acts on metastases as well as the primary.

Whilst the aim of treatment is generally cure, in practice, prolonging the disease-free survival or optimal management of metastatic disease is a more realistic goal. The effectiveness of various treatments has been evaluated in randomised clinical trials and the results have helped formulate national and international guidelines for treatment (see later). For patients with advanced disease, palliation is the main objective, with particular emphasis on optimising quality of life.

STAGING

Once the diagnosis of cancer has been made, the disease should be staged to define the extent of tumour spread. This enables optimal treatment to be planned and the prognosis estimated in terms of disease-free survival and overall survival. Staging commences with a full blood count, liver function tests and a chest X-ray. Ultrasound scans of the abdomen and isotope bone scans are used selectively to look for substantial distant metastatic disease. Micrometastases cannot be detected with any degree of reliability by current methods, but the presence of malignant disease in axillary lymph nodes is the strongest predictor of micrometastases at distant sites such as the liver, lungs and bone.

The TNM system (Fig. 45.15 and Table 45.2) classifies breast cancer according to the size of the primary Tumour,

Table 45.2 **American Joint Committee on Cancer staging system based on TNM status (6th edition 2003)**

T status	N status	M status	AJCC stage
Tis (in situ)	N0		Stage 0
T1	N0		Stage I
T0 T1 T2	N1 N1 N0		Stage IIA
T2 T3	N1 N0		Stage IIB
T0 T1 T2 T3 T3	N2 N2 N2 N1 N2	M0	Stage IIIA
T4	N0 N1 N2		Stage IIIB
any T	N3		Stage IIIC
any T	any N	M1	Stage IV

the pathological Nodal status and the presence or absence of distant Metastases. The American Joint Committee on Cancer (AJCC) uses TNM grading to generate an overall stage for individual patients. This stage lies between 0 and IV (see Table 45.2) and correlates well with observed rates

---

Box 45.5 Primary treatment for breast cancer

Note that surgery and radiotherapy constitute loco-regional treatment

Surgery
- Mastectomy (radical, modified radical, simple)
- Breast conservation (lumpectomy, wide local excision, quadrantectomy)

Radiotherapy
- Breast radiotherapy (post breast conservation surgery)
- Chest wall (post mastectomy)

Systemic therapy
- Hormonal therapy
- Chemotherapy
- Biological therapy

Box 45.6 Principles of management of breast cancer

- Establish the diagnosis
- Control disease in the affected breast and chest wall
- Prevent and treat local and regional disease in early breast cancer
- Control advanced and disseminated disease

---

of freedom from distant metastases at 5 years: 84% for stage I, 72% for stage II, 47% for stage III and 18% for stage IIIC tumours. For further details, see http://poptop. hypermart.net/brcastg.html. Note that as a result of screening, the proportion of small tumours detected has increased. Several subcategories of T1, mainly based on tumour size, have been introduced to refine the predictive value. Universal use of the TNM system means that the outcome of treatment for patients at any given stage can be compared in different trials.

LOCO-REGIONAL TREATMENT

The purpose of loco-regional treatment is to control disease within the breast and underlying chest wall. For patients with small tumours of favourable grade and some screen-detected lesions, loco-regional treatment alone is potentially curative. These treatments involve surgery or radiotherapy or a combination of the two. Complete removal of the breast (**mastectomy**) was previously the standard operation for invasive breast cancer, but over the past 30 years **breast conservation surgery** has become more prevalent.

Box 45.7 Selection criteria for breast conservation surgery

- Single lesion clinically and mammographically
- Tumour not larger than 3 cm (4 cm in larger breast)
- No extensive in situ component
- Tumours more than 2 cm away from nipple/areola
- Lesion of lower histological grade
- No extensive nodal involvement

BREAST CONSERVATION SURGERY

This involves removing the tumour with a margin of surrounding breast tissue, followed by radiotherapy to the breast to reduce local recurrence. The axillary nodes are biopsied and treated by surgery or radiotherapy if positive. Several long-term clinical trials have shown that overall survival is comparable with mastectomy. Despite this, some patients still opt for mastectomy even if suitable for breast conservation surgery. In parts of the world where radiotherapy is not available or is feared, mastectomy remains the treatment of choice.

Selection criteria for conservative surgery are shown in Box 45.7. A **lumpectomy** removes the tumour and a narrow rim of normal breast tissue of around 1 cm, but carries the risk of positive resection margins. **Wide local excision** is commonly practised in the UK and aims to remove the tumour and a 2–3 cm macroscopic margin of normal breast tissue. Skin is not usually excised unless there is tethering. A **quadrantectomy** removes the tumour as part of a quadrantic-shaped resection. This excises a greater volume of tissue but often yields a less good cosmetic result. In all cases, the specimen needs to be marked (e.g. with a suture) to orientate it for the pathologist so that the appropriate area can be re-excised if any margin contains malignant cells.

Patients undergoing breast conservation surgery generally report better body image and sexual functioning than those undergoing mastectomy, but it is not surprising that levels of anxiety and depression are similar given the diagnosis.

MASTECTOMY

There are several types of mastectomy in current use. **Radical mastectomy** was devised by William Halsted in the 1880s in the USA. At that time, many patients presented with large tumours invading pectoralis major muscle; his operation involved removal of the breast, axillary lymph nodes and pectoralis major and minor muscles.

Patey later devised a less mutilating operation in which the pectoralis major was preserved but pectoralis minor was removed to facilitate lymph node clearance. This is

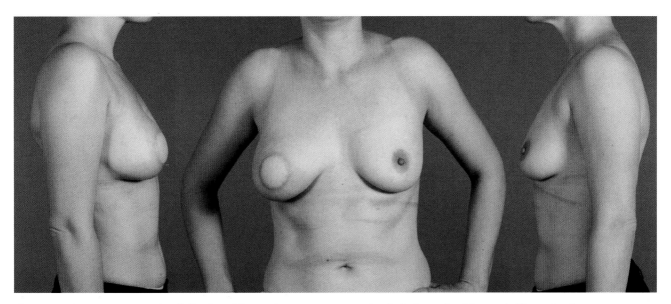

Fig. 45.16 Breast reconstruction following skin-sparing mastectomy using latissimus dorsi flap and silicone implant
Via a circumareolar incision, the entire breast tissue including the nipple–areolar complex is excised and the axillary node dissection performed. The latissimus dorsi muscle is mobilised as a pedicle flap together with an ellipse of overlying skin and tunnelled anteriorly to lie in the breast cavity. Excess skin is trimmed from the flap to leave a circular disc to replace the excised nipple. A silicone implant is sandwiched between the latissimus dorsi and pectoralis muscles to provide bulk and reshape the breast.

known as a **modified radical mastectomy**. Modern practice has moved towards preserving both pectoralis muscles and this form of mastectomy is now standard for invasive breast cancer.

In some patients, **immediate breast reconstruction** is practicable. A **skin-sparing mastectomy** is first performed, removing all of the breast tissue via a peri-areolar incision. The breast mound is reconstructed from prosthetic material only, the patient's own tissues (TRAM or transverse rectus abdominis myocutaneous flap) or a combination of both (LD or latissimus dorsi flap—Fig. 45.16). Immediate reconstruction is intended to improve psychological well-being but the magnitude of the operation is greater and it carries greater morbidity even though it does not compromise clearance of the cancer. Not all patients elect for immediate reconstruction even if offered, preferring mastectomy alone, whilst some choose late reconstruction.

Simple mastectomy is employed as a curative procedure for widespread ductal carcinoma in situ or as a palliative or 'toilet' procedure for locally advanced tumours.

The cosmetic effects of mastectomy are of great psychological importance to patients and their families. Careful attention to this can alleviate distress and improve acceptance of disfigurement. Preoperative counselling by medical or specially trained nursing staff should prepare the patient for treatment. After mastectomy, patients who do not undergo reconstruction should be fitted with a life-like breast prosthesis which is incorporated into the cup of a bra. Wherever possible, this should start with a temporary prosthesis in the immediate postoperative period.

AXILLARY SURGERY

Axillary nodal status is the most important prognostic factor in breast cancer. Thus axillary lymph nodes are excised for staging as well as for therapeutic purposes in mastectomy and breast conserving surgery. The **surgical levels** of axillary nodes are defined in relation to the pectoralis minor muscle. Most nodes are at level I, which is below the lower edge of the muscle. Level II is at the level of the muscle and level III is above the muscle. There is nearly always progressive spread of malignant cells from level I to level II to level III, with 'skip' metastases in only about 3% (i.e. involving higher levels without involving lower levels).

Standard axillary procedures include lymph node sampling and various levels of axillary dissection. Only about 25% of breast cancer patients now have nodal involvement at presentation, and this has prompted attempts to minimise axillary dissection in the remainder. **Lymph node sampling** involves excising at least 4 nodes from the axillary tail or low anterior axilla (level I); however, involved nodes are not necessarily palpable at operation and may be missed, giving a false negative result. If the sampled nodes are tumour free, no further treatment is given. When nodes contain tumour, completion dissection or irradiation of the axilla is performed later.

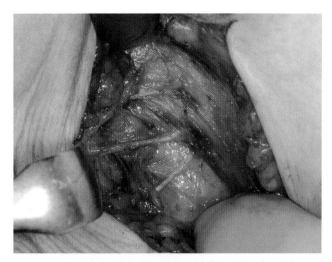

Fig. 45.17 Sentinel node biopsy
The sentinel node is usually the first axillary node to receive lymphatic drainage from the tumour. Before operation, a blue dye and a radiotracer are injected into subareolar area and at operation the sentinel node is identified visually and by using a device to detect radioactivity.

Targeted or **sentinel node biopsy** has been introduced to try to improve the sensitivity of node sampling (Fig. 45.17). The sentinel node is the first to receive lymphatic drainage from the tumour, so before operation a blue dye and a radiotracer are injected into subareolar area of the breast. At operation the sentinel node is identified visually and by detecting radioactivity. The node can be located in more than 90% of cases but there is still a false negative rate of 5–10%. Continuing trials will show whether this technique adversely affects loco-regional control or mortality compared with more radical node dissection, i.e. whether involved nodes are missed by sentinel node biopsy.

When more extensive axillary dissection is indicated, either as a first step or after finding positive nodes on sampling, level II dissection involving removing at least 10 nodes is the current standard. Level III dissection increases morbidity including lymphoedema of the arm, pain and paraesthesia and restricted shoulder mobility and is not generally indicated.

RADIOTHERAPY

Radiotherapy to the breast improves loco-regional control after breast conserving surgery, reducing tumour recurrence by 65%; it is also believed to reduce mortality from distant metastases by up to 5%. Treatment is by external beam irradiation (40–50 Gy administered over 3 or 5 weeks); patients with larger tumours or a narrow margin of normal tissue may receive a booster dose of 12–16 Gy.

Radiotherapy is also given to about a quarter of patients who, after mastectomy, are shown to have large poorly differentiated tumours with lymphovascular invasion and 4 or more nodes involved. In these, the supraclavicular nodes and sometimes the internal mammary chain are also irradiated. This post-mastectomy radiotherapy reduces local recurrence by up to 50% and is believed to improve survival by about 10% but does increase the risk of lymphoedema of the arm.

ADJUVANT SYSTEMIC TREATMENT

The unexpectedly low cure rate for apparently early breast cancer is due to occult metastatic spread. Many patients receive some form of systemic therapy intended to destroy or retard growth of these micrometastases and any circulating tumour cells. In planning systemic therapy, some form of prognostic index (see Table 45.4, p. 656) is often used as a guide, although this is more reliable for predicting short-term rather than long-term survival. Patients in the best prognostic group are unlikely to have micrometastases and do not generally require systemic treatment. For the rest, the choice of adjuvant therapies (or none) often involves detailed discussion between the patient and doctor about the balance of benefit and risk of side effects and sometimes cost. Table 45.3 summarises current thinking about adjuvant systemic therapies for the different categories of breast cancer patient. An American web-based system called adjuvantonline (www.adjuvantonline.com) is becoming widely used internationally to estimate the risk of cancer-related mortality or relapse without adjuvant therapy in individual patients, and the likely benefits and side effects of different therapies. Data are entered about the patient and their cancer (e.g. age, tumour size, nodal involvement, histological grade) and estimates can then be printed in graphical and text formats to inform consultations.

CHEMOTHERAPY

Several pulses of systemic adjuvant chemotherapy have been shown to improve survival in certain groups of patients. This may result from destroying early metastases or malignant cells capable of metastasising. Some clinicians believe, however, that the benefit results from the chemotherapy inducing ovarian ablation. Adjuvant chemotherapy certainly gives greater benefit in pre-menopausal women. For example, in women under 50 years with oestrogen receptor (ER) negative tumours chemotherapy gives an odds reduction in mortality at 10 years of 35% ± 9%. In women over 50, the equivalent odds reduction is 14% ± 4%.

If chemotherapy is to be considered, the choice depends on the likely benefits, given the woman's age, menopausal status and the hormone receptor status of the tumour. The benefits must be weighed against the toxicity of therapy, which in the short term includes nausea, vomiting, alo-

Table 45.3 Criteria for selection of adjuvant therapies*

Premenopausal			
Node negative	ER positive	Low risk Intermediate risk High risk, i.e. tumour > 2 cm, grade III	No adjuvant therapy Tamoxifen Chemotherapy + tamoxifen Consider ovarian ablation
	ER negative		Chemotherapy
Node positive	ER positive		Chemotherapy + tamoxifen Consider ovarian ablation
	ER negative		Chemotherapy
Postmenopausal			
Node negative	ER positive	Low risk Intermediate risk High risk, good general health	None or tamoxifen Tamoxifen ± chemotherapy Tamoxifen + chemotherapy
	ER negative		Consider chemotherapy
Node positive	ER positive		Tamoxifen/aromatase inhibitor + chemotherapy (calculate and discuss potential benefits)
	ER negative		Chemotherapy if general health good

*Low, intermediate and high risk refer to the chances of developing distant disease and relapse and are based on the criteria of tumour size, histological grade and nodal status

pecia, mucositis and neutropenia. Long-term complications include premature ovarian failure and as a result, induction of early menopause. There is also the possibility of inducing a cardiomyopathy if an anthracycline is used.

Combination chemotherapy is usual and most current regimens contain the alkylating agent cyclophosphamide. One of the first regimens, **CMF**, contains cyclophosphamide, methotrexate and 5-fluorouracil, and continued to be used for many years. This has largely been superseded by regimens that still contain cyclophosphamide but with an anthracycline such as **doxorubicin**. Anthracyclines are antibiotics that prevent cell division by disrupting the structure of DNA. Other combinations are the subjects of large-scale trials. **Taxanes** are a new class of agents which promote microtubule polymerisation leading to cell death. They work in a different way from anthracyclines and give additional response rates in metastatic disease of over 50%. Continuing trials are evaluating taxanes combined with or given sequentially with anthracyclines. Note that high-dose chemotherapy regimens should only be given in the context of clinical trials so that the risks and benefits can be properly evaluated.

Adjuvant chemotherapy is currently recommended for most premenopausal women shown to have high-grade tumours and axillary nodal spread but with no evidence of distant metastases. Treatment in premenopausal women gives an average proportional increase in survival of approximately 30% irrespective of nodal status. Systemic chemotherapy is used less frequently in node negative patients and in postmenopausal women, but the absolute benefits are less.

HORMONAL THERAPY

It is now recognised that hormonal therapy only benefits patients with oestrogen receptor (ER) positive tumours, in whom it can bring mortality reductions of up to 36%. Hormonal therapy gives the greatest benefit to postmenopausal women, reducing 10-year mortality by 28%. Similar benefits occur in premenopausal women but menopausal symptoms of oestrogen withdrawal may be troublesome.

Hormonal therapy includes ovarian ablation, selective oestrogen receptor modulators such as tamoxifen, and aromatase inhibitors. **Ovarian ablation** yields benefits comparable to chemotherapy in oestrogen receptor positive premenopausal women, and can be achieved with either LHRH analogues or oophorectomy, the latter usually performed laparoscopically.

Tamoxifen helps preserve bone density and a favourable lipid profile because of its selective action in blocking oestrogen receptors. However, the drug carries moderately increased risks of thromboembolism, endometrial cancer and visual disturbances. **Aromatase inhibitors** are a novel and important class of hormonal agents. In postmenopausal women, the principal source of oestrogen is adipose tissue; these drugs selectively inhibit the enzyme aromatase, thus blocking the peripheral synthesis of oestrogens in adipose tissue generally and in tumour tissue rather than competitively binding to oestrogen receptors.

BIOLOGICAL THERAPIES

These novel forms of therapy target growth factor pathways and are beginning to show promise when used in combination with conventional therapies. **Trastuzumab (Herceptin)** is a humanised monoclonal antibody to the HER/neu (cerbB2) transmembrane receptor which is overexpressed in 30% of breast cancers. It has demonstrated clinical response rates of about 35% in metastatic breast cancer in carefully selected cases. More recently trastuzumab has shown striking effects when used as adjuvant treatment, with a 50% reduction in the risk of recurrence and a substantial survival benefit. It should be emphasised that the drug has not been available for long enough for long-term evaluation, although it is generally well tolerated with few side effects.

CONTROL OF ADVANCED AND DISSEMINATED DISEASE

All patients presenting with clinically early breast cancer are treated with curative intent. About two-thirds of patients now survive for at least 20 years, but many eventually succumb from micrometastatic disease which progresses to clinically evident metastases. In reality, about 60% of patients presenting with early breast cancer will eventually succumb to the disease despite the best treatments, though this may be as long as 35 years later. Once metastases have appeared, treatment is palliative, but very worthwhile prolongation of life and improved quality of life can often be achieved.

Some cancers become locally advanced with involvement of most of the breast tissue (see Fig. 45.18). The skin becomes infiltrated and eventually ulcerates and the tumour can invade the chest wall. Ultimately much of the chest wall may become involved, when it is known as **carcinoma en cuirasse**. It is likely that the early stages have been neglected in such cases. Locally advanced disease of breast and axilla may appear to be inoperable but, after histological diagnosis, neoadjuvant chemotherapy (i.e. before surgery) often downsizes the cancer so that it becomes operable. Radiotherapy alone can be employed for palliation of advanced skin, breast, chest wall and lymph node disease.

Poorly differentiated lesions in younger women tend to spread to visceral organs. Recurrent **pleural effusions** result from **pulmonary metastases** (Fig. 45.19) and are

Fig. 45.18 Advanced breast cancer

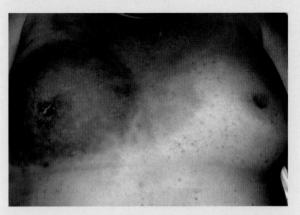

This 60-year-old woman had been aware of a lump in her right breast for over a year before she could be persuaded to seek treatment. The whole breast is involved and malignancy has spread through the skin widely across the chest wall. Palliative treatment was given with radiotherapy and tamoxifen.

managed with aspiration or pleurodesis. Pleurodesis involves obliterating the pleural cavity by instilling tetracycline or bleomycin or performing surgical pleurectomy. **Ascites** occurs secondary to **liver** involvement. Lymphangitis carcinomatosa (widespread dissemination in skin or lung lymphatics) and fulminant liver metastases may occur in the terminal stage of the disease.

Bone metastases are more likely in postmenopausal women with well-differentiated, hormone receptor positive tumours. More than 90% of patients with metastatic disease have bone lesions. These are usually lytic and commonly affect the ribs and vertebrae. These are painful and can lead to pathological fractures (Fig. 45.20). Luckily, they often respond to palliative radiotherapy.

Lobular carcinoma can metastasise to unusual sites such as skin (Fig. 45.21) and the gastrointestinal tract.

LONG-TERM FOLLOW-UP

Women who have had one breast cancer have a 15% lifetime risk of developing a second tumour in the other breast. The risk is higher if the original lesion was a lobular carcinoma. The breast tissue in these women may have an increased susceptibility to cancer, or else breast cancer may arise at the same time in multiple foci. Thus patients with breast cancer should be followed up clinically and by mammography for 3–5 years after initial treatment. There is no evidence that more prolonged follow-up improves outcomes. Patients should be instructed in how to examine themselves and to return if they notice new symptoms or signs.

Fig. 45.19 Chest manifestations of metastatic breast carcinoma

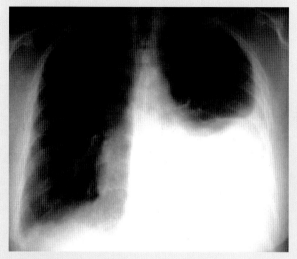

(a)

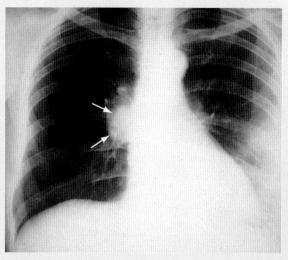

(b)

(a) This 38-year-old woman had undergone a right mastectomy for ductal carcinoma 7 years before and presented with increasing shortness of breath. This chest X-ray shows a large left pleural effusion confirmed on cytology to be malignant. It was palliated by drainage and pleurodesis.

(b) A different patient who had been treated 5 years before for lobular carcinoma of the breast. She presented with a chronic non-productive cough and was found to have a mass of lymph nodes at the right hilum (arrowed) and a right recurrent laryngeal nerve palsy due to invasion in the region of the carina.

Fig. 45.20 Skeletal metastases from carcinoma of the breast

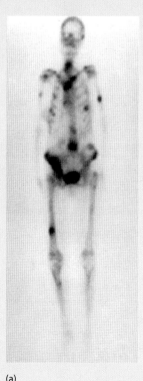

(a)

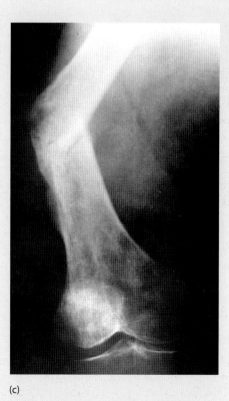

(b)

(c)

(a) Anterior view of radioisotope bone scan of a 48-year-old woman complaining of pain in the neck and right hip. She had undergone a mastectomy for carcinoma 8 years previously. The scan shows large metastatic deposits in the lower cervical and lumbar spine, right pelvis, right femur and left humerus as well as several smaller deposits in the ribs and elsewhere in the skeleton. (b) X-ray of the lower femur in a 79-year-old woman presenting with a fungating breast carcinoma and pain in the left knee. The X-ray shows radiolucencies (arrowed) in the distal femur and elevation of the periosteum P medially, indicating bony metastasis. Radiotherapy was arranged to alleviate the symptoms. (c) Some weeks later, despite treatment, the patient returned with this pathological fracture of the femur.

LIFE EXPECTANCY AND PROGNOSIS

When long-term survival curves have been examined statistically, there is no evidence of 'cure' in the normally accepted sense (Fig. 45.22), although a 'personal cure' is achieved in about 50% of patients who die from some other disease. Micrometastatic foci can remain dormant for 35 years or more and become 'kick started' for unknown reasons into progressive metastatic disease and death. Loco-regional relapse often occurs within the first 5 years, but distant disease tends to occur much later.

Breast cancer survival calculated from prognostic scoring systems is only useful for up to about 10 years, and since estimates are based on group analyses, they are of doubtful relevance for an individual patient. A commonly used tool is the Nottingham prognostic index (NPI) which divides patients into 5 prognostic groups (see Table 45.4).

Adjuvantonline (www.adjuvantonline.com) is another system that is becoming popular for estimating prognosis. It is also a valuable decision-support tool for calculating the potential benefits of adjuvant therapies for individuals.

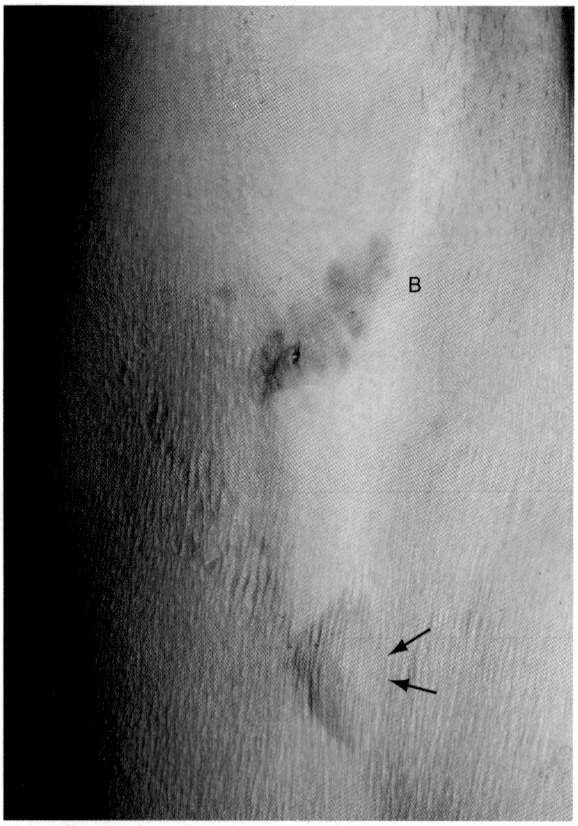

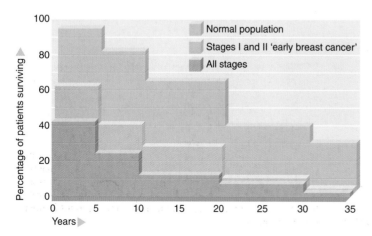

Fig. 45.21 Skin secondaries following simple mastectomy and radiotherapy
This patient presented with painless, slightly elevated nodules in the skin below the axilla 3 years after treatment for lobular carcinoma of the breast. In this photograph, the arm is elevated and one skin secondary can just be made out (arrowed); the site of excision biopsy of another is seen at **B**.

Table 45.4 Nottingham prognostic index (NPI) for breast cancer

Nottingham prognostic group	NPI score	Estimated 10-year survival
Excellent	≤ 2.4	95%
Good	≤ 3.4	83%
Moderate I	≤ 4.4	70%
Moderate II	< 5.4	51%
Poor	> 5.4	19%

The NPI is calculated as follows: 0.2 × tumour size in cm + histological grade + lymph node status (node negative scores 1; 1–3 positive nodes scores 2, and 4 or more positive scores 3.

Fig. 45.22 Life expectancy after diagnosis of breast cancer (after Brinkley and Haybittle)
Note that 5- and 10-year survival has improved in recent years as a result of better diagnosis and treatment but it is uncertain that long-term survival will also improve.

BENIGN BREAST DISORDERS

Most patients referred to breast clinics are found to have benign breast disorders. These include fibrocystic change (fibroadenosis), fibroadenoma, duct papilloma, fat necrosis, breast infections and mammary duct ectasia. The first two conditions are the most common and much time and effort is spent distinguishing these from more sinister lesions.

ABNORMALITIES OF NORMAL DEVELOPMENT AND INVOLUTION (ANDI)

Pathology

In women of reproductive age, breast tissue is constantly undergoing physiological changes in response to circulating hormones. This produces a spectrum of proliferative and regressive changes within the breast parenchyma including distortion and overgrowth of the main structural components—the ducts, lobules and fibrous tissue. These changes result in areas of general or focal **nodularity** associated with varying degrees of pain and tenderness. The term **fibrocystic change** or **fibroadenosis** has historically been applied to this condition. The main components are cyst formation, epitheliosis, fibrosis and proliferation of lobular acini, known as **adenosis**. Fibrosis may occur within areas of adenosis, splitting acini; this is known as **sclerosing adenosis**. A number of these features are often present within a single lesion, or in different areas of the same or the contralateral breast. The concept of 'abnormalities of normal development and involution (ANDI)' encompasses a variety of clinicopathological features which histologically include fibrosis, adenosis, apocrine metaplasia, epithelial hyperplasia and macro- and microcyst formation. By definition, the hyperplastic element is not histologically atypical and there is no increased risk of malignancy associated with this complex of benign breast changes (see Fig. 45.23).

Clinical presentation and management

Fibrocystic change (fibroadenosis) presents as either a single lump or areas of lumpiness which are painful and tender premenstrually, i.e. cyclically (see Fig. 45.24). These changes may be difficult to distinguish clinically from carcinoma, and florid fibrocystic change can mask a cancer both clinically and radiologically. Fibrocystic change is most common between the ages of 35 and 45 years.

Cyst formation is more prevalent over the age of 40 years and in perimenopausal women. Cysts may present symptomatically as single or occasionally multiple lumps (Fig. 45.23a). Cysts develop from lobules and are fluid-filled spaces. **Microcysts** are part of the involutionary process and may coalesce to produce a larger cyst which presents as a smooth, round palpable lump. Larger cysts may be tense, tender and fluctuant with the texture of a table tennis ball. Cysts can usually be diagnosed clinically and can be readily confirmed with ultrasonography; they are usually recognisable on a mammogram. Modern B-mode ultrasound accurately diagnoses simple cysts, which can be aspirated under ultrasound control or freehand. Provided the cyst fluid is not blood-stained, there is no residual lump post aspiration and there are no sonographically suspicious features, patients can be discharged without further follow-up, although cysts can recur or new cysts develop (see Fig. 45.25). Cysts are uncommon over the age of 60 years unless the patient is using HRT. Under these

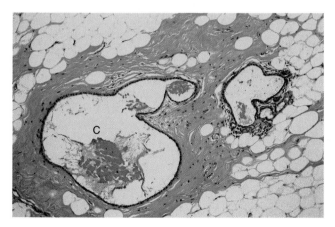

(a)

(a) Dilated ducts form cysts **C** of various sizes, from microscopic to large palpable lesions measuring several centimetres. Often a cyst is lined by flattened ductal epithelium; however, this may also show secretory features, known as **apocrine metaplasia**.

Fig. 45.23 Fibrocystic change (fibroadenosis)—histopathology

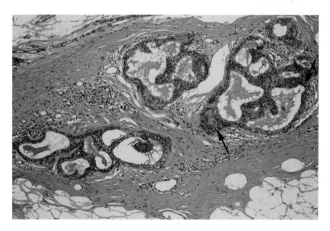

(b)

(b) Ducts show epithelial proliferation (arrowed), known as **epitheliosis**, which may give rise to single or multiple papillomas. The degree of hyperplasia within epitheliosis varies and may be associated with cytological atypia; this can indicate an increased risk of developing breast adenocarcinoma. At the extreme end of the spectrum, extreme ductal proliferation may amount to ductal carcinoma in situ.

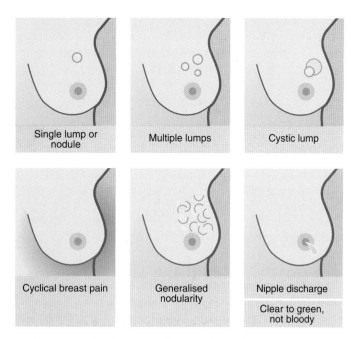

Single lump or nodule

Multiple lumps

Cystic lump

Cyclical breast pain

Generalised nodularity

Nipple discharge
Clear to green, not bloody

Fig. 45.24 Clinical presentation of fibroadenosis (fibrocystic change)

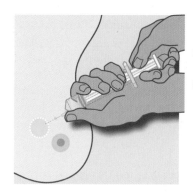

1 Fluid should not be blood-stained

2 Lump should disappear

3 Cyst should not recur

Fig. 45.25 Cyst aspiration and criteria for exclusion of cancer associated with a cyst

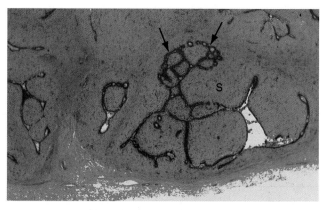

Fig. 45.26 Fibroadenoma—histopathology
This benign lesion shows proliferation of both glands (arrowed) and stroma **S**. In the variant illustrated, gland lumina are compressed by stroma. Fibroadenoma typically has a histologically well-defined edge.

circumstances it is important to exclude an intracystic papilloma, intracystic carcinoma or a cystic carcinoma.

Managing fibrocystic change

Once the patient has been reassured she does not have cancer, the symptoms of pain and tenderness associated with fibrocystic change can be treated. **Gamolenic acid (GLA)** relieves cyclical symptoms in more than half the cases and needs to be used at the optimum dosage for a minimum of 3 months. More than 90% of patients with mild to moderate breast pain can be satisfactorily managed with reassurance and GLA. For those with moderate to severe cyclical pain, danazol or bromocriptine offers relief in 70% of women, but both these drugs have substantial side effects which reduce compliance. Danazol inhibits pituitary gonadotrophin secretion and has androgenic side effects of acne and hirsutism. Bromocriptine inhibits pituitary prolactin release and can produce dizziness.

FIBROADENOMA

PATHOLOGY

Fibroadenoma is a localised form of ANDI rather than a benign tumour. These lesions arise from a single lobule and are composed of epithelial and fibrous components. The epithelium forms glandular structures lined by mammary ductal cells and the connective tissue forms a loose cellular stroma (see Fig. 45.26). Fibroadenomas undergo involution in the perimenopausal years but can persist into old age and become calcified.

CLINICAL PRESENTATION AND MANAGEMENT

Fibroadenomas are most common between the ages of 15 and 30 and thus occur in a younger age group than fibroadenosis. They present as a single rounded mass which is smooth, firm and highly mobile. Smaller lesions are sometimes described as **breast mice** since they slip away from beneath the palpating fingers. Fibroadenomas are occasionally multiple and bilateral and are more frequent in an Afro-Caribbean population. Larger fibroadenomas should be distinguished from benign **phyllodes tumours** which have similar features clinically, radiologically and on core biopsy. Where suspicion of phyllodes exists or a fibroadenoma is enlarging, excision biopsy is indicated, otherwise the lesions regress spontaneously in 85–90% of cases and do not require excision. Confirmatory tissue biopsy is unnecessary under the age of 21, but is advisable over this age. Certainly above the age of 40 there must be complete concordance of the diagnosis on triple assessment if excision is to be avoided.

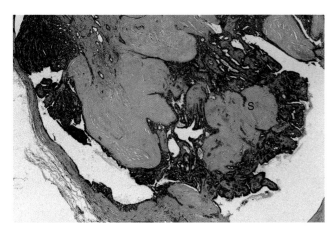

Fig. 45.27 Duct papilloma
This is essentially a localised form of epitheliosis. Papilloma in a larger duct must be distinguished from papillary carcinoma, which lacks the well-defined stromal cores **S**. Both lesions can present with blood-stained nipple discharge.

DUCT PAPILLOMA

Intraduct papillomas are localised areas of epithelial proliferation. They are villous lesions composed of a fibrovascular core covered by a double layer of epithelium. They usually occur as solitary lesions in the main lactiferous ducts close to the nipple but multiple papillomas can occur more peripherally. Papillomas usually have areas of epithelial hyperplasia but there is no cellular atypia and the lesions are not premalignant (see Fig. 45.27). They present as spontaneous blood-stained or clear watery nipple discharge, often from a single duct; a retroareolar mass may be palpable. These lesions are best imaged with ultrasound and the diagnosis confirmed on core biopsy. Ductography is no longer used for investigation. Papillomas are treated by excision of the affected duct (microdochectomy) or a group of ducts (wedge resection). If the causative lesion cannot be found at operation, a subareolar excision of all the ducts may be necessary.

TRAUMATIC FAT NECROSIS

Trauma to the breast can produce an area of fat necrosis that may mimic carcinoma clinically and radiologically. The episode may have been trivial; in more than half the cases, patients cannot recollect a history of breast trauma. There is typically an injury causing bruising, followed a few weeks later by a lump. Fat necrosis may also result from an iatrogenic procedure, for example following percutaneous needle biopsy, surgery or anticoagulant therapy plus mild trauma. There is an initial acute inflammatory response but necrotic adipose tissue can persist, provoking chronic inflammation and a fibrotic reaction. This produces a hard irregular lump which may have skin dimpling. Mammography may show a stellate area of dis-

Fig. 45.28 Breast abscess

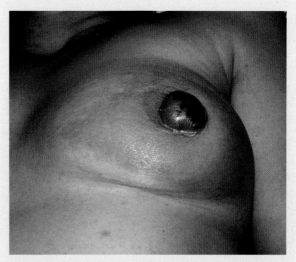

This woman of 40 presented with a neglected left breast abscess a few weeks after ceasing breast-feeding. The abscess was drained at open operation but had destroyed much of the breast tissue. The organism was *Staph. aureus* as is commonly the case.

tortion with calcification. Core biopsy distinguishes fat necrosis from carcinoma.

INFECTIONS OF THE BREAST

Infections of the breast lobules present as **diffuse cellulitis** or as an **abscess** (see Fig. 45.28). An abscess is often the result of inadequately treated cellulitis. Less commonly, infections arise in the sebaceous glands of the areola where they resemble skin boils. Deep infections occur most commonly during late pregnancy and lactation (**puerperal abscess**). The organism responsible is almost always *Staph. aureus*. It gains access to the breast tissue via cracked nipple skin, an inverted nipple or through the bloodstream. Retention of breast secretions causing ductal engorgement may be a predisposing factor. Abscesses can also occur in non-lactating women with nipple inversion.

The diagnosis of an abscess is usually obvious, with local and systemic signs of acute inflammation. The patient is generally unwell with a tachycardia and fever. The affected segment of the breast is painful and tender, red and warm. If the infection is inadequately treated, a large amount of breast tissue is destroyed and a great amount of pus forms. The lesion then becomes fluctuant and eventually 'points' to the surface and discharges.

The early cellulitic phase is reversible if treated with appropriate antibiotics. Flucloxacillin is usually the antibiotic of choice on a 'best-guess' basis. If antibiotics are started too late or the wrong antibiotic is chosen, tissue damage and accumulating polymorphs cause multiple loculi of pus to form. These can only be effectively treated by surgical drainage. The need for surgical drainage has declined in recent years because of prompt and appropriate antibiotic treatment, sometimes aided by needle aspiration.

At operation to drain an abscess, a skin incision is made over the most fluctuant area and the loculi are explored and broken down with a finger. If there is extensive damage, the wound should be closed around a corrugated drain, and if there is substantial residual cellulitis antibiotics should be prescribed.

Inflammatory carcinomas may be difficult to distinguish from infective conditions of the breast. The appearance can be similar mammographically, with both types of lesion showing a circumscribed opacity with an irregular, poorly defined margin. A breast abscess often contains necrotic debris simulating a solid mass on imaging. Chronic **mastitis during pregnancy** may mask an underlying inflammatory carcinoma and delay diagnosis.

DUCT ECTASIA

Mammary duct ectasia refers to dilatation and shortening of the major lactiferous ducts. It is a common involutional change that appears around the menopause and is seen in almost half of all women over the age of 60 years. Patients typically present with spontaneous multiple duct discharges which range from creamish to blue-green. Nipple retraction or a palpable mass may also be present. The nipple appears slit-like and an eczematous reaction caused by secretions may resemble Paget's disease. When an ectatic duct ruptures, a chronic inflammatory process occurs in the surrounding breast tissue. Figure 45.29 illustrates typical mammographic changes. Plasma cells are a characteristic feature on histology; this is described as **plasma cell mastitis**. An acute inflammatory response

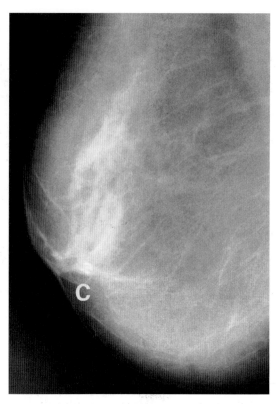

Fig. 45.29 Mammary duct ectasia
Radiopaque mass of dilated ducts with no features of malignancy. Large duct calcification **C** is also seen. Note the skin indentation caused by fibrosis. Clinically, this condition can be mistaken for carcinoma.

may occur with localised tenderness and reddening, but without overt signs of abscess formation. This should be managed with antibiotics as surgical intervention can lead to a chronic mammary fistula with recurrent episodes of infection. Troublesome discharge with soiling of undergarments can be treated by subareolar excision of the major ducts (Hadfield's or Adair's operation).

MALE BREAST DISORDERS

The two main breast conditions in males are gynaecomastia and cancer.

GYNAECOMASTIA

Gynaecomastia is an abnormal overdevelopment of the male breast with hypertrophy of the breast disc (see Fig. 45.30); the term literally means 'female breast'. Gynaecomastia is becoming more common and appears to result from an imbalance of oestrogens and androgens acting on the male breast 'bud'. Most cases are idiopathic, i.e. with no identifiable cause, but there are three recognised aetiological factors:

- **Physiological**—gynaecomastia may be present **at birth** in response to maternal oestrogens crossing the placenta; the condition resolves spontaneously over several weeks. The changing hormonal environment of **puberty** can result in enlargement of one (or sometimes both) breasts which can be a source of embarrassment. This usually settles by the late teenage years, but may warrant surgery if persistent
- **Medication**—several drugs affect metabolic and hormonal pathways and can produce gynaecomastia. These include cimetidine, spironolactone, digoxin and isoniazid. The causative drug should be discontinued when possible
- **Pathological**—liver disease interferes with the metabolism of oestrogens whilst testicular tumours may secrete oestrogens. Atherosclerosis affecting the

Fig. 45.30 Gynaecomastia

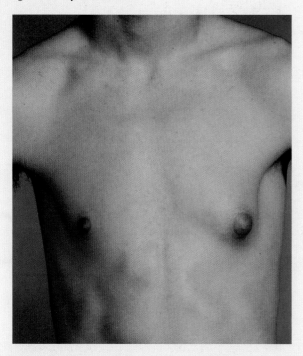

This 17-year-old was concerned about excess breast development on the left side. The breast tissue was removed via a subareolar incision.

testicular artery is believed to impair testosterone production and cause 'senile' gynaecomastia

In patients beyond middle life, imaging and needle biopsies should be performed to look for malignancy. Surgery for gynaecomastia is usually performed in younger males for cosmetic purposes. A complete subcutaneous mastectomy should be performed rather than central excision of breast tissue which can lead to unsightly 'saucerisation'.

MALE BREAST CANCER

Between 0.5 and 1% of breast cancers occur in males, who are an average of 10 years older than women at the time of presentation (usually 60–70 years). Male breast cancer is more common in carriers of *BRCA2* mutations and in states of hyperoestrogenism such as liver disease and Klinefelter's syndrome. Tumours are usually at an advanced stage, with infiltration of skin and underlying muscle (T_{4c}) and involvement of axillary lymph nodes. The patient may present late because the diagnosis has not been considered. The tumour is relatively large compared to the breast, so that mastectomy is the usual surgical option. Tamoxifen is prescribed for hormone receptor positive tumours (80–90% are oestrogen and progesterone receptor positive). Stage for stage, the prognosis is similar for breast cancer in men and women; male breast cancer tends to behave like postmenopausal disease in women.

46 Disorders of the skin

INTRODUCTION

Only a small proportion of the enormous variety of skin disorders are surgically important; unsightly lumps and possible malignant lesions fall into this category. **Ulcers** of the lower limb are common and usually of vascular or diabetic neuro-ischaemic origin. Some venous ulcers are managed by dermatologists, but most of the remainder are managed by surgeons and specialist nurses; these are discussed in Chapter 43. Ulceration also characterises many important, often malignant, skin lesions.

In general, the initial diagnostic referral is made to a dermatologist, who sees many more skin conditions than the general surgeon. However, skin disorders still comprise about 15% of new outpatient general surgical referrals. Many only require excision biopsy under local anaesthesia. A few patients are referred for further advice after a skin lesion has been excised by a family practitioner.

A small proportion of skin lesions have a potentially sinister course, particularly malignant melanoma. These must of course be accurately diagnosed and treated. Suspected malignant skin lesions are often managed jointly by dermatologists or surgeons (including plastic surgeons) and oncologists. Malignant melanomas comprise only 2% of all skin cancers in Northern Europe but, like basal cell and squamous cell carcinomas, their incidence closely correlates with sun exposure and fair skin. Skin malignancies and their premalignant stages are much more common in sunny countries like Australia where they have reached epidemic proportions; also the frequency of all skin cancers is rising with increasing foreign travel.

Finally, the nails, which are specialised skin appendages, pose surgical problems in the form of infected **ingrowing toenails** and **onychogryphosis**. The rare **sub-ungual melanoma** is an important diagnosis which must not be missed.

STRUCTURE OF NORMAL SKIN

The skin is made up of three main layers, the **epidermis**, the **dermis** and the **hypodermis**:

- The epidermis consists of four main layers—the basal layer, the prickle-cell layer, the granular layer and the keratin layer. Cell division normally occurs only in the basal layer

- The underlying dermis consists of dense, tough interlacing collagen fibres; their orientation determines the lines of tension in the skin known as **Langer's lines**. These are surgically important because incisions parallel to them heal with minimal scarring
- The deepest layer of the skin is the **hypodermis**, which consists of loose fibro-fatty tissue. The

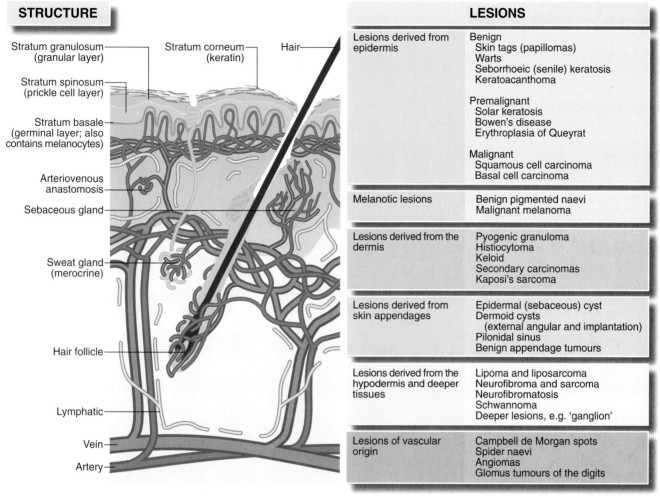

STRUCTURE

Stratum granulosum (granular layer)
Stratum corneum (keratin)
Hair
Stratum spinosum (prickle cell layer)
Stratum basale (germinal layer; also contains melanocytes)
Arteriovenous anastomosis
Sebaceous gland
Sweat gland (merocrine)
Hair follicle
Lymphatic
Vein
Artery

LESIONS

Lesions derived from epidermis	Benign
	  Skin tags (papillomas)
	  Warts
	  Seborrhoeic (senile) keratosis
	  Keratoacanthoma
	
	Premalignant
	  Solar keratosis
	  Bowen's disease
	  Erythroplasia of Queyrat
	
	Malignant
	  Squamous cell carcinoma
	  Basal cell carcinoma

Melanotic lesions	Benign pigmented naevi Malignant melanoma
Lesions derived from the dermis	Pyogenic granuloma Histiocytoma Keloid Secondary carcinomas Kaposi's sarcoma
Lesions derived from skin appendages	Epidermal (sebaceous) cyst Dermoid cysts (external angular and implantation) Pilonidal sinus Benign appendage tumours
Lesions derived from the hypodermis and deeper tissues	Lipoma and liposarcoma Neurofibroma and sarcoma Neurofibromatosis Schwannoma Deeper lesions, e.g. 'ganglion'
Lesions of vascular origin	Campbell de Morgan spots Spider naevi Angiomas Glomus tumours of the digits

Fig. 46.1 Structure of the skin and lesions of surgical importance

hypodermis contains the skin appendages—sweat glands, hair follicles and their associated sebaceous glands. The hypodermis is only loosely connected to the **superficial fascia**, which makes the skin mobile over the deeper structures. The exceptions are the palms of the hands, the soles of the feet and the scalp, where the skin is tightly bound to the fascial layer

A working classification of surgically important skin lesions based on site of origin is given in Figure 46.1.

SYMPTOMS AND SIGNS OF SKIN DISORDERS

The most common surgical skin complaint is a lump. This may be tender or painful, and it may have begun to bleed, discharge or ulcerate. The lesion may be pigmented or have changed colour. It may have appeared suddenly or enlarged rapidly, or there may have been some change in a longstanding lesion. The other main reason for surgical referral is hyperhidrosis or excessive sweating.

Any one of these symptoms may prompt the patient to seek medical advice, but the most frequent seem to be the ugliness or inconvenience of a lesion to the patient (e.g. getting in the way of a strap). Elderly patients may only come reluctantly and at the insistence of younger rela-

tives. Some patients do not present until a lesion is huge, while others present with trivial lesions. Both types of patient may be worried by the thought of malignancy.

In practice (and in clinical exams) the diagnosis of skin lesions rarely follows the conventional pattern of history taking, physical examination and investigations. Rather, the lesion is thrust before the doctor's eyes and a 'spot' diagnosis or differential diagnosis is made. History and examination are then used to see whether they confirm the diagnosis or narrow the differential possibilities. Table 46.1 summarises the important clinical features of skin lesions and their diagnostic significance.

Table 46.1 Symptoms and signs of skin disorders

Symptoms and signs	Diagnostic significance
1. Lump in or on the skin *Size, shape and surface features* Revealed by inspection—is the lesion smooth-surfaced, irregular, exophytic (i.e. projecting out of the surface)?	Epidermal lesions such as warts usually have a surface abnormality but deeper lesions are usually covered by normal epidermis. A **punctum** suggests the abnormality arises from an epidermal appendage, e.g. epidermal (sebaceous) cyst
Depth within the skin Superficial and deep attachments. Which tissue is the swelling derived from?	Tends to reflect the layer from which lesion is derived and therefore the range of differential diagnosis (i.e. epidermis, dermis, hypodermis or deeper)
Character of the margin Discreteness, tethering to surrounding tissues, three-dimensional shape	A regular shaped, discrete lesion is most likely cystic or encapsulated (e.g. benign tumour). Deep tethering implies origin from deeper structures (e.g. ganglion). Immobility of overlying epidermis suggests a lesion derived from skin appendage (e.g. epidermal cyst)
Consistency Soft, firm, hard, 'indurated', rubbery	Soft lesions are usually lipomas or fluid-filled cysts. Most cysts are fluctuant unless filled by semi-solid material (e.g.epidermal cysts), or the cyst is tense (e.g. small ganglion). Malignant lesions tend to be hard and irregular ('indurated') with an ill-defined margin due to invasion of surrounding tissue. Bony-hard lesions are either mineralised (e.g. gouty tophi) or consist of bone (e.g. exostoses)
Pulsatility	Pulsatility is usually transmitted from an underlying artery which may simply be tortuous or may be abnormal (e.g. aneurysm or arteriovenous fistula)
Emptying and refilling	Vascular lesions (e.g. venous malformations or haemangiomas) empty or blanch on pressure and then refill
Transilluminability	Lesions filled with clear fluid such as cysts 'light up' when transilluminated
Temperature	Excessive warmth implies acute inflammation, e.g. pilonidal abscess
2. Pain, tenderness and discomfort	These symptoms often indicate acute inflammation. Pain also develops if a non-inflammatory lesion becomes inflamed or infected (e.g. inflamed epidermal cyst). Malignant lesions are usually painless
3. Ulceration (i.e. loss of epidermal integrity with an inflamed base formed by dermis or deeper tissues)	Malignant lesions and keratoacanthomas tend to ulcerate as a result of central necrosis. Surface breakdown also occurs in arterial or venous insufficiency (e.g. ischaemic leg ulcers), chronic infection (e.g. TB or tropical ulcers) or trauma, particularly in an insensate foot
Character of the ulcer margin	Benign ulcers—the margin is only slightly raised by inflammatory oedema. The base lies below the level of normal skin Malignant ulcers—these begin as a solid mass of proliferating epidermal cells, the centre of which eventually becomes necrotic and breaks down. The margin is typically elevated 'rolled' and indurated by tumour growth and invasion
Behaviour of the ulcer	Malignant ulcers expand inexorably (though often slowly), but may go through cycles of breakdown and healing (often with bleeding)
4. Colour and pigmentation *Normal colour*	If a lesion is covered by normal-coloured skin then the lesion must lie deeply in the skin (e.g. epidermal cyst) or deep to the skin (e.g. ganglion)
Red or purple	Redness implies increased arterial vascularity, which is most common in inflammatory conditions like furuncles. Vascular abnormalities which contain a high proportion of arterial blood such as Campbell de Morgan spots or strawberry naevi are also red, whereas venous disorders such as port-wine stain are darker. Vascular lesions blanch on pressure and must be distinguished from purpura which does not
Deeply pigmented	Benign naevi (moles) and their malignant counterpart, malignant melanomas, are nearly always pigmented. Other lesions such as warts, papillomata or seborrhoeic keratoses may become pigmented secondarily. Hairy pigmented moles are almost never malignant. Rarely, malignant melanomas may be non-pigmented (**amelanotic**). New darkening of a pigmented lesion should be viewed with suspicion as it may indicated malignant change

(continued)

Table 46.1 Symptoms and signs of skin disorders—cont'd

Symptoms and signs	Diagnostic significance
5. Rapidly developing lesion	Keratoacanthoma, warts and pyogenic granuloma may all develop rapidly and eventually regress spontaneously. When fully developed, these conditions may be difficult to distinguish from malignancy. Spontaneous regression marks the lesion as benign
6. Multiple, recurrent and spreading lesions	In certain rare syndromes, multiple similar lesions develop over a period. Examples include neurofibromatosis and recurrent lipomata in Dercum's disease. Prolonged or intense sun exposure predisposes a large area of skin to malignant change. Viral warts may appear in crops. Malignant melanoma may spread diffusely (**superficial spreading melanoma**) or produce satellite lesions via dermal lymphatics
7. Site of the lesion	Some skin lesions arise much more commonly in certain areas of the body. The reason may be anatomical (e.g. pilonidal sinus, external angular dermoid or multiple pilar cysts of the scalp) or because of exposure to sun (e.g. solar keratoses or basal cell carcinomas of hands and face)
8. Age when lesion noticed	Congenital vascular abnormalities such as strawberry naevus or port-wine stain may be present at birth. Benign pigmented naevi (moles) may be detectable at birth, but only begin to enlarge and darken after the age of 2

HISTORY TAKING AND EXAMINATION

As the patient describes the problem, the lesion is usually offered for examination. The clinician then has the questionable advantage of having seen the lesion; this may then guide the direction and emphasis of history taking. The patient should be questioned about sun exposure and about other similar lesions or any regional lumps. Detailed inspection and palpation follow, and by this time a definite diagnosis or narrow differential diagnosis should have been established.

A **general history** must be taken at some point to establish whether there are any relevant systemic symptoms (e.g. weight loss suggesting malignant cachexia), concurrent disorders (e.g. diabetes predisposes to infection and may influence surgical management), any history of previous similar lesions, surgical treatment or trauma to the affected area. For example, a history of previous rodent ulcers (basal cell carcinoma) makes this diagnosis more likely another time. Previous surgery or trauma can lead to implantation epidermoids or a chronic inflammatory response to a foreign body.

Family history is occasionally valuable in rare genetic disorders such as neurofibromatosis. **Social history** should include occupational details as these may be relevant. For example, natal cleft pilonidal sinus is more common in truck drivers. Exposure to carcinogens such as lubricating oils persistently spilt on the same area of clothing may result in squamous carcinoma. Outdoor workers, especially those from the tropics, are predisposed to all types of skin cancer. Chronic ulcers may be contracted during **foreign travel**, e.g. tropical ulcers, Madura foot, tuberculous or atypical mycobacterial ulcers. Occasionally, patients deliberately injure themselves, producing mysterious chronic 'artefactual' lesions; a **psychiatric history** is valuable here, though rarely forthcoming.

Drug history is rarely relevant to 'surgical' skin lesions. Agents applied topically, e.g. silver nitrate stick, caustic agents and mechanical interference with wounds or lesions, can distort the clinical picture. It is also important to check if the patient is taking warfarin or aspirin since they may increase the risk of peroperative and postoperative haemorrhage.

The lesion is examined in detail, looking for the points described in Table 46.1. In addition, general clinical examination should search for other similar lesions, regional lymphadenopathy or a primary malignancy arising elsewhere and metastasising to skin. For example, if inguinal lymph nodes are enlarged, rectal and genital examination should be carried out to exclude concealed carcinoma. The lower limbs, including the soles of the feet, should also be examined, looking especially for malignant melanoma.

PRINCIPLES OF MANAGEMENT OF SKIN LESIONS

Many skin lesions can be diagnosed from the history and clinical examination, but wherever there is doubt, some form of biopsy is needed. This is particularly true if there is any risk of malignancy. Biopsy is performed as part of the treatment process if the lesion is small. Incision and excision biopsy techniques are illustrated in Chapter 11, and Box 46.1 summarises the options in the surgical management of skin conditions.

For axillary **hyperhidrosis**, the most effective and least risky option is injections of botulinum toxin into axillary skin. This needs to be repeated at 6–9-monthly intervals. For palmar hyperhidrosis unresponsive to dermatological management, thoracoscopic destruction of upper thoracic sympathetic nerves is highly effective.

LESIONS ORIGINATING IN THE EPIDERMIS

BENIGN EPIDERMAL LESIONS

SKIN TAGS (SQUAMOUS CELL PAPILLOMAS)

Skin tags are small benign polypoid lesions up to about 5 mm in diameter. They consist of a loose connective tissue core covered by normal, often excessively pigmented, keratinised epithelium. They are common in adults and may occur on any part of the body, particularly the trunk, neck, axillae and groins. In these locations, they may be irritated by clothing and bleed. Unsightly or inconvenient lesions may be easily removed by cryotherapy (freezing), cautery or excision (under local anaesthesia), or by tying a fine thread around the stalk (also under local anaesthesia) which leads to ischaemic atrophy.

WARTS

Warts are small, virus-induced epidermal tumours. They are characterised pathologically by irregular thickening of the epidermis with grossly excessive keratinisation and exaggerated dermal papillae. The morphology of the lesion depends on its location on the skin.

The **common wart** (verruca vulgaris), a papilliferous lesion up to 1 cm in diameter, is most common on the fingers and back of the hands. In children, warts are often multiple and commonly occur on the face. Facial lesions

are often less keratotic with a smoother, more dome-like shape. They are often called **juvenile or plane warts** (verruca plana juvenilis). Lesions on the sole of the foot, **plantar warts** (verruca plantaris), become extremely keratotic and flattened as a result of pressure. They may extend deeply into the foot, causing considerable pain. Warts may also occur on the genitalia, perineum and perianal area, usually spread by sexual contact. Genital warts sometimes grow to a large size; these are then known as **condylomata acuminata**.

Warts grow and regress spontaneously over several months, but they often require treatment to relieve pain, irritation or inconvenience. Many are treated for aesthetic reasons. Keratolytic applications (salicylic acid or podophyllin resin preparations), cryosurgery (liquid nitrogen application) or topical imiquimod are often the first choice of treatment. If unsuccessful, electrocautery (with or without curettage) and simple excision can be used.

SEBORRHOEIC KERATOSIS

Seborrhoeic keratoses (**seborrhoeic warts**) are extremely common skin lesions in elderly patients but occasionally appear in younger people (Fig. 46.2). The lesions are most often seen on the chest, face, neck and arms. There are often many lesions of different sizes with different intensities of pigmentation. They may be up to several centimetres in diameter. The lesions are slightly raised, sharply demarcated and plaque-like; they look and feel irregular and waxy. Sometimes they are so darkly pigmented that they cannot be distinguished clinically from superficial spreading malignant melanomas.

Histologically, a seborrhoeic keratosis is a localised proliferation of the basal layer of the epidermis. There is often hyperkeratosis in the surface crypts, resulting in

---

Box 46.1 Principles of management of 'surgical' skin lesions

Simple excision or other physical methods, e.g. electrocautery, laser therapy or cryotherapy—for small, obviously innocent lesions

Excision biopsy—if there is any risk of malignancy or the clinical diagnosis is doubtful (only for small lesions)

Biopsy—for large lesions. Definitive therapy is then planned according to the histology

Wide local excision with or without skin grafting—for malignant melanomas and sometimes for other large malignant lesions

Radiotherapy—an alternative to excision for basal cell carcinoma and primary squamous cell lesions. Also sometimes used if regional lymph nodes are involved in squamous cell carcinoma

Topical chemotherapy—with 5-fluorouracil cream for certain skin malignancies

Photodynamic therapy—for certain skin malignancies. Malignant cells absorb a photosensitising chemical which reacts with light of a particular wavelength to destroy the cells

Surgical lymph node clearance—if nodes are involved by malignant melanoma or squamous carcinoma

---

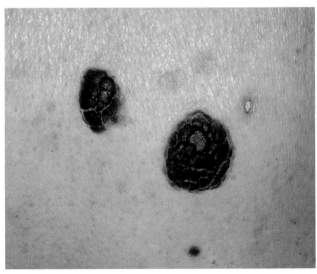

Fig. 46.2 Seborrhoeic keratoses

round keratin nests. Seborrhoeic keratoses are sometimes called **basal cell papillomas** because of their origin, but they are not true neoplasms and are unrelated to basal cell carcinoma.

Treatment is only required for unsightly or easily traumatised lesions. As they are so superficial, they can be 'scraped off' with a curette or scalpel under local anaesthesia. Another common treatment is cryotherapy but caution is needed, particularly in patients with dark coloured skin, since excessive cryotherapy can lead to the permanent loss of skin pigmentation.

KERATOACANTHOMA

A keratoacanthoma is a nodular, usually single skin lesion, up to 2 cm in diameter (Fig. 46.3 (b), (c)). It has an irregular central crater containing keratotic debris. As its name implies, the histological lesion consists of localised

tumour-like epidermal proliferation, with a thick prickle cell layer (**acanthosis**) and marked keratinisation. Some epithelial cells are large and have atypical nuclei; the underlying dermis exhibits marked chronic inflammatory cell infiltration.

The importance of this benign lesion is that it can be difficult to distinguish clinically or even histologically from squamous carcinoma. Keratoacanthomas, however, tend to have a short life cycle, appearing rapidly and regressing spontaneously over 2–3 months, whereas squamous cell carcinomas continue to enlarge. Keratin horns may also look similar but rarely regress. The cause of keratoacanthoma is unknown but its behaviour suggests a viral origin.

Diagnosis and treatment is by local excision unless the lesion is obviously regressing. If there is still diagnostic doubt, the patient should be followed up as for squamous carcinoma.

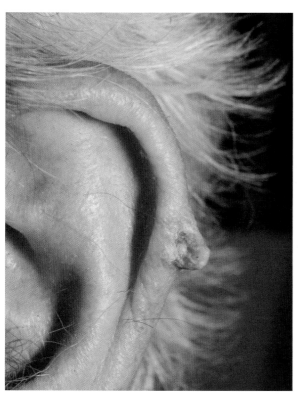

(a) Keratin horn on the pinna of an elderly man. If untreated, these can grow large.

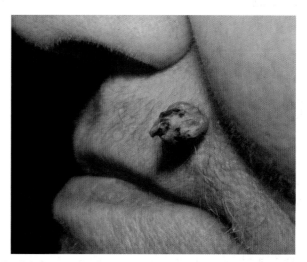

(b) This alarming looking lesion is a benign keratoacanthoma. The central keratin plug is characteristic. Resolution is spontaneous after a few weeks.

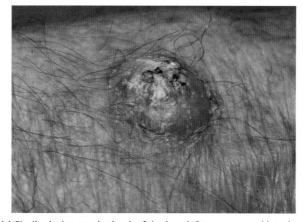

(c) Similar lesion on the back of the hand. Squamous and basal cell carcinoma need to be excluded.

Fig. 46.3 Keratin horn and keratoacanthoma

MELANOTIC LESIONS

BENIGN NAEVI

The deeper layers of the epidermis contain scattered melanocytes which synthesise melanin. This pigment is then transferred to nearby epidermal cells where it is responsible for skin colour. The concentration of melanocytes in the skin is similar in all races but the degree of skin pigmentation depends on the amount of melanin produced. Although skin colour is mainly determined by genetic factors, it is enhanced by exposure to the ultraviolet rays of sunlight (tanning).

Melanocytes originate from the neural crest and migrate to the ectoderm during embryological development. Hamartomatous accumulations of melanocytes may appear in the epidermis or dermis or both to form raised, variably pigmented lesions known as **naevi** or **moles**.

Lesions range in diameter from about 3 to 30 mm. The surface may be smooth or irregular and may contain hairs. According to clinical and histological features, naevi can be subdivided into five types: **junctional, intradermal, compound, blue** and **Spitz or spindle cell (juvenile) naevi**. The first three are closely related pathologically. (See Fig. 46.4 for histopathology.)

Junctional, intradermal and compound naevi

Junctional and intradermal naevi

Junctional naevi develop at or before puberty by accumulation of small clumps of melanocytes deep in the epidermis. The naevi manifest as small, slightly raised papules which are deeply pigmented because the melanocytes are close to the surface. After puberty, the **intradermal** variety of naevi predominates; the junctional naevus cells are thought to proliferate and migrate into the dermis

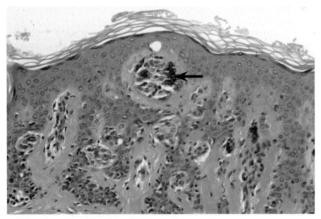

(a) Nests of naevus cells (arrowed) at the dermo-epidermal junction, known as a **junctional naevus.**

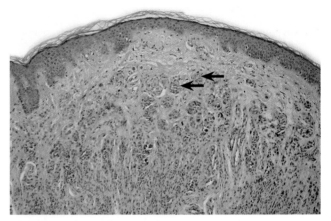

(b) Intradermal naevus showing naevus cells (arrowed) within the upper and mid-dermis. A compound naevus is made up of both junctional and intradermal components.

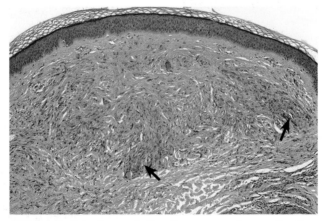

(c) Naevus cells having a spindle cell appearance (arrowed), rather than forming nests. This entity, known as **blue naevus,** may extend into deeper dermis. Sometimes a blue naevus component may be seen in association with the other types of naevi, a so-called **combined naevus.**

Fig. 46.4 Melanocytic naevi—histopathology. Increased numbers of melanocytes (naevus cells) may occur at various levels within the skin as illustrated

to form a mass of cells. These also present as raised papules but are larger than junctional naevi and paler, as the melanin is masked by the thickness of overlying skin.

Some intradermal naevi continue to enlarge; pilosebaceous elements become exaggerated to produce fleshy, dome-shaped or polypoid skin nodules often with protruding hairs. These slightly pigmented naevi are probably the most common skin lumps occurring on the face and are particularly seen in the elderly and in women (see Fig. 46.8, the lateral lesion).

Compound naevi

These uncommon moles contain junctional and intradermal components and look like something between the two, i.e. slightly raised, moderately pigmented papules. Compound naevi are probably a late transition from junctional to intradermal naevi occurring in early adulthood (see juvenile naevi below). Compound naevi are believed to be susceptible to transformation into **aggressive malignant melanomas**.

Blue naevi

Blue naevi are dark, blue-black, often flat moles formed by clumps of heavily pigmented melanocytes located deep in the dermis. The blue colour is an optical effect caused by the thick layer of overlying skin. Blue naevi occur at any age but are more common in the young; because of their dark colour they may be mistaken for malignant melanomas.

Spitz naevi

Spitz naevi (also known as spindle cell or juvenile naevi) are most common in the young but may occur at any age. Histologically, they are compound naevi. The cells are spindle-shaped, large and pleomorphic. In adults these characteristics would suggest malignancy but despite this, the lesions are benign.

Lentigo

Lentigines (the plural of lentigo) are benign pigmented lesions that may need to be considered in the differential diagnosis of potentially malignant melanotic lesions. They are large, heavily pigmented plaques which develop on the face and hands of the elderly. Melanocytes are more numerous, and melanin production is excessive but there is no accumulation of naevus cells. Lentigines are benign but predispose to the superficial spreading variety of malignant melanoma.

MANAGEMENT OF PIGMENTED LESIONS

People generally are becoming more aware that pigmented lesions can be malignant, and large numbers now seek medical advice. Fortunately, only a small proportion have malignant melanomas. With any suspicion of malignancy,

specialist opinion should be sought. A dermatologist is usually the first choice, but a surgeon will be involved if more than simple excision or biopsy is necessary.

Clinically it is not easy to distinguish between the different types of benign naevi, nor to be sure that a lesion is not malignant; however **dermoscopy** (dermatoscopy), i.e. examining the skin using surface microscopy, is a great help in expert hands in distinguishing between benign and malignant pigmented lesions. Note that if there is a history of recent change in a lesion or any doubt about its nature, excision biopsy is mandatory. In practice, if the patient or doctor is worried about a pigmented lesion, no matter how benign it looks, it is usually removed. Lesions subject to chronic irritation (e.g. at the waist, neck or palm) or in a site that is difficult to observe (e.g. sole of foot or genitalia) should certainly be removed. A fusiform incision removes the lesion together with a narrow margin of normal tissue (2–3 mm), enabling the skin edges to be readily opposed. All excised pigmented lesions should be examined histologically because a few benign-looking lesions will turn out to be malignant.

PREMALIGNANT AND MALIGNANT EPIDERMAL CONDITIONS

SOLAR (SENILE) KERATOSIS AND INTRA-EPIDERMAL CARCINOMA

Pathology and clinical features

Solar keratoses are flat, well-demarcated, brown, scaly or crusty lesions with an erythematous base (Fig. 46.5). They bleed easily if traumatised or scratched. Solar keratoses are often multiple and are most common in middle-aged or elderly patients on sun-exposed parts of the body such as face, neck, arms and hands. The incidence is higher in farm workers, fishermen and other outdoor

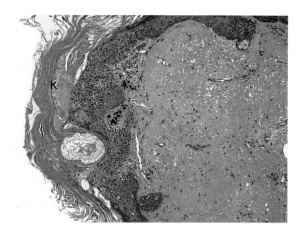

Fig. 46.5 Solar keratosis—histopathology
Occurring in sun-exposed areas, this lesion typically shows thickening of the keratin layer **K**. Epidermal cells can show a range of atypia, which may amount to squamous cell carcinoma in situ. The dermis shows severe solar damage.

workers. Solar keratoses are especially common in fair-skinned people living in tropical or subtropical regions such as Australia or the southern USA.

The characteristic histological features are marked thickening of the keratin layer (**hyperkeratosis**) and the prickle cell layer (**acanthosis**). Deep in the epidermis, there is a variable degree of dysplastic change and abnormal mitotic activity. These features suggest malignant transformation but, most importantly, the basal layer remains intact.

The epidemiology and pathology of solar keratosis suggest that it is a premalignant condition which predisposes to squamous carcinoma. Any lesions in which the dysplastic changes extend from the basal layers to the surface are considered to be malignant. They are termed **carcinoma in situ** or **intra-epidermal carcinoma**. Clinically, these are more erythematous than the premalignant type and are sometimes described as **Bowen's disease**. Bowen's disease occurring on the glans penis is known as **erythroplasia of Queyrat**.

Management

Management of solar keratoses depends on the number, size and distribution of the lesions, the age of the patient, and whether or not the skin type predisposes to cancer. Isolated lesions are best excised. For multiple keratoses, excision biopsy of representative lesions should be performed initially to confirm the diagnosis. This is followed by topical treatments such as 5-fluorouracil cream, diclofenac gel or imiquimod cream, or by excision biopsy, curettage or cryotherapy of suspicious lesions. Patients should be advised repeatedly to minimise exposure to ultraviolet rays by wearing protective clothing and hats and applying high factor total (UVA + UVB) sunscreen creams. These patients should also be regularly examined for squamous cell carcinomas, basal cell carcinomas and melanomas, which are all more common in patients with marked sunshine exposure.

SQUAMOUS CELL CARCINOMA

Pathology

Squamous cell carcinomas (Fig. 46.6) may occur anywhere on the skin or on stratified squamous epithelium of the mouth, tongue, oesophagus, anal canal, glans penis or uterine cervix. Squamous cell carcinoma also occurs in metaplastic squamous epithelium in the bronchus or bladder.

Squamous cell carcinoma of the skin usually occurs in older age groups, in areas of skin exposed repeatedly to ultraviolet light. Often, carcinoma develops from a pre-existing **solar (senile) keratosis**.

Much less commonly, squamous carcinoma develops in skin areas chronically exposed to **industrial carcinogens** such as ionising radiation, arsenic or chromium compounds, soot, tar, pitch or mineral oils. For example,

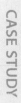

Fig. 46.6 Squamous carcinoma

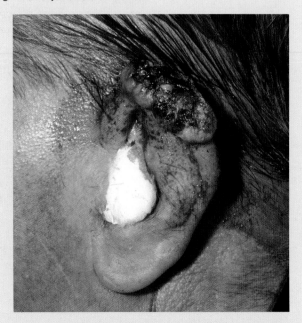

(a)

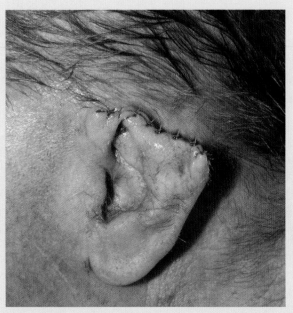

(b)

(a) This 70-year-old farmer had worked in the fields exposed to the sun all his life. He presented with this obviously malignant lesion on the upper part of the pinna. It was confirmed on biopsy to be a well-differentiated squamous cell carcinoma **(b)** after local resection.

carcinoma of the scrotum was common in chimney sweeps in the nineteenth century; the recognition of soot as the predisposing factor was a milestone in understanding carcinogenesis.

Chronic inflammation also predisposes to squamous carcinoma, which may develop at the margins of osteomyelitic sinuses or longstanding ulcers. These are common in developing countries where burns are poorly treated. A chronic burns ulcer in which carcinoma arises is known as a **Marjolin's ulcer**.

Histologically, squamous cell carcinomas of the skin are usually well differentiated, and the tumour cells resemble normal prickle cells. Keratin pearls and individual cell keratinisation are common features.

Clinical presentation

Squamous cell carcinoma usually presents as an enlarging painless ulcer with a rolled, indurated margin. Other lesions have an exophytic (outward growing, proliferative) cauliflower-like appearance with areas of ulceration, bleeding or serous exudation. Squamous cell carcinomas invade the dermis and deeper tissues such as bone or cartilage; further spread is usually to regional lymph nodes. Distant metastases are uncommon.

Management of squamous cell carcinoma (SCC)

Management involves first confirming the diagnosis by biopsy. This is followed by local radiotherapy or by excision of the carcinoma with a margin of normal tissue. For certain SCCs, including recurrences, tumours at sites where conserving normal tissue is important for cosmetic or functional reasons and for SCCs whose edges cannot be clearly defined, a special technique known as **Mohs' micrographic surgery** is often employed. This is performed under local anaesthesia and involves frozen section histology of horizontal sections. If malignant cells remain, further horizontal sections are removed until clear of malignancy.

Infiltrated lymph nodes are treated with **radiotherapy** or sometimes **block dissection** (i.e. removing all the regional lymph nodes in a single block of tissue). In general, these tumours respond favourably to radiotherapy and recurrence is unusual.

The prognosis is less good for tumours larger than 2 cm across, recurrent lesions, lesions arising in pre-existing scars, lesions on the skin of the lips, ears and scrotum, and lesions with poor differentiation or perineural invasion. Such patients are usually reviewed regularly for about 5 years after initial treatment.

BASAL CELL CARCINOMA

Pathology and clinical features

Basal cell carcinomas are common and nearly always result from exposure to excess ultraviolet sunlight. White-skinned people in tropical and sub-tropical regions have an extremely high incidence. Up to 50% of this group are affected at some time, often with multiple lesions. As with squamous cell carcinomas, basal cell carcinomas usually develop from middle age onwards, but their incidence is rising in younger 'sun-worshippers'. Males are affected at least twice as often as females, reflecting their greater occupational and recreational exposure to the sun.

Most basal cell carcinomas arise on the upper part of the face as shown in Figure 46.7, although any part of the skin can be involved. Most patients present early rather than late because the lesions are so visible.

Basal cell carcinomas begin as small pearly-white nodules with visible telangiectatic blood vessels (Fig. 46.8). Early lesions may ulcerate, bleed and then heal again, but as they grow larger they form irregular ulcers (**rodent ulcers**) with a pearly rolled margin. Although basal cell carcinomas almost never metastasise they are definitely malignant, invading underlying bone and cartilage. Neglected lesions on the scalp or neck may even invade the brain or spinal cord.

Histologically, the tumour cells have strongly basophilic nuclei and little cytoplasm. The cells at the periphery are arranged in a palisade pattern reminiscent of normal basal cells.

Management of basal cell carcinomas

Small lesions are usually treated by cryotherapy. Other treatment options used include topical chemotherapy with 5-fluorouracil cream or with imiquimod cream, local radiotherapy or 2–3 cycles of curettage combined with electrocautery. Excision biopsy may be appropriate for isolated or suspicious lesions. Radiotherapy must be avoided on the nose or ear where cartilage is susceptible to radiotherapy damage and may undergo necrosis. Larger

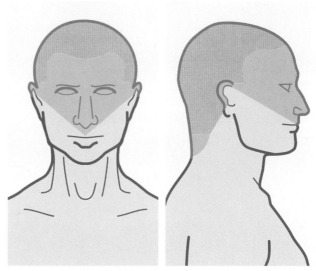

Fig. 46.7 Highest risk area for basal cell carcinomas shown in pink

Fig. 46.8 Basal cell carcinoma (BCC)

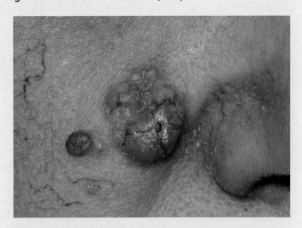 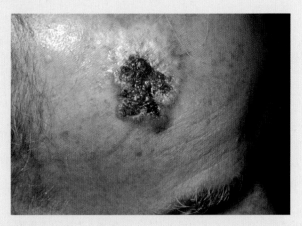

(a) The larger nodular lesion on the cheek of this woman aged 77 is a typical BCC. Note the pearly appearance of the lesion which is beginning to ulcerate. In this position, treatment with radiotherapy avoids distortion of the nasolabial fold. The smaller lesion lateral to the BCC is a benign naevus.

(b) Large BCC on the scalp of an elderly farm worker. Again, the typical pearly edge can be seen. After confirming the diagnosis on an incision biopsy of the edge, this was treated with radiotherapy.

destructive lesions are likely to require reconstructive plastic surgery involving skin grafts or flaps.

Photodynamic therapy (PDT) employs topical methyl amino-levulinate cream and light therapy. The drug is selectively absorbed into cancer cells and converted into photoactive porphyrins. When cancer cells loaded with porphyrins are exposed to light of wavelength 570–670 nm, a molecular reaction destroys the cancer cells. This treatment selectively targets tumour cells whilst leaving normal cells unharmed. It is recommended for solar keratoses and basal cell carcinomas situated on the mid-face or ears, those on severely sun-damaged skin, large lesions or recurrent lesions. Clinical trials have shown it gives cure rates at least as good as cryotherapy and surgery. It leaves minimal scarring and excellent cosmetic results.

As with squamous cell carcinomas, Mohs' micrographic surgery may be indicated for recurrent BCCs at sites where conservation of normal tissue is important or for BCCs where the edges cannot be clearly defined.

MALIGNANT MELANOMA

Introduction and pathology

Malignant melanoma (Fig. 46.9) arises by malignant transformation of melanocytes originating from the neural crest. Most malignant melanomas are poorly differentiated with numerous mitotic figures. The histological presence of melanin is diagnostic but suspected **amelanotic** (non-pigmented) **melanomas** may need to be confirmed by appropriate immunohistochemical tests.

Malignant melanoma is a common malignancy. The world incidence is rising substantially; in the UK, the

Fig. 46.9 Malignant melanoma

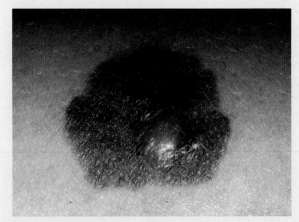

Pigmented lesion of the forearm in a 33-year-old woman. A small black lesion had been present for many years before starting to spread to reach its present diameter of 2.5 cm. Histologically, this proved to be a mixed type of malignant melanoma with both 'superficial spreading' and nodular elements.

number of new cases diagnosed rose by 50% between 1990 and 2000. The peak incidence is in the fourth decade. There has been an overall improvement in 5-year survival for melanoma patients from about 40% in the 1940s to about 80% now. In particular, melanomas of less than 1 mm Breslow thickness (see later) have a 95–100% 5-year survival rate. Improved survival may be due to greater public awareness, earlier detection and better treatment.

Risk factors

The epidemiology of malignant melanoma is fascinating. About 80% occur in white-skinned people and the disease is extremely common in albinos of all races. Until recent times, malignant melanoma was quite rare in northern Europe but the incidence has risen dramatically over the last three decades. Overall, about 1 in 100 Americans will be affected at some time in their lives. The highest incidence in the world is in northern and western Australia and it is certain that ultraviolet radiation is the essential aetiological factor. Whilst a cumulative sun effect is the main factor for other skin malignancies, short periods of intense sun exposure causing blistering sunburn, for example on a 2-week holiday, appear to be more important for malignant melanoma. There is evidence that unaccustomed exposure to strong sunlight can suppress general immunological responses and, by implication, immunological tumour surveillance. This might explain malignant melanomas on parts of the skin not generally exposed to the sun, for example the soles of the feet.

Other risk factors include a family history of malignant melanoma, freckling of the upper back, red or blond hair, blue or green or grey eyes and the presence of solar (actinic) keratoses. Each of these factors increases risk by about 3.5 times.

Melanoma subtypes

Melanomas may be classified as growing radially (**superficial spreading type**) or vertically (**nodular type**). About 80% are the superficial spreading type. These grow slowly and usually arise in pre-existing pigmented naevi. The lesions are flat with a variegated border and often have patches of regression. Nodular melanomas are more common in men and demonstrate an early vertical growth phase. They develop more rapidly and behave more aggressively than superficial spreading melanomas and tend to arise de novo in normal skin. Five per cent of nodular melanomas are **amelanotic**.

Lentigo maligna melanoma is uncommon and presents as large (> 3 cm) lesions on the face or neck of elderly women. It has a low metastatic potential but is locally invasive; it is distinct from **lentigo maligna**, which is its benign but precancerous counterpart.

Acral melanoma occurs on the palms or soles or under the nails. This is the only type that occurs in dark-skinned individuals and has a low incidence in white people. They occur at a mean age of 60 years (see Fig. 46.23 below). Note that malignant melanomas in less obvious areas of skin such as this have a reputation for aggressive behaviour but this may be because of late diagnosis.

Mucosal melanoma occurs on any mucosal surface from mouth to anus, pharynx or paranasal sinuses or in the vagina. They tend to behave particularly aggressively. **Ocular melanoma** arises from uveal melanocytes and is the most common ocular malignancy. It is unique in metastasising to the liver, often years after treatment of the primary lesion.

Clinical features of malignant melanoma

Most malignant melanomas are black or dark brown, flat or nodular lesions which may bleed or ulcerate. If a pre-existing or new mole enlarges, darkens, bleeds or becomes inflamed, ulcerated or itchy, it should be regarded with great suspicion (see Fig. 46.10). Superficial spreading melanoma can easily be mistaken for a seborrhoeic keratosis. In general, spread to regional lymph nodes occurs

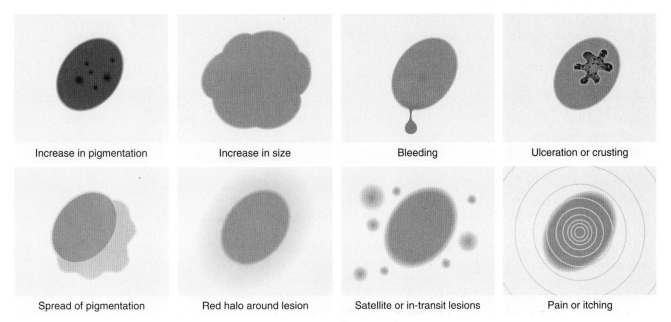

| Increase in pigmentation | Increase in size | Bleeding | Ulceration or crusting |

| Spread of pigmentation | Red halo around lesion | Satellite or in-transit lesions | Pain or itching |

Fig. 46.10 Clinical features in a pigmented lesion that suggest malignant melanoma

Tumour thickness	Risk of regional metastases	Risk of distant metastases	10-year survival without nodal or distant metastases
Less than 1 mm	3–5%	3–5%	95%
1–4 mm	25–60%	10–20%	60–75%
More than 4 mm	> 60%	70%	45%

Table 46.2 Risk of regional and distant metastasis in malignant melanoma according to Breslow thickness

early. Lateral spread in dermal lymphatics may produce **satellite lesions** around the primary nodule and 'in transit' lesions may appear along the course of the lymph node drainage.

Haematogenous spread occurs later, involving lung, liver, bone, brain and other tissues. The behaviour of malignant melanoma in an individual patient is unpredictable, although lesions arising before puberty or in the elderly tend to be less aggressive. Rarely, disseminated lesions undergo complete spontaneous regression, suggesting that immunological factors are involved. Melanomas that exhibit marked lymphocytic infiltration on histology have a better prognosis.

Prognostic factors

Measured tumour thickness on histological examination (Breslow) is the most useful guide to prognosis (Table 46.2) and has proved more accurate than the previously used 'level of invasion' (Clark's levels). Tumour thickness correlates well with the likelihood of regional and distant metastases as shown in Table 46.2. Other factors affecting prognosis include:

- The presence of 'satellite lesions' around the primary or 'in transit' lesions between the primary and its lymph node field—these make the prognosis worse
- Ulceration of the primary lesion—increases the likelihood of metastases and reduces survival
- Site of the primary—lesions of the head carry a worse prognosis than others
- Gender—with thick lesions, females fare better than males
- Pathological stage—nodal or distant involvement. The number and size of lymph node metastases has a bearing on survival—a single positive node is associated with a 40% 10-year survival, falling to 13% with two or more positive nodes. If distant metastases are present, 2-year survival is only about 25%
- Certain histopathological characteristics indicate a likely good or poor prognosis

Management of malignant melanoma

The first objective in managing a pigmented lesion is to establish whether it is malignant. Unless malignancy is clinically obvious, small lesions should be removed by excision biopsy and more extensive lesions sampled by incision biopsy. As a result of controlled trials, there have been two major changes in recent years in managing the local lesion. Firstly, it is no longer necessary to excise the lesion with a 5 cm margin all around and, secondly, split skin grafting is no longer regarded as essential to achieve skin cover and provide early warning of local recurrence. For thin melanomas, less than 1 mm thick, a clear margin of 1 cm is sufficient. For thicker melanomas (1.1–4 mm), wider excision with a 2 cm clearance is needed to achieve optimum survival. For lesions thicker than 4 mm, a 3 cm clearance is believed desirable. In most cases, primary closure or the use of local rotational flaps can safely achieve skin cover.

As regards lymph nodes, **elective lymph node dissection** of palpable regional lymph nodes undoubtedly improves survival; the same applies to removal of involved lymph nodes detected by ultrasonography. There has been an upsurge of interest in sentinel node biopsy for thicker lesions. Lymphatic dye is injected to locate 'sentinel' nodes for frozen section biopsy, proceeding to node dissection if positive. A large controlled trial comparing this approach with 'watchful waiting' and excision of palpable nodes that appear, however, showed no survival advantage.

Adjuvant therapy is largely ineffective but modified radiotherapy is under trial and may reduce local recurrence rates and even improve survival. Melanoma cells are sensitive to higher dose fractions than are usual (600 rad as opposed to 180 rad). Systemic cytotoxic chemotherapy has given disappointing results, but where there is locally advanced limb melanoma with 'in-transit' lesions and regional spread not amenable to surgical excision, hyperthermic local or limb perfusion chemotherapy techniques may provide effective control (but not cure).

LESIONS ORIGINATING IN THE DERMIS

CYSTS

In true pathological terms, cysts are epithelium-lined cavities; most represent ducts dilated by retained secretion, usually due to obstruction. In contrast, breast cysts may show epithelial hyperplasia, excessive secretion and structural distortion. Some cysts arise from ectopic epithelial remnants (dermoids) or as a result of necrosis in the centre of a malignant epithelial mass. Cysts commonly require surgical removal (or drainage) for aesthetic reasons or to exclude malignancy.

Cysts are common in the skin. Most arise from elements of hair follicles in the dermis and consist of an epithelium-lined cavity filled with viscous or semi-solid epithelial degradation products. These are **epidermal cysts** and **pilar cysts**. Occasionally, cysts arise from developmental epithelial remnants (**dermoid cysts**) or by traumatic implantation of epithelial fragments (**implantation (epi)dermoids**).

Epidermal cysts

These are by far the most common skin cysts, and are often incorrectly described as '**sebaceous cysts**'. They are usually solitary and may be found anywhere on the body (except the palms or soles), most commonly on the scalp, trunk, face and neck. They range up to several centimetres in diameter. Epidermal cysts are smooth and rounded, and covered by normal epidermis in which a blocked duct (**punctum**) may be visible (Fig. 46.11b). On palpation, they have a doughy, fluctuant consistency and are usually not tender. An important diagnostic feature is that since they originate in the skin, they are attached to it but are mobile over deeper tissues. Multiple small epidermal cysts sometimes develop on the scrotal skin or areola and cause embarrassment.

Histologically, an epidermal cyst has a stratified squamous lining epithelium and is filled with keratin; this is consistent with its derivation from a hair follicle. The cyst contents are thick and waxy, and were originally thought to be sebaceous material. This gave rise to the erroneous name of sebaceous cyst.

Surgical removal (see Ch. 11)

Epidermal cysts (Fig. 46.11) are mainly removed because of recurrent inflammation. Others are removed for cosmetic reasons or sometimes because they interfere with clothing or combing the hair. An incision is made over the cyst beside the punctum, taking care not to puncture the cavity. The cyst is then enucleated by blunt dissection and delivered from the wound in its entirety. This ensures all the epithelium is removed and prevents recurrence.

Inflamed epidermal cysts

Trauma to epidermal cysts (often unnoticed) may cause some of the contents to escape into the surrounding tissues, exciting an intense foreign-body inflammatory response. The patient may complain of pain, swelling, redness and even spontaneous discharge of liquefied cyst contents; this looks like pus but is in fact sterile. These inflamed epidermal cysts are often described as 'infected' but this is rarely the case and antibiotic therapy is not indicated.

It is unwise to attempt removal of an acutely inflamed epidermal cyst because the tissue planes cannot be recognised and some of the epithelial lining is likely to be left. If pain is severe, liquefied cyst contents should just be drained by simple incision under local anaesthesia; this provides rapid relief of symptoms. Culture of this material rarely yields any growth. The residual cyst should be excised later in the usual way as it is almost certain to flare up repeatedly if left.

Pilar cysts

Some individuals develop multiple epidermal cysts on the scalp known as pilar cysts. Multiple cysts occur less commonly on the face or neck. These range from a few millimetres to many centimetres in diameter, but grow very slowly. They can easily be excised under local anaesthesia.

INFECTIVE LESIONS

PYOGENIC GRANULOMA

Pyogenic granuloma (Fig. 46.12) is a common inflammatory lesion of the skin which arises in response to minor penetrating foreign bodies such as splinters or thorns. Lesions are most common on the hands and feet but may also occur on the lips and gums. Pathologically, a pyogenic granuloma consists of a mass of exuberant granulation tissue containing numerous polymorphs. It usually develops over a period of about a week but does not often regress spontaneously.

Clinically, pyogenic granulomas are solitary, reddish-blue fleshy nodules which may be polypoid. The surface may be ulcerated, in which case the lesion may be clinically indistinguishable from amelanotic malignant melanoma. Pyogenic granulomas should be excised and the base curetted or cauterised to prevent recurrence.

FURUNCLE (BOIL) AND CARBUNCLE

A furuncle is a staphylococcal abscess that develops in a hair follicle in the dermis. Diabetes mellitus can be a predisposing factor. The lesion rapidly enlarges and eventually 'points' at the surface, spontaneously discharging pus. The centre often contains a core of necrotic tissue. Once the pus has discharged and the necrotic

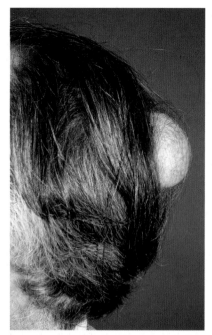

(a) This large epidermal (pilar) cyst of the scalp was clearly visible but several more were also palpable in the scalp hair of this 55-year-old man.

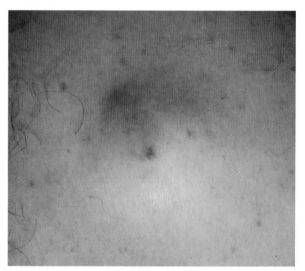

(b) Non-inflamed epidermal cyst of the skin of the buttock.

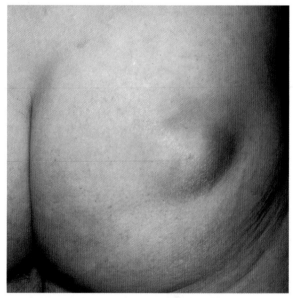

(c) Inflamed epidermal cyst of buttock.

Fig. 46.11 Epidermal cysts

tissue has been shed, the lesion heals spontaneously; however, the necrotic core may need excision to speed the healing process. Drainage may be encouraged with poultices or dressings, such as magnesium sulphate paste, which are said to draw the pus to the surface by osmosis. Furuncles are most common in young men with acne, especially on the face, the back of the trunk and the lower limbs. Axillary furuncles are common in middle-aged females, and tend to recur. Surgical drainage is necessary if a chronic abscess develops. A furuncle may be the source of systemic sepsis, especially in uncontrolled diabetes. **Cavernous sinus thrombosis** is a rare but very serious (and often fatal) complication of a furuncle on the lateral aspect of the nose or infra-orbital area. This area drains into the cavernous sinus via the facial vein and inferior ophthalmic veins (see Fig. 46.17, p. 680).

A **carbuncle**, also staphylococcal in origin, is larger than a furuncle and consists of a honeycomb of abscesses, often draining (inadequately) via multiple sinuses. The back of the neck is the usual site (Fig. 46.13); here the skin is tightly bound by interlacing bundles of fibrous tissue. Carbuncles are more common in diabetic patients, and may bring the diabetes to light. Treatment is with anti-staphylococcal antibiotics such as flucloxacillin as early as possible. The aim is to minimise pus formation and necrosis that would lead to skin loss and delay healing. If pus has formed, thorough desloughing and drainage of the abscesses is required, usually leaving wounds open to heal by secondary intention.

Fig. 46.12 Pyogenic granuloma—case study

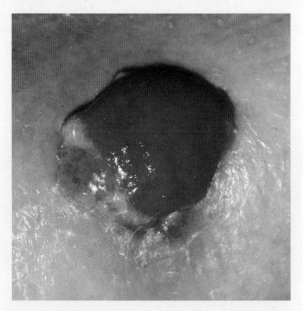

This man of 29 suffered a minor penetrating injury to his forearm from a piece of sharp metal. The wound did not heal as normal but produced this friable proliferative lesion. The appearance is typical of a pyogenic granuloma, composed largely of granulation tissue. It was removed by curettage under local anaesthesia and healing afterwards was uninterrupted.

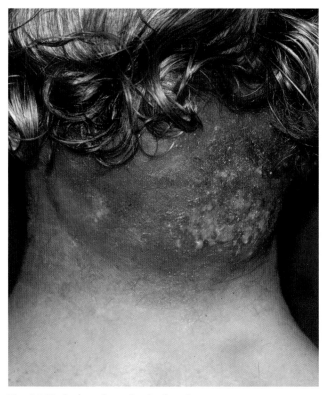

Fig. 46.13 Carbuncle on back of neck

ERYSIPELAS

Erysipelas is now an uncommon primary skin infection caused by group A streptococci. In this condition, the infection is more superficial than cellulitis, involving only the dermis. The spreading inflamed area is very well demarcated, with the margin raised above the normal skin.

NECROTISING FASCIITIS

This serious and alarming condition is usually a complication of surgery or traumatic wounds and is covered in Chapters 3 (microbiology) and 12 (clinical aspects)

MISCELLANEOUS BENIGN LESIONS

SEBACEOUS HYPERPLASIA

Localised hyperplasia of sebaceous glands on the nose and in nearby skin creases is common in both men and women. Sebaceous glands are plentiful in this area. The condition probably reflects a mildly abnormal response to sex hormones.

Apart from their unsightly appearance, these small nodular lesions may on occasion be clinically indistinguishable from basal cell carcinomas; the diagnosis is made on histology after excision biopsy.

In **rhinophyma**, an extreme manifestation of sebaceous hyperplasia, the nose becomes enlarged and lumpy. It is mainly seen in older men, and is (unreliably) said to occur in heavy drinkers. Rhinophyma is treated by surgical correction, carbon dioxide laser or dermabrasion.

KELOID SCARS

Keloids are formed by excessive deposition of collagen in the dermis during wound healing. The result is an elevated nodular lesion covered by normal epidermis. The chest and neck are particularly susceptible. The problem is much more common in black people.

Keloid formation may cause poor cosmetic results after injury, minor surgery, or even ear-piercing. Simply excising the lesion often makes scarring worse. Treatment is generally unsatisfactory; silicone gel under an occlusion dressing and/or intralesional steroids usually causes some regression. In extreme cases, excision of the scar followed by a low dose of local radiotherapy may suppress further keloid formation.

HISTIOCYTOMA

Histiocytomas (also known as **dermatofibromas**) are common painless skin lesions occurring mainly on the limbs. They are firm nodules, usually about 5 mm in diameter and deep reddish-brown in colour. They are clinically important because they may be mistaken for malignant melanoma. Histologically, they contain numerous lipid-filled macrophages (**histiocytes**). One histological variant contains prominent vascular elements and has given rise to the confusing term **sclerosing angioma**.

DERMOID CYSTS

True dermoid cysts are pathologically similar to epidermal cysts in that they are lined by stratified squamous epithelium. As well as keratin, however, they can contain hair, sebaceous glands and other ectodermal structures. Dermoids arise from cystic change in epithelial remnants left behind at lines of embryological fusion. They are usually found in the midline of the scalp, neck and lower jaw and at the outer angle of the eyebrow (**external angular dermoid**). Treatment is by excision.

IMPLANTATION (EPI)DERMOIDS

These small keratin-filled cysts arise from epidermal fragments implanted in the dermis by minor penetrating injuries. Though not derived from epidermal appendages, they are pathologically similar to epidermal cysts but may contain small foreign bodies. Implantation dermoids are most often seen on the fingers, often under the scar of a previous laceration.

MALIGNANT LESIONS

SECONDARY (METASTATIC) CARCINOMA

Metastatic tumour deposits may present as small hard painless nodules in the skin. They are usually located in the dermis and covered by normal epidermis. Visceral malignancy, e.g. pancreatic or colon cancer, may present with a metastasis at the umbilicus (Sister Joseph's nodule). With skin metastases, there is usually a history of a treated malignancy elsewhere. Lobular breast carcinomas are the most common cause, but carcinomas of stomach, uterus, lungs, large bowel and kidneys can also metastasise to skin. Occasionally, biopsy of a mysterious skin lesion leads to the diagnosis.

True skin metastases are a different entity from local spread of tumour or local implantation of cells during surgery, which are a particular feature of carcinoma of the breast. Laparoscopic surgery for malignancy acquired a bad reputation, partly because of local recurrences at port sites, but improved surgical techniques have virtually eliminated this problem.

Management of skin secondaries depends on the primary diagnosis but the prognosis is usually poor. Treatment is by local excision, radiotherapy or chemotherapy, depending on the severity of symptoms and the size, number and location of secondaries.

KAPOSI'S SARCOMA

This once rare condition has leapt to prominence as one of the most frequent presentations of **acquired immune deficiency syndrome** (AIDS). Kaposi's sarcoma (KS) has been shown to be associated with human herpes virus 8. The condition appears as multiple blueish-red to brown nodules or plaques, all of which are primary tumours (Fig. 46.14). They most commonly occur on the limbs.

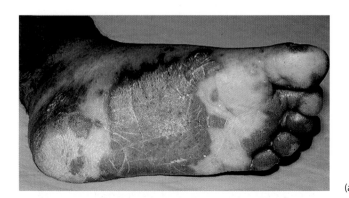

(a)

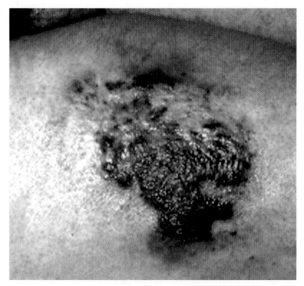

(b)

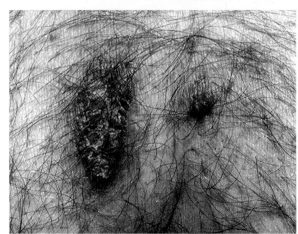

(c)

Fig. 46.14 Kaposi's sarcoma in various sites

Excision biopsy confirms the diagnosis. KS tumours are characterised by proliferating dysplastic fibroblasts, accompanied by chronic inflammation, endothelial proliferation and haemorrhage. Treatment varies: classical type KS usually does not need treatment but larger lesions respond to radiotherapy. Endemic KS is treated by chemotherapy and AIDS-related KS is controlled by highly active antiretroviral therapy.

LESIONS OF THE HYPODERMIS AND DEEPER TISSUES

CELLULITIS

Cellulitis is a diffuse spreading infection of the subcutaneous tissues and deeper layers of the skin. It may be acute or chronic. Beta-haemolytic streptococci, usually Lancefield group A (*S. pyogenes*), are commonly responsible. These bacteria produce fibrinolysins and hyaluronidase which break down the protective intercellular barriers and promote spread of infection through the tissue planes. Although an intense neutrophil inflammatory response develops, pus rarely accumulates. Rather, the tissues become red and oedematous. If the skin surface is broken, a serous exudate is released.

Any part of the skin may develop cellulitis (Fig. 46.15), the organisms usually gaining entry via a traumatic or surgical wound, although a wound is not always found. Clinically, the skin is greatly thickened, tense, hot, red and painful; the margins are fairly clearly demarcated from adjacent normal skin. Lymphatics draining the affected area become inflamed and **lymphangitis** develops. The inflamed lymphatics are visible as red streaks passing towards the regional lymph nodes, which are also swollen and tender (**lymphadenitis**). Systemic features such as fever and tachycardia indicate bacteraemia or even septicaemia.

Acute cellulitis was a serious infection in earlier times, not least as a complication of surgery. It is now readily treated with antibiotics.

CELLULITIS OF THE LOWER LIMB

Low-grade cellulitis may occur in the lower limb without evidence of any wound. This form of cellulitis is usually found in older women and presents as a localised, but not clearly demarcated, brawny inflammation of the leg, usually without regional lymph node involvement or systemic features of infection. Predisposing factors are lymphatic obstruction or oedema from any cause. These infections often recur and are difficult to document bacteriologically because there is no wound and no infected exudate. Nevertheless, they usually respond to antibiotics (such as tetracycline), rest, elevation of the limb and compression stockings when the inflammation has settled. Recurrence is common at intervals of months or years.

A similar low-grade cellulitis may occur in the upper limb or chest wall as a result of lymphatic obstruction following lymph node excision or radiotherapy for breast cancer.

LIPOMA AND LIPOSARCOMA

Lipomas are benign tumours of fat. They may occur anywhere that fat is normally present, most often in the hypodermis of the trunk and limbs. The aetiology is unknown, although mild trauma may be a factor. Typically, they present on the forearms (often multiple), in the supraclavicular fossa (Fig. 46.16), over the deltoid muscle or over the scapula. Lipomas can also be found within the peritoneal cavity, including the bowel submucosa, and within muscles or joints. They may also sometimes arise beneath the periosteum.

Pathologically, lipomas consist of a multilobular mass of fatty tissue with thin fibrous septa. A tenuous fibrous capsule usually defines the lesion clearly from the surrounding tissue. Lipoma cells are histologically indistinguishable from normal adipocytes. Lipomas vary in size

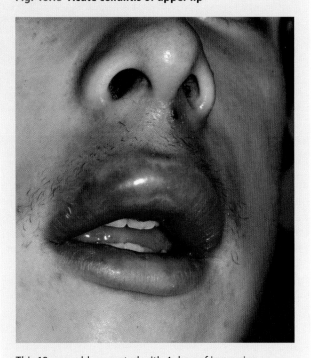

Fig. 46.15 Acute cellulitis of upper lip

This 18-year-old presented with 4 days of increasing swelling and pain affecting the upper lip following 'picking' of an acne spot. This infection lies in the 'danger triangle' involving the nose and upper lip where serious infection can be complicated by cavernous sinus thrombosis. This patient responded rapidly to intensive antibiotic therapy. The organism proved to be *Strep. pyogenes*.

Fig. 46.16 Lipoma

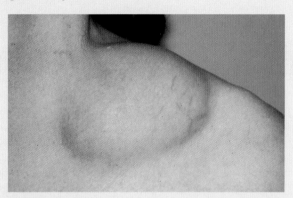

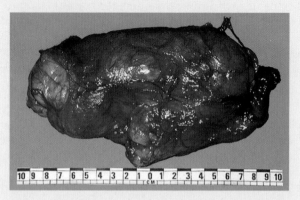

(a) Large soft lipoma overlying the supraclavicular fossa in a 46-year-old woman. This is a common site for lipomas. It had been present for many years but had recently started to enlarge.

(b) The surgical specimen. Note that it is larger than its clinical appearance would suggest.

from about 2–20 cm and are shaped like a flattened dome. The overlying skin is normal. Their consistency is soft and almost fluctuant. Lipomas are removed if they are inconvenient or unsightly. If the margin is poorly defined at operation, recurrence is likely.

Liposarcoma is a rare malignant variant. It tends to occur in the retroperitoneal area and mediastinum rather than in the skin.

NEUROFIBROMA, NEUROFIBROMATOSIS AND SCHWANNOMA

Neurofibromas are benign tumours arising from the supporting fibroblasts of peripheral nerves. The tumour cells are loosely arranged in a gelatinous (myxomatous) intercellular material which often makes the lesion soft and pulpy to palpation. In the skin, neurofibromas may present as solitary sessile or pedunculated lesions in the vicinity of peripheral nerves. They are sometimes very tender to palpation.

The autosomal dominant inherited syndrome called **neurofibromatosis** (von Recklinghausen's disease) is characterised by multiple neurofibromas and café-au-lait spots (coffee-coloured skin patches). Sometimes, the neurofibromas are extremely numerous, and occasionally there is gross hypertrophy of subcutaneous tissues and skin folds. This extreme variant was once thought to be the diagnosis of the famous 'elephant man' of Sir Frederick Treves, however it is now believed that he suffered from another inherited condition, Proteus syndrome. A small proportion of neurofibromas undergo malignant change into sarcomas.

Schwannomas are benign tumours arising from the Schwann cells supporting peripheral nerves. They present

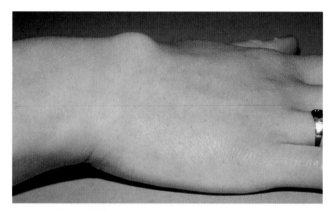

Fig. 46.17 Ganglion
This ganglion is in a common site, the dorsum of the hand.

as firm, nodular lesions tethered to a nerve, and pressure on the tumour may cause pain in the area of distribution of the nerve. Treatment is by careful excision, attempting to preserve the affected nerve. This usually requires an operating microscope and microsurgical manipulation.

GANGLION

This extremely common and inappropriately named condition is a cyst-like lesion derived from the lining of a synovial joint, tendon sheath or embryological remnants of synovial tissue. The 'cystic' space does not usually communicate with the associated joint or tendon sheath, and like synovial joint cavities, is not lined by epithelium. It contains a colourless, gelatinous fluid. Ganglia present as superficial lumps, usually about 1–2 cm in diameter, though sometimes larger. They are most common on the dorsum of the forearm and hand (Fig. 46.17) and around the ankle. They are rarely painful but sometimes cause mechanical problems or interference with footwear. Ganglia are easily recognised by their smooth, hemispherical surface, and firm but slightly fluctuant 'cyst-like' consistency. The overlying skin is normal and mobile and the ganglion weakly transilluminable.

The age-old treatment for a ganglion was a sharp blow with a family bible, which dissipated the cyst contents into the tissues. Recurrence almost inevitably followed. Needle aspiration or surgical excision are the accepted methods of treatment now, but recurrence is still common.

LESIONS OF VASCULAR ORIGIN

CAMPBELL DE MORGAN SPOTS

Campbell de Morgan spots are small, bright-red spots which appear on the trunk, usually in older patients. They represent highly localised capillary proliferation and have no clinical significance except for the titillation of bored examiners! Like other vascular lesions they blanch when compressed and then refill when pressure is removed.

SPIDER NAEVI

Spider naevi or telangiectases are small red lesions consisting of a central arteriole from which radiate dilated capillaries. This appearance explains their name. Isolated spider naevi may be found in normal individuals on the trunk, neck and face. Their numbers markedly increase in chronic liver disease, especially cirrhosis, and occasionally in pregnancy. Treatment is rarely required but, when needed, laser therapy is probably the treatment of choice.

ANGIOMAS

Despite their name, angiomas are not true neoplasms but rather congenital hamartomas. They arise from localised excessive development of thin-walled blood vessels which may be of small diameter (**capillary haemangiomas**) or hugely dilated (**cavernous haemangiomas**). The histological appearance is often ambiguous, with most angiomas containing capillary and cavernous elements, as well as arteriovenous or even lymphatic components.

'PORT-WINE STAINS'

The most common haemangiomas are port-wine stains. These can occur anywhere on the body, but especially the face, neck and scalp, and cause considerable cosmetic distress. They are present from birth and remain unchanged throughout life. Lesions are flat or slightly

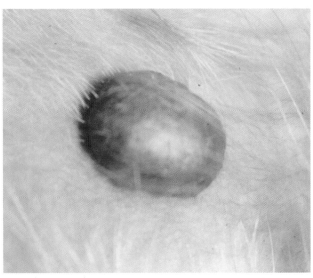

Fig. 46.18 Strawberry naevus
Strawberry naevus on the back of the neck in a 4-month-old infant. This was present at birth and can be expected to grow with the child for up to two years, then atrophy spontaneously, leaving no scar.

elevated and reddish-blue. They have an asymmetrical outline and range up to many centimetres in diameter. Trauma may cause bleeding or ulceration.

Surgical treatment, often urged by anguished patients, is rarely successful except for small lesions. Sclerosing agents can be injected to promote thrombosis, organisation and progressive devascularisation, but results are disappointing. Lasers such as the pulse dye laser, that are tuned to the colour frequency of haemoglobin, and other high-energy light sources are encouraging innovations and give promising results in some patients. Regrettably, the use of covering cosmetic preparations remains the best advice for most.

STRAWBERRY NAEVI

The strawberry naevus (Fig. 46.18) is a distinct type of angioma. These occur in early childhood as bright-red fleshy lesions and grow for a few years before involuting spontaneously. Almost all will resolve without scarring. Surgery is not indicated except to deal with redundant skin left after involution.

CYSTIC HYGROMA

Cystic hygroma is a lymphangioma that presents as a lump in the neck, usually during childhood; it is described in more detail on page 697. Characteristically, the lesion is highly transilluminable.

Fig. 46.19 Klippel–Trenaunay syndrome

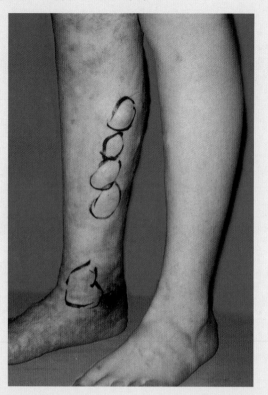

Klippel–Trenaunay syndrome affecting the right leg in a male aged 19. The three characteristic features are **gigantism** due to multiple congenital arterio-venous fistulae, gross **varicose veins** (outlined in marking pen on the skin) and cutaneous **capillary naevi**. In addition, this patient also had a varicose ulcer, seen below the medial malleolus.

CONGENITAL SYNDROMES

Gross vascular malformations form part of a number of rare congenital syndromes. These include **Sturge–Weber syndrome** (angiomas of the face and intracranial contents) and **Klippel–Trenaunay syndrome** (Fig. 46.19). Klippel–Trenaunay syndrome is characterised by the triad of port-wine stain, varicose veins and bone and soft tissue hypertrophy involving one lower limb; it may include the pelvis. Parks–Weber syndrome is probably another name for the same condition. The primary abnormality is believed to be multiple microscopic arterio-venous communications. These lead to hypertrophy of the limb (gigantism), which is warm to palpation. The venous abnormalities include gross varicose veins, deep venous abnormalities and persistent atypical veins. Venous abnormalities often lead to venous ulceration.

GLOMUS TUMOUR

This is a benign tumour derived from a glomus body, small arterio-venous communications normally found in the peripheries. The glomus bodies are thought to play a part in controlling local blood flow. Glomus tumours occur singly, usually in the fingers and often beneath the nail. They are tiny (1–3 mm) red flat lesions which are exquisitely tender to the touch. Treatment is by surgical excision.

LESIONS DERIVED FROM SKIN APPENDAGES

BENIGN APPENDAGE TUMOURS

A variety of benign tumours arise from skin appendages. The most common is the **cylindroma**, which is derived from sweat glands. Diagnosis is usually made unexpectedly on histological examination of an excised nondescript skin lump.

Pilonidal sinus and abscess are described in Chapter 30.

DISORDERS OF THE NAILS

INGROWING TOENAIL

Pathophysiology

An ingrowing toenail (Fig. 46.20) occurs when the distal edge of the nail persistently cuts into the adjacent nail fold. The problem almost exclusively affects the great toe. In effect there is a laceration which cannot heal because of the presence of a foreign body (the toenail). Superimposed infection by a mixture of local bacterial and fungal flora complicates the picture. The combination of acute inflammation and attempts at tissue repair results in the formation of exuberant granulation tissue around the laceration and surrounding inflammatory swelling. Swelling aggravates trauma caused by the nail edge.

Ingrowing toenail is mainly confined to teenagers and young adults, particularly males. It probably results from a combination of factors, including inadequate hygiene, unsuitable footwear, cutting the nails too short at the corners and the macerating effect of sweat on the skin. High levels of circulating testosterone, as found in adolescence, may be an important aetiological factor.

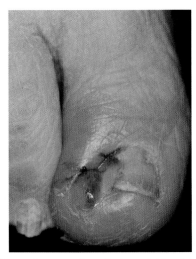

(a) Infected ingrowing toenail on the lateral side of the toe. This patient had suffered recurrent attacks over many years which prevented him playing football. Note the swelling of the lateral side of the toe, the overgrowth of granulation tissue caused by chronic irritation and the purulent discharge. Surgical treatment was employed once the acute inflammation had settled with saline soaks and antibiotics.

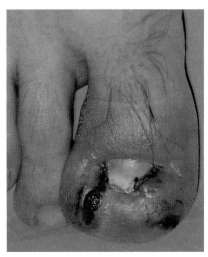

(b) Inflamed ingrowing toenail affecting medial and lateral sides. There is a great amount of hypertrophy, making suitable footwear hard to find.

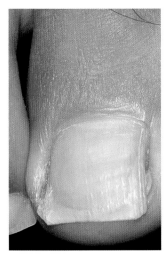

(c) Congenitally wide toenails. This man of 32 had suffered many bouts of inflammation over the years.

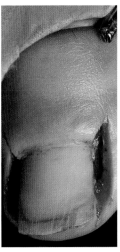

(d) and **(e)** The same patient undergoing wedge resection and phenolisation of both sides of the nail. Note the use of a tourniquet.

Fig. 46.20 Ingrowing toenail

Management

The main objective of treatment is to prevent persistent trauma by the nail edge. Surgical operations result in a week or more of discomfort and immobility, so conservative treatment should be tried first.

Conservative treatment

In all cases, simple conservative measures include regular bathing, frequent changes of socks (which should be made of cotton), avoiding tight or narrow shoes and avoiding trauma to the toe when inflamed, for example from kicking a football.

For an inflamed ingrowing toenail, foot soaks in warm saline should be carried out twice daily for at least 10 minutes. Surgical spirit applied twice daily may also help.

A useful further measure, once inflammation is settling, is to pack a small pledget of cotton wool beneath the corner of the nail to lift the nail out of the laceration. At the same time, the nail fold can be pushed away by packing a small elongated pledget between the nail fold and the nail edge. These tiny packs can be left in place for days but need to be increased in size as the corner of the nail rises away from its bed.

These conservative measures, all undertaken by the patient, are often successful in even severe cases but require perseverance. Systemic antibiotics should only be used if infection is spreading; topical antibiotics are of little use.

Surgical treatment

Urgent surgical treatment involves avulsion of the whole nail, or one side of the nail. This immediately removes the 'foreign body' and permits rapid resolution. For recurrent ingrowing toenails, particularly if abnormal nail morphology is a contributory factor, part of the nail bed is best removed. The more popular procedures are illustrated in Figure 46.21. The operations are usually performed under local anaesthesia using a ring block and tourniquet. Local anaesthetic incorporating a vasoconstrictor such as adrenaline must *never* be used in the digits because of the risk of ischaemic necrosis.

ONYCHOGRYPHOSIS

Onychogryphosis ('ram's horn nail') (Fig. 46.22) is a gross abnormality of nail growth. It most commonly affects the great toenail, which becomes greatly thickened and distorted. Nail cutting with ordinary nail scissors then becomes impossible. Onychogryphosis is usually seen only in elderly patients and probably results from previous trauma to the nail bed. This condition usually presents when it interferes with wearing shoes. A chiropodist (podiatrist) can treat onychogryphosis by using grinding instruments at regular intervals. Surgical removal

Removal of nail alone

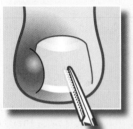

If badly infected and unresponsive to conservative treatment, 'first aid' is to remove the whole nail without disturbing the nail bed, under a local anaesthetic ring block
The nail can be lifted out by firmly grasping with artery forceps
Removal of the 'foreign body' allows inflammation to settle

Zadik's operation for permanent ablation of nail and nail bed

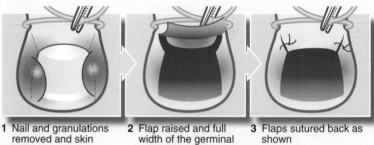

1 Nail and granulations removed and skin incised as shown (dotted lines)

2 Flap raised and full width of the germinal matrix treated by phenolisation as in 6 below

3 Flaps sutured back as shown

Wedge resection/phenolisation for permanent narrowing of nail

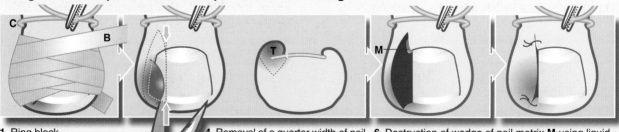

1 Ring block

2 Exsanguination of toe with 'mini-Esmark' bandage **B** (i.e. rubber bandage spirally applied)

3 Application of tourniquet **C** (e.g. thin rubber tube) around toe base before removing Esmark

4 Removal of a quarter width of nail using pointed scissors to cut from distal to proximal (between arrows) and lifting out fragment

5 Excision of a wedge of hypertrophic/inflamed tissue **T**

6 Destruction of wedge of nail matrix **M** using liquid 60% phenol. Undersides of the skin flaps are protected with paraffin jelly and a cotton pledget moistened with phenol placed on nail bed for 2 minutes

7 Skin closure with absorbable sutures if necessary

8 Pressure dressing. Leave toe tip visible and check for ischaemia. Non-adherent dressing and crepe bandage; then release tourniquet

9 Redress at 24 hours

Fig. 46.21 Operations for ingrowing toenail

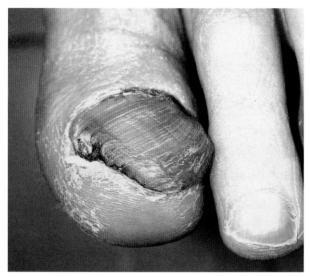

(a) Moderate degree of nail thickening and 'heaping up'.

Fig. 46.22 Onychogryphosis

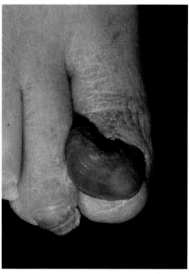

(b) More advanced and neglected case. Both of these were treated by chiropody, with careful and regular grinding down of the nails, but nail bed ablation is an alternative treatment.

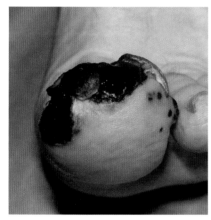

Fig. 46.23 Subungual malignant melanoma
Aggressive malignant melanoma arising from beneath the nail of the first toe. Note the large main lesion and the satellite lesions nearby. This patient died of melanomatosis one year after this picture was taken.

of the nail and ablation of the bed is sometimes performed.

SUBUNGUAL MELANOMA

Malignant melanomas sometimes develop beneath finger- or toenails (Fig. 46.23). Because of their location, they are difficult to diagnose. Pigmented melanomas are easily mistaken for old subungual haematomas, and amelanotic melanomas appear even more innocuous, resembling pyogenic granulomas. Subungual melanomas often present early as a changing pigmented nail streak or **longitudinal melanonychia**. Advanced or clinically aggressive nail unit melanomas tend to present as a tumourous growth. Any suspicious lesion under the nail should therefore be biopsied to avoid the disaster of missing a potentially curable malignant melanoma.

47

Lumps in the head and neck and salivary calculi

INTRODUCTION

Nearly all head and neck disorders that reach the general surgeon are lumps of one sort or another, including abscesses. The main reason for referral is the need to exclude malignancy. In some cases the patient is referred for consideration of surgical treatment of a metabolic disorder such as thyrotoxicosis or hyperparathyroidism. In this anatomical area, there is a large overlap with other specialties, particularly ENT, dental surgery, oral and maxillo-facial surgery, plastic and reconstructive surgery and dermatology.

Swellings of the thyroid gland may be confused with other swellings in the front of the neck. Thus, a complete examination of the head and neck should include the thyroid area, as described in Chapter 49.

Although problems in the mouth are usually managed by dental or oral and maxillo-facial surgeons, patients will often seek initial advice from another clinician. For this reason, most doctors, particularly those working in an accident department, should understand the essentials of oral and dental disease and their management (see also Ch. 48).

HISTORY AND EXAMINATION IN THE HEAD AND NECK

There are many different tissues concentrated in the head and neck and this is responsible for the profusion of conditions causing lumps in this area. Box 47.1 provides a simple classification.

SPECIAL POINTS IN THE HISTORY AND EXAMINATION

As is usually the case, the history provides important clues as to the diagnosis. Specific points such as the patient's age, the rate of growth of the lump and any associated symptoms such as pain, discharge or swelling related to eating ('mealtime syndrome') may lead quickly to the diagnosis.

Most lumps in the head and neck are best examined with the patient sitting in a chair. This allows the examiner to palpate the lump from in front and from behind. The examiner should establish the **characteristics of the lump** as summarised in Box 47.2. At the same time, he or she should try to determine the **relationship of the lump** to overlying or underlying anatomical structures. For example, a lump in the cheek may originate in the skin, in the superficial part of the parotid, the buccinator muscle, the oral mucosa or the parotid duct. In clinical examinations, it is often useful to describe the characteristics of the lesion as if to someone who cannot see the patient.

In the case of a lump or swelling, the whole of the scalp, the back of the neck and the skin behind and in the ears should be examined carefully. Endoscopic examination of the upper airways and pharynx may also be necessary. It is important to exclude primary tumours or infected lesions that underlie the presenting complaint of **lymph node enlargement**. The lymph nodes of the head and neck must also be palpated. A simple method is to think of them as lying in two planes, the horizontal and the vertical, as shown in Figure 47.1. The nodes in each plane can then be examined with two or three simple manoeuvres. For any lump in the lower half of the face or submandibular region, the **oral cavity** should be examined to exclude salivary gland lesions, oral malignancies or sources of infection such as a dental abscess. For any lump in the parotid region, the integrity of the **facial nerve** should be formally tested since malignant tumours often cause neurological deficits.

Examination of the oral cavity

For many doctors, asking the patient to open his or her mouth represents the entire oral examination. The following simple technique, illustrated in Figure 47.2a–d,

1. **Thyroid disorders** (classified in Table 49.1)
2. **Lymph node enlargement:**
   —Local inflammatory lymphadenopathy from acute infections of the head and neck
   Inflammatory lymphadenopathy as part of a generalised lymphadenopathy, e.g. glandular fever or AIDS-related lymphadenopathy
   —Local inflammatory lymphadenopathy from chronic infections, e.g. tuberculosis
   —Lymphomas
   —Secondary tumour deposits (metastases)
3. **Congenital cysts**—thyroglossal, branchial and pre-auricular cysts, external angular dermoids and cystic hygroma
4. **Salivary gland disorders**—adenoma, carcinoma, stones, rare autoimmune disorders such as Sjögren's syndrome
5. **Lumps in the skin**—any skin lesion may occur in the head and neck but the main problem is one of differential diagnosis, e.g. lipomas and epidermal cysts
6. **Rare tumours**—carotid body tumours, carcinoma of the maxillary sinus (antrum), tumours and cysts of the jaw
7. **Actinomycosis** (very rare)

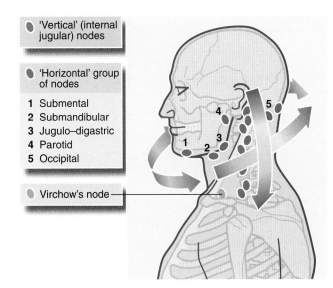

'Vertical' (internal jugular) nodes

'Horizontal' group of nodes

1 Submental
2 Submandibular
3 Jugulo–digastric
4 Parotid
5 Occipital

Virchow's node

Fig. 47.1 Simple technique for palpating head and neck lymph nodes

| Box | 47.2 | Characteristics of any lump on clinical examination |

- Site
- Size
- Shape
- Surface characteristics
- Fixation (superficial and deep)
- Anatomical origin
- Consistency
- Fluctuance
- Pulsatility
- Temperature
- Transilluminability
- Bruit
- Local lymphadenopathy

will enable most significant lesions to be seen without any special instruments or lighting.

First, the patient should remove his or her dentures. The lips and their mucosal lining, and the lining of the cheeks and gums are then inspected. To do this, the lips are retracted by the examiner's gloved fingers or a wooden spatula and the mouth illuminated with a pen torch. At the same time, the teeth are inspected for gross decay and gingival inflammation. Painful inflammation is com-

monly related to a flap of gum over a partially erupted lower wisdom tooth (Fig. 48.7).

If there is any suspicion of parotid disease, the orifice of the parotid duct should be identified and palpated. This lies opposite the upper second molar tooth. If the patient wears dentures or has irregular teeth, inspect for scarring around the parotid duct that could be causing obstruction. The palate is examined easily if the patient tilts his or her head backwards. Finally, the tongue and floor of the mouth are inspected for mucosal lesions. To assist the examination, the patient first protrudes, then elevates, the tongue inside the mouth.

Lumps in the floor of the mouth, submandibular area and cheeks should be palpated bimanually as shown in Figure 47.2f. Lumps in these areas are often mobile and tend to move away from an examining finger.

TUMOURS OF THE SALIVARY GLANDS

There are three pairs of major salivary glands, the **parotid**, **submandibular** and **sublingual** glands. The parotid produces serous (watery) saliva, the submandibular produces a mixed sero-mucous saliva and the sublingual produces a mucous secretion. The parotid and submandibular glands each drain into the mouth via their individual long ducts, whereas the sublingual glands drain via many small ducts into the floor of the mouth.

The surgical disorders of the major salivary glands are benign and malignant tumours, stones, bacterial infections and rare autoimmune disorders, all of which present as salivary gland lumps. The oral mucosa also contains numerous small 'minor' salivary glands, any of which can undergo neoplastic change. Their main disorders are tumours and retention cysts.

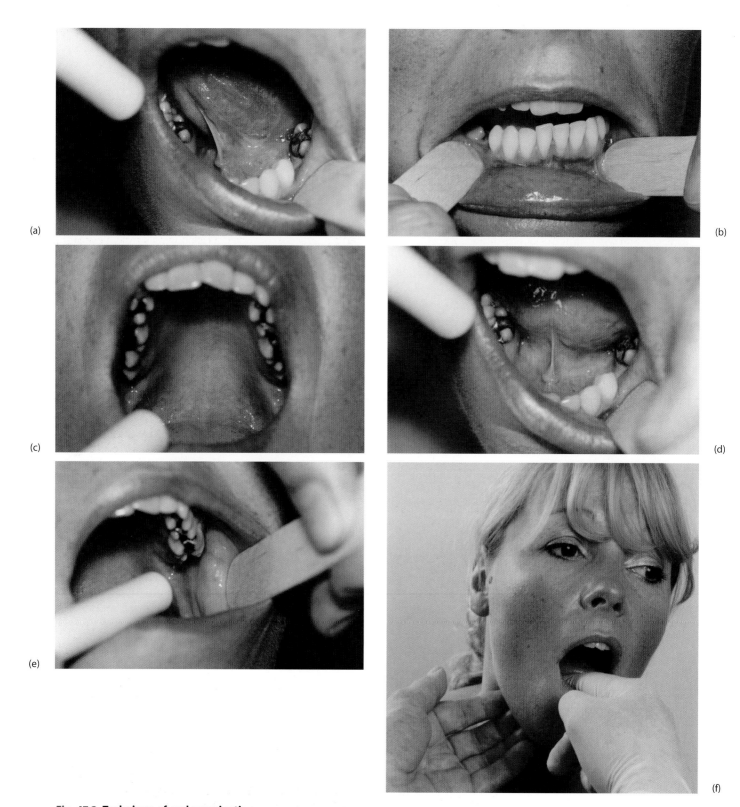

(a)

(b)

(c)

(d)

(e)

(f)

Fig. 47.2 Technique of oral examination
Teeth, gums and buccal sulci can be inspected by retracting the lips with wooden spatulas or fingers **(a)** and **(b)**. The palate is inspected by tilting the patient's head back and retracting the lips **(c)**, and the floor of the mouth and movements of the tongue examined as shown in **(d)**. The parotid papilla is demonstrated in **(e)**. Finally, bimanual palpation of the submandibular area, including the course of the submandibular duct, is performed with a gloved finger inside the mouth, as shown in **(f)**.

SALIVARY GLAND TUMOURS

Pleomorphic adenoma

Pleomorphic adenoma is by far the most common of the salivary gland neoplasms. It is also the most common cause of a lump in the parotid or submandibular gland. Most pleomorphic adenomas present in middle age or later, and both sexes are equally affected.

Pleomorphic adenomas are derived from salivary gland epithelium and are regarded as benign. Despite this, they show varying degrees of differentiation. The name **pleomorphic adenoma** was acquired from the varied histological appearance. Columns and islands of neoplastic epithelial cells are separated by a myxomatous connective tissue stroma which may contain areas resembling immature cartilage. This led early pathologists to believe that the tumour contained neoplastic tissue of both epithelial and connective tissue origin, thus generating the misleading name of **mixed salivary tumour**. Some tumours have no myxomatous tissue and are described as **monomorphic** variants.

Although they do not metastasise, pleomorphic adenomas are often poorly demarcated from the surrounding tissue. There is usually a well-defined thin capsule, but the surface is usually nodular rather than smooth, an important point when attempting removal. True malignant transformation occasionally takes place, usually to **squamous cell carcinoma**, with metastasis potentially occurring to cervical nodes and sometimes the lungs.

Clinically, a pleomorphic adenoma presents as a very slowly growing, painless lump (see Fig. 47.3). Most are in the parotid, some in the submandibular gland, and a few in minor salivary glands.

Most parotid gland tumours occur in the superficial part of the gland, external to the plane of the facial nerve branches. Occasionally, they occur in the deep part of the gland in more intimate association with the facial nerve. In either case, the tumour can extend between the branches of the facial nerve. As the tumour is benign, it does not invade the nerve to cause a facial palsy. Facial nerve damage is, however, a risk during surgical excision, especially of deeper lesions. Patients should be warned of this possibility before operation.

If an older patient has a slowly growing solid parotid lump without a facial palsy, it is best to assume it is a pleomorphic adenoma. Definitive diagnosis can usually be made by ultrasonography and fine needle aspiration cytology and then confirmed histologically after excision. If malignancy is suspected, CT scanning may be needed.

Treatment

Treatment of pleomorphic adenoma is by excision. For superficial lesions, the standard operation has long been **superficial parotidectomy**, which involves excising all

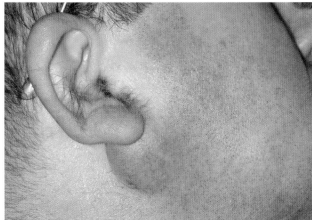
(a)

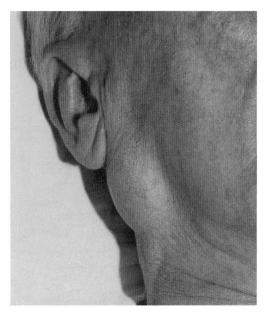
(b)

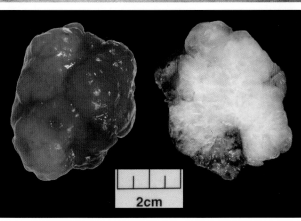
(c)

Fig. 47.3 Pleomorphic adenomas of the parotid
(a) Small lesion in the typical position below the ear lobe, between the posterior border of the ramus of the mandible and the upper end of the sternomastoid. **(b)** Larger lesion in an older man. This had been present at least 4 years before the patient presented. **(c)** Pathological specimen of large pleomorphic adenoma removed by extracapsular dissection. On the left the specimen has been freshly removed and shows the typical knobbly surface. On the right, the fixed and cut specimen shows the variegated and predominantly myxomatous appearance.

glandular tissue superficial to the plane of the facial nerve. An alternative and more logical approach is meticulous **extracapsular dissection** of the lump alone. This has been shown to be as effective in curing the problem in benign disease. It also carries a lower rate of side effects, particularly facial nerve damage and **Frey's syndrome** of gustatory sweating (see below). With either procedure, recurrence is uncommon. For deeper lesions, an attempt should be made to excise the entire lesion, carefully identifying and preserving the branches of the facial nerve. Again, extracapsular dissection may be the safer option. If there is doubt about whether excision has been complete, postoperative radiotherapy may be advisable.

Complications

The main complication of parotidectomy is damage to branches of the facial nerve. Damage to the temporal or upper zygomatic branches may prevent complete closure of the eye, leading to corneal drying and damage. Division of the mandibular branch causes drooping of the angle of the mouth and salivary dribbling, which is embarrassing. Nerve damage may also complicate submandibular gland excision. The mandibular branch is vulnerable if the incision is incorrectly sited and the hypoglossal nerve lies close to the deep surface of the gland. Damage causes unilateral tongue wasting.

Salivary fistula is an occasional complication following parotid surgery, causing saliva to leak onto the face at mealtimes. The fistula usually resolves spontaneously after several weeks.

Frey's syndrome is a late complication of superficial parotidectomy in 25% or more cases. It probably results from divided parasympathetic secretomotor fibres regenerating in the skin where they assume control of sweat gland activity. Facial sweating then occurs in response to salivatory stimuli; this is known as **gustatory sweating** and can also be embarrassing. It is virtually unknown after extracapsular dissection.

Adenolymphoma (Warthin's tumour)

This unusual benign lesion constitutes less than 10% of salivary neoplasms, and occurs almost exclusively in the parotid glands. These tumours usually arise after middle age and there is a strong male predominance. There is a strong association with cigarette smoking. They sometimes occur bilaterally, either at the same time or at different times.

Histologically, the tumour is composed of large glandular acini. The epithelium, similar to large salivary ducts, is embedded in dense lymphoid tissue in which lymphoid follicles may be seen. The histogenesis is not understood, but the glandular part may be hamartomatous salivary duct tissue within a normal parotid lymph node.

Adenolymphomas are invariably benign. They present as a parotid lump, clinically indistinguishable from pleo-morphic adenoma. The diagnosis can sometimes be made by fine needle aspiration cytology, in which case simple enucleation can be performed to remove the tumour or it can be left alone. Adenolymphomas do not recur, but a satellite lesion may enlarge and present as another tumour.

Malignant primary salivary tumours

Malignant tumours comprise only a small proportion of neoplasms of major salivary glands but form the greater proportion of tumours of the minor (accessory) salivary glands scattered throughout the oral mucosa. With parotid lumps, facial nerve weakness is diagnostic of malignancy. The majority of malignant tumours are **adenocystic carcinomas** (also known as adenoid cystic carcinomas, and less accurately as cylindromas). The remainder include rare epithelial tumours such as **acinic cell carcinoma** and **squamous cell carcinoma**. In Australia, the most common parotid tumour is a malignant melanoma invading from the skin.

Adenocystic carcinomas have a characteristic cribriform (sieve-like) microscopic appearance due to numerous small spaces in the tightly packed tumour cell mass. These tumours are highly invasive with early regional and systemic metastasis. Treatment involves wide mutilating surgery which usually destroys the facial nerve. Unfortunately, recurrence is very common and may occur as long as 5 years after apparently successful eradication. The tumours are unresponsive to radiotherapy and prognosis is almost uniformly poor.

Secondary tumours in salivary glands

The superficial part of the parotid gland contains lymph nodes which may become involved by secondary deposits from tumours of the face or scalp. In the same way, lymph node secondaries from the mouth may develop in the nodes within the submandibular gland. The finding of a parotid or submandibular lump should therefore prompt a search for a primary tumour locally, including the pharynx. Lymphomas also affect lymph nodes within salivary glands on occasions.

SALIVARY GLAND STONE DISEASE (SIALOLITHIASIS)

PATHOPHYSIOLOGY

The submandibular gland and duct are prone to form calcified stones (calculi) which obstruct salivary outflow and predispose to infection. Calculi also occur in the parotid duct but this is much less common. The aetiology of salivary calculi is not known, but the submandibular gland may be vulnerable because of its more viscid secretion and its elongated duct.

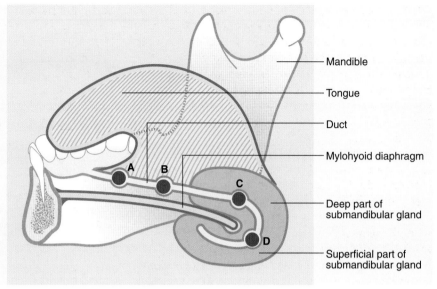

Note how the submandibular duct slopes downwards as it passes posteriorly. Thus the more posterior stones are increasingly difficult to remove from inside the mouth (**A→B**). **C** and **D** within the gland can only be removed by removing the gland via the skin surface.

Note also how the gland is in two parts, superficial and deep, wrapped around the posterior border of myohyoid

Mandible

Tongue

Duct

Mylohyoid diaphragm

Deep part of submandibular gland

Superficial part of submandibular gland

A B C D

Fig. 47.4 Submandibular gland and duct showing common sites for stones

Stones are not the only cause of salivary duct obstruction causing gland swelling. In both the parotid and submandibular gland, trauma to the duct orifice may result in stenosis and salivary stasis.

Submandibular stones may be found anywhere along Wharton's duct (see Fig. 47.4), including its course within the gland. Stones vary from several millimetres to a centimetre in diameter. Those in the distal part of the duct tend to have an elongated 'date stone' shape (see Fig. 47.5a,b).

CLINICAL FEATURES

Salivary calculi rarely cause complete obstruction but the patient usually experiences intermittent swelling or pain at mealtimes when salivary flow is high. The swelling then subsides over the next hour or so. Acidic foods such as lemon juice stimulate rapid salivary flow, and can be used as a test in clinic. Pain is not usually a prominent feature; rather, patients describe a sensation of fullness. Salivary calculi occasionally present with acute or chronic bacterial infection (**sialadenitis**). Secondary infection in the obstructed system leads to rapidly worsening symptoms and even spreading cellulitis of the floor of the mouth (**Ludwig's angina**, Fig. 47.6).

Most of the submandibular gland lies deep to the mandible and so there may be little to see on external examination. In symptomatic submandibular stone disease, palpation of the submandibular area usually confirms that the gland is moderately enlarged and firm. On intraoral examination, the tip of a stone may be visible if it impacts at the orifice of Wharton's duct. Bimanual palpation involves a gloved finger palpating the floor of the mouth with the other hand below the jaw. Any abnormal swelling can then be felt between the two. This is the only

clinical way to assess the size of the gland and will often confirm the presence of a stone in the duct. Palpation of the duct is performed from the back towards the front of the mouth to avoid displacing a mobile stone backwards into the gland.

MANAGEMENT OF SALIVARY CALCULI

Plain X-rays demonstrate most calculi. For the submandibular gland and duct, an **occlusal film** held between the teeth shows the floor of the mouth and a lateral oblique gives a second viewpoint. For the parotid, AP and lateral views are often used. Contrast radiography of the duct system (**sialography**) is sometimes indicated if the history suggests stone disease yet no stone is palpable or visible on plain X-ray. Sialography (Figs 47.7 and 47.8) requires cannulation of the salivary duct which itself may reveal a stenosis of the duct orifice and may relieve symptoms, at least temporarily. Stenosis alone of any part of the duct may produce symptoms similar to calculus obstruction.

The anterior two-thirds of the duct lie in the floor of the mouth and calculi here are removed via an intraoral (Fig. 47.5a,b) approach. Immediately before operation, the stone should be confirmed to be still present by palpation or X-ray. If the stone is palpable, operation may be performed under local or general anaesthesia. A longitudinal incision is made in the duct over the stone and the stone lifted out. If the stone is not palpable, the duct is incised from the orifice backwards and the stone can usually be removed with forceps. The incision is not usually sutured but left open to improve salivary drainage.

Less commonly, calculi lie within the gland where they are often multiple (Fig. 47.5e–g). The standard way to remove the obstruction is to excise the entire subman-

Fig. 47.5 Submandibular gland and duct calculi

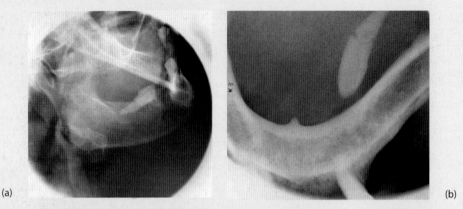

(a)

(b)

Submandibular duct calculus
(a) Lateral oblique plain X-ray, and (b) occlusal X-ray showing large 'date stone' calculus in the left submandibular duct. This was easily palpable bimanually in the floor of the mouth and then removed via the oral route.

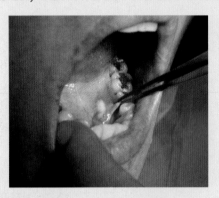

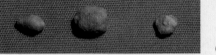

(d)

(c)

Submandibular duct stone—case study
(c) This photograph shows a stone visible in the anterior part of Wharton's duct; it was removed under local anaesthesia via a longitudinal incision in the duct. (d) Submandibular stones removed from a similar case.

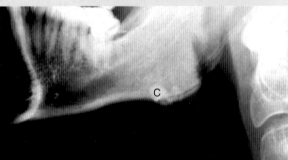

C

(e)

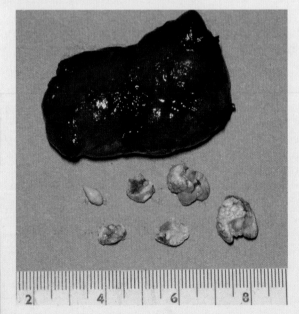

(g)

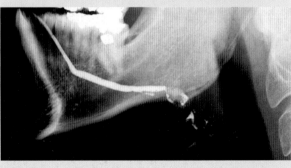

(f)

Submandibular gland stones—case study
This 43-year-old man suffered chronic swelling and intermittent infection of the right submandibular gland: (e) Lateral plain X-ray showing calculi **C** within the gland. (f) Sialogram showing a normal Wharton's duct (note how rapidly it descends from the floor of the mouth). The stones within the gland are represented by filling defects in the contrast material. (g) The only means of dealing with the problem was excision of the gland via an extraoral (submandibular) approach. The gland contained six calculi.

Fig. 47.6 Ludwig's angina

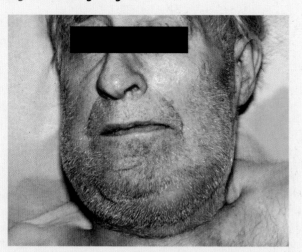

Spreading cellulitis of the submandibular region. This man of 70 had large obstructing stones of the left submandibular duct and this had led to infection in the duct and gland. This spread to the surrounding tissues. He was beginning to develop respiratory embarrassment as a result of laryngeal oedema but settled rapidly with antibiotics and removal of the stones from within the mouth.

Fig. 47.7 Parotid sialography showing stones

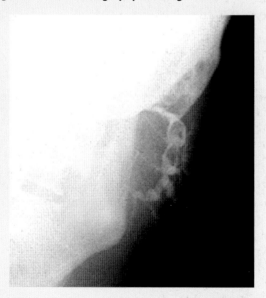

This man of 58 complained of intermittent swelling in the region of the left parotid gland, relieved on occasions by discharge of pus into the mouth. Contrast was injected into the orifice of the left parotid gland to outline the duct structure. The main duct is dilated and contains filling defects diagnosed as stones. This is an unusual finding as stones are much more common in the submandibular gland.

Fig. 47.8 Parotid sialography

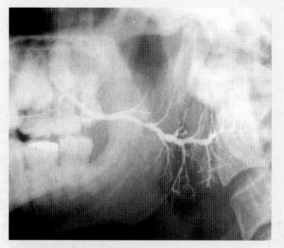

(a)

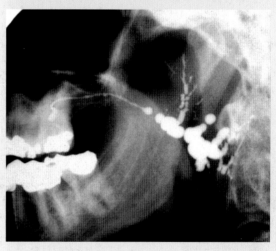

(b)

(a) Normal sialogram showing regular duct diameter and branching. **(b)** Case study—duct strictures and sialectasis. This 50-year-old man had recurrent bouts of parotid swelling complicated by infection. The sialogram shows several duct strictures with dilated ducts behind them. The dilatation is called sialectasis.

dibular gland via an incision below the mandible, carefully placed to avoid damaging the mandibular branch of the facial nerve and the hypoglossal nerve.

Parotid obstruction caused by orificial stenosis may respond to simple dilatation and attention to dentition causing trauma. If this fails, ductoplasty can be performed.

INFLAMMATORY DISORDERS OF THE SALIVARY GLANDS

The salivary glands are subject to infection by viruses (such as mumps) and by bacteria. Mumps is rare outside childhood and young adulthood, is usually bilateral, and resolves spontaneously. It is rarely a surgical problem unless secondary bacterial infection supervenes. The glands may also be affected by autoimmune disorders such as **Sjögren's syndrome**.

ACUTE BACTERIAL SIALADENITIS

This condition is now uncommon because of better mouth care in hospital; it almost always occurs in elderly, dehydrated or debilitated patients with poor oral hygiene. Occasionally it occurs in children, in which case the underlying cause is usually a suppurating lymph node within the parotid capsule. Dehydration and reduced salivary flow encourage ascending infection with resident oral flora, usually *Strep. viridans* or pneumococci; the parotid gland is usually involved, giving rise to acute parotitis. The result is a painful, unilateral swelling accompanied by **trismus** (reduced ability to open the mouth), pyrexia and tachycardia. On examination, the parotid gland is tender and diffusely enlarged and a purulent discharge can often be seen oozing (or can be 'milked') from the parotid duct orifice. **Acute parotitis** was once common in postoperative surgical patients because of dehydration and poor oral hygiene. Intravenous fluids and close nursing attention to mouth care have now made the condition rare.

Bacterial sialadenitis should be treated promptly with antibiotics. If a parotid abscess has already formed, external surgical drainage should be performed.

CHRONIC SIALADENITIS

Prolonged obstruction of a major salivary gland by a ductal calculus causes chronic inflammation of the gland. The glandular secretory elements progressively atrophy and are replaced by fibrous and adipose tissue. The duct system becomes dilated, fibrotic and infiltrated by chronic inflammatory cells. Chronic sialadenitis and salivary calculi usually involve the submandibular gland. The gland is swollen and there may be purulent discharge from the duct. The swelling is made worse by taking food. Treatment is by removing the duct obstruction; antibiotics may also be necessary. Gland function may be irreversibly damaged if the process has been prolonged, and the gland may have to be removed.

RECURRENT SIALADENITIS

This uncommon condition may occur at any age and usually affects the parotid gland. One or both glands are subject to recurrent attacks of painful swelling. This is caused by low-grade bacterial infection but duct obstruction is not usually evident. Recurrent attacks cause chronic swelling of the affected gland. Sialography shows dilatation of the duct system with terminal sacculation; this is described as **sialectasis**. The cause is often a duct orificial

stenosis, usually caused by trauma from poorly fitting dentures or displaced teeth, or stenoses of unknown origin more proximally in the duct.

Immediate treatment includes antibiotics, with the choice determined by culture of parotid duct discharge, as well as careful attention to oral hygiene. **Ductoplasty** to open the duct orifice is often successful. If sialography shows more remote duct stenoses, these can sometimes be dilated using balloons similar to angioplasty devices.

AUTOIMMUNE SALIVARY GLAND DISORDERS

The salivary glands occasionally become involved in a chronic inflammatory process characterised by diffuse lymphoid infiltration and fibrosis. This is part of poorly understood autoimmune disorders which also involve lachrymal glands and mucous glands of the mouth and upper respiratory tract. The parotid and submandibular glands become diffusely and symmetrically enlarged, and salivary production is curtailed. The resulting dry mouth (**xerostomia**) not only causes distress and dysphagia but predisposes to rampant dental caries. Diminished lachrymal secretion results in **keratoconjunctivitis sicca** affecting the eyes.

In isolation, the condition is known as **primary Sjögren's syndrome**. It may also occur in rheumatoid arthritis and other connective tissue disorders when it is known as secondary Sjögren's syndrome.

SALIVARY RETENTION CYSTS

Large retention cysts sometimes develop in the floor of the mouth. A cyst can reach several centimetres in diameter and is known as a **ranula** (frog mouth). The ranula typically appears as a blue-grey dome-like swelling beneath the tongue. It may burst spontaneously, discharging its contents and collapsing, but it almost invariably recurs. The condition is painless but occupies space in the mouth and treatment is often sought for this reason. Excision is difficult because of the tenuous lining and because of the proximity to vital structures in the floor of the mouth; incomplete removal leads to recurrence. The usual treatment, therefore, is excision of the sublingual gland, although **marsupialisation** remains an option, i.e. deroofing the cyst so that it opens into the floor of the mouth (see Fig. 47.9).

LYMPH NODE DISORDERS OF THE HEAD AND NECK

Patients are often referred to a surgeon for biopsy of an enlarged lymph node in the cervical region. Often there are no other symptoms or signs. **Isolated lymph node enlargement** may be caused by local disease within its field of drainage or as part of a more widespread lym-

Fig. 47.9 Marsupialisation of a ranula

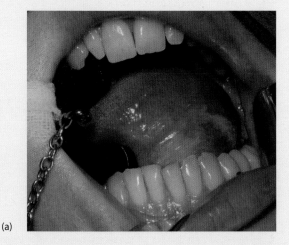 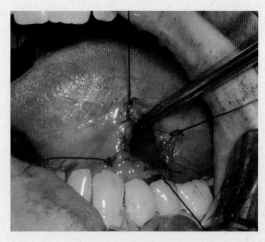

(a) (b)

(a) Large salivary retention cyst in the floor of the mouth displacing the tongue towards the opposite side. **(b)** Operative photograph showing the 'de-roofed' cyst and the edges being sutured to the oral mucosa. The cavity rapidly 'filled in' from the base, obliterating the defect.

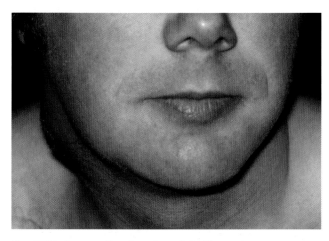

Fig. 47.10 Suppurating lymph node in the neck
This patient presented with a suppurating node in the neck which required external drainage. The primary site of sepsis was a dental abscess on a lower molar tooth.

phadenopathy. Examples of local disorders include tonsillitis or dental infection, tonsillar tuberculosis or a malignant oro-pharyngeal tumour. Nodes draining a bacterial infection may themselves suppurate, sometimes after the primary disorder has disappeared (see Fig. 47.10). An enlarged cervical lymph node may be part of a **systemic lymphadenopathy** caused by glandular fever, lymphoma or HIV. Thus, any patient presenting with an enlarged lymph node requires careful general examination as well as examination of the head, neck and mouth. The latter often includes thorough endoscopy of the whole pharyngeal area, usually by a specialist ENT surgeon (oto-rhino-laryngologist).

General clinical examination should pay particular attention to axillary and inguinal lymph nodes, liver and spleen. A chest X-ray should be taken to look for enlarged thoracic lymph nodes. If cervical lymph node biopsy is necessary, improved histological techniques mean it can now be performed using a fine needle or core needle, usually under ultrasound control, although some pathologists are not happy with the diagnostic value of needle biopsies in lymphoma. If surgical removal of a gland is required, this should always be performed under general anaesthesia if practicable since the operation is often unexpectedly difficult. This is because lymph nodes are intimately related to so many vital structures and, furthermore, preoperative palpation tends to underestimate the size and extent of lymph node involvement.

CERVICAL TUBERCULOSIS

Tuberculosis involving the cervical glands (**scrofula**) was once common, with the infection being acquired by drinking milk from cattle infected with bovine tuberculosis. Cervical tuberculosis is now extremely rare in developed countries but may be seen in recent immigrants from developing countries. The primary infection occurs in the tonsils but the condition presents with secondary involvement of the cervical nodes which become progressively enlarged and matted together. In advanced cases, liquefaction of the caseous material forms **cold abscesses**. If untreated, these eventually drain spontaneously onto the neck and leave disfiguring scars.

In the past, surgery was often required to drain and remove the affected glands. With modern chemotherapy this is now rarely necessary and surgery is mostly confined to excision biopsy for diagnosis.

LYMPHOMAS

An enlarged cervical lymph node is a common presentation of non-Hodgkin lymphoma or Hodgkin's disease. The disease is often at an early stage and there may be no other symptoms or clinical signs. The diagnosis is then made by histological examination of a biopsy specimen.

SECONDARY (METASTATIC) TUMOURS

Cervical lymph node metastases may originate from primary malignant tumours in the head or neck, chest or abdomen. An enlarged lymph node may be the first indication of a cancer or represent a recurrence following treatment.

Cancers of the head and neck usually metastasise to nodes in the submandibular region and upper part of the anterior triangle. The following head and neck tumours commonly metastasise to cervical lymph nodes:

- Squamous carcinoma and melanoma of the skin of the neck, face, scalp and ear
- Squamous carcinoma of the mouth and tongue
- Squamous carcinoma of the nasopharynx, oropharynx, larynx and paranasal sinuses. Note the primary tumour may be exceedingly small
- Adenocystic carcinoma of the major or accessory salivary glands
- Papillary (and occasionally medullary) carcinomas of the thyroid

In contrast, tumours from the chest and abdomen usually metastasise to the lower part of the posterior triangle, particularly to **Virchow's node** (Fig. 47.11) which lies deeply in the angle between the sternocleidomastoid and the clavicle on the left side.

MISCELLANEOUS CAUSES OF A LUMP IN THE NECK

CONGENITAL CYSTS AND SINUSES

A variety of cystic lesions of congenital origin occur in the head and neck and some of them may be associated with an external sinus opening. All are uncommon except in clinical 'short-case' examinations! They can be subdivided into thyroglossal cysts, branchial cysts, fusion-line dermoid cysts, pre-auricular cysts and sinuses, and cystic hygromas. All except for cystic hygroma are true epithelial cysts; cystic hygroma is a hamartomatous lymphatic or lympho-vascular malformation.

Fig. 47.11 Virchow's node

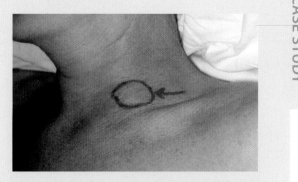

This 48-year-old woman noticed a painless lump in the left side of her neck. She had also lost a substantial amount of weight and had a poor appetite. Node biopsy revealed malignant adenocarcinoma cells and endoscopy showed that an advanced carcinoma of stomach was the cause. Palpation of a malignant node in this site is known as Troisier's sign, after the French physician who diagnosed gastric cancer in himself.

Branchial cysts, sinuses and fistulae

The precise embryological origin of these cysts is disputed but they probably arise from remnants of the second pharyngeal pouch or branchial cleft. **Branchial cysts** usually present in late adolescence or early adulthood but sometimes even later (Fig. 47.12). This late presentation is unusual for congenital lesions generally. The patient typically complains of a painless swelling in the side of the neck which may vary in size from time to time. Some patients present with the sudden appearance of a painful red swelling due to inflammation of a previously unnoticed cyst.

The lump lies deep to the sternocleidomastoid, at the junction of its upper third and lower two-thirds. It protrudes forwards into the anterior triangle of the neck. The lump is soft and fluctuant on palpation. Provided it is not inflamed, the cyst usually transilluminates. Treatment is by surgical excision; percutaneous drainage is rarely permanently successful. Inflamed cysts may require urgent drainage.

Branchial sinus and fistula presents as a discharging sinus near the lower end of the anterior border of the sternomastoid muscle. A **sinus** ends blindly on the lateral pharyngeal wall whereas a **fistula** communicates with the oropharynx near the tonsillar fossa. Surgical excision may be required.

Fusion-line dermoid cysts

Dermoid cysts of congenital origin arise from epithelial remnants along lines of embryological fusion in the head and neck.

Fig. 47.12 Branchial cyst

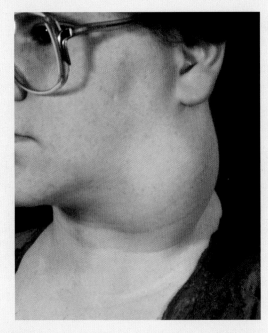

This 30-year-old woman reported the sudden appearance of this large swelling in her neck associated with moderate pain over the previous week. The swelling was non-tender and fluctuant. Ultrasound confirmed it contained fluid. It was aspirated several times but failed to resolve and was eventually excised. It is not known why branchial cysts often come to attention so suddenly.

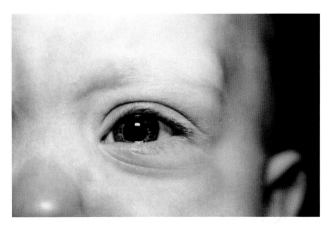

Fig. 47.13 External angular dermoid
This 4-month-old baby was noticed to have a swelling at the outer part of his left eyebrow. It was firm to palpation and was confidently diagnosed as a fusion-line dermoid.

anterior to the tragus of the ear and present either as a small lump or a tiny discharging sinus that occasionally becomes infected. There may be an obvious associated abnormality of the auricle. Treatment is usually by surgical excision.

Cystic hygromas

Cystic hygromas (Fig. 47.14) are not true cysts but lymphatic or lympho-vascular hamartomas which form multilocular cyst-like spaces. Cystic hygromas may be huge and disfiguring lesions present at birth. Smaller lesions may present in older children or adolescents as a painless lump in the neck just below the angle of the mandible. Cystic hygromas are soft and fluctuant and highly transilluminable.

Surgical excision may be difficult as these lesions often extend deeply into cervical and oro-facial tissues.

ACTINOMYCOSIS

Actinomycosis is a rare infection of the cervico-facial region. It is caused by *Actinomyces israelii*, an anaerobic Gram-positive bacterium with an unusual filamentous growth pattern similar to fungal mycelia. Actinomycosis is a chronic granulomatous infection which if untreated eventually forms multilocular abscesses that drain to the overlying skin via multiple sinuses. The pus exuding from the sinuses contains characteristic yellow clumps of organisms known as 'sulphur granules'. The infection stimulates much fibrosis.

The organism is an oropharyngeal commensal but gains access to the tissues via carious teeth, tooth extraction sockets or traumatic wounds. Initially, there is a painful intraoral swelling. Inflammation then spreads slowly into the tissues, causing firm swelling of the cheek, mandible and submandibular region ('lumpy

The most common are **external angular dermoids** (see Fig. 47.13), which are cystic swellings at the outer aspect of the supraorbital ridge. They are usually noticed soon after birth. On palpation these cysts are tense and firm and do not transilluminate because of their thick keratinous contents. They are deeply fixed and therefore immobile. External angular dermoids are usually removed surgically for cosmetic reasons during childhood.

Midline dermoid cysts are described as teratoid cysts because they contain a mixture of ectodermal, mesodermal and endodermal elements (e.g. nails and teeth, glands, blood vessels). As a rare phenomenon, dermoid cysts can arise in the midline of the head or neck, usually during the first year of life. They should be removed surgically.

Pre-auricular cysts and sinuses

Small cysts and sinuses may arise from developmental abnormalities of the first and second branchial arches which are involved in forming the external ear. The lesions become apparent in early childhood. They lie

Fig. 47.14 **Cystic hygroma**

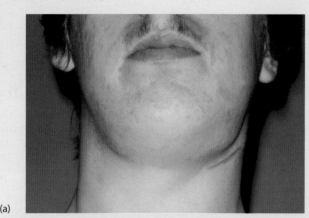
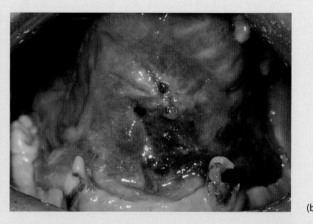

(a)   (b)

(a) This man of 23 had been born with a swelling under his left jaw which had not changed over recent years. The scar of a partial excision is visible. **(b)** Oral view of the same patient showing the haemangio-lymphangioma extending into the base of the tongue. It bleeds from time to time with minor trauma and this may have led him to neglect his teeth over the years.

jaw'). The infection eventually erodes into the salivary glands, jaws and adjacent structures. Suppurative foci drain onto the surface of the face forming chronic discharging sinuses.

Actinomycosis is treated with a prolonged course (4–6 weeks) of high-dose penicillin. If necessary, the abscess network is surgically explored and drained.

Cervico-facial actinomycosis was once common and its decline in developed countries is probably the result of better oral hygiene and dental care. Actinomycosis also occurs in the ileo-caecal area, gaining access from an appendiceal perforation. The infection is now most often encountered in the pelvis as a complication of an intra-uterine contraceptive device, although this remains rare.

Disorders of the mouth

48

DISORDERS OF THE ORAL CAVITY (EXCLUDING SALIVARY CALCULI)

The main disorders of the oral cavity are **dental caries** (tooth decay) and its sequelae, inflammations of the gums and supporting bone (**periodontal disease**), **tumours** and premalignant conditions of the oral mucosa (leukoplakia and squamous carcinoma) and **disorders of the accessory salivary glands** such as retention cysts. Disorders of the main salivary glands are covered in Chapter 47. The main symptoms and signs of oral disease are summarised in Box 48.1, page 701.

DENTAL CARIES

PATHOPHYSIOLOGY AND CLINICAL FEATURES

In developed countries, dental caries (dental decay) is one of the most common bacterial disorders. The process begins when the protective enamel surface of the tooth is breached by the demineralising action of lactic acid. This is generated by commensal oral bacteria as a by-product of carbohydrate metabolism, particularly of refined sugar products. The most vulnerable sites for decay are the areas of **enamel** just below the contact points of adjacent tooth crowns and the deep pits and fissures on the biting (occlusal) surface of molars and premolars. These sites are relatively inaccessible to the natural oral cleansing mechanisms and to tooth brushing.

Once the enamel is breached, proteolytic bacteria gain entry to the less densely calcified **dentine** beneath and cause its progressive destruction. The enamel remains intact until the supporting dentine beneath it is grossly undermined and the enamel fractures. Thus, dental caries may be well advanced before it is visible, even when examined with a dental mirror and probe, and may only be detectable on X-ray. In the meantime, the decay process is asymptomatic until close enough to the dental pulp to cause chemical inflammation and pain and, eventually, bacterial invasion and abscess formation. The usual pathological process and corresponding symptoms are outlined in Figure 48.1.

Once the pulp is **exposed**, inflammation and bacterial invasion usually destroy the dental pulp and then spread to the periapical region where an **abscess** develops. This causes painful oral and facial swelling, and if untreated, eventually drains into the mouth or occasionally onto the face (Fig. 48.2). However, since the initiating cause, the necrotic pulp, remains, a chronic abscess will develop and flare up from time to time or continue with a persistent discharge.

The pain of dental caries is usually well localised and recognised as a 'toothache' by the patient. Dental pain may, however, be poorly localised and cause non-specific facial pain. In the upper jaw, this may simulate sinusitis. Dental caries should always be considered before rarer diagnoses are accepted. Overall, however, a surprising amount of dental caries, even with periapical infection, is asymptomatic.

MANAGEMENT OF DENTAL CARIES

Provided the dental pulp has not been invaded by infection (i.e. become 'exposed'), a dentist can usually remove the carious enamel and dentine and restore it (Fig. 48.3) with a lining of silver amalgam, synthetic resin or gold. This is usually placed over a sedative insulating lining.

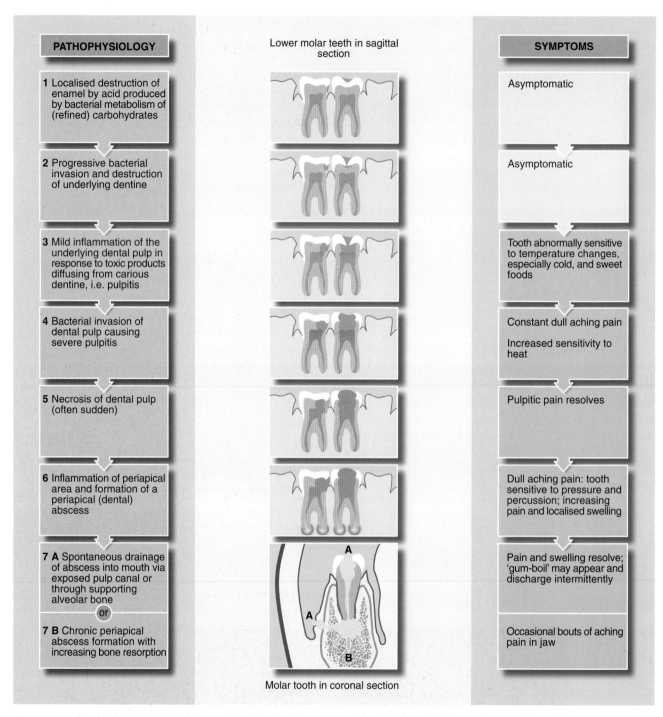

Fig. 48.1 Pathophysiology and symptoms of dental caries and its sequelae

Once bacteria have invaded the pulp, this necrotic tissue must be removed by **endodontic treatment**, and the pulp cavity filled; this is known as 'root filling'. In this way, the tooth can often be saved.

MANAGEMENT OF DENTAL ABSCESSES

A periapical abscess is the most common presentation of caries seen by the general medical practitioner or casualty officer. Primary treatment, as for other abscesses, is drainage of pus. Extracting the offending tooth is the most effective method, but if there is a chance of preserving the tooth, the abscess can be drained via the root canal after drilling into the tooth. Wherever possible, patients with periapical abscesses should be referred to a dentist for treatment.

Large acute abscesses which are 'pointing' within the mouth can be drained by incising the oral mucosa at the site of greatest fluctuation. Oral penicillin should be prescribed if there is spreading infection. Unless there is swelling or other signs of an acute abscess, antibiotics have no part in the management of toothache. A dental abscess occasionally presents on the face (Fig. 48.2) but will usually settle with extraction of the offending tooth. Dental abscesses are very rarely complicated by osteomyelitis.

TOOTH EXTRACTION AND POST-EXTRACTION PROBLEMS

Medical practitioners are rarely required to extract teeth except in geographically isolated places. Caries prevention and modern restorative and endodontic techniques have made the need for extraction much less common. Patients, however, often attend family practitioners or accident and emergency departments following tooth extraction or surgical tooth removal, with problems of bleeding, pain and swelling. These problems are described below.

Fig. 48.2 Dental abscess pointing on the face

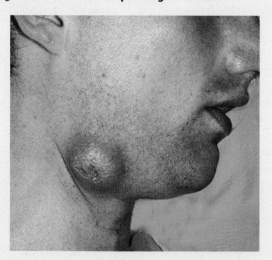

This young man presented to his doctor with an obvious abscess on the face; he was unaware that it arose from a tooth affected by dental caries. The abscess had to be drained externally and the tooth removed. The swelling then rapidly settled.

Box	48.1	Symptoms and signs of oral disease and their main causes

Pain—dental caries and its sequelae, acute gingival inflammation such as pericoronitis and Vincent's infection (acute ulcerative gingivitis)

Bleeding—chronic gingival inflammation

Halitosis—dental caries and chronic periodontal disease

White lesions—epithelial dysplasia (leukoplakia), lichen planus and candidal infection

Oral ulceration—aphthous ulcers, squamous carcinoma, retained tooth roots, chronic tooth or denture trauma, and rare epidermal disorders (e.g. lichen planus or Behçet's syndrome)

Discharging sinuses—periapical tooth abscess ('gum boil')

Bony lumps in the jaws—fibrous dysplasia, tumours, cysts, ectopic teeth

Salivary glands and duct-related lumps—retention cysts, submandibular duct stones, tumours

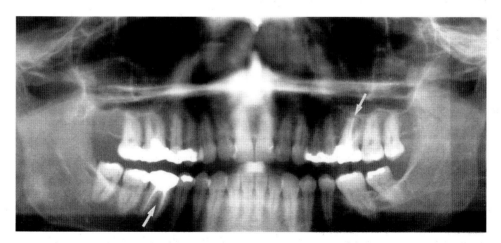

Fig. 48.3 Dental restorations and root fillings
This oral pantomograph (OPG) film shows silver amalgam restorations for caries in posterior teeth (shown as white radiopacities) and synthetic resin restorations in front teeth (shown as relative radiolucencies in the upper incisors). In addition, the upper left first molar and the lower right first molar (arrowed) have radiopaque root canal fillings, necessitated by dental caries invading the pulp.

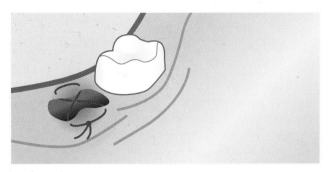

Fig. 48.4 Suture technique for bleeding tooth socket
A 'figure of eight' suture occludes bleeding gum edge on alveolar bone. The patient should bite for at least 10 minutes on a folded swab after suture to encourage clotting.

BLEEDING TOOTH SOCKET AFTER EXTRACTION

A small amount of blood mixed with saliva may look like a severe haemorrhage. The extraction site should be inspected for evidence of vigorous bleeding, which produces blood clots in the mouth. A normal extraction socket should be filled with firm clot but there may be an ooze from the gingival margin. This is made worse if the anxious patient continually disturbs the clot by rinsing the mouth or 'exploring' the socket with the tongue. Aspirin as an analgesic may also promote bleeding by interfering with platelet activity.

Oozing or minor bleeding is easily controlled by the patient biting on a small dry pack such as a folded gauze swab. Pressure should be maintained for 10–15 minutes. More persistent bleeding can usually be controlled by inserting one or more sutures through the gingival margins across the socket, partially closing the defect (Fig. 48.4). Afterwards, the patient should bite on a small dry gauze pad. Suturing is performed under local anaesthesia, a small amount of which is infiltrated into the gingiva on each side of the socket. Absorbable polyglactin sutures are preferred as they do not leave irritating sharp ends. Absorbable sutures dissolve in 5–10 days.

If bleeding continues after these simple measures, the patient should be investigated for a coagulation or platelet abnormality.

PAIN AFTER TOOTH EXTRACTION

Forceps extraction or surgical tooth removal may lead to a great deal of pain soon afterwards. Removal of lower molar teeth may cause **trismus** (masseteric spasm), making jaw movements painful and restricted. If there is no sign of infection, treatment is with analgesia, not antibiotics. Pain appearing several days after extraction is usually due to a superficial osteitis of exposed bone within the socket caused by failure of the socket to fill with organised clot. This condition, known as a **dry socket**, is intensely painful and requires dental treatment. Antibiotic therapy is not helpful.

SWELLING AFTER TOOTH EXTRACTION

Soft tissue swelling is not common after tooth extraction with the exception of surgically removed lower third molars ('wisdom teeth'). Extraction of these teeth often causes marked swelling around the angle of the mandible, with trismus and pain. This swelling represents a normal inflammatory response and interstitial haemorrhage rather than infection. The swelling subsides within a week or so postoperatively and again does not warrant antibiotic therapy.

INFLAMMATION OF THE PERIODONTAL TISSUES

GINGIVITIS AND PERIODONTITIS

Teeth are embedded in bony **alveolar ridges** in both upper and lower jaws. A thin layer of **cementum** (a bone-like material) on the root surface is joined to the bone of the socket by a tough collagenous tissue known as **periodontal membrane or ligament**. The oral mucosa is bound to the alveolar bone (the **gingiva** or gums) and normally forms a tight cuff around the tooth neck, protecting alveolar bone from bacteria and foreign material. A potential space between the gingival cuff and the enamel of the crown, known as the **gingival crevice**, extends down to the cemento-enamel junction. At the free margin of the gingiva, the tough stratified oral epithelium becomes a thin vulnerable layer lining the gingival crevice.

If oral hygiene is inadequate, commensal bacteria colonise the gingival margin and form a white gelatinous **plaque** on the enamel (Fig. 48.5). If allowed to persist, plaque becomes adherent to the tooth surface and becomes mineralised. This is known as **calculus**, and cannot be removed by tooth brushing. Bacterial toxins then cause inflammation of the gingiva, known as **marginal gingivitis**. This appears as swelling and redness of the gums and slight bleeding during tooth brushing.

As seen in Figure 48.6, gingivitis causes eversion of the gingival margin. This encourages more bacterial plaque and calculus to form in the gingival crevice and also results in greater trauma to the gum from food. These both lead to more extensive inflammation.

If untreated, inflammation gradually extends to involve the deeper supporting tissues. This causes progressive resorption of alveolar bone and destruction of the periodontal membrane, known as **periodontitis**. By this stage, the gingiva is thickened and inflamed with a purulent discharge from the gums. This explains the old term 'pyorrhoea' or flowing of pus. Despite this, the patient is remarkably pain free, although **halitosis** is obvious to others!

As periodontal inflammation progresses, more alveolar bone is destroyed and the gums recede. The root-surface becomes exposed to view, giving rise to the expression

(a) Normal gingiva

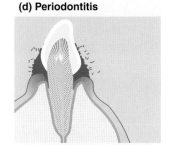

- Gingival crevice
- Gingiva
- Alveolar bone

Healthy pink gingiva forming tight cuff around base of crown

(b) Marginal gingivitis

Plaque accumulates around gingival margins. Toxins are produced by bacteria causing marginal inflammation; marginal gingiva becomes red, slightly swollen and bleeds easily

(c) Moderate gingivitis

More severe gingival inflammation: loss of tight protective cuff of gingiva allows accumulation of bacterial plaque and calculus in gingival crevice

(d) Periodontitis

The inflammation involves the supporting alveolar bone, which is progressively resorbed so that adequate tooth support is eventually lost

Fig. 48.5 Pathogenesis of periodontal disease

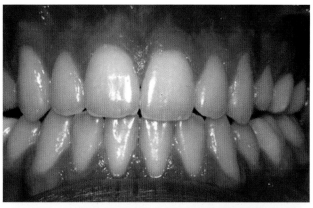

(a)

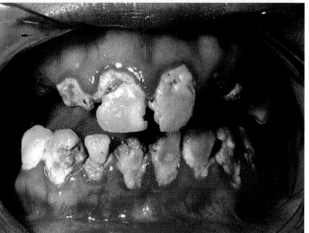

(b)

Fig. 48.6 Gingivitis and periodontitis
(a) Normal healthy gingivae. **(b)** Chronic gingivitis showing accumulated plaque and calculus around the gingival margins. At this stage, there has been no alveolar bone destruction and the inflammatory process is potentially reversible. Many of these teeth had to be extracted, however, because of rampant caries.

'long in the tooth', once thought to be inevitable with advancing age. Teeth gradually become more mobile until they fall out or can be extracted with the fingers!

An acute **periodontal abscess** may develop at some point. On the whole, however, periodontal disease is an insidious process commencing in early adulthood, but it is almost entirely preventable. In adults, **periodontitis** (not dental decay, as is commonly supposed) is responsible for most lost teeth. Inflammatory destruction of alveolar bone makes it difficult to construct satisfactory dentures for many of these patients, due to the lack of a retaining alveolar ridge.

Management of gingivitis and periodontitis

Gingivitis and periodontitis is almost entirely preventable by thorough and regular tooth brushing and use of dental floss, plus periodic dental scaling to remove inaccessible plaque and calculus.

Initial dental scaling, and careful oral hygiene instruction and supervision will cure gingivitis, which is a reversible condition. During the early stages of improved oral hygiene, bleeding will increase through brushing inflamed

tissues. This soon subsides unless further periodontal treatment is needed.

Once established, periodontitis requires even more meticulous oral hygiene once the teeth have been thoroughly cleaned of plaque and calculus. Lost bone is never replaced, and the gingival contour remains abnormal, making effective oral hygiene difficult. Surgical recontouring of the gingiva and underlying bone (**gingivoplasty**) may sometimes be appropriate. It must be emphasised that antibiotics play no part in the treatment of chronic gingivitis and periodontitis. Antibiotics may, however, be useful for acute gingival conditions such as pericoronitis and Vincent's infection (**acute ulcerative gingivitis**), described below.

PERICORONITIS

This condition occurs when a lower third molar (wisdom tooth) is impacted against the second molar or the ramus of the mandible so that its eruption into the mouth is

Fig. 48.7 Impacted lower third molars and pericoronitis

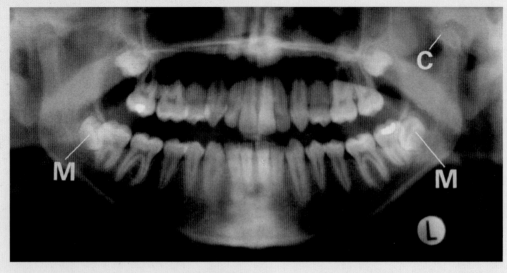

(a)

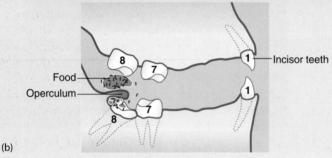

(b)

This OPG radiograph of a 16-year-old girl shows the whole lower jaw 'opened out'. Both lower third molars **M** are seen to be angled towards the second molars and impacted against them. The roots are not fully formed and there is little chance of these teeth erupting normally. These were an incidental finding, the X-rays having been taken to demonstrate a fracture of the neck of the left mandibular condyle **C**.

prevented (see Fig. 48.7). If a flap (**operculum**) of gingival tissue partly overlies the impacted tooth, this creates a space around the buried tooth crown (Fig. 48.7b). Food and bacterial plaque collect here and lead to acute infection, which may extend into surrounding tissues and even into the parapharyngeal area.

The patient complains of severe, poorly localised pain near the angle of the mandible. Pain is aggravated by closing the jaw because the opposing tooth bites on the swollen gingival flap. On examination, the pericoronal tissues of the affected tooth are red and swollen with a purulent discharge exuding from beneath the gingival flap. Oral examination may be difficult because of trismus. Externally, the submandibular lymph nodes are enlarged and tender.

Management of pericoronitis

Pericoronitis is a cellulitis with incipient abscess formation. It is caused by a mixture of organisms which are usually sensitive to penicillin. It is treated locally by irrigating beneath the flap with hydrogen peroxide and the

patient is also advised to rinse the mouth several times daily with warm salty water. Rapid relief can be obtained by removing the upper wisdom tooth if it impinges on the flap over the lower wisdom tooth. Oral penicillin is required if the patient is systemically unwell. Once the acute infection is over, the lower wisdom tooth may need to be removed surgically, especially if attacks are recurrent.

ACUTE ULCERATIVE GINGIVITIS (VINCENT'S INFECTION)

This is an acute inflammatory condition with necrotising ulceration of the gingival margin. It is caused by a mixture of Gram-negative organisms which are normal oral commensals. The most prominent bacteria are *Fusobacterium fusiformis*, *Borrelia vincentii* and *Bacteroides melaninogenicus*. Acute ulcerative gingivitis most commonly occurs in young adults who 'burn the candle at both ends' and become generally run down. Poor oral hygiene, pericoronitis and smoking may contribute. Acute ulcerative gingivitis is now uncommon, but was widespread among

Fig. 48.8 Acute ulcerative gingivitis

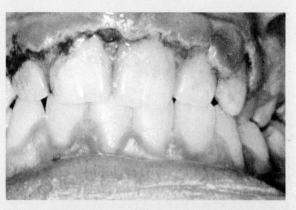

This shows the typical appearance of acute ulcerative gingivitis (Vincent's infection); there is ulceration of the whole gingival margin with destruction of the interdental papillae, giving a ragged but almost straight gum margin. Compare this with Fig. 48.6b.

soldiers in the First World War when it gained the name 'trench mouth'.

There is an abrupt onset of gingival pain and bleeding, accompanied by a foul, often metallic taste and marked halitosis. Cervical lymph nodes are enlarged and tender, and there may be fever, malaise and anorexia. Oral examination reveals characteristic ragged, punched-out ulceration of the gingival margin, especially between the teeth (see Fig. 48.8). Ulceration elsewhere in the mouth is rare, except in severe cases where the pharyngeal mucosa becomes inflamed and ulcerated (**Vincent's angina**). Acute ulcerative gingivitis is easily distinguished from **herpetic gingivo-stomatitis**, the other acute ulcerative condition with systemic symptoms, as the former is confined to the gingival margin, whereas herpetic ulcers are scattered all over the oral mucosa.

Management of acute ulcerative gingivitis

Vincent's infection rapidly responds to metronidazole tablets, usually with full recovery of gingival morphology; penicillin is also effective. Tooth brushing is extremely painful during an attack and the mouth should be frequently rinsed with warm water or weak hydrogen peroxide to keep it clean. Afterwards, careful attention to oral hygiene will usually prevent recurrence.

TUMOURS OF THE ORAL MUCOSA

PATHOPHYSIOLOGY AND AETIOLOGY

The whole oral cavity including the tongue is invested by stratified squamous epithelium. Squamous cell carcino-

mas of the mouth account for about 3% of all malignancies. Like their counterparts on the skin, squamous carcinomas in the mouth usually occur in older patients. Men are affected twice as often as women.

Tobacco products are the usual cause in developed and in developing countries. Pipe and cigar smokers appear to be at greatest risk. The tongue and lower lip are the common sites of oral cancer, each accounting for about 25% of cases. Chronic irritation by ill-fitting dentures, jagged tooth restorations or alcohol abuse may contribute to the aetiology.

In India, Sri Lanka and Papua New Guinea and other countries, the habit of chewing a small package of betel leaf, tobacco and lime causes a very high incidence of carcinoma of the buccal mucosa.

Leukoplakia is a premalignant dysplastic condition found in 50% of patients with oral carcinoma.

CLINICAL FEATURES OF ORAL CANCER

Oral cancer usually presents as a chronic indurated ulcer which slowly enlarges and fails to heal (Fig. 48.9b and c). An early lesion may present as a non-ulcerated mucosal swelling. Lesions are usually painless unless they become secondarily infected, although advanced lesions may cause pain as they invade deeply. Carcinoma of the tongue, for example, may cause pain referred to the ear or pharynx.

Oral squamous carcinomas are generally well differentiated. They invade locally but metastasise to submandibular and cervical lymph nodes only at a late stage. Spreading tumours of the posterior floor of mouth and tongue interfere with speech, mastication and swallowing. These are particularly distressing symptoms.

MANAGEMENT OF ORAL CANCER

A chronic oral ulcer which fails to heal after the removal of possible aggravating factors (such as ill-fitting dentures) should undergo incision biopsy to exclude cancer.

Oral cancers are excised with a margin of normal tissue. This may not be possible anatomically or cosmetically and often necessitates a major reconstructive surgical operation. Involved regional lymph nodes are removed by **block dissection**.

If excision is impractical, most of these tumours respond to radiotherapy. This may employ external beam treatment or radioactive implants. A disadvantage of radiotherapy, however, is that it damages salivary glands, resulting in **xerostomia** (dry mouth). Apart from the discomfort, this predisposes to salivary gland infection.

Carcinoma of the lip has the best prognosis. The 5-year survival rate is over 60%, but for tumours of the tongue and floor of the mouth, this falls to only about 25%.

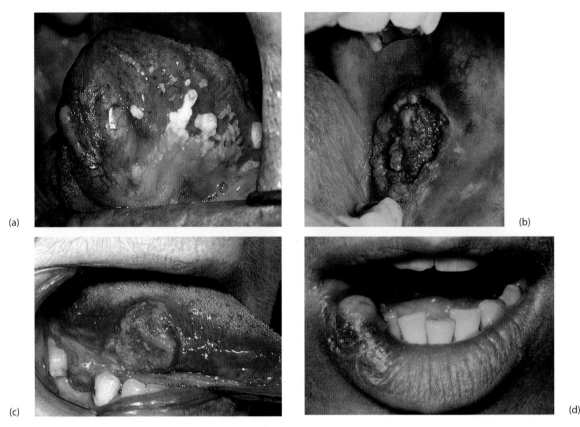

Fig. 48.9 Premalignant and malignant conditions of the mouth
(a) Leukoplakia under tongue. **(b)** Ulcerating squamous cell carcinoma (SCC) of the cheek. **(c)** Ulcerating SCC of the tongue. **(d)** Case study—squamous cell carcinoma of the lip. This man of 60 had smoked a pipe most of his life. He tended to keep the pipe constantly in his mouth while he worked. He presented with a non-healing ulcer of the lip, proven to be a well-differentiated SCC on biopsy. A wedge resection of the lip was performed and produced a cure.

LEUKOPLAKIA

Leukoplakia means 'white plaque', and the term is used to describe white patches on the oral mucosa which cannot readily be scraped off (see Fig. 48.9a). This distinguishes them from candidal infections. White plaques may be caused by oral lichen planus or lupus erythematosus, but the main importance of leukoplakia is that it may represent epithelial dysplasia or even carcinoma in situ.

The cheeks and tongue are most often affected, although dysplastic patches may develop anywhere in the oral mucosa. An innocent white line which is not leukoplakia is often seen along the inside of the cheek; this corresponds to the line of biting surfaces of the teeth and is caused by frictional hyperplasia.

Severe or extensive leukoplakia should be referred for specialist oral surgical opinion and biopsy. Areas of severe dysplasia require surgical removal, which may necessitate grafting.

EPULIS

An epulis is a benign, localised gingival swelling. Two types are recognised: fibrous epulis and giant cell epulis.

A **fibrous epulis** is simply a benign fibrous tissue tumour arising from the periodontal membrane or nearby periosteum. It forms a smooth, firm, slowly growing lump, covered with normal gingiva. A fibrous epulis usually emerges between two teeth, which may be slightly pushed apart by pressure. Treatment is by local excision with curettage of the origin. Otherwise, the lesion may recur (Fig. 48.10).

A **giant cell epulis** arises in a similar location but grows much faster. It forms an irregular red fleshy mass which ulcerates and bleeds. The lesion consists of numerous giant cells in a highly vascular stroma, which may invade local bone. Treatment involves extracting associated teeth and excising and curetting bone. This is the only way to avoid recurrence (Fig. 48.10).

Pyogenic granulomas may occur on the gums or oral mucosa of the lips. They have a similar appearance to pyogenic granulomas of the skin (see Ch. 46).

Fig. 48.10 Lumps and bumps around the mouth

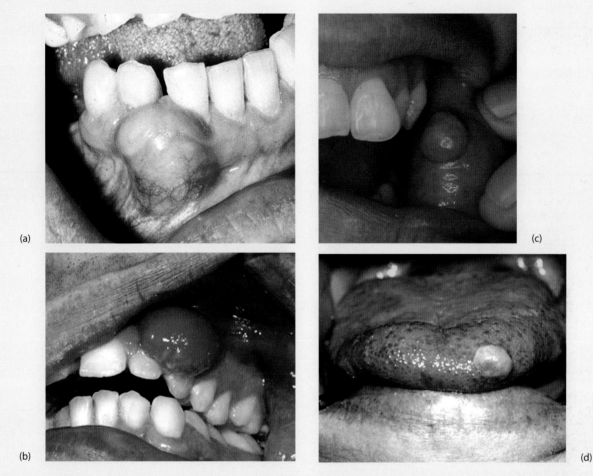

(a)

(b)

(c)

(d)

(a) Fibrous epulis. This can be seen to be moving the nearby tooth out of alignment. **(b)** Giant cell epulis. Both of these are in typical interdental location. The fibrous epulis is the same colour as the gum, while the giant cell epulis is a deeper red. **(c)** Fibroepithelial polyp inside cheek. These lesions are common and are probably initiated by minor biting trauma to the cheek or lip. They are often inadvertently chewed upon and gradually become larger. Excision is usually straightforward. **(d)** Pyogenic granuloma of the tongue. These are probably initiated by injury and maintained by an excessive healing response. They can occur on the gum or anywhere else in the mouth.

MISCELLANEOUS DISORDERS CAUSING INTRAORAL SWELLING

RETENTION CYSTS OF THE ACCESSORY SALIVARY GLANDS

The oral mucosa contains numerous accessory mucous and serous salivary glands. Small retention cysts probably develop as a result of minor trauma to the duct. Most retention cysts are smaller than 1 cm in diameter. They commonly occur in the lower lip mucosa where they cause annoyance and are readily traumatised during speech or chewing. Retention cysts are blue-grey and are extremely soft to palpation. They often rupture spontaneously but usually reform. Small retention cysts can usually be completely enucleated under local anaesthesia; larger ones may need marsupialisation.

TUMOURS OF ACCESSORY SALIVARY GLANDS

Tumours occasionally arise in the accessory salivary glands. These are often malignant **adenocystic carcinomas**. They present as small, firm lumps in the oral mucosa or posterior palate, and are often noticed before invading deeply or metastasising. Treatment is by wide excision but the prognosis is often poor.

BONY EXOSTOSES

Local outgrowths of the jaw bones are common and may produce an intraoral lump. To the uninitiated doctor, this

707

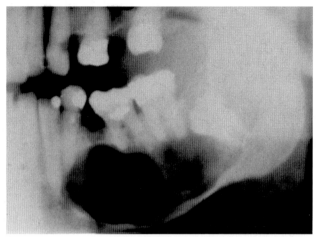

(a)

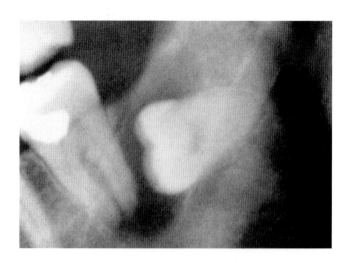

(b)

Fig. 48.11 Dental cyst and dentigerous cyst
(a) Large dental cyst in the mandible. This arose from tooth-forming epithelial remnants in the apical area of the lower left second premolar tooth which was extracted several months beforehand due to chronic periapical infection. **(b)** Dentigerous cyst associated with the crown of an unerupted lower third molar. These cysts originate from epithelial remnants of the tooth bud.

may be suspicious of neoplasia. The most common site is the centre of the hard palate, where it is known as a **torus palatinus**. A similar exostosis, usually bilateral, occurs inside the mandible, opposite the premolar teeth and is known as **torus mandibularis**.

These lesions are of course bony hard and are covered by normal oral mucosa. Excision is rarely needed unless there are problems in wearing a removable denture.

CYSTS AND TUMOURS OF THE JAWS

Various cystic lesions and tumours arise in the jaws. Many are abnormalities of tooth-forming epithelium, either developmental or acquired. Figure 48.11b shows a dentigerous cyst of the mandible, a developmental cyst originating from epithelial remnants of the tooth bud. Most are rare and can usually be diagnosed radiologically. The jaws are occasionally the site of benign or malignant bone tumours, as found elsewhere. Examples are osteosarcomas and osteoclastomas.

Growth disorders of bone such as fibrous dysplasia and Paget's disease of bone may also affect the jaw.

Disorders of the thyroid and parathyroid glands

49

INTRODUCTION

Patients with disorders of the thyroid gland presenting to a surgeon usually have a **lump in the neck**. This may be asymptomatic but the patient often fears malignancy. In some cases, the mass may be causing pressure symptoms or cosmetic deformity. When examined, a discrete thyroid lump may be found or the whole gland may be enlarged. A large thyroid swelling of either type is known in lay terms as a **goitre**, from the Latin for throat *'guttur'*. In most cases, the patient is clinically euthyroid (i.e. with normal thyroid hormone activity) and biochemical tests of thyroid function are normal. Occasionally patients are referred with **hyperthyroidism** when medical treatment has failed, radioisotope treatment is unsuitable or where the patient has an overactive nodule. These may require some form of thyroidectomy.

Parathyroid disorders usually reach the surgeon because of symptomatic or asymptomatic (biochemically detected) **hypercalcaemia** caused by excess parathormone secretion. This can only be successfully treated by surgical removal of the cause. In most cases, this is a solitary parathyroid adenoma; less commonly there is multigland hyperplasia and, very rarely, carcinoma.

DISORDERS OF THE THYROID

Diseases of the thyroid can be considered in four broad pathological categories:

- Developmental abnormalities
- Inflammatory and autoimmune disorders
- Hyperplastic and metabolic disorders
- Neoplasms

The main pathophysiological and clinical features are summarised in Table 49.1, except for thyroid malignancy, which is outlined later in Table 49.2.

MAIN CLINICAL PRESENTATIONS OF THYROID DISEASE IN SURGICAL PRACTICE

DIFFUSE OR GENERALISED ENLARGEMENT OF THE THYROID

The term **goitre** is often used to describe any substantial enlargement of the thyroid but the expression is descriptively and pathologically imprecise. Most large generalised thyroid swellings seen in developed countries are caused by simple, non-toxic **colloid goitre**, i.e. idiopathic diffuse or multinodular hyperplasia. **Multinodular goitres** usually develop from diffuse goitres over a period of years.

Where the condition is *endemic* (often in isolated, mountainous and underdeveloped regions such as Nepal), iodine deficiency is the usual cause, though this is less common now where iodine is added to the diet. These goitres are often asymmetrical and soft to palpation. They are composed of many large hyperplastic nodules and can reach enormous sizes (see Fig. 49.1). Although unsightly, endemic goitres cause surprisingly few symptoms and the patient is usually euthyroid.

Anaplastic carcinomas may also cause fairly large thyroid swellings in elderly patients (see Fig. 49.2), usually accompanied by symptoms of invasion into nearby structures. These include **hoarseness** if there is recurrent laryngeal nerve involvement, and **stridor**, particularly at

Table 49.1 Benign diseases of the thyroid

Condition (relative frequency in developed countries)	Pathophysiology	Clinical features
1. Developmental abnormalities		
a. Thyroglossal cyst (*uncommon*)	Cyst formation anywhere along the midline thyroglossal tract. This marks the line of embryological descent of the thyroid from the foramen caecum via the hyoid bone to the normal position in the neck	Smooth, rounded swelling in midline of neck anywhere between the submental area and isthmus of thyroid. Usually found in children and young adults
b. Thyroglossal fistula (*rare*)	Incision into or incomplete removal of a thyroglossal cyst can cause a fistula	Fistulous (or sinus) opening near midline of neck. Intermittently discharges clear fluid or becomes infected and discharges pus
c. Ectopic thyroid (*uncommon*)	Part or all of the thyroid lying anywhere along the thyroglossal tract	Usually symptomless but may present as an unusual swelling near foramen caecum at junction of anterior two-thirds and posterior third of tongue
2. Inflammatory and autoimmune disorders		
a. Hashimoto's thyroiditis (*common*)	Diffuse lymphocytic infiltration of thyroid gland with progressive destruction of thyroid follicles. Over a period of years, leads to progressive atrophy and fibrosis. Various anti-thyroid antibodies usually present in plasma in high titres. Polygenic inherited disorder which may be associated with other autoimmune disorders, e.g. pernicious anaemia. Focal lymphocytic thyroiditis is probably a milder variant of the same condition	Presents in adulthood with mild, diffuse, sometimes tender thyroid enlargement. Often the thyroid is not enlarged. Patient usually euthyroid or hyperthyroid at outset, but later becomes hypothyroid. Affects females much more frequently than males
b. Graves' disease (*fairly common*)	Diffuse thyroid hyperplasia due to the action of a circulating immunoglobulin 'long-acting thyroid stimulator' (LATS). This binds to thyroid acinar cells mimicking the effects of TSH and producing excess thyroid hormone	Diffuse thyroid enlargement, sometimes with a bruit, but main feature is marked hyperthyroidism (thyrotoxicosis) causing weight loss, heat intolerance, tachycardia, hyper-reflexia, tremor and sometimes exophthalmos
c. De Quervain's acute thyroiditis (*uncommon*)	Diffuse inflammation of thyroid gland, probably viral in origin. Neutrophilic and later lymphocytic and histiocytic infiltration of gland occurs	Very tender, diffuse moderate thyroid enlargement, with or without systemic symptoms. Episodes last weeks to months and are often recurrent. Patient usually euthyroid but may be hyperthyroid in acute phase
d. Riedel's thyroiditis (*very rare*)	Dense fibrosis of thyroid gland. Possibly an autoimmune process	Extremely hard ('woody goitre') often asymmetrical thyroid mass suspicious of tumour. Sometimes produces symptoms of compression
3. Hyperplastic and metabolic disorders		
a. Simple non-toxic colloid goitre (*very common*)	Benign, diffuse or multinodular hyperplasia of thyroid follicles. Cause is unknown but possibly minor abnormality of thyroid hormone synthesis	Diffuse or sporadic multinodular thyroid enlargement or single 'adenomatous' nodule or cyst. Patient clinically euthyroid and all thyroid function tests normal. Affects females much more than males
b. Endemic goitre (*very rare in UK*)	Diffuse hyperplasia of thyroid follicles due to dietary iodine deficiency or goitrogenic foods. Endemic in inland, developing countries, especially in mountainous areas	Diffuse, often massive thyroid enlargement which may later become nodular. T4 is low or normal and TSH tends to be elevated
c. Drug-induced goitre (*uncommon*)	Diffuse thyroid hyperplasia secondary to interference with thyroid hormone synthesis. Drugs causing this are anti-thyroid drugs used in therapy (e.g. carbimazole) or others like lithium and aminoglutethimide	Diffuse thyroid enlargement. Patient usually euthyroid. Can be prevented by using replacement dose of T4 concurrently with blocking drugs ('block and replace')
d. Dyshormonogenesis (*very uncommon*)	Diffuse thyroid hyperplasia caused by a variety of uncommon genetic (recessive) defects affecting thyroid hormone synthesis	Presents at birth or in childhood with thyroid enlargement and severe hypothyroidism (cretinism). In developed countries, these defects are usually diagnosed at birth by neonatal screening tests before any goitre has developed
e. Physiological (*common*)	Diffuse thyroid hyperplasia often associated with pregnancy and puberty	Mild diffuse thyroid enlargement. Patient euthyroid

Fig. 49.1 Endemic goitre

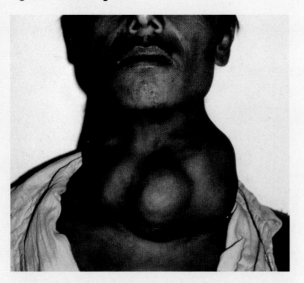

This condition, caused by iodine deficiency, is extremely common in isolated mountain regions. The thyroid can reach an enormous size, yet the patient suffers only minimal symptoms and is usually euthyroid. This typical example in a Nepalese man is only of moderate size by local standards!

Fig. 49.2 Anaplastic carcinoma

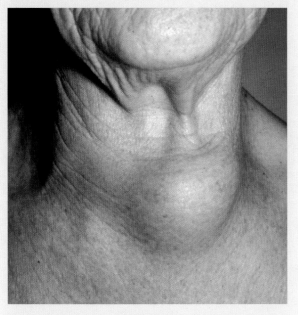

Rapidly enlarging hard thyroid mass in an elderly woman. The mass was firmly tethered to strap muscles and deeper structures. Treatment was purely palliative as this tumour does not respond to any current therapy.

Fig. 49.3 Solitary thyroid nodule

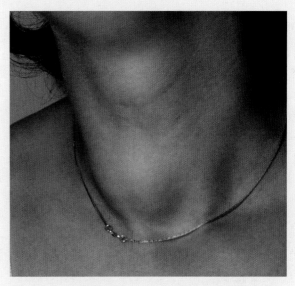

This asymptomatic nodule had been present for several years. It proved histologically to be a thyroid adenoma.

night, if there is tracheal displacement or compression. The gland is hard on palpation. The uncommon **lymphomas** of the thyroid also present with diffuse thyroid enlargement.

In **Graves' disease** (primary hyperthyroidism) there is usually a degree of smooth thyroid enlargement (see Fig. 49.3), often increased by drug treatment. This is almost never the main presenting feature, however. Similarly, in **Hashimoto's** thyroiditis, the thyroid may be moderately enlarged but firmer and finely nodular on palpation.

SOLITARY THYROID NODULE

A common presentation of thyroid disease is a clinically solitary thyroid nodule (see Fig. 49.4). This is an apparently isolated lump in the thyroid, although 50% turn out on imaging to be multinodular. When small, these lumps are not usually obvious and are found incidentally by the patient or the doctor. They may first be noticed by someone else when the patient swallows. Less than 10% of true solitary nodules are malignant although this rises to about 40% in patients who have undergone previous neck irradiation. Almost all nodules developing in the thyroid in **childhood** are malignant. Fallout from the nuclear meltdown at Chernobyl produced huge numbers of thyroid cancers in irradiated children. In any patient with a solitary nodule, malignancy needs to be excluded by investigation, and fine needle aspiration cytology or needle core biopsy is the first step in doing so.

An isolated lesion is most commonly a nodule of idiopathic hyperplasia which may be so discrete as to be

CASE STUDY

Fig. 49.4 Multinodular goitre

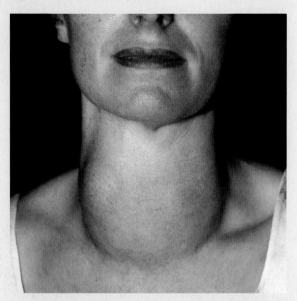

Longstanding multinodular goitre in a woman of 40 with a strong family history of thyroid disorders. The thyroid is multinodular on palpation, and on ultrasound there are multiple nodules of various sizes plus some small cysts. Any change in a multinodular goitre may herald malignancy.

CASE STUDY

Fig. 49.5 Hyperthyroidism

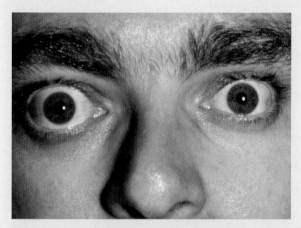

Exophthalmic eye signs of hyperthyroidism in 43-year-old man with 6-month history of hyperthyroidism. His family had noticed his increasingly staring eyes. He had proptosis and lid lag.

Box 49.1	Clinical manifestations of thyrotoxicosis

Metabolic—heat intolerance, increased appetite with weight loss, diarrhoea, menorrhagia
Cardiovascular—palpitations, tachycardia even while asleep, atrial fibrillation
Neuropsychiatric—hyperkinesis, insomnia, emotional instability, tremor, proximal myopathy
Ocular—exophthalmos including proptosis, lid retraction and eventually ophthalmoplegia
Cutaneous—pretibial myxoedema

described as a **thyroid adenoma**. **Thyroid cysts** are fairly common. Both of these fall within the spectrum of the pathological entity 'simple or multinodular colloid goitre'.

As mentioned earlier, an apparent solitary nodule may prove to be a focal accentuation of a generalised thyroid enlargement such as simple multinodular hyperplasia (colloid goitre) or, less often, Hashimoto's thyroiditis.

OTHER FEATURES ASSOCIATED WITH THYROID ENLARGEMENT

A new area of enlargement in an existing goitre may be caused by haemorrhage into a cyst or nodule, an enlarging hyperplastic nodule or a developing carcinoma. If the thyroid extends behind the sternum into the anterior mediastinum (see Fig. 49.7, below), the trachea may be compressed or displaced by this **retrosternal goitre** and cause **stridor**. Stridor may only become obvious when the neck is in certain positions, for example, sleeping on one side at night. Hoarseness or stridor may also result from **invasion** of trachea or recurrent laryngeal nerve by an anaplastic carcinoma.

Pain and tenderness are uncommon presenting features in thyroid disease, but characterise the rare infective **de Quervain's thyroiditis**. Sometimes the thyroid is painful and tender in Hashimoto's thyroiditis.

HYPERTHYROIDISM

The clinical manifestations of hyperthyroidism are summarised in Box 49.1. Excessive thyroid hormone production is a feature of Graves' disease, when it is often described as **thyrotoxicosis**. Mild hyperthyroidism may also occur in the early stages of Hashimoto's thyroiditis, with the condition burning out later and the patient becoming hypothyroid. A solitary hyperplastic (adenomatous) nodule may produce so much thyroid hormone that it causes hyperthyroidism. This is known as a **toxic or hot nodule**. More often, the patient is euthyroid but blood tests show the thyroid stimulating hormone (TSH) is low, suppressed by the autonomous production of thyroid hormones by the nodule.

In general, thyroid adenocarcinomas are non-secreting but very occasionally a well-differentiated carcinoma may cause hyperthyroidism.

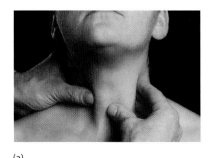 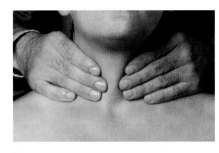 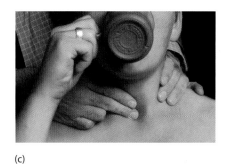

(a)　　　　　　　　　　　　　　　(b)　　　　　　　　　　　　　　　(c)

Fig. 49.6 Examination of the thyroid gland
The patient should be sitting upright in a chair with room for the examiner to approach from behind. **(a)** Gentle palpation from the front with slight sideways pressure from the left hand whilst palpating with the right. This is repeated for the right side of the gland. **(b)** General palpation of the gland from behind. Is there enlargement? Is it a single nodule or multinodular? How big is it? **(c)** Palpation of the gland while the patient swallows. Does the gland rise with swallowing? Is there retrosternal extension?

HYPOTHYROIDISM

Hypothyroidism is usually the result of late Hashimoto's thyroiditis or primary thyroid atrophy, or else previous treatment for hyperthyroidism. In either case, the gland is small and fibrous and as such does not present to the surgeon. Hypothyroidism is a late complication in up to 25% of patients after subtotal thyroidectomy and even more after radioiodine therapy for thyrotoxicosis, and is inevitable after total thyroidectomy for any reason including carcinoma. Hypothyroidism should be considered in surgical patients presenting with constipation and has also been implicated in abdominal aortic thrombosis in middle-aged women.

SPECIAL POINTS IN EXAMINING A THYROID SWELLING

Examining for a suspected thyroid swelling should begin by seating the patient in a chair (Fig. 49.6) with space to palpate from behind and ensuring there is a glass of water for the patient to swallow. First, general examination should look for signs of hyperthyroidism (tachycardia, atrial fibrillation, fine tremor, sweaty palms and hyperreflexia) and for signs specific to Graves' disease (exophthalmos and ophthalmoplegia). Next, the front of the neck is inspected while the patient swallows. The characteristic rise and fall of a thyroid swelling results from the gland being invested in the **pretracheal fascia** which is attached to the larynx above. A normal thyroid is not visible even on swallowing, and is not normally palpable.

The thyroid area is next palpated from behind with the patient seated. This position is best for examining the size, shape and consistency of the gland. It also allows the lower edge of the swelling to be palpated to identify any retrosternal extension. The lobes of the thyroid wrap around the larynx and lie deep to the sternomastoid muscles which tend to conceal thyroid enlargement and make it difficult to examine the whole gland.

Box	49.2	Principles of investigation of a thyroid mass

General thyroid status—thyroid function tests and thyroid autoantibodies
Morphology of the gland, i.e. size, shape and physical consistency, effects upon surrounding structures—ultrasound, plain X-rays of thoracic outlet, CT scanning
Tissue diagnosis—fine needle aspiration cytology or needle biopsy, incision or excision biopsy

---

The jugular chain of **lymph nodes** should be palpated for evidence of node metastases, since this may be the sole presenting feature of papillary carcinoma. In thyrotoxicosis, auscultation of the thyroid may reveal a **bruit** because of increased vascularity.

If there is any suspicion of recurrent laryngeal nerve palsy because of **hoarseness**, tests of vocal cord function should be performed. The patient is asked to cough and to pronounce the sound 'ee', both of which are likely to be abnormal if there is nerve damage. In this case, or if surgery is contemplated, formal assessment of cord function should be performed by indirect laryngoscopy, usually in an ENT department.

APPROACH TO INVESTIGATION OF A THYROID MASS

The questions to be answered in investigating a thyroid mass are summarised in Box 49.2 and are described in detail below. Patients who have undergone previous radiotherapy to the neck should be considered at high risk of thyroid carcinoma.

GENERAL THYROID STATUS

It should be established whether the patient is **euthyroid**, **hyperthyroid** or **hypothyroid**. Initially, this is performed

Fig. 49.7 Retrosternal goitre

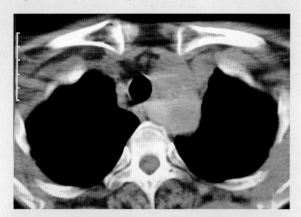

(a)

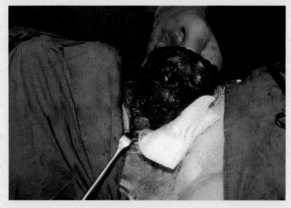

(b)

This 38-year-old woman had suffered stridor at night for several months. On palpation, the thyroid was not particularly large but the trachea was markedly deviated (Fig. 49.8) and the thyroid did not rise on swallowing, both providing evidence of substantial retrosternal extension. **(a)** CT scan at the level of the clavicles showing enlargement of the left side of the thyroid gland with moderate deviation but no compression of the trachea. **(b)** At operation, this huge retrosternal extension was drawn up out of the anterior mediastinum. As this was a multinodular goitre, a total thyroidectomy was performed. Histopathology confirmed a benign multinodular goitre.

Fig. 49.8 Tracheal displacement by a goitre

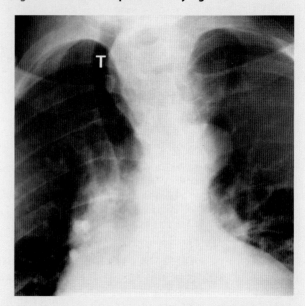

This chest X-ray shows gross displacement of the trachea **T** to the right by a large retrosternal goitre. The patient presented with nocturnal stridor when she lay on her left side.

clinically but estimations of free thyroxine (fT4) as well as thyroid stimulating hormone (TSH) are usually performed in most cases. Thyroid-binding globulin is elevated in pregnancy and puberty; the free thyroxine level takes account of this and avoids misleading interpretation of results. Tri-iodothyronine (T3) levels are occasionally measured if the patient is clinically hyperthyroid but the fT4 is normal. TSH level is usually low in hyperthyroidism and elevated in hypothyroidism. Some laboratories prefer to measure just the TSH level initially and perform more detailed tests if this is abnormal.

Thyroid autoantibodies are assayed if autoimmune disease is a possibility. Although not usually measured clinically, the presence of long-acting thyroid stimulating factor (LATS) is diagnostic of Graves' disease. Hashimoto's thyroiditis is characterised by elevation of other anti-thyroid antibodies such as anti-thyroglobulin or anti-mitochondrial antibodies (anti-thyroid M).

MORPHOLOGY OF THE GLAND

Ultrasound scanning is a useful method of establishing the morphology of the gland and reliably diagnoses cysts. It can also indicate retrosternal extension. CT scans of the neck and thoracic outlet are taken if there is suspicion of malignancy or if there appears to be tracheal displacement or compression (Figs 49.7, 49.8).

TISSUE DIAGNOSIS

Tissue diagnosis using fine needle aspiration cytology (FNA) or core needle biopsy is usually performed for solitary nodules or recently changed nodules in multinodular goitres. This can be performed without ultrasound, but ultrasound gives a fuller picture and guides biopsies. Given a competent and interested thyroid cytologist, up to 90% of thyroid nodules can be successfully categorised by this method. Needle core biopsy gives larger specimens with a greater diagnostic potential. If a **colloid nodule** is diagnosed, operative excision is not necessary unless the nodule causes compressive symptoms or cosmetic deformity. Lesions which are obviously malignant require operation. These include **papillary**, **medullary** and early **anaplastic carcinomas**. However, most **lymphomas** are inadequately sampled by FNA and core biopsy. In addition, **follicular carcinomas** cannot be distinguished cytologically from **benign follicular adenomas**; both display sheets of follicular cells. Lesions with this appearance should be removed, although most will be benign.

Incision biopsy at open operation is occasionally used for diagnosing generalised thyroid enlargement where the chances of malignancy are low or lymphoma is suspected.

FUNCTIONAL ACTIVITY OF GLANDULAR TISSUE

Injected radionuclides of iodine are avidly taken up by functioning thyroid tissue and were at one time employed widely for thyroid scanning. The isotope ^{131}I was found to deliver a high dose of radioactivity to the gland and was replaced by technetium-99m or ^{123}I, either of which delivers much lower doses. The increasing use of ultrasound and needle cytology and the knowledge that only 10% of cold nodules are malignant have greatly reduced the indications for thyroid radionuclide scanning.

When scanning is employed, the gland is imaged after isotope injection to identify the distribution of isotope activity. This may fall into one of four patterns:

- **Diffuse, homogeneous uptake**—this is found in the normal gland or where there is diffuse hyperactivity, e.g. Graves' disease
- **Generalised but patchy uptake**—this occurs in multinodular goitre where the hyperplastic nodules are less active than the surrounding normal tissue
- **The cold nodule**—an isolated area devoid of isotope uptake indicates non-secreting tissue, i.e. tumour, inactive adenomatous nodule or cyst. This requires tissue diagnosis, usually using fine needle aspiration cytology
- **The hot nodule**—or toxic adenoma. This represents an autonomous focus of excess T4 secretion. The secretory activity of the surrounding normal thyroid tissue is suppressed. The patient is usually euthyroid but sometimes thyrotoxic ('toxic nodule')

Very occasionally, **thyroid malignancies** secrete thyroid hormones and show up as warm or hot nodules on isotope scanning. Isotope scanning can also identify and localise **ectopic thyroid tissue** (in the tongue or along the course of the thyroglossal duct), **retrosternal extension** of a thyroid swelling and **metastases** of functioning thyroid carcinomas, provided the thyroid has been removed or ablated.

SPECIFIC CLINICAL PROBLEMS OF THE THYROID AND THEIR MANAGEMENT

THYROTOXICOSIS (HYPERTHYROIDISM)

Two percent of women and 0.2% of men in the UK have hyperthyroidism. Untreated, the condition causes weight loss, anxiety, tachycardia, palpitations and an increased risk of cardiovascular death. Most cases are caused by Graves' disease, some by toxic multinodular goitre and a few by toxic adenoma. Carcinoma is a very rare cause of thyrotoxicosis and is occasionally diagnosed incidentally when a hot nodule is examined histologically. Graves' disease is an autoimmune disorder in which circulating antibodies bind to TSH receptors in the thyroid gland and thus stimulate follicular cells to secrete thyroid hormones; this is independent of pituitary feedback. Hashimoto's thyroiditis may produce mild hyperthyroidism in its early stages but is self limiting. When in doubt, the aetiology can be determined by radioisotope scanning.

Treatment of hyperthyroidism

There are three main options for treating hyperthyroidism: **anti-thyroid drugs**, **radioisotope destruction** of functioning thyroid tissue and **subtotal (or total) thyroidectomy**. Anti-thyroid drugs are the first-line therapy except in the elderly and unfit, and patients with arrhythmias, angina and osteoporosis are usually treated with radioiodine from the outset. Only one randomised trial of all three modes of treatment has been published. Of those treated with drugs, 34% developed recurrent hyperthyroidism. In the radioiodine group, half needed more than one dose but all became hypothyroid within a year. In those treated by surgery, 8% recurred and needed further therapy. All groups reported 95% satisfaction and there was no difference in quality of life between the groups.

Thyrotoxic eye disease

Half of thyrotoxic patients develop eye disease. This is known as thyrotoxic ophthalmopathy and it can arise or regress independently of thyroid function. Eye disease does not occur in multinodular or adenoma thyrotoxicity. Eye disorders range from minor inflammation of conjunctiva with mild prominence of the globe to severe, debilitating and disfiguring eye disease that occurs in 3–5% of thyrotoxic patients.

Radioactive iodide therapy

Radioactive iodide (^{131}I or ^{125}I) may be used to treat thyrotoxicosis. It is administered as capsules or solution by mouth in doses 100 times higher than are used for diagnostic scanning (see Fig. 49.9). This treatment is appropriate for middle-aged or elderly patients but is contraindicated in pregnancy because of the risk of thyroid damage and genetic disruption in the fetus. Patients should avoid pregnancy for six months after treatment. Iodide is avidly taken up by the gland, and emission of beta particles destroys the most active thyroid tissue over a period of weeks or months. Note that anti-thyroid drug treatment usually needs to be continued until the radioiodine

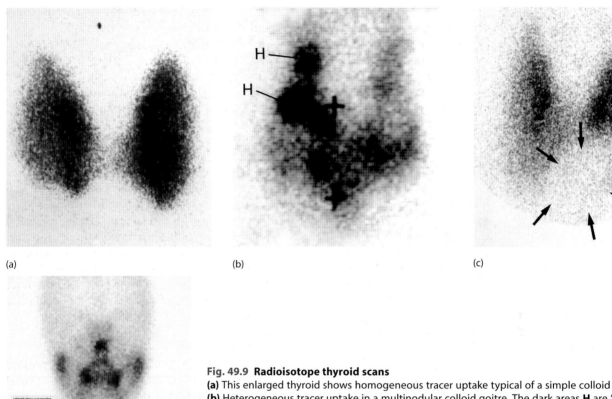

(a)

(b)

(c)

(d)

Fig. 49.9 Radioisotope thyroid scans
(a) This enlarged thyroid shows homogeneous tracer uptake typical of a simple colloid goitre.
(b) Heterogeneous tracer uptake in a multinodular colloid goitre. The dark areas **H** are 'hot nodules'; to maintain the euthyroid state, the rest of the gland exhibits diminished uptake. The + signs indicate the positions of the thyroid cartilage and the suprasternal notch.
(c) Solitary 'cold' thyroid nodule. The area of low uptake (outline arrowed) at the lower left pole of the thyroid corresponds with a palpable nodule. In the case of a solid lesion (as confirmed by ultrasound), a cold nodule may indicate malignancy. **(d)** Solitary 'hot' thyroid nodule. The area of high uptake in the lower part of the right lobe corresponds to a palpable mass. This patient was hyperthyroid and the lesion could be described as a 'toxic nodule'. Activity of the rest of the gland is suppressed by pituitary-mediated negative feedback from the high serum thyroxine level. The rectangle marked **BG** measures the background radiation in order to quantify the thyroid uptake.

reaches its greatest effect. After treatment, the rest of the isotope is excreted via the kidney, faeces, sweat, saliva and breath. Gamma rays are emitted from the patient's body and may be absorbed by others nearby.

Different radioiodide doses are used in different units, with higher doses giving a better chance of eliminating hyperthyroidism but giving a higher rate of hypothyroidism.

Ten to twenty per cent of patients need a second dose but once treatment is effective, recurrence is unlikely. Most patients treated eventually become hypothyroid (about 2–3% each year), especially those who are older, those previously treated with anti-thyroid drugs or those given a high dose. Many units now aim electively to make patients hypothyroid within six months and routinely provide levothyroxine replacement. This eliminates the risk of missing hypothyroidism 20 or more years later and may lower the risk of cardiovascular death in euthyroid patients after treatment. There is also a small theoretical risk of inducing malignancy and so radioiodine treatment is not advisable in the young.

Toxic multinodular disease and toxic adenoma also respond to this treatment; these patients rarely become hypothyroid afterwards.

Unwanted effects

There is a risk of exposing others to radiation after treatment. Current advice is that treated patients should keep 1 m away from anyone over 5 years for 11 days, from children aged 3–5 for 16 days and from those under 3 for 21 days.

Radioiodine tends to make thyrotoxic ophthalmopathy worse whereas anti-thyroid drugs and surgery do not affect its natural course. There is no increase in overall cancer death rate in treated patients, and the absolute risk of dying from thyroid cancer death is only 0.1%.

Anti-thyroid drugs

Most cases of thyrotoxicosis are initially managed with anti-thyroid drugs which block the synthesis of thyroid hormones. This treatment is not suitable for nodular toxicity because hyperactivity inevitably recurs. **Carbimazole** is the most popular drug of this type and is generally well tolerated. Carbimazole restores plasma hormone levels to normal over 4–8 weeks and treatment is continued for 12–18 months. Unfortunately, hyperthyroidism recurs in about half within 2 years. Five to ten per cent of patients develop a rash and there are rare cases of agranulocytosis, which is usually reversible. The white blood count should be monitored during treatment; a sore throat or other infection should alert the patient and the doctor to this possible complication. **Propylthiouracil** is an effective anti-thyroid drug that does not share these side effects. However, poor control, frequent relapses, side effects and non-compliance lead to eventual referral for definitive treatment in up to 40% of patients. In some patients in whom stable control cannot be achieved, and hypothyroidism alternates with hyperthyroidism, a **block and replace** regimen may succeed. Patients are given a higher dose of carbimazole to block thyroid hormone production altogether, together with a standard replacement dose of thyroxine.

Beta-adrenergic blocking drugs such as **propranolol** rapidly control the distressing and dangerous effects of thyrotoxicosis. These drugs may be used initially in extremely toxic patients until anti-thyroid drugs take effect, or if a patient urgently needs to be stabilised before thyroidectomy.

Surgical management

Indications for surgery
Surgery for thyrotoxicosis may be indicated as follows:

- When a quick and effective cure is desired which avoids long-term drug therapy and its drawbacks. It is often the best treatment for Graves' disease, particularly in younger patients, where the disease is not expected to burn itself out for many years
- When anti-thyroid drugs have proved unsatisfactory and radioiodide treatment is unsuitable
- Surgery is usually the most appropriate treatment for toxic multinodular goitre. Response to drug treatment in this condition is variable, and surgery also deals with the cosmetic deformity
- Toxic solitary nodules ('hot nodules') may be best excised to allow the suppressed normal thyroid to recover

Preoperative assessment and management of thyrotoxicosis
For all thyroid operations, preoperative assessment often includes indirect or direct **laryngoscopy** to demonstrate vocal cord function. This evaluates preoperative recurrent laryngeal nerve function should there later be a question of operative damage. Even without demonstrable cord damage, there is often a subtle change in voice quality after thyroidectomy, sometimes due to external laryngeal nerve damage. Patients should be warned of this before operation, especially if they are singers or politicians!

Wherever possible, thyroid function should be brought into the normal range before operation. The thyrotoxic state carries significant anaesthetic risks, especially of cardiac arrhythmias. Furthermore, manipulation of the gland may provoke massive release of thyroid hormone, precipitating a potentially lethal **thyrotoxic crisis** or 'thyroid storm'. Control of thyroid function is usually achieved with anti-thyroid drugs in the weeks preceding operation. If this fails, or if operation is very urgent, then beta-adrenergic blocking drugs such as propranolol can be used.

Anti-thyroid drugs increase the vascularity of the gland and this may add to surgical difficulty in toxic enlargement. It is standard practice to administer **Lugol's iodine** solution orally for 10 days before operation while continuing anti-thyroid therapy. This is believed to reduce vascularity and increase the firmness of the gland, making the operation easier.

Subtotal thyroidectomy
Surgery (Fig. 49.10) for hyperthyroidism aims to remove enough thyroid tissue to render the patient euthyroid whilst preserving sufficient of the gland to prevent hypothyroidism. For Graves' disease or toxic multinodular goitre, about 5–8 g of the gland is left intact. The technique of **subtotal thyroidectomy** leaves the posterior rim of each lobe in situ, thus minimising the risk of parathyroid or recurrent laryngeal damage. However, the risk of permanent hypoparathyroidism is 1–4% and that of permanent recurrent laryngeal nerve damage 1–5%. Patients need to be warned of these risks before giving their consent to operation. A low transverse collar incision along a skin crease gives the best cosmetic result but there is a 5% risk of a keloid scar in the long term. Meticulous care is required in ligating the **inferior thyroid artery** (after the recurrent laryngeal nerve has been identified) and the **upper pole vessels**. Primary or reactionary haemorrhage is a potentially serious complication causing major blood loss and laryngeal compression. To avoid suffocation from a postoperative bleed, instruments for emergency reopening of the wound should be kept at the patient's bedside after operation. The potential complications of thyroidectomy are summarised in Box 49.3.

THYROID MALIGNANCIES

Thyroid malignancies are uncommon, comprising less than 1% of all malignant tumours. Nearly all originate from thyroid follicular cells and form three distinct pathological entities: **papillary**, **follicular** and **anaplastic carcinomas**. Each has a characteristic pattern of behaviour and prognosis. Papillary and follicular carcinomas are usually well differentiated with low metastatic potential whereas anaplastic carcinomas behave aggressively. With

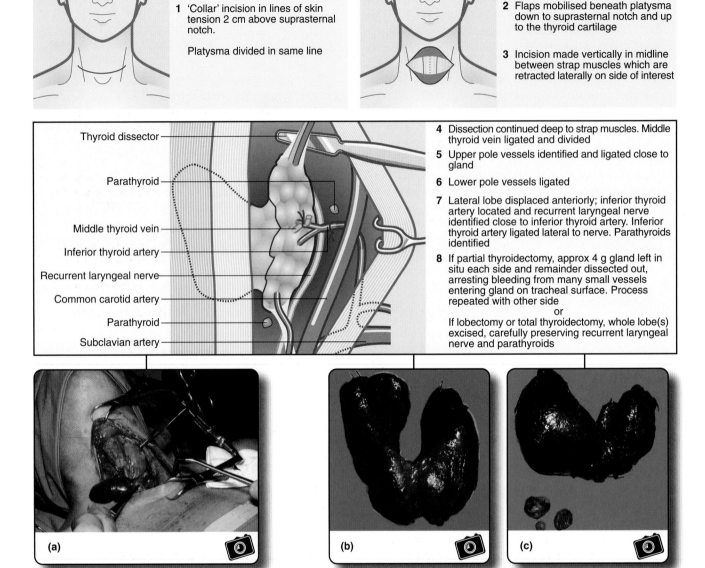

1   'Collar' incision in lines of skin tension 2 cm above suprasternal notch.

    Platysma divided in same line

2   Flaps mobilised beneath platysma down to suprasternal notch and up to the thyroid cartilage

3   Incision made vertically in midline between strap muscles which are retracted laterally on side of interest

Thyroid dissector
Parathyroid
Middle thyroid vein
Inferior thyroid artery
Recurrent laryngeal nerve
Common carotid artery
Parathyroid
Subclavian artery

4   Dissection continued deep to strap muscles. Middle thyroid vein ligated and divided
5   Upper pole vessels identified and ligated close to gland
6   Lower pole vessels ligated
7   Lateral lobe displaced anteriorly; inferior thyroid artery located and recurrent laryngeal nerve identified close to inferior thyroid artery. Inferior thyroid artery ligated lateral to nerve. Parathyroids identified
8   If partial thyroidectomy, approx 4 g gland left in situ each side and remainder dissected out, arresting bleeding from many small vessels entering gland on tracheal surface. Process repeated with other side
                            or
    If lobectomy or total thyroidectomy, whole lobe(s) excised, carefully preserving recurrent laryngeal nerve and parathyroids

(a)

(b)

(c)

Fig. 49.10 Thyroid and parathyroid operations
The drawings show the standard neck exploration approach to thyroid and parathyroid operations, and the structures at particular danger—the recurrent laryngeal nerve and parathyroid glands. In the photographs, **(a)** shows neck exploration for hyperparathyroidism. A collar incision has been made and upper and lower flaps are held apart with the specially designed Joll's retractor. A single large parathyroid adenoma is clearly visible. **(b)** Subtotal thyroidectomy specimen after operation for hyperthyroidism. **(c)** Total thyroidectomy specimen after operation for right-sided medullary carcinoma. Involved lymph nodes were 'cherry picked' and are also shown.

rare exceptions, these tumours do not secrete thyroid hormones.

In addition, about 7% of thyroid carcinomas arise from APUD C-cells which secrete calcitonin. These tumours are known as **medullary carcinomas** of the thyroid. **Lymphomas** occasionally involve the thyroid gland, usually in patients with pre-existing Hashimoto's disease.

Exposure to ionising radiation during childhood predisposes to thyroid carcinoma. This includes radiotherapy (once popular for treating 'status thymolymphaticus' and other benign disorders) and radioactive fallout. Many people exposed at the Hiroshima and Nagasaki bombings

and the Bikini atoll nuclear tests developed thyroid tumours and, more recently, children exposed to the fallout from Chernobyl had a high rate of thyroid cancer. In most cases of thyroid cancer, however, no aetiological factor can be identified.

Papillary carcinoma

Papillary carcinoma constitutes about two-thirds of thyroid malignancies in adults and nearly all thyroid malignancies in children. Females are affected at least three times as often as males and the peak incidence is

Table 49.2 Malignant diseases of the thyroid

Condition (relative frequency in developed countries)	Pathophysiology	Clinical features
Adenocarcinomas		
a. Papillary carcinoma *(relatively common—two-thirds of all thyroid carcinomas and 90% in children)*	Papillary adenocarcinoma forms a complex branching structure with a fibrous stroma (papillary pattern) and **psammoma** (sand grain) bodies. Variable degree of dysplasia. Commonly metastasises to cervical nodes but distant metastases rare	Slowly growing firm thyroid lump or cervical lymph nodes or both. Occurs in adults and sometimes children, 3F : 1M. Excellent prognosis even with local metastases—90% survival at 10 years
b. Follicular carcinoma *(relatively uncommon)*	Tumour forms a well-developed follicular pattern reminiscent of normal thyroid. Generally well differentiated but metastasis is usually distant, e.g. lungs and bone	Similar presentation to papillary carcinoma but does not involve cervical nodes. Affects slightly older age group than papillary carcinoma, 3F : 1M
c. Anaplastic carcinoma *(relatively uncommon)*	Aggressive tumour rapidly spreading beyond the confines of the gland	Diffuse, hard thyroid enlargement, often with symptoms of tracheal or recurrent laryngeal nerve involvement. Affects elderly patients. Very poor prognosis
d. Medullary carcinoma *(very uncommon)*	Well-differentiated tumour derived from parafollicular calcitonin-secreting cells (C-cells). Tumour contains deposits of amyloid	Stony hard thyroid lump, possibly with secondaries in cervical nodes. Often associated with MEN II. Poor prognosis. Calcitonin in blood is a tumour marker
Lymphoma *(rare)*	Diffuse lymphoid infiltration of thyroid gland	Diffuse thyroid enlargement. Patient euthyroid. Usually occurs in Hashimoto's disease

Box 49.3 Complications of thyroidectomy

Complications during operation

- *Uncontrollable haemorrhage*—uncommon, usually results from a slipped ligature on the upper pole vessels which then retract
- *Unilateral or bilateral recurrent laryngeal nerve damage*—bilateral nerve damage presents as laryngeal obstruction after tracheal extubation and necessitates immediate tracheostomy. Unilateral damage causes hoarseness and a weak voice and impairs coughing, see below
- *Inadvertent damage to other structures*—tracheal or oesophageal perforation or damage to laryngeal muscles or nerves

Early postoperative complications (within the first 12 hours)

- *Major haemorrhage*—presents as rapid swelling of the neck or a large volume of blood loss via the wound drain. This requires emergency surgical exploration of the wound to release the clot (to prevent laryngeal oedema) and then achieve haemostasis
- *Mediastinal haemorrhage*—presents with hypovolaemic shock
- *Laryngeal oedema*—presents as stridor, rapidly progressing to respiratory obstruction. This requires endotracheal intubation
- *Thyrotoxic crisis*—presents with abrupt onset of extreme agitation and confusion, hyperpyrexia, profuse sweating and rapid tachycardia or other arrhythmia. This requires

emergency beta-adrenergic blockade, intravenous hydrocortisone and potassium iodide therapy. The mortality of thyrotoxic crisis is 10% from coma, pulmonary oedema or circulatory collapse. The condition is very rare if the patient has been rendered euthyroid before operation by drug treatment.
- *Tracheomalacia*—removal of a longstanding lesion compressing the trachea may lead to tracheal collapse and stridor

Later postoperative complications

- *Hypoparathyroidism* due to inadvertent parathyroid damage—presents with muscle cramps, paraesthesiae and tetany within 36 hours of operation. Treatment is with calcium and vitamin D analogues
- *Unilateral recurrent laryngeal nerve damage*—presents with hoarseness of voice and defective cough
- *External laryngeal nerve damage*—changes the quality of the voice

Long-term complications

- *Hypothyroidism*—often overlooked because it develops insidiously. Features are loss of energy, weight gain, depression and intellectual deterioration and intolerance of cold weather
- *Recurrent thyrotoxicosis*—insufficient gland removed

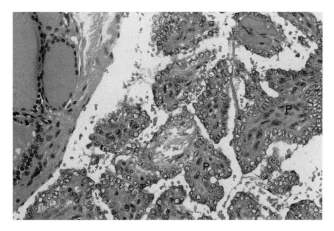

Fig. 49.11 Papillary carcinoma of the thyroid—histopathology
Tumour shows well-defined papillae **P** with many cells having large, clear nuclei. Despite its name, the diagnosis is based on these nuclear features, not on the presence of papillae. Normal thyroid tissue is also present.

between 30 and 45 years. Histologically, the tumour forms a complex branching papillary structure with a fibrovascular stroma, often containing characteristic calcified 'psammoma bodies'. Tumours vary over a wide range of epithelial dysplasia between apparently benign and obviously malignant. Whatever the degree of dysplasia, the tumours grow slowly. Papillary carcinomas are microscopically multicentric in about 80% of cases and about one-third affect both lobes; this is important in planning treatment. The tumour occasionally invades locally into trachea or oesophagus. Metastasis is to central cervical and later lateral cervical **lymph nodes** and only rarely to distant sites such as lung or bone. By the time of presentation, lymph nodes are involved in about 40% of patients (90% in children). Lymph node enlargement is often the sole presenting feature and the histology of involved lymph nodes is so close to normal thyroid tissue that at one time this condition was known as '**lateral aberrant thyroid**'. The prognosis of papillary carcinoma is the best of all thyroid carcinomas with only about 10% of patients dying of the tumour after 10 years (of remote metastases); it is remarkable that survival is hardly prejudiced by the presence of lymph node metastases. The prognosis is even better for '**minimal papillary carcinoma**', defined as a single tumour less than 1 cm in diameter in a young patient with no local invasiveness or metastases.

Symptoms and signs

Clinically, papillary carcinoma presents as a slow-growing solitary thyroid nodule or else an enlarged cervical lymph node close to the gland. The patient is euthyroid. If isotope scanning is performed, it usually shows no uptake in the palpable nodule. Sometimes, other tumour foci in the gland are large enough to also manifest as 'cold nodules'. The diagnosis is usually made nowadays by fine needle aspiration cytology of a solitary thyroid nodule. A patient presenting with just an enlarged cervical lymph node may be diagnosed unexpectedly as papillary carcinoma after excision biopsy and histological examination of the node.

Management

The standard management of papillary carcinoma is **total thyroidectomy** because of the high risk of other foci within the gland. Palpable cervical nodes are removed at the same operation. Technically, the operation is no more difficult than subtotal thyroidectomy but carries a higher risk of postoperative hypoparathyroidism. Total thyroidectomy has the added advantage that recurrent local disease, lymph node or distant metastases can then effectively be treated with radioiodine (^{131}I). This requires a very high TSH level, which only occurs if no normal thyroid tissue remains. A further advantage is that plasma thyroglobulin can then be used as a **tumour marker** to detect recurrent disease. After treatment, hormone replacement with oral thyroxine is always necessary at levels necessary to keep TSH close to zero to minimise the risk of stimulating any residual malignant cells. This treatment rarely causes problems. Tumour recurrence in cervical nodes is treated by excision and even this has little adverse effect on prognosis. External radiotherapy may be employed for local recurrence, or chemotherapy with doxorubicin for remote metastases.

Since papillary carcinomas progress so slowly and only about 15% develop contralateral lobe recurrence, some surgeons prefer to retain one thyroid lobe if the primary tumour is small and there are no palpable or isotope-detectable nodules. Their reasoning is that any further tumours can be removed later without reducing life expectancy.

Follicular carcinoma

Follicular carcinoma is another well-differentiated thyroid malignancy. Histologically, the neoplastic cells form a well-developed **follicular pattern** which is impossible to distinguish from benign adenomatous hyperplasia on fine needle aspiration cytology; even on histology of the surgical specimen, it may also be difficult to diagnose malignancy unless there is evident capsular or vascular invasion. Unlike papillary carcinoma, multicentricity is far less common. The peak incidence of follicular carcinoma is between 40 and 50 years of age, older than for papillary carcinoma, but it is still three times more common in women. Generally, follicular carcinoma grows slowly and metastasises at a late stage. In contrast to papillary carcinoma, metastasis tends to occur via the bloodstream to the lungs, bone and other remote sites rather than to local lymph nodes.

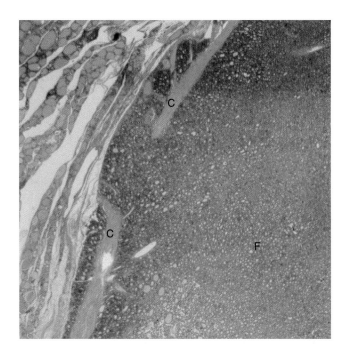

Fig. 49.12 Follicular carcinoma of the thyroid—histopathology
The tumour is made up of numerous small follicles **F** that are cytologically bland. Diagnosis of malignancy requires the demonstration of capsular and/or vascular invasion. In this higher power view, tumour can clearly be seen extending through the capsule **C**.

Since follicular carcinoma is rarely multicentric, management depends on the extent of local invasion (Fig. 49.12). A tumour with only microinvasion of the capsule has a very good prognosis and only requires removal of the thyroid lobe containing the tumour. If, however, there is gross capsular invasion or vascular invasion (or known remote metastases), total thyroidectomy is performed. The purpose of this is not to treat the local tumour but to enhance radioiodine uptake by metastatic lesions should this be required later for diagnosis, or any consequent treatment with high-dose radioiodine (as with papillary carcinoma).

Prognosis can be predicted by the degree of capsular and vascular invasion by the primary lesion and on histology. If there is no invasion, 10-year survival is close to 100% but this falls to about 30% if there is extensive local invasion.

Anaplastic carcinoma

Anaplastic carcinomas are extremely aggressive tumours with an appalling prognosis. Most patients die within a year of diagnosis. The tumours are found almost exclusively in the elderly. Most other cancers are less aggressive in this age group but for reasons unknown, thyroid carcinomas of this type are more aggressive.

Anaplastic carcinoma consists of sheets of very poorly differentiated cells which proliferate rapidly. The result is a diffuse, hard thyroid enlargement. The tumour soon invades surrounding structures, causing symptoms of tracheal and oesophageal obstruction and recurrent laryngeal nerve damage. There is also early dissemination to regional lymph nodes and haematogenous spread to the lungs, skeleton and brain.

Anaplastic carcinomas respond poorly to both radiotherapy and chemotherapy. The distressing symptoms of tracheal obstruction can sometimes be relieved by placing a luminal metal thyroid stent. This avoids the need for surgery but does nothing to slow the tumour growth.

Medullary carcinoma

This uncommon malignancy arises from parafollicular or C-cells. The tumour often secretes abnormal quantities of **calcitonin**, which can be used as a marker of tumour recurrence after excision. Tumours may also secrete other peptides and amines such as **serotonin** and **ACTH-like peptide**. Medullary carcinoma usually arises sporadically but may be transmitted genetically as part of the **multiple endocrine neoplasia syndrome type II (MEN II)**. This is an autosomal dominant trait with 50% penetrance and is associated with other APUD cell tumours, particularly **phaeochromocytoma** and **parathyroid adenomas**. Thus patients with medullary carcinoma of thyroid should be examined for these conditions before surgery as a phaeochromocytoma would take operative precedence.

Medullary carcinoma is of particular pathological interest because the stroma contains extensive deposits of **amyloid**. These make the tumour mass stony hard to palpation.

Medullary carcinoma grows relatively slowly, metastasising first to regional lymph nodes and later to lungs, bone, liver and elsewhere. The tumour does not take up radioiodine and is resistant to radiotherapy; hence an aggressive surgical approach is required. The standard treatment is total thyroidectomy and clearance of involved anterior cervical and superior mediastinal lymph nodes. Without metastases, operation is often curative but when nodes are involved, 10-year survival falls to about 50%. During follow-up, calcitonin levels are monitored and raised levels indicate tumour recurrence. Surgical re-exploration of the neck may be undertaken to remove involved lymph nodes.

Thyroid lymphoma

Lymphomas of the thyroid are rare and usually arise in pre-existing autoimmune (Hashimoto's) thyroiditis. Most are non-Hodgkin lymphomas. Diagnosis can only be made histologically, either by core needle biopsy or open biopsy, as FNA is not usually adequate. Treatment is with radiotherapy, and survival depends on whether spread has occurred beyond the thyroid capsule. For lesions confined within the capsule, 5-year survival is 85%, falling to 40% when local spread has occurred.

GOITRES AND THYROID NODULES

As indicated earlier in Table 49.1, several hyperplastic and metabolic disorders cause diffuse or nodular thyroid enlargement.

Idiopathic non-toxic thyroid hyperplasia

Most goitres referred to surgeons in developed countries are caused by simple, idiopathic hyperplasia of thyroid follicles. The condition probably begins with diffuse micronodular enlargement, and the nodules later become heterogeneously enlarged to form a **multinodular colloid goitre**. Within the same spectrum of disease are **solitary hyperplastic nodules** (which may actually be benign thyroid adenomas) and **thyroid cysts**, which are simply huge colloid-filled follicles or else contain straw-coloured fluid.

The aetiology of simple thyroid hyperplasia is unknown, but is probably related to disordered sensitivity to TSH. In this sense, the condition may be analogous to fibroadenosis of the breast. The patient is usually clinically euthyroid and thyroid function tests are normal. Sometimes, thyroid hormone secretion escapes from hypothalamic control so the patient becomes hyperthyroid and occasionally thyrotoxic.

Within the gland, secretory activity is heterogeneous, explaining the patchy distribution of radioiodine uptake on thyroid scanning. Focal hormone secretion from 'hot' adenomatous nodules may be so great as to completely suppress the rest of the gland. The overall hormone secretion may still be within the euthyroid range; this may be considered the most extreme form of secretory heterogeneity.

Diffuse or multinodular idiopathic goitres develop slowly and cause little trouble until they have been present for many years.

The reasons patients present to surgeons with thyroid enlargement are:

- A goitre has become so large as to be cosmetically unacceptable
- A localised lump has appeared in the thyroid region. This may be a solitary adenomatous nodule, a solitary cyst or, in 10% of cases, thyroid cancer. Alternatively, the apparent solitary lump may be part of an asymmetrical multinodular or multicystic enlargement
- A pre-existing multinodular goitre has undergone rapid asymmetric change. There are several possible causes, i.e. haemorrhage into a cyst or a degenerate area of hyperplasia, or malignant change

- The patient has become hyperthyroid
- The patient has developed stridor from tracheal compression caused by enlargement of a retrosternal extension of the thyroid

Surgical management of goitre

The indications for surgery in idiopathic goitre are:

- A lump suspicious of malignancy
- A retrosternal thyroid causing compression
- A solitary toxic nodule
- Toxic multinodular goitre
- Cosmetic deformity

In principle, only enough thyroid tissue is removed to achieve the objective, but in multinodular goitre recurrence is likely in the long term and a better mode of treatment is total thyroidectomy, with lifetime thyroxine replacement.

Patients presenting for cosmetic reasons with only moderate thyroid enlargement have often been treated with thyroxine. The theory is that when TSH is suppressed the gland may shrink to an acceptable size. Unfortunately, clinical trials have not shown this approach to be effective. Hyperthyroidism caused by idiopathic thyroid hyperplasia is unresponsive to anti-thyroid drugs and ineffectively treated with radioiodine; hence surgery is required if treatment is needed.

Thyroid cysts are diagnosed as fluid-filled lesions on ultrasound or by aspiration. Cytology should be performed to exclude malignancy. Large or recurrent cysts are best treated surgically.

CONGENITAL THYROID DISORDERS

Embryology

The thyroid originates as a diverticulum in the midline between the first two branchial pouches. Its origin is represented in the adult by the **foramen caecum**, visible at the junction of the anterior two-thirds and the posterior third of the tongue. The thyroid diverticulum forms the **thyroglossal duct** which extends caudally through the developing tongue musculature. It passes down in relation to the hyoid bone (in front of, through or behind it) to reach its normal position below the larynx. By this time, it has become a bilobed structure with the lobes connected by a narrow central **isthmus**. The thyroglossal duct later degenerates. The calcitonin-secreting C-cells originate from the **ultimobranchial body** of the fifth pouch.

Thyroglossal cyst and 'fistula'

Part of the thyroglossal duct may persist and become cystic. A thyroglossal cyst presents in children and occasionally adolescents as a smooth, rounded, anterior midline swelling in the neck. Most thyroglossal cysts occur below the hyoid, although rarely they are found in the submental region. A diagnostic feature is that the cyst rises when the patient swallows or protrudes the tongue. Most thyroglossal cysts are asymptomatic but they are prone to inflammation which causes pain and increased swelling. If an inflamed cyst is surgically drained, it may become an intermittently discharging sinus, often incorrectly described as a **thyroglossal fistula** (Fig. 49.13).

Thyroglossal cysts are usually excised along with the thyroglossal tract up to the base of the tongue. This requires removing the middle third of the hyoid bone (**Sistrunk's operation**). A persistent sinus or a recurrent cyst is likely to complicate incomplete excision.

Ectopic thyroid tissue

An ectopic thyroid gland is a rare congenital abnormality which results from interruption of normal descent. It may present in the same way as a thyroglossal cyst or as a lump in the tongue. As this may be the patient's only thyroid tissue, isotope scanning should be performed to check if there is thyroid tissue in the normal position before proceeding to excision.

Fig. 49.13 Thyroglossal 'fistula'

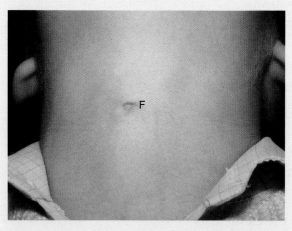

This photograph shows the front of the neck in a 14-year-old boy. An attempt had been made to remove a thyroglossal cyst several years previously. The inevitable result of incomplete surgical removal was an intermittently discharging fistula **F** in the midline of the neck.

DISORDERS OF PARATHYROID GLANDS

HYPERPARATHYROIDISM

Hyperparathyroidism is a disease characterised by excessive secretion of PTH, a polypeptide hormone containing 84 amino acids. Primary hyperparathyroidism (PHPT) is caused by excessive production of parathyroid hormone. It usually occurs in adults and is slightly more common in females. Increased parathormone increases osteoclastic activity, causing reduced bone density and hypercalcaemia. Many cases remain undetected but estimates from 'routine' calcium estimations suggest that about 1% of the adult population has primary hyperparathyroidism. About 80% of these are due to benign parathyroid adenoma. Most of the rest are due to hyperplasia of multiple parathyroid glands and less than 1% are due to parathyroid cancer.

SYMPTOMS AND SIGNS

Hyperparathyroidism is the most common clinical disorder of the parathyroid glands. Patients are usually referred to a surgeon after discovery of hypercalcaemia during investigation of **musculoskeletal pain** or **recurrent urinary tract calculi**. About half the affected people are likely to have the classical signs and symptoms of hypercalcaemia in addition to non-specific muscle weakness, thirst, polyuria, anorexia, weight loss and constipation. Classical clinical features are bone pain (with or without radiological changes of osteomalacia or osteitis fibrosa cystica), urinary tract stones, abdominal pain (caused by peptic ulcer or recurrent pancreatitis), and mental changes such as confusion, depression or even psychosis. These can be remembered by the aide mémoire **bones, stones, abdominal groans and psychic moans**.

In multiple endocrine neoplasia type I (MEN I), primary hyperparathyroidism may be associated with other hyperplastic endocrine disorders such as pancreatic islet cell tumours secreting insulin or gastrin or pituitary tumours. In MEN II, it may be associated with medullary carcinoma of the thyroid and/or phaeochromocytomas.

Hypercalcaemia is frequently found incidentally on biochemical screening and if patients are then shown to have raised parathormone levels, a diagnosis of hyperparathyroidism can be made. Many of these apparently asymptomatic patients turn out to have suffered non-specific symptoms of fatigue and malaise for years or have signs of hypertension or renal failure.

Secondary hyperparathyroidism occurs in renal failure and vitamin D deficiency (see below). In addition to osteomalacia and osteitis fibrosa cystica, patients also develop ectopic calcification, for example around joints and in arteries.

Raised plasma calcium levels cannot be tolerated for long without causing serious systemic problems or damage to bone. From Figure 49.14, it might seem paradoxical that urinary tract calculi are a common presenting feature of hyperparathyroidism, since parathormone *reduces* urinary calcium excretion. The probable reason for stone

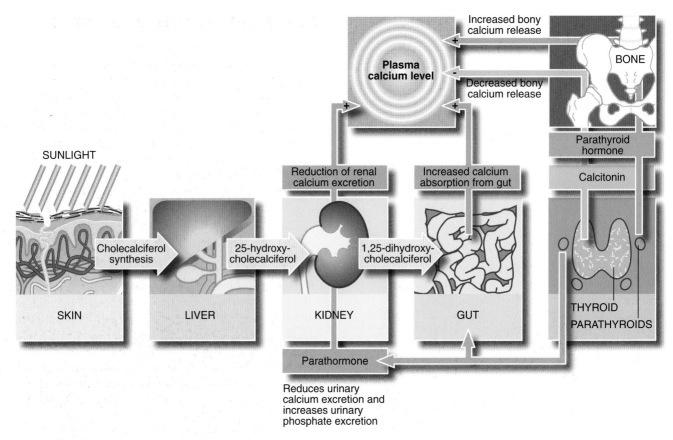

Fig. 49.14 Main control mechanisms for plasma calcium

formation is the excess phosphate excretion. This is associated with excessive urinary alkalinity, which predisposes to the precipitation of calcium salts.

CONTROL OF PLASMA CALCIUM (Fig. 49.14)

The plasma calcium level is normally maintained within a very narrow range by the combined effects of parathormone and vitamin D. The secretion rate of parathormone is governed directly by the plasma concentration of ionised calcium. If parathormone is overproduced, this raises the plasma calcium and causes phosphaturia, thereby decreasing serum phosphate.

Parathormone raises plasma calcium levels in the following ways:

- Increases osteoclastic activity and release of calcium from the bone matrix; this liberates calcium into the circulation
- Enhances renal tubular reabsorption of calcium and diminishes reabsorption of phosphate thereby increasing the renal clearance of phosphate
- In the presence of vitamin D, it promotes calcium absorption from the small intestine

Vitamin D (as cholecalciferol) is produced by the action of sunlight on cholesterol derivatives in the skin. Cholecalciferol is then converted to 25-hydroxycholecalciferol in the liver, and is further hydroxylated by the renal tubules to the active compound **1,25-dihydroxycholecalciferol**. This active compound is required for calcium absorption from the intestine. Calcitonin, produced by the C-cells of the thyroid gland, probably plays little part in normal calcium homeostasis.

Calcium homeostasis is thus dependent on normal functioning of parathyroids, liver and kidney, together with an adequate dietary intake of calcium and suitable quantities of vitamin D from diet or exposure to sunlight.

TYPES OF HYPERPARATHYROIDISM

Hyperparathyroidism is classified as follows:

Primary hyperparathyroidism

a. Single parathyroid adenoma
This is the most common cause of primary hyperparathyroidism, found in 80% of cases. One of the four parathyroid glands becomes replaced by an enlarged benign neoplasm which secretes parathormone in excessive amounts. Secretion by the other parathyroids is suppressed.

b. Diffuse parathyroid hyperplasia
This is an uncommon cause of primary hyperparathyroidism. The secretory cells of two or more of the glands

undergo idiopathic hyperplasia, resulting in excess hormone production.

c. Parathyroid carcinoma

This is extremely rare (1% of primary hyperparathyroidism) and involves only one of the parathyroid glands. These tumours are often palpable and cause gross elevation of plasma calcium.

Secondary and tertiary hyperparathyroidism

In **secondary hyperparathyroidism**, there is a chronic abnormal stimulus to parathormone production and the parathyroid glands undergo **diffuse hyperplasia**. This occurs most commonly in chronic renal failure (including nearly all patients on dialysis to some degree) but may also occur in vitamin D deficiency. The altered calcium/phosphate physiology in chronic renal insufficiency includes:

- Damage to the glomerulus causing phosphate retention which leads to hyperphosphataemia
- Hyperphosphataemia inhibits calcium absorption by the gut, thus reducing absorption of calcium to a minimum
- Renal tubular injury leads to reduced renal production of 1,25-dihydroxycholecalciferol (1,25-DHCC)
- The low blood calcium that results causes the negative feedback system to increase elaboration of parathormone. This promotes osteoclastic activity, restoring calcium levels but causing the bone disorders of osteomalacia and osteitis fibrosa cystica
- The raised product of calcium and phosphate in the blood leads to ectopic calcification in a variety of abnormal sites

After renal transplantation, hyperparathyroidism may persist if the hypertrophied parathyroid glands fail to return to normal. The glands continue to oversecrete parathormone in an autonomous fashion in the face of normal or even elevated serum calcium levels. This is described as **tertiary hyperparathyroidism** with clinical effects similar to secondary hyperparathyroidism.

Malignant hypercalcaemia

Hyperparathyroidism is only one cause of hypercalcaemia; the other main cause is malignant disease of various types. In 70%, this is due to secretion of **parathormone-related protein (PTH-rP)** and in the rest to widespread bone destruction from **lytic bone metastases**. The most common tumours to secrete PTH-rP are squamous cell carcinoma of the lung, renal cell carcinoma and bladder cancer. Tumours causing hypercalcaemia by bone destruction include breast cancer, leukaemias and multiple myeloma.

MANAGEMENT OF HYPERPARATHYROIDISM

Corrected plasma calcium levels are elevated in primary hyperparathyroidism but precise diagnosis was difficult before the advent of immunoassay for parathormone (PTH). Modern immunoassays use polyclonal antibodies marked by radioactive, luminescent or enzyme labels to recognise the PTH molecule. Elevated plasma calcium and PTH levels confirm the diagnosis of hyperparathyroidism in virtually all patients who do not have renal failure or metastatic disease.

In primary hyperparathyroidism, an **adenoma** can often be identified by radioisotope scanning using **sestamibi**, which is 2-methoxy isobutyl isonitrile labelled with technetium-99m. This is taken up by thyroid and any active parathyroid tissue but persists longer in the parathyroid, enabling an adenoma or sometimes a carcinoma to be localised. Normal or even hyperplastic parathyroids are so small that they are not detected by this method. In practice, ultrasound is usually employed in addition to look for an enlarged adenoma or carcinoma. **Diffuse hyperplasia** is best dealt with by surgical exploration of the neck and examination of all four parathyroid glands. Preoperative localisation can also be valuable prior to re-exploratory operations for recurrent hypercalcaemia.

Surgical management

Surgery is the only definitive treatment for primary and tertiary hyperparathyroidism. Secondary hyperparathyroidism is managed by treating renal failure and giving phosphate absorbent agents, although parathyroidectomy may be necessary if there is severe bone resorption. Hypercalcaemia due to ectopic parathormone production is managed medically as it is rarely possible to resect a tumour secreting parathormone-like protein.

There are normally two pairs of parathyroid glands, superior and inferior on each side, lying close to the thyroid. The superior pair usually lie close to where the inferior thyroid artery enters near the middle of the gland. The inferior pair are usually located below the lower poles of the thyroid or sometimes within the thymus gland retrosternally. They may be located elsewhere in a variety of sites including as low down as the aortic arch.

Parathyroid surgery is exacting and time-consuming, often interrupted by histological examination of several frozen section biopsies during the course of the operation. The surgical access is the same as for thyroidectomy. The likely anatomical position of each parathyroid is then meticulously explored in the search for parathyroid tissue. Although the parathyroids have a characteristic yellow-brown colour, they are often difficult to distinguish from thyroid tissue, especially if the tissues have been traumatised.

If one of the parathyroid glands is enlarged and the others are normal, the diagnosis is **parathyroid adenoma** or, rarely, **adenocarcinoma**. In either case, the abnormal gland is completely removed and the other glands left in situ. If an adenoma can be localised before operation, there is a trend to minimal surgery, simply removing the enlarged gland without exploring the rest of the neck.

If no individual gland is disproportionately enlarged, a diagnosis of diffuse hyperplasia can be made. In this case, there is a trend towards total parathyroidectomy rather than incomplete removal, now that plasma calcium can be controlled better medically. Some surgeons remove three and a half glands, while still others remove all the parathyroid tissue and reimplant a small mass of tissue in a forearm muscle pouch. If hyperparathyroidism persists, this parathyroid tissue is more readily removed than from the neck. The main problem with surgery for diffuse hyperplasia is that some parathyroid tissue may remain unidentified, however meticulous the surgery. In some units, plasma PTH is measured intraoperatively to ensure the operation is complete.

Complications of parathyroidectomy are similar to those of thyroid surgery (see Box 49.3 earlier). Hypoparathyroidism is more likely, however, and plasma calcium levels must be carefully monitored in the early postoperative period and treated if abnormally low.

HYPOPARATHYROIDISM

The most common cause of hypoparathyroidism is surgical removal or devascularisation of the parathyroid glands during thyroid or parathyroid surgery. It may also be a transient occurrence after excision of a parathyroid adenoma or subtotal parathyroidectomy, lasting until the remaining suppressed parathyroid tissue recovers normal function. Autoimmune hypoparathyroidism also occurs occasionally.

Hypoparathyroidism presents clinically with the effects of hypocalcaemia. A fall in the plasma calcium level increases neuromuscular excitability causing cramps or even **tetany** in severe cases. An early symptom of hypocalcaemia is paraesthesia, especially around the lips. After thyroid or parathyroid operations, patients should be asked if they have experienced any tingling around the mouth, and plasma calcium estimations should be performed the morning after operation, and again 24 hours later.

Clinical tests for hypocalcaemia include tapping over the parotid gland. This provokes transient contraction of the facial muscles and is known as **Chvostek's sign**. A further test involves inflating a sphygmomanometer cuff on the upper arm to above systolic pressure. This induces carpal spasm within about 3 minutes ('*main d'accoucheur*' or obstetrician's hand).

Early postoperative hypocalcaemia is treated with intravenous calcium gluconate. Persistent hypocalcaemia is controlled by oral administration of high doses of calcium and vitamin D.

Acute surgical problems in children

50

INTRODUCTION

A **neonate** is a newborn infant less than 28 days old, an **infant** is aged less than a year, a **child** is 1–15 years old and an **adult** is 16 or older. A large number of surgical conditions in children are treated by general surgeons with a special interest in paediatric surgery, but surgical problems in infants, major congenital abnormalities at any age and malignant tumours are usually managed in regional centres by specialist paediatric surgeons and urologists. Not only does the range of conditions seen in children differ from that seen in adults but the conditions themselves vary between different age groups. This is particularly true for conditions which present as acute emergencies. Reflecting this, paediatric emergencies are considered here under the headings of the **newborn** (the first few days of life, including premature babies), **infants and young children** (up to about 2 years) and **older children** (up to puberty). During puberty, the disorders merge with those of adulthood. Non-emergency and urogenital disorders tend to be less age specific and are discussed separately in the next chapter.

PHYSIOLOGICAL DIFFERENCES BETWEEN INFANTS AND ADULTS

Infants are not small adults and successful surgical management depends on understanding their physiological norms. For example, the **basal metabolic rate** is particularly high in the newborn, with an oxygen demand of 5–8 ml/kg/min. In older children and adults this falls to 2 ml/kg/min. The **blood volume** in a baby is only 80 ml per kg body weight, so operative technique needs to be meticulous to minimise blood loss. In an adult, the loss of 100 ml is negligible but to a small child it can be life threatening; even small blood losses need to be accurately measured and replaced if necessary during surgery.

FLUID AND ELECTROLYTE PROBLEMS

Fluid deficiency and **electrolyte imbalances** occur rapidly in children because each compartment has such a small fluid volume; in addition, paediatric fluid requirements are relatively greater than in adults. This is because the kidneys have a lower concentrating ability and the obligatory urine output is greater. Faecal fluid losses are also higher, particularly in children under 2 years; in severe diarrhoea, dehydration and electrolyte disturbances occur with frightening speed. Signs of fluid depletion are also somewhat different from adults. Young fluid-depleted children are often lethargic or drowsy and may even be comatose. The eyes and anterior fontanelle may be sunken but skin turgor is not lost. Tachycardia is usually present, but hypotension is a late sign because of efficient compensatory mechanisms. Urine output is likely to be low. The normal rate should be at least 1 ml per kg body weight per hour.

BLOOD GLUCOSE

Hypoglycaemia readily occurs because a baby's glycogen stores are meagre and there needs to be a constant supply of glucose by feeding or by intravenous infusion. Adrenergic responses to trauma and stress also increase glucose requirements. Hypoglycaemia is particularly likely to occur when a baby is fasted before surgery but is not given intravenous dextrose, or when a blood transfusion temporarily replaces intravenous dextrose. All small children undergoing surgery should have close monitoring of blood glucose to prevent hypoglycaemic brain damage.

TEMPERATURE REGULATION

Temperature regulation in infants is less robust than in older patients and **hypothermia** can be a real hazard. This is so for several reasons. Infants have a relatively large surface area, poor vasomotor control of skin blood vessels and an inability to generate heat by shivering. A controlled, heated environment is therefore necessary for operating upon and nursing newborn infants. For those under 1 kg, for example, the temperature is set between 34.5 and 35.5°C, and for those over 3 kg, between 31.5 and 34.5°C. For operations, a specially heated operating theatre is essential, with the infant placed on a heated mattress and all parts of the body except those close to the operating site kept insulated. Intravenous fluids and skin preparation antiseptics are warmed and anaesthetic gases humidified and warmed to prevent heat loss. Skin preparation should be aqueous rather than alcohol-based to prevent cooling by vaporisation.

LIVER FUNCTION

Liver function is immature during the newborn period. The common occurrence of physiological jaundice is caused by a high level of unconjugated bilirubin resulting from immaturity of the liver in synthesising the enzyme **glucuronyl transferase**. There is also a reduced ability to detoxify analgesic drugs; these must be used in greatly reduced doses compared with adults and the dose should be checked in a paediatric formulary before use. Another reason for reducing doses is that many drugs cross the blood–brain barrier more readily in young infants and are more likely to cause cerebral side effects. A further consequence of liver immaturity is reduced production of **prothrombin**. If prophylactic vitamin K was not given after the baby's birth, this can be rectified by giving intravenous vitamin K in the perioperative period. All babies undergoing major surgery should have clotting studies performed beforehand.

IMMUNITY

Infection can be rapidly fatal in small babies, particularly premature and immature small-for-dates babies who are likely to have defective immune mechanisms. Infection can be minimised by good surgical technique, meticulous haemostasis to avoid haematomas, and prophylactic antibiotics where appropriate.

MANAGING SURGERY IN INFANTS

The survival of babies undergoing complex surgery has steadily improved as their specific problems are better understood and better managed, often with surgeons and paediatricians working together. Examples include effective **total parental nutrition** to prevent babies dying from malnutrition whilst waiting for paralytic ileus to resolve, and an improved understanding of how mechanical ventilation should be managed. Specialised understanding of fluid and electrolyte balance, drug effects and nutritional needs is necessary for safe pre- and postoperative care of these small patients.

ABDOMINAL EMERGENCIES IN THE NEWBORN

The widespread use of **antenatal ultrasound** has meant that many congenital abnormalities that need surgical correction can be diagnosed before birth. Detectable abnormalities that require surgical correction soon after the baby is born include diaphragmatic hernia, abdominal wall defects such as gastroschisis and exomphalos, and cystic adenomatous lung malformations (CCAM). Once forewarned, parents can be counselled in advance and preparations made for operation. Most surgery is best done soon after birth but only very few conditions such as malrotation, gastroschisis or a tracheo-oesophageal fistula in a ventilated baby need truly urgent surgery. For these urgent cases, the delivery should be organised to take place at the hospital where the surgery will be carried out. Less urgent cases, such as a baby with exomphalos, can safely be left until the next day if born during the night, and posterior urethral valves simply need a bladder catheter before being investigated and then operated upon.

The more common abdominal emergencies in neonates are summarised in Box 50.1. All are congenital disorders with the exception of necrotising enterocolitis.

INTESTINAL OBSTRUCTION

Intestinal obstruction is the underlying phenomenon in most neonatal abdominal emergencies and occurs approximately once in every 2000 live births. Most causes of neonatal intestinal obstruction are not detectable by ultrasound before delivery. Complete obstruction, particularly of the proximal portion of the intestinal tract, prevents the fetus from swallowing amniotic fluid and this may result in **maternal polyhydramnios**. Just as in adults, intestinal obstruction presents with vomiting, constipation and abdominal distension.

In a baby, signs pointing to intestinal obstruction include poor feeding, failure to pass meconium and bile-stained vomiting. Abdominal distension may not occur at all in upper gastrointestinal tract obstruction. In lower gastrointestinal obstruction, distension may not be

> **Box 50.1 Main non-urological abdominal emergencies occurring in the newborn**
>
> - Incarcerated or strangulated inguinal hernia
> - Gastrointestinal atresias and stenoses
> - Midgut malrotation with volvulus
> - Anorectal abnormalities
> - Meconium ileus and other problems with meconium
> - Hirschsprung's disease
> - Congenital diaphragmatic hernia
> - Deficiencies in the abdominal wall (gastroschisis, exomphalos and ectopia vesicae)
> - Necrotising enterocolitis

obvious unless the baby is completely undressed. Meconium is normally passed within the first 24 hours in 80% of babies and delay beyond this is a cause for concern. Vomiting small amounts of milk, known as **posseting**, is normal in babies and simply reflects an immature gastro-oesophageal valve mechanism. However, **green vomiting** should be treated very seriously. Bile is normally yellow but when mixed with gastric juice for more than a short time, it turns green. Green vomitus is therefore a sign of gastric stasis and is caused by mechanical obstruction, paralytic ileus, or immaturity of the gut in a premature baby. Sepsis in babies from any source may cause a paralytic ileus.

The important causes of upper intestinal obstruction in babies are **duodenal atresia** and **malrotation with volvulus**. Causes of low obstruction include **Hirschsprung's disease** and **meconium ileus**. In addition, **small bowel atresia** may affect jejunum or ileum, causing high or low obstruction respectively. Confirming the diagnosis of intestinal obstruction after birth is usually possible with plain abdominal X-rays. When obstruction is high, there is a lack of intestinal gas (Fig. 50.1a); when low, there

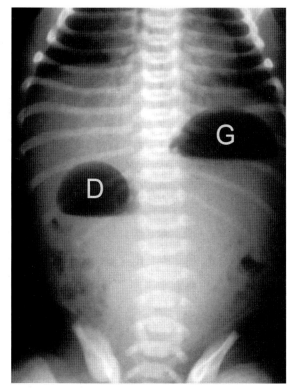

(a)

(a) Erect plain abdominal X-ray of a baby with 'high' intestinal obstruction, showing the typical 'double bubble' appearance of gas in the dilated stomach **G** and the first part of the duodenum **D**. The differential diagnosis includes duodenal atresia, malrotation with volvulus obstructing the duodenum and a very high jejunal atresia. Fluid levels are seen in this erect film.

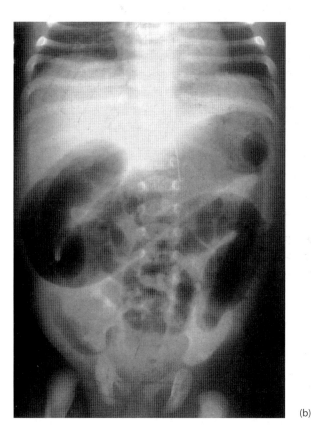

(b)

(b) Abdominal X-ray of a baby with a 'low' intestinal obstruction, showing several dilated loops of bowel. The differential diagnosis includes Hirschsprung's disease, meconium ileus and ileal atresia.

Fig. 50.1 Intestinal obstruction

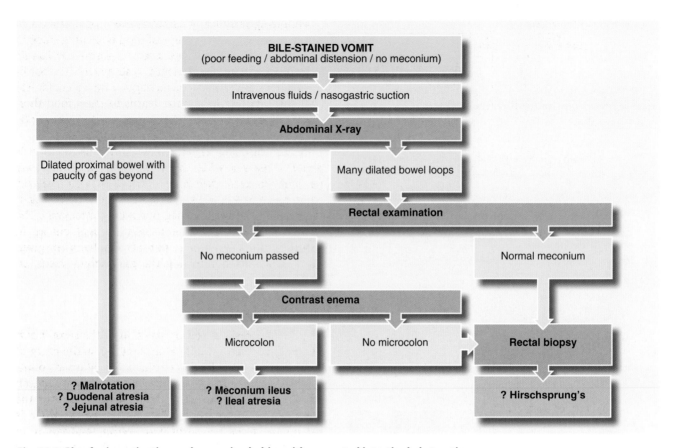

Fig. 50.2 Plan for investigating and managing babies with suspected intestinal obstruction

are numerous dilated loops of bowel (Fig. 50.1b). If malrotation is suspected, an upper gastrointestinal contrast study can determine the abnormal position of the duodeno-jejunal flexure. Other causes of obstruction such as an incarcerated inguinal hernia or imperforate anus can be detected by clinical examination without need for X-ray. A plan for investigating and managing babies with suspected obstruction is outlined in Figure 50.2.

If transfer to a specialist paediatric centre is necessary, the newborn infant must be placed in a portable incubator to maintain body temperature. Oxygen and suction must be available on the journey, and frequent gastric aspiration via a nasogastric tube reduces the risk of inhalation pneumonitis. Endotracheal intubation is vital for infants with respiratory insufficiency.

GASTROINTESTINAL ATRESIAS AND STENOSES

Atresia is defined as complete obliteration of a segment of the gastrointestinal tract, which is thus totally obstructed. In some cases of obstruction, a web partially or completely occludes the lumen. A **stenosis** is an indistensible narrowing causing partial obstruction. These problems are most common in the oesophagus, the small intestine, and in the colon following necrotising enterocolitis.

Oesophageal and duodenal atresias and ano-rectal malformations are true embryological abnormalities and are often associated with other congenital abnormalities. For example major cardiac, vertebral or renal abnormalities are found in 40% of babies with oesophageal atresia, and 30% of cases of duodenal atresia are found in infants with Down's syndrome. In contrast, small bowel atresias result from intrauterine **mesenteric vascular accidents** or failure of canalisation of the bowel and are rarely associated with other congenital abnormalities.

Oesophageal abnormalities

Potentially lethal oesophageal abnormalities occur in 1 in 3000 live births and there is associated **polyhydramnios** in nearly 30%. Oesophageal atresia with a distal tracheo-oesophageal fistula (TOF; Fig. 50.3) accounts for 90% of these, pure oesophageal atresia without a fistula accounts for 5% and several other variations account for the other 5%. Babies with oesophageal atresia may have other congenital abnormalities as part of a spectrum of disorders, the **VACTERL** association. This may include one or more V—vertebral, A—anorectal, C—cardiac, T—TOF, E—'esophageal' atresia, R—renal and L—limb abnormalities.

The diagnosis of oesophageal atresia may be suspected before birth if there is an absent gastric bubble on ultrasound scan, together with polyhydramnios, however these are not reliable signs. If a newborn infant has exces-

Following technically successful reconstruction, dysphagia can occur, with lumps of food becoming stuck in the oesophagus. This is because the normal peristaltic wave carrying food from mouth to stomach is uncoordinated after surgery. It can be managed with a diet of finely chopped food until the child learns to chew food thoroughly; this is often well after the age of 4. Anastomotic strictures can also occur and need dilatation.

In pure **oesophageal atresia without a fistula** there is almost always a wide gap between upper and lower oesophagus. Reconstruction is carried out using a gastric, colonic or small bowel conduit when the baby is bigger. Until then, feeding is carried out via a gastrostomy. The end of the upper pouch is usually brought out as an oesophagostomy in the neck so that the baby can be given **sham feeds** when receiving the gastrostomy feeds, so swallowing can be learnt.

Duodenal obstruction

Duodenal atresia causes obstruction of the second part of the duodenum, usually at a point below the entry of the common bile duct; this results in **bile-stained vomiting**. The anomaly is either a complete or incomplete web across the lumen or else a complete separation of the bowel ends. If the web contains an opening, there is usually an initial period of poor feeding and failure to thrive until some time later when a milk curd becomes impacted causing complete obstruction. Duodenal atresia presents in a similar manner.

Plain abdominal X-ray in either condition shows a **double bubble** appearance, with one air–fluid interface in the stomach and another in the first part of the duodenum (Fig. 50.1a).

Provided there is no malrotation or volvulus, surgical reconstruction does not have to be done immediately. Surgery involves joining proximal duodenum to duodenum distal to the obstruction to form a duodeno-duodenostomy. The two ends can easily be brought together without tension so a bypass procedure is never necessary. At one time, gastrojejunostomy was the procedure of choice but this often led to complications. These included bacterial colonisation of the defunctioned loop causing failure to thrive, stomal ulceration and gastrointestinal bleeding. Recovery after duodeno-duodenostomy is often slow because the proximal duodenum is atonic and peristalsis is slow to start, even though the obstruction has been relieved.

Jejuno-ileal atresias

The mechanisms of obstruction in jejunal or ileal atresia are similar to duodenal atresia, with a gap between the bowel ends or an intraluminal web. A gap is often the result of a vascular accident to the mesentery in utero. Obstructions occur at any level and are sometimes multiple. Bile-stained vomiting and abdominal distension are

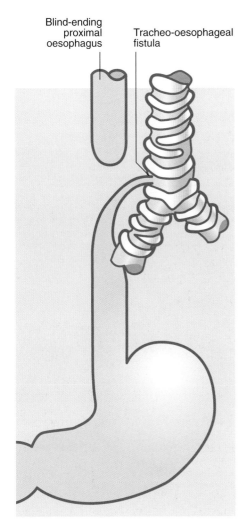

Blind-ending proximal oesophagus   Tracheo-oesophageal fistula

Fig. 50.3 Oesophageal atresia with tracheo-oesophageal fistula
The most common variant of oesophageal atresia, found in 90% of cases. Air enters the gastrointestinal tract via the fistula and may be seen on plain X-ray. 'Frothy' breathing may occur because the mouth and pharynx are full of saliva.

sive frothy saliva around the mouth, this diagnosis must be excluded before feeding. This is to prevent choking or cyanotic attacks and fluid entering the lungs by aspiration from the blind upper pouch or by regurgitation of gastric acid from the stomach via the fistula. Aspiration pneumonia is a serious complication. The diagnosis of oesophageal atresia is made by passing a nasogastric tube (10 F gauge) through the mouth. If gastric contents are not aspirated, a plain X-ray showing the tube in the upper oesophageal pouch confirms the diagnosis. If the oesophagus is obstructed but there is gas present in the stomach, this indicates there must be a fistula between the distal oesophagus and the trachea.

Operation is performed soon after diagnosis and after a search for any other congenital abnormalities. The majority are corrected by division of the fistula and primary oesophageal anastomosis. Oral feeding can be started a few days after surgery in uncomplicated cases.

often associated with **visible peristalsis** and hypertrophied proximal bowel. The diagnosis is usually evident from the plain abdominal X-ray.

Obstruction in jejunal or ileal atresia may be present from birth or may be delayed a few days if a web has an opening that allows passage of some intestinal contents. Signs at presentation depend on the level of obstruction. A high jejunal obstruction presents in a similar manner to duodenal atresia or malrotation with bile-stained vomiting and a lack of gas on the abdominal X-ray (Fig. 50.1a). A low ileal obstruction presents in a similar manner to meconium ileus or Hirschsprung's disease, with failure to pass meconium, poor feeding, abdominal distension and numerous dilated loops of intestine on the abdominal X-ray. Small bowel atresia is sometimes associated with cystic fibrosis, and babies with atresia should have a genetic screen and a sweat test to exclude cystic fibrosis.

Surgical treatment involves resecting the segment containing the web or the blind ends and reconstruction by end-to-end anastomosis. As with duodenal atresia, return of intestinal function may be slow, but may be accelerated if the segment of most dilated and atonic proximal bowel is resected at the operation (Fig. 50.4).

MIDGUT MALROTATION WITH VOLVULUS
(Fig. 50.5)

Pathophysiology

During early embryological development, the midgut develops outside the abdominal cavity. By the end of the third month, it has normally taken up its place within the abdominal cavity, having rotated 270° anti-clockwise in the process. When rotation is complete, there is a normally formed duodeno-jejunal (DJ) flexure and the caecum lies in the right iliac fossa. This produces a wide

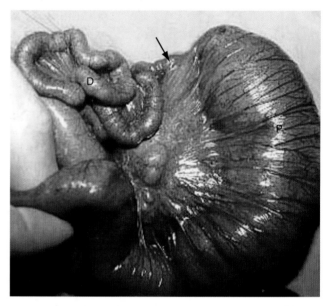

Fig. 50.4 Jejunal atresia
Findings at laparotomy on a neonate presenting with intestinal obstruction. The proximal jejunum **P** is greatly dilated whilst the distal jejunum is collapsed **D**. In between is an atretic segment without a lumen (arrow). This was resected and the bowel ends joined. The infant thrived soon afterwards.

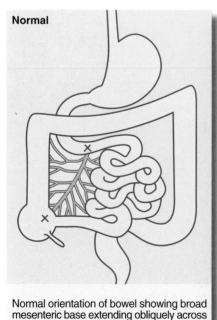

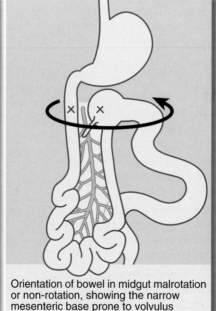

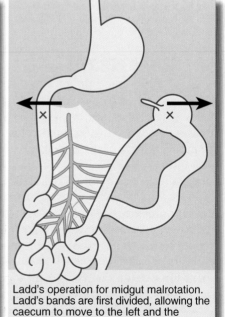

Normal orientation of bowel showing broad mesenteric base extending obliquely across the posterior abdominal wall

Orientation of bowel in midgut malrotation or non-rotation, showing the narrow mesenteric base prone to volvulus

Ladd's operation for midgut malrotation. Ladd's bands are first divided, allowing the caecum to move to the left and the duodeno-jejunal flexure to the right, the opposite of normal

Fig. 50.5 Midgut malrotation and volvulus

base to the midgut mesentery which stretches obliquely across the posterior abdominal wall so that volvulus does not occur. If rotation is **incomplete**, the duodeno-jejunal flexure lies to the right of the midline whereas it normally lies to the left; the fixation of the mesentery to the posterior abdominal wall is narrow and volvulus is likely to occur (Fig. 50.5). At one time **Ladd's bands** (local peritoneal folds stretching across the duodenum) were believed to be responsible for the obstruction but it is now known that volvulus is the usual cause.

Acute volvulus

Children born with malrotation may undergo **acute volvulus** at any time. In this condition, the mass of bowel can twist on its axis, occluding the superior mesenteric vessels (the vessels of the midgut), causing intestinal ischaemia and infarction. This is a surgical emergency presenting as high intestinal obstruction with bile-stained vomiting. There are features on plain radiographs similar to any other cause of high obstruction such as duodenal atresia (Fig. 50.1a). Previously well babies or children who present acutely with a sudden onset of duodenal obstruction, particularly if associated with signs of peritonitis, should have very urgent surgery so as to improve the chances of preventing midgut infarction. At operation, the bowel is untwisted and any gangrenous bowel resected. Note that if there is insufficient small bowel remaining, **short bowel syndrome** is likely, resulting in inadequate absorption of nutrients later. Surgery also involves dividing the Ladd's bands stretching across the duodenum. This broadens the base of the mesentery by moving the duodenum to the right and the caecum to the left (Fig. 50.5c). A stable situation is thus created without risk of volvulus.

Intermittent obstruction

If an older child has a history of intermittent bile-stained vomiting, an upper gastrointestinal contrast study can demonstrate an abnormal position of the duodeno-jejunal flexure. Elective surgery may then be appropriate to broaden the base of the mesentery.

ANORECTAL ABNORMALITIES

The primitive hindgut forms the **cloaca** in the early embryo and a septum then divides it into an **anterior compartment** from which the urinary tract and part of the genital tract are formed, and a **posterior compartment** from which the rectum and upper part of the anal canal are formed. The lower portion of the anal canal is developed from an invagination of ectoderm.

There is a wide spectrum of congenital anorectal disorders (imperforate anus) that has led authors to construct complex classifications. However, from a clinical standpoint it is sufficient to separate imperforate anus into **high and low varieties** according to whether the bowel terminates above or below levator ani. In nearly all cases, there is a fistula from the end of the bowel. When the malformation is low, the fistula opens to skin anterior to the sphincter muscle complex and meconium may emerge from it; because of this, the abnormality may not be immediately recognised (Fig. 50.6). Newborn babies need to be carefully examined to ensure the anus is situated correctly. In high malformations, there may also be a fistula. This communicates with the urethra in the male and the vagina in the female. **Urinary tract malformations** and lower vertebral anomalies are commonly associated with anorectal abnormalities and should be sought in affected babies.

In suspected anorectal abnormalities, the perineum is carefully examined for the presence of a fistula. If one is not found, it is worth waiting for 24 hours and then examining the perineum under anaesthesia for a fistula. If one is not found then the anomaly is treated as high and a colostomy performed as a first stage.

Treatment depends on the level of the distal pouch. In **low lesions**, the main pelvic muscle of continence

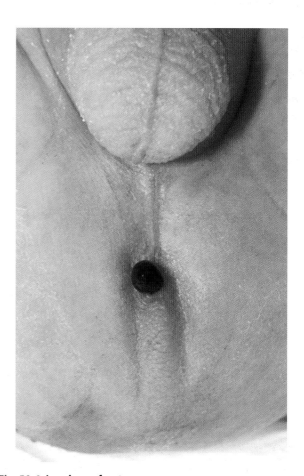

Fig. 50.6 Low imperforate anus
This shows an infant's perineum with an anterior fistula through which meconium has passed; the sphincter complex lies posterior to the fistula. The presence of visible meconium makes the diagnosis easy to miss.

(puborectalis) is well formed and operations via the perineum are often sufficient. An **anoplasty** is performed, increasing the calibre of the fistula and moving the opening to within the sphincter complex. **High lesions** require a preliminary colostomy to allow the baby to feed and empty the bowel, followed by complicated reconstruction later; these involve mobilising the bowel end and reconstructing the sphincter mechanism around it. The essence of the operation is the accurate apposition and repair of the levator muscles and the external anal sphincter. Long-term faecal continence and bowel control is imperfect in many children with both low and high anomalies, and constipation can be a problem in both groups.

FAILURE TO PASS MECONIUM

MECONIUM ILEUS

In meconium ileus, the distal ileum is obstructed by abnormal thick, viscid meconium and mucus plugs. About 95% of babies with this condition have **cystic fibrosis** and all babies with meconium ileus must be tested for this condition. The colon and rectum distal to the obstruction are of very small calibre. This microcolon results from the fact that no bowel contents have passed down it rather than any inherent abnormality (Fig. 50.7).

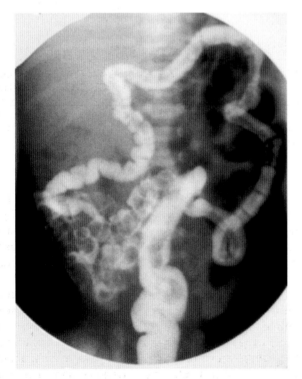

Fig. 50.7 Gastrografin enema in meconium ileus
Gastrografin enema X-rays in a baby with meconium ileus, showing the microcolon and the filling defects caused by abnormal meconium obstructing the distal ileum.

The condition presents soon after birth with lower intestinal obstruction; the diagnosis is suspected when rectal examination reveals a patent but very narrow rectum. An enema examination with Gastrografin may demonstrate the inspissated meconium in the distal ileum and may also break up the material by a detergent-like action, thereby relieving the obstruction. Laparotomy is required for unrelieved obstruction or those who have signs of peritonitis. The maximally dilated loop of ileum containing the inspissated meconium is resected and a primary anastomosis performed in most cases.

Babies with cystic fibrosis have an abnormality of mucus-secreting glands which causes secondary changes in the lungs, liver, pancreas and small bowel. Pancreatic enzymes which normally liquefy meconium are deficient and the thick meconium causes intestinal obstruction. Pancreatic enzyme supplements are given to prevent malabsorption and in an attempt to prevent the equivalent of meconium ileus in older children. Regular physiotherapy is given to help prevent pulmonary complications.

HIRSCHSPRUNG'S DISEASE (CONGENITAL AGANGLIONOSIS)

Hirschsprung's disease (Harald Hirschsprung 1830–1916) is a congenital abnormality of part of the distal intestine which affects all of the intramural autonomic nerves and causes intestinal obstruction. Ganglion cells are absent from the inter-myenteric and submucosal plexuses, and the parasympathetic and sympathetic nerves are scattered in a disorderly way throughout the layers of the bowel wall. The aganglionosis always involves the rectum, extending into the sigmoid in 80% and reaching to the small bowel in 5%. The pathology is continuous without skip lesions.

Peristalsis is deficient in the affected bowel and the internal anal sphincter does not relax. The baby therefore has a **functional obstruction of the bowel** that usually presents soon after birth with intestinal obstruction, but can present in later childhood with constipation and failure to thrive (Fig. 50.8). About 80% of normal babies pass meconium within the first 24 hours but about 80% of babies with Hirschsprung's disease do not, and this is a diagnostic pointer.

Rectal examination may allow an explosive release of air and meconium. Rectal biopsy is the definitive investigation and should be carried out in all children in whom a diagnosis of Hirschsprung's disease is entertained; contrast radiology is unnecessary. Mucosal biopsies show absent ganglion cells in the myenteric plexus and an increase in cholinesterase-positive (parasympathetic) nerves. A severe form of enterocolitis may occur in infants where the diagnosis of congenital aganglionosis has been delayed, and death may result from profound circulatory collapse.

Definitive surgery for Hirschsprung's may be carried out at any time after birth but is often delayed until the

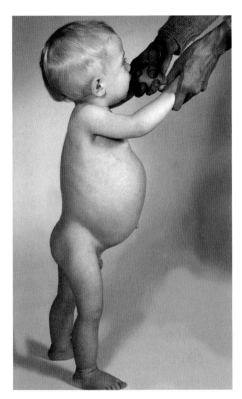

Fig. 50.8 Hirschsprung's disease
A historical photograph of a 3-year-old child with neglected Hirschsprung's disease demonstrating failure to thrive with buttock wasting and a dilated abdomen.

baby reaches 10 kg. In the first instance a colostomy is sited in normal ganglionic bowel to allow the baby to feed and grow. Definitive surgery involves removing the entire length of aganglionic bowel and joining normal bowel to the rectum at the level of the dentate line.

CONGENITAL DIAPHRAGMATIC HERNIA

The diaphragm is developed from a complex of embryological structures which include the mesoderm of the septum transversum, the lateral pleuroperitoneal folds and the dorsal mesentery of the embryo. The **phrenic nerve** arises from the area of origin of the septum transversum in the cervical region. Fusion of the various segments of the diaphragm takes place round about the eighth week of gestation.

Failure of closure of the **pleuroperitoneal canal** results in the most common type of congenital diaphragmatic hernia (Fig. 50.9b) which is postero-lateral in position. The incidence is 1 : 3500 live births and 80% are on the left side. Abdominal viscera lie in the chest, displacing the mediastinum to the contralateral side and interfering with lung development (Fig. 50.9a). The pulmonary hypoplasia may be so severe as to be incompatible with life.

Diagnosis is now frequently made before birth on antenatal ultrasound screening. The infants develop signs

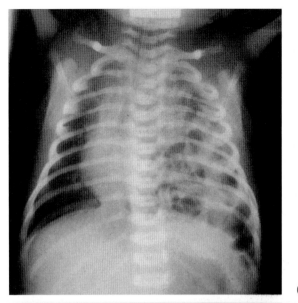

(a)

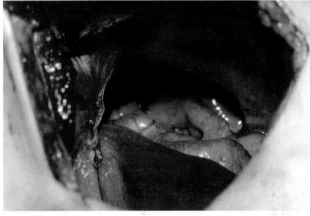

(b)

Fig. 50.9 Congenital diaphragmatic hernia
(a) Plain chest X-ray showing air-containing loops of bowel in the left chest and displacement of the mediastinum to the right. Note the endotracheal tube in place to allow assisted ventilation. **(b)** An operative picture viewed from the abdomen, showing the pleuro-peritoneal canal defect in the diaphragm. Some of the intestine had already been reduced from the thorax.

of respiratory distress soon after birth and survival depends on residual lung volume and its function. Cyanosis, mediastinal shift and an 'empty' (scaphoid) abdomen are the classic signs and the diagnosis is easily confirmed on a chest X-ray. Cardiac malformations may be associated with congenital diaphragmatic hernias.

The initial treatment is nasogastric decompression to prevent air entering the bowel in the chest so as to keep pulmonary compression to a minimum. Assisted ventilation is the mainstay of treatment to prevent the baby becoming hypoxic or acidotic. If this happens, the abnormally thick-walled pulmonary arterioles of the hypoplastic lung shut down, causing pulmonary hypertension and right-to-left shunting with a potential fatal outcome. Extra corporeal membrane oxygenation (ECMO) can be useful to maintain systemic oxygen saturation in the event of pulmonary hypertension.

Urgent surgery is rarely beneficial in the severely compromised child and is usually delayed until the baby is stable and requiring minimal ventilation. At operation, the diaphragmatic defect is closed via an abdominal incision. In many cases a complete diaphragm can be fashioned by suturing diaphragmatic remnants together after drawing the viscera out of the thoracic cavity. Large defects may require a patch of prosthetic material or a flap of abdominal wall muscle to achieve satisfactory closure. The position of the duodeno-jejunal flexure needs to be assessed, as **midgut malrotation** is present in 25% of babies born with a diaphragmatic hernia. Surgery to prevent volvulus is carried out if this is the case.

Despite advances in care, including better ventilation and ECMO, the mortality of babies born with a diaphragmatic hernia is high; survival has remained at between 60 and 70% for many years.

OTHER SURGICAL CONDITIONS CAUSING RESPIRATORY PROBLEMS IN THE NEWBORN

VASCULAR RING

This abnormality is caused by persistence of a double aortic arch or by abnormal configurations of the vessels that arise from the aortic arch. Either type of abnormality encircles the trachea and oesophagus resulting in compression. Symptoms include noisy breathing noted by the parents during the first few weeks of life and sometimes acute apnoeic events accompanied by cyanosis. Sometimes there is a history of persistent respiratory symptoms without frank stridor which have often been treated as asthma or bronchiolitis. In children with severe symptoms, treatment is essential and consists of dividing the smaller element of a double aortic arch or correction of the abnormal vessel anatomy. Children with only mild symptoms may improve spontaneously with growth. Oesophageal symptoms include vomiting, choking or dysphagia and tend to occur in older infants and children. Occasionally dysphagia or respiratory symptoms appear only later in childhood or adulthood.

CONGENITAL CYSTIC ADENOMATOUS MALFORMATIONS OF THE LUNG

The abnormality usually affects one part of the lung, most frequently one or other of the lower lobes. The cysts result from abnormal development of lung parenchyma. Large lesions can cause acute respiratory symptoms by compression of the normal lung and there is a risk of malignant change.

CONGENITAL LOBAR EMPHYSEMA

This condition usually affects an upper lobe of the right or left lung. A developmental weakness in a lobar bronchus allows air to enter the lobe, but bronchial collapse occurs during expiration and prevents deflation. Increasing lobar expansion compresses normal lung tissue and leads to deteriorating respiratory function. Surgical excision of the emphysematous lobe is relatively straightforward and curative.

ABDOMINAL WALL DEFECTS

Major deficiencies in the anterior abdominal wall are dramatically obvious at birth. They originate from a midline defect in the abdominal wall so that much of the bowel (and sometimes other viscera) lies outside the abdominal cavity, with or without a membranous covering. In **exomphalos** (Fig. 50.10), the viscera are invested with a layer of amnion whereas in **gastroschisis** (Fig. 50.11) coils of bare gut are exposed. **Ectopia vesicae** (exstrophy of the urinary bladder) is the rarest of the major abdominal wall defects and is more common in boys. It presents as a defect between the rectus muscles and the pubic bones with a failure of development of the entire anterior wall and neck of the bladder and urethra.

EXOMPHALOS

In exomphalos, the abdominal wall defect may be large (major) or small (minor). Babies with this problem may also have congenital cardiac problems, neural tube defects (spina bifida or anencephaly), chromosomal abnormalities or Beckwith–Wiedemann syndrome (gigantism, exomphalos, macroglossia, risk of neonatal hypoglycaemia and predisposition to intra-abdominal tumours, especially Wilms' tumours).

In **exomphalos major** there is a defect in the midline of the abdomen and part of the abdominal wall is missing. The defect may be up to 20 cm in diameter and can affect most of the anterior abdominal wall. At birth the bowel is covered with a sac of amnion and peritoneum; this ruptures spontaneously in utero and presents as a gastroschisis. Rupture after birth is rare in Western countries but may occur in developing countries where exomphalos is likely to be treated conservatively. Rupture allows evisceration of the bowel, predisposing to infection and sepsis. Treatment is described below, along with gastroschisis.

Exomphalos minor, herniation of the umbilical cord, does not exceed 5 cm in diameter. The bowel can be reduced with ease and the abdominal wall repaired as a primary surgical procedure.

GASTROSCHISIS

This is an abdominal wall defect characterised by herniation of bowel through a slit-like defect to the

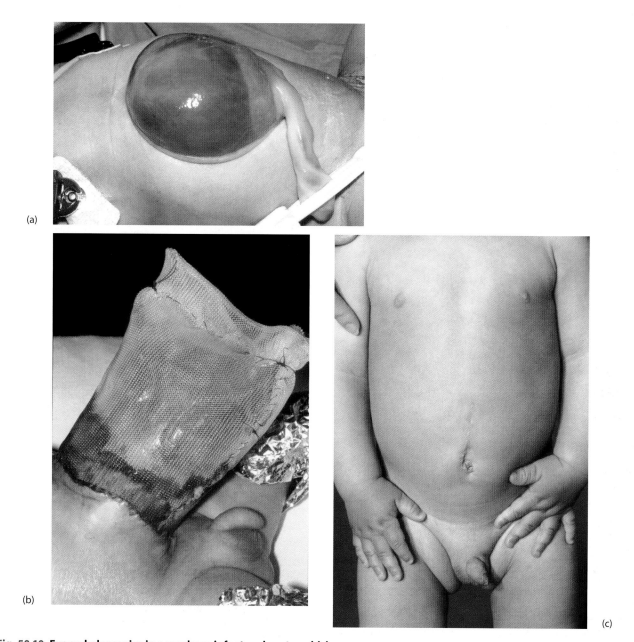

(a)

(b)

(c)

Fig. 50.10 Exomphalos major in a newborn infant and gastroschisis
(a) The amnion covering the liver and intestine can be clearly seen. Note the clamp on the umbilical cord. **(b)** In a different child with gastroschisis, the intra-abdominal volume was too small to contain the viscera so a silo was sutured in place to protect the viscera and to allow progressive reduction of the contents. **(c)** The child one year after reduction and abdominal wall closure.

right of the umbilicus. Unlike exomphalos there are few other associated congenital problems, although babies may be small and are often born prematurely. The defect is usually about 3 cm long and the bowel has no covering membrane (Fig. 50.11). The narrowness of the abdominal wall defect may impair the intestinal blood supply early on causing **small bowel atresias**. In addition, **malrotation** is usually present because the bowel has not fully assumed its correct position within the abdomen. Exposure to amniotic fluid before birth can cause widespread adhesions and shortened oedematous bowel loops.

Treatment of exomphalos major and gastroschisis

The aim of surgery is to reduce the viscera into the abdomen and close the abdominal wall. In gastroschisis, treatment is frequently possible by primary abdominal wall closure but this is possible less often in exomphalos where part of the abdominal wall is missing. Primary closure is often inadvisable here because the abdominal cavity has never expanded to its normal capacity and replacing the viscera would cause diaphragmatic splinting and inferior vena caval compression. In these cases, a **silo bag** covering the intestine can be sutured in place (Fig. **737**

Fig. 50.11 Gastroschisis

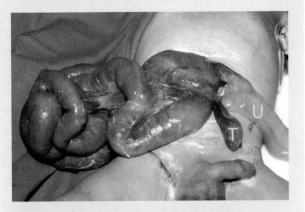

Gastroschisis in a newborn infant. The defect in the abdominal wall is small, lying to the right of the umbilicus. The intestine has no covering and loops are somewhat matted together by fibrinous adhesions. A testis **T** can be seen lying outside the abdomen on the left. The umbilical cord **U** is also visible. The treatment of this infant is shown in Figure 50.10b and c.

50.10b) and the bowel progressively reduced over several days by putting tucks into the silo, thus expanding the intra-abdominal volume. A formal repair of the abdomen is performed when this process is complete. Intravenous feeding is usually needed until normal bowel activity returns. The mortality rate for even these large lesions requiring a silo is low except where there are associated cardiac malformations.

ECTOPIA VESICAE

Ectopia vesicae is a very rare and complex abnormality which presents at birth with bladder mucosa exposed on the anterior abdominal wall and penile epispadias. The pubic bones may be widely separated causing posterior rotation of the hip joints. Treatment involves closure of the defect and repair of the epispadias, endeavouring to achieve urinary continence but without causing back-pressure on the kidneys. If continence fails to become established, urinary diversion to the abdominal wall via a bowel conduit may become necessary.

NECROTISING ENTEROCOLITIS

Necrotising enterocolitis (NEC) is a common condition that occurs in newborn babies. It may run a relatively benign course or it may be rapidly fatal. Babies affected are almost invariably premature, small-for-dates or seriously ill in special care baby units. The pathophysiology of this inflammatory condition is poorly understood but it involves diminution in blood flow to the intestine causing relative ischaemia of the bowel wall; the wall then becomes invaded by gas-producing bacteria. This may result in transmural inflammation, necrosis and perforation. The condition can affect small and large bowel and may be part of a more generalised illness with multisystem failure. The diagnosis can be made on clinical grounds if a neonate has bile-stained vomiting, passage of blood per rectum and abdominal distension; the diagnosis is confirmed on X-ray by finding intramural gas in the intestine. Necrotising enterocolitis may progress to bowel necrosis, perforation and generalised peritonitis.

Treatment involves vigorous resuscitation with intravenous fluids, nasogastric decompression and broad-spectrum antibiotics. Laparotomy and probable surgical resection is indicated if medical treatment is failing or if the intestine perforates and free intraperitoneal gas is seen on X-ray. Unfortunately mortality remains high in the severe cases.

CLEFT LIP AND PALATE

Cleft lip and palate are the most common congenital abnormalities of orofacial structure. A cleft upper lip is an obvious and unsightly deformity of facial appearance, causing great parental distress. Modern surgical techniques that concentrate on muscle repair give better cosmetic results than older ones but secondary cosmetic surgery is often required for the nose and lip. A cleft palate affects the child's ability to eat, speak, hear and breathe. Children with cleft palate may have trouble speaking, their voices sound nasal and do not carry well, and speech may be difficult to understand. Well-timed and skilled surgery together with speech therapy can help. Children with clefts often have missing, malformed or displaced teeth requiring dental and orthodontic treatment. They also often have a defective alveolar ridge that can displace or rotate permanent teeth and prevent permanent teeth from erupting. Both oral surgery and orthodontic tooth movement may be necessary at some stage.

Approximately half of all affected children have a cleft as the only congenital abnormality, but the other half have cardiac and other anomalies, or the cleft occurs as part of a congenital syndrome, e.g. Pierre Robin, Stickler or Treacher Collins. Ambroise Paré first wrote about repair of cleft palate in 1575 but the founder of modern cleft surgery was Philbert Joseph Roux of Paris in the early 1800s.

EMBRYOLOGY

The embryonic facial structure emerges between 4 and 7 weeks of gestation, from migration and fusion of the mesenchymal somite-derived facial elements, the frontonasal, bilateral maxillary and mandibular processes.

Facial clefts develop along embryonic fusion lines when the process is interrupted. The developing medial and lateral nasal processes and the maxillary prominences form the **primary palate** (lip and palate anterior to the primitive incisive foramen). The **secondary palate** (posterior two-thirds of the hard palate and the soft palate) develops separately at around 9 weeks; palatal clefts result when the palatal shelves of the maxillary processes fail to fuse. Palatal defects may be complete or involve only the posterior part; a **complete palatal cleft** involves primary and secondary palates, while an **incomplete cleft** involves only the secondary palate.

PRESENTATION

Cleft lip is readily diagnosed antenatally by ultrasound scanning but cleft palates are less easily demonstrated. The most common presentation is cleft lip and palate together (45%), followed by cleft palate alone (35%) and cleft lip alone (20%). Bilateral clefts occur in 15%. There is wide variation in the clinical presentation, with any degree or combination of lip and palatal involvement. Facial clefts affect 1 in 700 European babies and a similar proportion of Asians and Afro-Caribbeans; North American Indians have the highest rate at 3.75 per 1000.

AETIOLOGY

The aetiology of clefts is poorly understood but there appear to be genetic and environmental factors. Evidence for genetic causes includes clustering of cases in particular families (an affected first-degree relative increases the risk 20-fold) and the fact that clefts are associated with more than 150 congenital syndromes. Viral infections (e.g. rubella) and teratogens (e.g. steroids, anticonvulsants) during the first trimester have also been incriminated.

TREATMENT

When a cleft is recognised antenatally, explaining the likely future and counselling the parents can begin early. Once the child is born, restoring facial form and function is a complex task that may extend over several years. It includes attention to dentition, hearing, speech and breathing. Treatment planning and implementation needs to be sequenced according to the child's stage of development, with interventions balanced against their effect on growth. In practice, this can only be done effectively in a unit with substantial throughput and access to a range of experts working together as a team. With this in mind, the UK Clinical Standards Advisory Group (CSAG) produced a report in 1998 that set standards for cleft units, surgeons and training, and reduced the number of cleft units in the UK from 60 to 11.

Lip repair

Lip repair is the priority for most parents, but treatment begins with feeding techniques and orthodontic procedures to prepare the maxilla for repair. The need for long-term staged treatment and follow-up care from birth to adolescence also has to be explained.

An orthodontic palatal **obturator** is often employed to maintain arch width soon after birth. This decreases nasal regurgitation and helps oral suction; it also prevents arch collapse after the lip repair restores muscular forces on the malleable maxilla. At operation the most important goal is precise muscle repair. Most centres perform lip reconstruction at 2–4 months rather than earlier, as anaesthetic risks are lower and the larger lip elements permit more precise reconstruction. In bilateral clefts, the premaxilla protrudes and early external pressure with soft elastic tape helps maintain it within the arch; bilateral and extensive clefts often need two operations.

The overall aims of surgery are to achieve a normal symmetrical appearance of the lip, nose and face, to facilitate normal facial growth and to help normal speech. An ideal lip repair results in symmetrically shaped nostrils, adequate columellar length with a well-defined philtral groove and columns, a natural-appearing Cupid's bow and a deep upper labial sulcus. A good functional muscle repair allows a range and ease of movement that is close to normal.

Palate repair

Cleft palate is corrected surgically, usually between 9 and 18 months of age. Early surgery allows better speech development but takes place during a period of rapid growth. Bone grafts may be needed for extensive clefts. Secondary procedures are often required before the child attends school, including orthodontic surgery to allow expansion of the maxilla at around 10 years.

OTHER PROBLEMS ASSOCIATED WITH CLEFT LIP AND CLEFT PALATE

- Appearance—modern techniques with concentration on muscle repair give better cosmetic results than older ones but secondary cosmetic surgery is often required for the nose and lip
- Speech problems—children with cleft palate may have trouble speaking; their voices do not carry well and may sound nasal; speech may be difficult to understand. Well-timed and skilled surgery together with speech therapy can help
- Dental problems—children with clefts often have missing, malformed or displaced teeth requiring dental and orthodontic treatment. Children with cleft palate often have a defective alveolar ridge that can displace or rotate permanent teeth and prevent permanent teeth from erupting. Oral surgery and orthodontic tooth movement can be of assistance

ABDOMINAL EMERGENCIES IN INFANTS AND YOUNG CHILDREN

INCARCERATED INGUINAL HERNIA

PATHOPHYSIOLOGY

The description **incarcerated** means a hernia has become acutely irreducible whereas the term **strangulated** implies there is also impairment of the blood supply to the hernia contents. Strangulation can follow incarceration of a hernia but luckily is uncommon in young children, unlike in adults (Fig. 50.12).

Incarcerated inguinal hernia is a common cause of acute surgical admission in boys (and sometimes in girls) below the age of 2 years and may occur at any time from birth onwards. There is invariably a congenital **patent processus vaginalis**, i.e. the hernia is indirect, although an actual hernia may not have been evident beforehand. There is a particularly high incidence of incarceration of inguinal hernias in premature babies and 40% of hernias in the neonatal period are found because they become irreducible; the risk declines as a child becomes older. The high incidence of incarceration in young children is a strong argument in favour of operating upon any hernia in this age group soon after it has been discovered, with the need for surgery greatest in the very young.

CLINICAL FEATURES

When a hernia incarcerates it becomes painful, tender and irreducible. Classically, a mother discovers a firm lump in the groin of her crying (usually male) child. He may have vomited once or twice but the diagnosis is usually made before intestinal obstruction becomes established. On examination, the child is usually well. There is an obvious, irreducible lump in the groin (Fig. 50.12) which may extend into the scrotum. If the bowel becomes obstructed, fluid accumulates in the bowel and vomiting follows, causing fluid depletion and electrolyte disturbances. The blood supply of the incarcerated segment of intestine may become obstructed causing bowel infarction (Fig. 50.12b), but this is less common than in adults. Pressure on the spermatic cord may cause vascular obstruction to the testis, and rapid treatment is needed to avoid testicular infarction and irreversible damage.

MANAGEMENT

The typical child presenting early with an acutely irreducible hernia usually has an acutely tender painful groin swelling. The child is not systemically unwell and the hernia is neither tender nor red. At this stage, it is very unlikely that the incarcerated bowel has become infarcted. Emergency surgery is best avoided if possible, except in the unwell child with signs of intestinal obstruction, as the friable hernia sac makes surgery difficult and recurrence likely. Treatment should be directed at actively reducing the hernia with the intention of performing elective herniotomy 48 hours later when the oedema will have resolved.

Active reduction by gentle manipulation is carried out with the child sedated with intravenous opiates; it achieves its aim in about 80% of cases. Opiates can cause respiratory depression so the respiratory rate and oxygen saturation need to be monitored. After the procedure, it is important to be certain that the hernia has been fully reduced. If there is any doubt, or if the hernia proves irreducible, urgent surgery should be carried out. No child is too small to have surgery. It need be no more

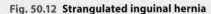

CASE STUDY

Fig. 50.12 Strangulated inguinal hernia

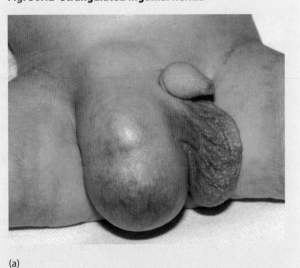

(a)

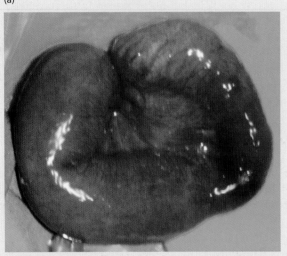

(b)

(a) Strangulated inguinal hernia in an infant. **(b)** At operation, an ileal loop trapped in the sac had undergone ischaemic necrosis and had to be resected.

dangerous than at any other age, even in the very young, provided the team has been trained in paediatric surgery and anaesthesia.

CONGENITAL HYPERTROPHIC PYLORIC STENOSIS

PATHOPHYSIOLOGY

This common condition of unknown aetiology commonly occurs between 2 weeks and 2 months of age. It presents with a gradual onset of progressive pyloric obstruction occurring over days or even a week or two, with projectile vomiting of milk following feeds. The underlying cause is marked hypertrophy of mainly circular muscle in the pyloric region of the stomach progressively occluding the gastric outlet. The disorder occurs in about 1 in 400 normal babies and there is a male predominance of 4 : 1; firstborn children are most commonly affected. Hereditary factors play a part since it is relatively common for siblings of affected children to develop the condition. It is also common for a parent or other close relative of an affected child to have had congenital pyloric stenosis.

The vomiting caused by pyloric obstruction results in fluid depletion. The baby has characteristic electrolyte disturbances, with the loss of hydrochloric acid causing a **hypochloraemic alkalosis**. In severe cases **hypokalaemia** may also occur as a result of hydrogen/potassium exchange in the kidney in which potassium irons are sacrificed to conserve hydrogen ions.

CLINICAL FEATURES

Typically, the infant thrives for the first 3 or 4 weeks and then begins to vomit after every feed. The vomiting characteristically becomes **projectile**, i.e. large amounts of vomitus are hurled from the mouth rather than running down the baby's front. The vomitus is not usually bile-stained and this readily distinguishes pyloric stenosis from duodenal stenosis or atresia. Apart from the vomiting, the child appears well and is eager for further milk. With sustained vomiting, however, the child becomes progressively dehydrated and electrolyte depleted and loses vigour. Standard examination often reveals no abdominal abnormality.

DIAGNOSIS

The persistent vomiting leads to hospital admission, where the child's response to feeding is observed. Diagnosis is made by carrying out a test feed, i.e. feeding the baby and palpating the abdomen at the same time. If pyloric stenosis is present, a hard mass about 2 cm in diameter is usually palpable deeply below the liver during the test feed and disappears after the feed. The condition can also be detected by abdominal ultrasound, but it is

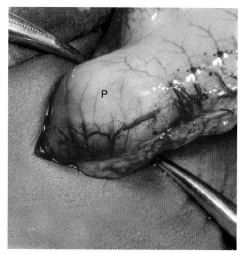

(a)

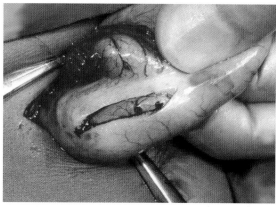

(b)

Fig. 50.13 Hypertrophic pyloric stenosis—Rammstedt's operation
(a) A small supra-umbilical incision has been made and the stomach and pyloric 'tumour' **P** delivered. **(b)** The serosa over the tumour has been incised and the hypertrophic muscle split with forceps. The mucosa is seen bulging through the muscle split.

unsafe to rely solely on ultrasound for the diagnosis. If the diagnosis remains in doubt, an upper gastrointestinal contrast study can reveal the typical very narrow pylorus and a small amount of contrast in the duodenum.

TREATMENT

Treatment is by **Rammstedt's pyloromyotomy**—Figure 50.13 (C. Rammstedt, 1912). Before operation, any fluid and electrolyte abnormalities must be corrected as the operation should only be performed on a well baby. In addition, the stomach is emptied by nasogastric aspiration and washed out with normal saline to prevent further vomiting. Surgery is carried out via an incision adjacent to the umbilicus. The hypertrophied pyloric muscle is incised longitudinally and then split without breaching the underlying mucosa (Fig. 50.13). Postoperative recovery is rapid, with full strength milk feeding started on the morning after surgery in reduced amounts, building up to full feeds by the following morning, when the baby

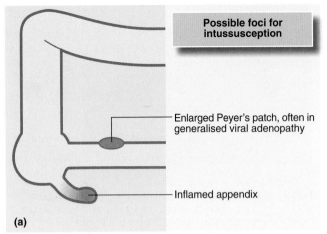

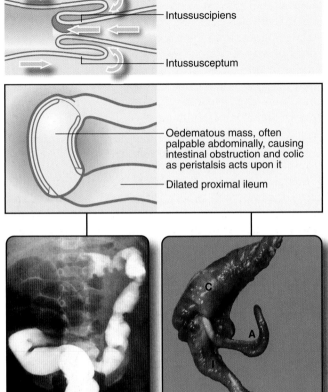

Fig. 50.14 Intussusception
(a) Mechanism of intussusception. **(b)** This 2-year-old child presented as an emergency with spasms of abdominal pain, having passed 'redcurrant jelly' rectally. This barium enema shows the typical appearance of large bowel obstruction by an intussusception of ileum which in this case has progressed to the transverse colon. The barium infusion pressure was increased, resulting in hydraulic reduction of the intussusception which did not recur. **(c)** In this case neither preoperative barium enema nor manual attempts at reduction were successful so the terminal ileum **I** and ascending colon **C** were resected. Note the appendix **A**.

can return home. The natural history of the disorder is that if an operation was not performed, the hypertrophy would gradually resolve over the course of several months. However, most children would die from electrolyte disturbances or malnutrition before this happened.

INTUSSUSCEPTION

PATHOPHYSIOLOGY

Intussusception is an acquired disorder that is most common between the ages of 6 weeks and 2 years. There appears to be a seasonal increase in incidence in the spring and autumn, probably because higher levels of microorganisms are present in the environment in these seasons leading to lymphatic swelling. The condition arises when a segment of bowel becomes telescoped into the bowel immediately distal to it (Fig. 50.14). The lead point (intussusceptum) that gives rise to the intussusception is commonly a thickening of the bowel wall caused by non-specific or viral hypertrophy of Peyer's lymphatic patches. The invaginated segment progressively elongates as it is propelled distally by peristalsis. **Ileocolic intussusception** is the most common variety and the intussusception commonly extends well into the transverse colon and may even present at the anus.

Intussusception presents with abdominal pain. If left untreated, the affected segment may undergo **venous infarction** over a period of hours or days. Intussusception sometimes occurs in older children and adults, when the initiating factor is a bowel wall tumour or polyp.

Pathology other than hypertrophy of Peyer's patches may initiate intussusception, and other causes should be suspected in a child presenting outside the usual age range or if intussusception recurs after radiological reduction. Meckel's diverticulum or even a lymphoma may present in this manner. Children with Henoch–Schönlein purpura (characterised by a purpuric rash on the extensor surface of the legs and buttocks) may sometimes develop ileo-ileal intussusception, i.e. the pathology is proximal to the colon.

CLINICAL FEATURES

Intussusception classically presents with bouts of severe colicky abdominal pain lasting for some minutes during which the child is doubled up and screaming. These episodes are separated by periods when the child appears entirely well. Within the first few hours, the child often passes a small amount of jelly-like blood per rectum. This is described as **redcurrant jelly stool**, which is almost pathognomonic of intussusception when the other clinical features are present. Vomiting begins later, consistent with distal bowel obstruction, but even without complete intestinal obstruction there may be profound fluid depletion. Some children with intussusception may be very drowsy, and this can only partly be explained by fluid depletion.

Diagnosis should be made on clinical grounds. On examination, a sausage-shaped mass is usually palpable, lying across the upper abdomen. The rectum is empty but may contain a little blood. Ultrasound may detect an intussusception but a normal result does not exclude it; however, a diagnostic air enema is quick to carry out and reliably demonstrates the condition. Intussusception is potentially life threatening so a definite diagnosis must be made urgently with a view to treatment, even in children who appear well at presentation. In Henoch–Schönlein purpura, an air enema does not give the diagnosis because the colon is unaffected; ultrasound can be helpful in these cases.

MANAGEMENT

Intussusception is potentially dangerous and treatment needs to be prompt and active, even if the child seems well. Intravenous access should be secured as rapid deterioration may be imminent. The intussusception can usually be reduced radiologically using an air or fluid contrast enema with carefully controlled pressure, performed under X-ray screening (Fig. 50.14c). Radiological reduction is inappropriate if the child is unwell; in these cases, rapid resuscitation with intravenous fluids should be followed by laparotomy. At operation, the intussusception is reduced by gentle manipulation and the appendix can be removed. Resection becomes necessary if the intussuscepted intestine is ischaemic or if it proves impossible to completely reduce the lesion without causing major trauma to the bowel.

SWALLOWED FOREIGN BODY

Young children examine their environment with their mouths and frequently swallow foreign bodies such as

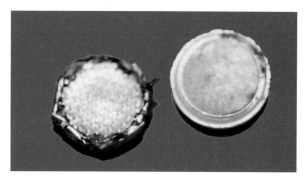

Fig. 50.15 Ingested foreign bodies
Mercury battery. Young children often put small hearing aid-type batteries into their mouths. They are at risk from inhalation and bronchial obstruction, and also from electrical activity burning through the stomach wall. Batteries can be removed without anaesthesia or sedation using a magnet on the end of a nasogastric tube.

coins, safety pins, buttons or small plastic objects. A potentially dangerous swallowed foreign body is a small button-shaped mercury battery (Fig. 50.15). The greatest danger is that electrical currents may allow it to burn its way through the stomach wall. There is also a danger of it disintegrating, releasing toxic mercury salts. Button batteries in the stomach are removed by means of a magnet on the end of a nasogastric tube. If they have passed beyond the stomach, gastrointestinal propulsive agents and laxatives are given and the child is admitted until the battery passes out of the gastrointestinal tract.

Foreign bodies commonly become arrested at the cricopharyngeus at the lower end of the pharynx or in the lower oesophagus above the gastro-oesophageal junction. All of these should be removed by endoscopy. Surprisingly, sharp foreign bodies rarely cause a problem but occasionally penetrate the bowel wall causing peritonitis. Sharp foreign bodies known to be in the stomach are usually removed by endoscopy. Blunt foreign bodies rarely cause trouble and only require intervention if they obstruct the bowel, usually at the terminal ileum or sometimes at the pylorus. If coins are present in the stomach, they are not removed but the parents are instructed to inspect the stools for the presence of the coin and to return with the child if there are signs of bowel obstruction. If the coin has not been found a month later, a further X-ray is taken and the coin removed if still there.

ABDOMINAL EMERGENCIES IN OLDER CHILDREN

THE ACUTE ABDOMEN

DIFFERENTIAL DIAGNOSIS (Box 50.2)

From childhood to adolescence, acute abdominal pain is a common cause of surgical admission. Usually **appendicitis** is suspected and this condition is described

in detail in Chapter 26. The major differential diagnoses are acute non-specific abdominal pain (which is common), closely followed by **mesenteric adenitis** (Box 50.2). Mesenteric adenitis sometimes causes a higher fever than appendicitis and the signs and symptoms usually settle within 24 hours; there is often a recent history of viral upper respiratory tract

> **Box 50.2 Differential diagnosis of acute abdominal pain in pre-adolescent children**
>
> - Acute non-specific abdominal pain
> - Acute appendicitis
> - Mesenteric adenitis
> - Extra-abdominal causes

infection and enlarged cervical lymph nodes may be palpable.

Less commonly, acute abdominal pain in this age group is caused by extra-abdominal causes such as:

- **Lower urinary tract infection** (although urinary symptoms are usually present)
- **Basal pneumonia**, usually right sided
- **Ear, nose or throat infection**
- **Torsion of the testis**—this sometimes presents solely with abdominal pain; the genitalia must always, therefore, be examined in boys with abdominal pain
- **Meningitis**

PRINCIPLES OF MANAGEMENT

If acute appendicitis is diagnosed when the child is first seen, operation should be performed without delay. More commonly, the diagnosis of appendicitis is uncertain. In these children, urinary tract infection should be excluded by urine microscopy. The child should be kept under close review and re-examined at intervals. Soon, a worsening or improving trend will become apparent. This approach may be used both in family practice and after surgical admission. It reduces the psychological trauma and the rate of unnecessary operations to a minimum and also ensures that appendicitis is not missed until peritonitis has become all too obvious.

Acute appendicitis (see also Ch. 26)

Acute appendicitis is uncommon in children less than 2 years of age. Anorexia is invariable and vomiting often starts after the onset of pain. Children with appendicitis find that movement exacerbates the pain and most find it impossible to walk without bending over. An inflamed appendix descending over the pelvic brim may cause secondary inflammation of the rectum or bladder, giving rise to diarrhoea or urinary symptoms. Pus cells may be found in the urine.

When assessing a child suspected of having appendicitis, it is important to consider other possible diagnoses. A full general examination must also be carried out in children with an acute abdomen. This includes a full ear and throat assessment, examination of the chest, testicular examination and a search for rashes and neck stiff-

ness. Otitis media, pharyngeal inflammation, basal pneumonia, testicular torsion or even meningitis can cause abdominal pain in children. Mesenteric adenitis can mimic appendicitis; a high fever and widespread lymphadenopathy suggest this diagnosis.

On examination the child's breath may be foul (foetor oris) and there may be signs of fluid depletion. The child may be pyrexial but a temperature of more than 38.5°C suggests a cause other than appendicitis, unless generalised peritonitis is present. The abdomen is tender in the right iliac fossa with localised guarding. Perforation of the appendix can lead to generalised peritonitis, with guarding over the whole abdomen.

A definitive diagnosis of appendicitis often cannot be made on initial assessment of a child with right iliac fossa pain. Investigations are of little help other than to exclude urinary tract infection and the child may find them frightening. The white blood count and CRP are unhelpful as these are raised in other inflammatory conditions, ultrasound is of some positive predictive value but cannot exclude appendicitis, and a CT scan is an expensive, arguably unnecessary, mode of investigation. Laparoscopy gives a precise diagnosis, but requires general anaesthesia; the procedure is better avoided if the appendix is not inflamed, as most children would agree.

The best way to make a diagnosis of appendicitis in the equivocal case is **active observation**. The child is admitted and allowed to eat (because fasting ameliorates the physical signs and so delays diagnosis). The child is examined every 2 hours or so, preferably by the same doctor, and this includes abdominal palpation. By the second or third examination it is usually apparent whether the physical signs are getting better or worse. The argument that active observation risks perforation, pelvic infection and infertility in girls is not borne out by fact. Active observation is able to select out those children with acute non-specific pain who have no detectable pathology and who need no active treatment, least of all surgical invasion of their peritoneal cavity.

TORSION OF THE TESTIS

Torsion can occur when there is a congenital abnormality of the fixation of the testis that predisposes to twisting of the testis on its vascular pedicle. The diagnosis must be considered in any male under about 25 years of age presenting with acute testicular pain. It is important to note, however, that torsion may also present with iliac fossa pain without testicular pain. Testicular torsion must not be missed as the testis undergoes necrosis within 4–6 hours. The predisposition to torsion is usually bilateral and both testes are therefore at risk; thus the non-torted testis should undergo corrective fixation at the same time as the torted testis (see Ch. 33).

Intrascrotal pathology that can mimic testicular torsion includes torsion of a hydatid of Morgagni and epididymitis. Palpating individual scrotal structures is often impossible because of extreme tenderness and sometimes oedema. When palpation is possible, a non-tender testis with an acutely tender epididymis (behind the testis) indicates epididymitis. Very localised tenderness at the superior pole of the testis is sometimes found in torsion of a hydatid of Morgagni.

Ultrasound with Doppler blood flow monitoring may be helpful in cases where the clinical picture makes torsion unlikely as it is reassuring to know there is good blood flow to the testis. However, if torsion is suspected, ultrasound can delay surgery and may compromise survival of the testis. Furthermore, ultrasound gives information on the testicular perfusion only at the time of examination and does not exclude intermittent torsion.

When a diagnosis of torsion cannot be excluded, the only safe option is to carry out urgent surgical exploration of the testis. If torsion is present and if the testis is viable, it should be untwisted and fixed to prevent re-torsion. A non-viable testis should be removed and the contralateral testis should also be fixed at the same time since the attachment abnormality is usually bilateral.

51 Non-acute abdominal and urological problems in children

INTRODUCTION

The acute conditions described in the previous chapter are largely congenital disorders presenting in the neonatal period, whereas non-acute conditions present across the whole age range of childhood. The most common reasons for non-acute surgical referral are hernias and associated problems, abnormalities of testicular descent and foreskin problems, mainly phimosis. Less often, surgeons are asked to manage chronic or recurrent abdominal pain, chronic constipation, rectal bleeding, an abdominal mass or rectal prolapse. Many of these children present first to a paediatrician and are then referred to a paediatric surgeon or general surgeon with an interest in paediatric surgery.

Finally, there is a range of **urological problems** that occur in infancy and childhood. Most of them are unique to young patients and are usually dealt with by specialist paediatric surgeons. Nowadays, congenital urological abnormalities can mostly be diagnosed by ultrasound in the antenatal period; they are then investigated and treated after delivery.

PROBLEMS WITH THE GROIN AND MALE GENITALIA

EMBRYOLOGY

The indifferent gonad (i.e. ovary or testis) begins to develop at the fifth week of intrauterine life in the **gonadal ridge**. This is part of the urogenital ridge derived from intermediate mesoderm that will also form the kidney and ureter and the genital ducts in the male or the uterus and uterine tubes in the female. At the lower pole of the putative testis, a strand of mesenchyme develops into the cord-like **gubernaculum** (the equivalent in females is the **round ligament** of the uterus). At about the eighth week, a prolongation of peritoneum known as the **processus vaginalis** appears along the gubernaculum (or round ligament), and extends down into the labioscrotal fold. The testis then migrates distally along the peritoneal canal.

HERNIAS AND ASSOCIATED PROBLEMS

The processus vaginalis normally closes spontaneously soon after birth. Persistence causes three very common problems in boys: patent processus vaginalis (PPV), hydrocoele and inguinal hernia. These conditions all present as inguinal or scrotal swellings, usually in babies and pre-school children. They are illustrated in Figure 51.1.

PATENT PROCESSUS VAGINALIS (PPV)

This term should be reserved for hydrocoeles that communicate with the peritoneal cavity via a remnant too narrow to admit bowel. Children with these **communicating hydrocoeles** present with a history of scrotal

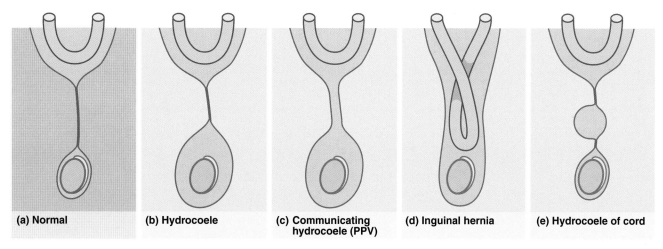

(a) Normal   (b) Hydrocoele   (c) Communicating hydrocoele (PPV)   (d) Inguinal hernia   (e) Hydrocoele of cord

Fig. 51.1 Abnormalities associated with the processus vaginalis

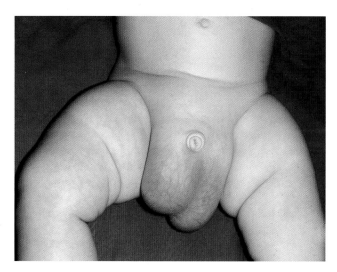

Fig. 51.2 Hydrocoeles
This 11-month-old boy had an enlarged scrotum confirmed by transillumination to be the result of hydrocoeles.

swelling that increases during the day as peritoneal fluid accumulates, and subsides during the night when the child lies flat. The condition is usually seen in toddlers up to the age of about 3 years. Treatment is surgical excision of the peritoneal remnant as in herniotomy (see below).

HYDROCOELE

Non-communicating hydrocoeles surrounding the testis are mostly seen in neonates and young babies (Fig. 51.2). The usual hydrocoele is a purely scrotal swelling that results from incomplete reabsorption of fluid from within the tunica vaginalis after closure of the processus vaginalis. There may also be a hernia present separately. These so-called 'primary hydrocoeles' sometimes appear following a viral illness. Much less commonly, a **secondary hydrocoele** results from testicular trauma or torsion, epididymitis or, rarely, a testicular tumour.

On examination, a primary hydrocoele is diagnosed if there is a fluid swelling surrounding a normal testis; the sac transilluminates brightly and the testis can be felt on the posterior wall. If this cannot be achieved, further investigation is needed to exclude a secondary hydrocoele. Inguinal hernias in neonates and infants may appear to transilluminate but the examiner cannot 'get above' the swelling, i.e. the swelling originates in the groin. Hydrocoeles also occur in the spermatic cord (hydrocoele of the cord) or in the round ligament in girls where they are known as **hydrocoeles of the canal of Nuck**. Most hydrocoeles resolve spontaneously between 18 and 24 months of age. A hydrocoele persisting beyond the age of 2 or appearing later probably requires surgical intervention.

INGUINAL HERNIA

Inguinal hernias in children arise because the processus vaginalis fails to close after testicular descent; they are therefore true congenital abnormalities. Anatomically, they are much the same as indirect inguinal hernias in adults (see Ch. 32) except that there is rarely a substantial abdominal wall defect. The incidence in infants ranges from 1 to 4.4% with a male preponderance of 4 : 1; 98% of these hernias are indirect. The incidence in **premature neonates** is much higher at 30%.

A hernia usually presents as a lump at the external inguinal ring that appears when the child cries or strains at stool but reduces spontaneously in between. When the child is seen electively by a surgeon, it is common for no abnormality to be found. However, most surgeons accept a parent's clear history that is consistent with a hernia and arrange surgical treatment. With larger defects, a lump is constantly present and expands during bouts of crying.

Inguinal hernias in neonates and infants may become **acutely irreducible** (obstructed) and painful, sometimes with obstructive symptoms such as vomiting. This condi-

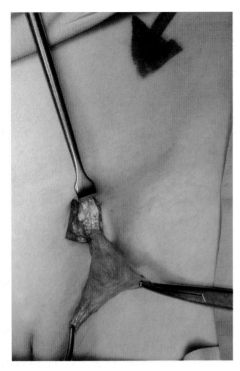

Fig. 51.3 Operation for inguinal hernia
At operation, the peritoneal sac is being held out before it is excised. No other procedure was necessary in this 4-year-old child. Unusually, the patient was female.

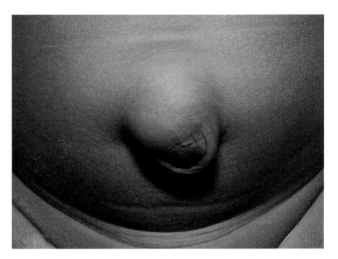

Fig. 51.4 Umbilical hernia in a 14-month-old boy
This was repaired surgically but smaller ones usually resolve spontaneously.

tion is covered in Chapter 50. In the acute case, there is a risk of testicular necrosis and of strangulation and isch-aemic necrosis of the contents of the hernia, e.g. bowel or ovary (see Fig. 50.12). If the hernia does not rapidly reduce with bed rest and analgesia, it should be repaired urgently. Asymptomatic inguinal hernias in children should also be electively repaired without delay to prevent acute obstruction.

The standard operation is **inguinal herniotomy** and this is one of the most common general paediatric surgi-cal procedures. In babies and children, the procedure involves isolating the peritoneal sac from the cord (or round ligament), ligating it at the external ring and removing it (**inguinal herniotomy**). There is rarely any need to perform a repair (herniorrhaphy); see Figure 51.3.

FEMORAL HERNIA

Femoral hernias are much less common than inguinal hernias in children and are located lower and more medi-ally in the groin. Note that enlarged lymph nodes can also occur in this position. Operation includes removing the sac and suturing the medial part of the inguinal ligament to the pectineus fascia to narrow the femoral canal.

UMBILICAL HERNIA

Many newborn babies have umbilical hernias, particu-larly if premature (Fig. 51.4), but the umbilical defect usually cicatrises and resolves during the first 2 years of life. Small umbilical hernias may still undergo spontane-ous closure up to 4–5 years. Rarely, umbilical hernias can become incarcerated (obstructed) or strangulate. Indica-tions for repair are symptomatic hernias, persistence beyond 5 years and perhaps social pressure to prevent teasing. A small subumbilical 'smile' incision allows emp-tying and ligation of the peritoneal sac and placement of a few absorbable repair sutures. The umbilical skin is usually sutured to the repair to restore its normal recessed appearance.

TESTICULAR MALDESCENT

There are several terms applied to testes that are not fully descended into the scrotum; **undescended** is not strictly accurate in that most missing testes have started along the normal pathway and have arrested in the inguinal region, a few have descended but to the wrong place and a few are missing altogether. The terms **maldescended** or **incompletely descended** cover all eventualities except the truly absent testis. Clinically, one or both testes fail to reach the scrotum in 3–4.5% of full-term newborn males. This percentage is greatly increased with prematu-rity. Full descent has occurred in most boys by the age of 6 months, leaving about 1.5% with maldescended testes and these rarely descend spontaneously later.

The normal mechanism of descent is not fully under-stood but appears to occur in two phases. Migration from the gonadal ridge to the internal inguinal ring depends on shortening of the gubernaculum, whilst descent from the internal ring to the scrotum is driven by circulating androgens. The maldescended testis may be arrested at any point on its path of descent. About 20% lie within the abdomen but 80% lie in the groin area, either in the inguinal canal or outside the external inguinal ring in the

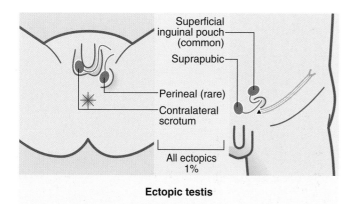

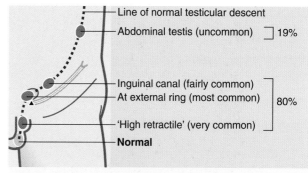

Fig. 51.5 Testicular maldescent

superficial inguinal pouch or upper scrotum. In addition, 1% of testes are deflected and come to lie in an ectopic position. There is some evidence that maldescent in this second phase can result from the testis being structurally abnormal, rather than any testicular abnormality being caused by maldescent. The main sites of incomplete descent or ectopia are shown in Figure 51.5.

The main concerns with maldescended testes are risk of torsion or traumatic injury, subfertility, and an increased risk of malignancy; the cosmetic appearance also has a bearing in later life.

- **Torsion**—incompletely descended testes are abnormally mobile. Torsion of the testis, which is actually torsion of the spermatic cord, causes strangulation of the testicular blood supply, resulting in necrosis and later atrophy. Torsion of an incompletely descended testis sometimes occurs during **intrauterine life** (said to be associated with high birth weight) but may happen at any age. The site of intrauterine and neonatal torsion is proximal to the reflection of the visceral and parietal components of the tunica vaginalis (i.e. it is **extravaginal**). Infarction results in atrophy and loss of the testis so that at laparoscopy only blind-ending testicular vessels and vas deferens are found. The condition occurs bilaterally in up to 30% of cases
- **Subfertility**—maldescended testes exhibit incomplete maturation of the seminiferous tubules, leading to the production of sperm abnormal in quantity, form or motility. This may be related in part to their being subject to normal body temperature instead of at least one degree cooler when correctly located in the scrotum. Early orchidopexy helps maturation of the tubules and spermatogenesis
- **Neoplasia**—carcinoma in situ is present in 2% of undescended testes and maldescent is associated with up to 10 times the normal risk of later testicular malignancy (although the risk is still small); surgical correction probably does not reduce this risk but enables the patient to perform self-examination and

report untoward lumps. Seminomas are the most common tumour (60%) and usually present between 20 and 40 years of age. Long-term follow-up after orchidopexy is desirable
- **Psychological**—normal genitalia are important in the development of body image, gender acceptance and personality in adolescence. Orchidopexy at an early age provides reassurance to the child and parents

Boys should be examined regularly from birth through school age to identify maldescent and allow timely surgical correction (**orchidopexy**). Periodic examination is needed because previously descended testes can later ascend and parents and doctors should be alert to this possibility.

With a history of a missing testis, the chief point on examination is whether the testis is palpable. If the testis is palpable at the scrotal neck, it should be gently manipulated into its correct position. If it then stays in the scrotum, it is termed **retractile** and requires no treatment provided it become less retractile as the boy grows. If the testis immediately returns to its previous position, it is maldescended and needs treatment.

If the testis is not palpable, investigations should be undertaken to locate it. Ultrasound is the first test and will demonstrate the testis if it lies in the inguinal canal or outside the external ring. If it is not found, then laparoscopy is the investigation of choice. At laparoscopy, the testis may be located intra-abdominally or the cord may be seen entering the deep ring; in either case, the testis is then mobilised and placed in the scrotum. Alternatively, a blind-ending spermatic cord may be found indicating that the testis is missing as a result of intrauterine torsion. No action is needed if this is unilateral but if bilateral, genetic screening is required together with possible hormonal treatment and testicular prostheses.

The optimum age for operation is between 18 months and 2 years so that fertility is not compromised, although some surgeons operate as early as 6 months. The usual technique of orchidopexy involves mobilising the testis and spermatic cord through a groin incision, separating and excising the processus vaginalis and placing the testis in a subcutaneous pouch outside the dartos muscle via a scrotal incision. For intra-abdominal testes, the operative technique is laparoscopic mobilisation and orchidopexy.

FORESKIN PROBLEMS

At birth the foreskin or prepuce is adherent to the glans penis and undergoes gradual separation between birth and 5 years of age. Parents should be advised not to attempt to retract an adherent foreskin as this may provoke a fibrotic response. Note that some adhesions may perfectly normally persist into adolescence. The prepuce protects the glans from ammoniacal dermatitis when the child is in nappies. By the time continence is achieved, 95% of boys have a retractile foreskin.

PHIMOSIS

Phimosis is a condition in which a tight fibrotic ring develops at the terminal part of the foreskin preventing retraction. **Primary phimosis** presents with chronic foreskin irritation or 'spraying' on micturition. 'Ballooning' on micturition is just a sign of a non-retractile foreskin and is not necessarily pathological. There is often a history of recent or recurrent **balano-posthitis** (infection beneath the foreskin); in these cases, urine should be analysed for glucose to exclude diabetes. Most boys with primary phimosis do not require circumcision; careful attention to hygiene (avoiding forcible retraction) allows the prepuce to retract normally in time. Attempts to simply dilate the phimosis under anaesthesia are unsuccessful as this causes further scarring and rapid relapse.

Circumcision is usually indicated in cases of recurrent infection or where the orifice is so tight that the meatus cannot be seen. In older boys, a non-retractile foreskin may cause sexual problems. For these, the lesser operation of **preputioplasty** may be appropriate if the phimosis is not too tight. This involves dividing the tight band longitudinally and suturing it transversely.

Secondary phimosis is usually due to **balanitis xerotica obliterans** (BXO) which is characterised by a thickened, whitish fibrotic non-retractile foreskin (Fig. 51.6).

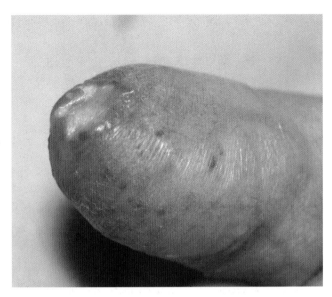

Fig. 51.6 Penis showing balanitis xerotica obliterans as a cause of phimosis
This condition is characterised by a scarred fibrotic foreskin. Circumcision is curative.

Plaques are formed on the deep surface which often adhere to the glans and may cause meatal stenosis. The peak incidence in children is around 8 years and the condition is a definite indication for a circumcision.

PARAPHIMOSIS

Paraphimosis sometimes occurs in children, especially if there is a degree of phimosis. The tip of the foreskin forms a tight band when retracted and this becomes trapped in the coronal sulcus behind the glans. The band inhibits venous return and causes swelling of the glans, which makes return of the prepuce even more difficult. Paraphimosis is painful and requires urgent reduction. This can sometimes be achieved using EMLA cream (local anaesthetic cream) or a penile local anaesthetic block. Manual compression of the glans often allows reduction but if this fails, general anaesthesia is needed. Sometimes the band needs dividing in a procedure known as a **dorsal slit**. Circumcision is usually performed later once the oedema has settled.

RENAL, VESICAL AND URETHRAL ABNORMALITIES

About a third of all congenital anomalies affect the genitourinary tract. These include abnormalities of the kidney, renal calyces, renal pelvis and ureters. Anomalies of the bladder and the urethra complete the spectrum of paediatric urogenital problems which may present at birth but need long-term follow-up, often well into adulthood. Many of these conditions can be diagnosed antenatally by ultrasound, allowing parents to be counselled and prepared for postnatal management. The common problems are pelviureteric junction (PUJ) obstruction, vesicoureteric reflux and hypospadias. Renal parenchymal disorders are less common. Not all congenital disorders of the urinary system present in childhood. The range of conditions that present later is long and includes unilateral renal agenesis, horseshoe kidney and polycystic kidneys (see Table 39.1). The congenital urinary tract dis-

Table 51.1 Congenital urinary tract disorders and their presentation

Nature of abnormality	Presentation
Kidney	
Multicystic dysplasia: dysplasia of kidney with multiple cysts; usually unilateral	Presents in the neonate as abdominal mass. Fatal if bilateral
Ectopic kidneys and *abnormalities of rotation* due to failure of developmental ascent	Found incidentally or during investigation of complications such as pelviureteric obstruction
Pelvicalyceal system and ureters	
Pelvic hydronephrosis: dilatation of pelvicalyceal system due to abnormal pelviureteric junction	Usually presents in childhood or adolescence with loin pain or mass
Megaureter: abnormality of peristalsis of lower ureter resulting in gross proximal dilatation	Presents in young children as recurrent urinary tract infections
Ureterocoele: cystic dilatation of intravesical part of ureter due to stenosis of ureteric orifice	Incidental finding or may cause infection or symptoms of obstruction, usually in adolescence
Vesicoureteric reflux: unilateral or bilateral abnormality of ureteric insertion into bladder	Presents as recurrent pyelonephritis—can cause severe damage to developing kidney
Ectopic ureter: ureter opens into part of the genital tract other than bladder, e.g. vagina	In females presents as dribbling incontinence and in males as recurrent urinary tract infections
Bladder and urethra	
Bladder hypoplasia: associated with some cases of hypospadias in boys or ectopic ureters in girls	Bladder distends once ureters or hypospadias are corrected
Urachal abnormalities, i.e. cyst, sinus, patent urachus: due to persistence of urachal remnants	Patent urachus presents in childhood with urine dribbling from umbilicus. Cysts and sinuses may present in adulthood. Adenocarcinoma sometimes develops in the urachal remnant
Bladder exstrophy: incomplete closure of lower abdominal wall in midline	Gross abnormality of genitourinary system with bladder open on abdominal wall; obvious at birth
Posterior urethral valves: cause varying degrees of bladder outlet obstruction	Severe cases present in the neonate with gross obstructive effects, renal failure and infection. Milder cases present later with recurrent infection
Epispadias: urethral meatus located in abnormal position somewhere on dorsum of penis. Often associated with major abnormality of penis	Obvious at birth
Hypospadias: urethra opens in abnormal position on ventral aspect of penis due to defective urethral fold. The prepuce is 'hooded' and incomplete ventrally. Distal urethra hypoplastic and shortened	Major cases obvious at birth. Minor cases have downward deviation of urinary stream. Sometimes a degree of *chordee* (downward bend of the penis)

orders that manifest in childhood and their clinical presentations are listed in Table 51.1 and the important remediable disorders are described below.

RENAL DYSPLASIA

Incomplete or abnormal differentiation during development causes dysplasia of one or both kidneys. Dysplasia is classified into **agenesis** (absent kidney), **hypoplastic** (underdeveloped) kidney and **multicystic dysplasia.** Bilateral agenesis is associated with other serious congenital abnormalities including pulmonary hypoplasia (Potter's syndrome) and is incompatible with life. Unilateral agenesis has an incidence of 1 in 1000 with a male preponderance. The contralateral kidney is usually normal and the disorder is not usually diagnosed until adulthood. Renal cystic disease is classified in Table 51.2.

A kidney affected by **multicystic dysplasia** contains many cysts of different sizes. The kidney is non-functional and there is ureteric atresia. The condition can be diagnosed antenatally but the priority postnatally is to determine the functional capacity of the opposite kidney and rule out vesicoureteric reflux (VUR). Most multicystic kidneys spontaneously involute (atrophy) without complication but nephrectomy is sometimes needed for a persistent cystic kidney suspected of malignancy or of causing hypertension.

In **renal ectopia** (see Fig. 39.6), the kidney comes to lie in an abnormal position in the pelvis or in the abdomen away from its normal retroperitoneal location. Renal ectopia can be discovered incidentally or it may be associated with congenital anomalies such as anorectal malformations.

Abnormal fusion of the developing metanephric masses during the first two months of fetal life results in the formation of a **horseshoe kidney** (see Fig. 39.5). This

Table 51.2 Classification of renal cystic disease

Pathology	Characteristics	Presentation
Genetic		
Polycystic kidney—autosomal recessive type	Often termed infantile polycystic disease. Incidence 1 : 10 000 to 1 : 40 000	Bilateral disorder. Neonates have grossly distended abdomens with nonfunctioning kidneys. Liver and pancreatic cysts are often present. The disease is fatal
Polycystic kidney—autosomal dominant type	The most prevalent major inherited disorder. Incidence in adults 1 : 1000	Manifests around 30 years of age with chronic renal failure, hypertension, haematuria and recurrent urinary tract infections
Cysts associated with multiple malformation syndrome	Involve several systems and viscera. Specific cyst-associated syndromes to be excluded	Genetic counselling and sonographic monitoring of subsequent pregnancies advisable
Non-genetic		
Multicystic dysplasia of the kidney	Incidence 1 in 4000 live births	Antenatal diagnosis, postnatally confirmed. Unilateral multicystic nonfunctional kidney
Solitary cyst	Involves upper or lower pole	Antenatal diagnosis. May present with loin pain and swelling. Sometimes found incidentally
Medullary sponge kidney (tubular ectasia)	Cystic dilatation of collecting ducts of one or more medullary pyramids in one or both kidneys	Incidental finding or diagnosed when investigating urinary tract infection or stones. Cysts calcify producing characteristic X-ray appearance

may cause hydronephrosis as a result of pelviureteric junction obstruction or it may be discovered incidentally at any age. Other congenital anomalies occur in at least a third of patients including skeletal and cardiovascular abnormalities; girls with Turner's syndrome often have a horseshoe kidney.

NEONATAL HYDRONEPHROSIS

Fetal urinary tract abnormalities occur in up to 1% of all pregnancies, and hydronephrosis accounts for half of these. Routine prenatal ultrasound often identifies this. Evaluation and management depend on the severity and whether it is unilateral or bilateral. Antenatal hydronephrosis may be caused by pelviureteric junction obstruction, vesicoureteric junction obstruction or reflux, multicystic kidney, primary obstructive megaureter and posterior urethral valves. The urgency and type of investigation depends on the size of the hydronephrosis. Small unilateral hydronephrosis requires no action, whereas larger lesions require ultrasound, micturating cystography and perhaps isotope renal scans repeated at intervals to decide if surgery is needed. In bilateral severe hydronephrosis, early investigation and surgery is essential.

VESICOURETERIC REFLUX

Any anatomical or functional abnormality of the urinary tract predisposes to urinary tract infections. This is particularly true in children, where the commonest predisposing abnormality is **vesicoureteric reflux** (VUR), i.e. retrograde flow of urine from the bladder to kidneys. This exposes the upper tracts to the greater range of pressure

Box 51.1 Causes of vesicoureteric reflux

Primary, i.e. maldevelopment of vesicoureteric junction

- Short submucosal tunnel
- Delayed maturity of vesicoureteric junction

Secondary

- Posterior urethral valves
- Duplex system and ureterocoele
- Ectopic ureters
- Congenital megaureters
- Detrusor instability
- Neurogenic bladder
- Surgical procedures to the lower end of the ureter

variation occurring in the lower urinary tract and to ascending infections. The causes are complex but in essence there is a faulty mechanism at the junction of ureter and bladder (vesicoureteric junction), see Box 51.1. Reflux is classified into a range of severities from I to V (see Table 51.3).

Vesicoureteric reflux in the neonatal period is due to anatomical abnormalities, with both sexes affected equally. Later, the condition appears predominantly in girls where **voiding disturbances** appear to play a large role. Dysfunctional voiding refers to abnormalities in the storage of urine or the emptying phase of micturition and is associated with urgency, frequency, incontinence and urinary tract infections. A vicious circle may develop with reflux leading to infection which then leads to bladder instability and further dysfunctional voiding.

Table 51.3 International classification of vesicoureteric reflux (VUR) and clinical classification

Grade of VUR	International classification	Clinical classification
I	Reflux into lower ureter on voiding	Mild non-dilating VUR on micturition
II	Reflux into ureter and renal pelvis on voiding but without dilatation	
III	Reflux into the ureter and renal pelvis on voiding with mild dilatation	
IV	Constant reflux with upper tract and ureteric dilatation	Constant severe dilating VUR
V	Constant reflux with blunted calyces and grossly dilated tortuous ureters	

PATHOPHYSIOLOGY

In the normal individual, the distal ureter takes an oblique course through the muscular bladder wall so that detrusor contraction during voiding acts as a sphincter, preventing urine from refluxing from the bladder into the ureters (the **anti-reflux mechanism**). This, together with contraction of the uretero-trigonal muscle (which draws the ureteric orifices together), prevents transmission of intermittent high bladder pressures. **Primary vesicoureteric reflux** is the most common form of reflux and usually results from a minor congenital (often familial) abnormality of ureteric insertion. Primary reflux may also be caused by other morphological abnormalities such as ectopic or duplex ureters or congenital megaureter (a peristaltic abnormality). **Secondary VUR** may be caused by bladder outlet obstruction, neuropathic bladder or previous surgical procedures to the lower end of the ureter.

Ascending infection of the upper tracts begins with bacteria reaching the bladder via the urethra and colonising it. Infected urine then refluxes into the upper tract but cannot be cleared from it effectively, thereby infecting the upper tract. Lower urinary tract infections can also cause inflammatory changes at the vesicoureteric junction, preventing it from closing effectively, resulting in further reflux.

Reflux of sterile urine into the pelvicalyceal system during early childhood probably causes impairment of normal renal development and function. Mild, non-dilating VUR (grades I to III; see Table 51.3) appears to cause little damage but severe, dilating VUR (grades IV and V) may cause renal scarring and reflux nephropathy, which, if untreated, may progress to irreversible renal damage (Fig. 51.7). If both kidneys are involved, this eventually results in renal insufficiency and hypertension.

CLINICAL PRESENTATION AND INVESTIGATION

Vesicoureteric reflux can be detected during antenatal ultrasound screening as fetal urinary tract dilatation. The other common presentation is a single or recurrent urinary tract infections occurring at any age. Girls are more prone to infections than boys, especially between the ages of 3 and 6 years, because of the short urethra and its proximity to the anus. Note that infants or young children with urinary tract infections may not exhibit symptoms and signs specific to the urinary tract and the diagnosis is often made on investigation of vomiting, fever or failure to thrive. Older children typically present with incontinence, frequency or dysuria, or abdominal pain and tenderness (mimicking appendicitis). In children with **symptomatic urinary tract infections**, the prevalence of vesicoureteric reflux is 50% in neonates and 30% in those aged 2–18 years. A single bacteriologically proven urinary tract infection in a boy, or two or more in a girl, is an indication for investigation.

In children with urinary tract infection, clinical examination seeks evidence of abnormal external genitalia, spina bifida and impaired perineal innervation (perineal sensation and anal sphincter tone). To demonstrate reflux, the sequential radiological investigations are ultrasound scan, micturating cystography, and isotope scans using DMSA and MAG3, coupled with indirect radionuclide cystography. **Micturating cystography** (Fig. 51.7) is the standard investigation and involves injecting contrast into the bladder via a urinary catheter. The urinary catheter is removed and X-rays taken during voiding to demonstrate reflux. The radiological grades of severity of reflux are shown in Table 51.3 and provide a useful guide to the likelihood of future renal damage. Severe dilating VUR requires **isotope studies**: ^{99m}Tc DMSA, bound to renal tubules, shows differential renal function and scarring within the renal parenchyma. In older children, an excretion MAG3 scan and indirect radionuclide cystogram would show differential function, reflux and sites of urinary tract obstruction.

MANAGEMENT OF VESICOURETERIC REFLUX

If there are no other anatomical abnormalities and the ureter is not dilated (i.e. grades I and II), there is an 85% chance of spontaneous resolution of vesicoureteric reflux as the child grows. In the meantime, the urinary tract must be kept free of infection. This is done by encouraging regular voiding and a high fluid intake including acidic fruit juices, avoiding constipation and maintaining perineal hygiene, together with medical management of bladder dysfunction. At the same time, the child is main-

Fig. 51.7 Vesicoureteric reflux

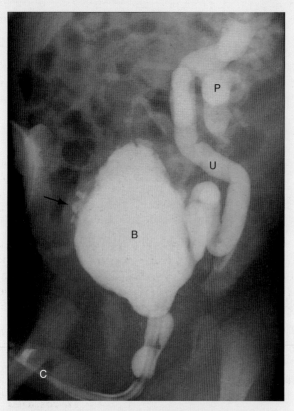

Micturating cysto-urethrogram (MCUG) in a child with recurrent urinary tract infections. The bladder **B** is trabeculated (diverticula arrowed). On voiding, the left ureter **U** and pelvicalyceal system **P** filled with contrast as a result of severe dilating vesicoureteric reflux. This is defined as grade V reflux.

tained on continuous **anti-bacterial chemotherapy** (such as trimethoprim) until the danger of reflux is past. The child is followed up regularly with serial ultrasound scans and charting the progress of growth and development, blood pressure and serum creatinine.

Surgical correction is indicated when there are recurrent break-through infections, deterioration of upper tract function or non-compliance to medical management. Otherwise, surgery is reserved for severe dilated VUR with complications and for other obvious anatomical abnormalities. The operations for reflux aim to **reimplant the ureter** in the bladder wall so that a length of it lies deep to the bladder mucosa; during voiding this is flattened by intraluminal pressure thus restoring an anti-reflux mechanism. Newer treatments include injection of PTFE or other agents such as bovine collagen into the submucosa of the ureter at the junction with the bladder; success rates of around 75% have been claimed for this type of therapy.

After operation, if there is no renal scarring, the child can be discharged from follow-up. If there is unilateral scarring, the blood pressure should be monitored lifelong because of the risk of hypertension. In bilateral scarring, the renal function must also be monitored because of the risk of deterioration.

PELVIURETERIC JUNCTION OBSTRUCTION

PATHOPHYSIOLOGY

Obstruction at the pelviureteric junction (PUJ) may be unilateral or bilateral, and can present at any age from birth through to the end of the fourth decade. It affects both sexes equally. PUJ obstruction is a congenital condition of unknown aetiology that manifests as dilatation of the renal pelvis and calyces (**hydronephrosis**). The cause of obstruction in most cases is a functional abnormality of the PUJ with an aperistaltic segment of ureter that lacks muscle. Aberrant lower pole vessels were once thought to cause mechanical obstruction but this is no longer believed. When the ureter contracts, the normal pelviureteric junction prevents reflux of urine into the kidney, but in PUJ obstruction, urine accumulates and causes dilatation of the pelvicalyceal system. This increases pressure in the renal collecting system which causes deterioration of renal function. Stasis also predisposes to infection.

CLINICAL PRESENTATION AND DIAGNOSIS

PUJ obstructions are often diagnosed antenatally. These are followed up regularly with postnatal ultrasound and those with persistent hydronephrosis are investigated for renal function, the effectiveness of urine drainage from the kidney and vesicoureteric reflux, and treated appropriately.

Many patients with PUJ obstruction go undetected. Many others are discovered by chance on ultrasound or urography during investigation of an apparently unrelated condition. Even in symptomatic patients, symptoms may be intermittent. Some patients complain of aching pain in the renal area; others suffer bouts of severe abdominal or loin pain (renal colic), sometimes with urinary tract infection or haematuria. Haematuria may be induced by exercise. No precipitating factor is usually found but symptoms can sometimes be exacerbated by drinking large volumes of fluid or by sudden changes in posture.

The initial diagnosis can be made by ultrasound, with detection of a dilated renal pelvis. The next step is to distinguish between static non-obstructive dilatation with preserved renal function and genuine PUJ obstruction causing stasis, dilatation and deteriorating function. **Radionuclide diuretic renography (^{99m}Tc MAG3 scan)** is the investigation of choice and gives a characteristic non-excretion curve with loss of function in classical PUJ obstruction. On a standard IVU, the typical changes on the affected side are a **prolonged nephrogram** and a **negative pyelogram** (i.e. contrast persists in the renal cortex without opacifying the pelvis), **delayed drainage of contrast** from an often dilated renal pelvis, or a combination of these features. The only reliable sign, however, is **spontaneous extravasation** of contrast into parenchymal lymphatics. This is seen as 'contrast streaking' in the renal cortex.

MANAGEMENT

PUJ obstruction with obstructive symptoms, stone formation, recurrent infections or progressive renal impairment, together with an obstructed isotope excretion curve, is an indication for intervention. Pyeloplasty is indicated unless the kidney has less than 10% of total renal function, in which case nephrectomy is indicated. Minimal invasive techniques include percutaneous antegrade endopyelotomy and laparoscopic pyeloplasty; the latter is now the treatment of choice where available. Standard operations have a high technical success rate and prevent further deterioration of renal function.

HYPOSPADIAS AND EPISPADIAS

Hypospadias is a common congenital abnormality of the penis and urethra. It occurs in about 1 in 300 male births. The distal urethra fails to develop normally, so that the urethral meatus lies somewhere along the ventral surface of the penis from the glans to the perineum (see Fig. 51.8). The remnant of urethral tissue distal to the meatus is fibrotic, often causing the penis to bend downwards or sideways on erection. This is known as **chordee**. The more proximal the urethral meatus, the worse the chordee. In addition, the ventral part of the foreskin is absent, giving rise to a hooded appearance. Distal hypospadias is more common, with the urethral opening between the glans and the mid-penile shaft and minimal chordee. The proximal variety is characterised by moderate to severe chordee.

Surgical correction is a highly specialised procedure and is required for both function and cosmesis. Functional correction enables voiding in a forward direction and forward ejaculation later. Since surgical repair utilises the hood of the foreskin, circumcision should **never** be

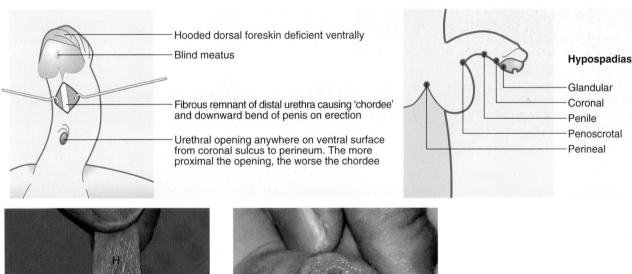

(a)

- Hooded dorsal foreskin deficient ventrally
- Blind meatus
- Fibrous remnant of distal urethra causing 'chordee' and downward bend of penis on erection
- Urethral opening anywhere on ventral surface from coronal sulcus to perineum. The more proximal the opening, the worse the chordee

Hypospadias
- Glandular
- Coronal
- Penile
- Penoscrotal
- Perineal

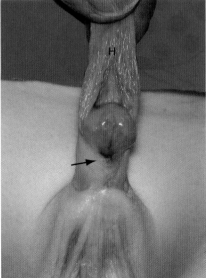

(b)

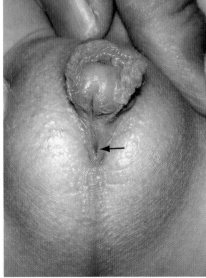

(c)

Fig. 51.8 Hypospadias
(a) Hypospadias.
(b) Distal coronal hypospadias. The urethral meatus is arrowed and **H** indicates the hooded foreskin. **(c)** Severe penoscrotal hypospadias. The urethral meatus is arrowed. Chordee, a marked downward bend of the penis, was prominent in this case but is not visible here.

carried out without specialist advice. The ideal age for surgery is between 6 and 12 months.

Epispadias is much less common and may be associated with other major genitourinary abnormalities. In epispadias, the urethral meatus is on the dorsal aspect of the penis.

POSTERIOR URETHRAL VALVES (PUV)

Urethral valves are congenital mucosal folds in the posterior urethra of a boy that impede or completely obstruct urinary flow. Standard antenatal fetal ultrasound scan screening usually detects the characteristic signs of oligohydramnios, a small thick-walled bladder and bilateral hydronephrosis and hydroureter. If not diagnosed antenatally, complete obstruction becomes apparent soon after birth but partial obstruction may be overlooked, and in untreated cases back-pressure effects soon lead to renal failure.

Severe oligohydramnios in this condition can be associated with pulmonary hypoplasia, which is incompatible with life. Neonates that are born with bladder outlet obstruction (Fig. 51.9) require urgent initial bladder drainage by suprapubic catheter. Investigations follow, including ultrasound scan, micturating cystography to establish the diagnosis of posterior urethral valves and isotope MAG3 scan to test differential renal excretory function.

Definitive treatment involves destroying the valves by diathermy using a paediatric resecting cystoscope. Long-term follow-up is imperative, as renal function may deteriorate to the point of needing renal transplantation. Sometimes a low-capacity high-pressure bladder persists, requiring drainage or a bladder augmentation procedure.

Fig. 51.9 Micturating cysto-urethrogram (MCUG) in a neonate with posterior urethral valves

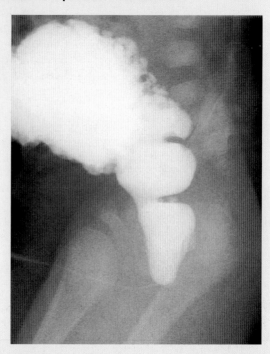

The X-ray shows bladder outlet obstruction which has caused detrusor muscle hypertrophy leading to a trabeculated low-capacity bladder.

ABDOMINAL PROBLEMS

CHRONIC AND RECURRENT ABDOMINAL PAIN

Chronic or recurrent abdominal pain is common in children of school age but in most, no cause is discovered and the problem gradually resolves (Box 51.2). These children are often managed by family practitioners or paediatricians but may be referred to a surgeon if an organic problem seems likely. Note that psychological factors are fairly common and should not be overlooked. The main organic causes are hydronephrosis (detailed in this chapter), inflammatory bowel disease and gallstones associated with haemolytic anaemia.

CHRONIC CONSTIPATION

Chronic constipation is among the most common abdominal problems in children; it may present as **faecal soiling**, i.e. faecal overflow incontinence. A detailed history including socio-psychological factors may reveal a cause but in most children the aetiology is unknown. The problem should not, however, be neglected as it may lead to lifelong problems. Early constipation usually responds to simple measures such as a high-fibre diet, adequate fluid intake, regular attempts at defaecation and, if necessary, appropriate combinations of osmotic and stimulant laxatives (e.g. lactulose or senna derivative).

In severe constipation, it is important to investigate for **cystic fibrosis, hypothyroidism** and **Hirschsprung's disease** (Ch. 50, p. 734). If these can be excluded, the child may end up requiring a surgical operation such as anterior resection for redundant non-functional rectum or the creation of a conduit into the colon to allow antegrade enemas to be given regularly.

Table 51.4 Common causes of gastrointestinal bleeding in children

Age	Upper gastrointestinal	Lower gastrointestinal
1–12 months	Oesophagitis Gastritis	Anal fissure Intussusception Necrotising enterocolitis Malrotation with volvulus Perianal abscess and fistula

1–2 years	Peptic ulcer disease associated with:
	  Burns (Curling's ulcer)
	  Head trauma (Cushing's ulcer)
	  Malignancy
	  Sepsis
		Anal fissure
		Polyps
		Rectal prolapse
		Meckel's diverticulum
		Perianal abscess and fistula

2–15 years	Oesophageal and gastric varices Portal hypertension with cirrhosis	Polyps Inflammatory bowel disease Trauma Sexual abuse Gastroenteritis—*Campylobacter* Arteriovenous malformations Miscellaneous lesions

---

Box 51.2 Organic causes of chronic or recurrent abdominal pain in children

- Chronic constipation—common
- Lower urinary tract infection—common
- Hydronephrosis—uncommon
- Sickle cell crises—uncommon
- Recurrent appendicitis—rare
- Crohn's disease
- Recurrent volvulus of small bowel—rare
- Gallstones—rare, sometimes associated with haemolytic anaemia
- Peptic ulceration—rare

GASTROINTESTINAL BLEEDING IN CHILDREN (Table 51.4)

UPPER GASTROINTESTINAL BLEEDING

In neonates, apparent vomiting of blood may result from swallowed maternal blood. In older infants, gastritis may be the cause. Less common causes are bleeding disorders and coagulopathy.

LOWER GASTROINTESTINAL BLEEDING

Rectal bleeding in neonates is most often due to anal fissure, necrotising enterocolitis or malrotation with volvulus. Rectal bleeding is a common problem in older infants and children, but it is rarely caused by tumour or haemorrhoids, the most common causes in adulthood. The common causes are summarised in Table 51.4 and include perianal abscess and fistula, anal fissures, large bowel polyps, rectal prolapse and Meckel's diverticulum.

Anal fissure

Anal fissure occurs at any age during infancy and childhood and is probably initiated by straining to pass a large hard stool. This splits the anal mucosa in the midline posteriorly or anteriorly. Anal fissures can also develop after an episode of severe diarrhoea. The main symptoms are pain at defaecation and a small amount of bright red blood on the stool or leaking immediately after defaecation. The condition is readily diagnosed when digital rectal examination is found to be impossible because of extreme tenderness; the posterior end of the fissure may sometimes be seen by parting the buttocks. Treatment involves gentle anal dilatation under general anaesthesia, followed by measures to prevent constipation.

Polyps

A **juvenile hamartomatous polyp** is a common cause of rectal bleeding in children. These polyps are nearly always solitary and usually occur in the rectum or sigmoid colon. Polyps may present with intermittent rectal bleeding in a child without constipation, as pain on defaecation that is not associated with an anal fissure, or by prolapsing through the anus. The polyp may be palpable on digital examination and is then confirmed on proctoscopy under general anaesthesia; it may then be suture ligated and resected. If no polyp is visible, colonoscopy is performed and any identified polyps removed by snare. Juvenile polyps are almost never malignant nor do they recur. **Familial adenomatous polyposis** may present in childhood with rectal bleeding. As described in Chapter 27, polyps of this type inevitably turn malignant from about the age of 16 onwards.

Rectal prolapse

Transient rectal prolapse is a common and alarming childhood problem, usually occurring during the first 2 years of life. The most common cause is excessive straining during defecation. Prolapse may be a presenting feature of cystic fibrosis because there is less mucus in the bowel and the mucus is thick and sticky. In addition, thick mucus often obstructs exocrine secretion from the pancreas impairing fat digestion. The majority of prolapses can be gently manipulated back into position without causing pain and will not recur if the stool is kept soft. If the problem is persistent or recurrent, proctoscopy and sigmoidoscopy are indicated. A rectal polyp is occasionally responsible, and can be removed by diathermy snare. If simple stool-softening measures fail to prevent recurrence, submucosal injections of phenol in oil are used to induce fibrosis. In the rare event of this failing, a circumanal subcutaneous suture may be inserted.

Perianal abscess

This is a common condition in infants and results from infection of an anal gland; the mechanism is the same as in adults. The abscess points 1–2 cm from the anal verge. Drainage alone would convert this into a **fistula** because of the persistent internal opening at the level of the anal valves. Proper treatment involves opening the fistulous tract entirely under general anaesthesia, as in adults.

Meckel's diverticulum

A Meckel's diverticulum is present in less than 2% of the population. It represents the embryological remnant of the **vitello-intestinal duct** which joined the fetal midgut and the yolk sac. The diverticulum is situated on the antimesenteric border (i.e. opposite the mesentery) of the distal ileum about 60 cm from the ileo-caecal junction. Meckel's diverticula are usually asymptomatic but may cause rectal bleeding or become inflamed and perforate.

Meckel's diverticula often contain a variety of gut-related tissues. These include **ectopic acid-secreting gastric mucosa**, which may cause peptic ulceration. In children below 2 years, this is an important cause of rectal bleeding which, if massive, may require transfusion. In older children, the ectopic gastric mucosa more often causes chronic occult bleeding, leading to iron deficiency anaemia. Much less commonly, **peptic ulceration** in a Meckel's diverticulum results in peptic ulcer **perforation** which presents with the signs of peritonitis.

If a Meckel's diverticulum is suspected to be the cause of rectal bleeding, an attempt may be made to confirm the diagnosis by performing a radionuclide Meckel's scan, employing an isotope concentrated in gastric mucosa. The test however has a relatively low negative **predictive value** and a laparoscopy or laparotomy often has to be performed to examine the bowel directly.

A Meckel's diverticulum with a narrow neck may become inflamed in the same way to be appendicitis and cause similar symptoms and signs (see Fig. 26.4, p. 394); the diagnosis is only made at operation. As with appendicitis, the complications of gangrenous inflammation are perforation and peritonitis. Unlike the complications of Meckel's peptic ulceration and bleeding, Meckel's diverticulitis is uncommon in children under 10 years of age and occurs in older children, adolescents and young adults.

At operation, the Meckel's diverticulum should be resected, together with 2 cm of normal ileum on each side, and primary ileo-ileal anastomosis performed. This is because ectopic gastric mucosa can extend beyond the diverticulum.

INFLAMMATORY BOWEL DISEASE
(see Ch. 28 for adult disease)

The incidence of Crohn's disease in children is increasing. The disease can involve any part of the gastrointestinal tract. Perianal disease is common, presenting with chronic indolent abscesses and fissures. These fissures are often located laterally, suggesting the diagnosis. Crohn's disease varies greatly in its presentation and this may cause substantial delay between the onset of symptoms and diagnosis. As in adults, there may be a history of recurrent abdominal pain and weight loss. The first presentation in adolescents may be growth retardation and delayed onset of puberty.

Ulcerative colitis presents with diarrhoea, malaise and weight loss; perianal disease and proctitis is uncommon. Management of both conditions is similar to that in adults.

ABDOMINAL MASS

An abdominal mass is an uncommon reason for surgical referral in children. It may be caused by a malignant embryonal tumour, most often a **nephroblastoma** (Wilms' tumour). Other causes of a mass include **hydronephrosis** and **post-traumatic pancreatic pseudocyst**.

NEPHROBLASTOMA (WILMS' TUMOUR)

Nephroblastoma presents in early childhood, with 80% presenting before the age of 5 at a median age of 3.5 years. The tumour arises from embryonal renal tissue in the kidney, hence its name. Tumours are locally invasive and metastasise to regional nodes, liver, lungs and bone. Often, a large abdominal mass is noticed by the mother as the child is bathed (see Fig. 51.10). The mass is sometimes so large as to obscure its site of origin. Less common

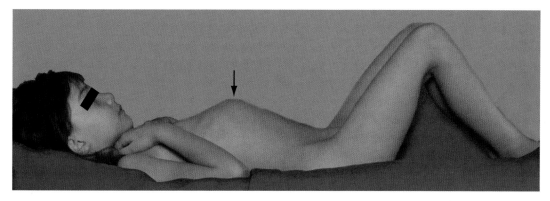

Fig. 51.10 Nephroblastoma
This 9-year-old girl presented with a large unilateral mass (arrowed), which was later confirmed to be arising from the left kidney (Wilms' tumour or nephroblastoma).

presenting features include haematuria, anorexia, weight loss, pyrexia and hypertension. Diagnosis is by ultrasonography, CT or MRI.

Treatment is by radical nephrectomy plus postoperative chemotherapy. Radiotherapy is employed for patients with residual tumour or lymphatic or pulmonary metastases. When surgery was the only treatment available the cure rate was only about 10%, but the modern combination of surgical resection, radiotherapy and chemotherapy gives an excellent chance of complete cure even when distant metastases are present.

NEUROBLASTOMA

This is another embryonal tumour occurring in early childhood. It is highly malignant and arises from embryonal sympathetic nervous tissue in the adrenal gland or sympathetic chain. The standard treatment is a combination of surgical resection, chemotherapy and radiotherapy, but the prognosis is poor. A less aggressive variant is the **ganglioblastoma**. This tumour sometimes presents as an abdominal mass but the usual presentation is failure to thrive.

Index

Note: Page numbers in *italics* refer to tables and figures.

763